Common haematology values *If outside this range, consult:*

Haemoglobin		p624
		p624
Mean cell volume, MCV		↓p626; ↑p632
Platelets	150–400 × 10⁹/L	p662
White cells (total)	4–11 × 10⁹/L	p630
neutrophils	40–75%	p630
lymphocytes	20–45%	p630
eosinophils	1–6%	p630

(barcode: KT-405-266)

Blood gases

	kPa	mmHg	
pH 7.35–7.45			p193, p198, p682
P_aO_2	>10.6	75–100	p193, p198, p682
P_aCO_2	4.7–6	35–45	p193, p198, p682
Base excess ±2mmol/L			p193, p198, p682

U&E etc (urea and electrolytes) *If outside this range, consult:*

sodium	135–145mmol/	p690
potassium	3.5–5mmol/L	p692
creatinine	70–150µmol/L	p272 & p276
urea	2.5–6.7mmol/L	p272 & p276
calcium	2.12–2.65mmol/L	p694–6
albumin	35–50g/L	p702
proteins	60–80g/L	p702

LFTs (liver function tests)

bilirubin	3–17µmol/L	p222
alanine aminotransferase, ALT	3–35iu/L	
aspartate transaminase, AST	3–35iu/L	p222
alkaline phosphatase	30–35iu/L *(adults)*	p222

'Cardiac enzymes' For troponins, see p120.

creatine kinase	25–195iu/L	p120 (p420)
lactate dehydrogenase, LDH	70–250iu/L	p120

Lipids and other biochemical values

cholesterol	<6mmol/L *desired*	p706
triglycerides	0.5–1.9mmol/L " "	p706
amylase	0–180*somorgyi* u/dL	p478
C-reactive protein, CRP	<10mg/L	p702
glucose, fasting	3.5–5.5mmol/L	p292
prostate specific antigen, PSA	0–4ng/mL	p705
T4 (total thyroxine)	70–140mmol/L	p302
TSH	0.5–~5mu/L	p302

For all other reference intervals, see p713–5

OXFORD HANDBOOK OF CLINICAL MEDICINE

SIXTH EDITION

OXFORD HANDBOOK OF CLINICAL MEDICINE

SIXTH EDITION

MURRAY LONGMORE
IAN B WILKINSON
SUPRAJ R RAJAGOPALAN

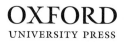

OXFORD
UNIVERSITY PRESS

OXFORD
UNIVERSITY PRESS

Great Clarendon Street, Oxford OX2 6DP.

Oxford University Press is a department of the University of Oxford.
It furthers the University's objective of excellence in research, scholarship,
and education by publishing worldwide in

Oxford New York

Auckland Bangkok Buenos Aires
Cape Town Chennai Dar es Salaam Delhi Hong Kong Istanbul
Karachi Kolkata Kuala Lumpur Madrid Melbourne Mexico City Mumbai
Nairobi São Paulo Shanghai Taipei Tokyo Toronto

Oxford is a registered trade mark of Oxford University Press
in the UK and in certain other countries

Published in the United States
by Oxford University Press Inc., New York

First published 1985 (Tony Hope and Murray Longmore)
Second edition 1989
Third edition 1993
Fourth edition 1998
Fifth edition 2001 (Murray Longmore and Ian Wilkinson)
Sixth edition 2004

British Library Cataloguing in Publication Data

Data available

Library of Congress Cataloging in Publication Data
ISBN 0 19 8525583

Typeset in Gill Sans
by Newgen Imaging Systems (P) Ltd., Chennai, India
Printed in China on acid-free paper

Contents

Each chapter's contents is detailed on each chapter's first page

Translations

French translation 1989, 1995
Spanish translation 1991, 2000
German translation 1991, 1994
Hungarian translation 1992
Polish translation 1993
Czech translation 1995
Slovac translation 1996
Romanian translation 1997
Italian translation 1999
Chinese translation 1999

For Judith

Preface to the sixth edition

There has seldom been a better time to be ill, one might think, on reviewing all the changes and developments since our last edition. From *Angina* to *Zollinger-Ellison syndrome*, the new developments, all detailed in this volume, seem universally bright or brightening—and overall death rates from the big killers such as coronary heart disease are declining faster than ever before. This superficial view hides darker forces which paint a more sombre picture. The pandemic of HIV has grown a pace or two or three. Diabetes is doubling its grip, and global warming is introducing new diseases to areas where local inhabitants have little immunity—these effects are described in Chapters 9 and 14. Once-trusted antibiotics are becoming useless in the face of pathogen development (p262); airlines are spreading completely new diseases around the world—eg SARS. Diseases caused by medicine have never been more common. Crucially, the world is no wealthier than when we first began to write on these topics.

While this book will doubtless prove indispensable in choosing correctly between self-destruction and passive extinction, some readers will point out that this received wisdom is wisdom subverted. Is SARS really an example of the darker prophesies being fulfilled? New diseases have always been appearing; what may be new about this epidemic was that is was caught early (albeit provisionally)—by the rapid dissemination of knowledge via electronic media. Often the people in white coats were waiting for the disease before it arrived. Information spread faster than the disease—and the organism's genome was sequenced almost as soon as it was identified. Similarly, with HIV, not all the news is bad. Rich countries are learning, painfully slowly, to share their expensive drugs with poorer populations. There is no alternative to altruism—*even if one takes a purely selfish view of one's own interests*. Altruism pays! (If the rich prosper only at the expense of others, the net result is not sustainable wealth—revolution, or something unknown, is more likely.)

These, and many other developments described in this book point to just what can be achieved by dialogue and teamwork. This edition sees a new beginning (our *Prologue*) in which we flesh out what teamwork really means by giving an example of when it all goes wrong. Evidence-based medicine is a prime example of teamwork going right—usually. The funding organizations, the investigators, the statisticians, and the clinicians work together to provide the best possible treatment for the patient. We detail more fruits of this collaboration than in all other editions. We are using a new disc sign, with a number below (⬤) to direct readers to the correct location on the web page of our references and their internet-enabled links at *www.oup.com/uk/medicine/handbooks*. Scholars among our readers may want to print these out to carry with them with our text to provide chapter and verse during tricky ward-rounds. Those who miss immediate access to our sources may remind themselves of Hagel's view in his *Aesthetics* that the purer the form, the less space it requires—and this economy of space has been one of our principal aims.⬤

Further changes include a short section on essential drugs; a new section on *Clinical Skills*; more ECGs; and many new algorithms to reflect current practice—as well as new topics from the all-encompassing (*Patient-centred care*) to rare minutiae (such as all the different types of *multiple endocrine neoplasia* and their nefarious genetic associations). There are new mnemonics—not too intrusive, and not too rude (usually). Much re-organization is in evidence (eg *Diabetes mellitus*). But the most important changes are the hardest to spot—thousands of small changes in the bodies of paragraphs. This incrementalism, accumulating like coral, amounts to whole new formations which, in this edition, take on a life of their own, set against backgrounds of rich tropical colours—a holiday for the eye, for which we thank the ever-creative staff at the Press.

JML IBW SRR 2004

From the preface to the first edition

This book, written by junior doctors, is intended principally for medical students and house officers. The student becomes, imperceptibly, the house officer. For him we wrote this book not because we know so much, but because we know we remember so little. For the student the problem is not simply the quantity of information, but the diversity of places from which it is dispensed. Trailing eagerly behind the surgeon, the student is admonished never to forget alcohol withdrawal as a cause of post-operative confusion. The scrap of paper on which this is written spends a month in the white coat pocket before being lost forever in the laundry. At different times, and in inconvenient places, a number of other causes may be presented to the student. Not only are these causes and aphorisms never brought together, but when, as a surgical house officer, the former student faces a confused patient, none is to hand.

This book is intended for use on the ward, in the lecture-theatre, library, and at home. Each subject only occupies 1 page, and opposite is a blank page for additions, updatings, and refinements. If they face the relevant page of print, they will be automatically indexed.

Clinical medicine has a habit of partly hiding as well as partly revealing the patient and his problems. We aim to encourage the doctor to enjoy his patients: in doing so we believe he will prosper in the practice of medicine. For a long time now, house officers have been encouraged to adopt monstrous proportions in order to straddle simultaneously the diverse pinnacles of clinical science and clinical experience. We hope that this book will make this endeavour a little easier by moving a cumulative memory burden from the mind into the pocket, and by removing some of the fears that are naturally felt when starting a career in medicine, thereby freely allowing the doctor's clinical acumen to grow by the slow accretion of many, many days and nights.

RAH
JML

Conflicts of interest

This volume has been critically appraised by 2 doctors (JML & JABC) who have no contact with commercial interests such as pharmaceutical companies. In order to reassure readers that there has been no covert pressure to exclude or include certain drugs in this text, they have adhered to a policy of not seeing representatives from any such commercial company, and neither are they in receipt of any gifts or hospitality from such companies.

Drugs (and how to keep abreast of changes)

While every effort has been made to check this text, it is still possible that errors have been missed. Also, dosage schedules are continually being revised and new side-effects recognized. Oxford University Press makes no representation, expressed or implied, that drug dosages in this book are correct. For these reasons, the reader is strongly urged to consult the most recently published *British National Formulary*, and the pharmaceutical company's *data sheet* (summaries of product characteristics/SPC; www.Medicines.org.uk) before administering any of the drugs recommended in this book. Unless stated otherwise, drug doses and recommendations are for the *non-pregnant adult* who is *not breast-feeding*.

Corrections and updatings are posted on the Internet at www.oup.com/uk/medicine/handbooks and www.emispdp.com. See also the *What's new* section of www.bnf.org.

Readers are also reminded of the need to keep up-to-date, and that this need can only ever be partly addressed by printed texts such as this.

Drug nomenclature[1]

This volume uses British[uk] approved names, followed, where there is a difference, by the recommended international non-proprietary name (rINN; usually there is no difference). A European Directive requires use of rINNs in the European Community. Exceptions to giving both names occur where the change is minute, eg amoxycillin[uk]/amoxicillin, where the rINN is used, to avoid tedious near-duplications. Among the new rINNs used are:

Alimemazine	(trimeprazine[uk])	Epinephrine	(adrenaline[uk])
Amoxicillin	(amoxycillin[uk])	Furosemide	(frusemide[uk])
Bendroflumethiazide	(bendrofluazide[uk])	Hydroxycarbamide	(hydroxyurea[uk])
		Lidocaine	(lignocaine[uk])
Ciclosporin	(cyclosporin[uk])	Chlormethine	(mustine[uk])
Clomifene	(clomiphene[uk])	Norepinephrine	(noradrenaline[uk])
Diethylstilbestrol	(stilboestrol[uk])	Sulfonamides (all)	(sulphonamides[uk])
Dosulepin	(dothiepin[uk])	Trihexyphenidyl	(benzhexol[uk])

rINNs for cephalosporins now all start with *cef* (not *ceph*). For consistency, and to avoid distracting variations in adjacent usages, we have spelt sulphur (and its derivatives) *sulfur* as all *sulphonamides* have a rINN starting *sulf...*

1 For a full list of recommended international non-proprietary names, see www.bnf.org

Acknowledgements

We would like to record our heartfelt thanks to our advisers on specific sections—each is acknowledged on each chapter's first page.

For checking the text we thank, and admire the fortitude of Dr J Collier, Dr Ghassanhamad, Dr H Jones, Dr P Lawson, Dr A Mafi, Dr R Wilkins. We also thank Suman Biswas for his comments on various sections. We particularly thank our drug reader, Dr Steve Emmett, for his painstaking work.

IBW would like to acknowledge his clinical mentors Jim Holt and John Cockcroft. SRR would like to extend particular thanks to the following consultants who have provided invaluable assistance on certain specialist surgical topics: Mr R Hardwick (*Upper GI*), Dr J Stevens (*Anaesthetics*), Mr K Varty (*Vascular*), Mr A Doble (*Urology*), and Dr C Wilson (*Surgical oncology*).

We also thank the team at Egton Medical Information Systems and the insights they have brought to this work: Dr H Thomas, Dr P Scott, Dr D Ward, Dr J Cox, Dr S Huins, Dr H Huins, Dr L Knott, Mr C Westerman, and Dr G Brooks (project director).

We also thank Dr P Scally and Dr J Harper for providing the x-ray plates, as well as for many thoughtful comments on the whole text. For further help we thank Dr J Burke and Professor J McCormack.

The British Lending Library, and staff at the Cairns Library, Oxford, and at Worthing Postgraduate Library have been most helpful in tracing references. Finally we would like to thank the staff of OUP for their help and support.

Readers' participation

Few authors can have been as fortunate in their readers' generosity and attention to detail as we have been in past editions. The long list below is proof that there is no alternative to the collaborative approach in medicine. We enjoy this collaboration (and the interesting verification work it entails) and the friendships it has brought. Taken all-in-all, our readers have more knowledge than our teachers and all the writers of the great medical tomes. It is a great pleasure to be able to coordinate this knowledge, and share it.

Thanks to this feedback on our readers' comments cards, we hope that this edition is keeping ever more nearly in step with our readers' needs. We have tried to write to all who have been kind enough to write to us, and apologize to anyone we have missed. In some instances comments were sent but either no name was given or we were unable to decipher their writing. We thank these anonymous people as well as the following for their interesting points and valuable help: Professor Tor Chiu (Hong Kong); Dr M Onwuamaegbu; Julie Thomas, cardiac nurse, St Richard's Hospital, Chichester; Milanovic Dusan, Fellow in Science, Mannheim, Germany; Huw J Davies, GP Principal, Port Talbot Wales; Laura Clipsham, medical student, Newark; Shayda Khoshnaw; Dr H S Livingston, Manguzi Hospital, Kwangwanase, South Africa; N Bhagrath, medical student, West Midlands; Dr Shakeel Ahmad, Resident ICU, Abdul-Aziz Hospital, Bisha; Jonathan C Yu Jin, University of Melbourne; Dr Edwin E Omohwo, SHO, Brighton; David Williams, medical student, Sheffield; Dr D B K Mistry, South Emsall, Yorkshire; Dr Meto Edgar Onwuamaegbu, Royal Brompton Hospital, Chelsea; M Thomas, Surrey; Pei Sze Liew, medical student, Kuala Lumpur; Marcelino Ruiz Martin, GP registrar, Stoke; Dr Sudad Sofi, Walsall; Michael Murray, Co Waterford, Ireland; Dr Asif H Osmani, Surgeon, Karachi, Pakistan; Tong Sheau Wann, medical student, Selangor, Malaysia; Professor Ng Tian Seng, Malaysia; Andrew Innes, medical student, Aberdeen, Nahla Al-Mansoori, medical student, United Arab Emirates; Dr Familus, Ireland; Dr Amii Asthana, GP, Ealing; Mr S Issa, medical student; Dr Abdul Nasis, Clinical Attachee, Pakistan; M Rafay; S Siddiqui, medical student, Ashford, Kent; E Monair, Student Nurse, Glasgow; Katrina Glasson, medical student, Australia; Bertrand Graz, Switzerland; Alexakis Lyk Ch, medical student, Greece; F Hodge, student, Brockley, London; Dr A Madkhana, Clinical Fellow, London; Dr Hossein Memarzadeh; London;

Cyrus C Chan, student, Dublin, Ireland; Dr Sarah Cox, Palliative Medicine Consultant, Chelsea and Westminster Hospital, London; Medhal Mohamed Madbouly, Cairo; Tariq Parvez, consultant oncologist, King Fahad Hospital, Saudi Arabia; Muhammad Azam Gill, house officer, Allama Iqbal Medical College, Lahore; Dr Glennis Roserson; Daniel Goodare, medical student, Coventry; Tasic Sas Juris, student, Slovenia; M Bevan, Nursing Lecturer, University of Leeds; Johan Wikner, MD, Stockholm; Professor Crispin Scully, Dean, Eastman Dental Institute, University College London; Artem Doletsky, Moscow; C I Buis, medical student, Netherlands; Dr Dilin G Ilapperuma, Sri Lanka; Dr Bansal, Warrington; Dr Ramaraj; Dr D J Grant, County Antrim; C Symeonides, medical student; Adrian Root, medical student, London; Linda Holmes, Nurse, Furness General Hospital, Barrow-in-Furness, Gerald Matiko, medical student, South Africa; Ngoo Kay Seong, medical student, Malaysia; Dr J Ngungu, SHO, London; Dr Jeffrey Boss, Stroud; Ingrid S Heaslip, medical student, County Meath, Ireland; D Clitherow, medical student, Sheffield; Jonathan Busst, Forensic Medical Criminologist, Surrey; Sarah Russ, SHO, Sheffield; Paresh Jogia, clinical pharmacist, Northern General Hospital, Sheffield; Ms Rozali, nurse, Malaysia; Williamson, Mowbray, Sue Littles, clinical nurse specialist, Essex; Sawers, Dumfries & Galloway Royal Infirmary, Dumfries; Dr J D Henderson Slate; Dr Botley; Dr R O'Shaughnessy, SHO, London; Chris Soper; Dr Hajro Shyti, Albania; C S C Hill; Dr Muhammad Asghar & Dr Gulnaz Ashgarai, Dublin; Dr C P Moxon, Birmingham; Katie J Adams, medical student, London; Antonia Kwan, medical student, London; Emily Hodkinson, medical student, Manchester; Miss Pauleen Pratt, Consultant Nurse, Leicester General Hospital, Leicester; Dr Mpmyint, SHO, Yorkshire; S Mohammad, medical student, London; P S Ireland, GP, Birmingham; Samir Khan Kabir, HO, Oldham; Ian McKay, SHO Surgery, Aberdeen; Brian Jordon, Principal GP, County Cork; K Guha, medical student, Coventry; A M E Englebrecht, Dietician, South Africa; Yusef Mahomed, King Edward Hospital, South Africa; Kedsheong Yong, medical officer, Malaysia; Kathy Gannon, Greenridge Surgery, Birmingham; Ahmed Abdelsalam Omran, HO, Cairo; Dr Matiul Haq, Pakistan; Dr Siuashumugam, Malaysia; Ahmed Sokwala, Istanbul; Arne Skulberg, Dublin, Dr A Hammodi, Wembley; Numan Alishah, medical student, High Wycombe; Kathryn Mair, Medical Student, Edinburgh. D Adams, G Adamson, R Adamson, A Adan, A Adiele, M M A Agbabiaka, A Agbobu, X Airton, N Ahmad, S Ahmad, A Alexandroff, M Al-Amin, L Alan, S Alan, A Aldridge, C Aldridge, A Alhashem, M Ali, A Alizai, B Alkani, M Allendorf-Burns, J Allport, S Al-Motari, R Al-Okaili, A Altaf, H Al-Tuiur, A Alvi, C Antonetti, M Anwar, R Armstrong, A Ashoush, R Asser, P Atack, M Azam, C Bache, D Baddeley, B Badgruddin, A Baig, N Balaswiya, D Bansevicius, M Barkham, M Barry, J Barth, H Bhatti, G Baumgartner, M Beirne, J Benbow, M Beranek, E Berinou, G Bhari, A Bhattarai, H Bhatti, A Bishop, J Bishop, I Bleenhen, K Boddu, M Bhagrath, V Bookhan, B Bourke, M Bowen, J Bradshaw, E Brewster, A Broadbent, J Brooks, J Brown, P Brykalski, H Bueckert, K Burn, M and G Butoi, P Buttery, A Byron, E Cameron, J Cameron, P Camosa, C Campbell, N Caporaso, D Carr, A Carvejal, R Casson, A Caulea, S Cembrowicz, R Chaira, E Chambers, V Char, M Charter, O Chaudhri, W Chicken, T Chin, P Chiquito, T Choudhry, A Chowdharay-Best, R Ciobanu, B Cleaver, L D Clark, J Collen, E Collier, M Collins, B Colvin, P Conway-Grim, S Cook, R Coull, J Cox, G Crockett, C Cuéllar, T Cuéllar, T Crockett, P Culliney, E Dankwa, A Das-Gupta, N David, G Davidson, H Davies, R Davies, Y de Boer, U Desai, A de silva, M de Silva, J Devine, G Dex, D Dey, E Dickinson, A Ditri, J Dobbie, J Donkin, P Dowds, M Dusan, N Duthie, T Eden, V Eden, D Elridge, N Elkan, D Ellis, R England, M Erlewyn-Lajeunesse, E Ersani, M Essa, G Evans, A Ezigweth, M Faragher, M Farooq, C Finfa, P Fisichella, E Fitzpatrick, P Flanagan, J Foust, M Gagan, J Ganane, I Ganans, M Gardarsdottir, J Germain, S Ghaem, J Gibson, K Gibson, M Gibson, J Gilbody, C Goddwin, S Gott, J Gotz, E Goudsmit, H Gray,

F Grima, J Grimley-Evans, D Groneberg, S Gupta, C Haase, D Habart, T Halbert, A Halitsky, J Haller, J Halpern, E Hammond, R Hanlon, C Hanna, R Haynes, J Hays, D Heath, G Heese, S Hjorleifsson, P Hollinshead, J Hopkinson, K Horncastle, A Horsfall, A Houghton, R Houghton, L Houlberg, P Hrincko, Z Htwe, M Hughes, M Huqit, M Hussian, I Ibrahim, J Iglesia, A Iqbal, S Jankovic, N Jayasekera, A Jennings, G Johnson, J de Jong, N Joshi, A Joshua, H Kan, Z Kango, R Karplus, E Katz, A Kelly, A Khalid, I Khan, M Klasa, W Klei, B Koh, Y Kontrobarsky, S Khoshnaw, N Kovacevic, M Kuepfer, H Kuralco, L Kwan, J Lagercranbe, G Lane, F Larkin, R Lawson, S Lee, G Lewis, J Lewis, J Lightowler, J Lima, J Linder, D Livingstone, F Lloyd, H Lockner, G Lomax, A Longmore, I Low, M Lowenthal, G Lyons, H MacDonald, P Mackey, C Maddok, P Maher, Y Mahomed, M Malkawi, D Mallett, C Martin, T Matteucci, G Matthes, E Mayer, J McAughan, A McCafferty, D McCandless, F McCormick, C McDaniel, A McDougall, J McGregor, H McIntosh, J McKenzie, F McLellan, K Marriott, D Meeking, B Melrad, M Melvan, E Merrens, W Mgaya, R Miller, K Mitchell, A Mohammed, S Monella, S Morariot, M Morgan, B Morton, D Moskopp, S Moultrie, M Moutoussis, M Muqit, M Musa, H Mutasa, K Muthe, S Muttu, T Mutwirah, N Naqui, A Naraen, J Nasir, M Nassar, M Nasson, B Naunton, E Neoh, M Nekhaila, M Newell, F Norman-Taylor, D Novitt, N Numan, K O'Driscoll, B Olalekan, O Olarinde, J Olson, S Otchirov, B Pait, F Palazzo, L Pang, L Pantanowitz, P Papanicolaou, B Parkin, C Patel, N Proho, E Pringle, M Procopiou, J Pryce, J Pryse, D Puxley, B Pynenburg, M Quaraishi, G Quiceno, H Raeder, R Raeder, H Rahman, A Ramachandran, C Ramyad, R Ranai, A Rasheed, R Rastogi, F Regan, J Revilla, D Rharmi, N Richmond, A Ritchie, M Robert, J Roberts, H Robertson-Ritchie, J Robinson, F Rosenberg, A Rosenthal, S Rothery, J Rudd, D Ryms, S-U Safer, J Salama, R Salib, A Samieh-Tucker, L Sarkozi, P Saunders, H Sayanvala, J Schmitt, J Schneider, H Schumacher, A Schutte, S Schwarz, F Scrase, M Scrase, P Seeley, F Sellers, Dr V Seshan, Christie Hospital, Manchester, D Steeples, V Sepe, A Shablak, Shahnaz-Hayat, T Shaikit, K Sheehan, D Shukla, I Silva, A Silverman, K Simpson, T Singh, S Sivananthan, E Smeland, R Smit, S Soran, G Spencer, P Spranh, K Spreadbury, K Sri-Ram, M Strahan, P Statham, D Stead, J Stern, A Stevenson, J Steyn, D Stredder, M Strachan, A Struber, R Szabo, A Taimoor, H Talat, J Tang, A Tavakkolizadeh, A Taylor, D Taylor, N Taylor, S Taylor, M Tengoe, F Toe, J Thomas, S Thomas, W Thomas, F Thompson, L Thomson, T Toma, S Topiwala, B Traynor, L Trieu, J Trois, P Trotman, T Tscherning, D Turner, M Turner, F Uddin, K Umanok, S Vaidya, C Vandenbussche, C van der Worp, J Van-Tam, M Vaughan, J Verghese, Y Wahowed, L Walker, S Walker, M Walsh, T Walton, T Wang, L Wasantu, J Watkins, L Watson, K Weerasinghe, H Weerasooriya, W Westall, P Whelan, T Whitehouse, J Wiesenfeldt, T Wiggin, J Wijbenga, P Wijingaarden, R Williams, J Williamsen, J Williamson, J Winkler, M Wong, S Wong, J Wood, X Xiong, D Yaniu, A Yawar, E Yeoh, N Yoo, K Yuet, A Zafiropoulos, R Zajdel, K Zarrabi, M Zeigler, M Zein, and M Zia.

Symbols and abbreviations

▶	this fact or idea is important
▶▶	don't dawdle!—prompt action saves lives
◆	incendiary (controversial) topic
🖫	reference available on our website www.oup.com/OHCM
♂:♀	male-to-female ratio (♂:♀ = 2:1 means twice as common in males)
@12345678	search Medline (www.ncbi.nlm.nih.gov/PubMed/) with this number to find the abstract referred to (don't include @ in the search)
∴ ~	on account of (∴ means *therefore*; ~ means *approximately*)
–ve; +ve	negative and positive, respectively
↑; ↓; ↔	increased, decreased, and normal, respectively (eg serum level)
Δ	diagnosis
ΔΔ	differential diagnosis
A₂	aortic component of second heart sound
A2A	angiotensin-2 receptor antagonist (p283; = AT-2, A2R, and AIIR)
Ab	antibody
ABC	airway, breathing, and circulation: basic life support (p766)
ABG	arterial blood gas measurement (P_aO_2, P_aCO_2, pH, HCO_3^-)
ABPA	allergic bronchopulmonary aspergillosis
ac	*ante cibum* (before food)
ACE(i)	angiotensin-converting enzyme (inhibitors)
ACTH	adrenocorticotrophic hormone
ADH	antidiuretic hormone
Ad lib	ad libitum; as much/as often as wanted (Latin for *at pleasure*)
ADL	activities of daily living
AF	atrial fibrillation
AFB	acid-fast bacillus
AFP	(and α-FP) alpha-fetoprotein
Ag	antigen
AIDS	acquired immunodeficiency syndrome
alk phos	alkaline phosphatase (also ALP)
ALL	acute lymphoblastic leukaemia
AMA	antimitochondrial antibody
AMP	adenosine monophosphate
ANA	antinuclear antibody
ANCA	antineutrophil cytoplasmic antibody
APTT	activated partial thromboplastin time
AR	aortic regurgitation
ARA	angiotensin receptor antagonist (p283; also AT-2, A2R, and AIIR)
ARDS	acute respiratory distress syndrome
ARF	acute renal failure
AS	aortic stenosis
ASD	atrial septal defect
ASO(T)	antistreptolysin O (titre)
AST	aspartate transaminase
AT-2	angiotensin-2 receptor blocker (p283; also AT-2, A2R, and AIIR)
ATN	acute tubular necrosis
ATP	adenosine triphosphate
AV	atrioventricular
AVM	arteriovenous malformation(s)
AXR	abdominal x-ray (plain)
azt	zidovudine
Ba	barium
BAL	bronchoalveolar lavage

BCR	British comparative ratio (≈INR)
bd	*bis die* (twice a day)
BKA	below-knee amputation
BMJ/BMA	*British Medical Journal/British Medical Association*
BNF	*British National Formulary*
BP	blood pressure
bpm	beats per minute (eg pulse)
ca	carcinoma
CABG	coronary artery bypass graft
cAMP	cyclic adenosine monophosphate (AMP)
CAPD	continuous ambulatory peritoneal dialysis
CBD	common bile duct
CC	creatinine clearance
CCF	congestive cardiac failure (ie left and right heart failure)
CCU	coronary care unit
CHB	complete heart block
CHD	coronary heart disease (related to ischaemia and atheroma)
CI	contraindications
CK	creatine (phospho)kinase (also CPK)
CLL	chronic lymphocytic leukaemia
CML	chronic myeloid leukaemia
CMV	cytomegalovirus
CNS	central nervous system
COC	combined oral contraceptive, ie (o)estrogen + progesterone
COPD	chronic obstructive pulmonary disease
CPAP	continuous positive airways pressure
CPR	cardiopulmonary resuscitation
CRF	chronic renal failure
CRP	C-reactive protein
CSF	cerebrospinal fluid
CT	computer tomography
CVP	central venous pressure
CVS	cardiovascular system
CXR	chest x-ray
d	day(s) (also expressed as ×/7)
DC	direct current
DIC	disseminated intravascular coagulation
DIP	distal interphalangeal
dL	decilitre
DoH (or DH)	Department of Health (United Kingdom)
DM	diabetes mellitus
DU	duodenal ulcer
D&V	diarrhoea and vomiting
DVT	deep venous thrombosis
DXT	deep radiotherapy
E-BM	evidence-based medicine (& its journal published by the BMA)
EBV	Epstein–Barr virus
ECG	electrocardiogram
Echo	echocardiogram
EDTA	ethylene diamine tetraacetic acid (eg in FBC bottle)
EEG	electroencephalogram
ELISA	enzyme linked immunosorbant assay
EM	electron microscope
EMG	electromyogram
ENT	ear, nose, and throat

ERCP	endoscopic retrograde cholangiopancreatography
ESR	erythrocyte sedimentation rate
ESRF	end-stage renal failure
EUA	examination under anaesthesia
FB	foreign body
FBC	full blood count
FDP	fibrin degradation products
FEV_1	forced expiratory volume in first second
FFP	fresh frozen plasma
F_iO_2	partial pressure of O_2 in inspired air
FROM	full range of movements
FSH	follicle-stimulating hormone
FVC	forced vital capacity
g	gram
GA	general anaesthetic
GAT^{sanford}	Sanford *guide to antimicrobial therapy* www.sanfordguide.com
GB	gall bladder
GC	gonococcus
GCS	Glasgow coma scale
GFR	glomerular filtration rate
GGT	gamma glutamyl transpeptidase
GH	growth hormone
GI	gastrointestinal
GP	general practitioner
G6PD	glucose-6-phosphate dehydrogenase
GTN	glyceryl trinitrate
GTT	glucose tolerance test (also OGTT: oral GTT)
GU	genitourinary
h	hour
HAV	hepatitis A virus
Hb	haemoglobin
HBsAg/HBV	hepatitis B surface antigen/hepatitis B virus
HCC	hepatocellular cancer
Hct	haematocrit
HCV	hepatitis C virus
HDL	high-density lipoprotein, p706
HDV	hepatitis D virus
HHT	hereditary haemorrhagic telangiectasia
HIDA	hepatic immunodiacetic acid
HIV	human immunodeficiency virus
HOCM	hypertrophic obstructive cardiomyopathy
HONK	hyperosmolar nonketotic (diabetic coma)
HRT	hormone replacement therapy
HSV	Herpes simplex virus
ICP	intracranial pressure
IDA	iron-deficiency anaemia
IDDM	insulin-dependent diabetes mellitus
IFN-α	alpha interferon
IE	infective endocarditis
Ig	immunoglobulin
IHD	ischaemic heart disease
IM	intramuscular
INR	international normalized ratio (prothrombin ratio)
IPPV	intermittent positive pressure ventilation
ITP	idiopathic thrombocytopenic purpura

ITU	intensive therapy unit
iu	international unit
IVC	inferior vena cava
IV(I)	intravenous (infusion)
IVU	intravenous urography
JAMA	*Journal of the American Medical Association*
JVP	jugular venous pressure
K	potassium
KCCT	kaolin cephalin clotting time
kg	kilogram
kPa	kiloPascal
L	litre
LAD	left axis deviation on the ECG
LBBB	left bundle branch block
LDH	lactate dehydrogenase
LDL	low-density lipoprotein, p706
LFT	liver function test
LH	luteinizing hormone
LIF	left iliac fossa
LKKS	liver, kidney (R), kidney (L), spleen
LMN	lower motor neurone
LP	lumbar puncture
LUQ	left upper quadrant
LV	left ventricle of the heart
LVF	left ventricular failure
LVH	left ventricular hypertrophy
µg	microgram
MAI	*Mycobacterium avium intracellulare*
MAOI	monoamine oxidase inhibitors
mane	morning (derived from the Latin)
MC & S	microscopy, culture and sensitivity
MCV	mean cell volume
MDMA	3,4-methylenedioxymethamphetamine
ME	myalgic encephalomyelitis
MET	maximal exercise test
mg	milligram
MI	myocardial infarction
min(s)	minute(s)
mL	millilitre
mmHg	millimetres of mercury
MND	motor neurone disease
MRI	magnetic resonance imaging
MRSA	methicillin-resistant *Staphylococcus aureus* (p590)
MS	multiple sclerosis (do not confuse with mitral stenosis)
MSU	midstream urine
NAD	nothing abnormal detected
NBM	nil by mouth
ND	notifiable disease
NEJM	*New England Journal of Medicine*
ng	nanogram
NG(T)	nasogastric (tube)
NHS	National Health Service (UK)
NICE	National[UK] Institute for Clinical Excellence (www.nice.org.uk)
NIDDM	noninsulin-dependent diabetes mellitus
NMDA	*N*-methyl-D-aspartate

NNT	number needed to treat, for 1 extra satisfactory result (p30)
Nocte	at night
NR	normal range—the same as reference interval
NSAIDs	non-steroidal anti-inflammatory drugs
N&V	nausea and/or vomiting
od	*omni die* (once daily)
OD	overdose
OGD	oesophagogastroduodenoscopy
OGS	oxogenic steroids
OGTT	oral glucose tolerance test
OHCS	*Oxford Handbook of Clinical Specialties*, 6ᵉ OUP, Collier & Longmore
om; on	*omni mane* (in the morning); *omni nocte* (at night)
OPD	out-patients department
ORh–	blood group O, Rh negative
OT	occupational therapist
OTM/S	*Oxford Textbook of Medicine* (OUP 4ᵉ, 2003)/*Surgery* (2000)
P_2	pulmonary component of second heart sound
P_aCO_2	partial pressure of carbon dioxide in arterial blood
PAN	polyarteritis nodosa
P_aO_2	partial pressure of oxygen in arterial blood
PBC	primary biliary cirrhosis
PCP	*Pneumocystis carinii* pneumonia
PCR	polymerase chain reaction (DNA diagnosis)
PCV	packed cell volume
PE	pulmonary embolism
PEEP	positive end-expiratory pressure
PERLA	pupils equal and reactive to light and accommodation
PEF(R)	peak expiratory flow (rate)
PID	pelvic inflammatory disease
PIP	proximal interphalangeal (joint)
PMH	past medical history
PND	paroxysmal nocturnal dyspnoea
PO	*per os* (by mouth)
PPF	purified plasma fraction (albumin)
PPI	proton pump inhibitor, eg omeprazole, lansoprazole, etc.
PR	*per rectum* (by the rectum)
PRL	prolactin
PRN	*pro re nata* (as required)
PRV	polycythaemia rubra vera
PSA	prostate specific antigen
PTH	parathyroid hormone
PTT	prothrombin time
PUO	pyrexia of unknown origin
PV	*per vaginam* (by the vagina; the route for pessaries)
qds	*quater die sumendus* (to be taken 4 times a day)
qid	*quater in die* (4 times a day); qqh: *quarta quaque hora* (every 4h)
R	right
RA	rheumatoid arthritis
RAD	right axis deviation on the ECG
RBBB	right bundle branch block
RBC	red blood cell
RFT	respiratory function tests
Rh	Rh; not an abbreviation, but derived from the rhesus monkey
RIF	right iliac fossa
RUQ	right upper quadrant

RV	right ventricle of heart
RVF	right ventricular failure
RVH	right ventricular hypertrophy
℞	*recipe* (treat with)
s or sec	second(s)
S1, S2	first and second heart sounds
SBE	subacute bacterial endocarditis (IE, *infective endocarditis*, is better)
SC	subcutaneous
SD	standard deviation
SE	side-effect(s)
SL	sublingual
SLE	systemic lupus erythematosus
SOB	short of breath (SOB(O)E: short of breath on exercise)
SPC	summary of product characteristics (/SPC; www.medicines.org.uk)
SR	slow-release (also called modified-release)
stat	*statim* (immediately; as initial dose)
STD/STI	sexually-transmitted disease or sexually-transmitted infection
SVC	superior vena cava
sy(n)	syndrome
T°	temperature
t½	biological half-life
T3	triiodothyronine
T4	thyroxine
TB	tuberculosis
tds	*ter die sumendus* (to be taken 3 times a day)
TFTs	thyroid function tests (eg TSH)
TIA	transient ischaemic attack
TIBC	total iron binding capacity
tid	*ter in die* (3 times a day)
TPR	temperature, pulse, and respirations count
TRH	thyroid-releasing hormone
TSH	thyroid-stimulating hormone
U	units
UC	ulcerative colitis
U&E	urea & electrolytes & creatinine in plasma, unless stated otherwise
UMN	upper motor neurone
URT	upper respiratory tract
URTI	upper respiratory tract infection
US(S)	ultrasound (scan)
UTI	urinary tract infection
VDRL	venereal diseases research laboratory
VE	ventricular extrasystole
VF	ventricular fibrillation
VMA	vanillyl mandelic acid (HMMA)
V̇/Q̇	ventilation/perfusion ratio
VSD	ventriculo-septal defect
VT	ventricular tachycardia
WBC	white blood cell
WCC	white cell count
wk(s)	week(s)
WR	Wassermann reaction
yr(s)	year(s)
ZN	Ziehl–Neelsen (stain for acid-fast bacilli, eg mycobacteria)

Other abbreviations are given on pages where they occur: consult the *index*.

The Old Hippocratic oath ~425BC

I swear by Apollo the physician, and Aesculapius and Health and All-heal, and all the gods and goddesses, that, according to my ability and judgment, I will keep this oath and stipulation—to reckon him who taught me this Art equally dear to me as my parents, to share my substance with him, and relieve his necessities if required; to look upon his offspring in the same footing as my own brothers, and to teach them this Art, if they shall wish to learn it, without fee or stipulation, and that by percept, lecture, and every other mode of instruction, I will impart a knowledge of the Art to my own sons, and those of my teachers, and to disciples bound by a stipulation and oath according to the law of medicine, but to none other.

I will follow that system of regimen, which, according to my ability and judgment, I consider for the benefit of my patients, and abstain from whatever is deleterious and mischievous.

I will give no deadly medicine to anyone if asked, nor suggest any such counsel; and in like manner I will not give to a woman a pessary to produce abortion. With purity and with holiness I will pass my life and practice my Art.

I will not cut persons labouring under the stone, but will leave this work to be done by men who are practitioners of this work.

Into whatever houses I enter, I will go into them for the benefit of the sick, and will abstain from every voluntary act of mischief and corruption; and, further, from the seduction of females, or males, of freemen or slaves.

Whatever, in connection with my professional practice, I see or hear, in the life of men, which ought not to be spoken of abroad, I will not divulge, as reckoning that all such should be kept secret.

While I continue to keep this oath unviolated, may it be granted to me to enjoy life and practice this Art, respected by all men, in all times. Should I violate this Oath, may the reverse be my lot.

A new Hippocratic oath ~2004AD

I promise that my medical knowledge will be used to benefit people's health; patients are my first concern. I will listen to them, and provide the best care I can. I will be honest, respectful, and compassionate towards them.

I will do my best to help anyone in medical need, in emergencies. I will make every effort to ensure the rights of all patients are respected, including vulnerable groups who lack means of making their needs known.

I will exercise my professional judgment as independently as possible, uninfluenced by political pressure or the social standing of my patient. I will not put personal profit or advancement above my duty to my patient.

I recognize the special value of human life, but I also know that prolongation of life is not the only aim of health care. If I agree to perform abortion,[1] I agree it should take place only within an ethical and legal context.

I will not provide treatments that are pointless or harmful, or which an informed and competent patient refuses. I will help[2] patients find the information and support they want to make decisions on their care.

I will answer as truthfully as I can, and respect patients' decisions, unless that puts others at risk of substantial[3] harm. If I cannot agree with their requests, I will explain why.

If my patients have limited mental awareness, I will still encourage them to participate in decisions as much as they feel able. I will do my best to maintain confidentiality about all patients.

If there are overriding reasons preventing my keeping a patient's confidentiality I will explain them. I will recognize the limits of my knowledge and seek advice from colleagues as needed. I will acknowledge my mistakes.

I will do my best to keep myself and my colleagues informed of new developments, and ensure that poor standards or bad practices are exposed to those who can improve them.

I will show respect for all those with whom I work and be ready to share my knowledge by teaching others what I know. I will use my training and professional standing to improve the community in which I work.

I will treat patients equitably and support a fair and humane distribution of health resources. I will try to influence positively authorities whose policies harm public health.

I will oppose policies which breach internationally accepted standards of human rights. I will strive to change laws that are contrary to patients' interests or to my professional ethics.

While I continue to keep this Oath unviolated, may it be granted to me to enjoy life and the practice of the Art, respected by all, in all times.

After the BMA's *Revised Hippocratic Oath*, with changes:

1 The BMA draft did not cater for those believing that abortion is unethical.

2 The BMA wording was stronger here, requiring us to *ensure* that patients actually *receive* this information (often an impossibility).

3 The word *substantial* has been added to prevent a serious breach of confidentiality in the name of a slight benefit to another party. Contrary to the BMA's version, the last paragraph about enjoying life has been inserted from the old Oath. Other changes are minor.

Prologue to clinical medicine: *Dag Hammarskjöld on teamwork*

All good doctors are good team players, because health care is complex, and nobody knows everything; and nobody knows how to relate to every patient and his or her unique needs. Because we are all fallible, we all see many examples of poor teams, where bad communication, power struggles, and personality clashes lead to poor outcomes. Stress, overwork, and resource restrictions contribute to this, but not inevitably. So it is worthwhile, at the outset of this journey through clinical medicine, to commit oneself to being a good team member. 3 rules help: (1) All members are valuable; none is irreplaceable, and members are valued for who they are, not just for the resources they bring. (2) 'Innocence is no excuse'—ie you may not be 'to blame' for a group's malfunction but in the end each member is responsible for everything. (3) Every member needs encouragement. Just how important this is, is shown by this comment from a well-known statesman[1]:

'He was impossible. It wasn't that he didn't attend to his work. But his manner brought him into conflict with everybody … When the crisis came, and the whole truth had to come out, he laid the blame on us: in his conduct there was nothing, absolutely nothing to reproach. His self-esteem was so strongly bound up, apparently, with the idea of his innocence, that one felt a brute as one demonstrated, step by step, the contradictions in his defence, and, bit by bit, stripped him naked before his own eyes. But justice to others demanded it.

When the last rag of a lie had been taken from him, and we thought there was nothing more to be said, out it came with stifled sobs.

"But why did you never help me? You knew that I always felt you were against me. And fear and insecurity drove me further and further along the course for which you now condemn me. It's been so hard—everything. One day, I remember, I was so happy: one of you said that something I had produced was quite good—"

So, in the end, we were, in fact, to blame. We had not voiced our criticisms, but we had allowed them to stop us from giving him a single word of acknowledgement, and in this way had barred every road to improvement. It is always the stronger one who is to blame.'

1 *Markings* p47 1964 *Dag Hammarskjöld* Translated by WH Auden, Faber.

Thinking about medicine

Contents

Ideals

Decision and *intervention* are the essence of action: reflection and conjecture are the essence of thought: the essence of medicine is combining these realms of action and thought in the service of others. We offer these ideals to stimulate both thought and action: like the stars, these ideals are hard to reach—but they serve for navigation during the night.

- *Do not blame the sick for being sick.*
- *If the patient's wishes are known, comply with them.*
- *Work for your patients, not your consultant.*
- *Use ward rounds to boost the patient's morale, not your own.*
- *Treat the whole patient, not the disease—or the ward sister.*
- *Admit people—not 'strokes', 'infarcts', or 'crumble'.*
- *Spend time with the bereaved*; you can help them shed their tears.
- *Question your conscience*—however strongly it tells you to act.
- *The ward sister is usually right*; respect her opinion.
- *Be kind to yourself*—you are not an inexhaustible resource.
- *Give the patient (and yourself) time*: time to ask questions, time to reflect, time to allow healing to take place, and time to gain autonomy.
- *Give the patient the benefit of the doubt.* If you can, *be optimistic*: optimistic patients who feel in charge live longer *and* feel better.

Ideal and less than ideal methods of care

A story illustrates the options: a man cut his hand and went round to his neighbour for help. This neighbour happened to be a doctor, but it was not the doctor but his 3-year-old daughter who opened the door. Seeing that he was hurt and bleeding, she took him in, pressed her handkerchief over his wound, and reclined him, feet up, in the nearest chair. She stroked his head and patted his hand, and told him about her marigolds, and then about her frogs, and, after some time, was starting to tell him about her father—when he eventually appeared. He quickly turned the neighbour into a patient, and then into a bleeding biohazard, and then dispatched him to Casualty 'for suturing'. (The neighbour had no idea what this was.) He waited 3h in Casualty, had 2 desultory stitches, and 1 interview, with a medical student who suggested a tetanus vaccination (to which he was allergic, as it turned out). He returned to his doctor next door a few days later, praising his young carer, but not the doctor (who had turned him into a patient), nor the hospital (who had turned him into an item on a conveyor belt), nor the student who turned him into a question mark (does a 50-year-old man with a full series of tetanus vaccinations need a booster at the time of injury?).

It was the 3-year-old who was his true nurse-and-physician and universal health worker, who took him in on his own terms, cared for him, and gave him time and dignity. Question her instinct for care as you will: point out that it could have led to harm, and is in any case inadequate for scientific medicine, and that the hospital was just a victim of its own success. But remember that the story shows that *there is*, as TS Eliot said, *at best, only a limited value in the knowledge derived from experience*[1]—eg the knowledge encompassed in this book. The child had the innate understanding and the natural compassion that we all too easily lose amid the science, the knowledge, and our stainless steel universe of organized health care.

---

1 Carl Jung's writings (*Memories, Dreams, Reflections*) support the same conclusion: acquiring knowledge removes us from the mythic world of instinctive understanding—but his life, in which he accumulated vast knowledge, teaches a different lesson: that both worlds are compatible, given a certain genius for reflective self-questioning. Herein lies the secret of the good life at the clinical, and the mythic, bedside.

The bedside manner and communication skills

Our bedside manner matters because it indicates to patients whether they can *trust* us. Where there is no trust there can be little healing. A good bedside manner is not static: it develops in the light of patients' needs, but it is grounded in the timeless clinical virtues of honesty, humour, and humility in the presence of human weakness and human suffering.

The following are examples from an endless variety of phenomena which arise whenever doctors meet patients. One of the great skills (and pleasures) in medicine is to learn how our actions and attitudes influence patients, and how to take this knowledge into account when assessing the validity and significance of the signs and symptoms we elicit. The information we receive from our patients is not 'hard evidence', but a much more plastic commodity, moulded as much by the doctor's attitude and the hospital or consulting room environment as by the patient's own hopes and fears. It is our job to adjust our attitudes and environment so that these hidden hopes and fears become manifest and the channels of communication are always open.

Anxiety reduction or intensification Simple explanation of what you are going to do often defuses what can be a highly charged affair. With children, try more subtle techniques, such as examining the abdomen using the child's own hands, or examining his teddy bear first.

Pain reduction or intensification Compare: 'I'm going to press your stomach. If it hurts, cry out' with 'I'm going to touch your stomach. Let me know what you feel' and 'Now I'll lay a hand on your stomach. Sing out if you feel anything'. The examination can be made to sound frightening, neutral, or joyful, and the patient will relax or tense up accordingly.

The tactful or clumsy invasion of personal space During ophthalmoscopy, eg we must get much nearer to the patient than is acceptable in normal social intercourse. Both doctor and patient may end up holding their breath, which neither helps the patient keep his eyes perfectly still, nor the doctor to carry out a full examination. Simply explain 'I need to get very close to your eyes for this.' (Not 'We need to get very close for this'—one of the authors was kissed repeatedly while conducting ophthalmoscopy by a patient with frontal lobe signs.)

The induction of a trance-like state Watch a skilful practitioner at work palpating the abdomen: the right hand rests idly on the abdomen, far away from the part which hurts. He meets the patient's gaze: 'Have you ever been to the seaside?' (His hand caresses rather than penetrates) . . . 'Imagine you are back on the beach now, perfectly at ease, gazing up at the blue, blue sky' (He presses as hard as he needs) . . . 'Tell me now, where were you born and bred?' If the patient stops talking and frowns only when the doctor's hand is over the right iliac fossa, he will already have found out something useful.

Communication Your skills are useless unless you communicate well. Be simple, and direct. Avoid jargon: 10% of patients think that jaundice means yellow vomit. 'Remission' and 'growth' are frequently misunderstood. See www.psychooncology.org . Give the most important details first. Be specific. 'Drink 6 cups of water per day' is better than 'Drink more fluids'. Give out videos or written information with easy readability. Flesch's formula quantifies this. Reading ease = $207 - 0.85W - S$. W is the mean number of syllables per 100 words, and S is the mean number of words per sentence. 100 is very easy; aim for >70. Do not assume your patient can read. Naming the pictures but not the words on our visual test chart (p63) helps find this out tactfully.

Ensure harmonization between your view of what should be done, and your patient's. We often talk of *compliance* with our regimens, when what we should talk of is *concordance*, for concordance recognizes the central role patient participation in all good plans of care.

Asking questions

No class of questions is 'correct'. Sometimes you need to ask one type of question; sometimes another. Get good at shifting from one kind to another, and you will soon learn to judge the most effective questions for the patient in front of you. The aim of asking questions is to *describe*, not from the point of view of intellectual imperialism ('If you can describe the world, you can have it'), but from the point of view of practical help: what cannot be described cannot be cured, and what is described but still cannot be cured can, at least, be shared, mitigated, and so partially overcome. Different kinds of questions either throw light on this issue, or obscure it, as in the 2 examples below.

Leading questions On seeing a bloodstained handkerchief you ask: 'How long have you been coughing up blood?' '6 weeks, doctor' so you assume haemoptysis for 6 weeks. In fact, the stain could be due to an infected finger, or to epistaxis (nose bleed). On finding this out later (and perhaps after expensive and unpleasant investigations), you will be annoyed with your patient for misleading you—whereas he was trying to be polite by giving the sort of answer you were obviously expecting. With such leading questions as these, the patient is not given an opportunity to deny your assumptions.

Questions suggesting the answer 'Was the vomit red, yellow, or black—like coffee grounds?'—the classic description of vomited blood. 'Yes, like coffee grounds, doctor.' The doctor's expectations and hurry to get the evidence into a pre-decided format have so tarnished the story as to make it useless.

Open questions The most open is 'How are you?' This suggests no particular answer, so the direction a patient chooses offers valuable information. Other examples are gentle imperatives such as 'Tell me about the vomit' 'It was dark' 'How dark?' 'Dark bits in it' 'Like…?' 'Like bits of soil in it.' This information is gold, although it is not cast in the form of 'coffee grounds'.

Patient-centred questions 'What do you think is wrong?' 'Are there any other aspects of this we might explore?' 'Are there any questions you want to ask? (a closed question).' Better still, try 'What are the other things on your mind?' How does having this affect you? What is the worst thing? It makes you feel…' (The doctor is silent.) ▶Unless you become patient-centred your patient may never be fully satisfied with you, or fully cooperative.

Casting your questions over the whole family This is particularly useful in revealing if symptoms are caused or perpetuated by psychological mechanisms. They probe the network of causes and enabling conditions which allow nebulous symptoms to flourish in family life. Who else is important in your life? … Are they worried about you? Who really understands you? Until this sort of question is asked, illness may be refractory to treatment. Eg: 'Who is present when your headache starts? Who notices it first—you or your wife? Who worries about it most (or least)? What does your wife do when (or before) you get it?' Think to yourself: *Who is his headache?* We note with fascination research showing that in clusters of hard-to-diagnose symptoms, it is the spouse's view of them that is the best predictor of outcome: if the spouse is determined that symptoms must be physical, the outcome is worse than if the spouse allows that some symptoms may be psychological.

Echoes Try repeating the last words said as a route to new intimacies, otherwise inaccessible, as you fade into the distance, and the patient soliloquizes '…I've always been suspicious of my wife.' 'Wife …' 'My wife … and her father together.' 'Together…' 'I've never trusted them together.' 'Trusted them together…' 'No, well, I've always felt I've known who my son's real father was… I can never trust those two together.' Without any questions you may unearth the unexpected, important clue which throws a new light on the history.

▶*If you only ask questions, you will only receive answers in reply*. If you interrogate a robin, he will fly away: treelike silence may bring him to your hand.

What is the mechanism? Finding narrative answers

Like toddlers, we should always be asking 'Why?'—not just to find ultimate causes, but to enable us to choose the simplest level for intervention. Some simple change early on in a chain of events may be sufficient to bring about a cure, whereas later on in the chain such opportunities may not arise.

For example, it is not enough for you to diagnose heart failure in your breathless patient. Ask: '*Why is there heart failure?*' If you do not, you will be satisfied with giving the patient an anti-failure drug—and any side-effects from these, such as uraemia or incontinence induced by diuretic-associated polyuria, will be attributed to an unavoidable consequence of necessary therapy.

If only you had asked '*What is the mechanism of the heart failure?*' you might have found an underlying cause, eg anaemia coupled with ischaemic heart disease. You cannot cure the latter, but treating the anaemia may be all that is required to cure the patient's breathlessness. But do not stop there. Ask: '*What is the mechanism of the anaemia?*' You find a low serum ferritin (p626)—and you might be tempted to say to yourself, I have the prime cause.

Wrong! Put aside the idea of prime causes, and go on asking '*What is the mechanism?*' Return to the patient (never think that the process of history-taking is over). Retaking the history shows a very poor diet. '*Why is the patient eating a poor diet?*' Is he ignorant or too poor to eat properly? You may find the patient's wife died a year ago, he is sinking into a depression, and cannot be bothered to eat. He would not care if he died tomorrow.

You now begin to realize that simply treating the patient's anaemia may not be of much help to him—so go on asking '*Why?*': '*Why did you bother to go to the doctor at all if you are not interested in getting better?*' It turns out that he only went to see the doctor to please his daughter. He is most unlikely to take your treatment unless you really get to the bottom of what he cares about. His daughter is what matters and, unless you can enlist her help, all your therapeutic initiatives will fail. Talk with his daughter, offer help for the depression, teach her about iron-rich foods and, with luck, your patient's breathlessness may gradually begin to disappear. Even if it does *not* start to disappear, you may perhaps have forged a friendship with your patient which can be used to enable him to accept help in other ways—and this dialogue may help you to be a more humane and a kinder doctor, particularly if you are feeling worn out and assaulted by long lists of technical tasks which you must somehow fit into impossibly overcrowded days and nights.

Constructing imaginative narratives yielding new meanings Doctors are often thought of as being reductionist and over-mechanistic—the above shows that always asking 'why' can sometimes enlarge the scope of our enquires rather than narrowing the focus. Another way to do this is to ask *What does this symptom mean?*—for this person, his family, and our world. For example, a limp might mean a neuropathy, or inability to meet mortgage repayments (if you are a dancer)—or it may represent a medically unexplained symptom which subtly alters family hierarchies both literally (during family walks through the country) and metaphorically. Science is about clarity, objectivity, and theory in modelling our external world. But there is another way of modelling the external world which involves subjectivity, emotion, ambiguity, and the seeking of arcane relationships between apparently unrelated phenomena. The medical humanities (p21) explore the latter—and have been burgeoning during the last decade —leading to the existence of two camps—humanities or science. If, while reading this you are getting impatient to get to the real nuts and bolts of technological medicine, you are in the latter camp. We are not suggesting that you leave it—only that you learn to operate out of both. If you do not, your professional life will be full of failures (which you may deny or remain in ignorance of). If you *do* straddle both camps, there will also be failures—but you will realize what these failures *mean*, and you will know how to *transform* them.

Death: diagnosis and management

Death is Nature's master stroke, albeit a cruel one, because it allows geno-types space and opportunity to try on new phenotypes. The time comes in the life of any organ or person when it is better to start again from scratch rather than carry on with the weight and muddle of endless accretions. Our bodies and minds are these perishable phenotypes—the froth, which always turns to scum, on the wave of our genes. These genes are not really *our* genes. It is us who belong to them for a few decades. It is one of Nature's great insults that she should prefer to put *all* her eggs in the basket of a defenceless, incompetent neonate rather than in the tried and tested custody of our own superb minds. But as our neurofibrils begin to tangle, and that neonate walks to a wisdom that eludes us, we are forced to give Nature credit for her daring idea. Of course, Nature, in her careless way, can get it wrong: people often die in the wrong order (one of our chief roles is to prevent this mis-ordering of deaths, not the phenomenon of death itself).

So we must admit that, on reflection, dying *is* a brilliant idea, and one that it is most unlikely we could have thought of ourselves.

Causes of death Homicide, suicide, misadventure, or natural causes.

Diagnosing death Apnoea with no pulse[1] and no heart sounds, and fixed pupils. If on a ventilator, brain death may be diagnosed even if the heart is still beating, via the *UK brain death criteria* which state that brain death is death of the brainstem, recognized by establishing:
- Deep coma with absent respirations (hence on a ventilator).
- The absence of drug intoxication and hypothermia (<35°C).
- The absence of hypoglycaemia, acidosis, and U&E imbalance.

Tests: All brainstem reflexes should be absent.
- Unreactive pupils. Absent corneal response.
- No vestibulo-ocular reflexes, ie no eye movement occurs after or during slow injection of 20mL of ice-cold water into each external auditory mea-tus in turn. Visualize the tympanic membrane first to eliminate false nega-tive tests, eg due to wax.
- No motor response within the cranial nerve distribution should be elicited by adequate stimulation.
- No gag reflex or response to bronchial stimulation, and no respiratory effort on stopping the ventilator and allowing P_CO_2 to rise to 6.7kPa.

Other considerations: Repeat the test after a suitable interval—usually 24h. Spinal reflexes are not relevant to the diagnosis of brain death. An EEG recording is not required, nor is a neurologist. The doctor diagnosing brain death must be a consultant (or his deputy registered for >5yrs). The opinion of one other doctor (any) should also be sought.

USA criteria for brain death are slightly different,[2] eg an EEG is required to confirm the absence of cerebral activity if brain death is to be diagnosed within 6h of apparent cessation of brain activity. Diagnosis of brain death is allowed in cases of intoxication if isotope angiography shows absent cerebral circulation, or if the intoxicant has been metabolized.

Organ donation: The point of diagnosing brain death is partly that this allows organs (kidney, liver, cornea, heart, or lungs) to be donated and removed with as little damage from hypoxia as possible. Do not avoid the topic with relatives. Many are glad to give consent and to think that some good can come after the death of their relative, that some part of the relative will go on living, giving a new life to another person.

After death Inform GP/consultant. See the relatives. Sign death certificates promptly. If the cause is violence, injury, neglect, surgery, anaesthesia, alcohol, suicide, or poisoning, or is unknown, inform the Coroner/Procurator Fiscal.

1 Length of absence of circulation (important for non-heart beating organ donation) before brain death occurs is controversial: 2 or 10min? *Lancet* 2000 **356** 528.
2 In USA, death of the *whole* brain is needed.

Facing death

People imagine that they are not afraid of death when they think of it while they are in good health (Marcel Proust). So, to get into the mood, as a thought experiment, place a finger in your left supraclavicular fossa, and feel there the craggy node of Virchow, telling of some distant gastric malignancy, as if it were your death warrant. Perhaps you have just 4 months left. Live with this 'knowledge' for the rest of the day, or rest of the week, and see how it changes your attitude to family and friends on the one hand, and the million irrelevances which clutter our minds on the other. As the week unfolds, you may experience thoughts and feelings that are new to you, but all too familiar to your patients. And as the months and years roll by, and you find yourself sitting opposite certain patients, put that finger once more on that metaphorical node and turn it over in your mind, and it will turn you, so you are sitting not opposite your patient but beside him. There is only so much comfort you can bring in this way, as, in the end, you cannot tame death.

Whenever you find yourself thinking *it is better for him not to know*, suspect that you mean: *it is easier for me not to tell*. We find it hard to tell for many reasons: it distresses patients; it may hold up a ward round; we do not like acknowledging our impotence to alter the course of diseases; telling reminds us of our own mortality and may unlock our previous griefs. We use many tricks to minimize the pain: *rationalization* ('He would not want to know'); *intellectualization* ('Research shows that 37% of people at stage 3 survive 2 years...'); *brusque honesty* ('You are unlikely to survive 1 month' and, so saying, the doctor rushes off to more vital things); *inappropriate delegation* ('Sister will explain it all to you when you are calmer'). Telling may help because:
- He already half knows but everyone shies away so he cannot discuss his fears (of pain, or that his family will not cope).
- There may be many affairs for the patient to put in order.
- To enable him to judge if unpleasant therapy is worthwhile.
- ▶Most patients are told less than they would like to know.

What are his worries likely to be? Put yourself in the patient's place.
- Give some information, and then the opportunity to ask for more.
- Be sensitive to hints that he may be ready to learn more. 'I'm worried about my son'. 'What is worrying you most?' 'Well, it will be a difficult time for him, (pause) starting school next year.' Silence, broken by the doctor 'I get the impression there are other things worrying you.' The patient now has the opportunity to proceed further, or to stop.
- Ensure that the GP and the nurses know what you have and have not said. Also make sure that this is written in the notes.

Stages of acceptance Accepting death takes time, and may involve passing through 'stages' on a path. It helps to know where your patient is on this path (but progress is rarely orderly and need not always be forwards: the same ground often needs to be recovered). At first there may be *shock* and *numbness*, then *denial* (which reduces anxiety), then *anger* (which may lead you to dislike your patient, but anger can have positive attributes, eg in energizing people—and it can trump fear and pain; it is different from hostility), then *grief*, and then, perhaps, *acceptance*. Finally there may be intense longing for death as the patient moves beyond the reach of worldly cares.[1]

Living wills/advance directives If a patient's views are known, comply with them. But these views change, are ambiguous, or hard to interpret, even if a *living will* exists. In one study of a will stating *...with the development of any life threatening medical situation I should not be given active treatment such as antibiotics or ventilation...* ' 6 out of 12 health professionals said they would give antibiotics for pneumonia, as the will was not clear enough (eg had quality of life deteriorated enough to trigger the will?). Assume that living wills *do* have legal status; get help from colleagues or a judge if in doubt.

1 JS Bach 1727 *Ich habe genug*, Cantata No. 82 composed for the Feast of the Purification.

The art and science of diagnosing

Diagnosis is (wrongly) held to be the central process of clinical medicine. We submit that the central processes of medicine are: relieving symptoms, providing reassurance and prognostic information, and lending a sympathetic ear. But it is very difficult to do this well, and to increase your rapport with your patient, unless you have a working diagnosis. How is this achieved?

We diagnose, it is held, by a 3-stage process: we take a history, we examine, and we do tests. We then collate this information, by a process which is never explained, and compare it with features of diseases we know. We then find the best match, and call this the diagnosis. Other nearly matching diseases then form the differential diagnosis (known as ΔΔ). This model ignores two factors: (1) Often no match can be found. (2) Doctors, in practice, hardly ever work like this. So how *are* diagnoses made?

Diagnosing by recognition For students, this is the most irritating method. You spend an hour asking all the wrong questions, and in waltzes a doctor who names the disease, and sorts it out before you have even finished taking the pulse. This doctor has simply recognized the illness like he recognizes an old friend (or enemy). But don't worry: you too will soon reach this position, if you spend enough time at bedsides with other doctors—and you too will just as effortlessly make all the errors that this approach is prone to.[1]

Diagnosing by probability theory Over our clinical lives we unconsciously build up a personal database of diagnoses and outcomes, and associated pitfalls. We unconsciously run each new 'case' through this personal and continuously developing fine-grained probabilistic algorithm—eventually with amazing speed and effortlessness.

Diagnosing by reasoning Like Sherlock Holmes, we exclude each differential diagnosis, then, whatever is left, *however unlikely*, must be the culprit. This process presupposes that your differential does include the culprit, and that we have methods for *absolutely* excluding diseases. All tests are statistical, rather than absolute—which is why the Holmes technique is, at best, fictional.

Diagnosing by WoE WoE stands for 'Wait on events'—and the notes of any good diagnostician will be littered with this injunction. Some doctors need to know immediately and definitively what the diagnosis is, while others can tolerate more uncertainty. With practice, one can sense that patients are not *in extremis*, and that the dangers and expense of exhaustive tests can be obviated by the skilful use of time. This cough *might* represent pneumonia, but I may choose not to prove this *now* by plating out a pulmonary aspirate in the microbiology department. Rather, I may say 'take this prescription if you get feverish, or your sputum becomes green—but you probably don't need anything from me, and your body will simply cure itself: wait and see.'

Diagnosing by hypothesizing We formulate a hypothesis and then try to disprove or prove it. Proof is elusive, but, in practice, who *does* doubt the blood's circulation, or the notion that humans are vertebrates?

Diagnosing by selective doubting Traditionally, patients are 'unreliable', signs are objective, and lab tests virtually perfect. When diagnosis is difficult, try inverting this hierarchy. The more you do so, the more you realize that there are no hard signs or perfect labs. But the game of medicine is unplayable if you doubt everything: so doubt selectively, bearing in mind Wittgenstein's dictum that unless you can *doubt* an entity, you can never be said to *know* it.

Diagnosing by computer Computing power is the only way of fully mapping the interrelatedness of diseases—eg $Na^+\downarrow$ with eosinophilia points to *Addison's disease*, but if there is oliguria too, a doctor with no computer may have to posit an unrelated disease; but the computer 'knows' that oliguria is a feature of shock, and shock is a complication of Addison's. *See* www.emispdp.com

---

1 Major errors are common (eg 20% on some categories), but use of tests such as ultrasound to validate diagnoses is reducing this rate—going from 1972→1982→1992: 30%→18%→14%. *Lancet* 2000 **355** 2027.

Diagnosis by iteration and reiteration

A brief history suggests looking for a few signs, whose assessment leads you to ask further questions, and do a few tests. These results lead to further questions and tests. The process of taking a history never ends on this view, and as this process reiterates, various diagnostic possibilities crop up, and receive more or less confirmation. 'I feel my heart racing'—and the doctor immediately puts his finger on the pulse, and feels it to be irregularly irregular, and infers atrial fibrillation (AF, p130). He wants to know *why* there is AF, so he asks about weight loss and preferring the cold weather. This suggests hyperthyroidism (p304) as the cause of the AF. While he takes the pulse he notices clubbing of the fingers, so he makes a mental note to do a chest x-ray to see if there are signs of cancer (could this cause the AF?—yes). This reminds him to ask about smoking: while in that parish he asks about alcohol, and elicits excessive drinking. 'Why now?' 'Because I lost my job.' 'Who cares about this more? You or your husband? . . .' In the time it takes to assess the pulse, the doctor has many promising leads to follow, and is starting to formulate a diagnosis in 3 dimensions: physical, psychological, and social. The patient's palms are clammy, and the pulse is weak, so the doctor knows he must be prompt and decisive, and gently explains that admission for various tests is needed. Whereupon the patient, who has been holding back tears, now weeps. Now holding her hand, as well as continuing to take her pulse, the doctor becomes aware of a change in rhythm. Is this sinus rhythm, brought on by the Valsalva-like manoeuvre of weeping? So the doctor now says 'Well . . . let's see how you get on over the next hour—you'll feel better for crying.' 'Yes: you're right, I feel better already.'

   This is a microcosm of the intuitive world of medicine which the systematic (or *only* systematic) doctor never knows. He would come on to the pulse only after a 'full history'—and would have missed everything. The doctor who is prepared to appear muddled, and who can work on many different levels simultaneously, will often be the first to know the diagnosis.

Prescribing drugs

▶Consult the *British National Formulary* (BNF) or your local equivalent before prescribing any drug with which you are not thoroughly familiar.

Before prescribing, ask if the patient is allergic to anything. The answer is often 'Yes'—but do not stop here. Find out what the reaction was, or else you run the risk of denying your patient a possibly life-saving, and very safe drug such as penicillin because of a mild reaction, eg nausea. Is the reaction a *true allergy* (anaphylaxis, p780, or a rash?), a *toxic effect* (eg ataxia is inevitable if given large quantities of phenytoin), or a *predictable adverse reaction* (eg GI bleeding from aspirin), or an *idiosyncratic reaction*?

Remember *primum non nocere*: first do no harm. The more minor the complaint, the more weight this dictum carries. The more serious, the complaint, the more its antithesis comes into play: *nothing ventured, nothing gained.*

Prescribing in renal failure See p277. In liver failure See p231.

Ten commandments ▶These should be written on every tablet.

1 Explore any alternatives to a prescription. Prescriptions lead to doctor-dependency, which in turn frequently leads to bad medicine. They are also expensive: over £5 billion/yr (UK); prices increase much faster than general inflation. There are 3 places to find alternatives: *The larder*: lemon and honey for sore throats, rather than penicillin.
The blackboard:—eg education about the self-inflicted causes of oesophagitis. Rather than giving expensive drugs, advise against too many big meals, smoking and alcohol excess, and wearing over-tight garments.
Lastly, look to yourself. Giving a piece of yourself, some real sympathy, is worth more than all the drugs in your pharmacopoeia to patients who are frightened, bereaved, or weary of life. One of us (JML) for many years looked after an old lady who was paranoid—monthly visits comprised an injection and a hug (no doubt always chaperoned)—until one day mental health nurses took over her care. She was seen by a different nurse on each occasion. They did not know about hugging, so after a while she stopped cooperating, and soon it fell to me to certify her death.

2 Are you prescribing for some minor ailment because you want to solve every problem? Patients may be happy just to know the ailment *is* minor. If he knows what it is, he may be happy to live with it. Some people do not believe in drugs, and you must find this out.

3 Decide if the patient is responsible. If he now swallows *all* the quinine pills you have so attentively prescribed for his cramps, death will be swift.

4 Know of other ways your prescription may be misused. Perhaps the patient whose 'insomnia' you so kindly treated is even now grinding up your prescription prior to injecting himself, desperate for a fix. Will you be suspicious when he returns to say he has lost your prescription?

5 Address these questions when prescribing off the ward:
 • How many daily doses are there? (1–2 is much better than 4.)
 • Are many other drugs to be taken? Can they be reduced?
 • The bottle: can the patient read the instructions—and can he open it?
 • How will you know if the patient forgets to return (follow-up)?
 • If the patient agrees, enlist the spouse's help in ensuring that he remembers to take the pills. Check, eg by counting the remaining pills at the next visit. List potential benefits of *this* drug to *this* patient.

6 List the risks (side-effects, contraindications, interactions, risk of allergy). Of any new problem, always ask yourself: *Is this a side-effect?*

7 Agree with the patient on the risk : benefit ratio's favourability. Try to ensure there is true concordance (p3) between you and your patient.

8 Record how you will review the patient's need for each drug.

9 Quantify progress towards specified, agreed goals, eg pulse rate to mark degree of β-blockade; or peak flow to guide steroid use in asthma.

10 Make a record of all drugs taken. Offer the patient a copy.

Prevention

Two mottoes: *The only good medicine is preventive medicine* and *If preventable…why not prevented?* During life on the wards you will have many opportunities for preventive medicine, and unconsciously you will pass most of them over, in favour of more glamorous tasks such as diagnosis, and clever interventions, involving probes, scalpels, and imaging. But if we imagine a ward where scalpels remain sheathed and the only thing being probed is our commitment to health, then preventive medicine comes to the fore, and it is our contention that such a ward might produce more health than some entire hospitals. The first step is to motivate your patient to take steps to benefit their own health by asking Socratic questions. 'Do you want to smoke?' 'What does your family think about smoking' 'Do you want your children to smoke?' 'Would there be any advantages in giving up?' 'Why is your health important to you?' 'Is there anything more important we can help with?' 'How would you spend the money you might save?' These types of questions along with specific strategies in prevention (p91) are more likely to produce change than withering looks and lectures on lung cancer. In summary: in any preventive activity…get the patient on your side—make him want to change. Once you have done this, preventive activities you might promote include:

Vaccination (eg 'flu if >65yrs)	General health:	Accidents in the home
Osteoporosis prevention if	• cervical cancer	Falls
on steroids (eg alendronate)	cytology	Household dangers
Aspirin if vascular disease	• mammography	Genetic counselling, eg if
Healthy eating	• smoking advice	family history +ve in 2
Cardiovascular risk reduction	• alcohol advice	1st degree relatives

Sometimes referral to other agencies is needed—eg for genetic counselling, contraception, and pre-conception advice (*OHCS* p94).

Ways of thinking about prevention Preventing a disease (eg by vaccination) is *primary prevention*. Controlling disease in an early form (eg carcinoma-*in-situ*) is *secondary prevention*. Preventing complications in those already symptomatic is *tertiary prevention*. The best way of thinking about prevention is *What can I do now with this patient in front of me?* On the wards this will often be secondary or tertiary prevention; eg blood pressure screening in diabetes, or colonoscopy in ulcerative colitis (looking for colon cancer), or endoscopic screening for oesophageal cancer in Barrett's oesophagus (p718). The more complicated or 'high-tech' the procedure, the less likely the aphorism that began this page will be true: the law of unintended consequences decrees that those whom you have to persuade the hardest to accept prevention by screening will be those to whom a complication befalls—such as colon perforation in the above example of colonoscopy. Or you will find an area of possible cancer in someone with Barrett's oesophagus—and a fit person dies of a post-op complication (oesophagectomy is dangerous). With this in mind, concentrate on those preventive activities which are simple, cheap, and have a complication rate approaching zero.

Individualized risk communication Risk communication which is done thoughtlessly and only dwelling on positive aspects can lead to bitterness, anger, and litigation.[8] If communication is based on a person's individual risk factors for a condition (eg age, family history, smoking status, cholesterol level eg using formulae such as that on p22), is risk communicated in ways that change behaviour? A 2003 Cochrane meta-analysis[9] suggests 'not necessarily' (although uptake of screening tests *is* improved). At least this technique promotes dialogue, and dialogue opens doors, minds, and possibilities for choice. *Informed participation* is the aim, not passive acceptance of advice. It does not make much difference whether information is given as an absolute risk, or as a risk score, or categorized as high, medium, or low risk.

Is this new drug any good? (analysis & meta-analysis)

This question frequently arises on reading journals.[10] Not only authors, but *all* clinicians, have to decide what new treatments to recommend, and which to ignore. In assessing the use of research, ask the following:

1 Does it give a clear, clinically significant answer as well as a statistically significant answer in patients similar to those I treat?

2 Is the journal peer reviewed? Experts vet the paper before release (an imperfect process, as they have unknown axes to grind ± competing interests).

3 Are the statistical analyses valid? Much must be taken on trust as many analyses depend on sophisticated computing. Few papers, unfortunately, present 'raw' data. Look out for obvious faults by asking questions such as:

- Is the sample large enough to detect a clinically important difference, say a 20% drop in deaths from disease X? If the sample is small, the chance of missing such a difference is high. In order to reduce this chance to less than 5%, and if disease X has a mortality of 10%, >10,000 patients would need to be randomized. If a small trial which lacks power (the ability to detect true differences) *does* give 'positive' results, the size of the difference between the groups is likely to be exaggerated. (This is type I error; a type II error applies to results which indicate that there is no effect, when in fact there is.) ▶So beware even quite big trials which purport to show that a new drug is equally effective as an established treatment.

- Were the compared groups chosen randomly? Did randomization produce groups that were well matched? Were the treatments being compared carried out by practitioners equally skilled in each treatment?

4 Was the study 'double blind' (both patient and doctor are unaware of which treatment the patient is having)? Could either have told which was given, eg by the metabolic effects of the drug?

5 Was the study placebo-controlled? Good research can go on outside the realm of double-blind, randomized trials, but you need to be more careful in drawing conclusions—eg for intermittent symptoms, a bad time (prompting a consultation) is followed by a good time, making any treatment given in the bad phase appear effective. *Regression towards the mean* occurs in many areas, eg repeated BP measurement: because of transitory or random effects, most people having a high value today will have a less high value tomorrow—and most of those having a low value today will have a less extreme value tomorrow. This concept works at the bedside: if someone who is drowsy after a head injury has a high BP, and the next measurements are *higher still*, ie no regression to the mean, then this suggests a 'real' effect, such as ICP↑.

6 Has time been allowed for criticism of the research to appear in the correspondence columns of the journal in question?

7 If I were the patient, would I want the new treatment?

8 What has the *National Institute for Clinical Excellence*[UK] (NICE) said? Note that NICE quite often changes its mind—a problem with all intelligent organizations.

Meta-analyses Systematic merging of similar trials can help resolve contentious issues and explain data inconsistencies. It is quicker and cheaper than doing new studies, and can establish generalizability of research.[7] *Be cautious!* In one study looking at recommendations of meta-analyses where there was a later 'definitive' big trial, it turned out that meta-analyses got it wrong 30% of the time, and 20% of even good meta-analyses fail to avoid bias.[12] ◆ Don't assume that all meta-analyses, even those from the best stables, such as Cochrane, are free of bias owing to pharmaceutical funding.[13]

▶A well-planned large trial may be worth centuries of uncritical medical practice; but a week's experience on the wards may be more valuable than years reading journals. This is the central paradox in medical education. How can we trust our own experiences knowing they are all anecdotal; how can we be open to novel ideas but avoid being merely fashionable? A stance of wary open-mindedness may serve us best.

Surviving house jobs

If some fool or visionary were to say that our aim should be to produce the greatest health and happiness for the greatest number of our patients, we would not expect to hear cheering from the tattered ranks of midnight house officers: rather, our ears are detecting a decimated groan—because these men and women know that there is something at stake in house-officership far more elemental than health or happiness: namely survival. Here we are talking about our own survival, not that of our patients. It is hard to think of a greater peacetime challenge than these first months on the wards. Within the first weeks, however, brightly your armour shone, it will now be smeared and splattered if not with blood, then with the fallout from very many decisions which were taken without sufficient care and attention. Not that you were lazy, but *force majeure* on the part of Nature and the exigencies of ward life have, we are suddenly stunned to realize, taught us to be second-rate: for to insist on being first-rate in all areas is to sign a kind of death warrant for many of our patients, and, more pertinently for this page, for ourselves. Perfectionism cannot survive in our clinical world. To cope with this fact, or, to put it less depressingly, to flourish in this new world, don't keep re-polishing your armour (what are the 10 causes of atrial fibrillation—or are there 11?), rather furnish your mind—and nourish your body (regular food and drink make those midnight groans of yours less intrusive). Do not voluntarily deny yourself the restorative power of sleep.

We cannot prepare you for finding out that you do not much like the person you are becoming, and neither would we dream of imposing on our readers a recommended regimen of exercise, diet, and mental fitness. Finding out what can lead you through adversity is the art of living. What will you choose: physical fitness, martial arts, poetry, karate, the sermon on the mount, juggling, meditation, yoga, a love affair—or will you make an art form out of the ironic observation of your contemporaries?

Many nourish their inner person through a religious belief, and attend mosque, church, synagogue, or temple. A multicultural society provides diversity and room for all branches of expression. Bear in mind not to compare yourself with your contemporaries. Those who make the most noise are often *not waving but drowning*. Plan your recreation in advance. Start thinking about senior house officer jobs, and speak to the Regional Postgraduate Advisor in the specialty you select. Such enquiries supply energy to get you through the darker hours of house jobs, and may motivate you if the going gets tough. Not that this is any guarantee that the plans will work, but if your yoga, your sermons, and your fitness regimens turn to ashes in your mouth, then at least you will know the direction in which to spit.

House jobs are not just a phase to get through and to enjoy where possible (there are frequently *many* such possibilities); they are also the anvil on which we are beaten into a new and perhaps rather uncomfortable shape. Luckily not all of us are made of iron and steel so there is a fair chance that, in due course, we will spring back into something resembling our normal shape, and, in so doing, we may come to realize that it was our weaknesses, not our strengths, which served us best.

House jobs can encompass tremendous up-and-down swings in energy, motivation, and mood, which can be precipitated by small incidents. If you are depressed for more than a day, speak to a sympathetic friend, partner, or counsellor to help you put it in perspective. ▶When in doubt, communicate.

13

Quality, QALYs, and the interpretation of dreams

Resource allocation: how to decide who gets what Resource allocation is about cutting the health cake—whose size is *given*. What slice should go to transplants, new joints, and services for dementia? Cynics would say that this depends on how vociferous is each group of doctors. But others try to find a rational basis for allocating resources. Health economists (econocrats) have invented the QALY for this purpose.

Making the cake Focusing on how to cut the cake diverts attention from the central issue: how large should the cake be? The answer may be that more needs to be spent on our health service, not at the expense of some other health gain but at the expense of something else.

What is a QALY? The essence of a QALY (Quality Adjusted Life Year) is that it takes a year of healthy life expectancy to be worth 1, but regards a year of unhealthy life expectancy to be worth <1. Its exact value is lower the worse the quality of life of the unhealthy person. If a patient is likely to live for 8yrs in perfect health on an old drug, he gains 8 QALYs; if a new drug would give him 16yrs but at a quality of life rated by him at only 25% of the maximum, he would gain only 4 QALYs. The dream of health economists is to buy most QALYs for his budget. As a rule of thumb, some heath assessment organizations (NICE[UK], controversially) *sometimes* keep an arbitrary figure in their head (such as £30,000/QALY). If an intervention costs more than this, the reasons for recommending it have to be all the more explicit.

Cost per QALY *In various studies, with undeclared assumptions, this was (£):*

GP advice to stop smoking	220	Kidney transplant	4710
Preventing stroke by BP treatment	940	Breast cancer screening	5780
Pacemaker implantation	1100	Infliximab in Crohn's	6700
Valve replaced	1140	Heart transplant	7840
(eg for aortic stenosis)		Home dialysis	17,260
Hip replacement (♀ aged 60–69)	1470	Brain tumour surgery	107,780
CABG for LAD stenosis (p151)	2090	Interferon in MS (p384)	834,000

QALYs *are* helpful in guiding rationing, but problems include accurate pricing, the invidiousness of choosing between the welfare of different patients—and the problem of QALYs not adding up: if a vase of flowers is beautiful, are 10 vases (or QALYs) 10 times as beautiful—or might the scent be overpowering?[1]

The inverse care law and distributive justice

Availability of good medical care tends to vary inversely with the need for it in the population served. This operates more completely where medical care is most exposed to market forces...The market distribution of medical care exaggerates maldistribution of medical resources.

There is much evidence in support of this thesis formulated by Tudor Hart, and there is no doubt that if one wants to make a positive contribution to health, it is no good just discovering pathways, blocking receptors, and inventing drugs. The more this is done, the more urgent the need for distributive justice—that unyielding and perpetually problematic benchmark against which all civilizations must, sometime or other, come to measure themselves.

If those who shout loudest get heard first, we need to know when to train our ears to be deaf—eg when deciding who to put on the urgent list and who to put on the routine list—or who to investigate and who to leave alone. Unconsciously, we calibrate our lives to reduce stress. If we can learn the art of selective deafness, this need for the quiet life becomes less pressing, and, in the silence, we may come to know our professional values a little better.

---

1 This is an example of a non-parametric statistic—ie a numerical system where simple ordering is valid, but not operations such as addition or multiplication. Most medical statistics are assumed to be parametric, but this assumption is often false, invalidating much research. www.statsoft.com/textbook/stnonpar.html

Psychiatry on medical and surgical wards

►Psychopathology is common in colleagues, patients, and relatives. ►Seek help for your own problems. Find a sympathetic GP and register with her. You are not the best person to plan your assessment, treatment, and referral.

Current mental state ►*OHCS* p324. 'Move gently through her thoughts, as one might explore a new garden.[1,20] What is in bloom now? Where do those paths lead? What is under that stone? *Focus on:* Appearance; behaviour (anxious? suspicious?); speech (rate; content); mood; beliefs; hallucinations; orientation; memory (current affairs recall, monarch's name); concentration. Note the patient's insight and degree of your rapport. Non-verbal behaviour.

Depression This is common, and often ignored, at great cost to well-being. 'I would be depressed in her situation. . .', you say to yourself, and so you do not think of offering treatment. The usual biological guides (early morning waking, ↓appetite, ↓weight, loss of interest in sex and hobbies) are of little help in diagnosing depression as they are very common on general wards. *The 2 'best questions' are:*[21] *'Have you been bothered by feeling down, depressed, or hopeless in the last month?'* If so, ask *'Have you been bothered by lack of interest or pleasure in doing things?'* If yes, assume depression is likely. There may also be guilt and feelings of worthlessness. ►*Don't think it's not your job to recognize and treat depression.* It is as important as pain. Try to arrange activities to boost the patient's morale and confidence, and keep him in touch with his fellows. Communicate your thoughts to other members of the team: nurses, physio- and occupational therapists—as well as relatives (if the patient wishes). Among these, your patient may find a kindred spirit who can give insight and support. ►If in doubt, try an antidepressant, and see if it helps—eg lofepramine[2] 70mg/8–12h PO, if no hepatic or severe renal impairment. For *selective serotonin reuptake inhibitors* (eg fluoxetine, 20mg/24h), see *OHCS* p340.

Alcohol This is a common cause of problems on the ward (both the results of abuse and the effects of withdrawal). See p254.

The violent patient Ensure your own and others' safety. Do not tackle violent patients until adequate help is to hand (eg hospital porters or police). Common causes: *alcohol intoxication*, *drugs* (recreational or prescribed), *hypoglycaemia*, *acute confusional states* (p372). Once help arrives, try to talk with the patient to calm him—and to gain an understanding of his mental state. If this fails, consider restraining him. English law allows this. Measure blood glucose, or give IV dextrose stat (p820). If not hypoglycaemic, before further investigation is possible, drugs may be needed, eg haloperidol ~2mg IM (up to 10 or, rarely, 18mg stat; monitor vital signs closely).

Prevent violence by being aware of its early signs, eg restlessness, earnest pacing, clenched fists, morose silences, chanting, shouting. Try to keep your own intuitions alert to developing problems. Find a nurse who knows the patient.

If a rational adult refuses vital treatment, it may be as well to respect this decision, provided he is 'competent', ie he is able to understand the consequences of his actions, and what you are telling him, and is able to retain this information, and form the belief that it is true. Competence is rarely all or nothing, so don't hesitate to get the opinion of a senior doctor. Enlist the persuasive powers of someone the patient respects.

Mental Health Acts Familiarize yourself with local procedures and laws pertaining to your country before your period of duty starts. In England, Common Law allows restraining a patient who is being violent on the ward.

---

1 Ian McEwan 2001 *Atonement* Vintage, 150.
2 Be cautious if history of heart disease, epilepsy, blood dyscrasias, prostatism, glaucoma, hyperthyroidism, or porphyria. SE: drowsiness, confusion, BP↓, pulse↑, vomiting, rash, LFT↑, marrow↓ ± anticholinergic SEs (dry mouth, constipation, vision↓, urine retention, sweating, tremor). Interactions: alcohol, anaesthetics (arrhythmias). Despite this, lofepramine is well tolerated compared with some of the older tricyclic antidepressants. Expect to wait 3wks for benefits to start.

The elderly patient in hospital

▶It is only in the last 200yrs that life-expectancy has risen much above 40yrs. *An ageing population is a sign of successful social, health, and economic policies.*

Healthy ageing is not a contradiction as health is not just '*complete mental and physical wellbeing* (WHO) but also a *process of adaptation, to changing environments, to growing up and ageing, to healing when damaged, to suffering, and death. Health embraces the future so includes anguish and the inner resources to live with it.*' (Illich, OHCS p414). ▶Ageing is a continuum and is malleable, representing the cumulative effects of stressors (eg free radicals) and acquired mechanisms for dealing with them (at least as important as genetic effects).

Beware of ageism Old age is associated with disease but doesn't cause it *per se.* Any deterioration is from treatable disease *until proved otherwise.*

1 Contrary to stereotype, most old people are fit. 95% of those over 65yrs and 80% of those over 85yrs old do not live in institutions; about 70% of the latter can manage stairs and can bathe without help.
2 With any problem, find the cause; don't always be thinking: *this is simply ageing.* Look (within reason) for treatable disease, ↓fitness, and social factors.
3 Do not restrict treatment simply because of age. Old people vary. Age alone is a poor predictor of outcome and should not be used as a substitute for careful assessment of each patient's potential for benefit and risk.

Characteristics of disease in old age There are differences of emphasis in the approach to old people compared with young people.

1 *Multiple pathology:* Several disease processes may coincide: find out which impinge on each complaint (eg senile cataract + arthritis = falls).
2 *Multiple causes:* One problem may have several causes. Treating each alone may do little good; treating all may be of much benefit.
3 *Non-specific presentations:* Some presentations are common in old people—eg the 'geriatric giants': incontinence (p500); immobility; instability (falls); and dementia/confusion (p374 & p372). Any disease may present with these. Also, typical signs and symptoms may be absent (myocardial infarction without chest pain; pneumonia, but no cough, fever, or sputum).
4 *Rapid worsening if treatment is delayed:* Complications are common.
5 *More time is required for recovery:* Points 4–6 reflect impairment in homeostatic mechanisms and loss of 'physiological reserve'.
6 *Impaired metabolism and excretion of drugs:* Doses may need lowering, not least because there is often less tolerance to side-effects.
7 *Social factors:* These are central in aiding recovery and return to home.

Special points *In the history:* Assess all disabilities, then:
• Obtain home details (eg stairs; access to toilet? can alarm be raised?).
• Medication What? When? Assess understanding and concordance (p3). How many different tablets can he cope with? Probably not many more than two. So which are the most important drugs? You may have to ignore other desirable remedies, or enlist the help of a friend, a spouse, or a pharmacist (who can batch morning, noon, and night doses in compartmentalized containers so complex regimens may be reduced to 'take the morning compartment when you get up, the noon compartment before lunch, etc.').
• Social network (regular visitors; family and friends).
• Care details: what services are in operation?—meals delivered; community psychiatric or district nurse—who else is involved in the care?
• Speak to others (relatives; neighbours; carers; GP).
• Make a ***care plan***. Include nutrition. If food is dumped beside a blind man, and no one helps cut it up, he may starve. A passing doctor may arrange CT 'for cachexia', when what he needs is food and cataract surgery.

On examination: Do BP lying and standing (postural drop ≈ falls). Rectal exam: impaction ≈ overflow incontinence. Detailed CNS examination is often needed, eg if presentation is non-specific. This tires patients, so consider doing in batches.

Beyond the hospital: planning successful discharges
(How to live and be frail in the community)

▶*Start planning discharge from day 1.* A very common question on ward-rounds is: 'Will this patient get on OK at home?—we've got him as good as we can, but is discharge safe?' In answering this take into account:

- Does the patient live alone? Does the carer have family support? Is he/she already exhausted by other duties (eg a handicapped toddler)?
- Most patients want to go home promptly. If not, find out why.
- Is the accommodation suitable? Stairs? Toilet on same floor?
- If toilet access is difficult, can he transfer from chair to commode?
- Can he open a tin, use the phone, plug in a kettle, cook soup?
- Is the family supportive—in theory or in practice?
- Are the neighbours friendly? 'But I would not trouble them'. Explore the validity of this sentiment by asking if they would want to know if they were reasonably fit, and a neighbour were in need.
- Are social services and community geriatric services well integrated? Or will the person who provides the lunch ignore the patient if she cannot gain access? Proper *case management programmes* with defined responsibilities, entailing integration of social and geriatric services really can help *and* save money (~20%).[20] Such integration is rare[ ] but is possible in the UK thanks partly to the advent of Primary Care Trusts with overarching responsibilities for *both* medical *and* social care.

17

UK NHS national service framework for older people

There are 8 standards of care   http://bmj.com/cgi/content/full/326/7402/1300

1 *Rooting out age discrimination:* NHS services are to be provided regardless of age, on the basis of need alone. Social services will not use age in eligibility criteria or policies, to restrict access to available services.
2 *Person-centred care:* NHS services treat older people as individuals and enable them to make choices about their own care.
3 *Intermediate care:* Older people will have access to intermediate care services at home or in designated care settings, to promote their independence by providing enhanced services from the NHS and councils to prevent unnecessary hospital admission. Rehabilitation services will enable early discharge from hospital and prevent premature or unnecessary admission to long-term residential care.
4 *General hospital care:* Older people's care in hospital is delivered through appropriate specialist care and by hospital staff who have the rights set of skills to meet their needs.
5 *Stroke:* People who are thought to have had a stroke have access to diagnostic services, are treated appropriately by a specialist stroke service, and subsequently, with their carers, participate in a multidisciplinary programme of secondary prevention and rehabilitation.
6 *Falls:* The NHS, working in partnership with councils, is required to take action to prevent falls and reduce fractures in older people and provide advice on fall prevention, through a specialist falls service.
7 *Mental health in older people* is to be promoted by access to integrated mental health services (from the NHS or councils) to ensure effective diagnosis, treatment, and support, for them and their carers.
8 *The promotion of health and active life in older age:* The health and well-being of older people are promoted through a coordinated programme of action led by the NHS with support from councils.

On being busy: Corrigan's secret door

Unstoppable demands, increasing expectations as to what medical care should bring, the rising number of elderly patients, coupled with the introduction of new and complex treatments all conspire, it might be thought, to make doctors ever busier. In fact, doctors have always been busy people. Sir James Paget, for example, would regularly see more than 60 patients each day, sometimes travelling many miles to their bedside. Sir Dominic Corrigan was so busy 150 years ago that he had to have a secret door made in his consulting room so that he could escape from the ever-growing queue of eager patients.

We are all familiar with the phenomenon of being hopelessly over-stretched—and of wanting Corrigan's secret door. Competing, urgent, and simultaneous demands make carrying out any task all but impossible: the house officer is trying to put up an intravenous infusion on a shocked patient when his 'bleep' sounds. On his way to the phone a patient is falling out of bed, being held in, apparently, only by his visibly lengthening catheter (which had taken the house officer an hour to insert). He knows he should stop to help but, instead, as he picks up the phone, he starts to tell Sister about 'this man dangling from his catheter' (knowing in his heart that the worst will have already happened). But he is interrupted by a thud coming from the bed of the lady who has just had her varicose veins attended to: however, it is not her, but her visiting husband who has collapsed and is now having a seizure. At this moment his cardiac arrest 'bleep' goes off, summoning him to some other patient. In despair, he turns to Sister and groans: 'There must be some way out of here!' At times like this we all need Corrigan to take us by the shadow of our hand, and walk with us through his metaphorical secret door, into a calm inner world. To enable this to happen, make things as easy as possible for yourself.

First, however lonely you feel, you are not usually alone. Do not pride yourself on not asking for help. If a decision is a hard one, share it with a colleague. Second, take any chance you get to sit down and rest. Have a cup of coffee with other members of staff, or with a friendly patient (patients are sources of renewal, not just devourers of your energies). Third, do not miss meals. If there is no time to go to the canteen, ensure that food is put aside for you to eat when you can: hard work and sleeplessness are twice as bad when you are hungry. Fourth, avoid making work for yourself. It is too easy for junior doctors, trapped in their image of excessive work and blackmailed by misplaced guilt, to remain on the wards reclerking patients, rewriting notes, or rechecking results at an hour when the priority should be caring for themselves. Fifth, when a bad part of the rota is looming, plan a good time for when you are off duty, to look forward to during the long nights.

Finally, remember that however busy the 'on take', your period of duty will end. For you, as for Macbeth:

Come what come may,
Time and the hour runs through the roughest day.

Health and medical ethics

In our public medical personas, we often act as though morality consisted only in following society's conventions: we do this not so much out of laziness but because we recognize that it is better that the public think of doctors as old-fashioned or stupid, than that they should think us evil. But in the silences of our consultations, when it is we ourselves who are under the microscope, then, wriggle as we may, we cannot escape our destiny, which is to lead as often as to follow, in the sphere of ethics. To do this, we need to return to first principles, and put society's expectations temporarily on one side.

Our analysis starts with our aim: to do good by making people healthy. *Good*[1] is the most general term of commendation, and entails four chief duties:

1 Not doing harm. We owe this duty to all people, not just our patients.
2 Doing good by positive actions. We particularly owe this to our patients.
3 Promoting justice—ie distributing scarce resources fairly (p14) and respecting rights: legal rights, rights to confidentiality, rights to be informed, to be offered all the options, and to be told the truth.
4 Promoting autonomy. (This is not universally recognized; in some cultures facing starvation, it may be irrelevant, or even be considered subversive.)

Health entails being sound in body and mind, and having powers of growth, development, healing, and regeneration. *How many people have you made healthy (or at least healthier) today?* And in achieving this, *how many cardinal principles have you ignored?* Herein lies a central feature of medicine. We cannot spend long on the wards or in our surgeries trying to 'make people healthy' before we have breached every cardinal duty—particularly (3) and (4). Does it matter? What is the point of having principles if they are regularly ignored? The point of having them is to provide a context for our negotiations with patients. If we want to be better doctors, there are many worse places to start than by trying to put these principles into action. Inevitably, when we try to, there are times when they conflict with each other. What should guide us when these principles conflict? It is not just a case of deciding off the top of one's head on the basis of the above analysis. It may be worthwhile aspiring to a synthesis—if you have the time (time will so often be what you do *not* have; but so often, in retrospect, when things have gone wrong, you realize that they would not have done so if you had *made* time).

Synthesis When we must act in the face of 2 conflicting duties, one of the duties is *not* a duty. How do we tell which one? Trying to find out involves getting to know our patients, and asking some questions:

- Are the patient's wishes being complied with?
- What do your colleagues think? What do the relatives think? Ask the patient's permission first. Have they his or her best interests at heart?
- Is it desirable that the reason for an action be universalizable? (That is, if I say this person is too old for such-and-such an operation, am I happy to make this a general rule for everyone?—Kant's 'law'.)[2]
- If an investigative journalist were to sit on a sulcus of mine, having full knowledge of my thoughts and actions, would she be bored or would she be composing vitriol for tomorrow's newspapers? If so, can I answer her, point for point? Am I happy with my answers? Or are they tactical cerebrations designed to outwit her?
- What would a patient's representative think—eg the elected chairman of a patient's participation group (*OHCS* p440)? These opinions are valuable as they are readily available (if a local group exists) and they can stop decision-making from becoming dangerously medicalized.

---

1 Don't think of good and evil as forever opposite; good can come out of evil, and vice versa: this fundamental mix-up explains why we learn more from our dissolute patients than we do from saints.
2 There are problems with universalizability: only intuition can suggest how to resolve conflicts between competing universalizable principles. Also, there is a sense in which all ethical dilemmas are unique, so no moral rules are possible or required—so they *cannot* be universal. (Sartre, Nietzsche)

Difficult patients

'Unless both the doctor and the patient become a problem to each other, no solution is found.'[1]

Jung's aphorism is untrue for half our waking lives: for an anaesthetist, eg there is no need for the patient to become a problem in order for the anaesthetic to work. But, as with all the best aphorisms, being untrue is the least of their problems. Great aphorisms signify because they unsettle. Our settled and smug satisfaction at finishing a period of duty without any problems is so often a sign of failure. We have kept the chaos at bay, whereas, if we were greater men or women, we would have embraced it. Half our waking professional lives we spend as if asleep, on automatic, following protocols or guidelines to some trite destination—or else we are dreaming of what we could do if we had more time, proper resources, and perhaps a different set of colleagues. But if we had Jung in our pockets he would be shaking us awake, derailing our guidelines, and saluting our attempts to risk genuine interactions with our patients, however much of a mess we make of it, and however much pain we cause and receive. (Pain, after all, is the inevitable companion to lives led authentically.[2]) To the unreflective doctor, and to all average minds, this interaction is anathema, to be avoided at all costs, because it leads us away from anaesthesia, to the unpredictable, and to destinations which are unknown.

So, every so often, try being pleased to have difficult patients: those who question us, those who do not respond to our treatments, or who complain when these treatments *do* work. Very often, it will seem that whatever you say it is wrong: misunderstood, misquoted, and mangled by the mind you are confronting—perhaps because of fear, loneliness, or past experiences which you can only guess at. If this is happening, *shut up*—but don't *give up*. Stick with your patient. Listen to what he or she is saying and not saying. And when you have understood your patient a bit more, negotiate, cajole, and even argue—but don't bully or blackmail ('If you do not let your daughter have the operation she needs, I'll tell her just what sort of a mother you are . . .'). When you find yourself turning to walk away from your patient, turn back and say 'This is not going very well, is it? Can we start again?' And don't hesitate to call in your colleagues' help: not to win by force of numbers, but to see if a different approach might bear fruit. By this process, you and your patient may grow in stature. You may even end up with a truly satisfied patient. And a satisfied patient is worth a thousand protocols.

20

1 Carl Jung, *Memories, Dreams, Reflections*, 166 www.jelder.com/quotations/woundedhealer.html.
2 'Some say that the world is a vale of tears. I say it is a place of soul making'—John Keats—the first medical student to formulate these ideas about pain. They did not do him much good, because he died shortly after expressing them. But his ideas can do us good—perhaps if each day we try at least once for authentic interactions with a patient, unencumbered by professionalism, research interests, defensive medicine, a wish to show off to our peers, or to get though the day with the minimum of fuss.

Medicine, art, and the humanities

Let us start with an elementary observation: *there are no justly famous living doctors*; indeed *there are no famous dead doctors*. The most famous doctors are those immortalized in literature—eg Dr Watson, Dr Frankenstein, and Dr Faustus.[1] Hereby we demonstrate the power of the written word. And it *is* an extraordinary power. When we curl up in an armchair and read for pleasure, we open the portals of our minds because we are alone. While we are reading, there is no point in dissembling. We confront our subject matter with a steady eye because we believe, that, while reading to ourselves, we cannot be judged. Then, suddenly, when we are at our most open and defenceless, literature takes us by the throat—and that eye which was so steady and confident a few minutes ago is now perhaps misting over, or our heart is missing a beat, or our skin is covered in a goose-flesh more popular than ever a Siberian winter produced. Once we have been on earth for a few decades, not much in our mundane world sends shivers down our spines, but the power of worlds of literature and art to do this ever grows.

There are, of course, doctors who are quite well known: Arthur Conan Doyle, William Carlos Williams, Somerset Maugham, and Anton Chekhov, and they are all artists. What about Sigmund Freud? Here is the exception which proves the rule—proves in the sense of testing, for he is not really an exception. We can accept him among the great only in so far as we view his oeuvre as an artistic oeuvre, rather than as a scientific one. Science has progressed for years without Freud but, as art, his work and insights will survive: and survival, as Bernard Shaw pointed out, is the only test of greatness.

The reason for the ascendancy of art over science is simple. We scientists, in our humble way, are only interested in explaining reality. Artists are good at explaining reality too: but they also *create* it. Our most powerful impressions are produced in our minds not by simple sensations but by the association of ideas. It is a pre-eminent feature of the human mind that it revels in seeing something as, or through, something else: life refracted through experience, light refracted through jewels, or a walk through the woods transmuted into a Pastoral Symphony. Ours is a world of metaphor, fantasy, and deceit.

What has all this to do with the day-to-day practice of medicine? The answer lies in the word 'defenceless' above. When we read alone and for pleasure, our defences are down—and we hide nothing from the great characters of fiction. In our consulting rooms, and on the ward, we so often do our best to hide everything, beneath the white coat, or the avuncular bedside manner. So often, a professional detachment is all that is left after all those years inured to the foibles, fallacies, and frictions of our patients' tragic lives. It is at the point where art and medicine collide, that doctors can re-attach themselves to the human race and re-feel those emotions which motivate or terrify our patients. We all have an Achilles heel: that part of our inner self which was not rendered forever invulnerable to mortal cares when we were dipped in the waters of the river Styx as it flowed down the wards of our first disillusion. Art and literature, among other things, may enable this Achilles heel to be the means of our survival as thinking, sentient beings, capable of maintaining a sympathetic sensibility to our patients.

The American approach is to create Professors of Literature-in-Medicine and to conjure with concepts such as *the patient as text*, and most American medical schools do courses in literature in an attempt to inculcate ethical reasoning and speculation. Here, we simply intend to demonstrate, albeit imperfectly, in our writings and in our practice of medicine, that *every* contact with patients has an ethical and artistic dimension, as well as a technical one.

---

1 Of course Dr Faust, that famous charlatan, necromancer, and quack from medieval Germany, did have a real existence. In fact, there may have been two of them, who together gave rise to myth of devil-dealing, debauchery, and the undisciplined pursuit of science, without the constraints of morality.

Epidemiology

Contents

See also QALYS, p14

An example of epidemiology at work

Some decades ago, epidemiologists tested the hypothesis that smoking and hypertension were associated with cardiovascular disease. Painstaking cohort studies confirmed that these were indeed *risk markers* (a term that does not imply causality). Over the years, as evidence accumulates, the term 'risk marker' may give way to *risk factor*, which implies causation, and the separate idea that risk-factor modification will cause a reduction in disease. Demonstrating a dose–response relationship (with the correct time sequence) is good evidence of a causal relationship—eg showing that the greater the number of cigarettes smoked, the greater the risk, or the higher the blood pressure, the greater the cardiovascular mortality. It is still possible that BP is a risk marker of some other phenomenon, but this is less likely if the relationship between BP and cardiovascular mortality is found to correlate *while keeping other known risk factors constant*. The work of the epidemiologist does not stop here. He or she can use actuarial statistics to weigh the relative merits and interactions of a number of risk factors, to give an overall estimate of risk for an individual. It is then possible to say things like: 'If the 5-yr risk of a serious cardiac event in people with no overt cardiac disease is >15%, then drug treatment of hyperlipidaemia may begin to be cost-effective—and a 10% 5-yr risk may be a sufficient point to trigger antihypertensive treatment in someone with, say, a BP of 150/90'. These figures are a guide only: only ~60% of those in the top 10% of the risk distribution will have an adverse coronary event in the 5-yr period. Nevertheless, this is more accurate than taking into account risk factors singly—and so we are led to our first important conclusion: *epidemiology improves and informs our dialogue with our patients*. We can give patients good evidence on which to base their choices.

Risk equations (ideally as part of computerized medical records) may be given as follows (a, m, μ, and σ are variables relating risk factors):

If $a = 11.1122 - [0.9119 \times \ln(\text{BP})] - (0.2767 \times \text{SMO}) - [0.7181 \times \ln(\text{FAT})] - (0.5865 \times \text{LVH})$

and for males $m = a - [1.4762 \times \ln(\text{AGE})] - 0.1759 \times \text{DIAB}$

and for females $m = a - 5.8549 + [1.8515 \times \ln(\text{AGE}/74)^2] - (0.3758 \times \text{DIAB})$

and $\mu = 4.4181 + m$

and $\sigma = e^{-(0.3155 - 0.278m)}$ and $v = [\ln(5) - \mu/\sigma]$

then **5-yr risk** $\approx 1 - (e^{-(e^v)})$ if AGE is 30–74yrs, BP is the mean systolic, eg 3 readings—and SMO, DIAB, and LVH are each 1 if the patient is a smoker, has diabetes or left ventricular hypertrophy, eg on ECG; if not present, each is 0. FAT is the ratio of total cholesterol to HDL. This is the EMIS formulation of the 'Dundee equations'; see also J Robson 1997 *BMJ* **ii** 277 & the corrected Sheffield tables for primary prevention of heart disease, *Lancet* 1996 **348** 1251.

▶Note that results from these equations are approximations only: beware spurious accuracy. Also, populations differ: figures taken from American cohorts in the past tend to over-estimate risk of MI in English males.

The essence of epidemiology

Epidemiology is the study of the distribution of clinical phenomena in populations. Its chief measures are prevalence and incidence.

Definitions The *period prevalence* is the number of cases, at any time during the study period, divided by the population at risk. If the population at risk is unclear, then the population must be specified—eg the prevalence of uterine cancer varies widely, depending on whether you specify the general population (men, women, boys, and girls) or only women, or women who have not already had a hysterectomy.

The *incidence* is the number of new cases within the study period which must be specified, eg annual incidence. *Point prevalence* is the prevalence at a point in time. The *lifetime* prevalence of hiccups is ~100%; the (UK) incidence is millions/year—but the point prevalence may be 0 at 3AM today if no one is actually having hiccups.

Association Epidemiological research is concerned with comparing rates of disease in different populations, eg rates of lung cancer in a population of men who smoke, compared with men who do not. A difference in rates points to an association (or dissociation) between the disease and factors which distinguish the populations (in this case, smoking or not). If the rates are equal, association is still possible, with a confounding variable (eg both groups share the same smoky environment).

Ways of accounting for associations: A may cause B; B cause A; a 3rd unknown agent, P, causes A and B; or it may be a chance finding.

There are 2 types of studies which explore causal connections:

1 *Case-control (retrospective) studies:* The study group consists of those with the disease (eg lung cancer); the control group consists of those without the disease. The previous occurrence of the putative cause (eg smoking) is compared between each group. Case–control studies are retrospective in that they start after the onset of the disease (although cases may be collected prospectively).

2 *Cohort (prospective) studies:* The study group consists of subjects exposed to the putative causal factor (eg smoking); and the control group consists of subjects not exposed. The incidence of the disease is compared between the groups over time. ►A cohort study generates incidence data, whereas a case–control study does not.

Matching An association between A and B may be due to another factor P. To eliminate this possibility, matching for P is often used in case–control studies. One powerful, but unreliable (if numbers are small), way to do this in clinical trials is for the subjects to be allocated to groups randomly; check important Ps have been distributed evenly between groups.

Overmatching If unemployment causes low income, and low income causes depression, then matching study and control groups for income would mask the genuine causal link between unemployment and depression. ►Avoid matching factors which may intervene in the causal chain linking A and B.

Blinding If the subject does not know which of two trial treatments she is having, the trial is single blind. To further reduce risk of bias, the experimenter should also not know (double blind).

►In a good treatment trial, the blind lead the blind.

Further reading: D Sackett *Clinical Epidemiology*, 2nd edn, Little, Brown, Boston; and D Sackett *Evidence-based Medicine: How to Practise and Teach EBM*, Churchill.

Evidence-based medicine (EBM)

This is the conscientious and judicious use of current best evidence from clinical research in the management of individual patients.

The problem 2,000,000 papers are published each year. Patients benefit directly from a tiny fraction of these papers. How do we find them?

A partial solution 50 journals are scanned not by experts in a specialized field, but by searchers trained to identify papers which have a direct message for clinical practice, and meet predefined criteria of rigour (below). Summaries are then published, eg in *Evidence-based Medicine*.

Questions used to evaluate papers:

1 Are the results *valid*? Randomized? Blinded? Were all patients accounted for who entered the trial? Was follow-up complete? Were the groups similar at the start? Were the groups treated equally, apart from the experimental intervention?

2 What *are* the results? How large was the treatment effect? How precise was the treatment effect?

3 Will the results help my patients (cost/benefit sum).

Problems with the solution ►*The concept of scientific rigour is opaque.*
What do we want? The science, the rigour, the truth, or what will be most useful to patients? These may overlap, but they are not the same.

- Will the best be the enemy of the good? Are useful papers rejected due to some blemish? Answer: appraise *all* evidence (often impossible).
- By reformulating in terms of answerable questions, EBM risks missing patient's reason for consulting. He may only want to express his fears, rather than be used as a substrate for an intellectual exercise.
- Is the standard the same for the evidence for *all* changes to our practice? We might avoid prescribing drug X for constipation if there is any chance that it might cause colon cancer, when there are many other drugs to choose from. More robust evidence may be needed to persuade us to do something rather counter-intuitive, eg giving heparin in DIC (p650). There is no science to tell us how robust the data need to be: we decide off the top of our head (albeit a wise head, we hope).
- What about the correspondence columns of the journals from which the winning papers are extracted? It takes years for unforeseen but fatal flaws to surface, and be reported in correspondence columns.
- There is a danger that by always asking 'What is the evidence ...' we will divert resources from hard-to-prove areas (eg physiotherapy, which may be very valuable) to easy-to-prove services. The unique personal attributes of the therapist may be as important as the objective regimen: she is impossible to quantify. It is an easier decision to transfer resources to some easy-to-quantify activity, eg neonatal screening.
- EBM can never be always up-to-date. Reworking meta-analyses in the light of new trials takes time, if it is ever done at all.
- 'My increased knowledge gradually permeated or repressed the world of intuitive premonitions ...' (*Carl Jung*). These premonitions may be vital!

Advantages of EBM

- Our reading habits improve.
- It leads us to ask questions, and then to be sceptical of the answers.
- As taxpayers, we should like it (wasteful practices can be abandoned).
- EBM presupposes that we keep up to date, and makes it worthwhile to take trips around the perimeter of our knowledge.
- EBM opens decision-making processes to patients.

There is little doubt that, *where available*, EBM can be better than what it is superseding. It may not have as much impact as we hope, as gaining unimpeachable evidence is time-consuming and expensive, and perhaps impossible. Despite these caveats, EBM is here to stay, so we may as well subscribe to its ideals—and to its journal.

Six to five against

Your surgical consultant asks whether Gobble's disease is more common in men or women. You have no idea, and make a guess. What is the chance of getting it right? Common sense decrees that it is even chances; 'Sod's Law' predicts that whatever you guess, your answer will always be wrong. A less pessimistic view is that the balance is slightly tipped against you: according to Damon Runyon, 'all life is six to five against'.

Do new symptoms suggest a new disease, or are they from an existing disease?
The answer is often counter-intuitive. Suppose s is quite a rare symptom of Gobble's disease (seen in 5% of patients), but that it is a very common symptom of disease A (seen in 90%). If we have a man whom we already know has Gobble's disease and who goes on to develop symptom s, is not s more likely to be due to disease A, rather than Gobble's disease? The answer is usually no: *it is generally the case that s is due to a disease which is already known, and does not imply a new disease.*

The 'odds ratio' makes this clearer, ie the ratio of [the probability of the symptom, given the known disease] to [the probability of the symptom given the new disease × *the probability of developing the new disease*]. This ratio is, usually, vastly in favour of the symptom being due to the old disease because of the prior odds of the two diseases.

Doctors as gamblers Patients are sometimes alarmed to learn that we doctors gamble with their lives. For example, one of us (JML) has just finished consulting with 20 patients. Not too many, perhaps: it might be argued that each of their symptoms, especially their *serious* symptoms, should be taken at face value and investigated until the cause is found. Let us look at this view critically. What counts as a serious symptom? One that, if left undiagnosed, might mean death, disfigurement, or disability. Some of these patients offered 5 separate symptom groups before being gently dissuaded from going on. During full elucidation of these symptoms others would emerge, and with a potentially endless cycle of investigation. Certainly some of these patients might not seem too serious ('this pain in my toe …'). But on reflection toe pain might be dangerous if caused by emboli or osteomyelitis. Fingernail problems with a slight rash might mean arsenic poisoning; lethargy may mean cancer, and so on. So medicine is not for pessimists—almost anything can be made to seem fatal, so that a pessimistic doctor would never get any sleep at night for worrying about the meanings of his patients' symptoms.

Medicine is not for blind optimists either, who too easily embrace a fool's paradise of false reassurance. Rather, **medicine is for gamblers**: gamblers who are happy to use subtle clues to change their outlook from pessimism to optimism and vice versa. Sometimes the gambling is scientific, rational, and methodical (odds-ratio analysis): sometimes it is not, as when the gambling is based on prior knowledge (vital but ill-defined) of one's patient, or the faint apprehension of terror in this new patient's eyes which shows you that there is something wrong, and that you don't yet know what it is.

Being lucky in both types of gambling is a requisite for being a successful doctor: after all we would all rather have a lucky doctor than a wise one. In this game, especially when it gets deadly serious, the chips are not just financial (the most cost-effective next step). They betoken time (for you are spending yourself as surely as you are spending money, as you walk the wards), your reputation, and the health or otherwise of your patient. So do not worry about the fact of gambling: *gambling is your job.* But make sure you assemble sufficient evidence to maximize your chances of being lucky.

Example of the odds ratio at work

A 50-yr-old man with known carcinoma of the lung has some transient neurological symptoms and a normal CT scan. Are these symptoms due to secondaries in the brain or to transient ischaemic attacks (TIAs)?

- The chance of secondaries in the brain which cause transient neurological symptoms is 0.045 given carcinoma of the lung.
- The chance of such secondaries not showing up on a CT scan is 0.1.
  ∴ the chance of this cluster of symptoms is 0.0045 (ie 0.045 × 0.1).
- The chance of a normal CT + transient CNS symptoms given a TIA is 0.9.
- The chance of a 50-yr-old man developing TIA is 0.0001.
  ∴ the odds ratio is 0.0045/(0.9 × 0.0001). This equals 50.

That is, the odds ratio is ~50 to 1 in favour of secondaries in the brain.

NB: It is only very rarely that the prior odds of a new disease are so high that the new disease is more likely, eg someone presenting with anaemia already known to have breast cancer, who lives in an African community where 50% of people have hookworm-induced anaemia, is likely to have anaemia due to hookworm *as well as* breast carcinoma.

Investigations change the odds

Only rarely does a single test provide a definitive diagnosis. More often tests alter the odds of a diagnosis. When taking a history and examining patients, we make various wagers with ourselves (often barely consciously) as to how likely various diagnoses are. Further test results simply affect these odds. A test is worthwhile if it alters diagnostic odds in a clinically useful way.

The effect of an investigation on the diagnostic odds To work this out you need to know the *sensitivity* and *specificity* of the test. All tests have false positive and false negative rates, as summarized below:

Test result	Patients with the condition	Patients without the condition
Subjects appear to have the condition	True +ve (*a*)	False +ve (*b*)
Subjects appear *not* to have the condition	False −ve (*c*)	True −ve (*d*)

Specificity: How reliably is the test −ve in health? $d/d+b$.
Sensitivity: How reliably is the test +ve in the disease? $a/a+c$. Screening tests need to have a high sensitivity: we know that 3–6% of chest pain patients sent home from casualty departments on the basis of a single ECG actually have myocardial infarction (MI). A single ECG is specific (77–100%), but not very sensitive for MI (56%). Troponin tests (p120) are more sensitive. So a doctor might use sensitivity/specificity data to act as follows. If history and ECG suggest MI, admit (thrombolysis, p782). If story and ECG are not typical of MI, do a troponin test 6h after onset of chest pain—only send home if 'normal'.[1] This strategy reduces inappropriate discharge to ~1%.[2] Note that studies showing these effects are *very* dependent on the local prevalence of MI. A few more MIs in the 'troponin normal' group would radically alter these results.

Suppose we have a test of sensitivity 0.8 and specificity 0.9. The *likelihood ratio* of the disease given a positive result (LR+) is the ratio of the chance of having a positive test if the disease is present to the chance of having a positive test if the disease is absent [0.8/(1−0.9)]; ie 8 : 1 in the above example.
In general: LR+ = sensitivity/(1−specificity)
    LR− (likelihood ratio of the disease given a negative result) = (1−sensitivity)/specificity. (1−0.8/0.9, ie 2 : 9 in the above example.)

Is there any point to this test? Work out the 'posterior odds' assuming a first a +ve and then a −ve test result—via the equation: *posterior odds* = (*prior odds*) × (*likelihood ratio*). If your clinical assessment of a man with exercise-induced chest pain is that the odds of this being due to coronary artery disease (CAD) are 4 : 1 (80%), is it worth his doing an exercise tolerance test (sensitivity 0.72; specificity 0.8)? If the test were positive, the odds in favour of CAD would be 4 × (0.72)/(1−0.8) = 14 : 1 (93%). If negative, they would be 4 × (1 − 0.72)/0.8 = 1.4 : 1 (58%), so the test has not in any way 'ruled out' CAD. Experienced doctors are likely to have higher prior odds for the most likely diagnosis. The above shows that with high prior odds, a test must have high sensitivity and specificity for a negative result to bring the odds below 50%.

Another example is John, who is a 40-yr-old (not on NSAIDs, with no prior peptic ulcer) referred for '?endoscopy' because of dyspepsia. Before the result of a bedside test for *Helicobacter pylori* is known, he has a 50% chance of harbouring this organism, which, if present, is the probable cause of an ulcer. The likelihood ratio for a −ve test result is 0.13 (sensitivity 0.88, specificity 0.91). *If the test is negative*, the chance of John having *H. pylori* is <11%—and it may be OK to send him home with symptomatic treatment (eg ranitidine) without endoscopy—if there are no 'cancer symptoms' (weight loss, dysphagia, etc, p215). *If the test is +ve*, the probability of *H. pylori* is >90%, strongly suggesting the need for specific anti-ulcer (anti-helicobacter) therapy, p215 and endoscopy if this does not cure his symptoms.

---

1 Troponin T (TnT) ≤0.1µg/L (or troponin I ≤0.2µg/L; labs vary); what is normal is itself a statistical issue, p676—as is what counts as an MI. [@12554056]
2 Sensitivity: 97%; specificity: 93%; −ve predictive value: 99.6%; +ve predictive value: 66%; LR+: 13.9; LR−: 0.03.

Number needed to treat (NNT)

If the risk of dying from an MI after 'standard treatment' is 10%, and a new treatment reduces this to 8%, then the absolute risk reduction is 2% (10−8%). The effect of the new drug is often made to look more impressive by quoting the relative risk reduction, ie 20% [(10−8/10) × 100%]. However, if 100 people with MI receive the drug, only ~2 would be expected to derive any benefit. In terms of numbers needed to treat, we might say that 50 patients would need treating to save one additional life ([1/absolute risk reduction] × 100). NNTs provide a useful way of quantifying benefit, but do not take into account treatment costs or the degree of potential benefit. The converse of NNT is number needed to harm. This is the number of people who must receive a treatment in order to produce one adverse event.

In some preventive studies of mild hypertension in the young, ~800 people may need treating according to a certain regimen to prevent one stroke. When expressed like this, the treatment seems less wonderful.

One of the strengths of NNT is that it is context-dependent. If a new anti-hypertension regimen is being compared with an old regimen where the NNT was 800 and the new regimen is only marginally better, the NNT to prevent one death or stroke *by adopting the new regimen in place of the old* may run into many thousands, as will your drugs bill if the new drug is more expensive.

One problem with NNTs occurs if there is a large placebo effect, eg in pain relief. Say the placebo response rate is 40% and that of a new analgesic is 60%. NNT is 5. Perhaps it is better to say to patients starting the new drug that 60% respond. Also, one needs to be clear whether the mean or median is given as the length of follow-up. 🔟

Screening

Modified Wilson criteria for screening (1–10 spells *iatrogenic*[1]—to remind us that in treating healthy populations we have an especial duty to do no harm.)
1 The condition screened for should be an important one.
2 There should be an acceptable treatment for the disease.
3 Diagnostic and treatment facilities should be available.
4 A recognizable latent or early symptomatic stage is required.
5 Opinions on who to treat as patients must be agreed.
6 The test must be of *high discriminatory power* (see below), *valid* (measuring what it purports to measure, not surrogate markers which might not correlate with reality), and be *reproducible*—with safety guaranteed.
7 The examination must be acceptable to the patient.
8 The untreated natural history of the disease must be known.
9 A simple inexpensive test should be all that is required.
10 Screening must be continuous (ie not a 'one-off' affair).
Summary: screening tests must be cost-effective.

Problems These have all affected UK screening programmes.
1 Those most at risk do not present for screening, thus increasing the gap between the healthy and the unhealthy—the *inverse care law* (p14).
2 The 'worried well' overload services by seeking repeat screening.
3 Services for investigating those testing positive are inadequate.
4 Those who are false positives suffer stress while awaiting investigation, and remain anxious about their health despite reassurance.

▶Before screening, the chances of harming a patient (by anxiety or subsequent invasive tests), as well as any benefits must be quantified: this is *Rees' rule.* 🔢

---

1 From Greek: *iatros* (physician) + *genic*—denoting illness caused by us doctors. You will find this word etched on all our soles producing a malign imprint however lightly we try to tread. *Ways to reduce iatrogenic illness:* ● Use EBM if possible ● Involve patients in all decisions ● Check drug labels/dosages by reading them aloud ● Be aware of drug interactions: look it up—don't assume you know ● Explain to patients how to tell if things are going wrong, and what actions must follow ('if …tell me …').

Examples of NNTs

Study	Outcome	NNT
Statins (p114) for primary prevention[1]	Death (MI)	931 (78) for 5yrs
Statins for secondary prevention (4s)	Death (MI)	30 (15) for 5.4yrs
Mild hypertension (MRC trial)	Stroke	850 for 1yr
Systolic hypertension in elderly (SHEP)	Stroke	43 for 4.5yrs
Aspirin in acute MI (ISIS-1)	Death	40
Streptokinase in acute MI (ISIS2)	Death	40
ACE-i for CCF (NYHA class iv (p137))	Death	6 for 1yr

Keep your eye on the question NNTs can vary markedly if the question is slightly rephrased—eg from being about primary prevention to being about secondary prevention (as in the statin example above).

NNT confidence intervals Get these by taking reciprocals of the values defining the confidence interval for the absolute risk reduction (ARR). If ARR ≈ 10% with a 95% confidence interval of 5–15%, NNT ≈ 10 (ie 100/10) and the 95% NNT-confidence interval ≈ 6.7–20 (ie 100/15 to 100/5). Non-significant treatment effects are problematic as NNTs can only be positive; here, give NNT *without* confidence intervals (Altman's rule).

31

Examples of effective screening	Unproven/ineffective screening
Cervical smears for cancer	Mental test score (dementia)
Mammography for breast cancer	Urine tests (diabetes; kidney disease)
Finding smokers (+quitting advice)	Antenatal procedures (OHCS p95)
Looking for malignant hypertension	PSA screening (prostate cancer, p705)

NB: Screening for cervical cancer (OHCS p32) and mammography (p504) are far from perfect: both are liable to false negatives, and a negative result is interpreted as *'I'm fine'* (and may be seen as a licence to take risks). So signs of interval cancers (arising between screenings) may be wished away by patients who assume they are in the clear.

1 Meta-analysis *Bandolier* 17(7), 41(3), 50 (8)

Clinical skills[1]

Contents

Other relevant pages: Symptoms and signs (p64–p89); pre-op care (p446); acute abdomen (p474); lumps (p510–p518); hernias (p524 & p526); varicose veins (p528); urine (p258); peripheral nerves (p336); dermatomes (p338).

In OHCS: Vaginal and other gynaecological examinations (OHCS p2); abdominal examination in pregnancy (OHCS p84); the history and examination in children and neonates (OHCS p172–p174); examination of the eye (OHCS p476); visual acuity (OHCS p476); eye movements (OHCS p486); ear, nose, and throat examination (OHCS p528 & p530); facial nerve lesions (OHCS p566); skin examination (OHCS p576); examination of joints—see the contents page to *Orthopaedics and trauma* (OHCS p604).

▶The way to learn physical signs is at the bedside, with guidance from an experienced colleague. This chapter is not intended as a substitute for this process: it is simply an *aide-mémoire*.

▶We ask questions to get information to help with differential diagnosis. But we also ask questions to find out about the inner life and past exploits of our patients, so that they do not bore us, and so that we can respect them as individuals. The patient is likely to notice and reciprocate this respect, and this reciprocation is the foundation of most of our therapeutic endeavours. One of us (JML) happened to ask a routine 80-year-old 'geriatric' patient with renal failure what he did—meaning did in the past, and was surprised to learn that he commuted to London frequently and was a buyer of dried fruits from the Middle East—an area where he had unrivalled business contacts and knowledge of local produce. It was not long before he was having dialysis. The message is not that special people should get special services: rather that it is easy to like, and hence promote the interests of, patients with whom you can identify. The challenge is to identify with as broad a range of humanity as possible, without getting exhausted by the scale of this enterprise.

▶'Truth lies not only in what is said, but also in who says it, to whom, why, how, and under what circumstances.'   Vaclav Havel *Letters To Olga* (138)

Principle sources: *Clinical Examination*, 4th edn, NJ Talley and S O'Connor, Blackwell Science; *Aids to Undergraduate Medicine*, 6th edn, JL Burton and BJL Burton, Churchill Livingstone.

1 We thank Dr Bheeshma Rajagopalan who is our Specialist Reader for this chapter.

The patient now waiting for you in cubicle 9...

The first news of your next patient will often be via a phone call 'There's an MI on the way in'—or 'There's someone dementing in cubicle 9'—or 'Can you take the overdose in resus.?' On hearing such sanitized dehumanized descriptions, our minds will start painting pictures, and the tone of these messages have the habit of colouring these pictures. So when we arrive at the bedside, our mind is far from a *tabula rasa* or blank canvas on which the patient can paint his woes.

The mind is always painting pictures, filling in gaps—and falling into traps. Perception is an active process, for, as Marcel Proust, that life-long all-knowing patient, observed[1]:

> *We never see the people who are dear to us save in the animated system, the perpetual motion of our incessant love for them, which before allowing the images that their faces present to reach us catches them in its vortex, flings them back upon the idea that we have always had of them, makes them adhere to it, coincide with it.*

So if you want to know your patient, take snapshots of him from various angles, and briefly contemplate him in the round before Proust's vortex whisks you off track. You can prepare for these snapshots in the blinking of an eye, saying to yourself: 'When I open my eyes I'm going to see my patient face to face' and in that clinical blink, divest yourself of those prejudices and expectations which all good diagnosticians somehow ignore. When you open your eyes you will be all set for a Gestalt recognition of incipient myxoedema (the cause of the dementia in cubicle 9), jaundice, anaemia, or, perhaps more importantly, the recognition that the person in front of you is frightened, failing, or dying. What goes into enabling this moment of Gestalt recognition is described on p291.

33

1 *The Guermantes Way* **i** p187 trans. CK Scott Moncrieff.

Taking a history

Taking (or receiving) histories is what most of us spend most of our professional life doing: it is worth doing it well. An accurate history is the biggest step in making the correct diagnosis. History-taking, examination, and treatment of a patient begin the moment one reaches the bedside. (The divisions imposed by our page titles are somewhat misleading.) Try to put the patient at ease: a good rapport may relieve distress on its own. It often helps to shake hands. Always introduce yourself. Check whether the patient is comfortable. Be conversational rather than interrogative in tone. General questions (age, occupation, marital status) help break the ice and help assess mental functions.

Presenting complaint (PC) 'What has been the trouble recently?' Record the patient's own words rather than, eg 'dyspnoea'.

History of presenting complaint (HPC) When did it start? What was the first thing noticed? Progress since then. Ever had it before? 'Socrates' questions: site; onset (gradual, sudden); character; radiation; associations (eg nausea, sweating); timing of pain/duration; exacerbating and alleviating factors; severity (eg scale of 1–10, or compared to childbirth).

Direct questioning (DQ) Specific questions about the diagnosis you have in mind (+its risk factors, eg travel—p554) & a review of the relevant system.

Past medical history (PMH) Ever in hospital? Illnesses? Operations? Ask specifically about diabetes, asthma, bronchitis, TB, jaundice, rheumatic fever, high BP, heart disease, stroke, epilepsy, peptic ulcer, anaesthetic problems.

Drug history (DH) Any tablets, injections? Any 'off the shelf' drugs? Herbal remedies, the Pill? Ask the features of allergies; it may not have been one.

Social history (SH) Probe without prying. 'Who else is there at home?' Job. Marital status. Spouse's job and marital status. Housing—any stairs at home? Who visits—relatives, neighbours, GP, nurse? Mobility—any walking aids needed? Who does the cooking and shopping? What can the patient not do because of the illness? Age, health, and cause of death, if known, of parents, siblings, and children; ask about TB, diabetes, and other relevant diseases. The social history is all too often seen as a dispensable adjunct, eg while the patient is being rushed to theatre. But vital clues may be missed about the quality of life and it is too late to ask when the surgeon's hand is deep in the belly and he or she is wondering how radical a procedure to perform. It is worth cultivating the skill of asking a few searching questions of the admitting family doctor while you are conversing on the phone. If you are both busy, do not waste time on things you will shortly be verifying yourself but tap his knowledge of the patient and his 'significant others'. Remember that the GP is likely to be a specialist in his patients, whom he may have known for decades. He may even hold a 'living will' or advance directive to reveal your patient's wishes if he cannot speak for himself.

Family history (FH) Areas of the family history may need detailed questioning, eg to determine if there is a significant family history of heart disease you need to ask about the health of the patient's grandfathers' and male siblings, smoking, tendency to hypertension, hyperlipidaemia, and claudication before they were 60 years old, as well as ascertaining the cause of death. *Be tactful when asking about a family history of malignancy.*

Alcohol, recreational drugs, tobacco How much? How long? When stopped? The CAGE questionnaire is useful as a screening test for alcoholism (p61). Quantify smoking in terms of *pack-years*: 20 cigarettes smoked per day for 1 year equals 1 pack year. *Smoking is forbidden among Sikhs, so be tactful.* We all like to present ourselves well, so be inclined to double stated quantities (*Holt's 'law'*).

Functional enquiry (p36) To uncover undeclared symptoms. Some of this may already have been incorporated into the history.

▶Don't hesitate to retake the history after a few days: recollections change.

Drawing family trees to reveal dominantly inherited disease[1]

Advances in genetics are touching all branches of medicine. It is increasingly important for doctors to identify patients at high risk of genetic disease, and to make appropriate referrals. The key skill is drawing a family tree to help you structure a family history as follows:

1 Start with your patient. Draw a square for a male and a circle for a female. Add a small arrow (↗, see below) to show that this person is the *propositus* (the person through whom the family tree is ascertained).

2 Add your patient's parents, brothers, and sisters. Record basic information only, eg age, and if alive and well (a&w). If dead, note age and cause of death, and pass an oblique stroke through that person's symbol.

3 Ask the key question 'Has anybody else in your family had a similar problem as yourself?', eg heart attack/angina/stroke/cancer. Ask only about the family of diseases that relate to your patient's main problem. Do not record a potted medical history for each family member: time is too short.

4 Extend the family tree upwards to include grandparents. If you haven't revealed a problem by now, go no further—you are unlikely to miss important familial disease. If your patient is elderly it may be impossible to obtain good information about grandparents. If so, fill out the family tree with your patient's uncles and aunts on both the mother's and father's sides.

5 Shade those in the family tree affected by the disease. ● = an affected female; ■ = an affected male. This helps to show any genetic problem and, if there is one, will help demonstrate the pattern of inheritance.

6 If you have identified a familial susceptibility, or your patient has a recognized genetic disease, extend the family tree down to include children, to identify others who may be at risk, and who may benefit from screening. ►You must find out who is pregnant in the family, or may soon be, and arrange appropriate genetic counselling (*OHCS* p212).

The family tree below shows these ideas at work and indicates that there is evidence for genetic risk of colon cancer, meriting referral to a geneticist.

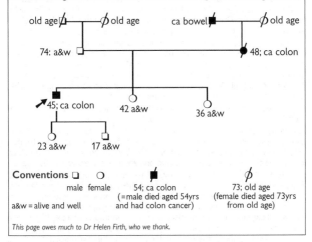

Conventions

male female

a&w = alive and well

54; ca colon (=male died aged 54yrs and had colon cancer)

73; old age (female died aged 73yrs from old age)

This page owes much to Dr Helen Firth, whom we thank.

1 Use a different approach in paediatrics, and for autosomal or sex-linked disease. Ask if parents are related (consanguinity ↑risk of recessive diseases).

Functional enquiry

Just as skilled acrobats are happy to work without safety nets, so also older clinicians may operate without the functional enquiry. But to do this you must be experienced enough to understand all the nuances of the presenting complaint.

General questions may be the most significant, eg in TB, endocrine problems, or cancer: • Weight loss • Night sweats • Any lumps • Fatigue • Sleeping pattern[1] • Appetite • Fevers • Itch • Recent trauma[2]

Cardio-respiratory symptoms Chest pain (p92). Exertional dyspnoea (=breathlessness; quantify exercise tolerance *and how it has changed*: eg stairs climbed, or distance walked, before onset of breathlessness). Paroxysmal nocturnal dyspnoea. Orthopnoea, ie breathlessness on lying flat (a symptom of left ventricular failure: quantify in terms of number of pillows the patient must sleep on to prevent dyspnoea). Oedema. Palpitations (awareness of heartbeats). Cough. Sputum. Haemoptysis (coughing up blood). Wheeze.

Gut symptoms Abdominal pain (constant or colicky, sharp or dull; site; radiation; duration; onset; severity; relationship to eating and bowel action; alleviating/exacerbating, or associated features). Other questions—think of symptoms throughout the GI tract, from mouth to anus:

- Swallowing
- Indigestion; nausea/vomiting
- Bowel habit
- Stool:
  – colour, consistency, blood, slime
  – difficulty flushing away (p252)
  – tenesmus or urgency

Tenesmus is the feeling that there is something in the rectum which cannot be passed (eg due to a tumour). Haematemesis is vomiting blood. Melaena is altered (black) blood passed PR (p224), with a characteristic smell.

Genitourinary symptoms Incontinence (stress or urge, p500). Dysuria (painful micturition). Haematuria (bloody micturition). Nocturia (needing to micturate at night). Frequency (frequent micturition) or polyuria (passing excessive amounts of urine). Hesitancy (difficulty starting micturition). Terminal dribbling.

Vaginal discharge (p588). Menses: frequency, regularity, heavy or light, duration, painful. First day of last menstrual period (LMP). Number of pregnancies. Menarche. Menopause. Any chance of pregnancy now?

Neurological symptoms *Special senses:* Sight, hearing, smell, and taste. Seizures, faints, 'funny turns'. Headache. 'Pins and needles' (paraesthesiae) or numbness. Weakness ('Do your arms and legs work?'), poor balance. Speech problems (p58). Sphincter disturbance. Higher mental function and psychiatric symptoms (p60 & p59). The important thing is to assess function: what the patient can and cannot do at home, work, etc.

Musculoskeletal symptoms Pain, stiffness, swelling of joints. Diurnal variation in symptoms (ie with time of day). Functional deficit.

Thyroid symptoms *Hyperthyroidism:* Prefers cold weather, bad tempered, sweaty, diarrhoea, oligomenorrhoea, weight↓ (though often ↑appetite), tremor, palpitations, visual problems. *Hypothyroidism:* Depressed, slow, tired, thin hair, croaky voice, heavy periods, constipation, dry skin, prefers warm weather.

▶History-taking may seem deceptively easy, as if the patient knew the hard facts and the only problem was extracting them; but what a patient says is a mixture of hearsay ('she said I looked very pale'), innuendo ('you know, doctor, down below'), legend ('I suppose I bit my tongue; it was a real fit, you know'), exaggeration ('I didn't sleep a wink'), and improbabilities ('The Pope put a transmitter in my brain'). The great skill (and pleasure) in taking a history lies not in ignoring these garbled messages, but in making sense of them.

1 Too sleepy? Think of myxoedema or narcolepsy. Early waking? Think of depression. Being woken by pain is always a serious sign. ▶For the significance of the other questions here listed, see chap 4.
2 Trauma is not just important because something may be broken, but because even if it seems trivial, it may provide the all-illuminating flash of insight which explains odd CNS features (eg post-traumatic subdural haemorrhage) or the vague prodromes of illnesses such as tetanus.

Presenting your findings—and the role of jargon

We are forever presenting patients to our colleagues, almost never questioning the mechanisms and unconscious motivations which permeate these oral exchanges—and sometimes send them awry. By some ancient right we assume authority to retell the patient's story at the bedside—not in our own words but in highly stylized medical code: 'Mr Hunt is a 19-year-old *Caucasian male*, a *known case of* Down's syndrome with little intelligible speech and an IQ of 60, *who complains of* paraesthesiae and weakness in his right *upper limb*... He *admits to drinking 21 units per week* and *other problems* are...'

Do not comfort yourself by supposing this ritualistic reinterpretation arises out of the need for brevity. If this were the reason, and we are speaking in front of the patient, all that is in italics above could be omitted, or drastically curtailed. The next easy conclusion to confront is that we purposely use this jargon to confuse or deceive the patient. This is only sometimes the case, and we must look for deeper reasons for why we are wedded to these medicalisms.

We get nearer to the truth when we realize that these medicalisms are used to sanitize and tame the raw data of our face-to-face encounters with patients—to make them bearable to us—so that we can *think* about the patient rather than having to *feel* for him or her. This is quite right and proper—but only sometimes. Usually what our patients need is sympathy, and this does not spring from cerebration. These medicalisms insulate us from the horrible unpredictability of experiential phenomena. We need the illusion that we are treading on well-marked-out territory when we are describing someone's pain—a fundamentally problematic enterprise, not least because if the description is objective it is invalid (pain is, *par excellence*, subjective), and if it is subjective, it is partly incommunicable.

These medicalisms enroll us into a half-proud, half-guilty brotherhood, cemented by what some call patronage and others call fear. This fear can manifest itself as intense loyalty so that, err as we may, we cling to our medical loyalties unto death (that of the patient, not our own). Language is the tool unwittingly used to defend this autocracy of fear. The modulations of our voice, the stylized vocabulary, and the casual neglect of logic and narrative order ensure, in the above example, that we take on board so little of our patient that we remain upright and afloat, above the whirlpools of our patients' lives. In this case, not a case at all, but a child, a family, a mother worried sick about what will happen to her son when she dies: a son who has never *complained* of anything, has never *admitted* to anything, expresses no *problems*—it is *our* problem that his hand is weak, and his mother's that he can no longer go riding for the disabled, because she can no longer be away from home and do her part-time job. So when you next hear yourself declaim in one breath that 'Mr Smith is a 50-year-old Caucasian male with crushing central chest pain radiating down his left arm', take heed—what you may be communicating is that you have stopped thinking about this person—and pause for a moment. Look into your patient's eyes: confront the whirlpool.

Physical examination

With a few exceptions (eg BP), physical examination is not a good screening test for detecting undisclosed disease. Plan your examination to emphasize the areas that the history suggests may be abnormal. A few well-directed, problem-orientated minutes can save hours of fruitless, but very thorough, physical examination. You will still be expected to examine all 4 major systems (cardiovascular, respiratory, abdominal, and neurological), but with time you will be adept at excluding any major undisclosed pathology. Practice is the key.

Look at your patient as a whole to decide how sick he seems to be. Is he well or *in extremis*? Try to decide *why* you think so. Is he in pain and does it make him lie still (eg peritonitis) or writhe about (eg colic)? Is his breathing laboured and rapid? Is he obese or cachectic? Is his behaviour appropriate? Can you detect any unusual smell eg hepatic fetor (p230), cigarettes, alcohol?

Specific diagnoses can often be made from the face and body habitus and these may be missed unless you stop and consider them: eg acromegaly, thyrotoxicosis, myxoedema, Cushing's syndrome, or hypopituitarism. Is there an abnormal distribution of body hair (eg bearded ♀, or hairless ♂) suggestive of endocrine disease? Is there anything about him to trigger thoughts about Paget's disease, Marfan's, myotonia, and Parkinson's syndrome? Look for rashes, eg the malar flush of mitral disease and the butterfly rash of SLE.

Assess the degree of hydration by examining the skin turgor (see BOX), the axillae, and mucous membranes. Sunken orbits may also occur in dehydration. Check peripheral perfusion (eg press the nose and time capillary return). Record the temperature, and BP (lying and standing may be compared to postural hypotension, a sign of shock).

Check for cyanosis (central and peripheral, p68). Is the patient jaundiced? Yellow skin is unreliable and may resemble the lemon tinge of uraemia, pernicious anaemia, carotenaemia (sclerae are not yellow), or caecal carcinoma. The sign of jaundice is yellow sclerae seen in good daylight. Pallor is a nonspecific sign and may be racial, familial, or cosmetic. Anaemia is assessed from the palmar skin creases and conjunctivae—usually pale if Hb <8–9g/dL: you cannot conclude anything from *normal* conjunctival colour; but if they are pale, the patient is probably anaemic. Koilonychia and stomatitis (redness around the mouth, particularly at its lateral edge) suggest iron-deficiency. Anaemia with jaundice suggests malignancy or haemolysis. Pathological hyperpigmentation is seen in Addison's, haemochromatosis (slate-grey) and amiodarone, gold, silver, and minocycline therapy.

Palpate for lymph nodes in the neck (from behind), axillae, groins, epitrochlear region, and abdomen (p76). Any subcutaneous nodules (p76)?

Don't forget to look at the results of urinalysis and urine output charts where indicated. Look at the temperature chart. Average temperature values are 36.8°C (mouth), 36.4°C (axilla), 37.3°C (rectum). *Hypothermia* is defined as a temperature <35°C; special thermometers may be needed to measure temperatures below this level. A morning[1] temperature ≥37.3°C (mouth) or >37.7°C (rectum) constitutes a *fever*. Note the periodicity of any fever (p552). Do not always believe the temperature chart—if you suspect that the patient has a fever (eg by back-of-the-hand on the forehead), take the temperature yourself.

---

1 The nadir is at 6 AM; with a zenith at 6 PM; the mean amplitude of variability is 0.5°C. [@1302471]

The hands

A wealth of information can be gained from shaking hands and rapidly examining the hands of the patient. Are they warm and well-perfused? Warm, sweaty hands may signal hyperthyroidism while cold, moist hands may be due to anxiety. Are the rings tight with oedema? Lightly pinch the dorsum of the hand—persistent ridging of the skin suggests loss of tissue turgor ie dehydration. Are there any nicotine stains? Does the patient have difficulty releasing your hand after shaking it (dystrophia myotonica, p398)? Reluctance to let go is also a sign of loneliness.

Nails *Koilonychia (spoon-shaped nails)* suggests iron deficiency (also fungal infection or Raynaud's). *Onycholysis (destruction of nails)* is seen with hyperthyroidism, fungal nail infection, and psoriasis. *Beau's lines* (PLATE 9) are transverse furrows that signify temporary arrest of nail growth and occur with periods of severe illness. As nails grow at ~0.1mm/d, by measuring distance from the cuticle it may be possible to date the stress. *Mees' lines* are single white, transverse bands sometimes seen in arsenic poisoning or renal failure. *Muehrcke's lines* are paired white, parallel transverse bands sometimes seen in hypoalbuminaemia. *Terry's nails:* Proximal portion of nail is white/pink, nail tip is red/brown (causes: cirrhosis, chronic renal failure). *Pitting* is seen in psoriasis & alopecia areata.

Splinter haemorrhages are fine longitudinal haemorrhagic streaks (under nails), which in the febrile patient may suggest infective endocarditis. They may be normal—being caused, eg by gardening, when their subconjunctival correlates will be *absent*.

Nail-fold infarcts are characteristically seen in vasculitic disorders.

Clubbing of the nails occurs with many disorders (see p68). There is an exaggerated longitudinal curvature and loss of the angle between the nail and the nail-fold (ie no dip). Also the nail feels 'boggy'. The cause is unknown but may be due to increased blood flow through multiple arteriovenous shunts in the distal phalanges.

Chronic paronychia is a chronic infection of the nail-fold and presents as a painful swollen nail with intermittent discharge. Treatment: keep nails dry; antibiotics, eg erythromycin 250mg/6h PO and nystatin ointment.

Changes occur in **the hands** in many diseases. *Palmar erythema* is associated with cirrhosis, pregnancy, and polycythaemia. *Pallor* of the palmar creases suggests anaemia. *Pigmentation* of the palmar creases is normal in Asians and Blacks but is also seen in Addison's. An odd rash on the knuckles (Gottren's papules) with dilated end-capillary loops at the nail-fold suggests dermatomyositis (p420). *Dupuytren's contracture* (fibrosis and contracture of palmar fascia, PLATE 23 and p722) is seen in liver disease, trauma, epilepsy, and ageing. Swollen proximal interphalangeal (PIP) joints with distal (DIP) joints spared suggests rheumatoid arthritis; swollen DIP joints suggests osteoarthritis, gout, or psoriasis. Look for *Heberden's* (distal) and *Bouchard's* (proximal) 'nodes' (osteophytes—bone overgrowth at a joint—seen with osteoarthritis).

The cardiovascular system

History Ask about age, occupation, hobbies, sport, and ethnic origin.

Presenting symptoms	Risk factors for IHD
Chest pain (p92 & p772)	Smoking
Dyspnoea (p70)—exertional? orthopnoea? PND?	Hypertension
	Diabetes mellitus
Ankle swelling	Hyperlipidaemia
Palpitations; dizziness; blackouts	Family history[1] (cardiovascular disease)

Past history	Past tests and procedures:	
Angina or MI	ECG	Echocardiography
Rheumatic fever	Angiograms	Scintigraphy
Intermittent claudication	Angioplasty/stents	CABG (bypass grafts)

Appearance Ill or well? In pain? Dyspnoeic? Are they pale, cold, and clammy? Is there corneal arcus or xanthelasma (hyperlipidaemia)? Is there a malar flush (mitral stenosis, low cardiac output)? Are there signs of Graves' disease (bulging eyes, goitre—p304)? Is the face dysmorphic, eg Down's syndrome, Marfan's syndrome (p730)—or Turner's, Noonan's, or William's syndromes (p157)? Can you hear the click of a prosthetic valve?

Hands Finger clubbing occurs in congenital cyanotic heart disease and endocarditis. Splinter haemorrhages, Osler's nodes (tender nodules in finger pulps) and Janeway lesions (red macules on palms) are signs of infective endocarditis. If found, examine the fundi for Roth's spots (retinal infarcts). Are there nail-fold infarcts (vasculitis, p424) or nailbed capillary pulsation (Quincke's sign, aortic regurgitation)? Is there arachnodactyly (Marfan's) or polydactyly (ASD)? Are there tendon xanthomata (hyperlipidaemia)?

Pulse (See p42.)

Blood pressure The *systolic* blood pressure is the pressure at which the pulse is first heard as the cuff is deflated; the *diastolic* is when the heart sounds disappear (Korotkov sound K5) or become muffled (K4—use, eg in the young who often have no K5; state which you use). The *pulse pressure* is defined as the difference between systolic and diastolic. It is narrow in aortic stenosis and wide in aortic regurgitation. *Defining hypertension* is problematic: see p140. Examine the fundi for hypertensive changes (p141). *Shock* may occur if systolic <100mmHg (p778). *Postural hypotension* is defined as a drop in systolic >15mmHg or diastolic >10mmHg on standing (p80).

Jugular venous pressure (See p42.)

Praecordium Inspect for *scars*: median stenotomy (CABG or valve replacement). Inspect for any pacemakers. Palpate the *apex beat*. Normal position: 5th intercostal space in the mid-clavicular line. Is it displaced laterally? Is it abnormal in nature: *heaving* (mitral or aortic regurgitation, VSD), *thrusting* (aortic stenosis), *tapping* (mitral stenosis), *diffuse* (LV failure, dilated cardiomyopathy) or *double impulse* (HOCM)? Is there dextrocardia? Feel for *left parasternal heave* (RV enlargement eg in pulmonary stenosis, cor pulmonale, ASD) or *thrills* (transmitted murmurs).

Auscultating the heart See BOX.

Lungs Examine the lung bases for crepitations and pleural effusions, indicative of cardiac failure.

Oedema Examine the ankles, legs, sacrum, torso for pitting oedema.

Abdomen Hepatomegaly and ascites may occur in right-sided heart failure. Pulsatile hepatomegaly occurs with tricuspid regurgitation. Splenomegaly may occur with infective endocarditis.

Peripheral pulses Palpate radial, brachial, carotid, femoral, popliteal, dorsalis pedis, and posterior tibial pulses. Feel for *radio-femoral* (coarctation of the aorta) and *radio-radial delay* (eg from aortic arch aneurysm). Auscultate for *bruits* over the carotids and elsewhere, particularly if there is inequality between pulses or absence of a pulse. Causes: atherosclerosis (elderly), vasculitis (young, p424).

---

1 1st degree relative <60yrs of age.

Auscultating the heart

▶If you spend time listening to the history, and feeling pulses, auscultation should hold few surprises: you will often already know the diagnosis.

• Listen with bell and diaphragm at the apex (mitral area). Identify 1st and 2nd *heart sounds*: are they normal? Listen for *added sounds* (p44) and *murmurs* (p46). Repeat at lower left sternal edge and in aortic and pulmonary areas (right and left of manubrium)—and in both the left axilla (radiation of mitral incompetence) and over the carotids (radiation of aortic stenosis).

• Reposition the patient in the left lateral position: again feel the apex beat (is it tapping, as in mitral stenosis?) and listen specifically for a diastolic rumble of mitral stenosis. Sit the patient up and listen at the lower left sternal edge for the blowing diastolic sound of aortic regurgitation—accentuated at the end of expiration.

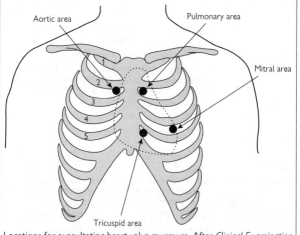

Locations for auscultating heart valve murmurs. After *Clinical Examination* 4th edn, N Talley and S O'Connor, Blackwell Science.

The jugular venous pressure

The internal jugular vein acts as a rather capricious manometer of right atrial pressure. Observe two features: the *height* (jugular venous pressure, JVP) and the *waveform* of the pulse. JVP observations are often difficult. Do not be downhearted if the skill seems to elude you. Keep on watching necks, and the patterns you see may slowly start to make sense.

The height Observe the patient at 45°, with his head turned slightly to the left. Look for the right internal jugular vein, which passes just medial to the clavicular head of sternocleidomastoid up behind the angle of the jaw to the ear lobes. The JVP is the vertical height of the pulse above the sternal angle. It is raised if >4cm. Pressing on the abdomen normally produces a transient rise in the JVP. If the rise persists throughout a 15 sec compression, it is a *positive abdominojugular reflux sign*.[1] This is a sign of right ventricular failure, reflecting inability to eject the increased venous return.

The waveform See BOX.

Abnormalities of the JVP

Raised JVP with normal waveform: Fluid overload, right heart failure.

Raised JVP with absent pulsation: SVC obstruction.

Large a wave: Pulmonary hypertension, pulmonary stenosis.

Cannon a wave: When the right atrium contracts against a closed tricuspid valve, large 'cannon' a waves result. *Causes:* complete heart block, atrial flutter, single chamber ventricular pacing, ventricular arrythmias/ectopics.

Absent a wave: Atrial fibrillation.

Large systolic v waves: Tricuspid regurgitation—look for earlobe movement.

Constrictive pericarditis: High plateau of JVP (which rises on inspiration— Kussmaul's sign) with deep x and y descents.

Pulses

▶Assess the radial pulse to determine *rate* and *rhythm*. *Character* and *volume* are best assessed at the brachials or carotids. A *collapsing pulse* may also be felt at the radials when the patient's arm is elevated above his head.

Rate Is the pulse tachycardic (>100bpm, p128) or bradycardic (<60bpm, p127)?

Rhythm An irregularly irregular pulse occurs in AF or multiple ectopics. A regularly irregular pulse occurs in 2° heart block and ventricular bigemini.

Character and volume

Bounding pulses are caused by CO_2 retention, liver failure, and sepsis.

Small volume pulses occur in aortic stenosis, shock, and pericardial effusion.

Collapsing pulses are caused by aortic incompetence, AV malformations, hyperdynamic circulation and patent ductus arteriosus.

Anacrotic (slow-rising) pulses occur in aortic stenosis.

Bisferiens pulses occur in combined aortic stenosis and regurgitation

Pulsus alternans (alternating strong and weak beats) suggests LVF, cardiomyopathy, or aortic stenosis.

Jerky pulses occur in HOCM.

Pulsus paradoxus (systolic pressure weakens in inspiration by >10mmHg) occurs in severe asthma, pericardial constriction, or cardiac tamponade.

Peripheral pulses (See p40.)

---

1 This sign was first described by Louis Pasteur in 1885, in the context of tricuspid incompetence. The term 'hepatojugular reflux' later arose, but was subsequently replaced by 'abdominojugular reflux', as pressure over the middle of the abdomen, as well as over the liver, can be used to elicit the sign.

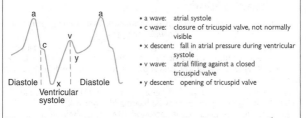

- a wave: atrial systole
- c wave: closure of tricuspid valve, not normally visible
- x descent: fall in atrial pressure during ventricular systole
- v wave: atrial filling against a closed tricuspid valve
- y descent: opening of tricuspid valve

The jugular venous pressure wave. After *Clinical Examination* 4th edn, ed Macleod, Churchill Livingstone.

Distinguishing arterial and venous pulses

In distinguishing venous from arterial pulses, note that the venous pulse:
- Is not usually palpable.
- Is obliterated by finger pressure on the vein.
- Rises transiently following pressure on the abdomen (*abdominojugular reflux*) or on the liver (*hepatojugular reflux*).
- Alters with changes in posture and respiration.
- Usually has a double pulse for every arterial pulse.

43

Arterial pulse waveforms

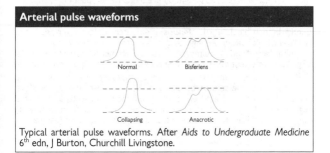

Typical arterial pulse waveforms. After *Aids to Undergraduate Medicine* 6th edn, J Burton, Churchill Livingstone.

The heart sounds

►Listen systematically: sounds then murmurs. While listening, palpate the carotid artery: S_1 is synchronous with the upstroke.

The heart sounds The 1st and 2nd sounds are usually clear. Confident pronouncements about other sounds and soft murmurs may be difficult. Even senior colleagues disagree with one another about the more difficult sounds and murmurs.

The 1st heart sound (S_1) represents closure of mitral (M_1) and tricuspid (T_1) valves. Splitting in inspiration may be heard and is normal.

In mitral stenosis, because the narrowed valve orifice limits ventricular filling, there is no gradual decrease in flow towards the end of diastole. The valves are therefore at their maximum excursion at the end of diastole, and so shut rapidly leading to a loud S_1 (the 'tapping' apex). S_1 is also loud if diastolic filling time is shortened eg if the P–R interval is short, and in tachycardia.

S_1 is soft if the diastolic filling time is prolonged eg if the P–R interval is long, or if the mitral valve leaflets fail to close properly (ie mitral incompetence).

The intensity of S_1 is variable in AV block, atrial fibrillation, and nodal or ventricular tachycardia.

The 2nd heart sound (S_2) represents aortic (A_2) and pulmonary valve (P_2) closure. The most important abnormality of A_2 is softening in aortic stenosis.

A_2 is said to be loud in tachycardia, hypertension, and transposition, but a loud A_2 is probably not a useful clinical entity.

P_2 is loud in pulmonary hypertension and soft in pulmonary stenosis. Splitting in inspiration is normal and is mainly due to the variation with respiration of right heart venous return, causing the pulmonary component to move. Wide splitting occurs in right bundle branch block, pulmonary stenosis, deep inspiration, mitral regurgitation, and VSD. Wide fixed splitting occurs in ASD. Reversed splitting (ie splitting increasing on expiration) occurs in left bundle branch block, aortic stenosis, PDA (patent ductus arteriosus), and right ventricular pacing. A single S_2 occurs in Fallot's tetralogy, severe aortic or pulmonary stenosis, pulmonary atresia, Eisenmenger syndrome (p161), large VSD, hypertension. NB: splitting is heard best in the pulmonary area.

A 3rd heart sound (S_3) may occur just after S_2. It is low pitched and best heard with the bell of the stethoscope. S_3 is pathological over the age of 30yrs. A loud S_3 occurs in a dilated left ventricle with rapid ventricular filling (mitral regurgitation, VSD) or poor LV function (post MI, dilated cardiomyopathy). In constrictive pericarditis or restrictive cardiomyopathy it occurs early and is more high pitched ('pericardial knock').

4th heart sound (S_4) occurs just before S_1. Always abnormal, it represents atrial contraction against a ventricle made stiff by any cause, eg aortic stenosis, or hypertensive heart disease.

Triple and gallop rhythms A 3rd or 4th heart sound occurring with a sinus tachycardia may give the impression of galloping hooves. An S_3 gallop sounds like 'Ken-tucky', whereas an S_4 gallop sounds like 'Tenne-ssee'. When S_3 and S_4 occur in a tachycardia, eg with pulmonary embolism, they may summate and appear as a single sound, a summation gallop.

An ejection systolic click is heard early in systole with bicuspid aortic valves, and if BP↑. The right heart equivalent lesions may also cause clicks.

Mid-systolic clicks occur in mitral valve prolapse (p146).

An opening snap precedes the mid-diastolic murmur of mitral stenosis. It indicates a pliable (noncalcified) valve.

Prosthetic sounds are caused by nonbiological valves, on opening and closing: rumbling sounds ≈ ball and cage valves (eg Starr–Edwards); single clicks ≈ tilting disc valve (eg single disc: Bjork Shiley; bileaflet: St Jude—usually quieter).[1]

1 Prosthetic mitral valve clicks occur in time with S_1, aortic valve clicks in time with S_2.

The cardiac cycle

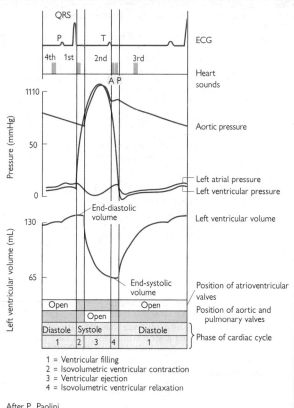

1 = Ventricular filling
2 = Isovolumetric ventricular contraction
3 = Ventricular ejection
4 = Isovolumetric ventricular relaxation

After P. Paolini.

Cardiac murmurs

▶Always consider other symptoms and signs before auscultation and think: what do I expect to hear? However, don't let your expectations determine what you hear.

▶Use the stethoscope correctly. The bell is good for low-pitched sounds (eg mitral stenosis) and should be applied gently to the skin. The diaphragm filters out low pitches, making higher pitched murmurs easier to detect (eg aortic regurgitation). NB: A bell applied tightly to the skin becomes a diaphragm.

▶Consider any murmur in terms of *character, timing, loudness, area where loudest, radiation*, and *accentuating manoeuvres*.

▶When in doubt, rely on echocardiography rather than disputed sounds.

Character and timing An *ejection-systolic murmur* (ESM, crescendo–decrescendo) usually originates from the outflow tract and waxes and wanes with the intraventricular pressures. ESMs may be innocent and are common in children and high output states (eg tachycardia, pregnancy). Organic causes include aortic stenosis and sclerosis, pulmonary stenosis, and HOCM.

A *pansystolic murmur* (PSM) is of uniform intensity and merges with S_2. It is usually organic and occurs in mitral or tricuspid regurgitation (S_1 may also be soft in these), or a ventricular septal defect (p160). Mitral valve prolapse may produce a late systolic murmur ± midsystolic click.

Early diastolic murmurs (EDM) are high pitched and easily missed: listen for the 'absence of silence' in early diastole. An EDM occurs in aortic and, though rare, pulmonary regurgitation. If the pulmonary regurgitation is secondary to pulmonary hypertension, which is itself due to mitral stenosis, then the EDM is called a Graham Steell murmur.

Mid-diastolic murmurs (MDM) are low pitched and rumbling. They occur in mitral stenosis (accentuated presystolically if heart still in sinus rhythm), rheumatic fever (Carey Coombs' murmur: due to thickening of the mitral valve leaflets), and aortic regurgitation (Austin Flint murmur: due to the fluttering of the anterior mitral valve cusp caused by the regurgitant stream).

Intensity Systolic murmurs are graded on a scale of 1–6 (see BOX). Diastolic murmurs, being less loud, are graded 1–4. Intensity is a poor guide to the severity of a lesion—an ESM may be inaudible in severe aortic stenosis.

Area where loudest Though an unreliable sign, mitral murmurs tend to be loudest over the apex, in contrast to the area of greatest intensity from lesions of the aortic (right 2nd intercostal space), pulmonary (left 2nd intercostal space) and tricuspid (left sternal edge) valves.

Radiation The ESM of aortic stenosis classically radiates to the carotids, in contrast to the PSM of mitral regurgitation which radiates to the axilla.

Accentuating manoeuvres *Movements* that bring the relevant part of the heart closer to the stethoscope accentuate murmurs (eg leaning forward for aortic regurgitation, left lateral position for mitral stenosis).

Expiration increases blood flow to the left-side of the heart and therefore accentuates left sided murmurs; *inspiration* has the opposite effect.

The *Valsalva manoeuvre* (forced expiration against a closed glottis) decreases systemic venous return, accentuating mitral valve prolapse and HOCM, but softening mitral regurgitation and aortic stenosis. *Squatting* has exactly the opposite effects. *Exercise* accentuates mitral stenosis.

Non-valvular murmurs A *pericardial friction rub* may be heard in pericarditis. It is a superficial scratching sound, not confined to systole or diastole. *Continuous murmurs* are present throughout the cardiac cycle and may occur with a patent ductus arteriosus, arteriovenous fistula, or ruptured sinus of Valsalva.

Heart murmurs in children (See *OHCS* p225.)

Common heart murmurs

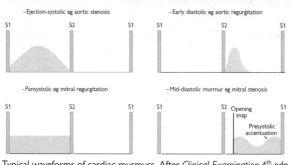

Typical waveforms of cardiac murmurs. After *Clinical Examination* 4th edn, N Talley and S O'Connor, Blackwell Science.

Grading intensity of heart murmurs

▶The following grading is commonly used for systolic murmurs:

Grade 1/6:   Very soft, only heard after listening for a while
Grade 2/6:   Soft, but detectable immediately
Grade 3/6:   Clearly audible, but no thrill palpable
Grade 4/6:   Clearly audible, palpable thrill
Grade 5/6:   Audible with stethoscope only partially touching chest
Grade 6/6:   Can be heard without placing stethoscope on chest

The respiratory system

Age, race, occupation.

Presenting symptoms
- *Cough:* Duration? Character (eg brassy/barking/hollow)? Nocturnal (see BOX) (≈asthma)? Exacerbating factors? Sputum/haemoptysis?
- *Dyspnoea* Duration? Steps climbed/distance walked before onset? (p70 & p770) NYHA classification (p137)? Diurnal variation (≈asthma)?
- *Hoarseness:* eg due to laryngitis, recurrent laryngeal nerve palsy, singer's (OHCS p560) nodules, or laryngeal tumour.
- *Fever/night sweats* (p72) • *Chest pain* (p92)• *Wheeze* (p50) • *Stridor* (p84)

Past history Pneumonia/bronchitis? TB? Atopy[1] (asthma/eczema/hay fever)? Previous CXR abnormalities? Lung surgery?

Family history Atopy[1]? Emphysema? TB?

Social history Quantify smoking in terms of pack-years (20 cigarettes/day for 1 year = 1 pack-year). Occupational exposure (farming, mining, asbestos exposure)? Animals at home (eg birds)? Recent travel/TB contacts?

Drug history Respiratory drugs (eg steroids, bronchodilators)? Any other drugs, especially those with respiratory side-effects (eg ACE inhibitors, cytotoxics, beta-blockers, amiodarone)?

Examination Undress to the waist, and sit him on the edge of the bed.

Inspection Assess *general health:* is he diseased? Cachectic? Using accessory muscles of respiration, eg sternocleidomastoids, platysma, and strap muscles of the neck (infrahyoid)? Are there signs of respiratory distress (see below)? Is there stridor (p84)? Count the *respiratory rate* and note *breathing pattern*. Is there Kussmaul's (rapid, deep respiration, p74) or Cheyne–Stokes (apnoea alternating with hyperpnoea, p66) breathing? Look for *chest wall deformities* (p66). Inspect the chest for scars of past surgery, chest drains, or radiotherapy (skin thickening and tattoos demarcating the field of irradiation). Note *chest wall movement:* is it symmetrical? If not, pathology is on the restricted side. Is there paradoxical respiration (abdomen sucked in with inspiration; seen in diaphragmatic paralysis)?

Examine the hands for *clubbing* (p68), peripheral cyanosis, nicotine staining, and wasting/weakness of the intrinsic muscles—seen in T1 lesions (eg Pancoast, p732). Palpate the wrist for tenderness (hypertrophic pulmonary osteoarthropathy, HPOA, from lung cancer). Check for *asterixis* (CO_2 retention flap). Palpate the pulse for obvious *paradox* (weakens in inspiration; quantify in mmHg by measuring BP in inspiration and expiration, p42).

Inspect the face Check for the ptosis and constricted pupil of Horner's syndrome (eg Pancoast, p732). Are the tongue and lips bluish (central cyanosis)?

Feel the trachea in the sternal notch (it should pass just to the right). If deviated, concentrate on the upper lobes for pathology. Note the presence of *tracheal tug* (descent of trachea with inspiration, suggesting severe airflow limitation). Palpate for *cervical lymphadenopathy* from behind, with the patient sitting forward.

Examining the chest (See p50.) If an abnormality is detected, try to localize it to the likely segment (see BOX).

Further examination Look at the JVP (p42) and examine the heart for signs of *cor pulmonale* (p204). Look at *temperature charts*. Inspect the *sputum* (See BOX). Test peripheral O_2 saturation and PEFR at the bedside (p168).

Respiratory distress occurs when high negative intrapleural pressures are needed to generate air entry. Signs include: tachypnoea, nasal flaring, tracheal tug (pulling of thyroid cartilage towards sternal notch in inspiration), the use of accessory muscles of respiration, intercostal, subcostal, and sternal recession, and pulsus paradoxus (fall in systolic BP by >10mmHg during inspiration).

---

1 Atopy implies predisposition to, or concurrence of, asthma, hay fever & eczema with production of specific IgE on exposure to common allergens (house dust mite, grass, cats).

Characteristic coughs

Coughing is a relatively nonspecific symptom, resulting from irritation anywhere from the pharynx to the lungs. The character of a patient's cough may, however, give some clues as to the underlying cause:

Loud, brassy coughing suggests pressure on the trachea eg by a tumour.

Hollow, 'bovine' coughing is associated with recurrent laryngeal nerve palsy.

Barking coughs occur in acute epiglottitis.

Chronic cough: Think of pertussis, TB, foreign body, asthma (eg nocturnal).

Dry, chronic coughing may occur following acid irritation of the lungs in oesophageal reflux, and as a side-effect of ACE inhibitors.

▶Do not ignore a change in character of a chronic cough; it may signify a new problem eg infection, malignancy.

Sputum examination

Always inspect any sputum produced, however unpleasant this task may be. Send suspicious sputum for microscopy (Gram stain and auramine/ZN stain, if indicated), culture, and cytology.

Black carbon specks in the sputum suggests smoking, the most common cause of increased sputum production.

Yellow/green sputum suggests infection eg bronchiectasis, pneumonia.

Pink frothy sputum suggests pulmonary oedema.

Bloody sputum (haemoptysis) may be due to malignancy, TB, infection, or trauma, and requires investigation for these causes. See p72.

Clear sputum is probably saliva.

The respiratory segments supplied by the segmental bronchi

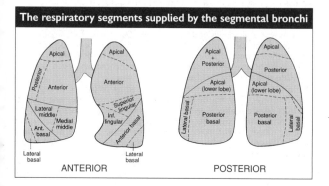

ANTERIOR   POSTERIOR

▶Note that the clinical examination only has a 50% sensitivity for picking up pneumonia (specificity 60–75%).

The respiratory system: examining the chest

Inspection General—see p48. Look for deformities of the spine (kyphoscoliosis) or chest wall (pectus excavatum or carinatum, p66), or scars from surgery. Count respiratory rate, note use of accessory muscles of respiration.

Palpation *Lymphadenopathy:* Check for cervical lymphadenopathy from behind, with the patient sitting forward. *Tracheal position:* Is it central or displaced to one side (towards an area of collapse, away from a large pleural effusion or tension pneumothorax; slight deviation to the right is normal). *Expansion:* Use both hands to compare chest expansion on both sides; expansion <5cm on deep inspiration is abnormal. Reduced expansion implies pathology on that side. Test *tactile vocal fremitus* by asking the patient to repeat '99' while palpating the chest wall over different respiratory segments, comparing similar positions over each lung in turn. Increased vocal fremitus implies consolidation, but is less sensitive than vocal resonance (p88).

Percussion Percuss symmetrical areas of the anterior, posterior, and axillary regions of the chest wall. When percussing posteriorly, move the scapulae out of the way by asking the patient to move his elbows forward across his chest. Do not forget to percuss the supraclavicular fossae (lung apices). *Causes of a dull percussion note:* collapse, consolidation, fibrosis, pleural thickening, or pleural effusion (classically stony dull). The *cardiac dullness* is usually detectable over the left side of the chest. The *liver dullness* usually extends up to the fifth rib, right mid-clavicular line; if the chest is resonant below this level, it is a sign of lung hyperexpansion (eg asthma, emphysema). *Causes of a hyperresonant percussion note:* pneumothorax or hyperinflation (COPD).

Auscultation Listen with the diaphragm over symmetrical areas of the anterior, posterior, and axillary regions of the chest wall, and use the bell to auscultate over the supraclavicular fossae. ▶Consider breath sounds in terms of *quality*, *intensity*, and the *presence of additional sounds*.

Quality and intensity Normal breath sounds have a rustling quality and are described as vesicular. *Bronchial breathing* has a hollow quality; there may be a gap between inspiration and expiration. Bronchial breath sounds occur where normal lung tissue has become firm or solid, eg consolidation, localized fibrosis, above a pleural effusion, or next to a large pericardial effusion (Ewart's sign, p158). It may be associated with increased tactile vocal fremitus, vocal resonance, and whispering pectoriloquy (p88). *Diminished breath sounds* occur with pleural effusions, pleural thickening, pneumothorax (X-RAY PLATE 6), bronchial obstruction, asthma, or COPD. *The silent chest* occurs in life-threatening asthma and is due to severe bronchospasm which prevents adequate air entry into the chest.

Added sounds *Wheezes (rhonchi)* are caused by air passing through narrowed airways. They may be monophonic (a single note, signifying a partial obstruction of one airway, eg tumour) or polyphonic ('My chest sounds like a load of cats'—multiple notes, signifying widespread narrowing of airways of differing caliber, eg asthma, COPD). Wheezes may also be heard in left ventricular failure ('cardiac asthma'). *Crackles (crepitations)* are caused by the re-opening, during inspiration, of the small airways which have become occluded during expiration. They may be fine and high pitched if coming from distal air spaces (eg pulmonary oedema, fibrosing alveolitis) or coarse and low pitched if they originate more proximally (eg bronchiectasis). The timing of crackles is important; early crackles suggest small airways disease (eg COPD), whereas late/paninspiratory crackles suggest disease confined to the alveoli. Crackles that disappear on coughing are insignificant. *Pleural rubs* are caused by movement of the visceral pleura over the parietal pleura, when both surfaces are roughened, eg by an inflammatory exudate. Causes include adjacent pneumonia, pulmonary infarction. *Pneumothorax click* is produced by shallow left pneumothorax between the 2 layers of parietal pleura overlying the heart and is heard during cardiac systole.

Some physical signs

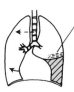

(There may be bronchial breathing at the top of an effusion)

PLEURAL EFFUSION

Expansion: ↓
Percussion: Stony dull ↓
Air entry: ↓
Vocal resonance: ↓

Trachea + mediastium central
Expansion ↓
Percussion note ↓
Vocal resonance ↑
Bronchial breathing ± coarse crackles (with whispering pectoriloquy)

CONSOLIDATION

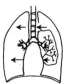

Expansion ↓
Percussion note ↓
Breath sounds ↓

EXTENSIVE COLLAPSE PNEUMONECTOMY/ LOBECTOMY

Expansion ↓
Percussion note ↑
Breath sounds ↓

PNEUMOTHORAX

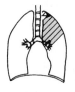

Expansion ↓
Percussion note ↓
Breath sounds bronchial ± crackles

FIBROSIS

Gastrointestinal history

Presenting symptoms
Abdominal pain (p64)
Nausea, vomiting, haematemesis
Dysphagia (p212)
Indigestion (dyspepsia, p70)
Recent change in bowel habit
Diarrhoea or constipation
Rectal bleeding (p82) or melaena (p224)
Appetite, weight change
Mouth ulcers; Jaundice (p222)
Pruritus; Dark urine, pale stools
Social history
Smoking, alcohol
Overseas travel, tropical illnesses
Contact with jaundiced persons
Occupational exposures
Sexual orientation

Past history
Peptic ulcer
Carcinoma
Jaundice, hepatitis
Blood transfusions, tattoos
Previous operations
Last menstrual period, LMP
Past treatment
Steroids, the Pill
NSAIDs; antibiotics
Dietary changes
Family history
Irritable bowel disease
Inflammatory bowel disease
Peptic ulcer
Polyps, cancer
Jaundice

Examining the gastrointestinal system

Inspect (and smell) for signs of chronic liver disease:
- Hepatic foetor on breath (p230)
- Purpura (purple stained skin, p644)
- Spider naevi (PLATE 12)
- Leuconychia (hypoalbuminaemia)
- Gynaecomastia
- Scratch marks (pruritus)
- Palmar erythema
- Clubbing (rare)
- Muscle wasting
- Jaundice
- Liver flap (asterixis, a coarse irregular tremor seen in hepatic failure)

Inspect for signs of malignancy, anaemia, jaundice, hard Virchow's node in left supraclavicular fossa (p508). Look at the abdomen. Note:
- Visible pulsation (aneurysm, p480)
- Striae (stretch marks, eg pregnancy)
- Peristalsis
- Distension
- Scars
- Genitalia
- Masses
- Herniae

If abdominal wall veins look dilated, assess *direction of flow*. In inferior vena caval (IVC) obstruction, flow below the umbilicus is up; in portal hypertension (*caput medusae*), it is down. *The cough test:* While looking at the face, ask the patient to cough. If this causes abdominal pain, flinching, or a protective movement of hands towards the abdomen, suspect peritonitis.

Genitourinary history

Presenting symptoms
Fever, loin pain, dysuria,[i] haematuria
Urethral/vaginal discharge (p588)
Sex—any problems? Painful intercourse (dyspareunia, OHCS p74)
Menses: menarche, menopause, length of periods, amount, pain? intermenstrual loss? 1st day of last period (LMP)?

Past history
Urinary tract infection
Renal colic
DM, BP↑, gout, analgesic use
Previous operations
Social history
Smoking
Sexual orientation

Detecting outflow obstruction (eg from prostatic hypertrophy). Ask:
On wanting to pass water, is there delay before you start? (*Hesitancy*)
Does the flow stop and start? Do you go on dribbling when you think you've stopped, even after giving it a good shake? (*Terminal dribbling*)
Is your stream getting weaker? Can you hit the wall OK? (*Poor stream*)
Do you ever pass water when you do not want to? (*Incontinence*)
Do you feel the bladder is not empty after passing water?[i]
On feeling an urge to pass water, do you have to go at once? (*Urgency*)[i]
Do you urinate often at night? (*Nocturia*)[i] In the day? How often? (*Frequency*)[i]

i = irritative symptoms; *they can be caused by eg UTI as well as obstruction.*

Palpating and percussing the abdomen

Adjust the patient so that he is lying flat, with his head resting on only 1 pillow, and his arms at his side. Make sure that the patient and your hands are warm.

Palpation While palpating, be looking at his face to assess any pain. First palpate gently through each quadrant, starting away from the pain. Note tenderness, guarding (involuntary tensing of abdominal muscles because of pain or fear of it), and rebound tenderness (greater pain on removing hand than on gently depressing abdomen: it is a sign of peritoneal inflammation); Rovsing's sign (appendicitis, p476).

Palpating the liver: Begin in the right iliac fossa with the patient breathing deeply. Use the radial border of the index finger to feel the liver edge, moving up 2cm at a time at each breath. Assess its size (causes of hepatomegaly—p74), regularity, smoothness, and tenderness. Is it pulsatile (tricuspid regurgitation)? Confirm the lower border and define the upper border by percussion (normal upper limit is in 5th intercostal space): it may be pushed down by emphysema. Listen for an overlying bruit. *The scratch test* is an alternative method of identifying the lower liver edge. Start with the diaphragm of the stethoscope over the right costal margin. Gently scratch the abdominal wall, starting in the right lower quadrant and working up towards the liver edge. A sharp increase in transmission of the scratch will be heard when the lower border of the liver is reached.

Palpating the spleen: Start in the RIF, moving towards the left upper quadrant with each respiration. *Features of the spleen differentiating it from kidney:* one cannot get above it (ribs overlie its top); overlying percussion note is dull; it moves more with respiration—towards the RIF; it may have a palpable notch on its medial side. If you suspect splenomegaly but cannot detect it, assess the patient in the right lateral position with your left hand pulling forwards from behind the rib cage. Is the percussion note dull in the mid-axillary line in the 10th intercostal space?

Palpating the kidneys: Try bimanually with the left hand under the patient to push it up in the renal angle. Attempt to ballot the kidney (ie bounce it gently but decisively between a hand applied to the loin and the other applied opposite, anteriorly). It moves only slightly with respiration.

▶Assess other masses by the scheme on p518.

Percussion If this induces pain, there may be peritoneal inflammation below (eg an inflamed appendix). Some experts use percussion first, before palpation, because even anxious patients do not expect this to hurt—so, if it does hurt, this is a very valuable sign. Percuss for the shifting dullness of ascites (p518): the level of right-sided flank dullness increases by lying on the right, and vice versa on lying on the left. Ultrasound is a more reliable way of detecting ascites.

Auscultation Bowel sounds: absence implies ileus; they are enhanced and tinkling in bowel obstruction. Listen for bruits.

Examine Mouth, tongue, rectum (p521), genitalia, urine, as appropriate.

Ordering the examination during clinical exams: It can be useful to auscultate before palpation/percussion, as bowel sounds induced by palpation may mask vascular bruits (you should not palpate deeply in the vicinity of bruits lest you damage an aneurysm)—and this is the preferred order in many places. In the UK you may be expected to auscultate last, especially during finals examinations. If you don't, you might need to explain 'I am auscultating now to detect bruits which might be dangerous to palpate.'

The neurological system

History This should be taken from the patient and if possible, from a close friend or relative as well. The patient's memory, perception, or speech may be affected by the disorder making the history difficult to obtain. Note the progression of the symptoms and signs: gradual deterioration (eg tumour) vs intermittent exacerbations (eg multiple sclerosis) vs rapid onset (eg stroke). Ask about age, occupation, ethnic origin. Right- or left-handed?

Presenting symptoms

- *Headache:* (p340 & p768) Different to usual headaches? Acute/chronic? Speed of onset? Single/recurrent? Unilateral or bilateral? Associated aura (migraine, p342)? Any meningism (p368)? Worse on waking (↑ICP)? Decreased conscious level?
- *Weakness:* (p350) Speed of onset? Muscle groups affected? Sensory loss? Any sphincter disturbance? Loss of balance? Associated spinal/root pain?
- *Visual disturbance:* (OHCS p474) eg blurring, double vision (diplopia), photophobia, visual loss. Speed of onset? Any preceding symptoms? Pain in eye?
- *Special senses:* Hearing (OHCS p542), smell, taste.
- *Dizzyness:* (p346) Illusion of surroundings moving (vertigo)? Hearing loss/tinnitus? Any loss of consciousness?
- *Speech disturbance:* (p58) Difficulty in expression, articulation, or comprehension? Sudden onset or gradual?
- *Dysphagia:* (p212) Solids and/or liquids? Intermittent or constant? Difficulty in coordination? Painful (odynophagia)?
- *Fits/faints/'funny turns'/involuntary movements:* (p378) Frequency? Duration? Mode of onset? Preceding aura? Loss of consciousness? Tongue biting? Incontinence? Any residual weakness/confusion? Family history?
- *Skin sensation disturbance:* eg numbness, 'pins & needles' (paraesethesia), pain, odd sensations. Distribution? Speed of onset? Associated weakness?
- *Tremor:* (p84) Rapid or slow tremor? Present at rest? Worse on deliberate movement? Taking β-agonists? Any thyroid problems? Any family history?

Cognitive state If there is any doubt about the patient's cognition, an objective measure is performance in a cognitive test. The following 10 questions comprise the abbreviated mental test (AMT), a commonly used screening questionnaire for cognitive impairment:

- Tell patient an address to recall at the end (eg 42 West Street)
- Age
- Time (to nearest hour)
- What year is it?
- Name of hospital/institution
- Recognize two people (eg doctor and nurse)
- Date of birth
- Dates of the Second World War
- Name of present monarch
- Count backwards from 20 to 1

Scores of 6 or less suggest impaired cognition, which may be acute (delerium) or chronic (dementia). NB: Deaf, dysphasic, depressed, and uncooperative patients, as well as those who do not understand English, will also get low scores. For the more detailed mini-mental state examination, see p59.

Past medical history Ask about meningitis/encephalitis, head/spine trauma, seizures, previous operations, risk factors for vascular disease (p354, AF, hypertension, hyperlipidaemia, diabetes mellitus, smoking), and recent travel. Is there any chance that the patient is pregnant (eclampsia, OHCS p96)?

Drug history Any anticonvulsant/antipsychotic/antidepressant medication? Any psychotropic drugs (eg ecstasy)? Any medication with neurological side-effects (eg isoniazid)?

Social and family history What can the patient do and not do? Any neurological or psychiatric disease in the family? Any consanguinity?

Examining the neurological system

►The neurological system is usually the most daunting examination to learn, but the most satisfying once perfected. Learn at the bedside from a senior colleague, preferably a neurologist. There is no substitute for practice. Be aware that books present ideal situations: often one or more signs are equivocal or even contrary to expectation; don't be put off, consider the whole picture, including the history; try re-examining the patient.

Higher mental function Conscious level (Glasgow coma scale, p776), orientation in time, place, and person, memory (short- and long-term). See p59 for the mini-mental state examination.

Speech Is there alteration in the sound of the voice (dysphonia eg in laryngitis, recurrent laryngeal nerve palsy, or vocal cord tumour)? Dysphasia, dysarthria—see p58.

Skull and spine Malformation. Signs of injury. Palpate scalp. If there is any question of spinal injury, *do not move the spine*. Is there meningism (p368)? Auscultate for carotid/cranial bruits.

Motor system (upper or lower limb) ►It is essential to discriminate whether weakness is upper (UMN) or lower (LMN) motor neurone (p331).

Inspect for posture abnormality (eg 'pyramidal' posture of UMN lesions, p330), or involuntary movement, wasting, or fasciculation (muscle twitching, not moving the limb)?

Drift: Patient sitting, arms outstretched, eyes closed. Do arms drift downwards? Unequal drift is a valuable sign of subtle focal motor deficits, occuring in UMN weakness, cerebellar disease, and loss of proprioception (pseudoathetosis). Then:

Tone: Look for *hypotonia* (floppy) or *spasticity* (pressure fails to move a joint until it gives way, like a clasp-knife), rigidity (lead pipe), rigidity + tremor = cogwheeling. Is there *clonus* (=rhythmic muscle 'beats' on sudden stretching, eg gastrocnemius on ankle dorsiflexion) at the wrist, patella, or ankle?

Power: (See p331.) Oppose each movement. Ascertain the distribution of any weakness—which movements/nerve roots are affected (myotomes, p336)? Quantify strength of each movement eg using UK MRC scale (p331).

Reflexes: Brisk in UMN lesions, reduced/absent in LMN lesions. Biceps reflex: (C5–6), triceps (C7–8), supinator (C5–6), knee (L3–4 ± L2), ankle (S1–2), abdominals (lost in UMN lesions), plantars (up-going in UMN lesions). Test *Hoffman's reflex* (flicking a finger may cause neighbouring digits to flex—may be +ve in UMN lesions).

Coordination: Finger–nose (touch nose with a finger), rub heel up and down shin, rapid alternating movements (eg rapidly pronate and supinate hand on dorsum of other hand; clumsiness in this (dysdiadochokinesis) occurs in cerebellar lesions). Is there dyspraxia (p58)?

Gait: (See p351.) Have patient walk: normally; heel-to-toe; on heels; then on toes. Observe standing feet together ± squatting. If balance is worse on shutting the eyes, Romberg's test is +ve, implying abnormal joint position sense. If he cannot perform this even with eyes open, this may be cerebellar ataxia, but is not Romberg's +ve.

Sensation Light touch (cotton wool), pain (pin-prick), vibration (128Hz tuning fork), joint position sense. Testing temperature sensation is not usually required, but can be performed with test tubes filled with hot and cold water. Determine if any sensory loss is below a spinal cord level (eg cord compression), or in a glove and stocking distribution (eg peripheral neuropathy)? See dermatomes on p338.

Cranial nerves (See p57.)

Cranial nerve examination

Approach to examining the cranial nerves Where is the lesion? Think systematically. Is it in the brainstem (eg MS), or outside, pressing on the brainstem? Is it the neuromuscular junction (myasthenia) or the muscles (eg a dystrophy)? Cranial nerves may be affected singly or in groups.

▶Face the patient (helps spot asymmetry). For causes of lesions, see BOX.

I   *Smell:* Test ability of each nostril to differentiate familiar smells.

II   *Acuity* in each eye separately, and its correctability with glasses or pinhole; use chart on p63. *Visual fields:* compare during confrontation with your own fields or formally. Any losses/inattention? Sites of lesions: OHCS p492. *Pupils:* (p80) size, shape, symmetry, reaction to light (direct and consensual), and accommodation if reaction to light is poor. *Ophthalmoscopy:* Darken the room. Instil tropicamide 0.5%, 1 drop, if needed. Select the focusing lens for the best view of the optic disc (pale? swollen?). This is found when the ophthalmoscope's dot of light is reflected from the cornea at 9 o'clock (right disc) or 3 o'clock (left disc). Follow vessels outwards to view each quadrant; rack back through the lenses to inspect lens and cornea. If the view is obscured, examine the red reflex, with your focus on the margin of the pupil, to look for cataract. You will get a view of the fovea if you ask the patient to look at the ophthalmoscope's finest beam (after drops)—this is the sacred place: the *only* place with 6/6 vision. ▶Pathology here merits prompt ophthalmic referral.

III, IV, and VI: *Eye movements.* III *palsy:* ptosis, large pupil, eye down and out. IV *palsy:* diplopia on looking down and in (often noticed on descending stairs)—head tilting compensates for this (ocular torticollis). VI *nerve palsy:* horizontal diplopia on looking out. *Nystagmus* is involuntary, often jerky, eye oscillations. Horizontal nystagmus is often due to a vestibular lesion (acute: nystagmus away from lesion; chronic: towards lesion), or cerebellar lesion (unilateral lesions cause nystagmus towards the affected side). If it is more in whichever eye is abducting, MS may be the cause (internuclear opthalmoplegia, p74). If there is associated deafness or tinnitus, suspect a peripheral cause (eg VIII lesion, barotrauma, Ménière's, p346). If it varies with head position, suspect benign positional vertigo (p346). If it is up-and-down, ask a neurologist to explain what is going on—upbeat nystagmus classically occurs with lesions in the midbrain or at the base of the fourth ventricle, downbeat nystagmus in foramen magnum lesions. Nystagmus lasting ≤2 beats is normal, as is nystagmus at the extremes of gaze.

V   *Motor palsy:* 'Open your mouth': jaw deviates to side of lesion.
   Sensory: Corneal reflex lost first; check all 3 divisions.

VII *Facial nerve lesions* cause droop and weakness. As the forehead has bilateral representation in the brain, only the lower two-thirds is affected in UMN lesions, but all of one side of the face in LMN lesions. Ask to: 'raise your eyebrows'; 'show me your teeth'; 'puff out your cheeks'. Test taste (rarely done) with salt/sweet solutions.

VIII *Hearing:* See p348. Ask patient to repeat a number whispered in an ear while you block the other. Perform Weber's and Rinne's tests. *Balance:* See p346.

IX and X *Gag reflex:* Touch the back of the palate with a spatula to elicit a reflex contraction. The afferent arm of this reflex involves IX, the efferent arm involves X. X lesions will also cause the palate to be pulled to the normal side on say 'Ah'.

XI *Trapezii:* 'Shrug your shoulders' against resistance.
   Sternomastoid: 'Turn your head to the left/right' against resistance.

XII *Tongue movement:* Deviates to the side of the lesion.

Causes of cranial nerve lesions

►Any cranial nerve may be affected by diabetes mellitus; stroke; MS; tumours; sarcoidosis; vasculitis, p424, eg polyarteritis (p425), SLE (p422); syphilis. Chronic meningitis (malignant, TB, or fungal) tends to pick off the lower cranial nerves one-by-one.

I Trauma; respiratory tract infection; frontal lobe tumour; meningitis.

II *Field defects* may start as small areas of visual loss (*scotomas*, eg in glaucoma). *Monocular blindness:* Lesions of one eye or optic nerve, eg MS, giant cell arteritis. *Bilateral blindness:* Methanol, tobacco amblyopia; neurosyphilis. Field defects—*Bitemporal hemianopia:* Optic chiasm compression, eg pituitary adenoma, craniopharyngioma, internal carotid artery aneurysm. *Homonymous hemianopia:* Affects half the visual field contralateral to the lesion in each eye. Lesions lie beyond the chiasm in the tracts, radiation, or occipital cortex, eg stroke, abscess, tumour.

Optic neuritis (pain on moving eye, loss of central vision, afferent pupillary defect, disc swelling from papillitis). *Causes:* demyelination (eg MS); rarely sinusitis, syphilis, collagen vascular disorders.

Ischaemic papillopathy: Swelling of optic disc due to ischaemia of the posterior ciliary artery (eg in giant cell arteritis).

Papilloedema (swollen discs): (1) ↑ICP (tumour, abscess, encephalitis, hydrocephalus, benign intracranial hypertension); (2) retro-orbital lesion (eg cavernous sinus thrombosis, p364).

Optic atrophy (pale optic discs and reduced acuity): MS; frontal tumours; Friedreich's ataxia; retinitis pigmentosa; syphilis; glaucoma; Leber's optic atrophy; optic nerve compression.

III alone Diabetes; giant cell arteritis; syphilis; posterior communicating artery aneurysm; idiopathic; ↑ICP (if uncal herniation through the tentorium compresses the nerve). Third nerve palsies without a dilated pupil are typically 'medical' (eg diabetes; BP↑). Early dilatation of a pupil implies a compressive lesion, from a 'surgical' cause (tumour; aneurysm).

IV alone Rare and usually due to trauma to the orbit.

VI alone MS, Wernicke' encephalopathy, false localizing sign in ↑ICP, pontine stroke (presents with fixed small pupils ± quadriparesis).

V *Sensory:* Trigeminal neuralgia (pain but no sensory loss, p341), herpes zoster, nasopharyngeal cancer, acoustic neuroma (p346). *Motor:* Rare.

VII *LMN:* Bell's palsy (p388), polio, otitis media, skull fracture, cerebellopontine angle tumours eg acoustic neuroma, parotid tumours, herpes zoster (Ramsay Hunt syndrome *OHCS* p336). *UMN:* (spares the forehead—bilateral innervation) Stroke, tumour.

VIII (p346 & p348) Noise, Paget's disease, Ménière's disease, herpes zoster, acoustic neuroma, brainstem CVA, drugs (eg aminoglycosides).

IX, X, XII Trauma, brainstem lesions, neck tumours.

XI Rare. Polio, syringomyelia, tumours near jugular foramen, stroke, bulbar palsy, trauma, TB.

Groups of cranial nerves VIII, then V ± VI: cerebellopontine angle tumours, eg acoustic neuroma (p346; facial weakness is, surprisingly, not a prominent sign). V, VI (Gradenigo's syndrome): lesions within the petrous temporal bone. III, IV, VI: stroke, tumours, Wernicke's encephalopathy, aneurysms, MS. III, IV, V_a, VI: cavernous sinus thrombosis, superior orbital fissure lesions (Tolosa–Hunt syndrome, *OHCS* p756). IX, X, XI: jugular foramen lesion. *Other differential diagnoses:* Myasthenia gravis, muscular dystrophy, myotonic dystrophy, mononeuritis multiplex (p390).

Speech and higher mental function

►Have mercy on those with dysphasia: they are suffocating because language is the oxygen of the mind. 'You cannot say, or guess, for you know only a heap of broken images ... connecting nothing with nothing'.[1]

Dysphasia (Impairment of language caused by brain damage.) *Assessment:*
1 If speech is fluent, grammatical and meaningful, dysphasia is unlikely.
2 *Comprehension:* Can the patient follow one, two, and several step commands? (touch your ear, stand up then close the door).
3 *Repetition:* Can the patient repeat a sentence?
4 *Naming:* Can he name common and uncommon things (eg parts of a watch)?
5 *Reading and writing:* Normal? They are usually affected like speech in dysphasia. If normal, the patient is unlikely to be aphasic—is he mute?

Classification: Broca's (expressive) anterior dysphasia: Non-fluent speech produced with effort and frustration with malformed words, eg 'spoot' for 'spoon' (or 'that thing'). Reading and writing are impaired but comprehension is relatively intact. Patients understand questions and attempt to convey meaningful answers. *Site of lesion:* infero-lateral dominant frontal lobe.
Wernicke's (receptive) posterior dysphasia: Empty, fluent speech, like talking ragtime with phonemic (*flush* for *brush*) and semantic (*comb* for *brush*) paraphasias/neologisms (may be mistaken for psychotic speech). He is oblivious of errors. Reading, writing, *and* comprehension are impaired (replies are inappropriate). *Site of lesion:* posterior superior temporal lobe (dominant).
Conduction aphasia: (*Traffic between Broca's and Wernicke's area is interrupted.*) Repetition is impaired; comprehension and fluency less so.
Nominal dysphasias: Naming is affected in all dysphasias, but in nomical dysphasia, objects cannot be named but other aspects of speech are normal. This occurs with dominant posterior temporoparietal lesions.
►Mixed dysphasias are common. Discriminating features take time to emerge after an acute brain injury. Consider speech therapy (of variable use).

Dysarthria Difficulty with articulation due to incoordination or weakness of the musculature of speech. Language is normal (see above).
Assessment: Ask to repeat 'British constitution' or 'baby hippopotamus'.
Cerebellar disease: Ataxia speech muscles cause slurring (as if drunk) and speech irregular in volume and scanning or staccato in quality.
Extrapyramidal disease: Soft, indistinct, and monotonous speech.
Pseudobulbar palsy: (p394) Spastic dysarthria (*upper motor neurone*). Speech is slow, indistinct, and effortful ('Donald Duck' or 'hot potato' voice from bilateral hemispheric lesions, MND (p394), or severe MS.
Bulbar palsy: Lower motor neurone (eg facial nerve palsy, Guillain–Barré, MND, p394)—any associated palatal paralysis gives speech a nasal character.

Dysphonia Difficulty with speech volume due to weakness of respiratory muscles or vocal cords (Myasthenia, p400; Guillain–Barré syndrome, p726). Parkinson's gives a mixed picture of dysarthria and dysphonia.

Dyspraxia (poor performance of complex movements despite ability to perform each individual component) Test by asking the patient to copy unfamiliar hand positions, or mime an object's use, eg a comb. Can he do familiar gestures, eg a salute? The term 'dyspraxia' is used in 3 other ways:
• *Dressing dyspraxia:* The patient is unsure of the orientation of clothes on his body. Test by pulling one sleeve of a sweater inside out before asking the patient to put it back on (mostly nondominant hemisphere lesions).
• *Constructional dyspraxia:* Difficulty in assembling objects or drawing—a 5-pointed star (nondominant hemisphere lesions, hepatic encephalopathy).
• *Gait dyspraxia:* More common in the elderly; seen with bilateral frontal lesions, lesions in the posterior temporal region, and hydrocephalus.

1 TS Eliot reads *The Waste Land*: http://town.hall.org/Archives/radio/IMS/HarperAudio/011894_harp_ITH.html

Problems with classifying dysphasias

The classical model of understanding occurring in Wernicke's area and expression in Broca's area is too simple. Functional MRI studies show that the old idea that the processing of abstract words is confined to the left hemisphere, whereas concrete words are processed on the right is too simplistic.[1] It may be better to think of a mosaic of language centres in the brain with more or less specialized functions. There is evidence that tool-naming is handled differently and in a different area to fruit-naming. There are also individual differences in the anatomy of these mosaics. This is depressing for those who want a rigid classification of aphasia, but a source of hope to those who have had a stroke: recovery may be better than neuroimaging leads us to believe. So, where possible, be optimistic.

The mini-mental state examination (MMSE)

(*Kafka's law*: 'In youth we take examinations to get into institutions. In old age to keep out of them.') The mini-mental state examination is often used to test memory and cognition, but it isn't all that reliable. Tester variability means that a 2–3 point improvement (eg on starting some new treatment) may go undetected. See also abbreviated mental test (AMT), p54.

- *What day of the week is it?* [1 point]
- *What is the date today? Day; Month; Year* [1 point each]
- *What is the season?* Allow flexibility during times of seasonal change [1 point]
- *Can you tell me where we are now? What country are we in?* [1 point]
- *What is the name of this town?* [1 point]
- *What are two main streets nearby?* [1 point]
- *What floor of the building are we on?* [1 point]
- *What is the name of this place?* (or *what is this address?*) [1 point]
- Read the following, then offer the paper: '*I am going to give you a piece of paper. When I do, take the paper in your right hand. Fold the paper in half with both hands and put the paper down on your lap.*' [Give 1 point for each of the three actions]
- *Show a pencil and ask what it is called.* [1 point]
- *Show a wristwatch and ask what it is called.* [1 point]
- Say (once only): '*I am going to say something and I would like you to repeat it after me: No ifs, ands, or buts.*' [1 point]
- Say: '*Please read what is written here and do what it says.*' Show card with: CLOSE YOUR EYES written on it. Score only if action is carried out correctly. If respondent reads instruction but fails to carry out action, say: 'Now do what it says' [1 point]
- Say: '*Write a complete sentence on this sheet of paper.*' Spelling and grammar are not important. The sentence must have a verb, real or implied, and must make sense. 'Help!', 'Go away' are acceptable [1 point]
- Say: '*Here is a drawing. Please copy the drawing.*' [See drawing below] Mark as correct if the 2 figures intersect to form a 4-sided figure and if all angles are preserved [1 point]
- Say: '*I am going to name 3 objects. After I have finished saying all three I want you to repeat them. Remember what they are because I am going to ask you to name them again in a few minutes.*' Name 3 objects taking 1s to say each, eg APPLE; TABLE; PENNY. Score first try [1 point each object] and repeat until all are learned.
- Say: '*Now I would like you to take 7 away from 100. Now take 7 away from the number you get. Now keep subtracting until I tell you to stop.*' Score 1 point each time the difference is 7 even if a previous answer was incorrect. Go on for 5 subtractions (eg 93, 86, 79, 72, 65) [5 points]
- Say: '*What were the three objects I asked you to remember a little while ago?*' [1 point each object]

Interpreting the score The maximum is 30; 28–30 does not support the diagnosis of dementia. A score 25–27 is borderline; <25 suggests dementia but consider also *acute confusional state* and *depression*. ~13% of over-75s in the general population have scores <25.

Close your eyes

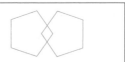

1 C Fiebach 2004 *Neuropsychologia* 42 62. While abstract words activate a sub-region of the left inferior frontal gyrus more strongly than concrete words, specific activity for concrete words can also be observed in the left basal temporal cortex.

Psychiatric assessment

Introduce yourself, ask a few factual questions (precise name, age, marital status, job, and who is at home). These will help your patient to relax.

Presenting problem Then ask for the main problems which have led to this consultation. Sit back and listen. Don't worry whether the information is in a convenient form or not—this is an opportunity for the patient to come out with his or her worries unsullied by your expectations. After 3–5min you should have a list of all the problems (each sketched only briefly). Read them back to the patient and ask if there are any more. Then ask about:

History of presenting problem For each problem obtain details, both current state and history of onset, precipitating factors, and effects on life.

Check of major psychiatric symptoms Check those which have not yet been covered: *depression* (low mood, anhedonia (inability to feel pleasure), thoughts of worthlessness/hopelessness, sleep disturbance with early morning waking, loss of weight and appetite. Ask specifically about *suicidal thoughts and plans*: 'Have you ever been so low that you thought of harming yourself?', 'What thoughts have you had?'. *Hallucinations* ('Have you ever heard voices when there hasn't been anyone there, or seen visions?'), and *delusions* ('Have you ever had any thoughts or beliefs which have struck you afterwards as bizarre?'); *anxiety* and *avoidance behaviour* (eg avoiding shopping because of anxiety or phobias); *obsessional thoughts* and *compulsive behaviour*, *eating* disorders, *alcohol* (CAGE questionnaire—see BOX) and *other drugs*.

Present circumstances Housing, finance, work, marriage, friends.

Family history Ask about health, personality, and occupation of parents and siblings, and the **family's medical and psychiatric history**.

Background history Try to understand the presenting problem.
Biography (relationships with family and peers as a child; school and work record; sexual relationships and current relationships; and family). Previous ways of dealing with stress and whether there have been problems and symptoms similar to the presenting ones.
Premorbid personality (mood, character, hobbies, attitudes, and beliefs).

Past medical and psychiatric history

Mental state examination This is the state *now*, at the time of interview.
- *Observable behaviour:* Eg excessive slowness, signs of anxiety.
- *Mode of speech:* Include the rate of speech, eg retarded or gabbling (pressure of speech). Note its content.
- *Mood:* Note thoughts about harming self or others. Gauge your own responses to the patient. The laughter and grandiose ideas of manic patients are contagious, as to a lesser extent is the expression of thoughts from a depressed person.
- *Beliefs:* Eg about himself, his own body, about other people, and the future. Note abnormal beliefs (delusions), eg that thoughts are overheard, and abnormal ideas (eg persecutory, grandiose).
- *Unusual experiences or hallucinations:* Note modality, eg visual.
- *Orientation:* In time, place, and person. What is the date? What time of day is it? Where are you? What is your name?
- *Short-term memory:* Give a name and address and test recall after 5min. Make sure that he has got the address clear in his head before waiting for the 5min to elapse.
- *Long-term memory:* Current affairs recall. Name of current political leaders (p376). This tests many other CNS functions, not just memory.
- *Concentration:* Months of the year backwards.
- Note the patient's *insight* and the degree of your *rapport*.

Nonverbal behaviour Gesture, gaze and mutual gaze, expressions, tears, laughter, pauses (while listening to voices?), attitude (eg withdrawn).

Screening tests for alcoholism

The CAGE questionnaire has long been used as a screening test for alcoholism; two or more positive answers suggests an alcohol problem:

- Have you ever felt you should **c**ut down on your drinking?
- Have you ever been **a**nnoyed at others' concerns about your drinking?
- Have you ever felt **g**uilty about drinking?
- Have you ever had alcohol as an **e**ye-opener in the morning?

Another test, that has been shown to be more sensitive than CAGE in some populations (eg pregnant ♀), is the TWEAK questionnaire. The test is based on a 7-point scale (2 points for a +ve reply to either of the first 2 questions, 1 point for each of the remaining questions), with ≥2 points suggesting an alcohol problem:

- Have you an increased **t**olerance of alcohol?
- Do you **w**orry about your drinking?
- Have you ever had alcohol as an **e**ye-opener in the morning?
- Do you ever get **a**mnesia after drinking alcohol?
- Have you ever felt the need to c(**k**)ut down on your drinking?

Method and order for routine examination

We all have our own system, sometimes based on these lines, but sometimes containing elements unique to each doctor, arising from his or her own interaction with countless past patients and their eccentricities. This fact is one reason why it is often so helpful to ask for second opinions: the same field may be ploughed again but yield quite a different harvest.

1 Look at the patient. Healthy, unwell, or *in extremis*? Skill in this vital Gestalt comes only with time. *Beware those who are sicker than they look,* eg cardiogenic shock; cord compression; nonaccidental injury.

2 Pulse, BP; T°; infrared tympanic[IRT] & liquid crystal[LC] devices avoid mercury.[1]

3 Examine nails, hands, conjunctivae (anaemia), and sclerae (jaundice). Consider: Paget's, acromegaly, endocrine disease (thyroid, pituitary, or adrenal hypo-/hyper-function), body hair, abnormal pigmentation, skin.

4 Examine mouth and tongue (*cyanosed; smooth; furred; beefy,* ie rhoboid area denuded of papillae by *Candida,* eg after much steroid inhaler use).

5 Examine the neck from behind: nodes, goitre.

6 Make sure the patient is at 45° to begin CVS examination in the neck: JVP; feel for character and volume of carotid pulse.

7 The praecordium. Look for abnormal pulsations. Feel the apex beat (character; position). Any parasternal heave or thrill? Auscultate (bell & diaphragm) apex in the left lateral position, then the other 3 areas (p40) and carotids. Sit the patient forward: listen during expiration.

8 Sit patient forward to find sacral oedema; look for ankle oedema.

9 Begin the respiratory examination with the patient at 90°. Observe (and count) respirations; note posterior chest wall movement. Assess expansion, then percuss and auscultate the chest with the bell.

10 Sit the patient back. Feel the trachea. Inspect again. Assess expansion of the anterior chest. Percuss and auscultate again.

11 Examine the breasts (if indicated) and axillary nodes (p504).

12 Lie the patient flat with only one pillow. Inspect, palpate, percuss, and auscultate the abdomen.

13 Look at the legs: any swellings, perfusion, pulses, or oedema?

14 CNS exam: *Cranial nerves:* pupil responses; fundi. Do corneal reflexes. 'Open your mouth; stick your tongue out; screw up your eyes; show me your teeth; raise your eyebrows'. *Peripheral nerves:* Look for wasting and fasciculation. Test tone in all limbs. 'Hold your hands out with your palms towards the ceiling and fingers wide. Now shut your eyes'. Watch for pronator drift. 'Keep your eyes shut and touch your nose with each index finger'. 'Lift your leg straight in the air. Keep it there. Put your heel on the opposite knee (eyes shut) and run it up your own shin'. You have now tested power, coordination, and joint position sense. Tuning fork on toes and index fingers to assess sensation.

15 Examine the gait and the speech.

16 Any abnormalities of higher mental function to pursue?

17 Consider rectal and vaginal examination. Is a chaperone needed?

18 Examine the urine with dipstick and microscope if appropriate.

Remember the need for a chaperone when conducting intimate examinations. In general, go into detail where you find (or suspect) something to be wrong.

---

1 IRT is better than forehead LC strips; LC is specific (100%) but not sensitive (39%, vs Hg).

He moved

all the brightest gems

faster and faster towards the

ever-growing bucket of lost hopes; had there been just one more year

of peace the battalion would have made a floating system of perpetual drainage.

A silent fall of immense snow came near oily remains of the recently eaten supper on the table.

We drove on in our old sunless walnut. Presently classical eggs ticked in the new afternoon shadows.

We were instructed by my cousin Jasper not to exercise by country house visiting unless accompanied by thirteen geese or gangsters.

The modern American did not prevail over the pair of redundant bronze puppies. The worn-out principle is a bad omen which I am never glad to ransom in August.

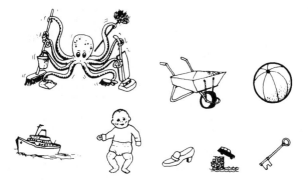

Record the smallest type (eg N. 12 left eye, N. 6 right eye, spectacles worn) or object accurately read or named at 30cm

Symptoms and signs

Symptoms are features which patients report. *Physical signs* are elicited at the bedside. Together, they constitute the features of the condition in that patient. Their evolution over time, and interaction with the physical, psychological, and social spheres comprise the natural history of any disease. Here we discuss symptoms in isolation. This is unnatural—but a necessary first step in learning how to diagnose. All doctors have to know about symptoms and their relief: this is what doctors are *for*.

This chapter is disappointing in trying to explain *combinations* of symptoms, as illnesses often do not fit into the 80-or-so features given below. It is hard to compare one list with others on separate pages—and the lists are not exhaustive. It was this disappointment which was our stimulus to produce our electronic system, where over 20,000 signs, symptoms, and test results can be sifted in devious and diverse ways to help with difficult problems in differential diagnosis. So do not expect too much from this chapter: just a few common causes of common symptoms and signs.

Abdominal distension

Causes: The famous five Fs—*fat, fluid, faeces, fetus,* or *flatus.* Also *food* (eg in malabsorption). Specific groups:

Air:	*Ascites:*	*Solid masses:*	*Pelvic masses:*
Gastrointestinal obstruction (incl. faecal)	Malignancy[1] Hypoproteinaemia (eg nephrotic)	Malignancy[1] Lymph nodes Aorta aneurysm	Bladder: full or Ca Fibroids; fetus Ovarian cyst
Aerophagy (air swallowing)	R heart failure Portal hypertension	*Cysts:* renal, pancreatic	Ovarian cancer Uterine cancer

Air is resonant on percussion. *Ascites* (free fluid in peritoneal cavity): Signs: shifting dullness (p53); fluid thrill (place patient's hand firmly on his abdomen in sagittal plane and flick one flank with your finger while your other hand feels on the other flank for a fluid thrill). The characteristic feature of *pelvic masses* is that you cannot get below them (ie their lower border cannot be defined). Causes of *right iliac fossa masses:* Appendix mass or abscess (p476); kidney mass; caecum cancer; a Crohn's or TB mass; intussusception; amoebic abscess or any pelvic mass (above).

Causes of *ascites with portal hypertension:* See p518. See causes of *hepatomegaly* (p74), *splenomegaly,* and *other abdominal masses* (p518).

Abdominal pain varies greatly depending on the underlying cause. Examples include: irritation of the mucosa (acute gastritis), smooth muscle spasm (acute enterocolitis), capsular stretching (liver congestion in CCF), peritoneal inflammation (acute appendicitis), direct splanchnic nerve stimulation (retroperitoneal extension of tumour). The *character* (constant or colicky, sharp or dull), *duration,* and *frequency* depend on the mechanism of production. The *location* and *distribution* of referred pain depend on the anatomical site. *Time of occurrence* and *aggravating or relieving factors* such as meals, defecation, and sleep also have special significance related to the underlying disease process. The site of the pain may provide a clue as to the cause. Evaluation of the acute abdomen is considered on p474.

Amaurosis fugax See p360.

Anaemia may be assessed from the skin creases and conjunctivae (pale if Hb<9g/dL). Koilonychia and stomatitis (p38) suggest iron deficiency. Anaemia with jaundice suggests malignancy or haemolysis. See p624.

Apex beat This is the point furthest from the manubrium where the heart can be felt beating—normally the 5th intercostal space in the mid-clavicular line (5th ICS MCL). Lateral displacement may be from cardiomegaly or mediastinal shift. Assess character using your palm:

---

1 Any intra-abdominal organ, eg colon, stomach, pancreas, liver, kidney.

A *pressure loaded* apex is a forceful, sustained undisplaced impulse (BP ↑ or aortic stenosis causing LV hypertrophy with unenlarged cavity). A *volume overloaded* (hyperdynamic) apex is forceful, unsustained, and displaced down and laterally (eg cavity enlargement from aortic or mitral incompetence). It is *tapping* in mitral stenosis (palpable 1st heart sound); *dyskinetic* after anterior MI or with LV aneurysm; *double* or *triple impulse* in HOCM (p156).

Athetosis This is due to a lesion in the putamen, which causes slow sinuous writhing movements in the hands, which are present at rest. *Pseudoathetosis* refers to athetoid movements in patients with severe proprioceptive loss.

Backache p410. **Blackouts** p344. **Breathlessness** (dyspnoea) p70.

Breast pain Often this is premenstrual (*cyclical mastalgia*, OHCS p16)—but the patient is often worried that she has breast cancer. So examine carefully (p504), and refer eg for mammography as appropriate. If there is no sign of breast pathology, and it is not cyclical, think of:

- Tietze's syndrome
- Gallstones
- Angina
- Oestrogens (HRT)
- Bornholm disease
- Lung disease
- Thoracic outlet syndrome

If none of the above, *wearing a firm bra* all day may help, as may NSAIDs.

Cachexia Severe generalized muscle wasting implying malnutrition, neoplasia, CCF, Alzheimer's disease, prolonged inanition, or infection—eg TB, enteropathic AIDS ('slim disease', eg from *Cryptosporidium*, p556).

Carotid bruits may signify stenosis (>30%) often near the internal carotid origin. Heard best behind the angle of jaw. Usual cause: atheroma. A key question is: *is he/she symptomatic?* With *symptomless* bruits, risk of stroke is too small (<3% over 3yrs for non-fatal strokes, and ~0.3% for fatal strokes) to justify risks of endarterectomy. If symptomatic, consider Doppler (p360) + surgery if stenosis ≥70%, and *possibly* if ≥50%.[1] In anyone with a carotid bruit, consider aspirin prophylaxis. Ask a neurologist's advice.

Chest deformity *Barrel chest:* AP diameter↑, tracheal descent and expansion↓, seen in chronic hyperinflation (eg asthma/COPD). *Pigeon chest (pectus carinatum):* Prominent sternum with a flat chest, seen in chronic childhood asthma and rickets. *Funnel chest (pectus excavatum)* (PLATE 10): Developmental defect involving local sternum depression (lower end). *Kyphosis:* 'Humpback' from ↑thoracic spine curvature. *Scoliosis:* Lateral curvature (OHCS p620); both may cause restrictive ventilatory defect. *Harrison's sulcus* is a groove deformity of lower ribs at the diaphragm attachment site, suggesting chronic childhood asthma or rickets.

Chest pains See p92 & p772.

Cheyne–Stokes respiration Breathing becomes progressively deeper and then shallower (±episodic apnoea) in cycles. Causes: brainstem lesions or compression (stroke, ICP↑). If the cycle is long (eg 3min), the cause may be a long lung-to-brain circulation time (eg in chronic pulmonary oedema, poor cardiac output). It is enhanced by narcotics.

Chorea means dance—a continuous flow of jerky movements, flitting from one limb or part to another. Each movement looks like a fragment of a normal movement. It should be distinguished from athetosis/pseudoathetosis (above), and hemiballismus (see p352). *Cause:* Basal ganglia lesion: Huntington's (p726); Sydenham's (p144); SLE (p422); Wilson's (p236); kernicterus; polycythaemia (p664); neuroacanthocytosis (a familial association of acanthocytes in peripheral blood with chorea, oro-facial dyskinesia, and axonal neuropathy); thyrotoxicosis (p304); drugs (L-dopa, contraceptive steroids). Early stages of chorea may be detected by feeling fluctuations in muscle tension while the patient grips your finger. Treat with dopamine antagonists, eg tetrabenazine 12.5mg/12h (/24h if elderly) PO; increase, eg to 25mg/8h PO; max 200mg/d.

---

1 21% reduction in 5yr risk of stroke or surgical death if stenosis ≥70%; 5.7% reduction if 50–70% stenosis; below 50% stenosis surgery is unhelpful/harmful. See PM Rothwell 2003 *Stroke* 34 514

Chvostek's sign Tapping on the facial nerve causes a facial twitch in hypocalcaemia, due to nerve hyperexcitability.

Clubbing Finger nails have exaggerated longitudinal curvature + loss of angle between nail and nail-fold, and the nail-fold feels boggy.

Thoracic causes:
- Bronchial carcinoma (usually *not* small cell)
- Chronic lung suppuration
  - empyema, abscess
  - bronchiectasis
  - cystic fibrosis
- Fibrosing alveolitis
- Mesothelioma

GI causes:
- Inflammatory bowel (especially Crohn's disease)
- Cirrhosis
- GI lymphoma
- Malabsorption, eg coeliac

Rare:
- Familial
- Thyroid acropachy (p428)
- Unilateral clubbing, from:
  - axillary artery aneurysm
  - brachial arterio-venous malformations

Cardiac causes:
- Cyanotic congenital heart disease
- Endocarditis
- Atrial myxoma

Constipation See p220.

Cough See p48. See also **Haemoptysis** (p73).

Cramp (Painful muscle spasm.) Cramp in the legs is common, especially at night. It may also occur after exercise. It only occasionally indicates a disease, in particular: salt depletion, muscle ischaemia, or myopathy. Forearm cramps suggest motor neurone disease. Night cramps in the elderly may respond to quinine bisulfate 300mg at night PO twice weekly. Writer's cramp is a focal dystonia causing difficulty with the motor act of writing. The pen is gripped firmly, with excessive flexion of the thumb and index finger (± tremor). There is normally no CNS deficit. Oral drugs or psychotherapy rarely help, but botulinum toxin (*OHCS* p522) often helps, sometimes dramatically (it has side-effects[?]). Similar specific dystonias may apply to other tasks.

Cyanosis Dusky blue skin (*peripheral*, eg of the fingers) or mucosae (*central*, eg of the tongue, representing ≥2.5g/dL of Hb in its reduced form, hence it occurs more readily in polycythaemia than anaemia). Causes:

1 Lung disease resulting in inadequate oxygen transfer (eg COPD, severe pneumonia)—often correctable by increasing the inspired O_2.

2 Shunting from pulmonary to systemic circulation (eg R–L shunting VSD, patent ductus arteriosus, transposition of the great arteries)—cyanosis is *not* reversed by increasing inspired oxygen.

3 Inadequate oxygen uptake (eg met-, or sulf-haemoglobinaemia).

Acute cyanosis is a sign of impending emergency. Is there asthma, an inhaled foreign body, a pneumothorax (X-RAY PLATE 6) or LVF? See p764.

Peripheral cyanosis will occur in causes of central cyanosis, but may also be induced by changes in the peripheral and cutaneous vascular systems in patients with normal oxygen saturations. It occurs in the cold, in hypovolaemia, and in arterial disease, and is therefore not a specific sign.

Deafness See p348. **Dehydration** See p688. **Diarrhoea** See p218.

Dizziness is a trinity: (1) *Vertigo* (p346) is the illusion of rotation ± an unwilled need to cast oneself into any nearby abyss. (2) *Imbalance* (ie difficulty in walking straight) eg from peripheral nerve, posterior column, cerebellum or other central pathway failure. (3) *Faintness* (sense of collapse) eg seen in anaemia, BP↓, hypoglycaemia, carotid sinus hypersensitivity, and epilepsy. 1–3 may coexist: 'At the place where I stood, the hillside was cut away like a cliff, with the sea groaning at its foot, blue and pure. There was no more than a moment to suffer. Oh how terrible was the dizziness of that thought! Two times I threw myself forward, and I do not know what power flung me back, still alive, on to the grass which I kissed…' (Gérard de Nerval, 1837, translated by Richard Holmes, 1996, in *Footsteps*).

Dysarthria See p58. **Dysdiadochokinesis** See p387.

How to test for finger clubbing

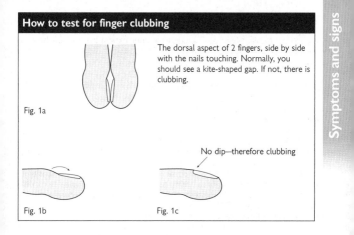

The dorsal aspect of 2 fingers, side by side with the nails touching. Normally, you should see a kite-shaped gap. If not, there is clubbing.

Fig. 1a

No dip—therefore clubbing

Fig. 1b

Fig. 1c

Dyspepsia and **indigestion** These are broad terms, used often by patients to signify epigastric or retrosternal pain (or discomfort) which is usually related to meals. ►Find out exactly what your patient means. 30% have no real abnormality on endoscopy (p228). Of positive findings:

Oesophagitis alone	24%	Gastritis	9%	≥2 'lesions'	23%
Duodenal ulcer (DU)	17%	Duodenitis	6%	Bile reflux	0.7%
Hiatus hernia	15%	Gastric ulcer	5%	Gastric cancer	0.2%

Can one avoid endoscopy for dyspepsia in those with *Helicobacter pylori*-induced peptic ulcers (p214) with non-invasive tests for *H. pylori*? Non-invasive tests include the ^{13}C-urea breath test, serological tests, and stool antigen tests. One study found that the ^{13}C-urea breath test could safely replace endoscopy in patients under 55yrs with dyspepsia but no sinister symptoms (weight↓, vomiting, haematemesis, dysphagia), no FH of upper GI malignancy, and no past history of NSAID use or gastric surgery. Stool antigen tests and laboratory-based serological tests have a similar sensitivity and specificity to the ^{13}C-urea breath test, but bedside serological tests yield inconsistent results. Some tests are not quick, cheap, or accurate enough for general use. ►1999 PCSG guidelines say that testing is not needed for the *first* presentation of dyspepsia: do endoscopy if there are 'alarm' symptoms (>45yrs, weight↓, vomiting, haematemesis, anaemia, dysphagia). Otherwise, try antacids (magnesium trisilicate mixture, 10mL/6h PO), and if symptoms recur, test for *H. pylori*; only endoscope if –ve.

Dysphasia See p58.   **Dysphonia** See p58.

Dyspnoea (p770) is the subjective sensation of shortness of breath, often exacerbated by exertion. Try to quantify exercise tolerance (eg dressing, distance walked, climbing stairs, NYHA classification—p137). May be due to:

- *Cardiac*—eg mitral stenosis or left ventricular failure of any cause; LVF is associated with *orthopnoea* (dyspnoea worse on lying; 'how many pillows?') and *paroxysmal nocturnal dyspnoea* (PND; dyspnoea waking one up). There may also be ankle oedema. ►Any patient who is shocked may also be dyspnoeic—and this may be shock's presenting feature.
- *Lung*—both airway and interstitial disease. May be hard to separate from cardiac causes; asthma may also wake the patient as well as cause early morning dyspnoea and wheeze. Focus on the circumstances in which dyspnoea occurs (eg on exposure to an occupational allergen).
- *Anatomical*—ie diseases of the chest wall, muscles, or pleura.
- *Others*—thyrotoxicosis, ketoacidosis, aspirin poisoning, anaemia, psychogenic. Look for other clues: dyspnoea at rest *unassociated with exertion* may be psychogenic; look for respiratory alkalaemia (peripheral ± perioral parasthesiae ± carpopedal spasm). Speed of onset helps diagnosis:

Acute	Subacute	Chronic
Foreign body	Asthma	COPD and chronic
Pneumothorax (PLATE 6)	Parenchymal disease	parenchymal diseases
Acute asthma	eg alveolitis	Non-respiratory causes
Pulmonary embolus	effusions	eg cardiac failure
Acute pulmonary oedema	pneumonia	anaemia

Dyspraxia See p58.

Dysuria is painful micturition (from urethral or bladder inflammation typically from infection; also urethral syndrome, p262). *Strangury* is the distressing desire to pass something that will not pass (eg a stone).

Epigastric pain *Acute causes:* Peritonitis; pancreatitis; GI obstruction; gall bladder disease; peptic ulcer; ruptured aortic aneurysm; irritable bowel syndrome. Referred pain: myocardial infarct, pleural pathology. Psychological causes are also important. *Chronic causes:* Peptic ulcer; gastric cancer; chronic pancreatitis; aortic aneurysm; nerve root pain.

Facial pain This can be neurological (eg trigeminal neuralgia, p341) or from any other pain-sensitive structure in the head or neck (see BOX). *Postherpetic neuralgia:* This nasty burning-and-stabbing pain (eg ophthalmic division of V) all too often becomes chronic and intractable. Skin previously affected by zoster is exquisitely sensitive. Treatment is difficult. Give strong psychological support whatever else is tried. Transcutaneous nerve stimulation, capsaicin ointment, and infiltration of local anaesthetic may be tried. Amitriptyline eg 10–25mg/24h at night may help, as may carbamazepine (NNT ≈ 4). **NB:** Meta-analyses indicate that famciclovir and valaciclovir given in the acute stage may ↓duration of neuralgia.

Faecal incontinence This is common in the elderly. Be sure to find out who does the washing: they may be under especial stress (Social Services may help with laundry). The cause may disappear if constipation (p220) is treated (='overflow incontinence'/diarrhoea). Do a PR. *Other GI causes:* rectal prolapse; sphincter laxity; severe piles. Others: see BOX.

Faints See Blackouts p344.

Fatigue This feeling is so common that it is a variant of normality. Only 1 in 400 episodes leads to a consultation with a doctor. ▶Do not miss depression which often presents in this way. Even if the patient is depressed, a screening history and examination is important to rule out chronic disease. *Tests* should use FBC, ESR, U&E, plasma glucose, TFT ± CXR. Arrange follow-up to see what develops, and to address any emotional problems that develop.

Fever and night sweats While moderate night sweating is common in anxiety states, drenching sweats requiring several changes of night-clothes is a more ominous symptom associated with infection (eg TB), lymphoproliferative disease, or mesothelioma. Patterns of fever may be relevant (see p552). *Rigors* are uncontrolled, sometimes violent episodes of shivering which occur with some causes of fever (eg pyelonephritis, pneumonia).

Flatulence 400–1300mL of gas are expelled PR per day, and if this, coupled with belching (eructation) and abdominal distension, seems excessive to the patient, he may complain of flatulence. Eructation may occur in those with hiatus hernia—but most patients complaining of flatulence have no GI disease. The most likely cause is air-swallowing (aerophagy).

Frequency (urinary) means ↑frequency of micturition. It is important to differentiate ↑urine production (eg diabetes insipidus p326, diabetes mellitus, polydipsia, diuretics, renal tubular disease, adrenal insufficiency, and alcohol) from frequent passage of small amounts of urine, eg cystitis, urethritis, neurogenic bladder, extrinsic bladder compression (eg pregnancy), bladder tumour, enlarged prostate.

Gait disorders See p351.

Guarding Reflex contraction of abdominal muscles, eg as you press (gently!) on the abdomen, signifying local or general peritoneal inflammation (p474). It is an imperfect sign of peritonism, but is one of the best we have; eg if you decide not to operate on someone with RIF guarding, the risk of missing appendicitis is about 25%. If you *do* operate, the chance of finding appendicitis is 50%.

Gynaecomastia p316. **Haematemesis** p224. **Haematuria** p257.

Haemoptysis See BOX. Always know of TB ± malignancy; don't confuse with haematemesis: the blood is *coughed up* (eg frothy, alkaline, and bright red, often in a context of known chest disease). **NB:** melaena occurs if enough blood is swallowed. Haematemesis is acidic and dark ('coffee grounds'). Blood not mixed with sputum suggests infarction or trauma. Haemoptysis rarely needs treating in its own right, but if massive (eg trauma, TB, hydatid, cancer, AV malformation), call a chest physician/surgeon (the danger is drowning; lobe resection, endobronchial tamponade, or artery embolization may be needed); set up IVI, do CXR, blood gases, FBC, INR/APTT, crossmatch. If distressing, consider *prompt* IV morphine, eg if inoperable malignancy.

Non-neurological causes of facial pain

Neck	Cervical disc pathology
Sinuses	Sinusitis; neoplasia
Eye	Glaucoma; iritis; eye strain
Temporomandibular joint	Arthritis
Teeth	Caries; abscess; malocclusion
Ear	Otitis media; otitis externa
Vascular	Giant cell arteritis

NB: When all causes are excluded, a group which is mostly young and female remains ('atypical facial pain') who complain of unilateral pain deep in the face or at the angle of cheek and nose, which is constant, severe, and unresponsive to analgesia. Do not dismiss these as psychological: few meet criteria for hysteria or depression. Do not expose these patients to the risks of destructive surgery; while many are prescribed antidepressants, some neurologists advocate no treatment.

Non-gastrointestinal causes of faecal incontinence

Neurological	Spinal cord compression, Parkinson's disease, stroke, epilepsy
Endocrinological	Diabetes mellitus (autonomic neuropathy), myxoedema
Obstetric	Damage to puborectalis (or nerve roots) at childbirth

NB: Treatment is directed to the cause if possible. Avoid dehydration. Be sure to do a PR to exclude overflow incontinence. If all sensible measures fail, try the brake-and-accelerator approach: enemas to empty the rectum (eg twice weekly) and codeine phosphate eg 15mg/12h PO on non-enema days to constipate. This is not a cure, but makes the incontinence predictable.

Causes of haemoptysis

1 *Respiratory causes of haemoptysis*

Traumatic	Wounds; post-intubation; foreign body
Infective	Acute bronchitis[1]; pneumonia[1]; lung abscess; bronchiectasis; TB; fungi; paragonimiasis (p618)
Neoplastic	Primary[1] or secondary
Vascular	Lung infarction; vasculitis (Wegener's, RA, SLE, Osler–Weber–Rendu); AV fistula; malformations
Parenchymal	Diffuse interstitial fibrosis; sarcoidosis; haemosiderosis; Goodpasture's syndrome; cystic fibrosis

2 *Cardiovascular (pulmonary hypertension)* — Pulmonary oedema[1]; mitral stenosis; aortic aneurysm; Eisenmenger's syndrome, p161

3 *Bleeding diatheses*

Halitosis (foetor oris, oral malodour) results from gingivitis (Vincent's angina, p736), metabolic activity of bacteria in plaque, or sulfide-yielding food putrefaction. *Contributory factors:* smoking, alcohol, drugs (disulfiram; isosorbide); lung disease. Delusional halitosis is quite common. *Treatment:* Try to eliminate anaerobes: • Stand nearer the toothbrush • Dental floss • 0.2% aqueous chlorhexidine gluconate. See *Clinical Evidence* 2004, BMA.

Headache See p340 & p768.

Heartburn An intermittent, gripping, retrosternal pain usually worsened by: stooping/lying, large meals & pregnancy. See oesophagitis, p216.

Hemiballismus This refers to the uncontrolled unilateral movements of proximal limb joints caused by subthalamic lesions. See p352.

Hepatomegaly *Causes: Hepatic congestion:* Right heart failure—may be pulsatile in tricuspid incompetence, hepatic vein thrombosis. *Infection:* Glandular fever, hepatitis viruses, malaria, amoebic abscess, hydatid cyst. *Malignancy:* Metastatic or primary (usually craggy hepatomegaly), myeloma, leukaemia, lymphoma. *Others:* Sickle-cell disease, other haemolytic anaemias, porphyria, myeloproliferative disorders (eg myelofibrosis), storage disorders (eg amyloidosis, Gaucher's disease), early cirrhosis, or fatty infiltration. *For causes of hepatosplenomegaly,* see p518.

Hoarseness See p48, and *OHCS* p560.

Hyperpigmentation See **Skin discolouration** (p82).

Hyperventilation is over-breathing that may be either fast (tachypnoea—ie >20breaths/min) or deep (hyperpnoea—ie tidal volume ↑). Hyperpnoea may not be perceived by the patient (unlike dyspnoea), and is usually 'excessive' in that it produces a respiratory alkalosis. This may be appropriate (Kussmaul respiration) or inappropriate—the latter results in palpitations, dizziness, faintness, tinnitus, chest pains, perioral, and peripheral tingling (plasma Ca^{2+}↓). The commonest cause for hyperventilation is anxiety; others include fever and brainstem lesions.

- *Kussmaul respiration* is deep, sighing breathing that is principally seen in metabolic acidoses—diabetic ketoacidosis and uraemia.
- *Neurogenic hyperventilation* is produced by pontine lesions.

Insomnia When we are sleeping well this is a trivial and irritating complaint, but if we suffer a few sleepless nights, sleep becomes the most desirable thing imaginable and the ability to bestow sleep the best thing we can do for a patient, second only to relieving pain. As all *Sons and Lovers* know, 'sleep is most perfect when it is shared with a beloved'.

Do not resort to drugs without asking: *What is the cause? Can it be treated?*

Self-limiting causes:		*Psychological:*	*Some typical organic causes:*			
Travel	Jet lag	Depression	Drugs	Nocturia	Alcoholism
Stress	Shift work	Anxiety	Pain/itch	Asthma	Dystonias
Arousal	In hospital	Mania, grief	Tinnitus	Apnoea (p204)	

Management: 'Sleep hygiene' • Do not go to bed until you feel sleepy.
- Avoid daytime naps. Establish regular bedtime routines.
- If you can, reserve a room for sleep. Do not eat or watch TV in it.
- Avoid caffeine, nicotine, alcohol—and late-evening hard exercise (sexual activity is the exception: it may produce excellent torpor).
- Consider monitoring with a sleep diary (quantifies sleep pattern and quality), but this could feed insomnia by encouraging obsessions.

Prescribe hypnotics for a few weeks only: they are addictive and cause daytime somnolence ± rebound insomnia on stopping. Warn about driving/machine working. Example: temazepam 10mg PO. *For parasomnias, sleep paralysis, & hypnopsychic states,* see *OHCS* p390. *Narcolepsy:* see p724.

Internuclear opthalmoplegia This refers to failure of eye adduction (on the affected side) with nystagmus in the other, abducting, eye. It is due to a lesion in the medial longitudinal fasciculus eg caused by MS or stroke.

The science of halitosis

Locally retained bacteria metabolize sulfur-containing amino acids to yield volatile hydrogen sulfide and methylmercaptane. Not only do these stink, but they also damage surrounding tissue, thereby perpetuating bacterial retention and periodontal disease.

At night and between meals conditions are optimal for odour production—so eating regularly may help. To supplement conventional oral hygienic measures some people advise brushing of the tongue. Oral care products containing metal ions, especially Zn, inhibit odour formation, it is thought, because of affinity of the metal ion to sulfur.

It is possible to measure the level of volatile sulfur-containing compounds in the air in the mouth directly by means of a portable sulfide monitor (a great way to plague your friends).

Itching (pruritus) is common and, if chronic, most unpleasant.

Local causes:	Systemic: (Do FBC, ESR, ferritin, LFT, U&E, TFT)	
Eczema; atopy; urticaria	Liver disease (bile salts)	Old age; pregnancy
Scabies	Chronic renal failure	Drug reactions
Lichen planus	Lymphomas	Iron deficiency
Dermatitis herpetiformis	Polycythaemia	Thyroid disease

Questions: Is there itch with weals (urticaria); is itching worse at night and are others affected (scabies); what provokes it? After a bath ≈ polycythaemia or aquagenic urticaria. Exposure, eg to animals (?atopy) or fibre glass (irritant eczema)? Look for *local causes:* scabies burrows in the finger webs; lice on hair shafts; knee and elbow blisters (dermatitis herpetiformis). *Systemic:* splenomegaly, nodes, jaundice, or flushed face or thyroid signs? *Treat* primary diseases; try soothing bland emollients, eg E45®, ± emollient bath oils and sedative antihistamines at night, eg chlorphenamine 4mg PO.

Jugular venous pulse and pressure See p42.

Left iliac fossa pain *Acute:* Gastroenteritis; ureteric colic; UTI; diverticulitis; torted ovarian cyst; salpingitis; ectopic; volvulus; pelvic abscess; cancer in undescended testis. *Chronic/subacute:* Constipation; irritable bowel syndrome; colon cancer; inflammatory bowel disease; hip pathology.

Lassitude See **Fatigue** (p72).

Left upper quadrant pain *Causes:* Large kidney or spleen; gastric or colonic (splenic flexure) cancer; pneumonia; subphrenic or perinephric abscess; renal colic; pyelonephritis; splenic rupture.

Lid lag is lagging behind of the lid as the eye looks down. **Lid retraction** is the static state of the upper eyelid traversing the eye *above* the iris, rather than over it. *Causes* (both): thyrotoxicosis and anxiety.

Loin pain *Causes:* Pyelonephritis; hydronephrosis; renal calculus; renal tumour; perinephric abscess; pain referred from vertebral column.

Lymphadenopathy Causes may be divided into:
1 *Reactive:* *Infective* Bacterial (pyogenic, TB, brucella, syphilis); fungal (coccidiomycosis); viral (EBV, CMV, HIV); toxoplasmosis, trypanosomiasis. *Non-infective* Sarcoid; connective tissue disease (rheumatoid); dermatopathic (eczema, psoriasis); drugs (phenytoin); berylliosis.
2 *Infiltrative:* *Benign* Histiocytosis (see OHCS p748); lipoidoses. *Malignant* Lymphoma (p658 & p660), metastases.

Musculoskeletal symptoms Chiefly *pain, deformity, reduced function*

Pain: Degenerative arthritis generally produces an aching pain worse with exercise and relieved by rest. Discomfort may be more in certain positions or motions. Cervical or lumbar spine degeneration may also produce subjective changes in sensation not following dermatome distribution. Both inflammatory and degenerative joint disease produce *morning stiffness* in the affected joints but in the former this generally improves during the day, while in the latter the pain is worse at the end of the day. The pain of *bone erosion* due to tumour or aneurysm tends to be deep, boring, and constant. The pain of *fracture* or *infection* of the bone is severe and throbbing and is increased by any motion of the part. *Acute nerve compression* causes a sharp, severe pain radiating along the distribution of the nerve. Joint pain may be referred, eg that from a hip disorder to anterior and lateral aspect of the thigh or to knee; shoulder to the lateral aspect of the humerus; cervical spine to the interscapular area, medial border of scapulae or tips of shoulders + lateral side of arms. (*Back pain*, p410; GALS locomotor assessment, p409.)

Reduced function: Causes: pain, bone or joint instability, or restriction of joint movement (eg due to muscle weakness, contractures, bony fusion or mechanical block by intracapsular bony fragments or cartilage).

Nodules *(subcutaneous)* Rheumatoid nodules; PAN; xanthomata; tuberose sclerosis; neurofibromata; sarcoid; granuloma annulare; rheumatic fever.

Oedema (p456). *Causes:* ↑*Venous pressure* (eg DVT or right-heart failure) or *lowered intravascular oncotic pressure* (plasma proteins↓, eg cirrhosis, nephrosis, malnutrition, or protein-losing enteropathy: here water moves down the osmotic gradient into the interstitium to dilute the solutes there, ↑entropy, according to the laws of thermodynamics). On standing, venous pressure at the ankle rises due to the height of blood from the heart (~100mmHg). This is short-lived if leg movement pumps blood through valved veins; but if venous pressure rises, or valves fail, capillary pressure rises, fluid is forced out (oedema), PCV rises locally, and microvascular stasis occurs. *Pitting oedema* (p456); *nonpitting oedema:* (ie non-indentible) ≈ poor lymph drainage (lymphoedema), eg primary (Milroy's syndrome, p730) or secondary (radiotherapy, malignant infiltration, infection, filariasis). The mechanism is complex.

Oliguria is defined as a urine output of <400mL/24h. This occurs in extreme dehydration, severe cardiac failure, urethral or bilateral ureteric obstruction, acute and chronic renal failure.

Orthopnoea See **Dyspnoea** above (p70).

Pallor is a non-specific sign and may be racial or familial. Pathology suggested by pallor includes anaemia, shock, Stokes–Adams attack, vasovagal faint, myxoedema, hypopituitarism, and albinism.

Palmar erythema *Causes:* pregnancy; polycythaemia; cirrhosis—eg via ↓inactivation of vasoactive endotoxins by the liver.

Palpitations represent to the patient the sensation of feeling his heart beat; to the doctor, the sensation of feeling his heart sink—because the symptom is notoriously elusive. Have the patient tap out the rate and regularity of the palpitations. • Irregular fast palpitations are likely to be paroxysmal AF, or flutter with variable block. • Dropped or missed beats related to rest, recumbency, or eating are likely to be atrial or ventricular ectopics. • Regular pounding is likely to be due to anxiety. • Slow palpitations are likely to be due to drugs such as β-blockers, or to bigeminus. Ask about associated pain, dyspnoea, and faints, suggesting haemodynamic compromise. Ask *when* symptoms occur: people often feel their (normal) heart beat in the anxious nocturnal silence of the bedroom:

> *At night on my pillow the syncopated stagger*
> *Of the pulse in my ear. Russian roulette:*
> *Every heartbeat a fresh throw of the dice . . .*
> *Hypochondria walked, holding my arm*
> *Like a nurse, her fingers over my pulse . . .*
> *The sudden lapping at my throat of loose blood . . .*   Ted Hughes, *Birthday Letters,*
> Faber & Faber, by kind permission

Often a clinical diagnosis of awareness of normal heart beats may be made, and reassurance is essential. If not, do TSH + transtelephonic event recording (better than 48h ECGs which may miss attacks).

Paraphimosis occurs when a tight foreskin is retracted and then becomes irreplaceable as the glans swells. It can occur when a doctor/nurse fails to replace the patient's foreskin after catheterization. Treat by asking the patient to squeeze the glans for half an hour. Or try soaking a swab in 50% dextrose, and applying it to the oedematous area for an hour, and the oedema may follow the osmotic gradient.

Pelvic pain *Causes:* UTI; urine retention; bladder stones; menses; labour; pregnancy; endometriosis (*OHCS* p52); salpingitis; endometritis (*OHCS* p36); ovarian cyst (eg torted). Cancer of: rectum, colon, ovary, cervix, bladder.

Percussion pain Pain on percussing the abdomen is a sign of peritonitis, and often less painful for the patient than testing **Rebound abdominal pain** (p82).

Phimosis The foreskin occludes the meatus, obstructing urine. Time (± trials of gentle retraction) usually obviates the need for circumcision.

Polyuria (eg urine >3.5L/24h). Causes: DM; over-enthusiastic IVI treatment; diabetes insipidus (p326); Ca^{2+} ↑; polydipsia; chronic renal failure.

Postural hypotension is defined as a drop in systolic or diastolic >15mmHg on standing for 3 minutes, compared with lying down. *Causes:* Hypovolaemia, Addison's disease (p312), hypopituitarism, autonomic neuropathy (eg diabetes, multisystem atrophy, p382), idiopathic orthostatic hypotension, drugs (eg vasodilators, diuretics).

Prostatism (p52 and p496) Symptoms of prostate enlargement are often termed 'prostatism', but it is better to use the terms *irritative* or *obstructive* bladder symptoms. Don't assume the cause is prostatic. (1) *Irritative bladder symptoms:* Urgency, dysuria, frequency, nocturia (the last two are also caused by UTI, polydipsia, detrusor instability, hypercalcaemia, or uraemia); (2) *Obstructive symptoms* (eg reduced size and force of urinary stream, hesitancy and interruption of stream during voiding)—may also be produced by strictures, tumours, urethral valves, or bladder neck contracture. Maximum flow rate of urine is normally ~18–30mL/s.

Pruritus See **Itching**, p76.

Ptosis is drooping of the upper eyelid. It is best observed with the patient sitting up, his head held by the examiner. The 3rd cranial nerve innervates the main muscle concerned (levator palpebrae), but nerves from the cervical sympathetic chain innervate the superior tarsal muscle, and a lesion of these nerves will cause a mild ptosis which can be overcome on looking up.

80

Causes: (1) Third nerve lesions usually causing unilateral complete ptosis. Look for other evidence of 3rd nerve lesion (ophthalmoplegia with outward deviation of the eye, pupil dilated and unreactive to light and accommodation). (2) Sympathetic paralysis usually causes unilateral partial ptosis. Look for other evidence of sympathetic lesion (constricted pupil, lack of sweating on same side of the face—Horner's syndrome). (3) Myopathy (dystrophia myotonica, myasthenia gravis). These usually cause bilateral partial ptosis. (4) Congenital (present since birth). May be unilateral or bilateral, is usually partial and is not associated with other neurological signs. (5) Syphilis.

Pulses See p42.

Pupillary abnormalities The key questions are: • Are the pupils equal, central, circular, dilated, or constricted? • Do they react to light, directly and consensually? • Do they constrict normally on convergence/accommodation? *Irregular pupils* are caused by iritis, syphilis, or globe rupture. *Dilated pupils* Causes: 3rd cranial nerve lesions and mydriatic drugs. But always ask: is this pupil dilated, or is it the other which is constricted? *Constricted pupils* are associated with old age, sympathetic nerve damage (Horner's syndrome, p726, and see **Ptosis** above), opiates, miotics (eg pilocarpine eye-drops for glaucoma), and pontine damage. *Unequal pupils (anisocoria)* may be due to a unilateral lesion, eye-drops, eye surgery, syphilis, or be a Holmes–Adie pupil (below). Some inequality is normal.

Reaction to light: Test by covering one eye and shining light into the other obliquely. Both pupils should constrict (one by the direct, the other by the consensual or indirect light reflex). Lesion site may be deduced by knowing the pathway: from the retina the message passes up the optic nerve to the superior colliculus (midbrain) and thence to the 3rd nerve nuclei bilaterally. The 3rd nerve causes pupillary constriction. If a light in one eye causes only contralateral constriction, the defect is 'efferent', as the afferent pathways from the retina being stimulated must be intact. Test for a *relative afferent pupillary defect* by moving the torch quickly from pupil to pupil. If an eye has severely reduced acuity (eg due to optic atrophy), the affected pupil will paradoxically dilate when the light is moved from the normal eye to the abnormal eye. This is because, in the face of reduced afferent input from the affected eye, the consensual pupillary relaxation response from the normal eye predominates. This phenomenon is also known as the Marcus Gunn sign.

Reaction to accommodation/convergence: If the patient first looks at a distant object and then at the examiner's finger held a few inches away, the eyes will converge and the pupils constrict. The neural pathway involves a projection from the cortex to the nucleus of the 3rd nerve.

Holmes-Adie (myotonic) pupil: This is a benign condition, which occurs usually in women and is unilateral in about 80% of cases. The affected pupil is normally moderately dilated and is poorly reactive to light, if at all. It is slowly reactive to accommodation; wait and watch carefully: it may eventually constrict more than a normal pupil. It is often associated with diminished or absent ankle and knee reflexes, in which case the Holmes–Adie syndrome is present. *Argyll Robertson pupil:* This occurs in neurosyphilis, but a similar phenomenon may occur in diabetes mellitus. The pupil is constricted. It is unreactive to light, but reacts to accommodation. The iris is usually patchily atrophied and depigmented. Pseudo-Argyll Robertson pupils may occur in Parinaud's syndrome (p732). *Hutchinson pupil:* This is the sequence of events resulting from rapidly rising unilateral intracranial pressure (eg in intracerebral haemorrhage). The pupil on the side of the lesion first constricts then widely dilates. The other pupil then goes through the same sequence.

Radio-femoral and radio-radial delay See p40.

Rebound abdominal pain is present if, on the sudden removal of pressure from the examiner's hand, the patient feels a *momentary increase* in pain. It signifies local peritoneal inflammation, manifest as pain as the peritoneum rebounds after being gently displaced.

Rectal bleeding Ascertain details about • Pain on defaecation? • Is blood mixed with stool, or just on surface? • Is blood just on toilet paper, or also in the toilet pan? *Causes and classical features:* Diverticulitis (painless, large volumes of blood in pan); colorectal cancer (blood mixed with stool); piles (bright red blood on paper and in pan); fissure-*in-ano* (painful, bright red blood on paper and surface of stool); inflammatory bowel disease (blood and mucus mixed with loose stool); trauma; polyps; angiodysplasia; ischaemic colitis; iatrogenic (radiation proctitis; post-polypectomy bleeding; aortoenteric fistula after aortic surgery).

Regurgitation Gastric and oesophageal contents are regurgitated effortlessly into the mouth—without contraction of abdominal muscles and diaphragm (so distinguishing it from true vomiting). Regurgitation is rarely preceded by nausea, and when due to gastro-oesophageal reflux, it is often associated with heartburn. An oesophageal pouch may cause regurgitation. Very high GI obstructions (eg gastric volvulus, p488) cause non-productive retching rather than true regurgitation.

Right iliac fossa pain *Causes:* All causes of left iliac fossa pain (see p76) plus appendicitis but usually excluding diverticulitis.

Right upper quadrant (hypochondrial) pain *Causes:* Gallstones; hepatitis; appendicitis (eg if pregnant); colonic cancer at the hepatic flexure; right kidney pathology (eg renal colic; pyelonephritis); intrathoracic conditions (eg pneumonia); subphrenic or perinephric abscess.

Rigors are uncontrolled, sometimes violent episodes of shivering which occur as a patient's temperature rises fast from normal. PUO: p552.

Skin discolouration Generalized hyperpigmentation due at least in part to melanin, may be genetic, or due to radiation, Addison's (p312), chronic renal failure (p276), pregnancy, oral contraceptive pill, any chronic wasting (eg TB, carcinoma), malabsorption, biliary cirrhosis, haemochromatosis, chlorpromazine, or busulfan. Hyperpigmentation due to other causes occurs in jaundice, carotenaemia, and gold therapy.

Splenomegaly Abnormally large spleen. *Causes:* See p518. If massive, think of: leishmaniasis, malaria, myelofibrosis, chronic myeloid leukaemia.

Sputum See p48.

Stertor is a poorly defined and inconsistently used term to describe a snoring sound heard over extrathoracic airways. Stertor does not have the musical quality of stridor. It may be heard in deeply unconscious patients.

Stridor is an inspiratory sound due to partial obstruction of the upper airways. That obstruction may be due to something within the lumen (eg foreign body, tumour, bilateral vocal cord palsy), within the wall (eg oedema from anaphylaxis, laryngospasm, tumour, croup, acute epiglottitis), or extrinsic (eg goitre, lymphadenopathy). It is a medical (or surgical) emergency if the airway is compromised.

Surgical emphysema Also known as subcutaneous emphysema, this is a crackling sensation felt on palpating the skin over the chest or neck, caused by air tracking from the lungs eg due to a pneumothorax. It may rarely occur due to a pneumomediastinum eg following oesophageal rupture.

Syncope See p344.

Tactile vocal fremitus See p50.

Tenesmus This is a sensation felt in the rectum of incomplete emptying following defecation—as if there was something else left behind, which cannot be passed. It is very common in the irritable bowel syndrome (p248), but can be caused by a tumour.

Terminal dribbling Dribbling at the end of urination, often seen in conjunction with incontinence following incomplete urination, is commonly associated with **prostatism** (p80).

84

Tinnitus See p348. **Tiredness** See **Fatigue** p72.

Tremor is rhythmic oscillation of limbs, trunk, head, or tongue. 3 types:

1 *Resting tremor*—worst at rest; feature of parkinsonism, but the tremor is more resistant to treatment than bradykinesia or rigidity. Usually a slow tremor (frequency: 3–5Hz)

2 *Postural tremor*—worst, eg if arms outstretched. Typically a rapid tremor (frequency: 8–12Hz). May be exaggerated physiological tremor (eg anxiety, thyrotoxicosis, alcohol, drugs), metabolic (eg hepatic encephalopathy, CO_2 retention), due to brain damage (eg Wilson's disease, syphilis) or *benign essential tremor* (BET). This is usually a familial (autosomal dominant) tremor of arms and head presenting at any age. It is suppressed by large-ish amounts of alcohol. Rarely progressive. Propranolol (40–80mg/8–12h PO) helps ~30%.

3 *Intention tremor*—worst during movement and occurs in cerebellar disease (eg in MS). No effective drug has been found.

See also **chorea** (p66), **athetosis** (p352), and **hemiballismus** (p352).

Trousseau's sign This is elicited by inflating a blood pressure cuff on an arm/leg to above systolic pressure. The hands and feet go into spasm (carpopedal spasm) in hypocalcaemia. The metacarpophalangeal joints become flexed and the interphalangeal joints are extended. See **Chvostek's sign**, p694.

Urinary changes *Cloudy urine* suggests pus (infection, UTI) but is often normal phosphate precipitation in an alkaline urine. *Pneumaturia* (bubbles in urine as it is passed) occurs with UTI due to gas-forming organisms or may signal an enterovesical (bowel bladder) fistula from diverticulitis or neoplastic diseases of the gut. *Nocturia* is seen in 'prostatism' (p80), diabetes mellitus, UTI, and reversed diurnal rhythm as occurs with renal and cardiac failure. *Haematuria* (RBC in urine) is due to neoplasia or glomerulonephritis until proven otherwise (p268).

Urinary frequency See **Frequency** p72.

Vaginal discharge See p588. **Vertigo** See p346.

Visual loss Get ophthalmic help. See *OHCS p498–500*. *If sudden, ask:*
- Is the eye painful/red (*glaucoma; iritis*, p426)? *Optic neuritis* may be painful.
- What is each eye's acuity? Is there a contact lens problem (eg *infection*)?
- History of trauma, migraine, *TIA*, *MS*, or *diabetes*; what is the blood sugar?
- Any flashes/floaters (*TIA*, *migraine*, *retinal artery occlusion; detachment*)?
- Is the cornea cloudy: *corneal ulcer* (*OHCS p496*); *glaucoma* (*OHCS p494*)?
- Is there a visual field problem/hemianopia (*stroke, space-occupying lesion, glaucoma*)? Formal field testing requires ophthalmic help.
- Any heart disease/bruits? (*emboli*); hyperlipidaemia (*xanthoma*, p706)?
- Is the BP raised or lowered? Measure it lying and standing.
- Are there focal CNS signs? Is there an afferent pupil defect (p80).
- Tender temporal arteries ± ESR ↑ ≈ *giant cell arteritis*: urgent steroids, p424.
- Any distant signs: *HIV* (causes retinitis), *SLE*, *sarcoid*, *Behçet's disease*, etc.?

Voice and disturbance of speech (p58) may be noted by the patient or the doctor. Assess if difficulty is with articulation (*dysarthria*, eg from muscle problems), or of word command (*dysphasia*—always central).

Vocal resonance See p48 and p50.

Vomiting Causes of nausea/vomiting include:

Gastrointestinal	*CNS*	*Metabolic/Endocrine*
Gastroenteritis	Meningitis/encephalitis	Uraemia
Peptic ulceration	Migraine	Hypercalcaemia
Pyloric stenosis	↑Intracranial pressure	Hyponatraemia
Intestinal obstruction	Brainstem lesions	Pregnancy
Paralytic ileus	Motion sickness	Diabetic ketoacidosis
Acute cholecystitis	Ménière's disease	Addison's disease
Acute pancreatitis	Labyrinthitis	Drugs:
	Psychiatric disorder:	– alcohol
Other	– self-induced	– antibiotics
Myocardial infarction	– psychogenic	– cytotoxics
Autonomic neuropathy	– bulimia nervosa	– digoxin
UTI		– opiates

The history is very important: ask about timing, relationship to meals, amount, and content (liquid, solid, bile, blood, 'coffee grounds'). Associated symptoms and previous medical history often indicate the cause. *Signs:* Look for signs of dehydration. Examine the abdomen for distension, tenderness, an abdominal mass, a succussion splash (pyloric stenosis), or tinkling bowel sounds (intestinal obstruction).

Walking difficulty ('Off my legs') In the elderly, this is a common and non-specific presentation: the reason may not be *local* (typically osteo- or rheumatoid arthritis, but remember fractured neck of femur), and it may not even be *systemic* (eg pneumonia, UTI, anaemia, drugs, hypothyroidism, renal failure, hypothermia)—but it may be a manifestation of depression or bereavement. *It is only rarely a manipulative strategy.*

More specific causes to consider are Parkinson's disease (p382), polymyalgia (very treatable, p424), and various neuropathies/myopathies. One of the key questions is 'Is there pain?'—another issue to address is whether there is muscle wasting and, if so, is it symmetrical?

If there is also ataxia, the cause is not always alcohol: other chemicals may be involved (cannabis, arsenic, thallium, mercury—or prescribed sedatives), or there may be a metastatic or non-metastatic manifestation of malignancy—or a CNS primary or vascular lesion.

Remember also treatable conditions, such as pellagra (p250), B₁₂↓, and beriberi, and infections such as encephalitis, myelitis, Lyme disease, brucellosis, or rarities such as botulism (p830).

Bilateral weak legs in an otherwise fit person suggests a cord lesion: see p350. If there is associated incontinence ± saddle anaesthesia, prompt treatment for cord compression may be needed.

Non-gastrointestinal causes of vomiting

▶Never forget these, as they can be a sign of serious disease. The following *aide-memoire* covers the most important non-gastrointestinal causes of vomiting: ABCDEFGHI

- **A**cute renal failure/**A**ddison's disease
- **B**rain (eg ↑ICP, p816)
- **C**ardiac (myocardial infarct)
- **D**iabetic ketoacidosis
- **E**ars (eg labyrinthitis, Ménière's disease)
- **F**oreign substances (alcohol, drugs eg opiates)
- **G**ravidity (eg hyperemesis gravidarum)
- **H**ypercalcaemia/**H**yponatraemia
- **I**nfection (eg UTI, meningitis)

Waterbrash refers to the excessive secretion of saliva, which suddenly fills the mouth. It typically occurs after meals, and may denote oesophageal disease. It is suggested that this is an exaggeration of the oesophago-salivary reflex. It should not be confused with **regurgitation** (p82).

Weight loss is a feature of chronic disease and depression—also of malnutrition, chronic infections, and infestations (eg TB, HIV/enteropathic AIDS), malignancy, diabetes mellitus, and hyperthyroidism (typically in the presence of increased appetite). Severe generalized muscle wasting is also seen as part of a number of degenerative neurological and muscle diseases and in cardiac failure (cardiac cachexia), although in the latter, right heart failure may not make weight loss a major complaint. Do not forget anorexia nervosa (*OHCS* p348) as a possible underlying cause of weight loss.

Focus on treatable causes, eg diabetes is easy to diagnose—TB can be very hard. For example, the CXR may look like cancer, so you may forget to send bronchoscopy samples for ZN stain and TB culture (to the detriment not just of the patient, but to the entire ward).

Wheeze See p50.

Whispering pectoriloquy This refers to the increased transmission of a patient's whispers heard when auscultating over consolidated lung. It is a manifestation of increased vocal resonance. See p50. **NB:** *Vocal resonance* is sound vibration of the patient's spoken or whispered voice transmitted to the stethoscope. *Tactile fremitus* is the sound vibration of the spoken or whispered voice transmitted via the lung fields and detected by palpation over the back.

Xanthomata These are localized deposits of fat under the skin surface, commonly occuring over joints, tendons, hands, and feet. They are a sign of hyperlipidaemia (p706). *Xanthelasma palpebra* is a xanthoma on the eyelid.

Unexplained signs and symptoms: how to refer a patient for an opinion

▶ *When you don't know: ask.*

▶ *If you find yourself wondering if you should ask: ask.*

Frequently, the skills needed will lie beyond the firm you are working on, so, during ward rounds, agree who should be asked for an opinion. You will be left with the job of making the arrangements. This can be a daunting task, if you are very junior and have been asked to contact an intimidating registrar or consultant. Don't be intimidated: perhaps this may be an opportunity to learn something new. A few simple points can help the process go smoothly.

• Have the patient's notes, observations, and drug charts to hand.
• Be familiar with the history: you may be interrogated.
• Ask if it is a convenient time to talk.
• At the outset, state if you are just looking for advice or if you are asking if the patient could be seen. Make it clear exactly what the question is that you want addressed, 'We wonder why Mr Smith's legs have become weak today . . .' This helps the listener to focus their thoughts while you describe the story and will save you wasting time if the switchboard has put you through to the wrong specialist.
• Give the patient's age and occupation, to give a snapshot of the person.
• Run through a brief history. Do not present the case as if you are in finals—it will take ages to get to the point and the listener will get more and more irritated.
• If you would like the patient to be seen, give warning if they will be going off the ward for a test at a particular time.
• It should not be necessary to write a long letter in the notes if you have given all the salient information available.
• The visiting doctor may be unfamiliar with your ward. When he or she arrives introduce yourself, get the notes and charts, and offer to introduce them to the patient. This will lead to all-round satisfaction and will make it easier to call the same doctor again.

We thank Martin Zeidler for providing the first draft of this page.

Cardiovascular medicine[1]

Contents

1 We thank Dr Rajesh Kharbanda who is our Specialist Reader for this chapter.

Ischaemic heart disease (IHD) is the most common cause of death worldwide. Encouraging cardiovascular health is not *only* about preventing IHD: health entails the ability to *exercise*, and enjoying vigorous activity (within reason!) is one of the best ways of achieving health, not just because the heart likes it (BP↓, 'good' high-density lipoprotein, HDL↑)—it can prevent osteoporosis, improve glucose tolerance, and augment immune function (eg in cancer and if HIV+ve). People who improve *and maintain* their fitness live longer: ►*age-adjusted mortality from all causes is reduced by >40%*. Avoiding obesity helps too, but it is a fallacy to suppose that because of this, fat people should try to slim. If they do, the evidence is that they will not live any longer[1] (it may *feel* longer given the lengthening intervals between ever more meagre meals)—although risk of diabetes *will* diminish if weight loss can be achieved.[2]

Moderate alcohol drinking may also promote cardiovascular health. Alcohol also reduces gastric infection with *Helicobacter pylori*, a known risk marker for cardiovascular disease.[3]

Smoking is the chief risk factor for cardiovascular mortality. You *can* help people give up, and giving up *does* undo much of the harm of smoking. *Simple advice works.* Most smokers want to give up (unlike the eaters of unhealthy diets who are mostly wedded to them by habit, and the pleasures of the palate). Just because smoking advice does not *always* work, do not stop giving it. Ask about smoking in consultations—especially those concerned with smoking-related diseases.

- Ensure advice is congruent with patient's beliefs about smoking.
- Concentrate on the benefits of giving up.
- Invite the patient to choose a date (when there will be few stresses) on which he or she will become a non-smoker.
- Suggest throwing away all accessories (cigarettes, pipes, ash trays, lighters, matches) in advance; inform friends of the new change; practise saying 'no' to their offers of 'just one little cigarette'.
- *Nicotine gum*, chewed intermittently to limit nicotine release: ≥ ten 2mg sticks may be needed/day. *Transdermal nicotine patches* may be easier. A dose increase at 1wk can help. Written advice offers no added benefit to advice from nurses. Always offer follow-up.
- *Bupropion* (=*amfebutamone*, p335) is said to ↑quit rate to 30% at 1yr vs 16% with patches and 15.6% for placebo (patches + bupropion: 35.5%):[4] consider if the above fails. *Dose:* 150mg/24h PO (while still smoking; quit within 2wks); dose may be twice daily from day 7; stop after 7wks. *Warn of SEs:* Seizures (risk <1 : 1000), insomnia, headache. *CI:* Epilepsy; cirrhosis; pregnancy/lactation; bipolar depression; eating disorders; CNS tumours; on antimalarials etc; alcohol or benzodiazepine withdrawal.

Lipids and BP (p706 & p140–142) are the other major modifiable risk factors (few can change their sex or genes).

To calculate how risk factors interact, see risk equation, p22.

►Apply preventive measures such as healthy eating (p208) *early* in life to maximize impact, when there are most years to save, and before bad habits get ingrained. **NB:** It's too early to recommend folate supplements, which lower plasma homocysteine, which is either a cause or a marker of ↑cardiovascular risk: randomized trials have been too small (but encouraging[5]).

For an example of implementation of cardiovascular health strategies, see the UK NHS national service framework: www.doh.gov.uk/nsf/coronary.htm

Cardiovascular symptoms

Chest pain ►Cardiac-sounding chest pain may have no serious cause, but always think *'Could this be a myocardial infarction (MI), dissecting aortic aneurysm, pericarditis, or pulmonary embolism?'*

Nature: *Constricting* suggests angina, oesophageal spasm, or anxiety; a *sharp* pain may be from the pleura or pericardium. A prolonged (>½h), dull, central crushing pain or pressure suggests MI.

Radiation: To shoulder, either or both arms, or neck/jaw suggests cardiac ischaemia. The pain of aortic dissection is classically instantaneous, tearing, and interscapular, but may be retrosternal. Epigastric pain may be cardiac.

Precipitants: Pain associated with cold, exercise, palpitations, or emotion suggest cardiac pain or anxiety; if brought on by food, lying flat, hot drinks, or alcohol, consider oesophageal spasm (but meals *can* cause angina).

Relieving factors: If pain is relieved *within minutes* by rest or glyceryl trinitrate (GTN), suspect angina (GTN relieves oesophageal spasm more slowly). If antacids help, suspect GI causes. Pericarditic pain improves on leaning forward.

Associations: Dyspnoea occurs with cardiac pain, pulmonary embolism, pleurisy, or anxiety. MI may cause nausea, vomiting, or sweating. In addition to coronary artery disease, angina may be caused by aortic stenosis (AS), hypertrophic obstructive cardiomyopathy (HOCM), paroxysmal supraventricular tachycardia (SVT) and be exacerbated by anaemia. Chest pain with *tenderness* suggests self-limiting costochondritis (Tietze's syndrome).

Differential diagnosis of chest pain: Pleuritic pain (ie exacerbated by inspiration) implies inflammation of the pleura secondary to pulmonary infection, inflammation, or infarction. It causes the patient to 'catch his breath'. *Musculoskeletal pain:* Exacerbated by pressure on the affected area. *Fractured rib:* Pain on respiration, exacerbated by gentle pressure on the sternum. *Subdiaphragmatic pathology* may also mimic cardiac pain.

Acutely ill patients: • Admit to hospital • Check pulse, BP in both arms, JVP, heart sounds and examine the legs for DVT • Give O₂ by face mask • Insert an IV line • Relieve pain (eg morphine 5–10mg IV slowly + an antiemetic) • Place on cardiac monitor; do 12-lead ECG • CXR • Arterial blood gas (ABG).

Famous traps: Aortic dissection; Herpes zoster (p568); ruptured oesophagus; cardiac tamponade (shock with JVP↑); opiate addiction.

Dyspnoea may be from LVF, pulmonary embolism, any respiratory cause, or anxiety. *Severity:* ►►Emergency presentations: p770. Ask about shortness of breath at rest or on exertion, exercise tolerance, and coping with daily tasks. *Associations:* Specific symptoms associated with heart failure are orthopnoea (ask about number of pillows used at night), paroxysmal nocturnal dyspnoea (waking up at night gasping for breath), and peripheral oedema. Pulmonary embolism is associated with acute onset of dyspnoea and pleuritic chest pain; ask about risk factors for DVT.

Palpitation(s) may be due to ectopics, AF, SVT and ventricular tachycardia (VT), thyrotoxicosis, anxiety, and rarely pheochromocytoma. See p78. *History:* Ask about previous episodes, precipitating/relieving factors, duration of symptoms, associated chest pain, dyspnoea, or dizziness. *Did the patient check his pulse?*

Syncope may reflect cardiac or CNS events. Vasovagal 'faints' are common (pulse↓, pupils dilated). The history from an observer is invaluable in diagnosis. *Prodromal symptoms:* Chest pain, palpitations, or dyspnoea point to a cardiac cause, eg arrhythmia. Aura, headache, dysarthria, limb weakness indicate CNS causes. *During the episode:* Was there a pulse? Was there limb jerking, tongue biting, or urinary incontinence? **NB:** Hypoxia from lack of cerebral perfusion may cause seizures. *Recovery:* Was this rapid (arrhythmia) or prolonged and associated with post-ictal drowsiness (seizure)?

How patients communicate ischaemic cardiac sensations

On emergency wards we are always hearing questions such as 'is your pain sharp or dull?', followed by an equivocal answer. The doctor goes on 'Sharp like a knife—or dull and crushing?' The doctor is getting irritated because the patient must know the answer, but is not saying it. A true story paves the way to being less inquisitorial, and having a more creative understanding of the nature of symptoms. A patient came to one of us (JML) saying 'Last night I dreamed I had a pain in my chest. Now I've woken up, and I'm not sure—have I got chest pain, doctor? What do you think?' How odd it is to find oneself examining a patient to exclude a symptom, not a disease. (It turned out that she *did* have serious chest pathology.) Odd, until one realizes that symptoms are often half-formed, and it is our role to give them a local habitation and a name. Dialogue can transform a symptom from 'airy nothingness' to a fact.[1] Patients often avoid using the word 'pain' to describe ischaemia: 'wind', 'tightening', 'pressure', 'burning', or 'a lump in the throat' (angina means to choke) may be used. He may say 'sharp' to communicate severity, and not character. So be as vague in your questioning as your patient is in his answers. 'Tell me some more about what you are feeling (long pause)... as if someone was doing *what* to you?' 'Sitting on me', or 'like a hotness' might be the response (suggesting cardiac ischaemia). Do not ask 'Does it go into your left arm'. Try 'Is there anything else about it?' (pause)... 'Does it go any-where?' Note down your patient's exact words.

Note also non-verbal clues: the clenched fist placed over the sternum is a telling feature of cardiac pain (Levine sign positive).

A good history, taking account of these features, is the best way to stratify patients likely to have cardiac pain. If the history is non-specific, and there are no risk factors for cardiovascular diseases, and ECG and plasma troponin T (p120) are normal (<0.2μg/L) 6–12h after the onset of pain, discharge will probably be OK. But when in doubt, get help.

Features making cardiac pain unlikely:
• Stabbing, shooting pain
• Pain lasting <30s, however intense
• Well-localized, left sub-mammary pain ('in my heart, doctor')
• Pains of continually varying location
• Youth.

Do not feel that you must diagnose every pain. *Chest pain with no cause* is common, even after extensive tests. Do not reject these patients: explain your findings to them. Some have a 'chronic pain syndrome' which responds to a tricyclic, eg imipramine 50mg at night (this dose does not imply any depression). It is similar to post-herpetic neuralgia.

---

1 Dialogue-transformed symptoms explain one of the junior doctors' main vexations: when patients retell symptoms to a consultant in the light of day, they bear no resemblance to what you originally heard. But do not be vexed: your dialogue may have helped the patient far more than any ward round.

ECG—a methodical approach

►First confirm the patient's name and age, and the ECG date. Then:

- *Rate:* At usual speed (25mm/s) each 'big square' is 0.2s; each 'small square' is 0.04s. To calculate the rate, divide 300 by the number of big squares per R–R interval (p95).

- *Rhythm:* If the cycles are not clearly regular, use the 'card method': lay a card along ECG, marking positions of 3 successive R waves. Slide the card to and fro to check that all intervals are equal. If not, note if different rates are multiples of each other (ie varying block), or is it 100% irregular (Atrial fibrillation (AF) or Ventricular fibrillation, VF)? *Sinus rhythm* is characterized by a P wave (upright in II, III, & aVF; inverted in aVR) followed by a QRS complex. AF has no discernible P waves and the QRS complexes are irregularly irregular. *Atrial flutter* has a 'sawtooth' baseline of atrial depolarization (~300/min) and regular QRS complexes. *Nodal rhythm* has a normal QRS complex but P waves are absent or occur just before or within the QRS complex. *Ventricular rhythm* has QRS complexes >0.12s with P waves following them.

- *Axis:* The mean frontal axis is the sum of all the ventricular forces during ventricular depolarization. The axis lies at 90° to the isoelectric complex (ie the one in which positive and negative deflections are equal). *Normal axis* is between −30° and +90°. As a simple rule of thumb, if the complexes in leads I and II are both 'positive', the axis is normal. *Left axis deviation* (LAD) is −30° to −90°. Causes: left anterior hemiblock, inferior MI, VT from LV focus, Wolff–Parkinson–White (WPW) syndrome (some types). *Right axis deviation* (RAD) is +90° to +180°. Causes: RVH, PE, anterolateral MI, left posterior hemiblock (rare), WPW syndrome (some types).

- *P wave:* Normally precedes each QRS complex. *Absent P wave:* AF, sinoatrial block, junctional (AV nodal) rhythm. Dissociation between P waves and QRS complexes indicates complete heart block. *P mitrale:* bifid P wave, indicates left atrial hypertrophy. *P pulmonale:* peaked P wave, indicates right atrial hypertrophy. Pseudo-P-pulmonale seen if K$^+$↓.

- *P-R interval:* Measure from start of P wave to start of QRS. *Normal range*: 0.12–0.2s (3–5 small squares). A *prolonged P-R interval* implies delayed AV conduction (1st degree heart block). A *short P-R interval* implies unusually fast AV conduction down an accessory pathway, eg WPW p128 (ECG p131).

- *QRS complex:* Normal duration: <0.12s. If ≥0.12s suggests ventricular conduction defects, eg a bundle branch block (p98 & p127). Large QRS complexes suggest *ventricular hypertrophy* (p98). *Normal Q wave* <0.04s wide and <2mm deep. *Pathological Q waves* may occur within a few hours of an acute MI.

- *QT interval:* Measure from start of QRS to *end* of T wave. It varies with rate. Calculate *corrected QT interval* (QT^c) by dividing the measured QT interval by the square root of the cycle length, ie QT^c = (QT)/($\sqrt{R-R}$). Normal QT^c: 0.38–0.42s. *Prolonged QT interval*: acute myocardial ischaemia, myocarditis, bradycardia (eg AV block), head injury, hypothermia, U&E imbalance (K$^+$↓, Ca^{2+}↓, Mg^{2+}↓), congenital (Romano–Ward & Jervell–Lange–Nielson syndromes); sotalol, quinidine, antihistamines, macrolides (eg erythromycin), amiodarone, phenothiazines, tricyclics.

- *ST segment:* Usually isoelectric. Planar elevation (>1mm) or depression (>0.5mm) usually implies infarction (p121) or ischaemia (p107), respectively.

- *T wave:* Abnormal if inverted in I, II, and V$_4$–V$_6$. It is peaked in hyperkalaemia (ECG 13, p693) and flattened in hypokalaemia.

ECG nomenclature (ventricular activation time, VAT)

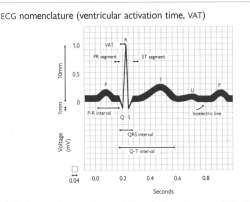

Calculating the R-R interval To calculate the rate, divide 300 by the number of big squares per R-R interval—if the UK standard ECG speed of 25mm/s is used (elsewhere, 50mm/s may be used: don't be confused!)

R-R duration (s)	Big squares	Rate (per min)
0.2	1	300
0.4	2	150
0.6	3	100
0.8	4	75
1.0	5	60
1.2	6	50
1.4	7	43

Determining the ECG axis

• The axis lies at 90° to the isoelectric complex (the one in which positive and negative deflections are equal in size).
• If the complexes in I and II are both predominantly positive, the axis is normal.

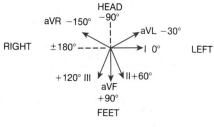

Causes of LAD	Causes of RAD
Left anterior hemiblock	RVH
Inferior MI	Pulmonary embolism
VT from LV focus	Anterolateral MI
WPW syndrome (some) p128	Left posterior hemiblock (rare)
	WPW syndrome (some)

ECG—abnormalities

Sinus tachycardia: Rate >100. Anxiety, exercise, pain, fever, sepsis, hypovolaemia, heart failure, pulmonary embolism, pregnancy, thyrotoxicosis, beri beri, CO_2 retention, autonomic neuropathy, sympathomimetics, eg caffeine, adrenaline, and nicotine (may produce abrupt changes in sinus rate, and other arrhythmias).

Sinus bradycardia: Rate <60. Physical fitness, vasovagal attacks, sick sinus syndrome, acute MI (esp. inferior), drugs (β-blockers, digoxin, amiodarone, verapamil), hypothyroidism, hypothermia, ↑intracranial pressure, cholestasis.

AF: (ECG p127) Common causes: IHD thyrotoxicosis, hypertension. See p130.

1ˢᵗ and 2ⁿᵈ degree heart block: Normal variant, athletes, sick sinus syndrome, IHD, acute carditis, drugs (digoxin, β-blockers).

Complete heart block: Idiopathic (fibrosis), congenital, IHD, aortic valve calcification, cardiac surgery/trauma, digoxin toxicity, infiltration (abscesses, granulomas, tumours, parasites).

ST elevation: Normal variant (high take-off), acute MI, Prinzmetal's angina (p732), acute pericarditis (saddle-shaped), left ventricular aneurysm.

ST depression: Normal variant (upward sloping), digoxin (downward sloping), ischaemic (horizontal): angina, acute posterior MI.

T inversion: In V_1–V_3: normal (Blacks and children), right bundle branch block (RBBB), pulmonary embolism. In V_2–V_5: subendocardial MI, HOCM, subarachnoid haemorrhage, lithium. In V_4–V_6 and aVL: ischaemia, LVH, associated with left bundle branch block (LBBB).

NB: ST and T wave changes are often non-specific, and must be interpreted in the light of the clinical context.

MI: (ECG p121.)
- Within hours, the T wave may become peaked, and the ST segment may begin to rise.
- Within 24h, the T wave inverts, as ST segment elevation begins to resolve. ST elevation rarely persists, unless a left ventricular aneurysm develops. T wave inversion may or may not persist.
- Within a few days, pathological Q waves begin to form. Q waves usually persist, but may resolve in 10%.

The leads affected reflect the site of the infarct: inferior (II, III, aVF), anteroseptal (V_{1-4}), anterolateral (V_{4-6}, I, aVL), posterior (tall R and ST↓ in V_{1-2}).

▶'Non-Q wave infarcts' (formerly called subendocardial infarcts) have ST and T changes without Q waves.

Pulmonary embolism: Sinus tachycardia is commonest. There may be RAD, RBBB (p95), right ventricular strain pattern V_{1-3} or AF. Rarely, the '$S_I Q_{III} T_{III}$' pattern occurs: deep S waves in I, pathological Q waves in III, inverted T waves in III.

Metabolic abnormalities: Digoxin effect: ST depression and inverted T wave in V_{5-6} (reversed tick). In *digoxin toxicity,* any arrhythmia may occur (ventricular ectopics & nodal bradycardia are common). *Hyperkalaemia:* Tall, tented T wave, widened QRS, absent P waves, 'sine wave' appearance (ECG 13, p693). *Hypokalaemia:* Small T waves, prominent U waves. *Hypercalcaemia:* Short QT interval. *Hypocalcaemia:* Long QT interval, small T waves.

Where to place the chest leads

V_1: right sternal edge, 4th intercostal space
V_2: left sternal edge, 4th intercostal space
V_3: half-way between V_2 and V_4
V_4: the patient's apex beat (p64)
   All subsequent leads are in the
   same horizontal plane as V_4
V_5: anterior axillary line
V_6: mid-axillary line (V_7: posterior axillary line)

Finish 12-lead ECGs with a long rhythm strip in lead II.

Disorders of ventricular conduction

Bundle branch block (p99, ECGs 1 and 2) Delayed conduction is evidenced by prolongation of QRS >0.12s. Abnormal conduction patterns lasting <0.12s are incomplete blocks. The area that would have been reached by the blocked bundle depolarizes slowly and late. Taking V_1 as an example, right ventricular depolarization is normally +ve and left ventricular depolarization is normally –ve.

In RBBB, the following pattern is seen: QRS >0.12s, 'RSR' pattern in V_1, dominant R in V_1, inverted T waves in V_1–V_3 or V_4, deep wide S wave in V_6. Causes: normal variant (isolated RBBB), pulmonary embolism, cor pulmonale.

In LBBB, the following pattern is seen: QRS >0.12s, 'M' pattern in V_5, no septal Q waves, inverted T waves in I, aVL, V_5–V_6. Causes: IHD, hypertension, cardiomyopathy, idiopathic fibrosis. ▶NB: If there is LBBB, no comment can be made on the ST segment or T wave.

Bifascicular block is the combination of RBBB and left bundle hemiblock, manifest as an axis deviation, eg LAD in the case of left anterior hemiblock.

Trifascicular block is the combination of bifascicular block and 1st degree heart block.

Ventricular hypertrophy There is no single marker of ventricular hypertrophy: electrical axis, voltage, and ST wave changes should all be taken into consideration. Relying on a single marker such as voltage may be unreliable as a thin chest wall may result in large voltage whereas a thick chest wall may mask it.

Suspect *left ventricular hypertrophy* (LVH) if the R wave in V_6 >25mm or the sum of the S wave in V_1 and the R wave in V_6 is >35mm (ECG 8 on p143).

Suspect *right ventricular hypertrophy* (RVH) if dominant R wave in V_1, T wave inversion in V_1–V_3 or V_4, deep S wave in V_6, RAD.

Other causes of *dominant R wave in V_1*: RBBB, posterior MI, some types of WPW syndrome (p128).

Causes of low voltage QRS complex: (QRS <5mm in all limb leads) Hypothyroidism, chronic obstructive pulmonary disease (COPD), ↑haematocrit (intracardiac blood resistivity is related to haematocrit), changes in chest wall impedance (eg in renal failure, subcutaneous emphysema but *not* obesity), pulmonary embolism, bundle branch block, carcinoid heart disease, myocarditis, cardiac amyloid, adriamycin cardiotoxicity, and other heart muscle diseases, pericardial effusion, pericarditis. [7]

See http://homepages.enterprise.net/djenkins/ecghome.html for MRCP-ish examples of ECGs.

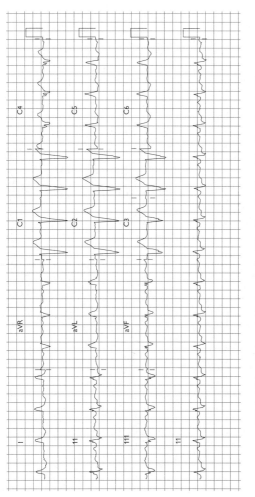

ECG 1—left bundle branch block: note the W pattern in C1 and the M pattern in C6.

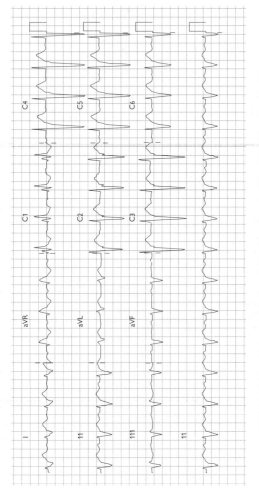

ECG 2—right bundle branch block—note the M pattern in C1 and the W pattern in C5.

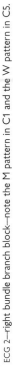

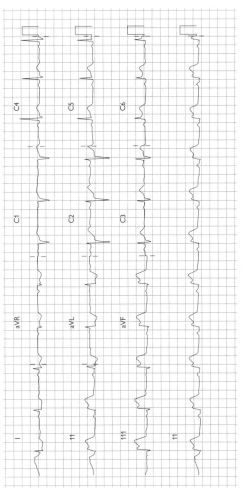

ECG 3—acute infero-lateral myocardial infarction: note the marked ST elevation in the inferior leads (II, III, aVF), but also in C5 and C6, indicating lateral involvement as well. There is also 'reciprocal change' ie ST-segment depression in leads I and aVL. The latter is often seen with a large myocardial infarction.

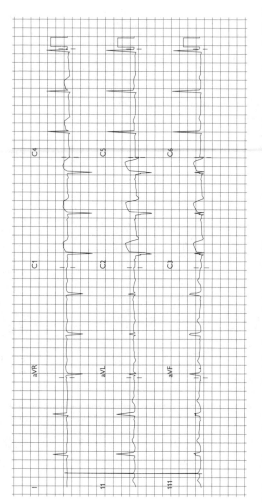

ECG 4—acute anterior myocardial infarction—note the marked ST segment elevation and evolving Q waves in leads C1–C4.

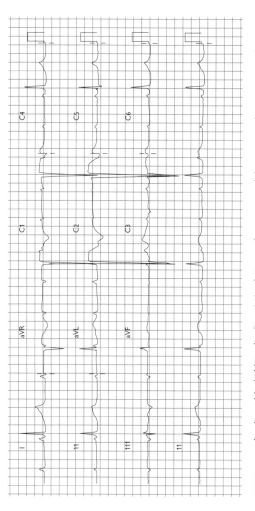

ECG 5—complete heart block. Note the dissociation between the P waves and the QRS complexes. QRS complexes are relatively narrow, indicating that there is a ventricular rhythm originating from the conducting pathway.

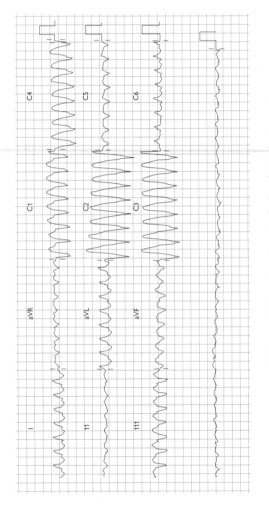

104

ECG 6—ventricular tachycardia—note the broad complexes.

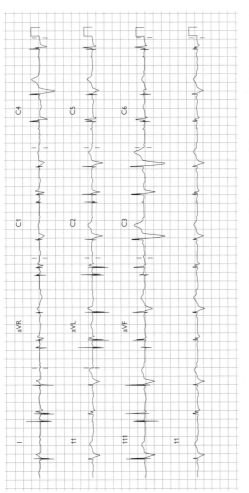

ECG 7—dual chamber pacemaker. Note the pacing spikes which occur before some of the P waves, and the QRS complexes.

Exercise ECG testing

The patient undergoes a graduated, treadmill exercise test, with continuous 12-lead ECG and blood pressure monitoring. There are numerous treadmill protocols; the 'Bruce protocol' is the most widely used.

Indications:
• To help confirm a suspected diagnosis of IHD.
• Assessment of cardiac function and exercise tolerance.
• Prognosis following MI. Often done pre-discharge (if +ve, worse outcome).
• Evaluation of response to treatment (drugs, angioplasty, coronary artery bypass grafting, CABG).
• Assessment of exercise-induced arrhythmias.

Contraindications:
• Unstable angina
• Recent Q wave MI (<5d)
• Severe AS
• Uncontrolled arrhythmia, hypertension, or heart failure.

Be cautious about arranging tests that will be hard to perform or interpret:
• Complete heart block, LBBB
• Pacemaker patients
• Osteoarthritis, COPD, stroke, or other limitations to exercise.

Stop the test if:
• Chest pain or dyspnoea occurs.
• The patient feels faint, exhausted, or is in danger of falling.
• ST segment elevation/depression >2mm (with or without chest pain).
• Atrial or ventricular arrhythmia (not just ectopics).
• Fall in blood pressure, failure of heart rate or blood pressure to rise with effort, or excessive rise in blood pressure (systolic >230mmHg).
• Development of AV block or LBBB.
• Maximal or 90% maximal heart rate for age is achieved.

Interpreting the test: A positive test only allows one to assess the *probability* that the patient has IHD. 75% with significant coronary artery disease have a positive test, but so do 5% of people with normal arteries (the false positive rate is even higher in middle-aged women, eg 20%). The more positive the result, the higher the predictive accuracy. Down-sloping ST depression is much more significant than up-sloping, eg 1mm J-point depression with down-sloping ST segment is 99% predictive of 2–3 vessel disease.

Morbidity: 24 in 100,000. *Mortality:* 10 in 100,000.

Ambulatory ECG monitoring

Continuous ECG monitoring for 24h may be used to try and pick up paroxysmal arrhythmias. However, >70% of patients will not have symptoms during the period of monitoring. ~20% will have a normal ECG during symptoms and only up to 10% will have an arrhythmia coinciding with symptoms. Give these patients a recorder they can activate themselves during an episode. Recorders may be programmed to detect ST segment depression, either symptomatic (to prove angina), or to reveal 'silent' ischaemia (predictive of re-infarction or death soon after MI).

Each complex is taken from sample ECGs (lead C5) recorded at 1-min intervals during exercise (top line) and recovery (bottom line). At maximum ST depression, the ST segment is almost horizontal. This is a positive exercise test.

This is an exercise ECG in the same format. It is negative because although the J point is depressed, the ensuring ST segment is steeply up-sloping.

Cardiac catheterization

This involves the insertion of a catheter into the heart via the femoral (or radial/brachial) artery or vein. The catheter is manipulated within the heart and great vessels to measure pressures. Catheterization can also be used to:

- Sample blood to assess oxygen saturation.
- Inject radiopaque contrast medium to image the anatomy of the heart and flow in blood vessels.
- Perform angioplasty (± stenting), valvuloplasty, and cardiac biopsies.
- Perform intravascular ultrasound to quantify arterial narrowing.

During the procedure, ECG and arterial pressures are monitored continuously. In the UK, 40% of cardiac catheters are performed as day-case procedures (provided the patient can rest lying down for 4h).

Indications:
- *Coronary artery disease:* diagnostic (assessment of coronary vessels and graft patency); therapeutic (angioplasty, stent insertion).
- *Valve disease:* diagnostic (to assess severity); therapeutic valvuloplasty (if the patient is too ill or declines valve surgery).
- *Congenital heart disease:* diagnostic (assessment of severity of lesions); therapeutic (balloon dilatation or septostomy).
- *Other:* cardiomyopathy; pericardial disease; endomyocardial biopsy.

Pre-procedure checks:
- Brief history/examination; **NB:** peripheral pulses, bruits, aneurysms.
- Investigations: FBC, U&E, LFT, clotting screen, group & save, CXR, ECG.
- Consent for angiogram ± angioplasty ± stent ± CABG. Explain reason for procedure and possible complications (below).
- IV access, ideally in the left hand.
- Patient should be nil by mouth (NBM) from 6h before the procedure.
- Patients should take all their morning drugs (& pre-medication if needed). Withhold oral antihypoglycaemics.

Post-procedure checks:
- Pulse, blood pressure, arterial puncture site (for bruising or swelling? false aneurysm), peripheral pulses.
- Investigations: FBC and clotting (if suspected blood loss), ECG.

Complications:
- *Haemorrhage.* Apply firm pressure over puncture site. If you suspect a false aneurysm, ultrasound the swelling and consider surgical repair.
- *Contrast reaction.* This is usually mild with modern contrast agents.
- *Loss of peripheral pulse.* May be due to dissection, thrombosis, or arterial spasm. Occurs in <1% of brachial catheterizations. Rare with femoral catheterization.
- *Angina.* May occur during or after cardiac catheterization. Usually responds to sublingual GTN; if not give analgesia and IV nitrates.
- *Arrhythmias.* Usually transient. Manage along standard lines.
- *Pericardial tamponade.* Rare, but should be suspected if the patient becomes hypotensive and anuric.
- *Infection.* Post-catheter pyrexia is usually due to a contrast reaction. If it persists for >24h, take blood cultures before giving antibiotics.

Mortality: <1 in 1000 patients, in most centres.

Intra-cardiac electrophysiology This catheter technique can determine types and origins of arrhythmias, and locate (and ablate) aberrant pathways (eg causing atrial flutter or ventricular tachycardia). Arrhythmias may be induced, and the effectiveness of control by drugs assessed.

Normal values for intracardiac pressures and saturations

Location	Pressure (mmHg)		Saturation (%)
	Mean	Range	
Inferior vena cava			76
Superior vena cava			70
Right atrium	4	0–8	74
Right ventricle			74
Systolic	25	15–30	
End-diastolic	4	0–8	
Pulmonary artery			74
Systolic	25	15–30	
Diastolic	10	5–15	
Mean	15	10–20	
Pulmonary artery	a	3–12	74
Wedge pressure	v	3–15	
Left ventricle			98
Systolic	110	80–140	
End-diastolic	70	60–90	
Aorta			98
Systolic	110	80–140	
Diastolic	70	60–90	
Mean	85	70–105	
Brachial			98
Systolic	120	90–140	
Diastolic	72	60–90	
Mean	83	70–105	

Gradients across stenotic valves

Valve	Normal gradient	Stenotic gradient (mmHg)		
	(mmHg)	Mild	Moderate	Severe
Aortic	0	<30	30–50	>50
Mitral	0	<5	5–15	>15
Prosthetic	5–10			

Coronary artery anatomy

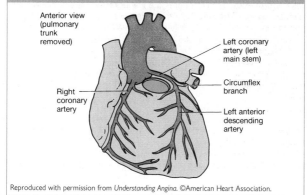

Anterior view (pulmonary trunk removed)

Left coronary artery (left main stem)

Circumflex branch

Right coronary artery

Left anterior descending artery

Reproduced with permission from *Understanding Angina*. ©American Heart Association.

Echocardiography

This non-invasive technique uses the differing ability of various structures within the heart to reflect ultrasound waves. It not only demonstrates anatomy but provides a continuous display of the functioning heart throughout its cycle. There are various types of scan:

M-mode (motion mode): Scans are displayed on light-sensitive paper moving at constant speed to produce a permanent single dimension (time) image.

2-dimensional (real time): A 2-D, fan-shaped image of a segment of the heart is produced on the screen, which may be 'frozen' and hard-copied. Several views are possible and the 4 commonest are: long axis, short axis, 4-chamber, and subcostal. 2-D echocardiography is good for visualizing conditions such as: congenital heart disease, LV aneurysm, mural thrombus, LA myxoma, septal defects.

Doppler and colour-flow echocardiography: Different coloured jets illustrate flow and gradients across valves and septal defects (p160).

Trans-oesophageal echocardiography (TOE) is more sensitive than transthoracic echocardiography (TTE) because the transducer is nearer to the heart. Indications: diagnosis aortic dissections; assessing prosthetic valves; finding cardiac source of emboli, and endocarditis. Don't do if oesphageal disease or cervical spine instability.

Stress echocardiography: Used to evaluate ventricular function, ejection fraction, myocardial thickening, and regional wall motion pre- and post-exercise. Dobutamine or dipyridamole may be used if the patient cannot exercise. Inexpensive and as sensitive/specific as a thallium scan (p112).

Uses of echocardiography

Quantification of global LV function: Heart failure may be due to systolic or diastolic ventricular impairment (or both). Echo helps by measuring end-diastolic volume. If this is large, systolic dysfunction is the likely cause. If small, diastolic. Pure forms of diastolic dysfunction are rare. Differentiation is important, as vasodilators are less useful in diastolic dysfunction as a high ventricular filling pressure is required.

Echo is also useful for detecting focal and global hypokinesia, LV aneurysm, mural thrombus, and LVH (echo is 5–10 times more sensitive than the ECG in detecting this).

Estimating right heart haemodynamics: Doppler studies of pulmonary artery flow allow evaluation of RV function and pressures.

Valve disease: Measurement of pressure gradients and valve orifice areas in stenotic lesions. Detecting valvular regurgitation and estimating its significance is less accurate. Evaluating function of prosthetic valves is another role.

Congenital heart disease: Establishing the presence of lesions and determining their functional significance.

Endocarditis: Vegetations may not be seen if <2mm in size. TTE with colour doppler is best for aortic regurgitation (AR). TOE is useful for visualizing mitral valve vegetations, leaflet perforation, or looking for an aortic root abscess.

Pericardial effusion is best diagnosed by echo. Fluid may first accumulate between the posterior pericardium and the left ventricle, then anterior to both ventricles and anterior and lateral to the right atrium. There may be paradoxical septal motion.

HOCM (p156): Echo features include asymmetrical septal hypertrophy, small LV cavity, dilated left atrium, and systolic anterior motion of the mitral valve.

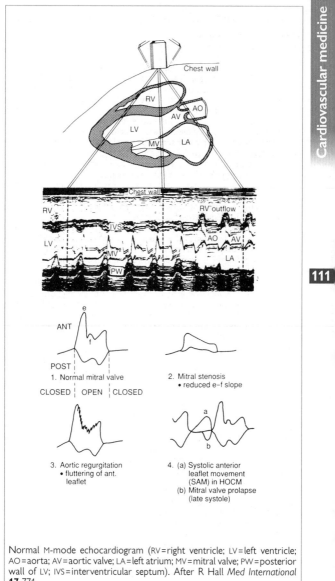

Normal M-mode echocardiogram (RV=right ventricle; LV=left ventricle; AO=aorta; AV=aortic valve; LA=left atrium; MV=mitral valve; PW=posterior wall of LV; IVS=interventricular septum). After R Hall *Med International* **17** 774.

Nuclear cardiology and other cardiac scans

Myocardial perfusion imaging

A non-invasive method of assessing regional myocardial blood flow and the cellular integrity of myocytes. The technique uses radionuclide tracers which cross the myocyte membrane and are trapped intracellularly.

Thallium-201, a K^+ analogue, is the most widely used agent. It is distributed via regional myocardial blood flow and requires cellular integrity for uptake. Newer *technetium-99* based agents are similar to thallium-201 but have improved imaging characteristics, and can also be used to assess myocardial perfusion and LV performance in the same study.

Myocardial territories supplied by unobstructed coronary vessels have normal perfusion whereas regions supplied by stenosed coronary vessels have poorer relative perfusion, a difference which is accentuated by exercise. For this reason, exercise tests are used in conjunction with radionuclide imaging to identify areas at risk of ischaemia/infarction. Exercise scans are compared with resting views: *reperfusion* (ischaemia) or *fixed defects* (infarct) can be seen and the coronary artery involved is reliably predicted. Drugs (eg adenosine and dipyridamole) can also be used to induce perfusion differences between normal and underperfused tissues.

Myocardial perfusion imaging has also been used in patients presenting with acute MI (to determine the amount of myocardium salvaged by thrombolysis) and in diagnosing acute chest pain in those without classical ECG changes (to define the presence of significant perfusion defects).

Positron emission tomography (PET)

Severely underperfused tissues, such as those supplied by a critically stenotic coronary artery, switch from fatty acid metabolism to glycolytic metabolism. Such altered cellular biochemistry may be imaged by PET using ^{18}F-labelled deoxyglucose (FDG), which identifies glycolytically active tissue that is viable. This phenomenon, severe resting ischaemia, occurs in up to 40% of fixed defects seen on thallium-201 scans.

Computer tomography (CT)

allows only limited assessment of cardiac structures. It can help evaluate cardiac disease (eg constrictive pericarditis). CT is also part of first line assessment for abnormalities of the ascending and descending aorta, especially in aortic dissection, and for detecting pulmonary emboli.

Magnetic resonance imaging (MRI)

MRI is used in assessing congenital heart disease, intra-cardiac structures, and the great vessels. Its advantages over CT are: the lack of exposure to radiation; the wide field of view and high-image resolution; the ability to orient images in multiple planes, and the ability to gate or trigger the MRI scanner, according to the cardiac cycle, allowing stop-frame imaging of the heart and great vessels. Spin-echo MRI has a high sensitivity for detecting false lumina and intra-mural flaps in aortic dissection compared with CT. Its main limitation, compared with TOE (p110) and CT, is its inability to image significantly unstable patients.

New uses of MRI include myocardial phosphorus-31 NMR spectroscopy (^{31}P-NMR) which may demonstrate ischaemia in the not-uncommon problem of women with chest pain but normal coronary angiograms. ('syndrome X' denotes this type of uncertain chest pain.) ^{31}P-NMR may suggest abnormal dilator responses of the microvasculature to stress.

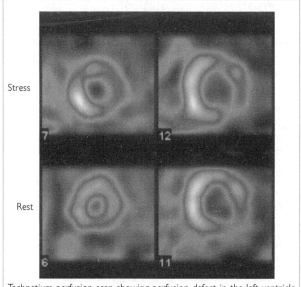

Stress

Rest

Technetium perfusion scan showing perfusion defect in the left ventricle anterior and lateral walls at stress which is reversible (difference between stress and rest images).

Atherosclerosis and 'statins'

Think of atheroma as the slow accretion of snow on a mountain. Nothing much happens until one day an avalanche devastates the community below. The snow is lipid and lipid-laden macrophages; the mountain is an arterial wall; the avalanche is plaque rupture; and the community below is, all too often, myocardium or CNS neurones. The devastation is infarction (Latin *farcire*, to stuff or obstruct). In assessing risk of thrombi, remember Rudolph Virchow's (1821–1902) triad of *changes in the vessel wall, changes in blood flow*, and *changes to the blood constituents*.

Plaque biology Atheroma is the result of cycles of vascular wall injury and repair, leading to the accretion of T lymphocytes, which produce growth factors, cytokines, and chemoattractants. Low-density lipoprotein (LDL) gains access by a process called transcytosis, where it undergoes modification by macrophage-derived oxidative free radicals—a process enhanced by smoking tobacco and hypertension. It is rupture of an atheromatous plaque which triggers most acute coronary events. These plaques have a core of lipid-laden macrophages, and a fibrous cap is all that separates them from endothelium. Many factors predispose to plaque formation, eg genetics, sex (♂), blood pressure, smoking, and diabetes mellitus. Plaques are not static, dead things. They can regress or accumulate, or get inflamed (eg in unstable angina). The balance between LDL efflux and influx is alterable, eg by diet or anti-lipid drugs. Neither is the vessel wall a non-participatory audience to these great events. A sclerotic arterial wall comprises areas of chronic inflammation, with monocytes, macrophages, and T lymphocytes—with smooth muscle proliferation, and elaboration of extracellular matrix. These macrophages make cholesterol, and also produce enzymes (eg interstitial collagenase, gelatinase, and stromelysin), which have been implicated in digesting the plaque cap. The thinner the cap, and the fewer smooth muscle cells involved, the more unstable the plaque. Endothelial cells also release a number of anti- and pro-atherogenic molecules including nitric oxide and endothelin-1. Normal endothelial function is lost early in the process of atherosclerosis with a shift to the production of pro-atherogenic molecules.

After plaque rupture, what happens to fibrinogen and passing platelets partly determines the extent of the impending catastrophe. Hypercholesterolaemia (if present) is associated with hypercoagulable blood and enhanced platelet reactivity at sites of vascular damage.

Disease prevention What can we do about plaques? First, try to prevent them: eat a healthy diet (p208, ?with vit E, p295), encourage *some* exercise, discourage smoking; treat high BP and diabetes. Once a plaque is there, it can be bypassed, ablated (physically removed or compressed), or stented (with a metal conduit). Angioplasty splits the plaque, causing an injury response: elastic recoil→thrombus formation→inflammation→smooth muscle proliferation→arterial remodelling. An alternative to this drastic change is to give a statin, even if the cholesterol is 'normal' since the whole process described above is favourably influenced by statins. Statins (eg simvastatin, pravastatin, p706) inhibit the enzyme HMG-COA reductase, which is responsible for the *de novo* synthesis of cholesterol in the liver. This leads to an increase in LDL receptor expression by hepatocytes and ultimately reduced circulating LDL cholesterol. More effective if given at night, but optimum dose, and target cholesterol are unknown. Besides this, statins have other favourable effects:

- Thrombotic state↓.
- Suppress inflammation (CRP↓).
- Plaque stabilization.
- Restoration of normal endothelial function.
- Reduction in cholesterol synthesis by within-vessel macrophages.
- Reduction of within-vessel macrophage proliferation and migration.

Other cardiovascular drugs

Antiplatelet drugs Aspirin irreversibly acetylates cyclo-oxygenase, preventing production of thromboxane A₂, thereby inhibiting platelet aggregation. Used in low dose (eg 75mg) for secondary prevention following MI, TIA/stroke, and for patients with angina or peripheral vascular disease. May have a role in primary prevention.[1] ADP receptor antagonists (eg clopidogrel) also block platelet aggregation, but may cause less gastric irritation. They have a role if intolerant of aspirin, and post-coronary stent insertion.

β-blockers Block β-adrenoceptors, thus antagonizing the sympathetic nervous system. Blocking β₁-receptors is negatively inotropic and chronotropic (pulse↓ by ↓firing of sinoatrial node), and β₂-receptors induce peripheral vasoconstriction and bronchoconstriction. Drugs vary in their β₁/β₂ selectivity (eg propranolol is non-selective, and bisoprolol relatively β₁ selective), but this does not seem to alter their clinical efficacy. *Uses:* Angina, hypertension, antidysrhythmic, post MI (↓mortality), heart failure (with caution). *CI:* Asthma/COPD, heart block. *Caution:* Peripheral vascular disease, heart failure/(but see carvedilol, p138). *SE:* Lethargy, impotence, *joie de vivre*↓, nightmares, headache.

Diuretics Loop diuretics (eg *Frusemide* = *furosemide*) used in heart failure, inhibit the Na/2Cl/K co-transporter. Thiazides used in hypertension inhibit Na/Cl co-transporter. *SE: Loop* dehydration, ↓K⁺, ↓Ca²⁺, ototoxic; *thiazides:* ↓K⁺, ↑Ca²⁺, ↓Mg²⁺, ↑urate (±gout), impotence (**NB:** small doses, eg bendrofluazide 2.5mg/24h rarely cause significant SEs); *Amiloride:* ↑K⁺, GI upset.

Vasodilators used in heart failure, IHD, and hypertension. Nitrates preferentially dilate veins & the large arteries, ↓ filling pressure (pre-load), while hydralazine primarily dilates the resistance vessels thus ↓ BP (after-load). Prazosin (an α-blocker) dilates arteries and veins.

Calcium antagonists These ↓cell entry of Ca²⁺ via voltage-sensitive channels on smooth muscle cells, thereby promoting coronary and peripheral vasodilatation and reducing myocardial oxygen consumption.
Pharmacology: Effects of specific Ca²⁺ antagonists vary because they have different effects on the L-Ca²⁺-type channels. The *dihydropyridines* eg nifedipine and amlodipine, are mainly peripheral vasodilators (they also dilate coronary arteries) and can cause a reflex tachycardia, so are often used with a β-blocker. They are used mainly in hypertension and angina. Verapamil and diltiazem (*non-dihydropyridines*) also slow conduction at the atrioventricular and sinoatrial nodes and may be used to treat hypertension, angina, and dysrhythmias. Don't give verapamil with β-blockers (risk of bradycardia ± LVF). *SE:* Flushes, headache, oedema (diuretic unresponsive), LV function↓, gingival hypertrophy. *CI:* heart block.

Digoxin[1][2] Blocks the Na⁺/K⁺ pump. It is used to slow the pulse in fast AF (p130; aim for <100). As it is a weak +ve inotrope, its role in heart failure in sinus rhythm may be best reserved if symptomatic despite optimal ACE-i therapy (p139);[3] here there is little benefit *vis-à-vis* mortality (but admissions for worsening CCF are ↓by ~25%).[4] Old people are at ↑risk of toxicity: use lower doses. Do plasma levels >6h post-dose (p711). Typical dose: 500µg stat PO, repeated after 12h, then 125µg (if elderly) to 375µg/d PO (62.5µg/d is almost never enough).[5] Toxicity risk↑ if: K⁺↓, Mg²⁺↓, or Ca²⁺↑. t½ ≈ 36h. If on digoxin, use less energy in cardioversion (start with 5J). *SE:* Any arrhythmia (supraventricular tachycardia SVT with AV block is suggestive), nausea, appetite↓, yellow vision, confusion, gynaecomastia. In toxicity, stop digoxin; check K⁺; treat arrhythmias; consider Digibind® by IVI (p830). *CI:* HOCM; WPW syndrome (p128 & p792).

ACE-inhibitors p139; **Nitrates** p118; **Antihypertensives** p142.

Angina pectoris

This is due to myocardial ischaemia and presents as a central chest tightness or heaviness, which is brought on by exertion and relieved by rest. It may radiate to one or both arms, the neck, jaw or teeth. *Other precipitants:* emotion, cold weather, and heavy meals. *Associated symptoms:* dyspnoea, nausea, sweatiness, faintness.

Causes Mostly atheroma. Rarely: anaemia, AS; tachyarrhythmias; HOCM; arteritis/small vessel disease. May be part of Syndrome X, p295.

Types of angina *Stable angina:* induced by effort, relieved by rest. *Unstable (crescendo) angina:* angina of increasing frequency or severity; occurs on minimal exertion or at rest; associated with ↑↑risk of MI. *Decubitus angina:* precipitated by lying flat. *Variant (Prinzmetal's) angina:* caused by coronary artery spasm (rare; may co-exist with fixed stenoses).

Tests ECG: usually normal, but may show ST depression; flat or inverted T waves; signs of past MI. If resting ECG normal, consider exercise ECG (p106), thallium scan (p112), or coronary angiography. Exclude precipitating factors: anaemia, diabetes, hyperlipidaemia, thyrotoxicosis, giant cell arteritis.

Management *Alteration of lifestyle:* Stop smoking, encourage exercise, weight loss. *Modify risk factors:* Hypertension, diabetes, etc., p91.
- *Aspirin* (75–150mg/24h) reduces mortality by 34%.
- *β-blockers:* eg atenolol 50–100mg/24h PO, unless contra-indications (asthma, COPD, LVF, bradycardia, coronary artery spasm).
- *Nitrates:* for symptoms, give GTN spray or sublingual tabs, up to every ½h. Prophylaxis: give regular oral nitrate, eg isosorbide mononitrate 10–30mg PO (eg bd; an 8h nitrate-free period to prevent tolerance) or slow-release nitrate (eg Imdur® 60mg/24h). Alternatives: adhesive nitrate skin patches or buccal pills. SE: headaches, BP↓.
- *Calcium antagonists:* amlodipine 5mg/24h; diltiazem-MR 90–180mg/12h PO.
- If total cholesterol >5mmol/L give a statin—see p122 & p706.
- Consider adding a K⁺ *channel activator,* eg nicorandil 10–30mg/12h PO.

▶Unstable angina requires admission & urgent treatment: *emergencies,* p784.

Indications for referral Diagnostic uncertainty; new angina of sudden onset; recurrent angina if past MI or CABG; angina uncontrolled by drugs; unstable angina. Some units routinely do exercise tolerance tests on those <70yrs old, but age alone is a poor way to stratify patients.

Percutaneous transluminal coronary angioplasty (PTCA) involves balloon dilatation of the stenotic vessel(s). *Indications:* poor response or intolerance to medical therapy; refractory angina in patients not suitable for CABG; previous CABG; post-thrombolysis in patients with severe stenoses, symptoms, or positive stress tests. Comparisons of PTCA vs drugs alone show that PTCA may control symptoms better but with more frequent cardiac events (eg MI and need for CABG⅙) and little effect on overall mortality. *Complications:* Restenosis (20–30% within 6 months); emergency CABG (<3%); MI (<2%); death (<0.5%). Stenting reduces restenosis rates and the need for bail out CABG. NICE recommends that >70% of angioplasties should be accompanied by stenting. Drug-coated stents reduce restenosis. Antiplatelet agents, eg clopidogrel reduce the risk of stent thrombosis. IV platelet glycoprotein IIb/IIIa-inhibitors (eg eptifibatide) can reduce procedure-related ischaemic events.⅐

CABG: Indications: Left main stem disease, multi-vessel disease; multiple severe stenoses; distal vessel disease; patient unsuitable for angioplasty; failed angioplasty; refractory angina; MI; pre-operatively (valve or vascular surgery). Comparisons of CABG vs PTCA have found that CABG results in better symptom control and lower re-intervention rate, but longer recovery time and length of inpatient stay.

Acute coronary syndromes (ACS)

Definitions ACS includes unstable angina and evolving MI, which share a common underlying pathology—plaque rupture, thrombosis, and inflammation. However, ACS may rarely be due to emboli or coronary spasm in normal coronary arteries, or vasculitis (p424). Usually divided into *ACS with ST-segment elevation* or new onset LBBB—what most of us mean by acute MI; and *ACS without ST-segment elevation*—the ECG may show ST-depression, T-wave inversion, non-specific changes, or be normal (includes non-Q wave or subendocardial MI). The degree of irreversible myocyte death varies, and significant necrosis can occur without ST-elevation. Cardiac troponins (T and I) are the most sensitive and specific markers of myocardial necrosis, and have become the test of choice in patients with ACS (see below).

Risk factors *Non-modifiable:* age, ♂ sex, family history of IHD (MI in first degree relative <55yrs). *Modifiable:* smoking, hypertension, DM, hyperlipidaemia, obesity, sedentary lifestyle. *Controversial* risk factors include: stress, type A personality, LVH, apoprotein A↑, fibrinogen↑, hyperinsulinaemia, homocysteine levels↑ (p91), ACE genotype, and cocaine use.

Incidence 5/1000 per annum (UK) for ST-segment elevation.

Diagnosis is based on the presence of at least 2 out of 3 of: typical history, ECG changes, and cardiac enzyme rise (WHO criteria).

Symptoms Acute central chest pain, lasting >20min, often associated with nausea, sweatiness, dyspnoea, palpitations. May present without chest pain ('silent' infarct) eg in elderly or diabetics. In such patients, presentations may include: syncope, pulmonary oedema, epigastric pain and vomiting, postoperative hypotension or oliguria, acute confusional state, stroke, diabetic hyperglycaemic states.

Signs Distress, anxiety, pallor, sweatiness, pulse↑ or ↓, BP↑ or ↓, 4th heart sound. There may be signs of heart failure (↑ JVP, 3rd heart sound and basal crepitations) or a pansystolic murmur (papillary muscle dysfunction/rupture, VSD). A low-grade pyrexia may be present. Later, a pericardial friction rub or peripheral oedema may develop.

Tests *ECG:* Classically, hyperacute (tall) T waves, ST elevation or new LBBB occur within hours of acute Q wave (transmural infarction). T wave inversion and the development of pathological Q waves follow over hours to days (p96). In other ACS: ST-depression, T-wave inversion, non-specific changes, or normal. ►*In 20% of MIs, the ECG may be normal initially.*

CXR: Look for cardiomegaly, pulmonary oedema, or a widened mediastinum (?aortic dissection). Don't routinely delay R whilst waiting for a CXR.

Blood: FBC, U&E, glucose↑, lipids↓, cardiac enzymes (CK, AST, LDH, troponin)↑[1], CK is found in myocardial and skeletal muscle. It is raised in: MI; after trauma (falls, seizures); prolonged exercise; myositis; Afro-Caribbeans; hypothermia; hypothyroidism. Check CK-MB isoenzyme levels if there is doubt as to the source (normal CK-MB/CK ratio <5%). Troponin T better reflects myocardial damage (peaks at 12–24h; elevated for >1wk). If normal ≥6h after onset of pain, and ECG normal, risk of missing MI is tiny (0.3%).[18] Peak post-MI levels also help risk stratification.[19]

Differential diagnosis (p92) Angina, pericarditis, myocarditis, aortic dissection (p480), pulmonary embolism, and oesophageal reflux/spasm.

Management See *emergencies*, p782. The management of ACS with and without ST-segment elevation varies. Likewise, if there is no ST-elevation, and symptoms settle without a rise in cardiac troponin, then no myocardial damage has occurred, the prognosis is good, and patients can be discharged. Therefore, the two key questions are: is there ST-segment elevation; and is there a rise in troponin?

Mortality 50% of deaths occur within 2h of onset of symptom.

---

1 If non ST-segment elevation ACS, cardiac enzymes (including troponin) *may* be normal.

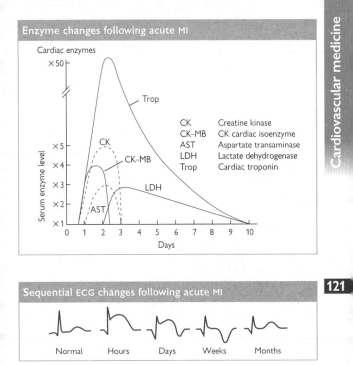

Enzyme changes following acute MI

Cardiac enzymes

Serum enzyme level

×50
×5
×4
×3
×2
×1

Trop

CK
CK–MB
AST
LDH

CK	Creatine kinase
CK–MB	CK cardiac isoenzyme
AST	Aspartate transaminase
LDH	Lactate dehydrogenase
Trop	Cardiac troponin

Days
0 1 2 3 4 5 6 7 8 9 10

Sequential ECG changes following acute MI

Normal   Hours   Days   Weeks   Months

Management of acute coronary syndrome

Pre-hospital Arrange emergency ambulance. Aspirin 300mg chewed (if no *absolute* CI) and GTN sublingual. Analgesia, eg morphine 5–10mg IV + metoclopramide 10mg IV (not IM because of risk of bleeding with thrombolysis).

In hospital O₂, IVI, morphine, aspirin ▶▶p782

Then the key question for subsequent management of ACS is whether there is ST-segment elevation (includes new onset LBBB or a true posterior MI).

ST-segment elevation
- *Thrombolysis*, if no contraindication, or primary angioplasty ▶▶p782.
- *β-blocker*, eg atenolol 5mg IV unless contraindicated; see e-bm 2000 5 12.
- *ACE-inhibitor*: Consider starting ACE-i (eg lisinopril 2.5mg) in all normotensive patients within 24h of acute MI, especially if there is clinical evidence of heart failure or echo evidence of LV dysfunction.

ACS without ST-segment elevation
- *β-blocker*, eg atenolol 5mg IV unless contraindicated; see e-bm 2000 5 12.
- *Low molecular weight heparin* (eg enoxaparin).
- *Nitrates*, unless contraindication (usually given intravenously).
- High-risk patients (persistent or recurrent ischaemia, ST-depression, diabetes, ↑ troponin) require infusion of a GPIIb/IIIa antagonist (eg tirofiban), and, ideally, urgent angiography. Clopidogrel may be useful in addition to aspirin.
- Low-risk patients (no further pain, flat or inverted T waves, or normal ECG, **and** negative troponin) can be discharged if a repeat troponin is negative. Treat medically and arrange further investigation eg stress test, angiogram.

Subsequent management Bed rest for 48h; continuous ECG monitoring.
- Daily examination of heart, lungs, and legs for complications (p124).
- Daily 12-lead ECG, U&E, cardiac enzymes for 2–3d.
- *Prophylaxis against thromboembolism*: eg heparin 5000U/12h SC until fully mobile. If large anterior MI, consider warfarin anticoagulation for 3 months as prophylaxis against systemic embolism from LV mural thrombus. Continue daily *low-dose aspirin* (eg 75–150mg) indefinitely. Aspirin reduces vascular events (MI, stroke, or vascular death) by 29%.
- Start oral *β-blocker* (eg metoprolol ~50mg/6h, enough to decrease the pulse to ≤60; continue for at least 1yr). Long-term β-blockade reduces mortality from all causes by ~25% in patients who have had a previous MI. If contraindicated, consider verapamil or diltiazem as an alternative.
- *Continue* ACE-i in all patients. ACE-i in those with evidence of heart failure ↓2yr mortality by 25–30%.
- *Start a statin.* Cholesterol reduction post-MI has been shown to be of benefit in patients with both elevated and normal cholesterol levels. Some treat all patients, others only if total cholesterol >4.8mmol/L[1] or LDL >3.2 mmol/L (p706).
- *Address modifiable risk factors:* Discourage smoking (p91). Encourage exercise. Identify and treat diabetes mellitus, hypertension, and hyperlipidaemia.
- *Exercise ECG.* May be useful in risk stratification post-MI after 3–4wks, and in subjects without ST-segment elevation or a troponin rise.
- *General advice.* If uncomplicated, discharge after 5–7d. *Work:* He may return to work after 2 months. A few occupations should not be restarted post-MI: airline pilots; air traffic controllers; divers. Drivers of public service or heavy goods vehicles may be permitted to return to work if they meet certain criteria. Patients undertaking heavy manual labour should be advised to seek a lighter job. *Diet:* A diet high in oily fish, fruit, vegetables, and fibre, and low in saturated fats should be encouraged. *Exercise:* Encourage regular daily exercise. *Sex:* Intercourse is best avoided for 1 month. *Travel:* Avoid air travel for 2 months.

Review at 5wks post-MI to review symptoms: Angina? dyspnoea? palpitations?
- If angina recurs, treat conventionally, and consider coronary angiography.

Review at 3 months
- Check fasting lipids. Is there a need for a statin (p706)?

---

1 Joint UK guidelines, but there is benefit if above ~4.2 (LIPID study).

Acute postero-lateral MI

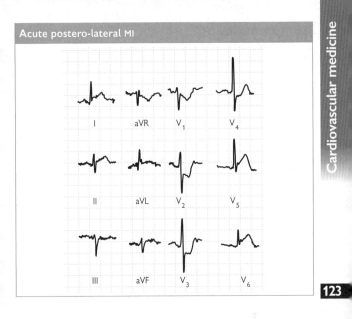

Complications of MI

- *Cardiac arrest* (p766); *cardiogenic shock* (p788).

- *Unstable angina:* Manage along standard lines (p784) and refer to a cardiologist for urgent investigation.

- *Bradycardias or heart block: Sinus bradycardia:* treat with atropine 0.6–1.2mg IV. Consider temporary cardiac pacing if no response, or poorly tolerated by the patient. *1st degree AV block:* Observe closely as approximately 40% develop higher degrees of AV block. *Wenckebach (Mobitz type I) block:* Does not require pacing unless poorly tolerated. *Mobitz type II block:* Carries a high risk of developing complete AV block; should be paced. *Complete AV block:* insert pacemaker; may not be necessary after inferior MI if narrow QRS and reasonably stable & pulse ≥40–50. *Bundle branch block:* MI complicated by trifascicular block or non-adjacent bifascicular disease should be paced.

- *Tachyarrhythmias:* **NB:** K^+↓, hypoxia and acidosis all predispose to arrhythmias and should be corrected. Regular broad complex tachycardia after MI is almost always VT. If haemodynamically stable, give lignocaine (= lidocaine) 100mg IV or amiodarone. If this fails, give a DC shock, then, if needed, procainamide 100mg IV over 2min (repeated at 5min intervals; max dose = 1g; monitor ECG). Consider maintenance antidysrhythmic therapy. Early VT (<24h): give lidocaine by infusion for 12–24h or amiodarone. Late VT (>24h) amiodarone and start oral therapy (amiodarone or sotalol). *SVT:* p128. *AF or flutter:* If compromised, DC cardioversion. Otherwise, control rate with digoxin (load with 0.5mg/12h PO for three doses; maintenance: 0.125–0.25mg/24h) ± β-blocker. In atrial flutter or intermittent AF, try amiodarone or sotalol (details p130).

- *Left ventricular failure (LVF):* p786.

- *Right ventricular failure (RVF)/infarction:* Presents with low cardiac output and JVP↑. Insert a Swan–Ganz catheter to measure right-sided pressures and guide fluid replacement. If BP remains low, give inotropes.

- *Pericarditis:* Central chest pain, relieved by sitting forwards. ECG: saddle-shaped ST elevation. Treatment: NSAIDs. Echo to check for effusion.

- *DVT & PE:* Patients are at risk of developing DVT & PE and should be prophylactically heparinized (5000U/12h sc) until fully mobile.

- *Systemic embolism:* May arise from a LV mural thrombus. After large anterior MIs, consider anticoagulation with warfarin for 3 months.

- *Cardiac tamponade:* (p788) Presents with low cardiac output, pulsus paradoxus, JVP↑, muffled heart sounds. Diagnosis: Echo. Treatment: Pericardial aspiration (provides temporary relief ▶▶see p757 for technique), surgery.

- *Mitral regurgitation:* May be mild (minor papillary muscle dysfunction) or severe (chordal or papillary muscle rupture or ischaemia). Presentation: Pulmonary oedema. Treat LVF (p786) and consider valve replacement.

- *Ventricular septal defect:* Presents with pansystolic murmur, JVP↑, cardiac failure. Diagnosis: Echo. Treatment: Surgery. 50% mortality in 1st wk.

- *Late malignant ventricular arrhythmias:* Occur 1–3wks post-MI and are the cardiologist's nightmare. Avoid hypokalemia, the most easily avoidable cause. Large MIs should have 24h ECG monitoring prior to discharge.

- *Dressler's syndrome:* (p722) Recurrent pericarditis, pleural effusions, fever, anaemia and ESR↑ 1–3wks post-MI. Treatment: NSAIDs; steroids if severe.

- *Left ventricular aneurysm:* This occurs late (4–6wks post-MI), and presents with LVF, angina, recurrent VT, or systemic embolism. ECG: Persistent ST segment elevation. Treatment: anticoagulate, consider excision.

Arrhythmias (Emergency management: **p790** & **p792**)

Disturbances of cardiac rhythm or arrhythmias are:
• Common
• Often benign (but may reflect underlying heart disease)
• Often intermittent, causing diagnostic difficulty
• Occasionally severe, causing cardiac compromise.

Causes *Cardiac:* MI, coronary artery disease, LV aneurysm, mitral valve disease, cardiomyopathy, pericarditis, myocarditis, aberrant conduction pathways. *Non-cardiac:* Caffeine, smoking, alcohol, pneumonia, drugs (β_2-agonists, digoxin, L-dopa, tricyclics, adriamycin, doxorubicin), metabolic imbalance (K^+, Ca^{2+}, Mg^{2+}, hypoxia, hypercapnia, metabolic acidosis, thyroid disease, phaeochromocytoma). Presentation is with palpitation, chest pain, presyncope/syncope, hypotension, or pulmonary oedema. Some arrhythmias may be asymptomatic and incidental, eg AF.

History Take a detailed history of palpitations (p78). Ask about precipitating factors, onset, nature (fast or slow, regular or irregular) duration, associated symptoms (chest pain, dyspnoea, collapse). Review drug history. Ask about past medical history or family history of cardiac disease.

Tests FBC, U&E, glucose, Ca^{2+}, Mg^{2+}, TSH. ECG: Look for signs of IHD, AF, short P–R interval (WPW syndrome), long QT interval (metabolic imbalance, drugs, congenital), U waves (hypokalaemia). 24h ECG monitoring; several recordings may be needed. Echo: To look for structural heart disease, eg mitral stenosis, HOCM. Provocation tests: Exercise ECG, cardiac catheterization, and electrophysiological studies may be required.

Treatment If the ECG is normal during palpitations, reassure the patient. Otherwise, treatment depends on the type of arrhythmia.

Bradycardia: (p127) If asymptomatic and rate >40bpm, no treatment is required. Look for a cause (drugs, sick sinus syndrome, hypothyroidism) and stop any drugs that may be contributing (β-blocker, digoxin). If rate <40bpm or patient is symptomatic, give atropine 0.6–1.2mg IV (up to maximum of 3mg). If no response, insert a temporary pacing wire (p762). If necessary, start an isoprenaline infusion or use external cardiac pacing.

Sick sinus syndrome: Sinus node dysfunction causes bradycardia ± arrest, sinoatrial block or SVT alternating with bradycardia/asystole (tachy–brady syndrome). AF and thromboembolism may occur. Pace if symptomatic.

SVT: (p128) Narrow complex tachycardia (rate >100bpm, QRS width <120ms). Acute management: Vagotonic manoeuvres followed by IV adenosine or verapamil (if not on β-blocker); DC shock if compromised. Maintenance therapy: β-blockers or verapamil.

AF/flutter: (p130) May be incidental finding. Control ventricular rate with digoxin: loading dose (~500µg/12h × 2) followed by maintenance dose (0.125–0.25mg/24h). Alternatives: Verapamil, β-blocker, or amiodarone. Flecainide for pre-excited AF. DC shock if compromised (p754).

VT: (p132) Broad complex tachycardia (rate >100bpm, QRS duration >120ms). Acute management: IV lignocaine (=lidocaine), or amiodarone IV, if no response or if compromised DC shock. Oral therapy: amiodarone loading dose (200mg/8h PO for 7d, then 200mg/12h for 7d) followed by maintenance therapy (200mg/24h). SE: Corneal deposits, photosensitivity, hepatitis, pneumonitis, lung fibrosis, nightmares, INR↑ (warfarin potentiation), T4↑, T3↓. Monitor LFT and TFT.

▶Finally, permanent pacing may be used to overdrive tachyarrhythmias, to treat bradyarrhythmias, or prophylactically in conduction disturbances (p134). Implanted automatic defibrillators can save lives.

Diagnosis of bradycardias and AV block

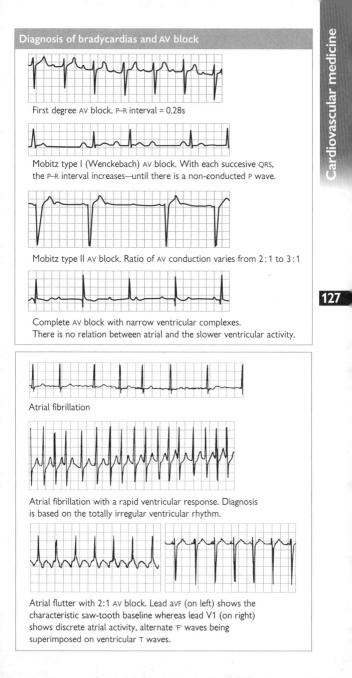

First degree AV block. P–R interval = 0.28s

Mobitz type I (Wenckebach) AV block. With each succesive QRS, the P–R interval increases—until there is a non-conducted P wave.

Mobitz type II AV block. Ratio of AV conduction varies from 2:1 to 3:1

Complete AV block with narrow ventricular complexes. There is no relation between atrial and the slower ventricular activity.

Atrial fibrillation

Atrial fibrillation with a rapid ventricular response. Diagnosis is based on the totally irregular ventricular rhythm.

Atrial flutter with 2:1 AV block. Lead aVF (on left) shows the characteristic saw-tooth baseline whereas lead V1 (on right) shows discrete atrial activity, alternate 'F' waves being superimposed on ventricular T waves.

Narrow complex tachycardia

ECG shows rate of >100bpm and QRS complex duration of <120ms.

Differential diagnosis
- Sinus tachycardia: normal P wave followed by normal QRS.
- SVT: P wave absent or inverted after QRS.
- AF: absent P wave, irregular QRS complexes.
- Atrial flutter: atrial rate usually 300bpm giving 'flutter waves' or 'sawtooth' baseline (p127), ventricular rate often 150bpm (2 : 1 block).
- Atrial tachycardia: abnormally shaped P waves, may outnumber QRS.
- Multifocal atrial tachycardia: 3 or more P wave morphologies, irregular QRS complexes.
- Junctional tachycardia: rate 150–250bpm, P wave either buried in QRS complex or occurring after QRS complex.

Principles of management See algorithm OPPOSITE.
- If the patient is compromised, use DC cardioversion (p754).
- Otherwise, identify the underlying rhythm and treat accordingly.
- Vagal manoeuvres (carotid sinus massage, Valsalva manoeuvre) transiently increase AV block, and may unmask an underlying atrial rhythm.
- If unsuccessful, give adenosine which causes transient AV block. It has a short half-life (10–15s) and works in 2 ways:
  by transiently slowing ventricles to show the underlying atrial rhythm;
  by cardioverting a junctional tachycardia to sinus rhythm.

Give 6mg IV bolus into a big vein; follow by saline flush, while recording a rhythm strip; if unsuccessful, give 12mg, then 12mg again at 2min intervals, unless on dipyridamole or post cardiac transplantation (see BNF). Warn of SE: transient chest tightness, dyspnoea, headache, flushing. CI: asthma, $2^{nd}/3^{rd}$ degree AV block, or sinoatrial disease (unless pacemaker). Drug interactions: potentiated by dipyridamole, antagonized by theophylline.

Specific management *Sinus tachycardia* Identify and treat the cause.

SVT: If adenosine fails, use verapamil 5–10mg IV over 2min, or over 3min if elderly (►not if already on β-blocker). If no response, give further dose of 5mg IV after 5–10min. Alternatives: atenolol 2.5mg IV at 1mg/min repeated at 5min intervals to a maximum of 10mg or sotalol 20–60mg IV. If no good, use DC cardioversion.

AF/flutter: Manage along standard lines (p130).

Atrial tachycardia: Rare. If due to digoxin toxicity, stop digoxin; consider digoxin-specific antibody fragments (p830). Maintain K^+ at 4–5mmol/L.

Multifocal atrial tachycardia: Most commonly occurs in COPD. Correct hypoxia and hypercapnia. Consider verapamil if rate remains >110bpm.

Junctional tachycardia: There are 3 types of junctional tachycardia: AV nodal re-entry tachycardia (AVNRT), AV re-entry tachycardia (AVRT), and His bundle tachycardia. Where anterograde conduction through the AV node occurs, vagal manoeuvres are worth trying. Adenosine will usually cardiovert a junctional rhythm to sinus rhythm. If it recurs, treat with a β-blocker or amiodarone. Radiofrequency ablation is increasingly being used in AVRT and in some patients with AVNRT.[25]

WPW syndrome (ECG p131) Caused by congenital accessory conduction pathway between atria and ventricles. Resting ECG shows short P–R interval and widened QRS complex due to slurred upstroke or 'delta wave'. 2 types: WPW type A (+ve δ wave in V_1), WPW type B (–ve δ wave in V_1). Patients present with SVT which may be due to an AVRT, pre-excited AF, or pre-excited atrial flutter. Refer to cardiologist for electrophysiology and ablation of the accessory pathway.

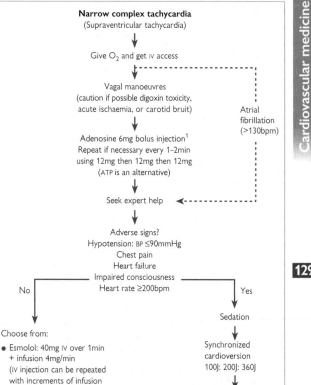

Narrow complex tachycardia
(Supraventricular tachycardia)

↓

Give O₂ and get IV access

↓

Vagal manoeuvres
(caution if possible digoxin toxicity,
acute ischaemia, or carotid bruit)

↓

Adenosine 6mg bolus injection[1]
Repeat if necessary every 1–2min
using 12mg then 12mg then 12mg
(ATP is an alternative)

↓

Atrial
fibrillation
(>130bpm)

Seek expert help ←----------

↓

Adverse signs?
Hypotension: BP ≤90mmHg
Chest pain
Heart failure
Impaired consciousness
Heart rate ≥200bpm

No ← | → Yes

No:

Choose from:

- Esmolol: 40mg IV over 1min
  + infusion 4mg/min
  (IV injection can be repeated
  with increments of infusion
  to 12mg/min)
- Digoxin: max IV dose 500µg
  over 30min ×2
- Verapamil: 5–10mg IV over 2min
- Amiodarone: 300mg over IV
  1h may be repeated once
  if necessary via a central
  line if possible
- Overdrive pacing—not AF

Yes:

Sedation

↓

Synchronized
cardioversion
100J: 200J: 360J

↓

Amiodarone 150mg IV
over 10min
then 300mg
over 1h if necessary
preferably by central
line and repeat
cardioversion

Atrial fibrillation (AF) and flutter

AF is a chaotic, irregular atrial rhythm at 300–600bpm. The AV node responds intermittently, hence the irregular ventricular rate. It is common in the elderly (≤9%). The main risk is of embolic stroke, which is preventable by warfarin (reducible to 1%/yr from 4%; higher risk if old, CCF, poor LV function, DM, past TIA or stroke, or large left atrium on echocardiogram).

Common causes: Heart failure; hypertension; cardiac ischaemia; MI (seen in 22%);[26] mitral valve disease; pneumonia; hyperthyroidism; alcohol.

Rare causes: Cardiomyopathy, constrictive pericarditis, sick sinus syndrome, bronchial carcinoma, atrial myxoma, endocarditis, haemochromatosis, sarcoidosis. 'Lone' AF means none of the above causes.

Signs & symptoms: It may be asymptomatic (found incidentally) or present with chest pain, palpitations, dyspnoea, or presyncope. On examination, the pulse is *irregularly irregular*, the apical pulse rate is greater than the radial rate and the first heart sound is of variable intensity. Look for signs of mitral valve disease or hyperthyroidism.

Tests: ECG shows absent P waves, irregular QRS complexes. *Blood tests:* U&E, cardiac enzymes, thyroid function tests. Echo to look for LA enlargement, mitral valve disease, poor LV function, and other structural abnormalities.

Acute AF (eg ≤72h):
- Treat any associated acute illness (eg MI, pneumonia).
- Control ventricular rate with digoxin PO (0.5mg/12h, 2 doses, then 0.125–0.25mg daily) or IV (0.75–1mg in 0.9% NaCl over 2h).
- If ventricular rate still too fast, and LV function is adequate, consider low-dose β-blocker (eg metoprolol 50mg/12h PO; use 10mg/8h if LV function is poor) and gradually increase dose. If AF does not resolve, consider drug or electrical cardioversion.
- Drug cardioversion: amiodarone IVI (5mg/kg over 1h then ~900mg over 24h via a central line max 1.2g in 24h) or PO (200mg/8h for 1wk, 200mg/12h for 1wk, 100–200mg/24h maintenance). Alternative (if haemodynamically stable and no known IHD): flecainide 2mg/kg IV over >25min (max 150mg) with ECG monitoring. 300mg stat PO may also work.
- DC cardioversion is indicated: (1) electively, following a first attack of AF with an identifiable cause; (2) as an emergency, if the patient is compromised. Protocol: 200J→360J→360J (100J may be tried first, but is successful in <20%).
- Anticoagulation is not required if AF is of recent onset with a structurally normal heart on echo, but aspirin may be given. Otherwise, anticoagulate with warfarin for 3wks before and 4wks after DC cardioversion.

Chronic AF:
- Control rate with digoxin PO: loading dose (0.5mg/12h, two doses) followed by maintenance (0.125–0.25mg/24h). In the elderly, load with 0.75mg in total and use 0.0625–0.125mg/24h.
- If rate still too fast, check compliance and serum level (take blood >6h after last dose), cautiously increase dose or consider low-dose β-blocker (eg metoprolol). Alternative: amiodarone PO.
- Anticoagulate with warfarin if INR is contraindication. Aim for an INR of 2.5–3.5.[27] For those aged <65 years with no other risk factors (eg hypertension, diabetes, LV dysfunction, increased LA size, rheumatic valve disease, MI), or those in whom warfarin is contraindicated, aspirin (300mg PO) is an alternative.

Paroxysmal AF:
- Sotalol 80mg/24h PO (after at least 48h, gradually ↑dose to 80mg/12h, then 160mg/12h; monitor QT interval).
- Alternative: amiodarone PO. Anticoagulate with warfarin.

Summary of treatment of AF

- Treat any reversible cause.
- Control ventricular rate.
- Consider cardioversion to sinus rhythm, if onset within last 12 months (do echo first; is heart structurally normal?).
- Prevent emboli: warfarin (or aspirin).

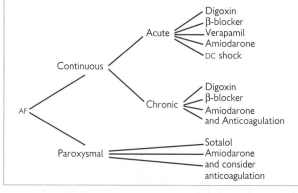

Note on atrial flutter

- ECG: Continuous atrial depolarization (eg ~300/min, but very variable) produces a sawtooth baseline ± 2:1 AV block (as if SVT at, eg 150bpm).
- Carotid sinus massage or IV adenosine transiently block the AV node and may unmask flutter waves.
- Treatment: Anti-AF drugs may not work; consider cavotricuspid isthmus ablation (this 'flutter isthmus' is low in the right atrium).[28]

See p127 for ECGs.

Wolff Parkinson White syndrome

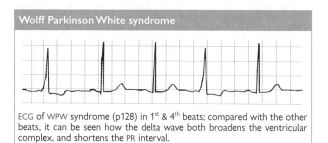

ECG of WPW syndrome (p128) in 1st & 4th beats; compared with the other beats, it can be seen how the delta wave both broadens the ventricular complex, and shortens the PR interval.

Broad complex tachycardia

ECG shows rate of >100 and QRS complexes >120ms (>3 small squares, p94). If no clear QRS complexes, it is VF or asystole, p766.

Principles of management

Identify the underlying rhythm and treat accordingly.
If in doubt, treat as VT (the commonest cause).

Differential diagnosis

VT; includes Torsade de pointes, below
SVT with aberrant conduction, eg AF, atrial flutter.

(**NB:** Ventricular ectopics should not cause confusion when occurring singly; but if >3 together at rate of >120, this constitutes VT.)

Identification of the underlying rhythm (see OPPOSITE) may be difficult, seek expert help. Diagnosis is based on the history (IHD increases the likelihood of a ventricular arrhythmia), a 12-lead ECG, and the lack of response to IV adenosine (p128). ECG findings in favour of VT:

• Positive QRS concordance in chest leads
• Marked LAD
• AV dissociation (occurs in 25%) or 2 : 1 or 3 : 1 AV block
• Fusion beats or capture beats (p133)
• RSR complex in V_1 (with positive QRS in V_1)
• QS complex in V_6 (with negative QRS in V_6)

Concordance means QRS complexes are all +ve or −ve. A *fusion beat* is when an 'normal beat' fuses with a VT complex to create an unusual complex, and a *capture beat* is a normal QRS between abnormal beats (see OPPOSITE).

Management Connect to a cardiac monitor; have a defibrillator to hand.

• Give high-flow oxygen by face mask
• Obtain IV access and take blood for U&E, cardiac enzymes, Ca^{2+}, Mg^{2+}
• Obtain 12-lead ECG
• ABG (if evidence of pulmonary oedema, reduced conscious level, sepsis).

VT: Haemodynamically stable

• Correct hypokalaemia and hypomagnaesemia
• Amiodarone 150mg IV over 10min, then 300mg over 1hr
• OR lignocaine 50mg over 2min repeated every 5min to 200mg max
• If this fails, or cardiac arrest occurs, use DC shock (p754; see also the *European Resuscitation Guidelines*, p767).
• After correction of VT, establish the cause from history/investigations.
• Maintenance antiarrhythmic therapy may be required. If VT occurs <24h after MI, give IV lidocaine or amiodarone IVI for 12–24h. If VT occurs >24h after MI, give IV lidocaine infusion and start oral antiarrhythmic: eg amiodarone.
• Prevention of recurrent VT: Surgical isolation of the arrhythmogenic area or implantation of tiny automatic defibrillators may help.

VF: (ECG, see OPPOSITE) Use asynchronized DC shock (p754): see also the *European Resuscitation Guidelines* (p767).

Ventricular extrasystoles (ectopics) are the commonest post-MI arrhythmia but they are also seen in healthy people (≥10/h). Post-MI they suggest electrical instability, and there is a risk of VF if the 'R on T' pattern (ie no gap before the T wave) is seen. If frequent (>10/min), treat with lignocaine 100mg IV as above. Otherwise, just observe patient.

Torsade de pointes: Looks like VF but is VT with varying axis (ECG, see OPPOSITE). It is due ↑QT interval (a SE of antiarrhythmics, so consider stopping). R: Mg sulfate, 8mmol over 15min (≈4mL of 50% solution) ± overdrive pacing.

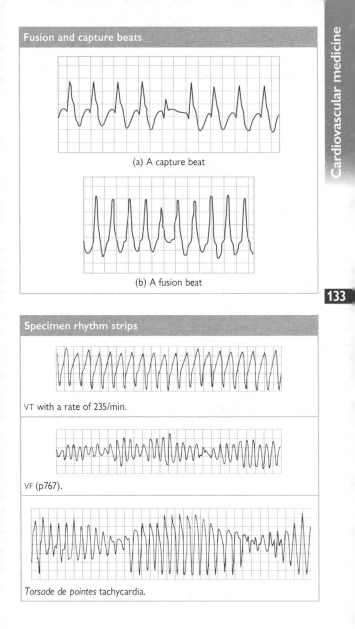

Fusion and capture beats

(a) A capture beat

(b) A fusion beat

Specimen rhythm strips

VT with a rate of 235/min.

VF (p767).

Torsade de pointes tachycardia.

Pacemakers

Pacemakers supply electrical initiation to myocardial contraction. The pacemaker lies subcutaneously where it may be programmed through the skin as necessary. Pacemakers usually last 7–15yrs.

Indications for temporary cardiac pacing ►See p762 for further details and insertion technique.

• Symptomatic bradycardia, unresponsive to atropine.
• Acute conduction disturbances following MI:
  After acute *anterior* MI, prophylactic pacing is required in:
    Complete AV block
    Mobitz type I AV block (Wenckebach)
    Mobitz type II AV block
    Non-adjacent bifascicular or trifascicular block (p98).
  After *inferior* MI, pacing may not be needed in complete AV block if reasonably stable, and rate is >40–50, and QRS complexes are narrow.
• Suppression of drug-resistant tachyarrhythmias, eg SVT, VT.
• Special situations: During general anaesthesia; during cardiac surgery; during electrophysiological studies; drug overdose (eg digoxin, β-blockers, verapamil).

Indications for a permanent pacemaker

• Complete AV block (Stokes–Adams attacks, asymptomatic, congenital)
• Mobitz type II AV block (p127)
• Persistent AV block after anterior MI
• Symptomatic bradycardias (eg sick sinus syndrome, p126)
• Drug-resistant tachyarrhythmias.

Some say persistent bifascicular block after MI requires a permanent system: this remains controversial.

Pre-operative assessment: FBC, clotting screen, HBsAg. Insert IV cannula. Consent for procedure under local anaesthetic. Consider pre-medication. Give antibiotic cover (eg flucloxacillin 500mg IM and benzylpenicillin 600mg IM) 20min before, and 1 and 6h after.

Post-procedure assessment: Prior to discharge, check wound for bleeding or haematoma; check position on CXR; check pacemaker function. During first week, inspect for wound haematoma or dehiscence. Count apical rate (p64): if this is six or more bpm less than the rate quoted for the pacemaker, suspect malfunction. Other problems: lead fracture; pacemaker interference (eg from patient's muscles). Driving rules: p162.

Types of pacemakers: 3-letter pacemaker codes enable the identification of the pacemaker: the 1st letter indicates the chamber paced (A = atria, V = ventricles, D = dual chamber); the 2nd letter identifies the chamber sensed (A = atria, V = ventricles, D = dual chamber, 0 = none), and the 3rd letter indicates the pacemaker response (T = triggered, I = inhibited, D = dual, R = reverse). VVI pacemakers are the most frequently used in the UK. DDD pacemakers are the only pacemakers that sense and pace both chambers. The 3-letter code is likely to be superseded by a 5-letter code to cope with programmable functions.

ECG of paced rhythm: (ECG 7 p105, and OPPOSITE for rhythm strip) If the system is on 'demand' of 60bpm, a pacing spike will only be seen if the intrinsic heart rate is <60bpm. If it is cutting in at a higher rate, its sensing mode is malfunctioning. If it is failing to cut in at slower rates, its pacing mode is malfunctioning, ie the lead may be dislodged, the pacing threshold is too high, or the lead (or insulation) is faulty. If you see spikes but no capture (ie no systole), suspect dislodgment.

Some confusing pacemaker terms

Fusion beat: Union of native depolarization and pacemaker impulse.

Pseudofusion: The pacemaker impulse occurs just after cardiac depolarization, so it is ineffective, but it distorts the QRS morphology.

Pseudopseudofusion beat: If a DVI pacemaker gives an atrial spike within a native QRS complex, the atrial output is non-contributory.

Pacemaker syndrome: In single-chamber pacing, retrograde conduction to the atria, which then contract during ventricular systole. This leads to retrograde flow in pulmonary veins, and ↓cardiac output.

Pacemaker tachycardia: In dual-chamber pacing, a short-circuit loop goes between the electrodes, causing an artificial WPW-like syndrome. Solution: Single-chamber pacing.

Web images: www.txt.co.uk/full.cfm?1074

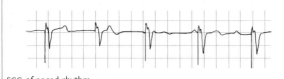

ECG of paced rhythm.

Heart failure—basic concepts

Definition Cardiac output and BP are inadequate for the body's requirements. Prognosis is poor with 82% of patients dying within 6yrs of diagnosis.

Classification LVF and RVF may occur independently, or together as *congestive cardiac failure (CCF)*. *Low-output cardiac failure:* The heart's output is inadequate (eg ejection fraction <0.35), or is only adequate with high filling pressures. Causes: Usually ischaemia, hypertension, valve disorders, or ↑alcohol use.

- *Pump failure due to:*
  Heart muscle disease: IHD; cardiomyopathy (p156).
  Restricted filling: Constrictive pericarditis, tamponade, restrictive cardiomyopathy. This may be the mechanism of action of fluid overload: an expanding right heart impinges on the LV, so filling is restricted by the ungiving pericardium (the mechanism invoking a 'hump in the Starling curve' is now said to be an error based on an artefact).
  Inadequate heart rate: β-blockers, heart block, post MI.
  Negatively inotropic drugs: eg most antiarrhythmic agents.
- *Excessive preload:* eg mitral regurgitation or fluid overload (eg NSAID causing fluid retention). Fluid overload may cause LVF in a normal heart if renal excretion is impaired or big volumes are involved (eg IVI running too fast). More common if there is simultaneous compromise of cardiac function and in the elderly.
- *Chronic excessive afterload:* eg AS, hypertension.

NB: High-output failure is rare. Here, output is normal or increased in the face of much increased needs. Failure occurs when cardiac output fails to meet needs. It will occur with a normal heart, but even earlier if there is heart disease. *Causes:* Heart disease with anaemia or pregnancy, hyperthyroidism, Paget's disease, arteriovenous malformation, beri beri. *Consequences:* Initially features of RVF; later LVF becomes evident.

Symptoms depend on which ventricle is more affected. *LVF:* Dyspnoea, poor exercise tolerance, fatigue, orthopnoea, paroxysmal nocturnal dyspnoea (PND), nocturnal cough (±pink frothy sputum), wheeze (cardiac 'asthma'), nocturia, cold peripheries, weight loss, muscle wasting. *RVF:* Peripheral oedema (up to thighs, sacrum, abdominal wall), abdominal distension (ascites), nausea, anorexia, facial engorgement, pulsation in neck and face (tricuspid regurgitation), epistaxis. In addition, patients may be depressed or complain of drug-related side effects.

Signs The patient may look ill and exhausted, with cool peripheries, and peripheral cyanosis. Pulse: resting tachycardia, pulsus alternans. Systolic BP↓, narrow pulse pressure, Raised JVP. Praecordium: displaced apex (LV dilatation), RV heave (pulmonary hypertension), Auscultation: S₃ gallop (p44), murmurs of mitral or aortic valve disease. Chest: tachypnoea, bibasal end-inspiratory crackles, wheeze ('cardiac asthma'), pleural effusions. Abdomen: hepatomegaly (pulsatile in tricuspid regurgitation), ascites, peripheral oedema.

Investigations According to NICE,[29] if ECG and BNP (b-type natriuretic peptide, p689) are normal, heart failure is unlikely and an alternative diagnosis should be considered; if either abnormal, an Echo is required.

Blood tests: FBC; U&E; BNP *CXR:* Cardiomegaly (cardiothoracic ratio >50%), prominent upper lobe veins (upper lobe diversion), peribronchial cuffing, diffuse interstitial or alveolar shadowing, classical perihilar 'bat's wing' shadowing, fluid in the fissures, pleural effusions, Kerley B lines (variously attributed to interstitial oedema[30] and engorged peripheral lymphatics[31]). *ECG* may indicate cause (look for evidence of ischaemia, MI, or ventricular hypertrophy). It is rare to get a completely normal ECG in chronic heart failure. *Echocardiography* is the key investigation.[32] It may indicate the cause (MI, valvular heart disease) and can confirm the presence or absence of LV dysfunction. *Endomyocardial biopsy* is rarely needed.

New York classification of heart failure: summary

I   Heart disease present, but no undue dyspnoea from ordinary activity.
II Comfortable at rest; dyspnoea on ordinary activities.
III Less than ordinary activity causes dyspnoea, which is limiting.
IV Dyspnoea present at rest; all activity causes discomfort.

The CXR in left ventricular failure   (see also x-ray Plate 2)

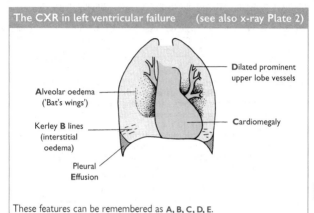

Dilated prominent upper lobe vessels

Alveolar oedema ('Bat's wings')

Kerley **B** lines (interstitial oedema)

Pleural **E**ffusion

Cardiomegaly

These features can be remembered as **A, B, C, D, E**.

137

Heart failure—management

Acute heart failure is a medical emergency (see p786).

Chronic heart failure Treat the cause (eg if arrhythmias; valve disease).

- Treat exacerbating factors (anaemia, thyroid disease, infection, ↑BP).
- Avoid exacerbating factors, eg NSAIDs (cause fluid retention), and verapamil (negative inotrope).
- Stop smoking. Eat less salt. Maintain optimal weight and nutrition.
- Drugs: the following are used:

    1 *Diuretics:* Loop diuretics routinely used to relieve symptoms eg *frusemide* (=furosemide) 40mg/24h PO; increase dose as necessary. SE: K⁺↓, renal impairment. Monitor U&E and add K⁺ sparing diuretic (eg *spironolactone*) if K⁺ <3.2mmol/L, predisposition to arrhythmias, concurrent digoxin therapy (K⁺↓ increases risk of digoxin toxicity), or pre-existing K⁺-losing conditions. If refractory oedema, consider adding *metolazone* 5–20mg/24h PO.

    2 *ACE-inhibitor:* Consider in all patients with left ventricular systolic dysfunction; improves symptoms and prolong life (see OPPOSITE). If cough is a problem an angiotensin receptor antagonist may be substituted (eg losartan 25mg/d; max 100mg PO).

    3 *β-blockers* (eg carvedilol) Recent randomized trials show that β-blockers ↓mortality in heart failure. These benefits appear to be additional to those of ACE-i in patients with heart failure due to LV dysfunction. Should be initiated after diuretic and ACE-i. Use with caution: 'start low and go slow'; if in doubt seek specialist advice first.

    4 *Spironolactone:* The RALES trial showed that spironolactone (25mg/24h PO) ↓mortality by 30% when added to conventional therapy. It should be initiated in patients who remain symptomatic despite optimal therapy as listed above. It improves endothelial dysfunction (↑nitric oxide bioactivity) and inhibits vascular angiotensin I/angiotensin II conversion. Spirono-lactone is K⁺-sparing, but there is little risk of significant hyperkalaemia, even when given with ACE-i.

    5 *Digoxin* improves symptoms even in those with sinus rhythm (data from the RADIANCE and other trials). Use it if diuretics, ACE-i, and β-blocker do not control symptoms, or in patients with AF. Dose: 0.125–0.25mg/24h PO. Monitor U&E and maintain K⁺ at 4–5mmol/L. Other inotropes are unhelpful in terms of outcome.

    6 *Vasodilators:* Long-acting nitrates ↓preload by causing venodilatation, eg isosorbide mononitrate MR 60mg/24h PO. 2ⁿᵈ line agents include arterial vasodilators, which reduce afterload (eg hydralazine, SE: drug-induced lupus) or α-blockers, which are combined arterial and venous vasodilators, eg prazosin. Vasodilators improve arterial haemodynamics and ↓mortality (so especially valuable if ACE-i is contraindicated).

Intractable heart failure Reassess the cause. Is he taking his drugs?—at maximum dose? Admit to hospital for:

- Strict bed rest.
- Metolazone & IV frusemide (p786).
- IV opiates and nitrates may relieve symptoms (p786).
- Daily weight & frequent U&E (K⁺↓).
- DVT prophylaxis: heparin 5000U/8h SC and TED stockings.
- *In extremis,* IV inotropes (p788) may be needed (it may be difficult to wean patients off them).
- Finally, consider a heart transplant. **NB:** reports of the Jarvik thumb-sized titanium axial-flow impeller pump seem promising. It is implanted in to the LV. A graft takes the blood to the descending aorta—making surgery hazardous.

Further reading:
B Pitt 1999 *NEJM* 1999 **341** 709 www.nejm.org/content/1999/0341/0010/0709.asp

How to start ACE-inhibitors

Check that there are no contraindications/cautions:
- Renal failure (serum creatinine >200µmol/L; but not an absolute CI)
- Hyperkalaemia: K$^+$ >5.5mmol/L
- Hyponatraemia: caution if <130mmol/L (relates to a poorer prognosis)
- Hypovolaemia
- Hypotension (systolic BP <90mmHg)
- AS or LV outflow tract obstruction
- Pregnancy or lactation
- Severe COPD or cor pulmonale (not an absolute CI)
- Renal artery stenosis[1] (Suspect if arteriopathic, eg cerebrovascular disease, IHD, peripheral vascular disease. ACE-inhibitors reduce GFR and may precipitate acute renal failure.)

Warn the patient about possible side effects:
- Hypotension, especially with 1st dose (so lie down after swallowing)
- Dry cough (1 : 10)
- Taste disturbance
- Hyperkalaemia
- Renal impairment
- Urticaria and angioneurotic oedema (<1 : 1,000)
- Rarely: proteinuria, leukopaenia, fatigue

Starting ACE-inhibitors:

Hypertensive patients can be safely started on ACE-inhibitors as outpatients. Warn them about postural hypotension and advise them to take the 1st dose on going to bed. Use a long-acting ACE-inhibitor, eg lisinopril 10mg PO per day, 2.5mg per day in the elderly.

Patients with CCF are best started on ACE-inhibitors under close medical supervision. Start with small dose and increase every 2wks until at target dose (equivalent of 30–35mg lisinopril a day) or side effects supervene (↓BP, ↑creatinine). Review in ~1wk for assessment; monitor U&E regularly. Patients on high doses of diuretics (>80mg frusemide a day) may need a reduction in their diuretic dose first—seek expert help.

139

---

1 If renovascular disease precludes the use of ACE-i and frusemide (=furosemide) is providing no answer, consider maximal vasodilatation with nitrates and hydralazine: seek expert advice.

Hypertension

▶Hypertension is a major risk factor for stroke and MI. It is usually asymptomatic, so screening is vital.

Defining hypertension Blood pressure has a skewed normal distribution within the population, and risk is continuously related to blood pressure. Therefore, it is impossible to define 'hypertension'. We choose to select a value above which risk is significantly increased, and the benefit of treatment is clear cut, see below. BP should be assessed over a period of time (don't rely on a single reading). The 'observation' period depends on the BP and the presence of other risk factors or end-organ damage.

Whom to treat All patients with malignant hypertension or a sustained pressure ≥160/100mmHg should be treated (see p141). For those ≥140/90, the decision depends on the risk of coronary events, presence of diabetes or end-organ damage; see the *Joint British Guidelines*, p141.

Systolic or diastolic pressure? For many years diastolic pressure was considered to be more important than systolic pressure. However, evidence from the Framingham and the MrFIT studies indicates that systolic pressure is the most important determinant of cardiovascular risk in the over 50s.

Systolic hypertension in the elderly: The age-related rise in systolic BP was considered part of the 'normal' ageing process, and isolated systolic hypertension (ISH) in the elderly was largely ignored. But evidence from 3 major studies indicates, beyond doubt, that benefits of treating are even greater than treating moderate hypertension in middle-aged patients.

'Malignant' hypertension: This refers to severe hypertension (eg systolic >200, diastolic >130mmHg) in conjunction with bilateral retinal haemorrhages and exudates; papilloedema may or may not be present. Symptoms are common, eg headache ± visual disturbance. Alone it requires urgent treatment. However, it may precipitate acute renal failure, heart failure, or encephalopathy, which are hypertensive emergencies. Untreated, 90% die in 1yr; treated, 70% survive 5yrs. Pathological hallmark is fibrinoid necrosis. It is more common in younger patients and in Blacks. Look hard for any underlying cause.

Causes

Essential hypertension (primary, cause unknown). ~95% of cases.

Secondary hypertension. ~5% of cases. Causes include:

- *Renal disease:* The most common secondary cause. ¾ are from *intrinsic renal disease:* glomerulonephritis, polyarteritis nodosa (PAN), systemic sclerosis, chronic pyelonephritis, or polycystic kidneys. ¼ are due to *renovascular disease,* most frequently atheromatous (elderly ♂ cigarette smokers, eg with peripheral vascular disease) or rarely fibromuscular dysplasia (young ♀), p282.
- *Endocrine disease:* Cushing's (p310) and Conn's syndromes (p314), phaeochromocytoma (p314), acromegaly, hyperparathyroidism.
- *Others:* Coarctation, pregnancy (OHCS p96), steroids, MAOI, 'the Pill'.

Signs & symptoms Usually asymptomatic (except malignant hypertension, above). Always examine the CVS system fully and check for retinopathy. Are there features of an underlying cause (phaeochromocytoma, p314 etc.), signs of renal disease, radiofemoral delay, or weak femoral pulses (coarctation), renal bruits, palpable kidneys, or Cushing's syndrome? Look for end-organ damage: LVH, retinopathy & proteinuria—indicates severity and duration of hypertension and associated with a poorer prognosis.

Investigations Basic: U&E, creatinine, cholesterol, glucose, ECG, urine analysis (for protein, blood). *Specific* (exclude a secondary cause): renal ultrasound, renal arteriography, 24-h urinary VMA × 3 (p314), urinary free cortisol (p311), renin, and aldosterone. ECHO and 24-h ambulatory BP monitoring may be helpful in some cases eg white coat or borderline hypertension.

Hypertensive retinopathy

Grade
I   Tortuous arteries with thick shiny walls (silver or copper wiring)
II A–V nipping (narrowing where arteries cross veins)
III Flame haemorrhages and cotton wool spots
IV Papilloedema.

Measuring blood pressure

- Use the correct size cuff. The width of the cuff should be at least 40% of the arm circumference. The bladder should be centred over the brachial artery, and the cuff applied snugly. Support the arm in a horizontal position at mid-sternal level.
- Inflate the cuff while palpating the brachial artery, until the pulse disappears. This provides an estimate of systolic pressure.
- Inflate the cuff until 30mmHg above systolic pressure, then place stethoscope over the brachial artery. Deflate the cuff at 2mmHg/s.
- *Systolic pressure:* The appearance of sustained repetitive tapping sounds (Korotkoff I).
- *Diastolic pressure:* Usually the disappearance of sounds (Korotkoff V). However, in some individuals (eg pregnant women) sounds are present until the zero-point. In this case, the muffling of sounds, Korotkoff IV, should be used. For children, see *OHCS* p304.

British Hypertension Society 2004 guidelines[1]

www.hyp.ac.uk/bhs/resources/guidelines.htm

Measure BP and other risk factors (plasma lipids, glucose)

SBP ≥160 and/or DBP ≥100	SBP 140–159 and/or DBP 90–99		SBP <140 and DBP <90
Lifestyle change + drugs if BP sustained at these levels on repeated measurements	CHD + stroke risk* ≥20% over 10yrs or target organ damage or diabetes	CHD + stroke risk* <20% and no target organ damage	Reassess in 5yrs Give advice on healthy lifestyle
	↓ Lifestyle and drug(s) if BP sustained on repeat measurements	↓ Lifestyle and reassess every year	

All values are mmHg; SBP=systolic; DBP=diastolic.

In diabetes mellitus, aim for <130/80mmHg (<125/75 if proteinuria).
In non-diabetics, the treatment goal is 140/85.

*To quantify this, see www.hyp.ac.uk/bhs/resources/guidelines.htm. **NB:** most sources older than 2004 just tabulate CHD risk, not CHD + stroke. The new CHD + stroke threshold of 20% ≈ 15% for CHD alone.

Examples of target (end-organ) damage:
- LVH
- PMH myocardial infarct
- PMH stroke/TIA
- Peripheral vascular disease
- PMH angina
- Renal failure.

1 See British Cardiac Society & British Hyperlipidaemia Association & British Hypertension Society (BHS) & British Diabetic Association 1998 *Heart* **80** suppl 2; see also USA Joint National Committee regimen (JNC 7) 2003 *JAMA* **289** 2560–72; BHS-IV *2004 Guidelines, BMJ* 2004 **328** 634.

Hypertension—management

Look for and treat underlying causes (eg renal disease, alcohol↑: see p140).

Treatment goal For most patients aim for BP <140/85,[1] but 130/80 in patients with diabetes. Reduce blood pressure gradually; a rapid reduction can be fatal, especially in the context of stroke.

Lifestyle changes ↓Concomitant risk factors: stop smoking; low-fat diet. Reduce alcohol and salt intake; increase exercise; reduce weight if obese.

Drugs Explain the need for long-term treatment. Essential hypertension is not 'curable'. The recent ALLHAT study suggests that adequate blood pressure reduction is more important than the specific drug used[38]. However, ACE-i may provide additional renal benefit if co-existing diabetes.

- *Thiazide diuretics:* Are 1st choice,[39] eg bendrofluazide (=bendroflumethiazide) 2.5mg/24h PO. Increasing the dose brings no benefit, and produces more SEs: hypokalaemia, hyponatraemia, postural hypotension, impotence.
- *β-blockers:* Eg atenolol 50mg/24h PO. Higher doses provide little additional benefit. SE: bronchospasm, heart failure, cold peripheries, lethargy, impotence. CI: asthma; caution in heart failure.
- *ACE-i:* Eg lisinopril 2.5–20mg/24h PO (max 40mg/d) or enalapril. ACE-i may be 1st choice if co-existing LVF, or in diabetics with microalbuminuria (p288) or proteinuria. SE: cough, K⁺↑, renal failure, angio-oedema. CI renal artery stenosis, AS.
- *Ca²⁺-channel antagonist:* Eg nifedipine MR 30–60mg/24h PO. SE: flushing, fatigue, gum hyperplasia, ankle oedema. Avoid short-acting drugs.
- *Others:* Angiotensin receptor antagonists (eg losartan), methyldopa (used in pregnancy), and doxazosin (an α-blocker). For refractory cases: clonidine, minoxidil, or hydralazine (causes a tachycardia unless given with a β-blocker and may cause an SLE-like syndrome).

The 4 main classes of agent happen to start with ABCD. There is some evidence that in monotherapy A&B are more effective in younger people and C&D in older individuals (and Blacks). This may guide initial therapy, and if one drug fails, switch between groups. When adding drugs, it makes sense to combine A or B with C or D eg a thiazide and ACE-i, or β-blocker and Ca²⁺—channel antagonist—the 'ABCD rule'. Remember that most drugs take 4–8 wks to produce their maximum effect, and don't assess efficacy on the basis of a single clinic blood pressure measurement.

Malignant hypertension Most patients can be managed with oral therapy, except for those with encephalopathy. The aim is for a controlled reduction in blood pressure over days, not hours. Avoid sudden drops in BP as cerebral autoregulation is poor (so stroke risk↑).

- Bed rest; start a loop diuretic, eg frusemide (=furosemide) 40–80mg daily ± a thiazide. There is no ideal antihypertensive therapy, but labetalol, atenolol, or long-acting calcium blockers may be used orally.
- Encephalopathy (headache, focal CNS signs, seizures, coma): aim to reduce blood pressure to ~110mmHg diastolic over 4h. Admit to monitored area. Insert intra-arterial line for pressure monitoring. Frusemide 40–80mg IV; then either IV labetalol (eg 50mg IV over 1min, repeated every 5min, max 200mg), or sodium nitroprusside infusion (0.5µg/kg/min IVI titrated up to 8µg/kg/min, eg 50mg in 1L dextrose 5%; expect to give 100–200mL/h for a few hours only, to avoid cyanide risk).

▶Never use sublingual (SL) nifedipine to reduce BP (it can cause an uncontrollable drop in BP and stroke).[40]

1 The lower the better, but *you cannot tell what is far enough without going too far*—see British Hypertension Society 2004 (*BHS-IV*) guidelines *BMJ* 2004 **328** 634. See also M Alderman 2000 *Lancet* **355** 159 & I Whie *Lancet* **356** 682 for further discussion

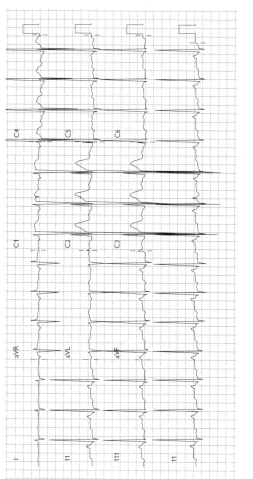

ECG 8—left ventricular hypertrophy—this is from a patient with malignant hypertension—note the sum of the S-wave in C2 and R-wave in C6 is greater than 35mm.

Rheumatic fever

This systemic infection is still common in the Third World, although increasingly rare in the West. Peak incidence: 5–15yrs. Tends to recur unless prevented. Pharyngeal infection with Lancefield Group A β-haemolytic streptococci triggers rheumatic fever 2–4wks later, in the susceptible 2% of the population. An antibody to the carbohydrate cell wall of the streptococcus cross-reacts with valve tissue (antigenic mimicry) and may cause permanent damage to the heart valves.

Diagnosis Use the *revised Jones criteria*. There must be evidence of recent strep infection plus 2 major criteria, or 1 major + 2 minor.

Evidence of streptococcal infection:
• Recent streptococcal infection
• History of scarlet fever
• Positive throat swab
• Increase in ASOT >200U/mL
• Increase in DNase B titre.

Major criteria:
• *Carditis:* Tachycardia, murmurs (mitral or AR, Carey Coombs' murmur, p46), pericardial rub, CCF, cardiomegaly, conduction defects (45–70%). An apical systolic murmur may be the only sign.[41]
• *Arthritis:* A migratory, 'flitting' polyarthritis; usually affects the larger joints (75%).
• *Subcutaneous nodules:* Small, mobile painless nodules on extensor surfaces of joints and spine (2–20%).
• *Erythema marginatum:* Geographical-type rash with red, raised edges and clear centre; occurs mainly on trunk, thighs, arms in 2–10% (p428).
• *Sydenham's chorea* (St Vitus' dance): Occurs late in 10%. Unilateral or bilateral involuntary semi-purposeful movements. May be preceded by emotional lability and uncharacteristic behaviour.[42]

Minor criteria:
• Fever
• Raised ESR or CRP
• Arthralgia (but not if arthritis is one of the major criteria)
• Prolonged P–R interval (but not if carditis is major criterion)
• Previous rheumatic fever.

Management
• Bed rest until CRP normal for 2wks (may be 3 months).
• Benzylpenicillin 0.6–1.2g IM stat then penicillin V 250mg/6h PO.
• Analgesia for carditis/arthritis: Aspirin 100mg/kg/d PO in divided doses (maximum 8g/d) for 2d, then 70mg/kg/d for 6wks. Monitor salicylate level. Toxicity causes tinnitus, hyperventilation, metabolic acidosis. Alternative: NSAIDs (p414).
• Steroids are thought not to have a major impact on sequelae, but they may improve symptoms.[43][44]
• Immobilize joints in severe arthritis.
• Haloperidol (0.5mg/8h PO) or diazepam for the chorea.

Prognosis 60% with carditis develop chronic rheumatic heart disease. This correlates with the severity of the carditis.[45] Acute attacks last an average of 3 months. Recurrence may be precipitated by further streptococcal infections, pregnancy, or use of the Pill. Cardiac sequelae affect mitral (70%), aortic (40%), tricuspid (10%), and pulmonary (2%) valves. Incompetent lesions develop during the attack, stenoses years later.

Secondary prophylaxis Penicillin V 250mg/12h PO until no longer at risk (>30yrs). Alternative: sulfadiazine 1g daily (0.5g if <30kg). Thereafter, give antibiotic prophylaxis for dental or other surgery (p154).

Mitral valve disease

Mitral stenosis *Causes:* Rheumatic; congenital, mucopolysaccharidoses, endocardial fibroelastosis, malignant carcinoid, prosthetic valve.

Presentation: Dyspnoea; fatigue; palpitations; chest pain; systemic emboli; haemoptysis; chronic bronchitis-like picture ± complications (below).

Signs: Malar (ie cheek) flush; low-volume pulse; AF common; tapping, undisplaced, apex beat (palpable S_1). On auscultation: loud S_1; opening snap (pliable valve); rumbling mid-diastolic murmur (heard best in expiration, as the patient lies on their left side). Graham Steell murmur (p46) may occur. *Severity:* The more severe the stenosis, the longer the diastolic murmur, and the closer the opening snap is to S_2.

Tests: ECG: AF; P-mitrale if in sinus rhythm; RVH; progressive RAD. *CXR:* left atrial enlargement; pulmonary oedema; mitral valve calcification. *Echocardiography* is diagnostic. Significant stenosis exists if the valve orifice is $<1\text{cm}^2/\text{m}^2$ body surface area. Indications for *cardiac catheterization:* previous valvotomy; signs of other valve disease; angina; severe pulmonary hypertension; calcified mitral valve.

Management: If in AF, use digoxin (p138); *rate control is crucial;* (add a β-blocker if needed to keep the pulse rate <90); anticoagulate with warfarin (p649). Diuretics ↓preload and pulmonary venous congestion. If this fails to control symptoms, balloon valvuloplasty (if pliable, non-calcified valve), open mitral valvotomy or valve replacement. SBE/IE prophylaxis for dental or surgical procedures (p154). Oral penicillin as prophylaxis against recurrent rheumatic fever if <30yrs old (p144).

Complications: Pulmonary hypertension; emboli, pressure from large LA on local structures, eg hoarseness (recurrent laryngeal nerve), dysphagia (oesophagus), bronchial obstruction; infective endocarditis (rare).

Mitral regurgitation *Causes:* Functional (LV dilatation); annular calcification (elderly); rheumatic fever, infective endocarditis, mitral valve prolapse, ruptured chordae tendinae; papillary muscle dysfunction/rupture; connective tissue disorders (Ehlers–Danlos, Marfan's); cardiomyopathy; congenital (may be associated with other defects, eg ASD, AV canal); appetite suppressants (eg fenfluramine, phentermine).

Symptoms: Dyspnoea; fatigue; palpitations; infective endocarditis. *Signs:* AF; displaced, hyperdynamic apex; RV heave; soft S_1; split S_2; loud P_2 (pulmonary hypertension) pansystolic murmur at apex radiating to axilla. *Severity:* The more severe, the larger the left ventricle.

Tests: ECG: AF ± P-mitrale if in sinus rhythm (may mean left atrial size↑); LVH. *CXR:* big LA & LV; mitral valve calcification; pulmonary oedema.

Echocardiogram to assess LV function (trans-oesophageal to assess severity and suitability for repair rather than replacement). *Doppler echo* to assess size and site of regurgitant jet. *Cardiac catheterization* to confirm diagnosis, exclude other valve disease, assess coronary artery disease.

Management: Digoxin for fast AF. Anticoagulate if: AF; history of embolism; prosthetic valve; additional mitral stenosis. Diuretics improve symptoms. Surgery for deteriorating symptoms; aim to repair or replace the valve before LV irreversibly impaired. Antibiotics to prevent endocarditis.

Mitral valve prolapse *Prevalence:* ~5%. Occurs alone or with: ASD, patent ductus arteriosus, cardiomyopathy, Turner's syndrome, Marfan's syndrome, osteogenesis imperfecta, pseudoxanthoma elasticum, WPW (p128). *Symptoms:* Asymptomatic—or atypical chest pain and palpitations. *Signs:* Mid-systolic click and/or a late systolic murmur. *Complications:* Mitral regurgitation, cerebral emboli, arrhythmias, sudden death. *Tests: Echocardiography* is diagnostic. ECG may show inferior T wave inversion. *Treatment:* β-blockers may help palpitations and chest pain. Give endocarditis prophylaxis (p154), if co-existing mitral regurgitation.

Aortic valve disease

Aortic stenosis (AS) *Causes:* Senile calcification is the commonest. Others: congenital (bicuspid valve, William's syndrome, p157).

Presentation: Angina; dyspnoea; dizziness; faints; systemic emboli if infective endocarditis; CCF; sudden death. *Signs:* Slow rising pulse with narrow pulse pressure (feel for diminished and delayed carotid upstroke—'parvus et tardus'); heaving, undisplaced apex beat; LV heave; aortic thrill; ejection systolic murmur (heard at the base, left sternal edge and the aortic area, radiates to the carotids). As stenosis worsens, A_2 is increasingly delayed, giving first a single S_2 and then reversed splitting. But this sign is rare. More common is a quiet A_2. In severe AS, A_2 may be inaudible (calcified valve). There may be an ejection click (pliable valve) or an audible S_4 (said to occur more commonly with bicuspid valves, but not in all populations).

Tests: ECG: P-mitrale, LVH with strain pattern; LAD (left anterior hemiblock); poor R wave progression; LBBB or complete AV block (calcified ring). CXR: LVH; calcified aortic valve; post-stenotic dilatation of ascending aorta. *Echo* is diagnostic (p110). *Doppler echo* can estimate the gradient across valves: severe stenosis if gradient ≥50mmHg and valve area <0.5cm². If the aortic jet velocity is >4m/s (or is increasing by >0.3m/s per year) risk of complications is increased. *Cardiac catheter* can assess: valve gradient; LV function; coronary artery disease; the aortic root.

Differential diagnosis: Hypertrophic obstructive cardiomyopathy (HOCM).

Management: Symptomatic patients have a poor prognosis: 2–3yr survival if angina/syncope; 1–2yr survival with cardiac failure. Prompt valve replacement (p150) is recommended. In asymptomatic patients with severe AS and a deteriorating ECG, valve replacement is also recommended. If the patient is not medically fit for surgery, percutaneous valvuloplasty may be attempted. Endocarditis prophylaxis (p154).

Aortic sclerosis is senile degeneration of the valve. There is an ejection systolic murmur, no carotid radiation, and a normal pulse and S_2.

Aortic regurgitation (AR) *Causes: Congenital. Valve disease:* rheumatic fever; infective endocarditis, rheumatoid arthritis; SLE; pseudoxanthoma elasticum; appetite suppressants (eg fenfluramine, phentermine). *Aortic root disease:* hypertension; trauma; aortic dissection; seronegative arthritides (ankylosing spondylitis, Reiter's syndrome, psoriatic arthropathy); Marfan's syndrome; osteogenesis imperfecta; syphilitic aortitis.

Symptoms: Dyspnoea; palpitations; cardiac failure. *Signs:* Collapsing (water-hammer) pulse; wide pulse pressure; displaced, hyperdynamic apex beat; high-pitched early diastolic murmur (heard best in expiration, with patient sitting forward). Associated signs: Corrigan's sign (carotid pulsation); de Musset's sign (head nodding); Quincke's sign (capillary pulsations in nail beds); Duroziez's sign (femoral diastolic murmur as blood flows backwards in diastole); Traube's sign ('pistol shot' sound over femoral arteries). In severe AR, an Austin Flint murmur may be heard (p46).

Investigations: ECG: LVH. CXR: cardiomegaly; dilated ascending aorta; pulmonary oedema. *Echocardiography* is diagnostic. *Cardiac catheterization* to assess: severity of lesion; anatomy of aortic root; LV function; coronary artery disease; other valve disease.

Management: Indications for surgery: increasing symptoms; enlarging heart on CXR/echo; ECG deterioration (T wave inversion in lateral leads); infective endocarditis refractory to medical therapy. Aim to replace the valve before significant LV dysfunction occurs. Endocarditis prophylaxis (p154).

Right heart valve disease

Tricuspid regurgitation *Causes:* Functional (pulmonary hypertension); rheumatic fever; infective endocarditis (IV drug abusers); carcinoid syndrome; congenital (eg ASD, AV canal, Ebstein's anomaly, *OHCS* p746). *Symptoms:* Fatigue; hepatic pain on exertion; ascites; oedema. *Signs:* Giant *v* waves and prominent *y* descent in JVP (p42); RV heave; pansystolic murmur, heard best at lower sternal edge in inspiration; pulsatile hepatomegaly; jaundice; ascites. *Management:* Treat underlying cause. Drugs: diuretics, digoxin, ACE-inhibitors. Valve replacement (20% operative mortality).

Tricuspid stenosis *Cause:* Rheumatic fever; almost always occurs with mitral or aortic valve disease. *Symptoms:* Fatigue, ascites, oedema. *Signs:* Giant *a* wave and slow *y* descent in JVP (p42); opening snap, early diastolic murmur heard at the left sternal edge in inspiration. *Diagnosis:* Doppler echo. *Treatment:* Diuretics; surgical repair.

Pulmonary stenosis *Causes:* Usually congenital (Turner's syndrome, Noonan's syndrome, William's syndrome, Fallot's tetralogy, rubella). Acquired causes: rheumatic fever, carcinoid syndrome. *Symptoms:* Dyspnoea; fatigue; oedema; ascites. *Signs:* Dysmorphic facies (congenital causes); prominent *a* wave in JVP; RV heave. In mild stenosis, there is an ejection click, ejection systolic murmur (which radiates to the left shoulder); widely split S_2. In severe stenosis, the murmur becomes longer and obscures A_2. P_2 becomes softer and may be inaudible. *Tests:* ECG: RAD, P-pulmonale, RVH, RBBB. CXR: post-stenotic dilatation of pulmonary artery; oligaemic lung fields; RV hypertrophy; right atrial hypertrophy. Cardiac catheterization is diagnostic. *Treatment:* Pulmonary valvuloplasty or valvotomy.

Pulmonary regurgitation is caused by any cause of pulmonary hypertension (p204). A decrescendo murmur is heard in early diastole at the left sternal edge (the Graham Steell murmur).

Cardiac surgery

Valvuloplasty can be used in mitral or pulmonary stenosis (pliable, noncalcified valve, no regurgitation). A balloon catheter is inserted across the valve and inflated.

Valvotomy Closed valvotomy is rarely performed now. Open valvotomy is performed under cardiopulmonary bypass through a median stenotomy.

Valve replacements *Mechanical valves* may be of the ball-cage (Starr–Edwards), tilting disc (Bjork–Shiley), or double tilting disc (St Jude) type. These valves are very durable but the risk of thromboembolism is high; patients require lifelong anticoagulation. *Xenografts* are made from porcine valves or pericardium. These valves are less durable and may require replacement at 8–10yrs. Anticoagulation is not required unless there is AF. *Homografts* are cadaveric valves. They are particularly useful in young patients and in the replacement of infected valves. *Complications of prosthetic valves:* systemic embolism, infective endocarditis, haemolysis, structural valve failure, arrhythmias.

CABG See OPPOSITE.

Cardiac transplantation Consider this when cardiac disease is *severely* curtailing quality of life, and survival is not expected beyond 6–12 months. Refer to a specialist centre.

Coronary artery bypass grafts

Indications for CABG: to improve survival
Left mainstem disease
Triple vessel disease involving proximal
  part of the left anterior descending

To relieve symptoms
Angina unresponsive to drugs
Unstable angina (sometimes)
If angioplasty is unsuccessful

NB: When CABG and percutaneous coronary intervention (PCI, eg angio-plasty) are both clinically valid options, NICE recommends that the avail-ability of new stent technology should push the decision towards PCI.

Procedure: Surgery is planned in the light of angiograms. Not all stenoses are bypassable. The heart is stopped and blood pumped artificially by a machine outside the body (cardiac bypass). (Minimally invasive thora-cotomies not requiring this are well-described,[49] but have not yet been validated in randomized trials.)

The patient's own saphenous vein or internal mammary artery is used as the graft. Several grafts may be placed.

>50% of vein grafts close in 10yrs (low-dose aspirin helps prevent this). Internal mammary artery grafts last longer (but may cause chest-wall numbness).

After CABG: If angina persists or recurs (from poor run-off from the graft, distal disease, new atheroma, or graft occlusion) restart anti-anginal drugs, and consider angioplasty (repeat surgery is dangerous). Mood, sex, and intellectual problems[50] are common early. Rehabilitation helps:

- Exercise: walk→cycle→swim→jog
- Drive at 1 month: no need to tell DVLA if non-HGV licences, p162
- Get back to work eg at 3 months
- Attend to: smoking; BP; lipids
- Aspirin 75mg/24h PO forever.

Infective endocarditis

▶ *Fever + new murmur = endocarditis until proven otherwise.*

Classification

• 50% of all endocarditis occurs on *normal valves*. It follows an *acute course*, and presents with acute heart failure.

• Endocarditis on *abnormal valves* tends to run a *subacute course*. Predisposing cardiac lesions: aortic or mitral valve disease; tricuspid valves in IV drug users; coarctation; patent ductus arteriosus; VSD; prosthetic valves. Endocarditis on prosthetic valves may be 'early' (acquired at the time of surgery, poor prognosis) or 'late' (acquired haematogenously).

Causes *Bacteria:* Any cause of bacteraemia exposes valves to the risk of bacterial colonization (eg dental work; UTI; urinary catheterization; cystoscopy; respiratory infection; endoscopy (controversial); colonic carcinoma; gall bladder disease; skin disease; IV cannulation; surgery; abortion; fractures). Quite often, no cause is found. *Streptococcus viridans* is the commonest (35–50%). Others: enterococci; *Staphylococcus aureus/epidermidis*; diphtheroids and microaerophilic streptococci. Rarely: HACEK group of Gram –ve bacteria (*Haemophilus–Actinobacillus–Cardiobacterium–Eikenella–Kingella*); *Coxiella burnetii*; *Chlamydia*. *Fungi:* These include *Candida, Aspergillus,* and *Histoplasma. Other causes:* SLE (Libman–Sacks endocarditis); malignancy.

Clinical features The patient may present with any of the following: *Signs of infection:* Fever, rigors, night sweats, malaise, weight loss, anaemia, splenomegaly, and clubbing. *Cardiac lesions:* Any new murmur, or a change in the nature of a pre-existing murmur, should raise the suspicion of endocarditis. Vegetations may cause valve destruction, and severe regurgitation, or valve obstruction. An aortic root abscess causes prolongation of the P–R interval, and may lead to complete AV block. LVF is a common cause of death. *Immune complex deposition:* Vasculitis (p424) may affect any vessel. Microscopic haematuria is common; glomerulonephritis and acute renal failure may occur. Roth spots (boat-shaped retinal haemorrhage with pale centre); splinter haemorrhages (on finger or toe nails); Osler's nodes (painful pulp infarcts in fingers or toes) and Janeway lesions (painless palmar or plantar macules) are pathognomonic. *Embolic phenomena:* Emboli may cause abscesses in the relevant organ, eg brain, heart, kidney, spleen, GI tract. In right-sided endocarditis, pulmonary abscesses may occur.

Diagnosis The *Duke* criteria⬚ for definitive diagnosis of endocarditis are given OPPOSITE. *Blood cultures:* Take 3 sets at different times and from different sites at peak fever. 85–90% are diagnosed from the first two sets; 10% are culture-negative. *Blood tests:* Normochromic, normocytic anaemia, neutrophil leucocytosis, high ESR/CRP. Also check U&E, Mg^{2+}, LFTs. *Urinalysis* for microscopic haematuria. *CXR* (cardiomegaly) and *ECG* (prolonged P–R interval) at regular intervals. *Echocardiography* TTE (p110) may show vegetations, but only if >2mm. TOE (p110) is more sensitive, and better for visualizing mitral lesions and possible development of aortic root abscess.

Management Liaise early with a microbiologist and a cardiologist.

• Antibiotics: see p153, OPPOSITE.

• Consider surgery if: heart failure, valvular obstruction; repeated emboli; fungal endocarditis; persistent bacteraemia; myocardial abscess; unstable infected prosthetic valve.⬚

Prognosis 30% mortality with staphylococci; 14% with bowel organisms; 6% with sensitive streptococci.

Duke criteria for infective endocarditis

Major criteria:
- Positive blood culture:
  - typical organism in 2 separate cultures or
  - persistently +ve blood cultures, eg 3, >12h apart (or majority if ≥4)
- Endocardium involved:
  - positive echocardiogram (vegetation, abscess, dehiscence of prosthetic valve) or
  - new valvular regurgitation (change in murmur not sufficient).

Minor criteria:
- Predisposition (cardiac lesion; IV drug abuse)
- Fever >38°C
- Vascular/immunological signs
- Positive blood culture that do not meet major criteria
- Positive echocardiogram that does not meet major criteria.

How to diagnose: Definite infective endocarditis: 2 major **or** 1 major and 3 minor **or** all 5 minor criteria (if no major criterion is met).

Antibiotic therapy for infective endocarditis

- Consult a microbiologist early. The following are guidelines only:
- *Empirical therapy:* benzylpenicillin[1] 1.2g/4h IV + gentamicin, eg 80mg/12h IV (p710). If acute, add flucloxacillin 2g/6h IV to cover staphylococci.
- *Streptococci:* benzylpenicillin[1] 1.2g/4h IV for 2–4wks; then amoxicillin 1g/8h PO for 2wks. Monitor minimum inhibitory concentration (MIC) and add gentamicin, eg 80mg/12h IV if MIC >0.01ng/mL. Monitor gentamicin levels (p710).
- *Enterococci:* amoxicillin[1] 1g/6h IV + gentamicin, eg 80mg/12h IV for 4wks. Monitor gentamicin levels (p710).
- *Staphylococci:* flucloxacillin[1] 2g/6h IV + gentamicin 80mg/12h IV. Treat for 6–8wks; stop gentamicin after 1wk.
- *Coxiella:* doxycycline 100mg/12h PO indefinitely + co-trimoxazole, rifampicin, or ciprofloxacin.
- *Fungi:* flucytosine 3g/6h IVI over 30 minutes followed by fluconazole 50mg/24h PO (a higher dose may be needed). Amphotericin if flucytosine resistance or *Aspergillus*. Miconazole if renal function is poor.

153

[1] For penicillin allergy, use vancomycin 1g/12h IV.

Prevention of endocarditis

Anyone with congenital heart disease, acquired valve disease, or prosthetic valves is at risk of infective endocarditis and should take prophylactic antibiotics before procedures which may result in bacteraemia. The recommendations of the *British Cardiac Society/Royal College of Physicians* are:

Which conditions?

Prophylaxis recommended
Prosthetic valve(s)
Previous endocarditis
Septal defects
Mitral prolapse with regurgitation
Acquired valve disease

Prophylaxis not recommended
Mitral prolapse (no regurgitation)
Functional/innocent murmur

Which procedures?

Prophylaxis recommended
Dental procedures[1]
Upper respiratory tract surgery
Oesophageal dilatation
Sclerotherapy of varices
Surgery/instrumentation of lower
  bowel, gall bladder, or GU tract

Prophylaxis not recommended
Flexible bronchoscopy
Diagnostic upper GI endoscopy
TOE (p110)
Caesarean or normal delivery
Cardiac catheterization
  (unless high-risk patient)

Which regimen?

• *Dental procedures*
  Local or no anaesthetic: Amoxicillin 3g PO, 1h before the procedure. Alternative (if penicillin allergy or >1 dose of penicillin in previous month): clindamycin 600mg PO.

  General anaesthetic, no special risk: amoxicillin 1g IV at induction, followed by 500mg PO 6h later *or* amoxicillin 3g PO 4h before induction, followed by 3g PO as soon as possible after procedure.

  General anaesthetic, special risk patients (prosthetic valve or previous endocarditis): amoxicillin 1g IV + gentamicin 120mg IV at induction, followed by amoxicillin 500mg PO 6h later. *Alternatives* (if penicillin allergy or >1 dose of penicillin in previous month): vancomycin 1g IV over 100min (+gentamicin 120mg IV at induction) *or* teicoplanin 400mg IV (+gentamicin 120mg IV at induction) *or* clindamycin 300mg IV over 10min at induction (followed by clindamycin 150mg IV or PO 6h later).

• *Upper respiratory tract procedures*
  As for dental procedures. Post-op dose may be given parenterally if swallowing is painful.

• *Genitourinary procedures*
  Antibiotics as for special risk dental patients above (except clindamycin). Prophylactic antibiotics should also cover any UTI.

• *Gastrointestinal, obstetric, and gynaecological procedures*
  Prophylaxis is only indicated if prosthetic valve or previous endocarditis; then as for genitourinary procedures.

---

1 Dental procedures involving extractions, scaling, polishing, or gingival surgery.

Diseases of heart muscle

Acute myocarditis *Causes:* Inflamed myocardium from viruses (coxsackie, polio, HIV, Lassa fever); bacteria (Clostridia, diphtheria, Meningococcus, Mycoplasma, psittacosis); spirochaetes (Leptospirosis, syphilis, Lyme disease); protozoa (Chagas' disease); drugs; toxins; vasculitis, p424.

Signs & symptoms: Fatigue, dyspnoea, chest pain, palpitations, tachycardia, soft S_1, S_4 gallop (p44).

Tests: ECG: ST segment elevation/depression, T wave inversion, atrial arrhythmias, transient AV block. Serology may be helpful.

Management: Treat the underlying cause. Supportive measures. Patients may recover or get intractable heart failure (p138).

Dilated cardiomyopathy A dilated, flabby heart of unknown cause. Associations: alcohol, ↑BP, haemochromatosis, viral infection, autoimmune, peri- or postpartum, thyrotoxicosis, congenital (X-linked). *Prevalence:* 0.2%. *Signs:*

Presentation: Fatigue, dyspnoea, pulmonary oedema, RVF, emboli, AF, VT. *Signs:* ↑Pulse, ↓BP, ↑JVP, displaced, diffuse apex, S_3 gallop, mitral or tricuspid regurgitation (MR/TR), pleural effusion, oedema, jaundice, hepatomegaly, ascites.

Tests: CXR: cardiomegaly, pulmonary oedema. ECG: tachycardia, non-specific T wave changes, poor R wave progression. *Echo:* globally dilated hypokinetic heart with low ejection fraction. Look for MR, TR, LV mural thrombus.

Management: Bed rest, diuretics, digoxin, ACE-inhibitor, anticoagulation. Consider cardiac transplantation. *Mortality:* Variable, eg 40% in 2yrs.

Hypertrophic cardiomyopathy HOCM ≈ LV outflow tract (LVOT) obstruction from asymmetric septal hypertrophy.

Prevalence: 0.2%. Autosomal dominant inheritance, but 50% are sporadic. 70% have mutations in genes encoding β-myosin, α-tropomyosin, and troponin T. May present at any age. Ask about family history or sudden death.

The patient: Angina; dyspnoea; palpitation; syncope; sudden death (VF is amenable to implantable defibrillators). Jerky pulse; *a* wave in JVP; double apex beat; systolic thrill at lower left sternal edge; harsh ejection systolic murmur.

Tests: ECG: LVH; progressive T wave inversion; deep Q waves (inferior + lateral leads); AF; WPW syndrome (p128); ventricular ectopics; VT. *Echo:* asymmetrical septal hypertrophy; small LV cavity with hypercontractile posterior wall; midsystolic closure of aortic valve; systolic anterior movement of mitral valve. *Cardiac catheterization* may provoke VT. It helps assess: severity of gradient; coronary artery disease or mitral regurgitation. Electrophysiological studies may be needed (WPW). Exercise test ± Holter monitor to risk stratify.

Management: β-blockers or verapamil for symptoms (p116). Amiodarone 100–200mg/day for arrhythmias (AF, VT). Anticoagulate for paroxysmal AF or systemic emboli. Dual-chamber pacing (p134) is used if symptomatic despite drugs. Septal myomectomy (surgical, or chemical, with alcohol, to ↓LV outflow tract gradient) is reserved for those with severe symptoms. Consider implantable defibrillator.

Mortality: 5.9%/yr if <14yrs; 2.5%/yr if >14yrs. *Poor prognostic factors:* age <14yrs or syncope at presentation; family history of HOCM/sudden death.

Restrictive cardiomyopathy *Causes:* Amyloidosis; haemochromatosis; sarcoidosis; scleroderma; Löffler's eosinophilic endocarditis, endomyocardial fibrosis. *Presentation* is like constrictive pericarditis (p158). Features of RVF predominate: ↑JVP, with prominent x and y descents; hepatomegaly; oedema; ascites. *Diagnosis:* Cardiac catheterization.

Cardiac myxoma Rare benign cardiac tumour. Prevalence ≤5/10,000, ♀:♂ ≈ 2:1. Usually sporadic, may be familial (autosomal-dominant). It may mimic infective endocarditis (fever, weight loss, clubbing, ↑ESR), or mitral stenosis (left atrial obstruction, systemic emboli, AF). A 'tumour plop' may be heard, and signs may vary according to posture. *Tests:* Echocardiography. *Treatment:* Excision.

The heart in various, mostly rare, systemic diseases

This list reminds us to look at the heart *and* the whole patient, not just in exams (where those with odd syndromes congregate), but always.

Acromegaly: (p324) BP↑; LVH; hypertrophic cardiomyopathy; high output cardiac failure; coronary artery disease.

Amyloidosis: (p668) Restrictive cardiomyopathy.

Ankylosing spondylitis: Conduction defects; AV block; AR.

Behçet's disease: (p718) AR; arterial ± venous thrombi.

Cushing's syndrome: (p310) Hypertension.

Down's syndrome: (OHCS p210) ASD; VSD; mitral regurgitation.

Ehlers-Danlos syndrome: (OHCS p746) Mitral valve prolapse + hyperelastic skin ± aneurysms and GI bleeds. Joints are loose and hypermobile; mutations exist, eg in genes for procollagen (COL3A1); there are 6 types.

Friedreich's ataxia: (p722) Hypertrophic cardiomyopathy.

Haemochromatosis: (p234) AF; cardiomyopathy.

Holt-Oram syndrome: ASD or VSD with upper limb defects. ♙

Human immunodeficiency virus: (p578) Myocarditis; dilated cardio-myopathy; effusion; ventricular arrhythmias; SBE/IE; non-infective thrombotic (marantic) endocarditis; RVF (pulmonary hypertension); me-tastatic Kaposi's sarcoma.

Hypothyroidism: (p306) Sinus bradycardia; low pulse pressure; pericardial effusion; coronary artery disease; low voltage ECG.

Kawasaki disease: (OHCS p750) Coronary arteritis similar to PAN; com-moner than *rheumatic fever* (p144) as a cause of acquired heart disease.

Klinefelter's syndrome:♂ (OHCS p752) ASD. Psychopathy; learning difficulties; libido↓; gynaecomastia; sparse facial hair and small firm testes. XXY.

Marfan's syndrome: (p730) Mitral valve prolapse; AR; aortic dissection. Look for long fingers and a high-arched palate.

Noonan's syndrome: (OHCS p754) ASD; pulmonary stenosis ± low-set ears.

PAN: (p425) Small and medium vessel vasculitis + angina; MI; arrhythmias; CCF; pericarditis and conduction defects.

Rheumatoid nodules: Conduction defects; pericarditis; LV dysfunction; AR; coronary arteritis. Look for arthritis signs, p414.

Sarcoidosis: (p198) Infiltrating granulomas may cause complete AV block; ventricular or supraventricular tachycardia; myocarditis; CCF; restrictive cardiomyopathy. ECG may show Q waves.

Syphilis: (p601) Myocarditis; ascending aortic aneurysm.

Systemic lupus erythematosus: (p422) Pericarditis/effusion; myocarditis; Libman-Sacks endocarditis; mitral valve prolapse; coronary arteritis.

Systemic sclerosis: (p420) Pericarditis; pericardial effusion; myocardial fibro-sis; myocardial ischaemia; conduction defects; cardiomyopathy.

Thyrotoxicosis: (p304) Pulse↑; AF ± emboli; wide pulse pressure; hyperdy-namic apex; loud heart sounds; ejection systolic murmur; pleuroperican-dial rub; angina; high output cardiac failure.

Turner's syndrome:♀ Coarctation of aorta. Look for webbed neck. XO.

William's syndrome: Supravalvular aortic stenosis (visuo-spatial IQ↓).

Pericardial diseases

Acute pericarditis Inflammation of the pericardium which may be primary or secondary to systemic disease.

Causes: • Viruses (coxsackie, 'flu, Epstein–Barr, mumps, varicella, HIV) • Bacteria (pneumonia, rheumatic fever, TB) • Fungi • Myocardial infarct • Dressler's (p722) • Uraemia • Rheumatoid arthritis • SLE • Myxoedema • Trauma • Surgery • Malignancy • Radiotherapy • Procainamide; hydralazine.

Clinical features: Central chest pain worse on inspiration or lying flat ± relief by sitting forward. A pericardial friction rub may be heard. Look for evidence of a pericardial effusion or cardiac tamponade (see below).

Tests: ECG classically shows concave (saddle-shaped) ST segment elevation, but may be normal or non-specific (10%). *Blood tests:* FBC, ESR, U&E, cardiac enzymes, viral serology, blood cultures, and, if indicated, autoantibodies (p421), fungal precipitins, thyroid function tests. Cardiomegaly on CXR may indicate a pericardial effusion. *Echo* (if suspected pericardial effusion).

Treatment: Analgesia, eg ibuprofen 400mg/8h PO with food. Treat the cause. Consider colchicine before steroids/immunosuppressants if relapse or continuing symptoms occur. 15–40% *do* recur.

Pericardial effusion Accumulation of fluid in the pericardial sac.

Causes: Any cause of pericarditis (see above).

Clinical features: Dyspnoea, raised JVP (with prominent x descent, p43), bronchial breathing at left base (Ewart's sign: large effusion compressing left lower lobe). Look for signs of cardiac tamponade (see below).

Diagnosis: CXR shows an enlarged, globular heart. ECG shows low voltage QRS complexes and alternating QRS morphologies (electrical alternans). *Echocardiography* shows an echo-free zone surrounding the heart.

Management: Treat the cause. Pericardiocentesis may be *diagnostic* (suspected bacterial pericarditis) or *therapeutic* (cardiac tamponade). See p757. Send pericardial fluid for culture, ZN stain/TB culture, and cytology.

Constrictive pericarditis The heart is encased in a rigid pericardium.

Causes: Often unknown (UK); elsewhere TB, or after *any* pericarditis.

Clinical features: These are mainly of right heart failure with ↑JVP (with prominent x and y descents, p42); Kussmaul's sign (JVP rising paradoxically with inspiration); soft, diffuse apex beat; quiet heart sounds; S_3; diastolic pericardial knock, hepatosplenomegaly, ascites, and oedema.

Tests: CXR: small heart ± pericardial calcification (if none, CT/MRI helps distinguish from other cardiomyopathies). *Echo*; cardiac catheterization.

Management: Surgical excision.

Cardiac tamponade Accumulation of pericardial fluid raises intrapericardial pressure, hence poor ventricular filling and fall in cardiac output.

Causes: Any pericarditis (above); aortic dissection; haemodialysis; warfarin; trans-septal puncture at cardiac catheterization; post cardiac biopsy.

Signs: Pulse↑, BP↓, pulsus paradoxus, JVP↑, Kussmaul's sign, muffled S_1 & S_2.

Diagnosis: Beck's triad: falling BP; rising JVP; small, quiet heart. CXR: big globular heart (if >250mL fluid). ECG: low voltage QRS ± electrical alternans. *Echo* is diagnostic: echo-free zone (>2cm, or >1cm if acute) around the heart ± diastolic collapse of right atrium and right ventricle.

Management: Seek expert help. The pericardial effusion needs urgent drainage (p757). Send fluid for culture, ZN stain/TB culture & cytology.

Pericarditis

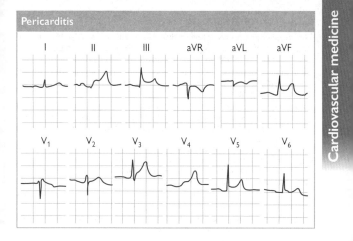

Congenital heart disease

The spectrum of congenital heart disease in adults is considerably different from that in infants and children; adults are unlikely to have complex lesions. The commonest lesions, in descending order of frequency, are:

Bicuspid aortic valve These function well at birth and go undetected. Most eventually develop AS (requiring valve replacement) and/or AR (predisposing to IE/SBE). See p148.

Atrial septal defect (ASD) A hole connects the atria. *Ostium secundum* defects (high in the septum) are commonest; *ostium primum* defects (opposing the endocardial cushions) are associated with AV valve anomalies. Primum ASDs present early. Secundum ASDs are often asymptomatic until adulthood, as the L→R shunt depends on compliance of the right and left ventricles. The latter decreases with age (esp. if BP↑). This augments L→R shunting causing dyspnoea and heart failure, eg at age 40–60. There may be pulmonary hypertension, cyanosis, arrhythmia, haemoptysis, and chest pain.

Signs: AF; ↑JVP; wide, fixed split S_2; pulmonary ejection systolic murmur. Pulmonary hypertension may cause pulmonary or tricuspid regurgitation.

Complications: Reversal of left to right shunt (Eisenmenger complex, see OPPOSITE), paradoxical embolism (rare).

Tests: ECG: RBBB with LAD and prolonged P–R interval (primum defect) or RAD (secundum defect). CXR: small aortic knuckle, pulmonary plethora, progressive atrial enlargement. Echocardiography is diagnostic. Cardiac catheterization shows step up in O_2 saturation in the right atrium.

Treatment: In children, surgical closure is recommended before age 10yrs. In adults, closure is recommended if symptomatic, or if asymptomatic but having pulmonary to systemic blood flow ratios of ≥1.5 : 1.

Ventricular septal defect (VSD) A hole connecting the 2 ventricles.

Causes: congenital (prevalence 2 : 1000 births); acquired (post-MI).

Symptoms: May present with severe heart failure in infancy, or remain asymptomatic and be detected incidentally in later life.

Signs: These depend upon the size and site of the VSD: smaller holes, which are haemodynamically less significant, give louder murmurs. Classically, a harsh pansystolic murmur is heard at the left sternal edge, accompanied by a systolic thrill, ± left parasternal heave. Larger holes are associated with signs of pulmonary hypertension.

Complications: AR, infundibular stenosis, infective endocarditis, pulmonary hypertension, Eisenmenger complex (OPPOSITE).

Tests: ECG: normal (small VSD), LAD + LVH (moderate VSD) or LVH + RVH (large VSD). CXR: normal heart size ± mild pulmonary plethora (small VSD) or cardiomegaly, large pulmonary arteries and marked pulmonary plethora (large VSD). Cardiac catheter: step up in O_2 saturation in right ventricle.

Treatment: This is medical, at first, as many VSDs close spontaneously. Indications for surgical closure: failed medical therapy, symptomatic VSD, shunt >3 : 1, SBE/IE. Give SBE/IE prophylaxis for untreated defects (p154).

Coarctation of the aorta Congenital narrowing of the descending aorta; usually occurs just distal to the origin of the left subclavian artery. More common in boys. *Associations:* Bicuspid aortic valve, Turner's syndrome. *Signs:* Radio-femoral delay, weak femoral pulse, BP↑, scapular bruit, systolic murmur (best heard over the left scapula). *Complications:* Heart failure, infective endocarditis. *Tests:* CXR shows rib notching. *Treatment:* Surgery.

Pulmonary stenosis may occur alone or with other lesions (p150).

Eisenmenger's syndrome

A congenital heart defect which is at first associated with a left to right shunt may lead to pulmonary hypertension and shunt reversal. If so, cyanosis develops (± heart failure and respiratory infections), and Eisenmenger's syndrome is present.

Driving and the heart[1] (Ordinary UK licences only)

UK licences are inscribed 'You are required by law to inform Drivers Medical Branch, DVLA, Swansea SA99 1AT at once if you have any disability (physical or medical), which is, or may become likely to affect your fitness as a driver, unless you do not expect it to last more than 3 months'. It is the responsibility of drivers to inform the DVLA, and that of their doctors to advise patients that medical conditions (and drugs) may affect their ability to drive and for which conditions patients should inform the DVLA. Drivers should also inform their insurance company of any condition disclosed to the DVLA. If in doubt, ask your defence union. The following are examples of the guidance for holders of standard licences. Different rules apply for group 2 vehicle licence-holders (eg HGV, buses).

Angina Driving must cease when symptoms occur at rest or at the wheel. Driving may recommence when satisfactory symptom control is achieved. DVLA need not be notified.

Angioplasty Driving must cease for 1wk, and may recommence thereafter provided no other disqualifying condition. DVLA need not be notified.

MI/CABG Driving must cease for >4wks. Driving may recommence thereafter provided there is no other disqualifying condition. DVLA need not be notified.

Arrhythmias *Sinoatrial:* Driving may recommence 1 month after successful control provided there is no other disqualifying condition.

Significant atrioventricular conduction defects: Driving may be permitted when underlying cause has been identified and controlled for >4wks.

AF/flutter: DVLA need not be notified unless there are distracting/disabling symptoms.

Pacemaker implant Stop driving for 1wk.

Implanted cardioverter/defibrillator The licence is subject to annual review. Driving may occur when these criteria can be met:
• The 1st device has been implanted for at least 6 months.
• The device has not administered therapy (shock and/or symptomatic anti-tachycardia pacing) within the last 6 months (except during testing).
• Any previous therapy has not been accompanied by *incapacity* (whether caused by the device or arrhythmia).
• A period of 1 month off driving must occur following any revision of the device (generator and/or electrode) or alteration of antiarrhythmics.
• The device is subject to regular review with interrogation.
• There is no other disqualifying condition.

Syncope *Simple faint:* no restriction. *Unexplained syncope* with low risk of recurrence 4wks off driving, high risk of recurrence 4wks off driving if cause identified and treated otherwise, 6 months off. See driving and epilepsy, OPPOSITE. Patients who have had a single episode of loss of consciousness (no cause found) still need to have at least 1yr off driving.

Hypertension Driving may continue unless treatment causes unacceptable side effects. DVLA need not be notified.

Other conditions: UK DVLA state they must be informed if:

- An epileptic event. A person who has suffered an epileptic attack while awake must not drive for 1yr from the date of the attack. A person who has suffered an attack while asleep must also refrain from driving for 1yr from the date of the attack, unless they have had an attack while asleep >3yrs ago and have not had any awake attacks since that asleep attack. In any event, they should not drive if they are likely to cause danger to the public or themselves.
- Patients with TIA or stroke should not drive for at least 1 month. There is no need to inform the DVLA unless there is residual neurological defect after 1 month eg visual field defect. If TIAS have been recurrent and frequent, a 3-month period free of attacks may be required.
- Sudden attacks or disabling giddiness, fainting, or blackouts. Multiple sclerosis, Parkinson's (any 'freezing' or on–off effects), motor neurone diseases are relevant here.
- Severe mental handicap. Those with dementia should only drive if the condition is mild (do not rely on armchair judgements: on-the-road trials are better). Encourage relatives to contact DVLA if a dementing relative should not be driving. GPs may desire to breach confidentiality (the GMC approves) and inform DVLA of demented or psychotic patients (tel. 01792 783686). Many elderly drivers (~1 in 3) who die in accidents are found to have Alzheimer's.
- A pacemaker, defibrillator, or antiventricular tachycardia device fitted.
- Diabetes controlled by insulin or tablets.
- Angina while driving.
- Parkinson's disease.
- Any other chronic neurological condition.
- A serious problem with memory.
- A major or minor stroke with deficit continuing for >1 month.
- Any type of brain surgery, brain tumour. Severe head injury involving inpatient treatment at hospital.
- Any severe psychiatric illness or mental disorder.
- Continuing/permanent difficulty in the use of arms or legs which affects ability to control a vehicle.
- Dependence on or misuse of alcohol, illicit drugs, or chemical substances in the past 3yrs (do not include drink/driving offences).
- Any visual disability which affects *both* eyes (do not declare short/long sight or colour blindness).

Vision (new drivers) should be 6/9 on Snellen's scale in the better eye and 6/12 on the Snellen scale in the other eye and (wearing glasses or contact lenses if needed) and 3/60 in each eye without glasses or contact lenses.

Chest medicine[1]

Contents

Signs:

Investigations:

Diseases and conditions:

Relevant pages in other sections:

---

1 We thank Dr Mark Pasteur, who is our Specialist Reader for this chapter.

Chest x-ray

Films are usually taken with the patient standing in front of the film with the x-ray source behind (PA film). Emergency films may be the other way (AP), which magnifies heart size. There are 4 radiographic densities: air, fat, water/soft tissue, bone. A border is only seen at an interface of 2 densities, eg heart (water) and lung (air); this 'silhouette' is lost if air in the lung is replaced by consolidation (water). This is the silhouette sign and helps localize pathology (eg middle lobe pneumonia or collapse causing loss of distinction of the right heart border).

Trachea should be central.

Heart is normally <½ the width of the thorax. It may appear tall and narrow if the chest is hyperinflated (chronic obstructive pulmonary disease, COPD) or larger, if an AP film is taken.

Mediastinum may be widened in many disorders: retrosternal thyroid, lymph node enlargement (sarcoidosis, lymphoma, metastases, TB), tumour (thymoma, teratoma, neurogenic tumours), aortic aneurysm, cysts (bronchogenic cyst, pericardial cyst), paravertebral mass (TB), oesophageal dilatation (achalasia, hiatus hernia).

Hila The left hilum is higher than the right. Hila may be pulled up or down by fibrosis or collapse. (1) *Enlarged hila:* nodes; pulmonary arterial hypertension; bronchial ca. (2) *Calcification:* past TB; silicosis; histoplasmosis (p612).

The diaphragm (Right side is usually slightly higher). *Causes of a raised hemidiaphragm:* lung volume loss, stroke, phrenic nerve palsy (from: trauma; MND, p394; cancer), hepatomegaly, subphrenic abscess; subpulmonic effusion and diaphragm rupture give apparent elevation. **NB:** bilateral palsies (polio, muscular dystrophy) cause hypoxia.

Lung fields Shadowing may be described as nodular, reticular (network of fine lines, interstitial), or alveolar (fluffy).

Nodular shadows:
• Neoplasia (metastases, lung carcinoma, adenoma, hamartoma)
• Infections (varicella pneumonia, hydatid, septic emboli)
• Granulomas (miliary TB, sarcoidosis, histoplasmosis, Wegener's, p738)
• Pneumoconioses (except asbestosis), Caplan's syndrome (p720)

Reticular shadows: Usually acute interstitial changes (cardiac or non-cardiac pulmonary interstitial oedema, atypical pneumonia, eg viral). Also:
• Fibrosis; TB; histoplasmosis   • Neoplasia (lymphangitis carcinomatosa)
• Sarcoidosis; silicosis; asbestosis • Fibrosing alveolitis; rheumatoid (p414)
• Extrinsic allergic alveolitis (EAA) • Wegener's (p738); SLE; PAN; CREST (p420)

Alveolar shadows: Usually pulmonary oedema from LVF (p786). Also:
• Pneumonia   • Renal or liver failure (p276 & p230)
• Haemorrhage   • ARDS (p190); DIC (p650)
• Drugs (heroin, cytotoxics, p440) • Head injury, or after neurosurgery
• Smoke inhalation (p835)   • Alveolar proteinosis
• O₂ toxicity   • Near-drowning (OHCS p682)
• Fat emboli, ~7 days post-fracture • Heat stroke (p778)

'Ring' shadows: Either airways seen end-on (pulmonary oedema, bronchiectasis), or cavitating lesions, eg abscess (bacterial, fungal, amoebic), tumour, or pulmonary infarct (triangular with a pleural base).

Linear opacities: Septal lines (Kerley's B lines, ie interlobular lymphatics seen with fluid, tumour, or dusts). Atelectasis.

Apparently normal CXR Check for apical pneumothorax, tracheal compression, absent breast shadow (mastectomy), rib pathology (fractures, metastases, or notching), air under diaphragm (perforated viscus), double left heart border (left lower lobe collapse), fluid level behind the heart (hiatus hernia, achalasia), and paravertebral abscess (TB).

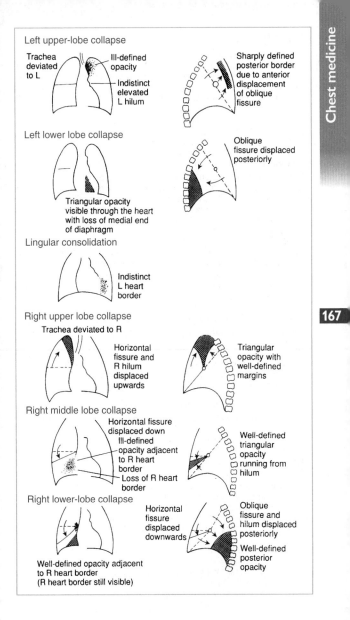

Left upper-lobe collapse

Trachea deviated to L — Ill-defined opacity — Indistinct elevated L hilum

Sharply defined posterior border due to anterior displacement of oblique fissure

Left lower lobe collapse

Triangular opacity visible through the heart with loss of medial end of diaphragm

Oblique fissure displaced posteriorly

Lingular consolidation

Indistinct L heart border

Right upper lobe collapse

Trachea deviated to R

Horizontal fissure and R hilum displaced upwards

Triangular opacity with well-defined margins

Right middle lobe collapse

Horizontal fissure displaced down Ill-defined opacity adjacent to R heart border Loss of R heart border

Well-defined triangular opacity running from hilum

Right lower-lobe collapse

Horizontal fissure displaced downwards

Oblique fissure and hilum displaced posteriorly Well-defined posterior opacity

Well-defined opacity adjacent to R heart border (R heart border still visible)

Bedside tests in chest medicine

Sputum examination Collect a good sample; if necessary ask a physio-therapist to help. Note the appearance: clear and colourless (chronic bron-chitis), yellow/green (pulmonary infection), red (haemoptysis), black (smoke, coal), or frothy white/pink (pulmonary oedema). Send the sample to the laboratory for microscopy (Gram stain and auramine/ZN stain, if indicated), culture, and cytology.

Peak expiratory flow (PEF) is measured by a maximal forced expiration through a peak flow meter. It correlates well with the forced expiratory volume in 1 second (FEV_1) and is used as an estimate of airway calibre. Peak flow rates should be measured regularly in asthmatics to monitor response to therapy and disease control.

Pulse oximetry allows non-invasive assessment of peripheral O_2 saturation. It provides a useful tool for monitoring those who are acutely ill or at risk of deterioration. On most pulse oximeters, the alarm is set at 90%. An oxygen saturation of ≤80% is clearly abnormal and action is required (unless this is normal for the patient, eg in COPD. Here, check arterial blood gases (ABG) as P_aCO_2 may be rising despite a normal P_aO_2). Erroneous readings may be caused by: poor perfusion, motion, excess light, skin pigmentation, nail varnish, dyshaemoglobinaemias, and carbon monoxide poisoning. As with any bedside test, be sceptical, and check ABG whenever indicated (p193).

Arterial blood gas (ABG) analysis Heparinized blood is taken from the radial, brachial, or femoral artery, and pH, P_aO_2, and P_aCO_2 are measured using an automated analyser. Remember to note the FiO_2 (fraction or percentage of inspired oxygen).

- *Acid–base balance:* Normal pH is 7.35–7.45. A pH <7.35 indicates *acidosis* and a pH >7.45 indicates *alkalosis*. For interpretation of abnormalities, see p682.
- *Oxygenation:* Normal P_aO_2 is 10.5–13.5kPa. Hypoxia is caused by one or more of the following reasons: ventilation/perfusion ($\dot{V}/\dot{Q}$) mismatch, hypoventilation, abnormal diffusion, right to left cardiac shunts. Of these, $\dot{V}/\dot{Q}$ mismatch is the commonest cause. Severe hypoxia is defined as a P_aO_2 <8kPa (see p192).
- *Ventilatory efficiency:* Normal P_aCO_2 is 4.5–6.0kPa. P_aCO_2 is directly related to alveolar ventilation. A P_aCO_2 <4.5kPa indicates *hyperventilation* and a P_aCO_2 >6.0kPa indicates *hypoventilation*. Type 1 respiratory failure is defined as P_aO_2 <8kPa and P_aCO_2<6.0kPa, whereas Type II respiratory failure is defined as P_aO_2 <8kPa and P_aCO_2 >6.0kPa.

Alveolar–arterial O_2 concentration gradient may be calculated from the FiO_2, P_aO_2, and P_aCO_2: see OPPOSITE.

Spirometry measures functional lung volumes. Forced expiratory volume in 1s (FEV_1) and forced vital capacity (FVC) are measured from a full forced expiration into spirometer (Vitalograph); exhalation continues until no more breath can be exhaled. FEV_1 is less effort-dependent than PEF. The FEV_1/FVC ratio gives a good estimate of severity of airflow obstruction; normal ratio is 75–80%.

- *Obstructive defect* (eg asthma, COPD) FEV_1 is reduced more than the FVC and the FEV_1/FVC ratio is <75%.
- *Restrictive defect* (eg lung fibrosis) FVC is reduced and the FEV_1/FVC ratio is normal or raised. Other causes: sarcoidosis; pneumoconiosis, interstitial pneumonias; connective tissue diseases; pleural effusion; obesity; kyphosco-liosis; neuromuscular problems.

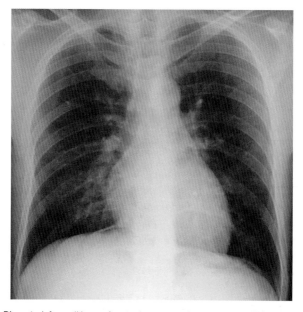

Plate 1. A few millilitres of gas in the peritoneal cavity can be difficult to see. The best way is with a CXR after remaining erect for 10 min. This may be a small pneumoperitoneum at the right cardiophrenic angle. Check with another view or a CT if necessary. If you strongly suspected a perforated ulcer and the CXR and AXR showed no signs of pneumoperitoneum, could you exclude the diagnosis? No. Only 75% of perforations have evidence of pneumoperitoneum.

The authors and publishers would like to thank Peter Scally for permission to use these plates taken from Scally, P. (1999) *Medical imaging: an Oxford core text*. Oxford University Press, Oxford

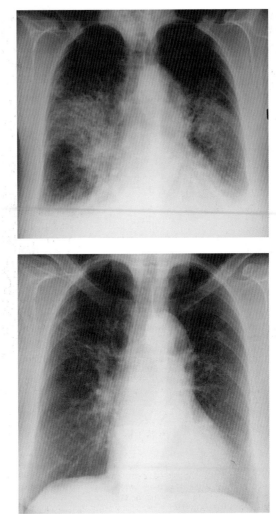

(a)

(b)

Plate 2. (a) (b) Two radiographs, 4 days apart. *Lungs*: The major abnormality in the initial film is in the lungs; perihilar opacities that are poorly defined. This is consolidation. But what is the cause? Pulmonary oedema, infection, or blood? The lungs are filled with fluid and unable to expand fully. *Pleura*: The hemidiaphragms are not visible because of pleural effusions, seen curving up the side walls. *Mediastinum*: The heart is enlarged. *Hila, bones, soft tissues*: normal. These are the changes of severe left heart failure. The pulmonary venous pressure has been so high that fluid has flowed from the capillaries, into the interstitium, and then into the alveoli. Look at how the lungs have expanded and the heart borders and hemidiaphragms have sharpened up after treatment.

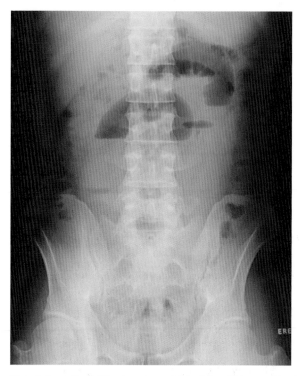

Plate 3. Erect. The fluid levels are immediately obvious in the erect film, but let's approach it in a systematic way. *Gas* can be seen in the colon from the rectum back to the caecum. The stomach bubble is barely visible. That leaves several loops with fluid levels to be explained. They must be small intestine, being centrally placed and with a few valvulae conniventes. The loops are dilated, 3 cm wide, and are probably ileum as the valvulae conniventes are less pronounced here than in the jejunum. By comparison, if the large bowel was obstructed it would show as a few peripheral loops, often over 5 cm in diameter, containing faeces and showing a haustral (scalloped) pattern. Folds in the mucosa of the colon do not extend completely across the lumen. No sign of *calcification in the biliary tree or urinary tract*. The *bones* and *soft tissues* are normal. We would be looking for evidence of a cause of small bowel obstruction: a hernia, surgical clips, or any other signs of surgery.

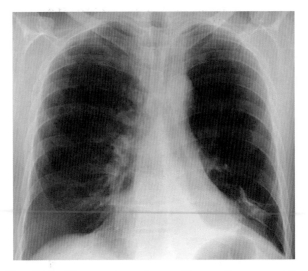

Plate 4. *Lungs*: These are of normal volume. Fewer markings are seen in the left lung except at the base. *Pleura*: Following the pleura reveals loss of the clarity of the left hemidiaphragm. *Mediastinum*: In the mediastinum the left main bronchus is pulled down and there is a triangular opacity behind the heart on the left. This is a collapsed left lower lobe. It also depresses the left *hilum*. *Bones*: Check the bones for metastatic disease because the left lower lobe bronchus may be obstructed by a neoplasm. *Soft tissues*: appear unremarkable.

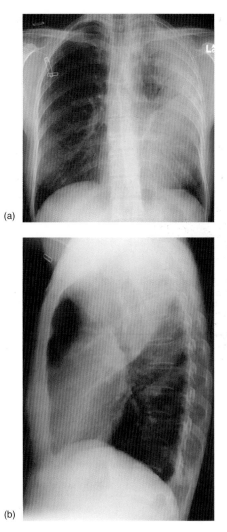

(a)

(b)

Plate 5. (a) (b) *Lungs*: Normal lung volumes. A poorly defined opacity in the left lung obliterates the left heart border and therefore is in the upper lobe. The air-bronchogram indicates consolidation. *Pleura*: The pleura in the right hemithorax seem normal. *Mediastinum*: This is central but the oblique fissure on the lateral film is bowed inferiorly because of a slight increase in volume. *Hila*: The left hilum is not visible. *Bones, soft tissues*: normal. Left upper lobe pneumonia (lobar pneumonia). Pneumonia is an infection of the lung, classified as lobar, broncho, and atypical. Usually the pathology progresses through four stages: congestion, red hepatization, grey hepatization, and resolution. This would be one of the stages of hepatization.

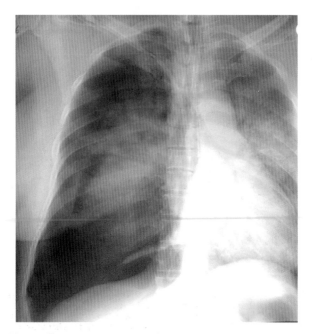

Plate 6. This is a great educational film from the intensive care unit. The inexperienced doctor could be distracted by the poor quality, badly centred film. The technicians do the best they can under difficult conditions. To ask for another in this instance would be a mistake. There is adequate information to make a life-saving decision. After checking the name of the patient, see that the tubes and lines are well positioned—the endotracheal and nasogastric tubes and the right subclavian central venous line. *Lungs*: The left lung shows consolidation. The right hemithorax is too black and hyperexpanded. Right hemidiaphragm is depressed. *Pleura*: The pleural recess is seen at the right base. *Mediastinum*: This is shifted to the left, obstructing venous return and decreasing cardiac output, a threat to life. Is it being pushed or pulled? *Hila, bones*, and *soft tissues*: Check these structures. Is the endotracheal tube down the right main bronchus, inflating the right lung and collapsing the left? No. Is the right lung collapsed? Yes. Right tension pneumothorax. Beware of the half-toning of the hemidiaphragm in a supine film. In the supine position, a pneumothorax will be anterior and the lung will fall posteriorly. A chest tube is needed immediately. The consolidation in the left lung could be a result of any of the causes of the acute respiratory distress syndrome (ARDS). Consolidation/collapse often occurs in intubated patients at the left base. Suction catheters to clear the lungs pass down the ETT and preferentially into the right main bronchus.

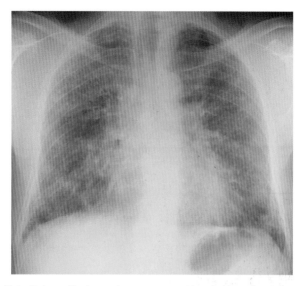

Plate 7. *Lungs*: The lung volumes are normal but the parenchyma shows increased markings that extend out to the chest wall. Normally vessels (arteries and veins) are only seen for 80% of the distance from hilum to pleura. The bronchi should barely be visible. *Pleura*: Following the pleura demonstrates that the heart borders are poorly defined, reflecting interstitial disease in the lung adjacent to the heart. *Mediastinum*: The mediastinal structures themselves are normal. *Hila*: The hila are difficult to interpret. So what? It is not unusual to be missing a piece of information when making a clinical decision. No need for wringing of hands and gnashing of teeth. Either go ahead without it or, if it is essential, find it. In this case, further information is available by comparison with old films or by requesting a CT. *Bone* and *soft tissues*: No abnormality. This is interstitial lung disease. It has a similar appearance to the interstitial oedema of moderate left heart failure but without a big heart. Check the previous film to see if it is acute. It was not. The diagnosis in this example is fibrosing alveolitis.

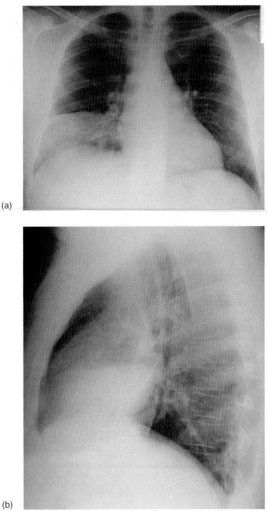

(a)

(b)

Plate 8. (a) (b) *Lungs*: An opacity can be seen at the base of the right lung. *Pleura*: The silhouette of the pleura over the right hemidiaphragm is lost because of adjacent lung disease. The right heart border is also unclear. *Mediastinum, hila, bones, soft tissues*: normal. The middle lobe has two segments. The consolidation of lobar pneumonia here involves principally the lateral segment. The medial segment is affected to a lesser extent, shown by the loss of clarity of the right heart border. Also well seen on the lateral projection, but the PA view has adequate information.

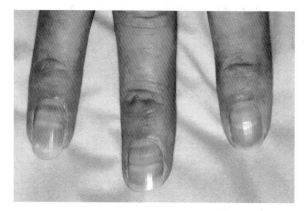

Plate 9. Beau's lines. See p39.

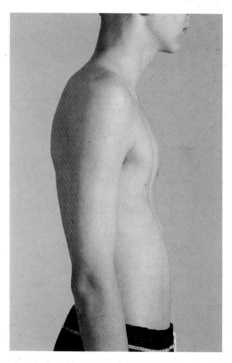

Plate 10. Pectus excavatum. The medical term for funnel or sunken chest. Associations: scoliosis; restrictive spirometry; Marfan's syndrome; Ehlers–Danlos syndrome (plate 24).

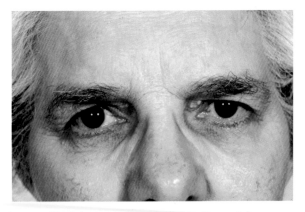

Plate 11. Xanthelasma. *Xanthos* is Greek for yellow, and *elasma* means plate. Xanthelasma are lipid-laden yellow plaques congregating around the lids. They are typically a few mm wide, and signify hyperlipidaemia, p706.

Plate 12. Spider naevi. These consist of a central arteriole, from which numerous vessels radiate (like the legs of a spider). These fill from the centre. They occur most commonly in skin drained by the superior vena cava. Up to 5 are said to be normal (they are common in young females). Causes include liver failure, contraceptive steroids, and pregnancy (ie changes in oestrogen metabolism).

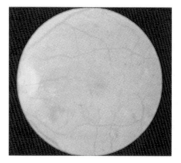

Plate 13. Diabetes, background retinopathy. There are scattered blot haemorrhages and sparse hard exudates but vision is normal.

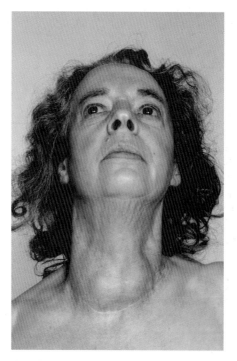

Plate 14. Nodular goitre. See p516.

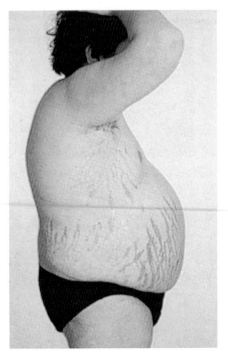

Plate 15. Cushing's disease. See p310. Signs of Cushings include purple abdominal striae and wasting, eg in the thighs.

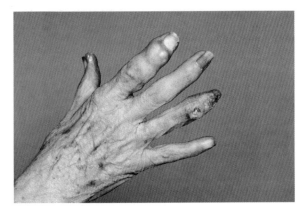

Plate 16. Tophaceous gout. See p416.

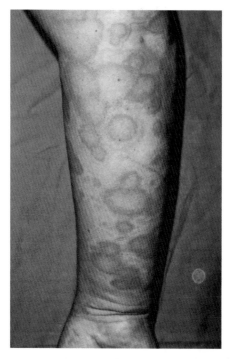

Plate 17. Erythema multiforme. Target lesions eg caused by drugs, herpes or mycoplasma. See p428.

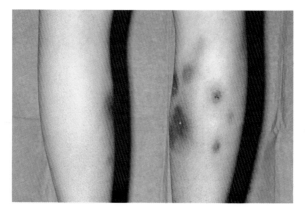

Plate 18. Erythema nodosum. See p428. Causes include sarcoidosis, drugs, streps, TB, and UC/Crohn's disease.

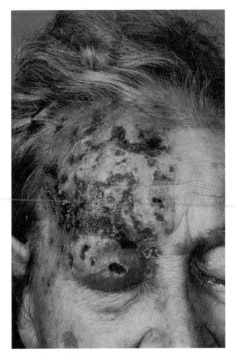

Plate 19. Shingles (herpes zoster) involving the ophthalmic (Vi) division of the trigeminal nerve.

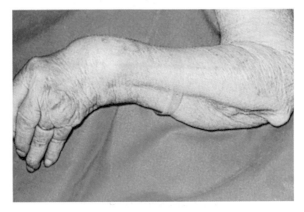

Plate 20. Rheumatoid arthritis. See p414. Note ulnar deviation of fingers.

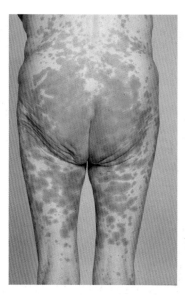

Plate 21. Drug reaction.

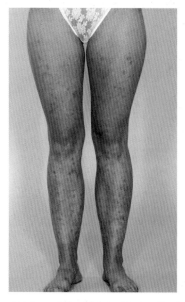

Plate 22. Vascultic skin rash from Behcet's disease. See p718.

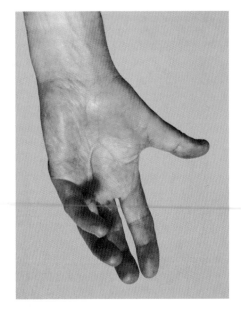

Plate 23. Dupuytren's contracture. See p722.

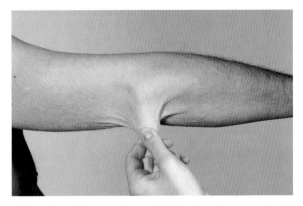

Plate 24. Ehlers–Danlos syndrome. Note the hyperelasticity of the skin. Associations: aneurysms; GI bleeds/perforations; hypermobile joints; flat feet. It is a disorder of collagen.

(Aa)PO$_2$: the Aveolar–arterial (Aa) oxygen gradient

This is the difference in the O_2 partial pressures between the alveolar and arterial sides. In type II respiratory failure it helps tell if hypoventilation is from lung disease or poor respiratory effort. $(Aa)PO_2 = P_AO_2 - P_aO_2$. How do we find P_AO_2, the partial pressure of oxygen in the alveoli? Respiratory physiology teaches that this depends on **R**, the respiratory quotient (≈ 0.8, nearer to 1 if eating all carbohydrates); barometric pressure ($P_B \approx 101$kPa at sea level), and P_{H_2O}, the water saturation of airway gas ($P_{H_2O} \approx 6.2$kPa as inspired air is usually fully saturated by the time it gets to the carina). P_AO_2 clearly depends on F_iO_2, the fractional concentration of O_2 in inspired air (eg F_iO_2 is 0.5 if breathing 50% O_2, and 0.21 if breathing room air). So...

$$P_AO_2 = (P_B - P_{H_2O}) \times F_iO_2 - P_aCO_2/R$$
$$= (101 - 6.2) \times F_iO_2 - P_aCO_2/0.8 \text{ (at sea level)}$$
$$= 94.8 \times F_iO_2 - 1.25 \times P_aCO_2$$

See A Williams *BMJ* 1998 **317** 1213

Breathing air and having a P_aCO_2 of 8kPa

In this case, $P_AO_2 = 94.8 \times 0.21 - (1.25 \times 8) = 10$kPa. *Aa normal ranges breathing air:* 0.2–1.5kPa at 25yrs old; increasing with age to 1.5–3.0 at 75yrs.

Examples of expected Aa gradients: 6.65 at an F_iO_2 of 0.5 ($P_AO_2 - P_aO_2 = 44.6 - 37.95 = 6.65$) and 16 for an F_iO_2 of 1.0 ($P_AO_2 - P_aO_2 = 89 - 73 = 16$).

Normal peak expiratory flow (PEF)

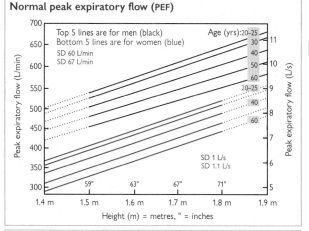

Examples of spirograms

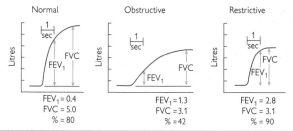

Normal	Obstructive	Restrictive
FEV$_1$ = 0.4	FEV$_1$ = 1.3	FEV$_1$ = 2.8
FVC = 5.0	FVC = 3.1	FVC = 3.1
% = 80	% = 42	% = 90

Further investigations in chest medicine

Lung function tests PEF, FEV$_1$, FVC (see p168). *Total lung capacity* (TLC) and *residual volume* (RV) are useful in distinguishing obstructive and restrictive diseases. TLC and RV are increased in obstructive airways disease and reduced in restrictive lung diseases and musculoskeletal abnormalities. The *gas transfer co-efficient* (KCO) across alveoli is calculated by measuring carbon monoxide uptake from a single inspiration in a standard time (usually 10s). Low in emphysema and interstitial lung disease, high in alveolar haemorrhage. KCO and DLCO (carbon monoxide diffusing capacity) need to be corrected for alveolar volume[1]. *Flow volume loop* measures flow at various lung volumes. Characteristic patterns are seen with intrathoracic airways obstruction (asthma, emphysema) and extrathoracic airways obstruction (tracheal stenosis).

Radiology *Chest x-ray* see p166. *Ultrasound* is used in the diagnosis and drainage of pleural effusions (particularly loculated effusions) and empyema. *Radionuclide scans Ventilation/perfusion (V̇/Q̇) scans* are used to diagnose pulmonary embolism (PE) (unmatched perfusion defects are seen). *Bone scans* are used to diagnose bone metastases. *Computer tomography* (CT) of the thorax is used for diagnosing and staging lung ca, imaging the hilar, mediastinum and pleura, and guiding biopsies. Thin (1–1.5mm) section high resolution CT (HRCT) is used in the diagnosis of interstitial lung disease and bronchiectasis. Spiral CT pulmonary angiography (CTPA) is used increasingly in the diagnosis of PE. *Pulmonary angiography* is also used for diagnosing PE and pulmonary hypertension.

Fibreoptic bronchoscopy is performed under local anaesthetic via the nose or mouth. *Diagnostic indications:* suspected lung ca, slowly resolving pneumonia, pneumonia in the immunosuppressed, interstitial lung disease. Bronchial lavage fluid may be sent to the lab for microscopy, culture, and cytology. Mucosal abnormalities may be brushed (cytology) and biopsied (histopathology). *Therapeutic indications:* aspiration of mucus plugs causing lobar collapse or removal of foreign bodies. *Pre-procedure investigations:* FBC, CXR, spirometry, pulse oximetry and arterial blood gases (if indicated). Check clotting if recent anticoagulation and a biopsy may be performed. *Complications:* respiratory depression, bleeding, pneumothorax (X-RAY PLATE 6).

Bronchoalveolar lavage (BAL) is performed at the time of bronchoscopy by instilling and aspirating a known volume of warmed, buffered 0.9% saline into the distal airway. *Diagnostic indications:* suspected malignancy, pneumonia in the immunosuppressed (especially HIV), suspected TB (if sputum negative), interstitial lung diseases (eg sarcoidosis, extrinsic allergic alveolitis, histiocytosis X). *Therapeutic indications:* alveolar proteinosis. *Complications:* hypoxia (give supplemental O$_2$), transient fever, transient CXR shadow, infection (rare).

Lung biopsy may be performed in several ways. *Percutaneous needle biopsy* is performed under radiological guidance and is useful for peripheral lung and pleural lesions. *Transbronchial biopsy* performed at bronchoscopy may help in diagnosing diffuse lung diseases, eg sarcoidosis. If these are unsuccessful, an *open lung biopsy* may be performed under general anaesthetic.

Surgical procedures are performed under general anaesthetic. *Rigid bronchoscopy* provides a wide lumen, enables larger mucosal biopsies, controlling bleeding, and removal of foreign bodies. *Mediastinoscopy* and *mediastinotomy* enable examination and biopsy of the mediastinal lymph nodes/lesions. *Thoracoscopy* allows examination and biopsy of pleural lesions, drainage of pleural effusions, and talc pleurodesis.

1 D Johnson 2000 *Respir Med* **94** 28–37 [@10714476]

Lung volumes: physiological and pathological[1]

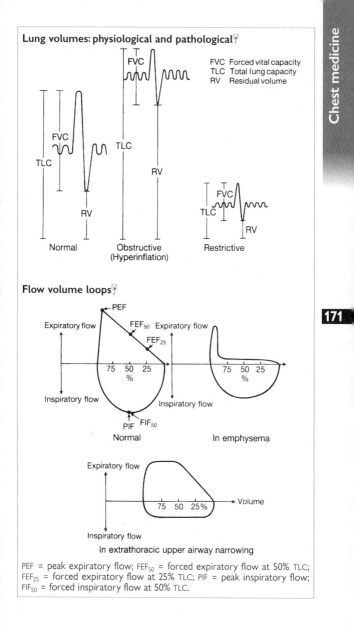

FVC Forced vital capacity
TLC Total lung capacity
RV Residual volume

Normal

Obstructive
(Hyperinflation)

Restrictive

Flow volume loops[2]

Expiratory flow

PEF
FEF$_{50}$ Expiratory flow
FEF$_{25}$

75 50 25
%

Inspiratory flow

Inspiratory flow

PIF FIF$_{50}$

Normal

In emphysema

Expiratory flow

Volume

75 50 25%

Inspiratory flow

In extrathoracic upper airway narrowing

PEF = peak expiratory flow; FEF$_{50}$ = forced expiratory flow at 50% TLC;
FEF$_{25}$ = forced expiratory flow at 25% TLC; PIF = peak inspiratory flow;
FIF$_{50}$ = forced inspiratory flow at 50% TLC.

An acute lower respiratory tract illness associated with fever, symptoms and signs in the chest, and abnormalities on the chest x-ray. Incidence: 1–3/1000 population. Mortality: 10% (patients admitted to hospital).

Classification and causes

1 *Community-acquired* pneumonia (CAP) may be primary or secondary to underlying disease. *Streptococcus pneumoniae* is the commonest cause, followed by *Haemophilus influenzae* and *Mycoplasma pneumoniae*. *Staphylococcus aureus*, *Legionella* species, *Moraxella catarrhalis*, and *Chlamydia* account for most of the remainder. Gram negative bacilli, *Coxiella burnetii* and anaerobes are rare. Viruses account for up to 15%.

2 *Hospital acquired (Nosocomial)* (>48h after hospital admission). Most commonly Gram negative enterobacteria or *Staph. aureus*. Also *Pseudomonas*, *Klebsiella*, *Bacteroides*, and *Clostridia*.

3 *Aspiration* Those with stroke, myasthenia, bulbar palsies, ↓consciousness (eg post-ictal or drunk), oesophageal disease (achalasia, reflux), or with poor dental hygiene, risk aspirating oropharyngeal anaerobes.

4 *Immunocompromised patient* Strep. pneumoniae, H. influenzae, Staph. aureus, M. catarrhalis, M. pneumoniae, Gram –ve bacilli and Pneumocystis carinii (p580–1). Other fungi, viruses (CMV, HSV), and mycobacteria.

Clinical features *Symptoms:* Fever, rigors, malaise, anorexia, dyspnoea, cough, purulent sputum, haemoptysis, and pleuritic chest pain. *Signs:* fever, cyanosis, confusion (may be the only sign in the elderly), tachypnoea, tachycardia, hypotension, signs of consolidation (diminished expansion, dull percussion note, increased tactile vocal fremitus/vocal resonance, bronchial breathing), and a pleural rub.

Tests aim to establish diagnosis, identify pathogen, and assess severity (see below). *CXR* (X-RAY PLATES 5 & 8): lobar or multilobar infiltrates, cavitation or pleural effusion. *Assess oxygenation:* oxygen saturation (ABGs if S_aO_2 <92% or severe pneumonia). *Blood tests:* FBC, U&E, LFT, CRP, blood cultures. *Sputum* for microscopy and culture. In severe cases, check for Legionella (sputum culture, urine antigen), atypical organism/viral serology (complement fixation tests acutely and paired serology) and some centres may check for pneumococcal antigen in urine, sputum, or blood. *Pleural fluid* may be aspirated for culture. Consider *bronchoscopy* and bronchoalveolar lavage if patient is immunocompromised or on ITU.

Severity Core adverse features: 'CURB' score: **C**onfusion (abbreviated mental test ≤8); **U**rea >7mmol/L; **R**espiratory rate ≥30/min; **B**P <90 systolic and/or 60mmHg diastolic). Score >1 indicates severe pneumonia. Other features increasing the risk of death are: age ≥50yrs; co-existing disease; bilateral/multilobar involvement; P_aO_2 <8kPa/S_aO_2 <92%.

Management ►►p800. *Antibiotics* (p173), orally if not severe and not vomiting. *Oxygen* keep P_aO_2 >8.0 or saturation ≥92%. *IV fluids* (anorexia, dehydration, shock). *Analgesia* if pleurisy—eg paracetamol 1g/6h. If severe pneumonia should have IV antibiotics and consider ITU if failure to improve quickly, shock, hypercapnia, or uncorrected hypoxia.

Complications (p176) Pleural effusion, empyema, lung abscess, respiratory failure, septicaemia, brain abscess, pericarditis, myocarditis, cholestatic jaundice. Repeat CRP and CXR in patients not progressing satisfactorily.

Preventing pneumococcal infection Offer pneumococcal vaccine (23-valent Pneumovax II® 0.5mL SC) to those with: • Chronic heart or lung conditions • Cirrhosis • Nephrosis • Diabetes mellitus • Immunosuppression (eg splenectomy, AIDS, or on chemotherapy). CI: pregnancy, lactation, fever. If high risk of fatal pneumococcal infection (asplenia, sickle-cell disease, nephrosis, post-transplant), re-vaccinate after 6yrs (3–5yrs in children >2yrs old), unless they had a severe vaccine reaction.

172

Empirical treatment of pneumonia

Clinical setting	Organisms	Antibiotic (further dosage details: p543 & p544)
Community acquired		
Mild not previously Rx	*Streptococcus pneumoniae* *Haemophilus influenzae*	Amoxicillin 500mg–1.0g/8h or erythromycin[1] 500mg/6h PO
Mild	*Streptococcus pneumoniae* *Haemophilus influenzae* *Mycoplasma pneumoniae*	Amoxicillin 500mg–1.0g/8h PO + erythromycin[1] 500mg/6h PO or fluoroquinolone if IV required: ampicillin 500mg/6h + erythromycin[1] 500mg/6h IVI
Severe	As above	Co-amoxiclav IV or cephalosporin IV (eg Cefuroxime 1.5g/8h IV) AND erythromycin[1] 1g/6h IVI
Atypical	*Legionella pneumophilia*	Clarithromycin 500mg/12h PO/IVI ± rifampicin
	Chlamydia species	Tetracycline
	Pneumocystis carinii	High-dose co-trimoxazole (see p580–1)
Hospital acquired		
	Gram negative bacilli Pseudomonas Anaerobes	Aminoglycoside IV + antipseudomonal penicillin IV or 3rd gen. cephalosporin IV (p544)
Aspiration		
	Streptococcus pneumoniae Anaerobes	Cefuroxime 1.5g/8h IV + metronidazole 500mg/8h IV
Neutropenic patients		
	Gram positive cocci Gram negative bacilli	Aminoglycoside IV + antipseudomonal penicillin IV or 3rd gen. cephalosporin IV
	Fungi (p180)	Consider antifungals after 48h

3rd gen = 3rd generation, eg cefotaxime, p545; gentamicin is an example of an aminoglycoside (p547).

1 Clarithromycin 500mg bd PO/IVI may be used in place of erythromycin throughout these recommendations.

Specific pneumonias

For antibiotic doses, see p543 & p546. TB: ►see p564 & p566.

Pneumococcal pneumonia is the commonest bacterial pneumonia. It affects all ages, but is commoner in the elderly, alcoholics, post-splenectomy, immunosuppressed, and patients with chronic heart failure or pre-existing lung disease. Clinical features: fever, pleurisy, herpes labialis. CXR shows lobar consolidation. Treatment: amoxicillin, benzylpenicillin, or cephalosporin.

Staphylococcal pneumonia may complicate influenza infection or occur in the young, elderly, intravenous drug users, or patients with underlying disease (eg leukaemia, lymphoma, cystic fibrosis, (CF)). It causes a bilateral cavitating bronchopneumonia. Treatment: flucloxacillin.

Klebsiella pneumonia occurs in the elderly and causes a cavitating pneumonia, particularly of the upper lobes. Treatment: cefuroxime.

Pseudomonas is a common pathogen in bronchiectasis and CF. It also causes hospital acquired infections, particularly on ITU or after surgery. Treatment: anti-pseudomonal penicillin, ceftazidime, meropenem, or ciprofloxacin.

Mycoplasma pneumoniae occurs in epidemics about every 4yrs. It presents insidiously with 'flu-like symptoms (headache, myalgia, arthralgia) followed by a dry cough. CXR shows bilateral patchy consolidation. Diagnosis: mycoplasma serology. Cold agglutinins may cause an autoimmune haemolytic anaemia. Complications: skin rash (erythema multiforme (PLATE 17), Stevens–Johnson syndrome), meningoencephalitis or myelitis; Guillain–Barré syndrome. Treatment: erythromycin/clarithromycin or tetracycline.

Legionella pneumophilia colonizes water tanks kept at <60°C (eg hotel air-conditioning and hot water systems) causing outbreaks of Legionnaire's disease. 'Flu-like symptoms (fever, malaise, myalgia) precede a dry cough and dyspnoea. Extra-pulmonary features include anorexia, D&V, hepatitis, renal failure, confusion, and coma. CXR shows bi-basal consolidation. Blood tests may show lymphopenia, hyponatraemia, and deranged LFTs. Urinalysis may show haematuria. Diagnosis: Legionella serology/urine antigen. Treatment: clarithromycin ± rifampicin or fluoroquinolone. 10% mortality.

Chlamydia pneumoniae is commonest chlamydial infection. Person-to-person spread occurs causing a biphasic illness: pharyngitis, hoarseness, otitis, followed by pneumonia. Diagnosis: *Chlamydia* serology (non-specific). Treatment: tetracycline.

Chlamydia psittaci causes psittacosis, an ornithosis acquired from infected birds (typically parrots). Symptoms include headache, fever, dry cough, lethargy, arthralgia, anorexia, and D&V. Extra-pulmonary features are legion but rare, eg meningoencephalitis, infective endocarditis, hepatitis, nephritis, rash, splenomegaly. CXR shows patchy consolidation. Diagnosis: *Chlamydia* serology. Treatment: tetracycline.

Viral pneumonia The commonest cause is influenza (p572). Other viruses that can affect the lung are: measles, CMV, and varicella zoster.

Pneumocystis carinii pneumonia (PCP) This causes pneumonia in the immunosuppressed (eg HIV). It presents with a dry cough, exertional dyspnoea, fever, bilateral crepitations. CXR may be normal or show bilateral perihilar interstitial shadowing. Diagnosis: visualization of the organism in induced sputum, bronchoalveolar lavage, or in a lung biopsy specimen. Drugs: high-dose co-trimoxazole (p580–1), or pentamidine by slow IVI for 2–3 weeks (p581). Steroids are beneficial if severe hypoxaemia. Prophylaxis is indicated if the CD4 count is <200 × 10⁶/L or after the 1st attack.

Complications of pneumonia

Respiratory failure (See p192.) Type 1 respiratory failure (P_aO_2 <8kPa) is relatively common. Treatment is with high-flow (60%) oxygen. *Transfer the patient to ITU if hypoxia does not improve with O_2 therapy or P_aCO_2 rises to >6kPa.* Careful O_2 administration is required in COPD patients; check arterial blood gases frequently and consider elective ventilation if rising P_aCO_2 or worsening acidosis. Aim to keep SaO_2 at 90–94%.

Hypotension may be due to a combination of dehydration and vasodilatation due to sepsis. If systolic BP is <90mmHg, give an intravenous fluid challenge of 250mL colloid/crystalloid over 15min. If BP does not rise, insert a central line and give intravenous fluids to maintain the systolic BP >90mmHg. If systolic BP remains <90mmHg despite fluid therapy, request ITU assessment for inotropic support (adrenaline, noradrenaline) .

Atrial fibrillation (p130) is quite common, particularly in the elderly. It usually resolves with treatment of the pneumonia. Digoxin may be required to slow the ventricular response rate in the short term.

Pleural effusion Inflammation of the pleura by adjacent pneumonia may cause fluid exudation into the pleural space. If this accumulates in the pleural space faster than it is reabsorbed, a pleural effusion develops. If this is small it may be of no consequence. If it becomes large and symptomatic, or infected (empyema), drainage is required (p196 & p750).

Empyema is pus in the pleural space. It should be suspected if a patient with a resolving pneumonia develops a recurrent fever. Clinical features and the CXR indicate a pleural effusion. The aspirated pleural fluid is typically yellow and turbid with a pH <7.2, glucose↓, and LDH↑. The empyema should be drained using a chest drain, preferably inserted under radiological guidance. Although intrapleural streptokinase (250,000U in 50mL 0.9% saline/12h for 3d) has been used to break down the adhesions (p196) the latest data indicate no benefit.

Lung abscess is a cavitating area of localized, suppurative infection within the lung.

Causes: • Inadequately treated pneumonia • Aspiration (eg alcoholism, oesophageal obstruction, bulbar palsy) • Bronchial obstruction (tumour, foreign body) • Pulmonary infarction • Septic emboli (septicaemia, right heart endocarditis, IV drug use) • Subphrenic or hepatic abscess.

Clinical features: Swinging fever; cough; purulent, foul-smelling sputum; pleuritic chest pain; haemoptysis; malaise; weight loss. Look for: finger clubbing; anaemia; crepitations. Empyema develops in 20–30%.

Tests: Blood: FBC (anaemia, neutrophilia), ESR, CRP, blood cultures. *Sputum* microscopy, culture, and cytology. *CXR:* walled cavity, often with a fluid level. Consider CT scan to exclude obstruction, and bronchoscopy obtain diagnostic specimens.

Treatment: Antibiotics as indicated by sensitivities; continue until healed (4–6 wks). Postural drainage. Repeated aspiration, antibiotic instillation, or surgical excision may be required.

Septicaemia may occur as a result of bacterial spread from the lung parenchyma into the bloodstream. This may cause metastatic infection, eg infective endocarditis, meningitis. Treatment is with intravenous antibiotic according to sensitivities.

Pericarditis and myocarditis may also complicate pneumonia.

Jaundice This is usually cholestatic, and may be due to sepsis or secondary to antibiotic therapy (particularly flucloxacillin and co-amoxiclav).

Bronchiectasis

Pathology Chronic infection of the bronchi and bronchioles leading to permanent dilatation of these airways. Main organisms: *H. influenzae*; *Strep. pneumoniae; Staph. aureus; Pseudomonas aeruginosa.*

Causes *Congenital:* CF; Young's syndrome; primary ciliary dyskinesia; Kartagener's syndrome. *Post-infection:* measles; pertussis; bronchiolitis; pneumonia; TB; HIV. *Other:* Bronchial obstruction (tumour, foreign body); allergic bronchopulmonary aspergillosis (ABPA p180); hypogammaglobulinaemia; rheumatoid arthritis; ulcerative colitis; idiopathic.

Clinical features *Symptoms:* persistent cough; copious purulent sputum; intermittent haemoptysis. *Signs:* finger clubbing; coarse inspiratory crepitations, wheeze (asthma, COPD, ABPA). *Complications:* pneumonia, pleural effusion; pneumothorax; haemoptysis; cerebral abscess; amyloidosis.

Investigations *Sputum* culture. *CXR:* cystic shadows, thickened bronchial walls (tramline and ring shadows). *HRCT chest:* to assess extent and distribution of disease. *Spirometry* often shows an obstructive pattern; reversibility should be assessed. *Bronchoscopy* to locate site of haemoptysis or exclude obstruction. *Other tests:* serum immunoglobulins; CF sweat test; *Aspergillus* precipitins or skin-prick test.

Management • *Postural drainage* should be performed twice daily. Chest physiotherapy may aid sputum expectoration and mucous drainage. • *Antibiotics* should be prescribed according to bacterial sensitivities. Patients known to culture *Pseudomonas* will require either oral ciprofloxacin or IV antibiotics. • *Bronchodilators* (eg nebulized salbutamol) may be useful in patients with asthma, COPD, CF, ABPA (p180). • *Corticosteroids* (eg prednisolone) for ABPA. • *Surgery* may be indicated in localized disease or to control severe haemoptysis.

Cystic fibrosis (CF)   See *OHCS* (Paediatrics, p192)

One of the commonest life-threatening autosomal recessive conditions (1 : 2000 live births) affecting Caucasians. Caused by mutations in the CF transmembrane conductance regulator (CFTR) gene on chromosome 7 (>800 mutations have now been identified). This leads to a combination of defective chloride secretion and increased sodium absorption across airway epithelium. The changes in the composition of airway surface liquid predisposes the lung to chronic pulmonary infections and bronchiectasis.

Clinical features *Neonate:* Failure to thrive; meconium ileus; rectal prolapse.

Children and young adults: Respiratory: cough; wheeze; recurrent infections; bronchiectasis; pneumothorax; haemoptysis; respiratory failure; cor pulmonale. *Gastrointestinal:* pancreatic insufficiency (diabetes mellitus, steatorrhea); distal intestinal obstruction syndrome (meconium ileus equivalent); gallstones; cirrhosis. *Other:* male infertility; osteoporosis; arthritis; vasculitis (p424); nasal polyps; sinusitis; and hypertrophic pulmonary osteoarthropathy (HPOA). *Signs:* Cyanosis; finger clubbing; bilateral coarse crackles.

Diagnosis *Sweat test:* sweat sodium and chloride >60mmol/L; chloride usually > sodium. *Genetics:* screening for known common CF mutations should be considered. *Faecal elastase* is a simple and useful screening test for exocrine pancreatic dysfunction.

Tests *Blood:* FBC, U&E, LFTS; clotting; vitamin A, D, E levels; annual glucose tolerance test (p294). *Bacteriology:* cough swab, sputum culture. *Radiology:* CXR; hyperinflation; bronchiectasis. *Abdominal ultrasound:* fatty liver; cirrhosis; chronic pancreatitis; *Spirometry:* obstructive defect. *Aspergillus serology/skin test* (20% develop ABPA, p180). *Biochemsitry:* faecal fat analysis.

Management

Patients with CF are best managed by a multidisciplinary team including physician, physiotherapist, specialist nurse, and dietician with attention to psychosocial as well as physical well-being. Gene therapy (transfer of CFTR gene using liposome or adenovirus vectors) is not yet possible.

Chest Physiotherapy regularly (postural drainage, active cycle techniques or forced expiratory techniques); Antibiotics are given for acute infective exacerbations (PO for *Staph. aureus*, IV for *P. aeruginosa*) and prophylactically PO (flucloxacillin) or nebulized (colomycin or tobramycin); Mucolytics may be useful (eg DNase 2.5mg daily nebulized, *OHCS* p193); Bronchodilators.

Gastrointestinal Pancreatic enzyme replacement; fat soluble vitamin supplements (A, D, E, K); ursodeoxycholic acid for impaired liver function; cirrhosis may require liver transplantation.

Other Treatment of CF-related diabetes; screening for and treatment of osteoporosis; treatment of arthritis, sinusitis, and vasculitis; fertility and genetic counselling.

Advanced lung disease Oxygen, diuretics (cor pulmonale); non-invasive ventilation; lung or heart/lung transplantation.

Prognosis Median survival is now over 30yrs.

Fungi and the lung

Aspergillus This group of fungi affects the lung in 5 ways:

1 *Asthma:* Type I hypersensitivity (atopic) reaction to fungal spores, p184.

2 *Allergic bronchopulmonary aspergillosis (ABPA):* This results from a Type I and III hypersensitivity reaction to *Aspergillus fumigatus*. Early on, the allergic response causes bronchoconstriction, but as the inflammation persists, permanent damage occurs, causing bronchiectasis. *Symptoms:* wheeze, cough, sputum (plugs of mucus containing fungal hyphae), dyspnoea, and 'recurrent pneumonia'. *Investigations:* CXR (transient segmental collapse or consolidation, bronchiectasis); *Aspergillus* in sputum; positive aspergillus skin test and/or aspergillus-specific IgE RAST; positive serum precipitins; eosinophilia; raised serum IgE. *Treatment:* Prednisolone 30–40mg/24h PO for acute attacks; maintenance dose 5–10mg/d. Sometimes itraconazole is used in combination with corticosteroids. Bronchodilators for asthma. Sometimes bronchoscopic aspiration of mucous plugs is needed.

3 *Aspergilloma (mycetoma):* A fungus ball within a pre-existing cavity (often caused by TB, sarcoidosis). It is usually asymptomatic but may cause cough, haemoptysis (may be torrential), lethargy ± weight loss. *Investigations:* CXR (round opacity within a cavity, usually apical); sputum culture; strongly positive serum precipitins; *Aspergillus* skin test (30% +ve). *Treatment* (only if symptomatic). Consider surgical excision for solitary symptomatic lesions or severe haemoptysis. Oral itraconazole and other antifungals have been tried with limited success. Local instillation of amphotericin paste under CT-guidance yields partial success in carefully selected patients, eg in massive haemoptysis.

4 *Invasive aspergillosis: Risk factors:* immunocompromise, eg HIV, leukaemia, burns, Wegener's (p738), and SLE, or after broad-spectrum antibiotic therapy. *Investigations:* sputum culture; serum precipitins; CXR (consolidation, abscess). Early chest CT and serial serum measurements of galactogamman (an *Aspergillus* antigen) can be very helpful. Diagnosis may only be made at lung biopsy or autopsy. *Treatment:* IV amphotericin B (see below). Alternatives: IV miconazole or ketoconazole (less effective). *Prognosis:* very poor.

5 *Extrinsic allergic alveolitis (EAA)* is caused by sensitivity to *Aspergillus clavatus* ('malt worker's lung'). Clinical features and treatment are as for other causes of EAA (p200). Diagnosis is based on a history of exposure and the presence of serum precipitins to *A. clavatus*. Pulmonary fibrosis may occur if untreated.

Using amphotericin B Test dose: 1mg in 20mL 5% dextrose IV over 20–30min. There are many different preparations. Consult BNF. *Do not give any other drug in the same IVI.* SE: anaphylaxis; fever; rash; anorexia; nausea; D&V; headache; myalgia; arthralgia; anaemia; ↓K⁺; ↓Mg²⁺; nephrotoxicity; hepatotoxicity; arrhythmias; hearing loss; diplopia; seizures; peripheral neuropathy; phlebitis. *Monitor U&E daily.* Ambisome® (liposomal amphotericin) has fewer SEs, but is expensive; it is indicated in systemic or deep mycoses where nephrotoxicity precludes conventional amphotericin; IV initial test dose: 1mg over 10min, then 1mg/kg/d, as a single IVI dose; gradually↑ if needed to 3mg/kg/d. Alternatives: Abelcet® & Amphocil®

Other fungal infections *Candida* and *Cryptococcus* may cause pneumonia in the immunosuppressed (see p612).

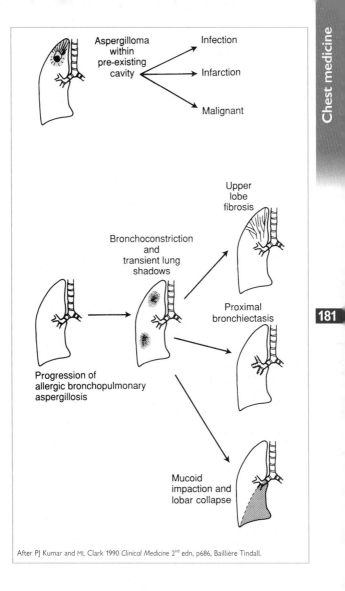

After PJ Kumar and ML Clark 1990 *Clinical Medicine* 2nd edn, p686, Baillière Tindall.

Lung tumours

Carcinoma of the bronchus Accounts for ≈19% of all cancers and 27% of cancer deaths (40,000 cases/yr in UK). Incidence is increasing in women.

Risk factors: Cigarette smoking is the major risk factor. Others: asbestos, chromium, arsenic, iron oxides, and radiation (radon gas).

Histology: Squamous (30%); adenocarcinoma (30%); small (oat) cell (25%); large cell (15%); alveolar cell carcinoma (rare, <1%).

Symptoms: Cough (80%); haemoptysis (70%); dyspnoea (60%); chest pain (40%); recurrent or slowly resolving pneumonia; anorexia; weight loss.

Signs: Cachexia; anaemia; clubbing; HPOA (hypertrophic pulmonary osteoarthropathy, causing wrist pain); supraclavicular or axillary lymphadenopathy. *Chest signs:* may be none; consolidation; collapse; pleural effusion. *Metastases:* bone tenderness; hepatomegaly; confusion; fits; focal CNS deficit; cerebellar syndrome; proximal myopathy; peripheral neuropathy.

Complications: Local: recurrent laryngeal nerve palsy; phrenic nerve palsy; SVC obstruction; Horner's syndrome (Pancoast's tumour); rib erosion; pericarditis; AF. *Metastatic:* brain; bone (bone pain, anaemia, $\uparrow Ca^{2+}$); liver (hepatomegaly); adrenals (Addison's). *Endocrine:* Ectopic hormone secretion, eg SIADH ($\downarrow Na^+$ and $\uparrow ADH$, p690) and ACTH (Cushing's) by oat cell tumours; PTH ($\uparrow Ca^{2+}$) by squamous cell tumours. *Non-metastatic neurological:* confusion; fits; cerebellar syndrome; proximal myopathy; peripheral neuropathy; polymyositis; Eaton–Lambert syndrome (p400). *Other:* finger clubbing, HPOA, dermatomyositis; acanthosis nigricans (p428); thrombophlebitis migrans (p428).

Tests: Cytology: sputum & pleural fluid. *CXR:* peripheral circular opacity; hilar enlargement; consolidation; lung collapse (X-RAY PLATE 4) pleural effusion; bony secondaries. Peripheral lesions and superficial lymph nodes may be amenable to *percutaneous fine needle aspiration/biopsy*. *Bronchoscopy:* to give histological diagnosis and assess operability. *CT:* to stage the tumour (OPPO-SITE). *Radionuclide bone scan:* for suspected metastases. *Lung function tests.*

Treatment: Non-small cell tumours: Excision is the treatment of choice for peripheral tumours, with no metastatic spread (~25%). *Curative radiotherapy* is an alternative in patients with inadequate respiratory reserve. *Small cell tumours* are almost always disseminated at presentation. They may respond to *chemotherapy* with a combination of cyclophosphamide, doxorubicin, vincristine, etoposide, or cisplatin. *Palliation: Radiotherapy* is used for bronchial obstruction, SVC obstruction, haemoptysis, bone pain, and cerebral metastases. *SVC stent + radiotherapy/dexamethasone* for SVC obstruction. *Endobronchial therapy* includes tracheal stenting, cryotherapy, laser therapy, and brachytherapy (a radioactive source is placed close to the tumour). *Pleural drainage/pleurodesis* for symptomatic pleural effusions. *Drug therapy:* analgesia; corticosteroids; antiemetics; cough linctus (codeine); bronchodilators; antidepressants.

Prognosis: Non-small cell: 50% 2yr survival without spread; 10% with spread. *Small cell:* median survival is 3 months if untreated; 1–1½yrs if treated.

Prevention: Actively discourage smoking (for practical help, see p91). Prevent occupational exposure to carcinogens.

Other lung tumours *Bronchial adenoma:* Rare, slow-growing tumour. 90% are carcinoid tumours; 10% are cylindromas. Treatment: surgery. *Hamartoma:* Rare, benign tumour. CT scan: lobulated mass with flecks of calcification. Often excised to exclude malignancy. *Mesothelioma* (p202).

Coin lesions of the lung

- Malignancy (1° or 2°)
- Abscesses (p174)
- Granuloma
- Carcinoid tumour
- Pulmonary hamartoma
- Arteriovenous malformation
- Encysted effusion (fluid, blood, pus)
- Cyst
- Foreign body
- Skin tumour (eg seborrhoeic wart)

TNM staging for lung cancer

Primary tumour (T)	TX	Malignant cells in bronchial secretions, no other evidence of tumour
	Tis	Carcinoma *in situ*
	T0	None evident
	T1	≤3cm, in lobar or more distal airway
	T2	>3cm and >2cm distal to carina *or* any size if pleural involvement *or* obstructive pneumonitis extending to hilum, but not all the lung
	T3	Involves the chest wall, diaphragm, mediastinal pleura, pericardium, or <2cm from, but not at, carina
	T4	Involves the mediastinum, heart, great vessels, trachea, oesophagus, vertebral body, carina, *or* a malignant effusion is present
Regional nodes (N)	N0	None involved (after mediastinoscopy)
	N1	Peribronchial and/or ipsilateral hilum
	N2	Ipsilateral mediastinum or subcarinal
	N3	Contralateral mediastinum or hilum, scalene, or supraclavicular
Distant metastasis (M)	M0	None
	M1	Distant metastases present

Stage	Tumour	Lymph nodes	Metastasis
Occult	TX	N0	M0
I	Tis, T1, or T2	N0	M0
II	T1 or T2	N1	M0
	T3	N0	M0
IIIa	T3	N1	M0
	T1–T3	N2	M0
IIIb	T1–T4	N3	M0
	T4	N0–N2	M0
IV	T1–T4	N0–N3	M1

Asthma

Asthma affects 5–8% of the population. It is characterized by recurrent episodes of dyspnoea, cough, and wheeze caused by reversible airways obstruction. Three factors contribute to airway narrowing: *bronchial muscle contraction*, triggered by a variety of stimuli; *mucosal swelling/inflammation*, caused by mast cell and basophil degranulation resulting in the release of inflammatory mediators; *increased mucus production*.

Symptoms Intermittent dyspnoea, wheeze, cough (often nocturnal) and sputum. Ask specifically about:
- *Precipitants:* Cold air, exercise, emotion, allergens (house dust mite, pollen, animal fur), infection, drugs (eg aspirin, NSAIDs, β-blockers).
- *Diurnal variation* in symptoms or peak flow. Marked morning dipping of peak flow is common and can tip the patient over into a serious attack, despite having normal peak flow at other times.
- *Exercise:* Quantify the exercise tolerance.
- *Disturbed sleep:* Quantify as nights per week (a sign of serious asthma).
- *Acid reflux:* This has a known association with asthma.
- *Other atopic disease:* Eczema, hay fever, allergy, or family history?
- *The home (especially the bedroom):* Pets? carpet? feather pillows or duvet? Floor cushions and other 'soft furnishings'?
- *Occupation:* If symptoms remit at weekends or holidays, something at work may be a trigger. Ask the patient to measure his peak flow at work and at home (at the same time of day) to confirm this.
- *Days per week off work or school.*

Signs Tachypnoea; audible wheeze; hyper-inflated chest; hyper-resonant percussion note; diminished air entry; widespread, polyphonic wheeze. *Severe attack:* Inability to complete sentences; pulse >110bpm; respiratory rate >25/min; PEF 33–50% of predicted. *Life-threatening attack:* silent chest; cyanosis; bradycardia; exhaustion; PEF <33% of predicted; confusion; feeble respiratory effort.

Tests *Chronic asthma:* PEF monitoring (p168): a diurnal variation of >20% on ≥3d a wk for 2wks. Spirometry: obstructive defect (↓FEV_1/FVC, ↑RV); usually ≥15% improvement in FEV_1 following $β_2$ agonists or steroid trial. CXR: hyper-inflation. Skin-prick tests may help to identify allergens. Histamine or methacholine challenge. *Aspergillus* serology. *Acute attack:* PEF, sputum culture, FBC, U&E, CRP, blood cultures. ABG analysis usually shows a normal or slightly reduced P_aO_2 and low P_aCO_2 (hyperventilation). If P_aO_2 normal but the patient is hyperventilating, watch carefully and repeat the ABG a little later. *If P_aCO_2 is raised transfer to high dependency unit or ITU for ventilation.* CXR (to exclude infection or pneumothorax).

Treatment Chronic asthma (p186). Emergency treatment (p794).

Differential diagnosis Pulmonary oedema ('cardiac asthma'); COPD (often co-exists); large airway obstruction (eg foreign body, tumour); SVC obstruction (wheeze/dyspnoea not episodic); pneumothorax; PE; bronchiectasis; obliterative bronchiolitis (suspect in elderly).

Associated diseases Acid reflux; polyarteritis nodosa (PAN, p425); Churg–Strauss syndrome (p425); ABPA (p180).

Natural history Most childhood asthmatics (see OHCS p270) either grow out of asthma in adolescence, or suffer much less as adults. A significant number of people develop chronic asthma late in life.

Mortality Death certificates give a figure of 2000/yr (UK): more careful surveys more than halve this figure. 50% are >65yrs old.

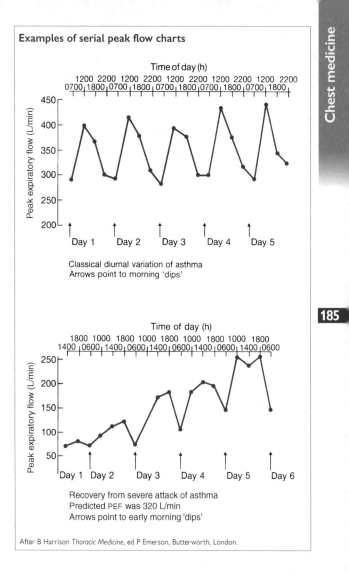

Examples of serial peak flow charts

Classical diurnal variation of asthma
Arrows point to morning 'dips'

Recovery from severe attack of asthma
Predicted PEF was 320 L/min
Arrows point to early morning 'dips'

After B Harrison *Thoracic Medicine*, ed P Emerson, Butterworth, London.

Management of chronic asthma

Behaviour Stop smoking and avoid precipitants. Check inhaler technique. Teach patients to use a peak flow meter to monitor PEF twice a day. Educate patients to manage their disease by altering their medication in response to changes in symptoms or PEF. Give specific advice about what to do in an emergency; provide a written action plan.

British Thoracic Society guidelines Start at the step most appropriate to severity; moving up if needed, or down if control is good for >3 months. Rescue courses of prednisolone may be used at any time.

Step 1 Occasional short-acting inhaled β₂-agonist as required for symptom relief. If used more than once daily, or night-time symptoms, go to Step 2.

Step 2 Add standard-dose inhaled steroid: beclometasone or budesonide 100–400µg/12h or fluticasone 50–200µg/12h.

Step 3 Add long-acting β₂-agonist (eg salmeterol 50µg/12h or formoterol 12µg/12h). If benefit—but still inadequate control—continue and ↑dose of beclometasone to 400µg/12h, (if no effect of long acting β₂-agonist stop it).

Step 4 Consider trials of: beclometasone up to 1000µg/12h; modified-release oral theophylline; modified-release oral β₂-agonist; or oral leukotriene receptor antagonist; in conjunction with previous therapy.

Step 5 Add regular oral prednisolone (1 daily dose, at the lowest possible dose). Refer to asthma clinic.

Drugs *β₂-adrenoreceptor agonists* relax bronchial smooth muscle, acting within minutes. Salbutamol is best given by inhalation (aerosol, powder, nebulizer), but may also be given PO or IV. SE: tachyarrhythmias, ↓K⁺, tremor, anxiety. Long-acting inhaled β₂-agonist (eg salmeterol, formoterol) can help nocturnal symptoms and reduce morning dips. They may be an alternative to ↑steroid dose when symptoms are uncontrolled. SE: as salbutamol, paradoxical bronchospasm (salmeterol). SE: paradoxical bronchospasm, tolerance, arrhythmias.

Corticosteroids are best inhaled, eg beclometasone via spacer (or powder), but may be given PO or IV. They act over days to ↓bronchial mucosal inflammation. Rinse mouth after inhaled steroids to prevent oral candidiasis. Oral steroids are used acutely (high-dose, short courses, eg prednisolone 30–40mg/24h PO for 7d) and longer term in lower dose (eg 5–10mg/24h) if control is not optimal on inhalers. Warn about SEs: p286.

Aminophylline (metabolized to theophylline) may act by inhibiting phosphodiesterase, thus ↓bronchoconstriction by ↑cAMP levels. Try as prophylaxis, at night, PO, to prevent morning dipping. Stick with one brand name (bioavailability variable). It is also useful as an adjunct if inhaled therapy is inadequate. In acute severe asthma, it may be given IVI. It has a narrow therapeutic ratio, causing arrhythmias, GI upset, and fits in the toxic range. Check theophylline levels (p711), and do ECG monitoring and check plasma levels after 24h if IV therapy is used.

Anticholinergics (eg ipratropium) may ↓muscle spasm synergistically with β₂-agonists. They may be of more benefit in COPD than in asthma. Try each alone, and then together; assess with spirometry.

Cromoglycate May be used as prophylaxis in mild and exercise-induced asthma (always inhaled), especially in children. It may precipitate asthma.

Leukotriene receptor antagonists (eg montelukast, zafirlukast) block the effects of cysteinyl leukotrienes in the airways.

Doses of some inhaled drugs used in bronchoconstriction

	Inhaled aerosol	Inhaled powder	Nebulized (*supervised*)
Salbutamol			
Dose example:	100–200µg/6h	200–400µg/6h	2.5–5mg/6h
(the same for **CFC** and **CFC**-free devices Salamol® is an example of a **CFC**-free inhaler Airomir® is **CFC**-free and breath-actuated)			
Terbutaline			
Single dose	250µg	500µg[1]	2.5mg/mL
Recommended regimen	≤500µg/4h	500µg/6h	5–10mg/6–12h
Salmeterol			
Dose/puff	25µg	50µg	—
Recommended regimen	50–100µg/12h	50–100µg/12h	—
Ipratropium bromide			
Dose/puff	20µg or 40µg	—	250µg/mL
Recommended regimen	20–80µg/6h	—	100–500µg/6h
Steroids			
(*Becotide® = beclometasone; Pulmicort® = budesonide[1]; Flixotide® = fluticasone*)			
Fluticasone (Flixotide®)			
Doses available/puff	25, 50, 125µg &	50–500µg	250µg/mL
(formulations with **CFC**s)	250µg		
Recommended regimen	100–250µg/12h	100–250µg/12h	½–2mg/12h
(formulations with **CFC**s)		max 1mg/12h	
Becotide 50 & 100®			
Doses available/puff	50 & 100µg	—	—
	(Becloforte = 250µg)		
Recommended regimen	100µg/12h		
(formulations with **CFC**s)	↓		
	200µg/12h		
	↓		
	250µg/12h		
	↓		
	500–1000µg/12h		

Any puff/dose ≥250µg≈significant steroid absorption: carry a steroid card; this recommendation is being widened, so that, eg *any* dose of Qvar (below) is said to merit a steroid card (manufacturer's information).

Changing to a CFC-free device (eg Qvar® beclometasone 50 or 100µg autohaler): doses of Qvar are lower than for **CFC** inhalers as particle size is smaller. If well-controlled pre-changeover, try half the daily dose of Qvar, if poorly controlled try the same dose, then ↓ as control is achieved.

100µg Qvar®≈100µg Flixotide® = 200–250µg Becotide® with **CFC**. Max Qvar dose: 400µg/12h. **NB**: soon *all* inhalers will be **CFC**-free. Tell patients their inhaler may taste different and that **CFC**s will not have harmed them. They may not like the new taste: anticipate this point, and reassure.

187

1 Available as a Turbohaler®; Autohalers® are an alternative (breath-actuated) and don't need breathing coordination eg Airomir[no cfc] (salbutamol) & Aerobec® & Qvar® (both beclometasone). Accuhalers deliver dry powders (eg Flixotide®, Serevent®).
Systemic absorption (via the throat) is minimized if inhalation is through a **large-volume device**, eg Volumatic® or Aero Chamber Plus (for Airomir & Qvar) devices. The latter is more compact. Static charge on some devices reduces dose delivery, so wash in water before dose and leave to dry. It is pointless to squirt many puffs into the device: it is best to repeat single doses—and be sure to inhale *as soon as the drug is in the spacer* (BMJ 1997 i 1061). **SE**: local (oral) candidiasis (p210); ↑rate of cataract if lifetime dose ≥2g beclometasone (EBM 1998 3 24). **NB**: CFC = **chlorofluorocarbon**.

Chronic obstructive pulmonary disease (COPD)

Definitions COPD is a common progressive disorder of airway obstruction (↓FEV₁, ↓FEV₁/FVC, p168–70) with little or no reversibility. COPD includes chronic bronchitis and emphysema (NICE states that COPD is the preferred term). Usually patients have *either* COPD *or* asthma, not both: COPD is favoured by:
• Age of onset >35yrs • Smoking related • Chronic dyspnoea • Sputum production • No marked diurnal or day-to-day FEV₁ variation. *Chronic bronchitis* is defined *clinically* as cough, sputum production on most days for 3 months of 2 successive years. There is no increase in mortality if lung function is normal. Symptoms improve in 90% if they stop smoking. *Emphysema* is defined *histologically* as enlargement of the air spaces distal to the terminal bronchioles, with destruction of the alveolar walls.

Prevalence ~1.5million. *COPD mortality:* 25,000 deaths/yr in England & Wales.

Pink puffers and blue bloaters (Two ends of a spectrum) *Pink puffers* have ↑alveolar ventilation, a near normal P_aO_2 and a normal or low P_aCO_2. They are breathless but not cyanosed. They may progress to Type I respiratory failure (p192). *Blue bloaters* have ↓alveolar ventilation, with a low P_aO_2 and a high P_aCO_2. They are cyanosed but not breathless and may go on to develop cor pulmonale. Their respiratory centres are relatively insensitive to CO_2 and they rely on their hypoxic drive to maintain respiratory effort (p192)—►*supplemental oxygen should be given with care.*

Clinical features *Symptoms:* Cough, sputum, dyspnoea, and wheeze. *Signs:* Tachypnoea; use of accessory muscles of respiration; hyper-inflation; ↓cricosternal distance (<3cm); ↓expansion; resonant or hyper-resonant note; quiet breath sounds (eg over bullae); wheeze; cyanosis; cor pulmonale. *Complications:* Acute exacerbations ± infection; polycythaemia; respiratory failure; cor pulmonale (oedema; JVP↑); pneumothorax (ruptured bullae); lung ca.

Tests *FBC:* PCV↑. *CXR:* Hyperinflation (>6 anterior ribs seen above diaphragm in mid-clavicular line); flat hemidiaphragms; large central pulmonary arteries; ↓peripheral vascular markings; bullae. *ECG:* Right atrial and ventricular hypertrophy (cor pulmonale). *ABG:* P_aO_2↓ ± hypercapnia. *Lung function* (p168–70): obstructive + air trapping (FEV₁ <80% of predicted—see below, FEV₁:FVC ratio <70%, TLC↑, RV↑, DLCO↓ in emphysema). Learn how to do FEV₁ and FVC from an experienced spirometrist: ensure *maximal* expiration of the full breath (it takes ≥4sec; it's *not* a quick puff out). *Trial of steroids:* See BOX.

Treatment *Chronic stable:* see BOX; ►►*Emergency Rx:* p796. Offer *smoking cessation advice* with cordial vigour (p91). BMI is often low: *diet advice ± supplements* may help, p466. *Mucolytics* (BNF 3.7) may help chronic productive cough (NICE 2004). Disabilities may cause serious, treatable *depression;* screen for this (p15). *Respiratory failure:* p192. 'Flu and pneumococcal vaccinations: p572.

Longterm O_2 therapy (LTOT): An MRC trial showed that if P_aO_2 was maintained ≥8.0kPa for 15h a day, 3yr survival improved by 50%. UK DoH guidelines suggest LTOT should be given for: (1) clinically stable non-smokers with P_aO_2 <7.3kPa—despite maximal Rx. These values should be stable on two occasions >3 wks apart. (2) If P_aO_2 7.3–8.0 **and** pulmonary hypertension (eg RVH; loud S_2) + cor pulmonale. O_2 can also be prescribed for terminally ill patients.

188

Predicted FEV₁ (Caucasian males; litres, ↓level in other races)[1]

Height cm	150	155	160	165	170	175	180	185	190	195
♂ Age(yr) 10	2.5	2.8	3.0	3.2	3.5	3.7	3.9	4.1	4.4	4.6
25	2.9	3.2	3.4	3.7	4.0	4.2	4.3	4.7	5.0	5.3
30	2.8	3.1	3.3	3.6	3.8	4.1	4.3	4.6	4.9	5.1
40	2.5	2.8	3.0	3.3	3.6	3.8	4.1	4.3	4.6	4.9
50	2.2	2.5	2.8	3.0	3.3	3.5	3.8	4.0	4.3	4.6
60	2.0	2.2	2.5	2.8	3.0	3.3	3.5	3.8	4.0	4.3
70	1.7	2.0	2.2	2.5	2.7	3.0	3.3	3.5	3.8	4.0
80	1.4	1.7	2.0	2.2	2.5	2.7	3.0	3.3	3.5	3.8

Height cm	145	150	155	160	165	170	175	180	185	190
10	2.1	2.2	2.3	2.5	2.6	2.7	2.9	3.0	3.1	3.3
25	2.6	2.7	2.9	3.0	3.1	3.3	3.4	3.5	3.7	3.8
30	2.5	2.6	2.8	2.9	3.0	3.2	3.3	3.4	3.6	3.7
40	2.3	2.4	2.5	2.7	2.8	3.0	3.2	3.3	3.5	
50	2.1	2.2	2.3	2.5	2.6	2.7	2.9	3.0	3.1	3.3
60	1.7	2.0	2.1	2.3	2.4	2.5	2.7	2.8	2.9	3.1
70	1.6	1.8	1.9	2.1	2.2	2.3	2.5	2.6	2.7	2.9
80	1.4	1.6	1.7	1.9	2.0	2.1	2.2	2.4	2.5	2.7

www.nationalasthma.org.au/publications/spiro/appc.html☆Mean

1 African FEV₁ is 10–15% lower; Chinese: 20% lower; Indian: 10% lower; note: PEF varies little between groups.

British Thoracic Society (BTS)/NICE 2004 COPD guidelines

Assessment of COPD	Spirometry
	Bronchodilator response
	Trial of oral steroids;[1] look for >15% ↑ in FEV_1
	CXR ?bullae ?other pathology
	ABG ?hypoxia ?hypercapnia
Severity of COPD	Mild FEV_1 60–80% predicted
	Moderate FEV_1 40–59% predicted
	Severe FEV_1 <40% predicted
Treating stable COPD	**NB:** air travel is risky if FEV_1 <50% or P_aO_2 <6.7kPa

Non-pharmacological Stop smoking, encourage exercise, treat poor nutrition or obesity, influenza and pneumococcal vaccination, pulmonary rehabilitation/palliative care.[2]

Pharmacological: Mild Eg antimuscarinic, ipratropium inhaled PRN.

Moderate Regular ipratropium or long-acting inhaled $β_2$ agonist (salmeterol) ± inhaled steroid (fluticasone) if FEV_1<50% and ≥2 exacerbations/yr. Seretide® combines these. Symbicort® is budesonide + formoterol; there is conflicting evidence on whether this improves quality of life and symptom scores; but it *may* ↓time to 1st exacerbation. *Drug Ther Bul 2004 18*

Severe Combination therapy with regular short-acting $β_2$-agonist and ipratropium.
Consider steroid trial;[1] assess for home nebulizers.

More advanced COPD
- Consider pulmonary rehabilitation[2] ± theophylline (monitor blood levels).
- Consider LTOT if P_aO_2 <7.3kPa (see OPPOSITE).
- Indications for surgery: recurrent pneumothoraces; isolated bullous disease; lung volume reduction surgery (selected patients).
- Assess home set-up and support needed. Treat depression (p15).

Indications for specialist referral
- Uncertain diagnosis.
- Suspected severe COPD or a rapid decline in FEV_1.
- Onset of cor pulmonale.
- Assessment for oral corticosteroids, nebulizer therapy, or LTOT.
- Bullous lung disease (to assess for surgery).
- <10 pack-years smoking (=PYS = the number of packs/day × number of years of smoking). Smokers have an excess loss of FEV_1 of 7.4–12.6mL/PYS for men and 4.4–7.2mL per pack year for women.[19]
- Symptoms disproportionate to lung function tests.
- Frequent infections (to exclude bronchiectasis).
- COPD in patient <40yrs (eg is the cause $α_1$-antitrypsin deficiency? p236).

189

1 Steroid trial: 30mg prednisolone/24h PO for 2wks. If FEV_1 rises by >15%, the COPD is 'steroid responsive' and benefit may be had by using longterm inhaled corticosteroids (p187). If this doesn't achieve the post-prednisolone FEV_1, do not simply give longterm oral prednisolone (side-effects may be lethal, p675); instead, request expert help. (BTS advice). **NB:** NICE says that 'reversibility testing is not necessary as a part of the diagnostic process or to plan initial therapy with bronchodilators or corticosteroids. It may be unhelpful or misleading because: (1) repeated FEV_1 measurements can show small spontaneous fluctuations; (2) results of a reversibility tests on different occasions can be inconsistent and not reproducible; (3) Over-reliance on a single reversibility test may be misleading unless the change in FEV_1 is >400 mL. (4) Definition of a significant change is arbitrary; (5) Response to long-term therapy is not predicted by acute reversibility testing.'
2 Palliative care involves referral to a multidisciplinary team ± use of benzodiazepines, antidepressants, opiates, major tranquillizers, and O_2 with a view to diminish symptoms in end-stage COPD.

Acute respiratory distress syndrome (ARDS)

ARDS, or acute lung injury, may be caused by direct lung injury or occur secondary to severe systemic illness. Lung damage and release of inflammatory mediators cause increased capillary permeability and non-cardiogenic pulmonary oedema, often accompanied by multiorgan failure.

Causes *Pulmonary:* Pneumonia; gastric aspiration; inhalation; injury; vasculitis (p424); contusion. *Other:* Shock; septicaemia; haemorrhage; multiple transfusions; DIC (p650); pancreatitis; acute liver failure; trauma; head injury; malaria; fat embolism; burns; obstetric events (eclampsia; amniotic fluid embolus); drugs/toxins (aspirin, heroin, paraquat).

Clinical features Cyanosis; tachypnoea; tachycardia; peripheral vasodilatation; bilateral fine inspiratory crackles.

Investigations FBC, U&E, LFT, amylase, clotting, CRP, blood cultures, ABG. CXR shows bilateral pulmonary infiltrates. Pulmonary artery catheter to measure pulmonary capillary wedge pressure (PCWP).

Diagnostic criteria One consensus requires these 4 to exist: (1) Acute onset. (2) CXR: bilateral infiltrates. (3) PCWP <19mmHg or a lack of clinical congestive heart failure. (4) Refractory hypoxaemia with P_aO_2 : FiO_2 <200 for ARDS. Others include total thoracic compliance <30mL/cm H_2O.

Management Admit to ITU, give supportive therapy, and treat the underlying cause.

- *Respiratory support* In early ARDS continuous positive airway pressure (CPAP) with 40–60% oxygen may be adequate to maintain oxygenation. But most patients need mechanical ventilation. Indications for ventilation: P_aO_2: <8.3kPa despite 60% O_2; P_aCO_2: >6kPa. The large tidal volumes (10–15mL/kg) produced by conventional ventilation plus reduced lung compliance in ARDS may lead to high peak airway pressures ± pneumothorax. Positive end-expiratory pressure (PEEP) increases oxygenation but at the expense of venous return, cardiac output, and perfusion of the kidneys and liver. Other approaches include inverse ratio ventilation (inspiration > expiration), permissive hypercapnia, and high-frequency jet ventilation, and other low-tidal-volume techniques.[20]
- *Circulatory support* Invasive haemodynamic monitoring with an arterial line and Swan–Ganz catheter aids the diagnosis and may be helpful in monitoring PCWP and cardiac output. Maintain cardiac output and O_2 delivery with inotropes (eg dobutamine 2.5–10µg/kg/min IV), vasodilators, and blood transfusion. Consider treating pulmonary hypertension with low-dose (20–120 parts per million) nitric oxide, a selective pulmonary vasodilator. Haemofiltration may be needed in renal failure and to achieve a negative fluid balance.[21]
- *Sepsis* Identify organism(s) and treat accordingly. If clinically septic, but no organisms cultured, use empirical broad-spectrum antibiotics (p173). Avoid nephrotoxic antibiotics.
- *Other:* Nutritional support: enteral is best: p466 & p468. Steroids don't ↓mortality in the acute phase, but may help later on (>7d), particularly if eosinophilia in blood or in fluid from broncho-alveolar lavage.

Prognosis Overall mortality is 50%–75%. Prognosis varies with age of patient, cause of ARDS (pneumonia 86%, trauma 38%), and number of organs involved (3 organs involved for >1wk is 'invariably' fatal).

Risk factors for ARDS

- Sepsis
- Hypovolaemic shock
- Trauma
- Pneumonia
- Diabetic ketoacidosis
- Gastric aspiration
- Pregnancy
- Eclampsia
- Amniotic fluid embolus
- Drugs/toxins
- Paraquat, heroin, aspirin
- Pulmonary contusion
- Massive transfusion
- Burns (p834)
- Smoke inhalation (p835)
- Near drowning
- Acute pancreatitis
- DIC (p650)
- Head injury
- ICP↑
- Fat embolus
- Heart/lung bypass
- Tumour lysis syndrome (p436)
- Malaria

Respiratory failure

Respiratory failure occurs when gas exchange is inadequate, resulting in hypoxia. It is defined as a P_aO_2 <8kPa and subdivided into 2 types according to P_aCO_2 level.

Type I respiratory failure is defined as hypoxia (P_aO_2 <8kPa) with a normal or low P_aCO_2. It is caused primarily by ventilation/perfusion ($\dot{V}/\dot{Q}$) mismatch. Causes include:
• Pneumonia
• Pulmonary oedema
• PE
• Asthma
• Emphysema
• Fibrosing alveolitis
• ARDS (p190).

Type II respiratory failure is defined as hypoxia (P_aO_2 <8kPa) with hypercapnia (P_aCO_2 is >6.0kPa). This is caused by alveolar hypoventilation, with or without $\dot{V}/\dot{Q}$ mismatch. Causes include:
• *Pulmonary disease:* asthma, COPD, pneumonia, pulmonary fibrosis, obstructive sleep apnoea (OSA, p204).
• *Reduced respiratory drive:* sedative drugs, CNS tumour, or trauma.
• *Neuromuscular disease:* cervical cord lesion, diaphragmatic paralysis, poliomyelitis, myasthenia gravis, Guillain–Barré syndrome.
• *Thoracic wall disease:* flail chest, kyphoscoliosis.

Clinical features are those of the underlying cause together with symptoms and signs of hypoxia, with or without hypercapnia.

Hypoxia: Dyspnoea; restlessness; agitation; confusion; central cyanosis. If longstanding hypoxia: polycythaemia; pulmonary hypertension; cor pulmonale.

Hypercapnia: Headache; peripheral vasodilatation; tachycardia; bounding pulse; tremor/flap; papilloedema; confusion; drowsiness; coma.

Investigations are aimed at determining the underlying cause:
• Blood tests: FBC, U&E, CRP, ABG
• Radiology: CXR
• Microbiology: sputum and blood cultures (if febrile)
• Spirometry (COPD, neuromuscular disease, Guillain–Barré syndrome).

Management depends on the cause:

Type I respiratory failure
• Treat underlying cause.
• Give oxygen (35–60%) by face mask to correct hypoxia.
• Assisted ventilation if P_aO_2 <8kPa despite 60% O_2.

Type II respiratory failure The respiratory centre may be relatively insensitive to CO_2 and respiration could be driven by hypoxia. ►*Oxygen therapy should be given with care.* Nevertheless, don't leave the hypoxia untreated.
• Treat underlying cause.
• Controlled oxygen therapy: start at 24% O_2.
• Recheck ABG after 20min. If P_aCO_2 is steady or lower, increase O_2 concentration to 28%, If P_aCO_2 has risen >1.5kPa and the patient is still hypoxic, consider a respiratory stimulant (eg doxapram 1.5–4mg/min IV) or assisted ventilation (eg NIPPV, p188, ie non-invasive positive pressure ventilation).
• If this fails, consider intubation and ventilation, if appropriate.

When to consider ABG (arterial blood gas) measurement

In these clinical scenarios:

Any unexpected deterioration in an ill patient.

Anyone with an acute exacerbation of a chronic chest condition.

Anyone with impaired consciousness.

Anyone with impaired respiratory effort.

Or if any of these signs or symptoms are present:

Bounding pulse, drowsy, tremor (flapping), headache, pink palms, papilloedema (signs of CO_2 retention).

Cyanosis, confusion, visual hallucinations (signs of hypoxia).

Or to monitor the progress of a critically ill patient:

Monitoring the treatment of known respiratory failure.

Anyone ventilated on ITU.

After major surgery.

After major trauma.

To validate measurements from transcutaneous pulse oximetry:

Pulse oximetry (p168) *sometimes* suffices when it is not critical to know P_aCO_2. Even so, it is wise to do periodic blood gas checks.

Learn arterial puncture from an expert (local anaesthesia *does* ↓pain).

Pulmonary embolism (PE)

Causes PEs usually arise from a venous thrombosis in the pelvis or legs. Clots break off and pass through the venous system and the right side of the heart before lodging in the pulmonary circulation. Rare causes include: right ventricular thrombus (post-MI); septic emboli (right-sided endocarditis); fat, air, or amniotic fluid embolism; neoplastic cells; parasites. *Risk factors:* Any cause of immobility or hypercoagulability:

- Recent surgery
- Thrombophilia/antiphospholipid syn. (p672)
- Recent stroke or MI
- Prolonged bed rest
- Disseminated malignancy
- Pregnancy; postpartum; the Pill/HRT

Clinical features These depend on the number, size, and distribution of the emboli; small emboli may be asymptomatic whereas large emboli are often fatal. *Symptoms:* Acute breathlessness, pleuritic chest pain, haemoptysis; dizziness; syncope. Ask about risk factors (above), past history or family history of thromboembolism. *Signs:* Pyrexia; cyanosis; tachypnoea; tachycardia; hypotension; raised JVP, pleural rub; pleural effusion. Look for signs of a cause, eg deep vein thrombosis; scar from recent surgery.

Tests

- *CXR* may be normal, or may show oligaemia of affected segment, dilated pulmonary artery, linear atelectasis, small pleural effusion, wedge-shaped opacities or cavitation (rare).
- *ECG* may be normal, or show tachycardia, right bundle branch block, right ventricular strain (inverted T in V_1 to V_4), The classical $S_IQ_{III}T_{III}$ pattern (p96) is rare.
- *ABG* may show a low P_aO_2 and a low P_aCO_2.

▶Further investigations are shown on p802.

194

Treatment ▶▶See p802. Anticoagulate with low molecular weight heparin (eg dalteparin 200U/kg/24h SC, max dose 18,000U/24h) and start oral warfarin 10mg (p648). Stop heparin when INR is >2 and continue warfarin for a minimum of 3 months (see p649); aim for an INR of 2–3. Consider placement of a *vena caval filter* in patients who develop emboli despite adequate anticoagulation (NB increased risk if placed without concomitant anticoagulation).

Prevention Give heparin (eg dalteparin 2500U/24h SC) to all immobile patients. Prescribe TED stockings and encourage early mobilization. Women should stop HRT and the Pill pre-op (if reliable with another form of contraception). Patients with a past or family history of thromboembolism should be investigated for thrombophilia (p672).

Pneumothorax

Management p798 & *X-RAY PLATE* 6.

Causes Often spontaneous (especially in young thin men) due to rupture of a subpleural bulla. Other causes: asthma; COPD; TB; pneumonia; lung abscess; carcinoma; cystic fibrosis; lung fibrosis; sarcoidosis; connective tissue disorders (Marfan's syndrome, Ehlers–Danlos syndrome), trauma; iatrogenic (subclavian CVP line insertion, pleural aspiration or biopsy, percutaneous liver biopsy, positive pressure ventilation).

Clinical features *Symptoms:* There may be no symptoms (especially in fit young people with small pneumothoraces) or there may be sudden onset of dyspnoea and/or pleuritic chest pain. Patients with asthma or COPD may present with a sudden deterioration. Mechanically ventilated patients may present with hypoxia or an increase in ventilation pressures. *Signs:* Reduced expansion, hyper-resonance to percussion and diminished breath sounds on the affected side. *With a tension pneumothorax, the trachea will be deviated away from the affected side.*

Management and tension pneumothorax see p798

▶▶Placing a chest drain, p750.

Investigation of suspected PE

- First assess the likely probability of a PE
  - Numerous scoring systems are available
  - One simple system is the presence of clinical features of a PE (SOB and tachypnoea, with or without pleuritic chest pain and haemoptysis) and either *a)* the absence of another reasonable explanation, or *b)* the presence of a major risk factor. If *a* and *b* co-exist, the probability is high; if only one exists, intermediate; if neither exist, low.
- *D-dimers* only perform in those patients **without** a high probability of a PE. A negative D-dimer test excludes a PE in those with a low or intermediate clinical probability, and imaging is NOT required. However, a positive test does not prove a diagnosis of a PE, and imaging is required.
- *Imaging* The conventional 1st-line, if the CXR is normal, is a $\dot{V}/\dot{Q}$ *scan* (p170 & p802; look for perfusion defects with no corresponding ventilation defects). If 'normal', a PE is reliably excluded. If non-diagnostic, further imaging is required, but may give some false positives. The recommended 1st-line imaging modality now is CT pulmonary angiography (CTPA), which can show clots down to 5th-order pulmonary arteries (after the 4th branching). This may also be useful for subjects with indeterminant isotope scans. Bilateral leg ultrasound (or rarely venograms) may also be sufficient to CONFIRM, but not exclude, a PE in patients with a co-existing clinical DVT.

Major risk factors for PE

- Surgery
  Major abdominal/pelvic
  Hip/knee replacement
- Obstetrics
  Late pregnancy; post-partum
  Caesarean section

- Lower limb problems
  Fracture
  Varicose veins
- Malignancy
- Reduced mobility
- Previous PE

Pleural effusion

Definitions A pleural effusion is fluid in the pleural space. Effusions can be divided by their protein concentration into *transudates* (<25g/L) and *exudates* (>35g/L), see OPPOSITE. Blood in the pleural space is a *haemothorax*; pus in the pleural space is an *empyema*, and chyle (lymph with fat) is a *chylothorax*. Both blood and air in the pleural space is called a *haemopneumothorax*.

Causes *Transudates* may be due to ↑venous pressure (cardiac failure, constrictive pericarditis, fluid overload), or hypoproteinaemia (cirrhosis, nephrotic syndrome, malabsorption). Also occur in hypothyroidism and Meigs' syndrome (right pleural effusion and ovarian fibroma). *Exudates* are mostly due to increased leakiness of pleural capillaries secondary to infection, inflammation, or malignancy. Causes: pneumonia; TB; pulmonary infarction; rheumatoid arthritis; SLE; bronchogenic carcinoma; malignant metastases; lymphoma; mesothelioma; lymphangitis carcinomatosis.

Symptoms Asymptomatic—or dyspnoea, pleuritic chest pain.

Signs *Decreased expansion; stony dull percussion note; diminished breath sounds* occur on the affected side. Tactile vocal fremitus and vocal resonance are ↓ (inconstant and unreliable). Above the effusion, where lung is compressed, there may be *bronchial breathing* and *aegophony* (bleating vocal resonance). With large effusions there may be *tracheal deviation* away from the effusion. Look for aspiration marks and signs of associated disease: malignancy (cachexia, clubbing, lymphadenopathy, radiation marks, mastectomy scar); stigmata of chronic liver disease; cardiac failure; hypothyroidism; rheumatoid arthritis; butterfly rash of SLE.

Tests *CXR* Small effusions blunt the costophrenic angles, larger ones are seen as water-dense shadows with concave upper borders. A completely horizontal upper border implies that there is also a pneumothorax.

Ultrasound is useful in identifying the presence of pleural fluid and in guiding diagnostic or therapeutic aspiration.

Diagnostic aspiration: Percuss the upper border of the pleural effusion and choose a site 1 or 2 intercostal spaces below it. Infiltrate down to the pleura with 5–10mL of 1% lidocaine. Attach a 21G needle to a syringe and insert it just above the upper border of an appropriate rib (avoids neurovascular bundle). Draw off 10–30mL of pleural fluid and send it to the lab for *clinical chemistry* (protein, glucose, pH, LDH, amylase); *bacteriology* (microscopy and culture, auramine stain, TB culture); *cytology* and, if indicated, *immunology* (rheumatoid factor, ANA, complement).

Pleural biopsy: If pleural fluid analysis is inconclusive, consider parietal pleural biopsy with an Abrams' needle. Thoracoscopic or CT-guided pleural biopsy increases diagnostic yield (by enabling direct visualization of the pleural cavity and biopsy of suspicious areas).

Management is of the underlying cause.
- *Drainage* If the effusion is symptomatic, drain it, repeatedly if necessary. Fluid is best removed slowly (≤2L/24h). It may be aspirated in the same way as a diagnostic tap, or using an intercostal drain (see p750).
- *Pleurodesis* with tetracycline, bleomycin, or talc may be helpful for recurrent effusions. Thorascopic talc pleurodesis is most effective for malignant effusions. Empyemas (p176) are best drained using a chest drain, inserted under ultrasound or CT guidance.
- *Intrapleural streptokinase* Probably no benefit.
- *Surgery:* Persistent collections and increasing pleural thickness (on ultrasound) requires surgery.

Pleural fluid analysis

Gross appearance | *Cause*
Clear, straw-coloured | Transudate, exudate
Turbid, yellow | Empyema, parapneumonic effusion
Haemorrhagic | Trauma, malignancy, pulmonary infarction

Cytology
Neutrophils ++ | Parapneumonic effusion, PE
Lymphocytes ++ | Malignancy, TB, RA, SLE, sarcoidosis
Mesothelial cells ++ | Pulmonary infarction
Abnormal mesothelial cells | Mesothelioma
Multinucleated giant cells | RA
Lupus erythematosus cells | SLE

Clinical chemistry
Protein <25g/L | Transudate
　　　　>35g/L | Exudate
　　　　25–35g/L | If pleural fluid protein/serum protein >0.5, effusion is an exudate

Glucose <3.3mmol/L | Empyema, malignancy, TB, RA, SLE
pH <7.2 | Empyema, malignancy, TB, RA, SLE
LDH↑(pleural:serum >0.6) | Empyema, malignancy, TB, RA, SLE
Amylase↑ | Pancreatitis, carcinoma, bacterial pneumonia, oesophageal rupture

Immunology
Rheumatoid factor | RA
Antinuclear antibody | SLE
Complement levels↓ | RA, SLE, malignancy, infection

Sarcoidosis

A multisystem granulomatous disorder of unknown cause. Prevalence in UK: $10–20/10^5$ population. Commonly affects adults aged 20–40yrs. Afro-Caribbeans are affected more frequently and more severely than Caucasians, particularly by extrathoracic disease.

Clinical features *Asymptomatic* In 20–40%, the disease is discovered incidentally, after a routine CXR. *Acute sarcoidosis* often presents with erythema nodosum (PLATE 18)[1] ± polyarthralgia. It usually resolves spontaneously.

Pulmonary disease 90% have abnormal CXRs with bilateral hilar lymphadenopathy (**BHL**) ± pulmonary infiltrates or fibrosis. *Symptoms:* Dry cough, progressive dyspnoea, ↓exercise tolerance and chest pain. In 10–20% symptoms progress, with concurrent deterioration in lung function.

Non-pulmonary manifestations are legion: lymphadenopathy; hepatomegaly; splenomegaly; uveitis; conjunctivitis; keratoconjunctivitis sicca; glaucoma; terminal phalangeal bone cysts; enlargement of lacrimal and parotid glands; Bell's palsy; neuropathy; meningitis; brainstem and spinal syndromes; space-occupying lesion; erythema nodosum (PLATE 18); lupus pernio; subcutaneous nodules; cardiomyopathy; arrhythmias; hypercalcaemia; hypercalciuria; renal stones; pituitary dysfunction.

Investigations *Blood tests:* ↑ESR, lymphopenia, abnormal LFT, ↑serum ACE, ↑immunoglobulins. *24h urine:* Ca^{2+}↑; hypercalciuria. *Tuberculin skin test* is –ve in two-thirds;. *CXR* is abnormal 90%. *Stage 0:* normal. *Stage 1:* BHL. *Stage 2:* BHL + peripheral pulmonary infiltrates. *Stage 3:* peripheral pulmonary infiltrates alone. *Stage 4:* progressive pulmonary fibrosis; bulla formation (honeycombing); pleural involvement.

ECG may show arrhythmias or bundle branch block. *Lung function tests* may be normal or show reduced lung volumes, impaired gas transfer, and a restrictive ventilatory defect. *Tissue biopsy* (lung, liver, lymph nodes, skin nodules. or lacrimal glands) is diagnostic and shows non-caseating granulomata.

Bronchoalveolar lavage (BAL) shows ↑lymphocytes in active disease; ↑neutrophils with pulmonary fibrosis.

Ultrasound may show nephrocalcinosis or hepatosplenomegaly.

Bone x-rays show 'punched out' lesions in terminal phalanges.

CT/MRI may be useful in assessing severity of pulmonary disease or diagnosing neurosarcoidosis. *Opthalmology assessment* (slit lamp examination, fluorescein angiography) is indicated in ocular disease. *Kveim tests* are obsolete.

Management ►*Patients with BHL alone do not require treatment since the majority recover spontaneously.* Acute sarcoidosis: Bed rest, NSAIDs, *Indications for corticosteroid therapy:*
- Parenchymal lung disease (symptomatic, static, or progressive)
- Uveitis
- Hypercalcaemia
- Neurological or cardiac involvement.

Prednisolone (40mg/24h) PO for 4–6 wks, then ↓dose over 1yr according to clinical status. A few patients relapse and may need a further course or long-term therapy. In severe illness, IV methylprednisolone or immunosuppressants (methotrexate, ciclosporin (=cyclosporin), cyclophosphamide) may be needed.

Prognosis 60% of patients with thoracic sarcoidosis show spontaneous resolution within 2yrs. 20% of patients respond to steroid therapy. In the remainder, improvement is unlikely despite therapy.

---

1 A detailed history and exam (including for synovitis) + CXR, 2 ASO-titres & a tuberculin skin test is usually enough to diagnose erythema nodosum: R Pugol 2000 *Arthr Rheu* **43** 584

Causes of BHL (bilateral hylar lymphadenopathy)

Infection	TB
	Mycoplasma
Malignancy	Lymphoma
	Carcinoma
	Mediastinal tumours
Organic dust disease	Silicosis
	Berylliosis
Extrinsic allergic alveolitis	

Differential diagnosis of granulomatous diseases

Infections	Bacteria	TB
		Leprosy
		Syphilis
		Cat scratch fever
	Fungi	*Cryptococcus neoformans*
		Coccidioides immitis
	Protozoa	Schistosomiasis
Autoimmune	Primary biliary cirrhosis	
	Granulomatous orchitis	
Vasculitis (p424)	Giant cell arteritis	
	Polyarteritis nodosa	
	Takayasu's arteritis	
	Wegener's granulomatosis	
Organic dust disease	Silicosis	
	Berylliosis	
Idiopathic	Crohn's disease	
	de Quervain's thyroiditis	
	Sarcoidosis	
Extrinsic allergic alveolitis		
Histiocytosis X		

199

Extrinsic allergic alveolitis (EAA)

In sensitized individuals, inhalation of allergens (fungal spores or avian proteins) provokes a hypersensitivity reaction. In the acute phase, the alveoli are infiltrated with acute inflammatory cells. With chronic exposure, granuloma formation and obliterative bronchiolitis occur.

Causes
- Bird fancier's and pigeon fancier's lung (proteins in bird droppings).
- Farmer's and mushroom worker's lung (*Micropolyspora faeni, Thermoactinomyces vulgaris*).
- Malt worker's lung (*Aspergillus clavatus*).
- Bagassosis (*Thermoactinomyces sacchari*).

Clinical features *4–6h post-exposure:* Fever, rigors, myalgia, dry cough, dyspnoea, crackles (no wheeze). *Chronic:* Increasing dyspnoea, weight↓, exertional dyspnoea, Type I respiratory failure, cor pulmonale.

Tests *Acute:* Blood: FBC (neutrophilia); ESR↑; ABGs; positive serum precipitins (indicate exposure only). *CXR:* mid-zone mottling/consolidation; hilar lymphadenopathy (rare). *Lung function tests:* reversible restrictive defect; reduced gas transfer during acute attacks.

Chronic: Blood tests: positive serum precipitins. *CXR:* upper-zone fibrosis; honeycomb lung. *Lung function tests:* persistent changes (see above). Bronchoalveolar lavage *(BAL)* fluid shows increased lymphocytes and mast cells.

Management *Acute attack:* Remove allergen and give O_2 (35–60%), then:
- Hydrocortisone 200mg IV.
- Oral prednisolone (40mg/24h PO), followed by reducing dose.

Chronic: Avoid exposure to allergens, or wear a face mask or +ve pressure helmet. Long-term steroids often achieve CXR and physiological improvement. Compensation (UK Industrial Injuries Act) may be payable.

Cryptogenic[1] fibrosing alveolitis   (X-RAY PLATE 7)

A disease of unknown cause, characterized by an inflammatory cell infiltrate and pulmonary fibrosis.

Symptoms Dry cough; exertional dyspnoea; malaise; weight↓; arthralgia.

Signs Cyanosis; finger clubbing; fine end-inspiratory crepitations.

Complications Type 1 respiratory failure; increased risk of lung cancer.

Tests *Blood:* ABG (P_aO_2↓; P_aCO_2↑); CRP↑; immunoglobulins↑; ANA (30% +ve), rheumatoid factor (10% +ve). *CXR:* (X-RAY PLATE 7) Lung volume↓; bilateral lower zone reticulo-nodular shadows; honeycomb lung (advanced disease). *Spirometry:* Restrictive (p168); ↓transfer factor. *BAL* may indicate activity of alveolitis: lymphocytes↑ (good response/prognosis) or neutrophils and eosinophils↑ (poor response/prognosis). **$^{99}Tc^m$-DTPA** scan: (diethylene-triamine-penta-acetic acid) may reflect disease activity. *Lung biopsy* may be needed for diagnosis.[24]

Management A large proportion of patients have chronic irreversible disease which is unresponsive to treatment. Prednisolone 60mg/24h PO for 6 wks, followed by a reducing dose. Alternative: cyclophosphamide 100–120mg/24h PO + prednisolone 20mg PO on alternate days. Monitor response with symptom enquiry, CXR, and lung function tests. The patient may be suitable for lung transplantation.[25]

Prognosis 50% overall 5yr survival rate (range 1–20yrs).

---

1 It is not called cryptogenic if associated with connective tissue disease (RA, SLE, systemic sclerosis, mixed connective tissue disease, Sjögren's, dermatomyositis); chronic hepatitis; renal tubular acidosis; autoimmune thyroid disease; ulcerative colitis.

Industrial dust diseases

Coal worker's pneumoconiosis (CWP) is the commonest dust disease in the UK. It results from inhalation of coal dust particles (1–3μm in diameter) over 15–20yrs. These are ingested by macrophages which die, releasing their enzymes and causing fibrosis.

Clinical features: Asymptomatic, but co-existing chronic bronchitis is common. CXR: many round opacities (1–10mm), especially upper zone.

Management: Avoid exposure to coal dust; treat co-existing chronic bronchitis; claim compensation (in the UK, *via* the Industrial Injuries Act).

Progressive massive fibrosis (PMF) is due to progression of CWP, which causes progressive dyspnoea, fibrosis, and eventually, cor pulmonale. CXR: upper-zone fibrotic masses (1–10cm).

Management: Avoid exposure to coal dust; claim compensation (as above).

Caplan's syndrome is the association between rheumatoid arthritis, pneumoconiosis, and pulmonary rheumatoid nodules.

Silicosis is caused by inhalation of silica particles, which are very fibrogenic. A number of jobs may be associated with exposure, eg metal mining, stone quarrying, sandblasting, and pottery/ceramic manufacture.

Clinical features: Progressive dyspnoea, ↑incidence of TB, CXR shows diffuse miliary or nodular pattern in upper and mid-zones and egg-shell calcification of hilar nodes. Spirometry: restrictive ventilatory defect.

Management: Avoid exposure to silica; claim compensation (as above).

Asbestosis is caused by inhalation of asbestos fibres. Chrysotile (white asbestos) is the least fibrogenic—crocidolite (blue asbestos) is the most fibrogenic. Amosite (brown asbestos) is the least common and has intermediate fibrogenicity. Asbestos was commonly used in the building trade for fire proofing, pipe lagging, electrical wire insulation, and roofing felt. Degree of asbestos exposure is related to degree of pulmonary fibrosis.

Clinical features: Similar to other fibrotic lung diseases with progressive dyspnoea, clubbing, and fine end-inspiratory crackles. Also causes pleural plaques, ↑risk of bronchial adenocarcinoma and mesothelioma.

Management Symptomatic. Patients are often eligible for compensation through the UK Industrial Injuries Act.

Malignant mesothelioma is a tumour of mesothelial cells which usually occurs in the pleura, and rarely in the peritoneum or other organs. It is associated with occupational exposure to asbestos but the relationship is complex.[26][27] 90% report previous exposure to asbestos, but only 20% of patients have pulmonary asbestosis. The latent period between exposure and development of the tumour may be up to 45yrs.

Clinical features include chest pain, dyspnoea, weight loss, finger clubbing, recurrent pleural effusions. If the tumour has metastasized there may be lymphadenopathy, hepatomegaly, bone pain/tenderness, abdominal pain/obstruction (peritoneal malignant mesothelioma).

Tests: CXR/CT: pleural thickening/effusion. Bloody pleural fluid.

Diagnosis is made on histology, following a pleural biopsy—Abrams' needle (p748), thoracoscopy. Often the diagnosis is only made post-mortem.

Management: Symptomatic, with industrial compensation, as above.

Prognosis is very poor (<2yrs, >650 deaths/yr in the UK).

Causes of pulmonary fibrosis

Granulomatous diseases	Tuberculosis
	Sarcoidosis
Drugs	Amiodarone
	Bleomycin
	Busulfan
	Nitrofurantoin
	Sulfasalazine
Connective tissue diseases	Ankylosing spondylitis
	Rheumatoid arthritis
	Systemic lupus erythematosus
	Systemic sclerosis
Extrinsic allergic alveolitis (EAA) (p200)	Bird fancier's lung
	Farmer's lung
	Malt worker's lung
	Mushroom picker's lung
	Pigeon fancier's lung
Industrial dust diseases	Asbestosis
	Berylliosis
	Pneumoconiosis
	Silicosis
Radiation	
Chronic pulmonary oedema (mitral stenosis)	
Bronchiolitis obliterans (organizing pneumonia)	
Cryptogenic fibrosing alveolitis	

Obstructive sleep apnoea syndrome

This disorder is characterized by intermittent closure/collapse of the pharyngeal airway which causes apnoeic episodes during sleep. These are terminated by partial arousal.

Clinical features The typical patient is a fat, middle-aged man (or a postmenopausal woman) who presents because of snoring or daytime somnolence. His partner often describes apnoeic episodes during sleep.

• Snorts loudly in sleep • Daytime somnolence • Poor sleep quality
• Morning headache • Decreased libido • Cognitive performance↓

Complications Pulmonary hypertension; Type II respiratory failure (p192). Sleep apnoea is also reported as an independent risk factor for hypertension.[28]

Investigations Simple studies (eg pulse oximetry, video recordings) may be all that are required for diagnosis. Polysomnography (which monitors oxygen saturation, airflow at the nose and mouth, ECG, EMG chest and abdominal wall movement during sleep) is diagnostic. The occurrence of 15 or more episodes of apnoea or hypopnoea during 1h of sleep indicates significant sleep apnoea.

Management
• Weight reduction
• Avoidance of tobacco and alcohol
• CPAP via a nasal mask during sleep is effective
• Surgical procedures to relieve pharyngeal obstruction (tonsillectomy, uvulopalatopharyngoplasty, or tracheostomy) are occasionally needed, but only after seeing a chest physician.

Cor pulmonale

Cor pulmonale is right heart failure caused by chronic pulmonary hypertension. Causes include chronic lung disease, pulmonary vascular disorders, and neuromuscular and skeletal diseases (see p205).

Clinical features Symptoms include dyspnoea, fatigue, or syncope. Signs: cyanosis; tachycardia; raised JVP with prominent *a* and *v* waves; RV heave; loud P_2, pansystolic murmur (tricuspid regurgitation); early diastolic Graham Steell murmur; hepatomegaly and oedema.

Investigations *FBC:* Hb and haematocrit↑ (secondary polycythaemia). *ABG:* hypoxia, with or without hypercapnia. *CXR:* enlarged right atrium and ventricle, prominent pulmonary arteries. *ECG:* P pulmonale; right axis deviation; right ventricular hypertrophy/strain.

Management
• *Treat underlying cause*—eg COPD and pulmonary infections.
• *Treat respiratory failure*—in the acute situation give 24% oxygen if P_aO_2 <8kPa. Monitor ABG and gradually increase oxygen concentration if P_aCO_2 is stable (p192). In COPD patients, long-term oxygen therapy (LTOT) for 15h/d increases survival (see p188). Patients with chronic hypoxia when clinically stable should be assessed for LTOT.
• *Treat cardiac failure* with diuretics such as frusemide (=furosemide, eg 40–160mg/24h PO). Monitor U&E and give amiloride or potassium supplements if necessary. Alternative: spironolactone.
• Consider *venesection* if the haematocrit is >55%.
• Consider *heart-lung transplantation* in young patients.

Prognosis Poor. 50% die within 5yrs.

Causes of cor pulmonale

- *Lung disease*
  Asthma (severe, chronic)
  COPD
  Bronchiectasis
  Pulmonary fibrosis
  Lung resection

- *Pulmonary vascular disease*
  Pulmonary emboli
  Pulmonary vasculitis
  Primary pulmonary hypertension
  ARDS
  Sickle-cell disease
  Parasite infestation

- *Thoracic cage abnormality*
  Kyphosis
  Scoliosis
  Thoracoplasty

- *Neuromuscular disease*
  Myasthenia gravis
  Poliomyelitis
  Motor neurone disease

- *Hypoventilation*
  Sleep apnoea
  Enlarged adenoids in children
  Cerebrovascular disease

Gastroenterology[1]

Contents

Relevant pages in other chapters: *Signs & symptoms:* Abdominal distension (p64); epigastric pain (p70); flatulence (p72); guarding (p72); heartburn (p74); hepatomegaly (p74); LIF and LUQ pain (p76); palmar erythema (p78); rebound tenderness (p82); regurgitation (p82); RIF pain (p82); RUQ pain (p82); skin discolouration (p82); splenomegaly (p518); tenesmus (p84); vomiting (p86); waterbrash (p88); weight loss (p88). *Surgical topics:* Contents to *Surgery* (p444). *Haematology:* Iron-deficiency anaemia (p626). *Infections:* Viral hepatitis (p576). *Emergencies:* Upper GI bleeding (p804); acute liver failure (p806).

1 We thank Dr Miles Parkes who is our Specialist Reader for this chapter.

Lumen

We learn about gastroenterological diseases as if they were separate entities, independent species collected by naturalists, each kept in its own dark matchbox—collectors' items collecting dust in a desiccated world on a library shelf. But this is not how illness works. Otto had diabetes, but refused to see a doctor until it was far advanced, and an amputation was needed. He needed looking after by his wife Aurelia. But she had her children Warren and Sylvia to look after too. And when Otto was no longer the bread-winner, she forced herself to work as a teacher, an accountant, and at any other job she could get. Otto's illness manifested in Aurelia's duodenum—as an ulcer. The gut often bears the brunt of other people's worries. Inside every piece of a gut is a lumen[1]—the world is in the gut, and the gut is in the world. But the light does not always shine. So when the lumen filled with Aurelia's blood, we can expect the illness to impact on the whole family. Her daughter knows where blood comes from ('straight from the heart ...pink fizz'). After Otto died, Sylvia needed long-term psychiatric care, and Aurelia moved to be near her daughter. The bleeding duodenal ulcer got worse when Sylvia needed electroconvulsive therapy. The therapy worked and now, briefly, Sylvia, before her own premature death, is able to look after Aurelia, as she prepares for a gastrectomy.

The story of each illness told separately misses something; but even taken in its social context, this story is missing something vital—the poetry, in most of our patients lived rather than written—tragic, comic, human, and usually obscure—but in the case of this family not so obscure. Welling up, as unstoppable as the bleeding from her mother's ulcer, came the poetry of Sylvia Plath.[2]

---

1 *Lumen* is Latin for light (hence its medical meaning of a tubular cavity open to the world at both ends), as well as being the SI unit of light flux falling on an object—ie the power to transilluminate. All doctors have this power, whether by insightfully interpreting patients' lives and illnesses to them, or by acts of kindness—even something so simple as bringing a cup of tea.

2 ...*And here you come, with a cup of tea*
Wreathed in steam.
The blood jet is poetry,
There is no stopping it.
You hand me two children, two roses.

Sylvia Plath, *Kindness*, Collected Poems, 1981, Faber; ISBN 0571118380.

Healthy, enjoyable eating

▶ *There's a lot of people in this world who spend so much time watching their health that they haven't the time to enjoy it.* Josh Billings (1818–85).

There are no good or bad *foods*, and no universally good or bad *diets*. We must not consider diet out of context with a desired lifestyle, and nor should we assume that everyone wants to be thin, healthy, and live for ever. If we are walking to the south pole, we need a diet as full of fat as possible: taking any other food would be a waste of space (fat is energy-rich). But if we live a sedentary life, the converse is not necessarily (or even probably) true.[1] The sad truth is that after decades of research, we do not know who should eat what, or when. Are 3 meals a day healthier than 1? Is fat bad if weight is normal? Is a balanced diet (BOX) best? Should we eat 3, 5, 7, or 9 fruits per day? The latter is one recommendation for men, but recent studies (2003; $n=1926$) find no benefit beyond 3.[?] The traditional answers to these questions is 'Yes'—and the more fruit the better, but evidence is far from complete, not just because of a few randomized trials, but because of complex interactions between eating and health—and all diets have unintended consequences. *An example of such an interaction:* The 'good' antioxidant epicatechin (a flavonoid) in dark chocolate is annulled by taking milk at the same time.[?]

Current recommendations must take into account 3 facts:

- Obesity is an escalating epidemic costing health services as much as smoking.
- Diabetes mellitus is burgeoning: in some places prevalence is >7% (p293).
- Past advice has not changed eating habits in large sections of the population.

Advice is likely to focus on the following:

1 *Body mass index:* Weight in kilogram/(height in metres)^2; aim for 20–25; ie *eat less*. Controlling quantity may be more important than quality. In hypertension, eating the 'right' things lowered BP by 0.6mmHg, but controlling weight (*OHCS* p470) caused a 3.7mmHg reduction in 6 months in 1 randomized trial.[3] [N≈810]

2 *Oily fish:* (Rich in omega-3 fatty acid, eg mackerel, herring, pilchards, salmon). This helps those with hyperlipidaemia. If tinned fish, avoid those in unspecified oils. Nuts are also valuable: walnuts lower total cholesterol and have one of the highest ratios of polyunsaturates to saturates (7:1). Soya protein lowers cholesterol, low-density lipoproteins, and triglycerides.

3 *Refined sugar:* (see BOX for its deleterious effects) Use fruit to add sweetness. Have low-sugar drinks. Don't add sugar to drinks or cereals. (In a thin, active, elderly, normoglycaemic person, sugar may be no great evil.)

4 *Eat enough fruit and fibre*—see BOX. *Reduce salt.*

5 *Enjoy moderate alcohol use (adults)* ♀: <15U/wk; ♂: <20U/wk (higher levels are controversial)—taken regularly, not in binges. Alcohol inhibits platelet aggregation and is an antioxidant (∴ cardioprotective). There is no evidence that spirit or beer drinkers should switch to wine. There is evidence that the benefit accrues *only* to those whose LDL cholesterol is ≥5.25mmol/L.

▶ *Avoid this diet if:* • <5yrs old • Need for low residue (Crohn's, UC, p246) or special diet (coeliac, p252) • If weight *loss* expected (eg HIV +ve). *Emphasis may be different in:* Dyslipidaemia (p706); DM (p293); obesity; constipation (p220); liver failure (p230); chronic pancreatitis (p252); renal failure (less protein); BP↑.[2]

Difficulties It is an imposition to ask us to change our diet (children often refuse point-blank); a more subtle approach is to take a meal we enjoy (eg crisps and Coke®) and make it healthier, eg caffeine-free Diet Coke® and crisps made from jacket potatoes, fried in sunflower oil.

1 Randomized trials (not without problems) show how an *Atkins-type diet* low in carbohydrate (∴ ↑fat & ↑protein) can *improve* lipid profiles and insulin resistance. Possible SEs: renal problems; excessive calcium excretion. Foster G 2003 *NEJM* 348 2082 & Samaha F 2003 *NEJM* **348** 2074
2 Dietary Approaches to Stop Hypertension *DASH diet* emphasizing fruits, vegetables, & ↓fat dairy items lowers BP and can make losartan more effective. Conlin P 2003 *Am J Hypertens* **16** 337

Traditional low-fat nutritional advice: *the balance of good health*

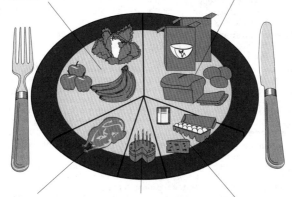

Fruits and vegetables

Bread, other cereals, and potatoes

Meat, fish, and alternatives

Foods containing fat
Foods containing sugar

Milk and dairy foods

The only way to keep your health is to eat what you don't want, drink what you don't like, and do what you'd rather not.
Mark Twain

This shows rough proportions of food types that make up the putatively ideal meal. It is a model against which other diets are compared. Don't fall into the trap of dismissing this model as a plateful of platitudes: there are some patients for whom it will be especially beneficial, eg in gallstones.

Starchy foods: Bread, rice, pasta, potatoes, etc. form the main energy source (especially wholemeal). ↑Fluid intake with a diet high in non-starch polysaccharide (NSP)—eg 8 cups (1–2½ pints) daily. Warn about bulky stools. NSP ↓calcium and iron absorption, so restrict main intake to 1 meal a day.

Fruit, vegetables: eg >6 different pieces of fruit (ideally with skins) or portions of pulses, beans, or lightly cooked greens per day.[1] This probably ↓cardiovascular and cancer mortality.[2] The term *fibre* is imprecise. Most is NSP (the preferred term).

Meat and alternatives: Meat should be cooked without additional fat. Lower fat alternatives, such as white meat (poultry, without skin), white fish, and vegetable protein sources (eg pulses, soya) are encouraged.

Dairy foods: Low-fat semi-skimmed milk/yoghurt; edam or cottage cheese.

Fat and sugary foods: Avoiding extra fat in cooking is advised ('grill, boil, steam, or bake, but don't fry'). Fatty spreads (eg butter) are kept to a minimum and snack foods (crisps, sweets, biscuits, or cake) are avoided.

Avoiding obesity: Excess sugar causes caries, diabetes, and obesity (this contributes to osteoarthritis, cancer,[3] and hypertension, and ↑oxidative stress—so raising cardiovascular mortality).[4]

Drugs for obesity? Orlistat lowers fat absorption (hence SE of oily faecal incontinence). Sibutramine increases post-ingestive satiety—see *OHCS p470.*

1 Children 2-6yrs: 5 servings/d; if >6yrs, eat 6/d; women & teens: 7/d; teen boys & men: 9/d—US Dept. Health & Human Services. Do potatoes/chips count? Probably not. [@10999025]
2 This may be why lifelong vegetarianism protects against some cancers. *Int J Cancer* 2002 **99** 238
3 R Sinha 2004 *Int J Cancer* **108** 287 & E Calle 2003 *NEJM* **348** 1625. ↑weight is associated with ↑death rates for all cancers combined and those at multiple specific sites. n = 900,000 USA adults followed for 16yrs.
4 Framingham 2003 data J Keaney *Arterioscler Thromb Vasc Biol* **23** 434

The mouth

Leucoplakia White thickening of the tongue or oral mucosa. It is potentially premalignant. ▶When in doubt, refer all intra-oral while lesions. *Causes:* Poor dental hygiene; smoking; sepsis; aphthous stomatitis; squamous papilloma; verucca vulgaris; secondary syphilis. ▶Oral hairy leucoplakia is a shaggy white patch on the side of the tongue due to EBV which is seen in HIV.

Mouth commensals 50% of us carry candida (eg *Candida albicans; C. Krusei*); 20% carry aspergillous (eg *Aspergillus flavus; A. niger*[1])—more if we don't brush our teeth.

Aphthous ulcers 20% of us get these shallow, painful ulcers on the tongue or buccal mucosa that heal without scarring. *Causes of severe ulcers:* Crohn's & coeliac diseases; Behçet's (p718); trauma; erythema multiforme (PLATE 17); lichen planus; pemphigus; pemphigoid; infections (herpes simplex, syphilis, Vincent's angina, p736). *Treatment* is difficult: hydrocortisone lozenges held on the ulcer may help, as may tetracycline mouthwash. ▶Biopsy any ulcer not healing after 3wks to exclude malignancy; refer to an oral surgeon if uncertain.

Candidiasis (thrush) causes white patches or erythema of the buccal mucosa. Patches may be hard to remove and bleed if scraped. *Risk factors:* extremes of age; DM; antibiotics; immunosuppression (long-term corticosteroids, including inhalers; cytotoxics; malignancy; HIV). ▶Oropharyngeal candidiasis in an apparently fit patient suggests underlying HIV infection *Treatment:* Nystatin suspension or pastilles or amphotericin lozenges. Fluconazole for oropharyngeal candidiasis.

Cheilitis (angular stomatitis) Fissuring of the mouth's corners is caused by denture problems, candidosis (above), or deficiency of iron or riboflavin.

Gingivitis Gum inflammation ± hypertrophy occurs with poor oral hygiene, drugs (phenytoin, ciclosporin, nifedipine), pregnancy, vitamin C deficiency (scurvy, p250), acute myeloid leukaemia (p654), or Vincent's angina (p736).

Microstomia The mouth is too small, eg from thickening and tightening of the perioral skin after burns or in epidermolysis bullosa (destructive skin and mucous membrane blisters ± ankyloglossia) or systemic sclerosis (p420; look for facial telangiectasia; sclerodactyly; Raynaud's; calcinosis).

Oral pigmentation Perioral brown spots characterize Peutz–Jeghers' syndrome (p732). Pigmentation anywhere in the mouth suggests Addison's disease or drugs (eg antimalarials). Telangiectasia may be seen in systemic sclerosis and Osler–Weber–Rendu syndrome (p732).

Teeth A blue line at the gum–tooth margin suggests lead poisoning. Prenatal or childhood tetracycline exposure causes a yellow–brownness.

Tongue This may be *furred* or *dry* in dehydration, if on tricyclics, etc.,[2] or in Sjögren's syndrome (p734 or related Mikulicz's syndrome) or Crohn's.

Glossitis means a smooth, red, sore tongue, eg caused by iron, folate, or B_{12} deficiency. If *local* loss of papillae leads to ulcer-like lesions that change in colour and size, use the term *geographic tongue* (harmless migratory glossitis). *Macroglossia:* The tongue is too big. *Causes:* Myxoedema; acromegaly; amyloid. A *ranula* is a bluish salivary retention cyst on one side of the frenulum, named after the bulging vocal pouch of frogs' throats (genus *Rana*).

Tongue cancer: This typically appears on its edge as a raised ulcer with firm edges and environs. Examine underneath of tongue and ask patient to deviate his extended tongue sideways. Spread: the anterior one-third of the tongue drains to the submental nodes; the middle one-third to the submandibular nodes, and the posterior one-third to the deep cervical nodes. Treatment: surgery or radiotherapy. 5yr survival (early disease): 80%. ▶When in doubt, refer all tongue ulcers.

---

1 *A niger* may cause a black tongue. The significance of aspergillus carriage is unknown. [@12212815]
2 Drugs causing xerostomia: ACE-i, antidepressants; antihistamines; antipsychotics; antimuscarinics/anticholinergics (benzhexol; hyoscine; ipratropium, tolterodine, oxybutynine, baclofen, procyclidine, propantheline); bromocriptine; diuretics; loperamide; nifedipine; opiates; prazocin; prochlorperazine, etc.

Dysphagia

Dysphagia is difficulty in swallowing. Progressive or new-onset dysphagia lasting >3wks needs urgent investigation to exclude a malignant stricture.

Causes may be oral, pharyngeal, or oesophageal:

Mechanical block
Malignant stricture
  Oesophageal cancer
  Gastric cancer
  Pharyngeal cancer
Benign strictures
  Oesophageal web or ring
  Peptic stricture
Extrinsic pressure
  Lung cancer
  Mediastinal lymph nodes
  Retrosternal goitre
  Aortic aneurysm
  Left atrial enlargement
Pharyngeal pouch

Motility disorders
Achalasia
Diffuse oesophageal spasm
Systemic sclerosis (p420)
Myasthenia gravis (p400)
Bulbar palsy (p394)
Pseudobulbar palsy (p394)
Syringobulbia (p404)
Bulbar poliomyelitis (p602)
Chagas' disease (p608)
Others
Oesophagitis
  Infection (*Candida*, HSV)
  Reflux oesophagitis
Globus hystericus

Clinical features There are a number of key questions to ask:

1 Was there difficulty swallowing solids *and* liquids from the start?
  Yes: Motility disorder (achalasia, neurological), or pharyngeal causes.
  No: Suspect a stricture (benign or malignant).
2 Is it difficult to make the swallowing movement?
  Yes: Suspect bulbar palsy, especially if he coughs on swallowing.
3 Is swallowing painful (odynophagia)?
  Yes: Suspect cancer, oesophagitis, achalasia, or oesophageal spasm.
4 Is the dysphagia intermittent or is it constant and getting worse?
  Intermittent: Suspect oesophageal spasm.
  Constant and worsening: Suspect malignant stricture.
5 Does the neck bulge or gurgle on drinking?
  Yes: Suspect a pharyngeal pouch.

▶Is the patient cachectic or anaemic? Examine the mouth; feel for supraclavicular nodes; look for signs of systemic disease, eg systemic sclerosis, CNS disease.

Investigations FBC (anaemia); U&E (dehydration); CXR (mediastinal fluid level, absent gastric bubble, aspiration); barium swallow; upper GI endoscopy and biopsy. Further investigations: oesophageal manometry (if normal barium swallow); ENT opinion if suspected pharyngeal cause.

Specific conditions *Oesophagitis* p216. *Diffuse oesophageal spasm* causes intermittent dysphagia ± chest pain. Barium swallow: abnormal contractions, eg corkscrew oesophagus.[1] *Achalasia* Failure of relaxation of the lower oesophageal sphincter (due to degeneration of the myenteric plexus) causes dysphagia, regurgitation, substernal cramps, and ↓weight. Barium swallow: dilated tapering oesophagus. Treatment: endoscopic balloon dilatation or Heller's cardiomyotomy—then proton pump inhibitors (PPIs, p216). *Benign oesophageal stricture:* Caused by gastro-oesophageal reflux disease (GORD) (p216), corrosives, surgery, or radiotherapy. ℞: endoscopic balloon dilatation. *Oesophageal cancer* (p508) Associations: GORD,🔖 tobacco, alcohol, Barrett's oesophagus (p718), achalasia, tylosis (palmar hyperkeratosis), Paterson-Brown-Kelly syndrome. *Paterson-Brown-Kelly (Plummer-Vinson) syndrome* Postcricoid web + iron-deficiency anaemia.

---

1 Non-propulsive contractions manifest as tertiary contractions or '*corkscrew oesophagus*' and suggest an underlying motility disorder and may lead to impaired acid clearance. [@1992626] *Nutcracker oesophagus* denotes distal peristaltic contractions >180mmHg. It causes pain; [@12526934] it has been found to be partly ameliorable by the smooth muscle relaxant sildenafil (p316). [@12010875]

Dyspepsia and peptic ulceration

Dyspepsia (indigestion) is a non-specific group of symptoms related to the upper GI tract. ΔΔ: Non-ulcer dyspepsia; duodenal ulcer (DU); duodenitis; gastric ulcer (GU); gastritis; gastric malignancy; gastro-oesophageal reflux; oesophagitis.

Symptoms Epigastric pain related to hunger, eating specific foods, or time of day; eg associated with bloating ± fullness after meals; heartburn (retrosternal pain that may or may not be associated with demonstrable acid reflux).

Signs Epigastric tenderness (non-specific). Feel for an abdominal mass; supra-clavicular lymph nodes ± hepatomegaly (?malignancy).

Management of dyspepsia[1] See BOX/NICE advice (it changes often). *If ≤ 55yrs old:* test for *Helicobacter pylori;* treat if +ve (below[2]). 'Test and treat' is more effective than acid suppression[?] (eg just lansoprazole 30mg/24h for 4wks; SE: D&V, oedema, bronchospasm, Stevens–Johnson syndrome, toxic epidermal necrolysis, alopecia, photosensitivity, interstitial nephritis, LFT↑, agranulocytosis). [13]C breath test for *H. pylori* is more reliable than other tests. *If ≥55:* Refer urgently for endoscopy. GI bleeding, dysphagia, weight↓, prolonged vomiting, Hb↓, platelets↑, ESR↑, and LFT↑ suggest an organic cause.

Duodenal ulcers (DU) are 4× commoner than GU. *Major risk factors:* H. pylori (~90%); drugs (aspirin; NSAIDs; steroids). *Minor risk factors:* ↑Gastric acid secretion; ↑gastric emptying (↓duodenal pH); blood group O; smoking. The role of stress is controversial. *Symptoms:* Epigastric pain typically before meals or at night, relieved by eating, or drinking milk. 50% are asymptomatic; others experience recurrent episodes. *Signs:* Epigastric tenderness (non-specific). *Diagnosis:* Upper GI endoscopy (stop anti-ulcer drugs 1wk before). Test for *H. pylori* (see BOX). Gastrin concentrations should be measured if Zollinger–Ellison syndrome (p740) is suspected. ΔΔ: Non-ulcer dyspepsia; duodenal Crohn's disease; TB; lymphoma; pancreatic cancer.

Gastric ulcers (GU) occur mainly in the elderly, on the lesser curve of the stomach. Ulcers elsewhere are more likely to be malignant. *Risk factors:* H. pylori (~80%); smoking; NSAID; reflux of duodenal contents; delayed gastric emptying; stress, eg neurosurgery (Cushing's ulcers) or burns (Curling's ulcers). *Symptoms:* May be asymptomatic—or cause epigastric pain (related to meals and relieved by antacids) and weight loss. May also present with complications, eg haematemesis or perforation. *Tests:* Upper GI endoscopy must be performed to exclude malignancy; take multiple biopsies from the rim and base of the ulcer (histology, *H. pylori*) and brushings (cytology).

Treatment of peptic ulcers *Lifestyle:* Avoid food that worsens symptoms. Stop smoking (slows healing in GU; ↑relapse rates in DU). *H. pylori eradication:* Triple therapy.[2] *Drugs to reduce acid:* PPI, eg lansoprazole 30mg/24h PO for 4 (DU) or 8 (GU) wks. *Alternative:* H[2]-receptor antagonists (H[2]RA): ranitidine 300mg PO *nocte* or cimetidine 800mg PO *nocte* for 8wks. *NSAID-associated ulcers:* Stop NSAID if possible (if not, use H[2]-receptor antagonist, PPI, or misoprostol for prevention). If symptoms persist, re-endoscope, recheck for *H. pylori*, and reconsider the differential diagnosis. *Surgery:* p530.

Nausea and vomiting

Causes: p86

Tests *Blood tests* FBC, U&E, LFT, Ca^{2+}, glucose, and amylase. A metabolic alkalosis (pH > 7.45, HCO_3^-↑) indicates severe vomiting. Request a plain AXR if suspected bowel obstruction. Consider upper GI *endoscopy* if persistent vomiting. Identify and *treat the underlying cause* if possible.

Treatment: *Drugs* Metoclopramide 10mg IV for GI causes (except intestinal obstruction). Prochlorperazine 12.5mg IM for metabolic or drug-induced vomiting. Cinnarizine 15–30mg PO or prochlorperazine 5mg/8h PO for vestibular disorders. Domperidone 20mg PO or 60mg PR is preferable in the elderly (less extrapyramidal SE). Avoid drugs in pregnancy. *Fluids* Give IV fluids if severely dehydrated or nil by mouth; monitor fluid balance.

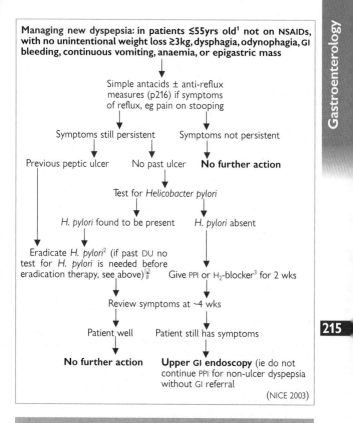

Managing new dyspepsia: in patients ≤55yrs old[1] not on NSAIDs, with no unintentional weight loss ≥3kg, dysphagia, odynophagia, GI bleeding, continuous vomiting, anaemia, or epigastric mass

Simple antacids ± anti-reflux measures (p216) if symptoms of reflux, eg pain on stooping

Symptoms still persistent   Symptoms not persistent

Previous peptic ulcer   No past ulcer   **No further action**

Test for *Helicobacter pylori*

H. pylori found to be present   *H. pylori* absent

Eradicate *H. pylori*[2] (if past DU no test for *H. pylori* is needed before eradication therapy, see above)

Give PPI or H$_2$-blocker[3] for 2 wks

Review symptoms at ~4 wks

Patient well   Patient still has symptoms

No further action   **Upper GI endoscopy** (ie do not continue PPI for non-ulcer dyspepsia without GI referral

(NICE 2003)

215

Why don't we give under 55s with dyspepsia antihelicobacter drugs without ^{13}C tests?

NNT (see p30) ≈ 9 for this strategy in non-ulcer dyspepsia, and peptic ulcers *are* prevented. But we do not know enough about the long-term effects of such a strategy for authoritative advice. We also know that non-ulcer dyspepsia often does not improve with eradication therapy. **NB:** ^{13}C-urea breath tests are a good non-invasive way to detect *H. pylori*. Serology is less good, as antibodies stay for months after eradication.

1 If ≥55, or weight loss, etc, refer urgently for endoscopy to rule out cancer. This age limit is arbitrary; use a lower age if resources allow, or the local prevalence of gastric ca is high.
2 *Triple therapy* for 7d: *(1)* PPI (eg lansoprazole 30mg dose twice daily) or 'ranitidine bismuth citrate' *(2)* amoxicillin 500–1g twice daily *(3)* clarithromycin 500mg twice daily. If this fails, some try *quadruple therapy*: PPI (as above, plus bismuth subcitrate 120mg/6h PO), *plus* metronidazole 400–500mg/8h, *plus* tetracycline 500mg/6h. ► Resistance causes eradication failure in >12% of patients in some studies—Eisig J 2004. [@14534667]
3 Cimetidine 800mg/d is the cheapest antisecretory therapy (antisecretory refers to acid production).

Gastro-oesophageal reflux disease (GORD)

Dysfunction of the lower oesophageal sphincter predisposes to the gastro-oesophageal reflux of acid. If reflux is prolonged or excessive, it may cause inflammation of the oesophagus (oesophagitis), benign oesophageal stricture, or Barrett's oesophagus (p718).

Associations Smoking, alcohol, hiatus hernia, pregnancy, obesity, tight clothes, big meals, surgery in achalasia, drugs (tricyclics, anticholinergics, nitrates); systemic sclerosis. GORD can also contribute to asthma.

Symptoms Heartburn (burning, retrosternal discomfort related to meals, lying down, stooping, and straining, relieved by antacids); belching; acid brash (acid or bile regurgitation); waterbrash (excessive salivation); odynophagia (painful swallowing, eg from oesophagitis or stricture); nocturnal asthma (cough/wheeze with apparently minimal inhalation of gastric contents).

Complications: Oesophagitis, ulcers, iron deficiency, anaemia, benign stricture, Barrett's oesophagus (p718), and oesophageal adenocarcinoma.

Differential diagnosis: Oesophagitis (corrosives, NSAID); infection (CMV, herpes, *Candida*); DU; gastric ulcers or cancers; non-ulcer dyspepsia.

Tests Isolated symptoms do not require investigation. *Indications for upper GI endoscopy:* age >55yrs; symptoms >4wks; dysphagia; persistent symptoms despite treatment; relapsing symptoms; weight loss. Barium swallow may show hiatus hernia. 24h oesophageal pH monitoring ± oesophageal manometry may be needed to distinguish GORD from other causes.

The Los Angeles (LA) classification: Minor diffuse changes (erythema, oedema; friability) are not included, and the term *mucosal break* is used to encompass the old terms erosion and ulceration. There are 4 grades.

1 One or more mucosal breaks <5mm long, not extending beyond 2 mucosal fold tops. A mucosal break is a well-demarcated area of slough/erythema.
2 Mucosal break >5mm long limited to the space between 2 mucosal fold tops.
3 Mucosal break continuous between the tops of 2 or more mucosal folds but which involves less than 75% of the oesophageal circumference.
4 Mucosal break involving ≥75% of the oesophageal circumference.

Record *complications of GORD* (above) as either present or absent.

Treatment See BOX.

Hiatus hernia

The proximal stomach herniates through the diaphragm into the thorax.

Sliding hiatus hernia (80%) where the gastro-oesophageal junction slides up into the chest. *Rolling hiatus hernia* (20%) where the gastro-oesophageal junction remains in the abdomen but a bulge of stomach herniates up into the chest alongside the oesophagus.

Clinical features Common: 30% of patients >50yrs, especially obese women. 50% have symptomatic gastro-oesophageal reflux.

Investigations Barium swallow is the best diagnostic test. Upper GI endoscopy allows visualization of the mucosa (?oesophagitis).

Management Lose weight. Treat reflux symptoms (see BOX). Indications for surgery (eg Nissen, see BOX): intractable symptoms; recurrent stricture.

Management of gastro-oesophageal reflux

1 *Lifestyle: Encourage:* Weight loss; raise bed head; small, regular meals *Avoid:* Hot drinks, alcohol, and eating <3h before bed. Avoid drugs affecting oesophageal motility (nitrates, anticholinergics, tricyclic antidepressants) or that damage the mucosa (NSAID, K⁺ salts, alendronate).

2 *Drugs: Antacids* eg magnesium trisilicate mixture (10mL/8h) or *alginates* eg Gaviscon® (10–20mL/8h PO pc) relieve symptoms. If symptoms persist for >4wks (or weight↓; dysphagia; excessive vomiting; GI bleeding), *refer for GI endoscopy*. If oesophagitis confirmed, try a *PPI* (the most effective and most expensive drug option) eg lansoprazole 30mg/24h PO. *Prokinetic drugs:* These help gastric emptying (eg metoclopramide, 10mg/8h PO; dystonias can be a serious side-effect).

3 *Surgery:* (Nissen fundoplication, p532) is not indicated unless symptoms are bad *and* there is radiological or pH-monitoring evidence of *severe* reflux. Laparoscopic repairs are gaining favour. **NB:** surgery is better than drugs at improving asthma (?less acid spill-over into the lung).[1]

NB: the role of *H. pylori* in GORD is controversial; some studies show benefit of *H. pylori* eradication in GORD patients needing long-term PPI therapy.[2]

---

1 In one randomized study (*n* = 62), surgery produced a 43% improvement in asthma symptom scores, compared with <10% in medical and control patients. There was a worsening of asthma in 12% of the surgical group, 36% of medical patients, and 48% of the control group. *Am J Gastroenterol* 2003 **98** 987
2 E Kuipers *Gut* 2004 **53** 12

Diarrhoea

Diarrhoea means increased stool water (hence ↑stool volume, eg >200mL daily), and this increases stool frequency and the passage of liquid stool. If it is the stool's fat content which is increased, use the term *steatorrhoea*. Distinguish both from *faecal urgency* (may be caused by cancers or UC, p244).

Common causes	Uncommon	Rare
Gastroenteritis	Microscopic colitis[1]	Autonomic neuropathy
– viral	Coeliac disease	Addison's disease
– bacterial	Chronic pancreatitis	Ischaemic colitis
– parasites/protozoa	Thyrotoxicosis	Amyloidosis
Irritable bowel	Laxative abuse; food allergy	Tropical enteropathy
Drugs (below)	Lactose intolerance	Gastrinoma, VIPoma[2]
Colorectal cancer	Ileal/gastric resection	Carcinoid syndrome
Ulcerative colitis (UC)	Bacterial overgrowth	Medullary thyroid cancer
Crohn's disease	Pseudomembranous colitis[3]	Pellagra

Clinical features It is important to take a detailed history:

Is it acute or chronic? Acute: suspect gastroenteritis. Ask about travel, change in diet, others affected in household. Chronic diarrhoea alternating with constipation suggests irritable bowel syndrome (IBS) (p248). Anorexia, weight↓, anaemia, or nocturnal diarrhoea suggest an organic cause.

• *Is there blood, mucus, or pus?* Bloody diarrhoea: Campylobacter, Shigella, Salmonella, E. coli, amoebiasis, ulcerative colitis, Crohn's disease, colorectal cancer, colonic polyps, pseudomembranous colitis, ischaemic colitis (p488). *Fresh rectal bleeding:* Haemorrhoids, diverticulitis, colorectal cancer, colonic polyps, radiation proctitis, trauma, anal fissure, angiodysplasia. *Mucus* occurs in IBS, colonic adenocarcinoma, polyps. *Pus* suggests inflammatory bowel disease or diverticulitis.

• *Is the large or small bowel to blame?* Large bowel symptoms: watery stool ± blood or mucus; pelvic pain relieved by defecation; tenesmus; urgency. Small bowel symptoms: periumbilical (or RIF) pain, not relieved by defecation; watery stool or steatorrhoea (p252).

• *Could there be a non-GI cause?* Think of drugs (antibiotics; PPIs; cimetidine; propranolol; cytotoxics; NSAIDs; digoxin; alcohol; laxative abuse) and medical conditions (thyrotoxicosis, autonomic neuropathy, Addison's disease).

Examination Look for weight↓, anaemia, dehydration, oral ulcer, clubbing, rashes, and abdominal scars. Feel for: enlarged thyroid or an abdominal mass. *Do a rectal examination:* Any rectal mass (rectal carcinoma), or impacted faeces (overflow diarrhoea)? Test stools for faecal occult blood.

Tests *Bloods:* FBC (iron deficiency; MCV↑ in coeliac disease, ↑alcohol use, ileal Crohn's); U&E (K⁺↓); ESR↑ (cancer, Crohn's/UC); CRP↑ (infection, Crohn's/UC). TSH↓ (thyrotoxicosis); coeliac serology (p252 ± duodenal biopsy).

Stool for pathogens & *Cl. difficile* toxin (pseudomembranous colitis). Faecal fat excretion or ¹³C-hiolein (highly labelled triolein) breath test (nicer and reliable) if symptoms of chronic pancreatitis, malabsorption, or steatorrhoea.

Rigid sigmoidoscopy + biopsy of normal and abnormal looking mucosa: ~15% of patients with Crohn's disease have *macroscopically* normal mucosa.

Colonoscopy/Barium enema: In colitis, and to exclude malignancy. If normal, consider small bowel radiology (Crohn's) ± endoscopic retrograde cholangio-pancreatography (ERCP) (p229, eg chronic pancreatitis).

Management Treat causes. Oral rehydration is preferable to IV rehydration. If severely dehydrated, give 0.9% saline + 20mmol K⁺/L IVI. Codeine phosphate 30mg/6h PO reduces stool frequency. Avoid antibiotics unless the patient has infective diarrhoea and is systemically unwell (see p219).

---

1 Think of microscopic colitis in any chronic diarrhoea; do biopsy (may be +ve on normal looking colon mucosa—reported as 'lymphocytic' or 'collagenous' colitis). Prognosis: good. Bismuth subsalicylate may help (eg Pepto-Bismol®). L Schiller 2000 *Lancet* **355** 1198 & *Gastrointest Dis* 2000 **10** 145
2 Vasoactive intestinal polypeptide-secreting tumour—suspect if hypokalaemic acidosis; Ca²⁺↑; Mg²⁺↓.

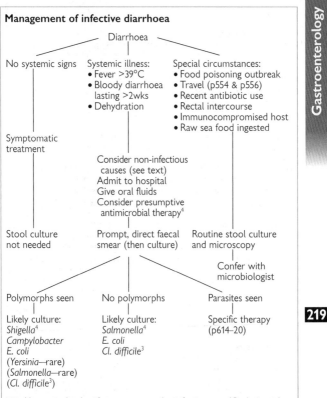

Management of infective diarrhoea

Diarrhoea

No systemic signs — Systemic illness: — Special circumstances:
  • Fever >39°C   • Food poisoning outbreak
  • Bloody diarrhoea   • Travel (p554 & p556)
    lasting >2wks   • Recent antibiotic use
  • Dehydration   • Rectal intercourse
                         • Immunocompromised host
                         • Raw sea food ingested

Symptomatic
treatment

Consider non-infectious
causes (see text)
Admit to hospital
Give oral fluids
Consider presumptive
antimicrobial therapy[4]

Stool culture   Prompt, direct faecal   Routine stool culture
not needed   smear (then culture)   and microscopy

                                                    Confer with
                                                    microbiologist

Polymorphs seen   No polymorphs   Parasites seen

Likely culture: Likely culture: Specific therapy
Shigella[4]   *Salmonella*[4]   (p614–20)
Campylobacter   *E. coli*
E. coli   *Cl. difficile*[3]
(*Yersinia*—rare)
(*Salmonella*—rare)
(*Cl. difficile*[3])

NB: Alternatively, classify into *secretory* (eg infections, UC/Crohn's etc.) or *osmotic* causes (if water drawn into the gut, as in laxative use).

219

3 Pseudomembranous colitis is caused by overgrowth of *Clostridium difficile*, following any antibiotic therapy—or a stay in hospital. *Treatment:* Metronidazole 400mg/8h PO (cheaper; more palatable than the other alternative—vancomycin 125mg/6h PO). Liaise with a microbiologist.
4 Prompt, specific treatment (eg ciprofloxacin, p556) may be needed before sensitivities are known. Be guided by likely diagnosis following microscopy.

Constipation

►Always ask the patient exactly what he means by 'constipation'. There are various formal (and different) definitions of constipation but the infrequent passage of stool (<3 times weekly) or difficulty in defecation, with straining or discomfort, is a reasonably practical working definition.

Causes of constipation are numerous (see BOX).

Clinical features Ask about frequency, nature, and consistency of the stool. Is there blood or mucus in/on the stools? Is there diarrhoea alternating with constipation? Has there been a recent change in bowel habit? Ask about diet and drugs. Rectal examination is essential.

Tests Most constipation do not need investigation, especially young, mildly affected patients. Indications for investigation: age >40yrs; recent change in bowel habit; associated symptoms (weight loss, rectal bleeding, mucous discharge, or tenesmus). *Blood tests:* FBC, U&E, Ca^{2+}, TFT. *Sigmoidoscopy* and biopsy of abnormal mucosa. *Barium enema* if suspected colorectal malignancy. Special investigations (eg transit studies; anorectal physiology) are rarely needed.

Treatment Treat the cause (see BOX). Advise exercise and a good fluid intake (a high-fibre diet is often advised, but this may cause bloating without helping the constipation).⬚ Consider drugs only if these measures fail, and try to use them for short periods only.[1] Often, a stimulant such as senna ± a bulking agent is more effective and cheaper than agents such as lactulose.⬚

Bulking agents ↑Faecal mass, so stimulating peristalsis. They must be taken with plenty of fluid. CI: difficulty in swallowing; intestinal obstruction; colonic atony; faecal impaction. *Bran powder* 3.5g 2–3 times/d with food (may hinder absorption of dietary trace elements if taken with every meal).⬚ *Ispaghula husk*, eg 1 Fybogel® 3.5g sachet after a meal, mixed in water and swallowed immediately (otherwise it becomes an unpleasant sludge). *Methylcellulose*, eg Celevac® 3–6 500mg tablets/12h with water. *Sterculia*, eg Normacol® granules, 10mL sprinkled on food once or twice a day.

Stimulant laxatives increase intestinal motility and should not be used in intestinal obstruction. Prolonged use should be avoided as it may cause colonic atony and hypokalaemia (but there are no good, long-term follow-up studies).⬚ Pure stimulant laxatives are *bisacodyl* tablets (5–10mg at night) or suppositories (10mg in the mornings) and *senna* (2–4 tablets at night). *Docusate sodium* and *danthron*[2] (=dantron) have stimulant and softening actions. *Glycerol suppositories* act as a rectal stimulant. *Sodium picosulfate* is useful for rapid bowel evacuation prior to procedures.

Stool softeners: Arachis oil enemas lubricate and soften impacted faeces. *Liquid paraffin* should not be used for a prolonged period (SE: anal seepage, lipoid pneumonia, malabsorption of fat-soluble vitamins).

Osmotic laxatives retain fluid in the bowel. *Lactulose*, a semisynthetic disaccharide, produces an osmotic diarrhoea of low faecal pH that discourages growth of ammonia-producing organisms. It is useful in constipation (dose: 15mL/12h) and hepatic encephalopathy (dose: 30–50mL/12h). *Magnesium salts* (eg magnesium hydroxide and magnesium sulfate) are useful when rapid bowel evacuation is required. *Sodium salts* (eg Microlette® and Micralax® enemas) should be avoided as they may cause sodium and water retention. *Phosphate enemas* are useful for rapid bowel evacuation prior to procedures.

What if laxatives don't help? A multi-disciplinary approach with behaviour therapy, psychological support, habit training ± sphincter-action biofeedback may help.⬚ 5HT$_4$ agonists are under development (tegaserod; prucalopride).⬚

---

1 Risks of laxative abuse have been overemphasized ('cathartic colon' is a questionable entity); stimulant laxatives may be used chronically when patients fail to respond adequately to bulk or osmotic laxatives alone. Wald A 2003 *J Clin Gastroenterol* **36** 386
2 Danthron causes colon & liver tumours in animals so reserve use for the *very elderly* or *terminally ill*.

Causes of constipation

Poor diet
Inadequate fluid intake or dehydration
Immobility (or lack of exercise)
Irritable bowel syndrome
Old age
Post-operative pain
Hospital environment (lack of privacy, having to use a bed pan)
Distant, squalid, or otherwise unsatisfactory toilets

Anorectal disease
Anal fissure
Anal stricture
Rectal prolapse

Intestinal obstruction
Colorectal carcinoma
Strictures (eg Crohn's disease)
Pelvic mass (eg fetus, fibroids)
Diverticulosis (rectal bleeding is a commoner presentation)
Congenital abnormalities
Pseudo-obstruction (p492)

Metabolic/endocrine
Hypothyroidism
Hypercalcaemia
Hypokalaemia
Porphyria
Lead poisoning

Drugs
Opiate analgesics (eg morphine, codeine)
Anticholinergics (tricyclics, phenothiazines)
Iron

Neuromuscular (slow transit with ↓propulsive activity)
Spinal or pelvic nerve injury
Aganglionosis (Chagas' disease, Hirschsprung's disease)
Systemic sclerosis
Diabetic neuropathy[1]

Other causes
Chronic laxative abuse (rare—diarrhoea is commoner)
Idiopathic slow transit
Idiopathic megarectum/colon
Psychological (eg associated with depression or abuse as a child).[22]

221

---

1 Deficiency of interstitial gut pacemaker cells of Cajal may be to blame. *J Gastroenterol Hepatol* 2002 **17** 666

Jaundice

Jaundice (icterus) refers to a yellow pigmentation of skin, sclerae, and mucosa due to a raised plasma bilirubin (visible at >35μmol/L). Jaundice may be classified by the type of circulating bilirubin (conjugated or unconjugated) or by the site of the problem (pre-hepatic, hepatocellular, or cholestatic/obstructive). *Bilirubin metabolism:* Bilirubin is formed from the breakdown of haemoglobin. It is conjugated with glucuronic acid by hepatocytes, making it water soluble. Conjugated bilirubin is secreted into the bile and passes out into the gut. Some is taken up again by the liver (enterohepatic circulation) and the rest is converted to urobilinogen by gut bacteria. Urobilinogen is either reabsorbed and excreted by the kidneys, or converted to stercobilin, which colours faeces brown.

Pre-hepatic jaundice If there is excess bilirubin production (haemolysis, ↓liver uptake or ↓conjugation), unconjugated bilirubin enters the blood. As it is water insoluble, it does not enter urine resulting in an *unconjugated (acholuric) hyperbilirubinaemia. Causes:* Physiological (neonatal); haemolysis; dyserythropoiesis; glucuronyl transferase deficiency (eg Gilbert's syndrome, p724; Crigler–Najjar syndrome, *OHCS* p744).

Hepatocellular jaundice There is hepatocyte damage ± some cholestasis. *Causes: Viruses:* hepatitis (p576, eg, A, B, C, etc.), CMV (p574), EBV (p570); drugs (see BOX); alcoholic hepatitis; cirrhosis; liver metastases/abscess; haemochromatosis; autoimmune hepatitis (AIH); septicaemia; leptospirosis; α₁-antitrypsin deficiency (p236); Budd–Chiari (p720); Wilson's disease (p236); failure to excrete conjugated bilirubin (Dubin–Johnson, p722, and Rotor syndromes, p734); right heart failure; toxins, eg carbon tetrachloride; fungi (*Amanita phalloides*).

Cholestatic (obstructive) jaundice If the common bile duct is blocked, conjugated bilirubin overspills into the blood causing a *conjugated hyperbilirubinaemia.* Being water soluble, it is excreted in urine, making it dark. Less conjugated bilirubin enters the bowel and the faeces become pale. *Causes:* Gallstones in the common bile duct; pancreatic cancer; lymph nodes at the porta hepatis; drugs (see BOX); cholangiocarcinoma; sclerosing cholangitis; primary biliary cirrhosis (PBC); choledochal cyst; biliary atresia.

Clinical features Ask about blood transfusions, intravenous drug use, body piercing, tattoos, sexual activity, travel abroad, jaundiced contacts, family history, alcohol consumption, and *all* medications (eg old drug charts; GP records). *Examine* for signs of chronic liver disease (p428), hepatic encephalopathy (p230), lymphadenopathy, hepatomegaly, splenomegaly, palpable gall bladder, and ascites. Pale stools & dark urine ≈ obstructive jaundice.

Tests *Urine:* Bilirubin is absent in pre-hepatic causes; urobilinogen is absent in obstructive jaundice (which then becomes a 'surgical problem' if US scan shows the bile ducts to be dilated). *Haematology:* FBC, clotting, blood film, reticulocyte count, Coomb's test. *Biochemistry:* U&E, LFT[1] (bilirubin, ALT, AST, alk phos, γ-GT, total protein, albumin). *Virology:* EBV, CMV, HAV, HBV, & HCV serology (p576). *Other specific tests,* eg for haemochromatosis (↑ferritin, ↑iron, ↓TIBC), α₁-antitrypsin deficiency (plasma for genetics), Wilson's disease (eg ↓serum copper, ↓caeruloplasmin: see p236), PBC (↑antimitochondrial antibodies, AMA) and AIH (↑anti-nuclear and anti-smooth muscle antibodies; IgG↑).🔲 *Ultrasound:* Are the bile ducts dilated (obstruction)? Are there gallstones, hepatic metastases or pancreatic masses? Request ERCP (p229) if bile ducts are dilated. Perform a *liver biopsy* (p228) if the bile ducts are normal. Consider abdominal CT or MRI scan.

---

1 Albumin and prothrombin time are the best indicators of hepatic synthetic function. Elevated transaminases (ALT, AST) indicate hepatocyte damage. ↑Alk phos is typical of obstructive jaundice, but also occurs in hepatocellular jaundice and malignant infiltration, Paget's disease, pregnancy, and childhood.

Drug-induced jaundice

Hepatitis	Paracetamol overdose
	Anti-TB (isoniazid, rifampicin, pyrazinamide)
	Statins (p114)
	Sodium valproate
	Monoamine oxidase inhibitors
	Halothane
Cholestasis	Antibiotics (flucloxacillin, fusidic acid,
	co-amoxiclav, nitrofurantoin)
	Anabolic steroids
	Oral contraceptives
	Chlorpromazine
	Prochlorperazine
	Sulfonylureas
	Gold

Causes of jaundice in a previously stable patient with cirrhosis

- Sepsis
- Alcohol
- Drugs
- Malignancy (eg hepatocellular carcinoma)
- GI bleeding

Upper gastrointestinal bleeding: 1

Haematemesis is vomiting of blood. It may be bright or look like coffee grounds. *Melaena* mean black motions, often like tar (signifying altered blood, which has a characteristic smell). Both indicate upper GI bleeding.

Causes

Common

Peptic ulcers
Gastritis/gastric erosions
Mallory–Weiss tear (p728)
Duodenitis
Oesophageal varices (p226)
Oesophagitis
Malignancy
Drugs (NSAIDs, steroids, thrombolytics, anticoagulants)

Rare

Bleeding disorders
Portal hypertensive gastropathy
Aorto–enteric fistula; angiodysplasia
Haemobilia (bleeding in biliary tree)
Dieulafoy lesion (rupture of an unusually big arteriole, eg in fundus)
Meckel's diverticulum (OHCS p754)
Peutz–Jeghers' syndrome (p732)
Osler–Weber–Rendu syndrome (p732)

Assessment Brief history and examination to assess severity.

History: Ask about previous GI bleed; dyspepsia or known ulcers (p214); known liver disease or oesophageal varices; dysphagia; vomiting; weight loss. Check drugs (NSAIDs; steroids; anticoagulants) and alcohol consumption. Is there serious concomitant disease, eg cardiovascular disease, respiratory disease, hepatic or renal impairment, or malignancy?

Examination: Look for signs of chronic liver disease (p232) and do a PR to check for melaena. Is the patient shocked?
• Peripherally shut down (cool and clammy).
• Tachycardic (pulse >100bpm, and JVP not raised).
• Hypotensive (systolic BP <100mmHg).
• Postural drop in BP.
• Poor urine output, eg <30mL/h.

Calculating the *Rockall risk score* (see BOX) may help to stratify risk.

Acute management (see p778). In summary:
▸▸ Protect airway and give high-flow oxygen.
▸▸ Insert 2 large-bore (14–16G) IV cannulae and take blood for FBC, U&E, LFT, clotting, cross-match 4–6 units (1 unit per g/dL <14g/dL).
▸▸ Give IV colloid (eg haemaccel 500–1000mL) while waiting for blood to be crossmatched. In a dire emergency, give group O Rh–ve blood.
▸▸ Transfuse until haemodynamically stable.
▸▸ Correct clotting abnormalities (vitamin K, FFP, platelets).
▸▸ Monitor pulse, BP, and CVP at least hourly until stable.
▸▸ Insert a urinary catheter and monitor hourly urine output if shocked.
▸▸ Consider a CVP line to monitor CVP and guide fluid replacement.
▸▸ Organize a CXR, ECG, and check arterial blood gases in high-risk patients.
▸▸ Arrange an urgent endoscopy (p226).
▸▸ Notify surgeons of all severe bleeds on admission.

Further management
• Re-examine after 4h and give FFP if >4 units transfused.
• Monitor pulse, BP, CVP, and urine output hourly; ↓frequency to 4hrly if haemodynamically stable.
• Check FBC, U&E, LFT, and clotting daily.
• Transfuse to keep Hb >10g/dL; always keep 2 units of blood in reserve.
• Keep 'nil by mouth' for 24h. Allow clear fluids after 24h and light diet after 48h, if no evidence of rebleeding (p226).
• Consider IV omeprazole (p805).

Rockall risk-scoring system for GI bleeds

Score	0	1	2	3
Age	<60yrs	60–79yrs	≥80yrs	
Shock: systolic BP pulse rate	BP >100mmHg <100/min	BP >100mmHg Pulse >100/min	BP <100mmHg	
Co-morbidity	No major	Cardiac failure Ischaemic heart disease	Renal failure Liver failure	Metastases
Diagnosis	Mallory– Weiss tear; no lesion; no sign of rec- ent bleeding	All other diagnoses	Upper GI malignancy	
Signs of recent haemorrhage on endoscopy	None, or dark-red spot		Blood in upper GI tract; Adherent clot; Visible vessel	

Rockall scores help predict risk of rebleeding and death after upper GI bleeding.[26] A score >6 is said to be an indication for surgery—but decisions relating to surgery are rarely taken on the basis of Rockall scores alone.

GI bleeding management plan: ►►Resuscitate (p778)

↓

Any suspicion of variceal bleeding? (See p226)

No — **Yes**

↓ ↓

Endoscopy (at <24h if shock) Emergency endoscopy (at <4h if shock)
Are there bleeding varices?

↓ ↓ ↓ ↓

Peptic ulcer   Other diagnosis   **Yes**   **No**

Are risk factors present?
- ≥6 units transfused
- Haematemesis *and* melaena
- Rebleeding
- Bleeding vessel seen on endoscopy, or clot in an ulcer.

Sclerotherapy/banding;
see p226

► No risk factors:→conservative treatment

► ≥1 risk factor→surgery (or endoscopic diathermy eg if frail); surgery is most relevant in the context of ongoing bleeding despite endoscopic therapy, and in rebleeding if ≥6U already transfused

Endoscopy should be arranged after resuscitation, within 4h if variceal haemorrhage is suspected, or bleeding is ongoing—and otherwise within 12–24h of admission. It can identify the site of bleeding, be used to estimate the risk of rebleeding, and to administer treatment, eg adrenaline, sclerotherapy, variceal banding. Signs associated with risk of rebleeding: active arterial bleeding (90% risk); visible vessel (70% risk); adherent clot/black dots (30% risk).

Rebleeding 40% of rebleeders will die of complications. Identify high-risk patients (p225); monitor closely for signs of rebleeding. IV omeprazole has a preventive role: p804. Get help; *inform a surgeon at once if:* • Haematemesis with melaena • ↑Pulse rate • ↓JVP (monitor CVP) • ↓BP • ↓Urine output.

Indications for surgery
• Severe bleeding or bleeding despite transfusing 6U if >60yrs (8U if <60yrs)
• Rebleeding
• Active bleeding at endoscopy
• Rockall score >6 (p225).

Varices Portal hypertension causes dilated collateral veins (varices) at sites of porto-systemic anastomosis. Varices most commonly occur in the lower oesophagus, but may also be found in the stomach (gastric varices), around the umbilicus (caput medusae—rare) and in the rectum (rectal varices). Varices develop in patients with cirrhosis once portal pressure (measured by hepatic venous pressure gradient) is >10mmHg; if >12mmHg, variceal bleeding may develop—associated with a mortality of 30–50% per episode.[1]

Other causes of portal hypertension *Pre-hepatic:* Portal vein thrombosis; splenic vein thrombosis. *Intrahepatic:* Cirrhosis (80% in UK); schistosomiasis (commonest worldwide); sarcoidosis; myeloproliferative diseases; congenital hepatic fibrosis. *Post-hepatic:* Budd–Chiari syndrome (p720); right heart failure; constrictive pericarditis; veno-occlusive disease.

Risk factors for variceal haemorrhage: ↑Portal pressure; variceal size, endoscopic features of the variceal wall, eg haematocystic spots and Child–Pugh score ≥8 (see BOX).[27]

Suspect varices as a cause of GI bleeding if there is alcohol abuse or cirrhosis. Look for signs of chronic liver disease, encephalopathy, splenomegaly ± ascites.

Prophylaxis—primary: Without treatment, ~30% of cirrhotic patients with varices bleed—reducible to 15% by: (1) β-blockers (propranolol 40–80mg/12h PO) ± nitrates (isosorbide mononitrate 10–40mg/12h PO). (2) Endoscopic ligation (banding) may be indicated for large varices. This ↓ risk of 1st bleeding when compared with propranolol. **NB:** Endoscopic sclerotherapy is not used as complications may outweigh benefits. *Secondary:* After an initial variceal bleed, risk of further bleeding is high. Options are (1) and (2) as above, + transjugular intrahepatic porto–systemic shunting (TIPS)[2] or surgical shunts. Endoscopic banding is better than sclerotherapy (lower bleeding rates & fewer complications). TIPS is also used in uncontrolled variceal hemorrhage. Consider surgical shunts if TIPS is impossible for technical reasons.

Acute variceal bleeding: Get expert help at the bedside from your senior.
➥ Resuscitate until haemodynamically stable (do not give 0.9% saline).
➥ Correct clotting abnormalities with vitamin K and FFP.
➥ Start IVI of octreotide (50µg/h for 2–5d)[28] or glypressin (=terlipressin 2mg bolus, then 2mg/4h for 3d).[29] These work in 83% of patients.
➥ Endoscopic sclerotherapy—only if vasoactive drugs fail (Cochrane meta-analysis).[30] **NB:** banding may be impossible (∴ limited visualization).
➥ If bleeding uncontrolled, a Minnesota tube or Sengstaken–Blakemore tube should be placed by someone with experience—or TIPS as above.[31]

NB *intensive sclerotherapy regimens* ↓risk of rebleeding but may not ↑survival.

1 Russo M 2002 *Curr Treat Options Gastroenterol* 2002 **5** 471
2 TIPS works by shunting blood away from the portal circulation.

Balloon tamponade with a Sengstaken–Blakemore tube

In life-threatening variceal bleeding, this can buy time to arrange transfer to a specialist liver centre or surgical decompression.

It uses balloons to compress gastric and oesophageal varices.

Before insertion, inflate balloons with a measured volume (120–300mL) of air giving pressures of 60mmHg (check with a sphygmomanometer).

• Deflate, and clamp exits.

• Pass the lubricated tube (try to avoid sedation) and inflate the gastric balloon with the predetermined volume of air. **NB:** The tube is easier to pass when it is cold, which is why it is kept in the fridge.

• Inflate the oesophageal balloon. Check pressures (should be 20–30mmHg greater than on the trial run). This phase of the procedure is dangerous: do not over inflate the balloon (risk of oesophageal necrosis or rupture).

• Tape to patient's forehead to ensure the gastric balloon impacts gently on the gastro-oesophageal junction.

• Place the oesophageal aspiration channel on continuous low suction and arrange for the gastric channel to drain freely.

• Leave *in situ* until bleeding stops. Remove after <24h.

Various other techniques of insertion may be used, and tubes vary in structure. *Do not try to pass one yourself if you have no or little experience:* ask an expert; if unavailable, transfer urgently to a specialist liver centre.

Endoscopy and biopsy

Upper GI endoscopy *Diagnostic indications* Haematemesis
Dyspepsia, especially if >55yrs old   Persistent vomiting
Gastric biopsy (suspected malignancy)   Iron-deficiency anaemia
Duodenal biopsy (eg coeliac disease)

Therapeutic: Mainly injecting/coagulating of bleeding lesions. Also:
- Sclerotherapy or banding of oesophageal varices
- Dilatation of strictures (oesophageal, pyloric)
- Palliation of oesophageal cancer (stent insertion, laser therapy).

Pre-procedure: Nil by mouth for 8h (but water up to 90min pre-op may be OK). Obtain written consent. Advise the patient not to drive for 24h if sedation is being given. Arrange follow-up.

Procedure: Sedation may be given (eg midazolam 2mg IV; monitor O_2 saturation with a pulse oximeter). The pharynx is sprayed with local anaesthetic and a flexible endoscope is swallowed. Continuous suction must be available to prevent aspiration. *Complications:* Transient sore throat; amnesia following sedation; perforation (<0.1%); cardiorespiratory arrest (<0.1%).
NB: Inform endoscopists of prior antisecretory use (eg PPI): these mask diagnosis of up to ~30% of adenocarcinomas.[32]

Duodenal biopsy is the gold standard for diagnosing coeliac disease. It is also useful in investigating unusual causes of malabsorption, eg giardiasis, lymphoma, Whipple's disease, amyloid, or microscopic colitis (p218).

Sigmoidoscopy views the rectum; rigid or flexible sigmoidoscopy should precede barium enema in suspected colorectal cancer. Flexible sigmoidoscopes gain better access than rigid ones, but ~25% of colon cancers are still out of reach.[33]

Pre-procedure: Give 2 phosphate enemas; get written consent. Do biopsies, as macroscopic appearances may be normal in certain diseases, eg inflammatory bowel disease, amyloidosis.

Colonoscopy *Diagnostic indications:* Rectal bleeding; iron deficiency; persistent diarrhoea; biopsy of a lesion seen on barium enema; to assess Crohn's or UC; colorectal cancer surveillance (sometimes); *Strep. bovis* endocarditis.[1]

Therapeutic indications: Polypectomy; diathermy to angiodysplasia (p482); treating pseudo-obstruction or volvulus.

Preparation: Prescribe sodium picosulfate (Picolax®) 1 sachet morning and afternoon, the day before the procedure. Obtain written consent.

Procedure: Sedation and analgesia are given before a flexible colonoscope is passed per rectum around the colon.

Complications: Abdominal discomfort; incomplete examination; perforation (0.2%); haemorrhage after biopsy or polypectomy.

Liver biopsy *Indications:* Abnormal LFT, chronic viral hepatitis; alcoholic hepatitis; auto-immune hepatitis (AIH); suspected cirrhosis; suspected carcinoma; biopsy of hepatic lesions; investigation of PUO.

Pre-procedure: Nil by mouth for 8h. Check clotting (INR <1.3) and platelet count (>100 × 10^9/L). Obtain written consent. Prescribe analgesia.

Procedure: Sedation (eg diazepam 5mg IV) may be given. The liver borders are percussed out and where there is dullness in the midaxillary line in expiration, local anaesthetic (lidocaine 2%) is infiltrated down to the liver capsule. Breathing is rehearsed and a needle biopsy is taken with the breath held in expiration. Afterwards the patient lies on the right side for 2h, then in bed for 6h while regular pulse and BP observations are taken.

Complications: Local pain; pneumothorax; bleeding (<0.5%); death (<0.1%).[34]

Endoscopy images: See www.gastrosource.com/kisweb/atlas.htm

---

1 The cancer is the portal of entry: think of this whenever *Strep. bovis* is cultured from the blood.

Abdominal ultrasound is used for the investigation of abdominal pain, abnormal LFT, jaundice, hepatomegaly or abdominal masses. Patients should be nil by mouth for 4h before the scan in order to allow visualization of the gall bladder. Pelvic ultrasound requires the bladder to be full. Ultrasound may also be used to guide diagnostic biopsy or therapeutic aspiration.

Endoscopic retrograde cholangiopancreatography (ERCP) *Diagnostic indications:* Useful when MRCP (below) is unavailable—eg in cholangitis; jaundice with dilated intrahepatic ducts; jaundice with normal calibre ducts and a non-diagnostic liver biopsy; recurrent pancreatitis; post-cholecystectomy pain. *Therapeutic indications:* Sphincterotomy for common bile duct stones; stenting of malignant strictures. *Pre-procedure:* Check clotting and platelet count. Prescribe antibiotic prophylaxis (eg ciprofloxacin 750mg PO 2h before), analgesia (eg morphine 5mg and metoclopramide 10mg IV 1h before) and sedation (eg midazolam 2.5–10mg IV). *Procedure:* A catheter is advanced from a side-viewing duodenoscope via the ampulla into the common bile duct. Contrast medium is injected and x-rays taken to show lesions in the biliary tree and pancreatic ducts. *Complications:* Pancreatitis; bleeding; cholangitis; perforation. *Mortality:* <0.2% overall; 0.4% if stone removal.

Small bowel follow through After bowel preparation, barium is ingested and serial x-ray films are taken every 30min until barium reaches the caecum. Enhanced films are taken of areas of interest, eg terminal ileum.

Small bowel enema After bowel preparation, barium is introduced via duodenal intubation. Although technically more demanding than a barium follow-through, this method results in better mucosal definition.

Barium enema Always do a PR first ± rigid sigmoidoscopy & biopsy. Preparation is as in colonoscopy (p228). For a double contrast barium enema, barium and air are introduced per rectum. Special views may be needed to visualize the areas of interest. Gastrograffin may be used instead of barium in suspected colonic obstruction. It may show diverticular disease, or cancers (eg an irregular 'apple-core' narrowing of the lumen). In Crohn's disease, look for 'cobblestoning', 'rose thorn' ulcers, colonic strictures with rectal sparing. *Disadvantages:* Significant radiation dose; no biopsy possible.

Computer tomography (CT) is indicated if ultrasound is technically difficult or non-diagnostic. It allows better visualization of retroperitoneal structures but requires skilled interpretation. Oral or IV contrast may be given to enhance definition. The main disadvantage is the high radiation dose.

Magnetic resonance imaging (MRI) provides superior soft tissue imaging and enables the distinction of benign and malignant lesions. The other advantage over CT is the lack of radiation. Disadvantages are that patients with pacemakers and certain metal implants cannot be scanned, and that the scanner itself can induce claustrophobia. *Magnetic resonance cholangiopancreatography (MRCP)* MRCP enables *in vivo* anatomic exploration of the main pancreatic duct. Horizontal sections provide helpful radio-anatomic information. The technique nevertheless remains limited by poor spatial resolution. MRCP had a sensitivity of 83% and a specificity of 99% for diagnosing common bile duct stones (p484), and, according to some authorities, is the investigation of choice—partly, no doubt, due to lack of side-effects.

Imaging via a wireless enteroscopy capsule This capsule is swallowed and sends images to a recorder worn by the patient. Currently it cannot take pictures fast enough to cope with rapid oesophageal transit—and by the time it gets to the colon its battery may have run out. It may be useful for imaging the small bowel when investigating occult GI bleeding (eg angiodysplasia). Robotic biopsy and therapeutic procedures are not yet possible.

Liver failure

Definitions Liver failure may occur suddenly in the previously healthy liver: *acute hepatic failure*. More commonly it occurs as a result of decompensation of chronic liver disease: *acute-on-chronic hepatic failure*. *Fulminant hepatic failure* refers to encephalopathy occurring within 8wks of symptoms of acute liver failure. *Late-onset hepatic failure* refers to encephalopathy occurring within 9–26wks.

Causes *Infections:* Viral hepatitis, yellow fever, leptospirosis.
Drugs: Paracetamol overdose, halothane, isoniazid.
Toxins: Amanita phalloides mushrooms, carbon tetrachloride.
Vascular: Budd–Chiari syndrome (p720), veno-occlusive disease.
Others: primary biliary cirrhosis, haemochromatosis, autoimmune hepatitis, α_1-antitrypsin deficiency, Wilson's disease, fatty liver of pregnancy (*OHCS* p158), malignancy.

Clinical features *Hepatic encephalopathy* is graded as follows:

Grade I   Altered mood or behaviour
Grade II   Increasing drowsiness, confusion, slurred speech
Grade III   Stupor, incoherence, restlessness, significant confusion
Grade IV   Coma.

Other features: Jaundice, fetor hepaticus (smells like pear drops), asterixis, constructional apraxia (ask the patient to draw a five-pointed star). Signs of chronic liver disease (p232) suggest acute-on-chronic hepatic failure.

Investigations
Blood tests: FBC (?infection,[1] ?GI bleed); U&E[2] (?renal failure); LFT (↑bilirubin, AST, and ALT); clotting (↑PT/INR); glucose (?hypoglycaemia), paracetamol level, hepatitis serology, ferritin, α_1-antitrypsin, caeruloplasmin.

Microbiology: Blood culture; urine culture; microscopy/culture of ascites; ascitic neutrophils >250/mm^3 indicates spontaneous bacterial peritonitis.

Radiology: CXR, abdominal ultrasound; Doppler flow studies of the portal vein (& hepatic vein, in suspected Budd–Chiari, p720).

Neurophysiological studies: EEG may show high-voltage slow waveforms.

Management Beware sepsis, hypoglycaemia, and encephalopathy: ▶▶see p806.
- Nurse with a 20° head-up tilt in ITU. Protect the airway and insert an NG tube to avoid aspiration and remove any blood from stomach.
- Monitor temperature; pulse; RR; BP; pupils; urine output hourly.
- Check FBC, U&E, LFTs, and INR daily.
- Give 10% dextrose IV, 1L/12h to avoid hypoglycaemia. Give 50mL 50% dextrose IV if blood glucose <3.5mmol/L (do every 1–4h in acute liver failure).
- Treat the cause, if known (eg paracetamol poisoning, p832).
- If malnourished, get dietary help (eg diet rich in carbohydrate- and protein-derived calories, preferably orally; in encephalopathy, avoid excessive protein in the diet (branched-chain amino acids may have a role in achieving a +ve nitrogen balance). Give thiamine and folate supplements as needed.
- Haemofiltration or haemodialysis, if renal failure develops (see BOX).
- Avoid sedatives or other drugs with hepatic metabolism (see *BNF*).
- Liaise early with your nearest transplant centre regarding the appropriateness of transfer (see BOX). Indications: see BOX.

Prognosis Poor prognostic factors: Grade III or IV encephalopathy, age >40yrs, albumin <30g/L, drug-induced liver failure, late-onset hepatic failure worse than fulminant failure. 65% survival post-transplantation.

---

1 Leucocytosis need not mean a secondary infection: hepatitis may itself be the cause.
2 As urea is synthesized in the liver, it is a poor test of renal function in liver failure; use creatinine instead.

Treating the complications of acute hepatic failure

Bleeding: Vit. K 10mg/d IV for 3d + platelets, FFP + blood as needed.

Infection: Until sensitivities are known, give ceftriaxone 1–2g/24h IV. Avoid gentamicin (↑risk of renal failure).

Ascites: Fluid restriction, low-salt diet, diuretics, daily weights.

Hypoglycaemia: Check blood glucose regularly and give 50mL of 50% glucose IV if levels fall below 2mmol/L. Watch plasma K^+.

Encephalopathy: Avoid sedatives; 20° head-up tilt in ITU; lactulose + neomycin 1g/6h PO to ↓numbers of bowel organisms. Aim for 2 soft stools/d.

Cerebral oedema: Give 20% mannitol IV. Hyperventilate.

Hepatorenal syndrome (HRS)[1]: HRS occurs in ~18% of cirrhotic patients with ascites—with intense renal vasoconstriction, ↓glomerular filtration rate, and *normal* renal histology. *Rx:* Albumin IV ± haemodialysis. **NB:** ↑levels of neuropeptide Y (NPY) occur in HRS worsening renal vasoconstriction—and terlipressin (=glypressin) may help.●⁴⁰ (NPY is a renal vasoconstrictor peptide released on stimulation of sympathetic nervous system.)⁴¹

King's College Hospital[UK] criteria for liver transplantation

Paracetamol liver failure	Arterial pH < 7.3 24h after ingestion *Or all of the following:* Prothrombin time (PT) > 100s Creatinine > 300µmol/L Grade III or IV encephalopathy
Non-paracetamol liver failure	PT > 100s *Or 3 out of 5 of the following:* **1** Drug-induced liver failure **2** Age <10 or >40 yrs old **3** >1wk between onset of jaundice and encephalopathy **4** PT > 50s **5** Bilirubin > 300µmol/L

Guidelines vary, see:
rcpe.ac.uk/public/gardennet.html

231

In some centres, transplantation is either *cadaveric* or from *live donors* (right lobe)—a procedure not without complications (eg biliary fistula). Gaining *valid consent* from the donor is difficult: the normal procedure sounds simple 'Use only words the patient understands; ensure that he believes your facts and can retain the pros and cons long enough to inform his decision—and make sure his choice is free from pressure from others'. But this last proviso is nearly impossible in live donation. There is evidence that altruistic donors make up their minds before the procedure, and only listen to information which endorses their decision. So 'donor advocate teams' have been developed, comprising a social worker, psychiatrist, and an independent examining physician uninvolved with the transplant team. This way of helping equipoise in communicating risks and benefits could be a model for consent in other contexts.⁴²

Prescribing in liver failure

Avoid opiates, diuretics (↑risk of encephalopathy), oral hypoglycaemics, and saline-containing IVIs. Warfarin effects are enhanced. Hepatotoxic drugs include: paracetamol, methotrexate, phenothiazines, isoniazid, azathioprine, oestrogen, 6-mercaptopurine, salicylates, tetracycline, mitomycin.

---

1 *Liver-kidney interactions* In cirrhosis ↓hepatic clearance of immune complexes leads to their trapping in the kidney (∴ IgA nephropathy ± hepatic glomerulosclerosis). *Viruses:* HCV can cause cryoglobulinaemia and membranoproliferative glomerulonephritis. HBV may cause membranous nephropathy and PAN. Membranoproliferative glomerulonephritis can occur in α_1-antitrypsin deficiency. [@12118395]

Cirrhosis

Cirrhosis implies irreversible liver damage. Histologically, there is loss of normal hepatic architecture with fibrosis and nodular regeneration.

Causes Chronic alcohol abuse, HBV, and HCV infection. Others: see BOX.

Presentation varies from asymptomatic with ↑LFTs to decompensated end-stage liver disease. *Chronic liver disease:* Leuconychia—white nails with lunulae undemarcated, from hypoalbuminaemia; Terry's nails—white proximally but distal 30% reddened by telangiectasias; ⚐ palmar erythema (hyperdynamic circulation); spider naevi; Dupuytren's contracture; gynaecomastia; testicular atrophy; parotids enlarged; clubbing; hepatomegaly, or small liver in late disease.

Complications *Hepatic failure:* Coagulopathy (↓factors II, VII, IX, & X causes ↑INR); encephalopathy—ie liver flap (asterixis) + confusion, coma; hypoalbuminaemia (oedema, leuconychia); sepsis (bacterial peritonitis)[1]; hypoglycaemia. *Portal hypertension:* Ascites; splenomegaly; portosystemic shunts including oesophageal varices (±life-threatening upper GI bleed) and 'caput medusae' (enlarged superficial periumbilical veins). ↑Risk of hepatocellular carcinoma.

Tests *Blood:* LFT: ↔ or ↑bilirubin, ↑AST, ↑ALT, ↑alk phos & ↑GGT. Later, with loss of synthetic function, look for ↓albumin ± ↑PT/INR. ↓WCC & ↓platelets indicate hypersplenism. *Find the cause:* Ferritin, iron/total iron-binding capacity (p234); hepatitis serology; immunoglobulins (p238); autoantibodies (ANA, AMA, SMA, p421); α-fetoprotein (p242); caeruloplasmin (p236); α₁-antitrypsin (p236).

Liver ultrasound may show hepatomegaly, splenomegaly, focal liver lesion(s), hepatic vein thrombi, reversed flow in the portal vein, or ascites. *MRI:* Caudate lobe size↑, smaller islands of regenerating nodules, and the presence of the right posterior hepatic notch are more frequent in alcoholic cirrhosis than in virus-induced cirrhosis.⚐ MRI scoring systems based on spleen volume, liver volume, and presence of ascites or varices/collaterals etc. can quantify severity of cirrhosis in a way that correlates well with Child grades (see BOX).⚐

Ascitic tap should be performed and fluid sent for urgent MC + S: an ascitic WCC of >250/mm³ indicates spontaneous bacterial peritonitis. *Liver biopsy* (p228) confirms the clinical diagnosis. This may be done percutaneously (if clotting is normal, see p228) or via the transjugular route with FFP cover.

Management *General:* Good nutrition (avoid protein excess, p230), low-salt diet (if ascites). Alcohol abstinence. Avoid NSAIDs, sedatives, and opiates. Colestyramine may help pruritus (4g/8h PO, 1h after other drugs). Consider ultrasound and α-fetoprotein every 3–6 months♦ to screen for HCC, p242.⚐

Specific treatments: Interferon-α (± ribavirin) improves liver biochemistry and may retard development of hepatocellular cancer (HCC) in HCV-induced cirrhosis (p576). Meta-analyses show little benefit of ursodeoxycholic acid in PBC.⚐ Penicillamine for Wilson's disease (p236).

Ascites: Bedrest, fluid restriction (<1.5L/d), low-salt diet (40–100mmol/d). Give spironolactone 100mg/24h PO; ↑dose every 48h, to 400mg/24h. Chart daily weight; aim for weight loss of ≤½kg/d. If response is poor, add in furosemide ≤120mg/24h PO; do U&E/creatinine often. Therapeutic paracentesis with concomitant albumin infusion (6–8g/L fluid removed) may be tried.

Spontaneous bacterial peritonitis: Treatment: eg cefuroxime 1.5g/8h + metronidazole 500mg eg daily (get help with dose; it depends on degree of liver failure, consult the *datasheet*) until sensitivities known. *Prophylaxis:* Ciprofloxacin 250mg PO or co-trimoxazole 960mg PO on weekdays only.⚐

Prognosis Overall 5yr survival is ~50%. Poor prognostic indicators: encephalopathy; serum Na⁺< 110mmol/L; serum albumin < 25g/L; ↑INR.

Liver transplantation (p231) is the only definitive treatment for cirrhosis.⚐ This increases 5yr survival from ~20% in end-stage disease to ~70%.⚐

---

1 Mattos A 2004 *Arq Gastroenterol* **40** 11. Other infections in cirrhosis: UTI; pneumonia; septicaemia.

Causes of cirrhosis

- Chronic alcohol abuse
- Chronic HBV or HCV infection[1]
- Autoimmune disease: PBC (p238)
  Primary sclerosing cholangitis (PSC) (p238)
  Autoimmune liver disease (p240)
- Genetic disorders: α_1-antitrypsin deficiency p236
  Wilson's disease (p236)
  Haemachromatosis (p234)
- Others: Budd–Chiari syndrome (p720, hepatic vein thrombosis)
- Drugs Eg amiodarone, methyldopa, methotrexate

Child-Pugh grading and risk of variceal bleeding

	1 point	2 points	3 points
Bilirubin (μmol/L)	<34	34–51	>51
Albumin (g/L)	>3.5	2.8–3.5	<2.8
Prothrombin ratio (seconds > normal)	1–3	4–6	>6
Ascites	None	Slight	Moderate
Encephalopathy	None	1–2	3–4

Risk ↑↑ if score ≥8

1 Clues as to which patients with chronic HCV are going on to get cirrhosis: platelet count ≤140,000/mm³, globulin/albumin ratio ≥ 1, and AST/ALT ratio ≥ 1—100% positive predictive value but lower sensitivity (~30%)—Luo J 2003 *Hepatogastroenterology* **49** 78

Hereditary haemochromatosis (HH)

This is an inherited disorder of iron metabolism in which increased intestinal iron absorption leads to its deposition in multiple organs (joints, liver, heart, pancreas, and pituitary). Middle-aged males are more frequently and severely affected than women, in whom the disease tends to present ~10yrs later (menstrual blood loss is protective).

Genetics HH is one of the commonest inherited disease in those of Northern European (especially Celtic) ancestry (carrier rate of ~1 in 10 and a frequency of homozygosity of ~1 : 200 – 1 : 400. The gene responsible for most HH is called HFE. 2 major mutations are termed C282Y and H63D. C282Y accounts for 60–100% of HH, and H63D accounts for 3–7%, with compound heterozygotes accounting for 1–4%. Penetrance is unknown but is clearly <100%.

Clinical features Asymptomatic early on—then tiredness and arthralgia (MCP and large joints). Later, look for: slate-grey skin pigmentation; diabetes mellitus ('bronze diabetes'); signs of chronic liver disease (p232); hepatomegaly; cirrhosis; cardiac failure (dilated cardiomyopathy); hypogonadism, p318 (pituitary dysfunction↓, or via cirrhosis) and associated osteoporosis. Other endocrinopathies include hyporeninaemic hypoaldosteronism.

Tests *Blood:* Abnormal LFT; ↑serum ferritin; ↑serum iron; ↓TIBC; transferrin saturation >80%. HFE genotyping. Blood glucose (?DM). *Joint x-rays* may show chondrocalcinosis. *Liver biopsy:* Perl's stain quantifies iron loading (hepatic iron index (HII)[1] >1.9μmol/kg/yr) and assesses disease severity. MRI also helps estimates hepatic iron loading. Do ECG & echo if you suspect cardiomyopathy.

Management *Venesect* ~1 unit/wk, until mildly iron-deficient. Iron will continue to accumulate, so maintenance venesection (1U every 2–3 months) is needed for life. Maintain haematocrit <0.5, serum ferritin <100mg/L, TIBC >50mmol/L, and transferrin saturation <40%. *Other monitoring:* Diabetes (p296). Hb_A1c levels may falsely low as venesection reduces the time available for Hb glycosylation. *Over-the-counter self-medication:* Make sure that vitamin preparations etc. contain no iron. *Screening:* Test serum ferritin and genotype in 1st-degree relatives. Prevalence of iron overload in asymptomatic C282Y homozygotes is ≤4.5 per 1000 persons screened. How many will go on to develop iron overload is unknown.

Prognosis Venesection returns life expectancy to normal if non-cirrhotic and non-diabetic. Arthropathy may improve or worsen. Gonadal failure is irreversible. In non-cirrhotic patients, venesection may improve liver histology. ►Cirrhotic patients have >10% chance of developing HCC. Sources vary on the exact risk: some authorities quote 30%; others 22%. One cause of variability is varying co-factors: age over 50yrs ↑risk by 13-fold; being HBsAg +ve by 5-fold and alcohol abuse by 2-fold.

Secondary haemochromatosis may occur in any haematological condition where many transfusions (~40L in total) have been given. To reduce need for transfusions, find out if the haematological condition responds to erythropoietin or marrow transplantation—before irreversible effects of iron overload become too great. See iron management in thalassaemia, p642.

---

1 The HII aims to separate HH from other causes of hepatic siderosis (eg HBV; alcoholic cirrhosis). It is less used now that genotyping is available. HII in μmol iron/gram liver/year = [Iron concentration (μg iron per gram dry weight of liver)/55.846 (atomic weight of Fe)]/patient's age. HII >1.9 in a non-rhotic liver strongly suggests HH. *Caveats:* • ~7% of those with HH have a HII <1.9. Using a threshold hepatic iron concentration of 71μmol/g as well as HII can detect most of these. [@9322522] • Cirrhotic livers can rapidly accumulate iron in non-HH liver disease making HII >1.9. Some say that an HII cut-off of ~4.2 is best in diagnosing HH in cirrhotics. [@9576576]. • Iron is not uniformly distributed in the liver (sampling variation). • Correlation among HII, phenotypic HH, & genotypic HH is not 100%.
http://tpis.upmc.edu/tpis/liver/Hepaticironindex.html

α₁-antitrypsin deficiency

α₁-antitrypsin is one of a family of **ser**ine **p**rotease **in**hibitors (deficiency is termed a 'serpinopathy') controlling inflammatory cascades. It is synthesized in the liver, making up 90% of serum α₁-globulin on electrophoresis (p703). α₁-antitrypsin deficiency is the chief genetic cause of liver disease in children. In adults, its lack causes emphysema (p188), chronic liver disease, and HCC (p242). *Other associations:* Asthma, pancreatitis, gallstones, Wegener's (p738). *Decreased* risk of stroke. *Prevalence:* 1 : 2000–1 : 7000.

Genetics *Carrier frequency:* 1 : 10. Genetic variants are typed by their electrophoretic mobility as *medium* (M), *slow* (S), or *very slow* (Z). S and Z types are due to single amino acid substitutions at positions 264 and 342, respectively. These result in ↓production of α₁-antitrypsin (S=60%, Z=15%). The normal genotype is PIMM, the homozygote is PIZZ; heterozygotes are PIMZ & PISZ.

Symptomatic patients (eg *cholestatic jaundice*/cirrhosis; *dyspnoea* from emphysema) usually have PIZZ genotype. **NB:** cholestasis often remits in adolescence. In adults, cirrhosis ± HCC affect 25% of α₁-antitrypsin-deficient adults >50yrs.

Tests *Serum α₁-antitrypsin* levels↓. *Liver biopsy:* (p228) Periodic acid Schiff (PAS) +ve; diastase-resistant globules. *Phenotyping* by isoelectric focusing requires expertise to distinguish SZ and ZZ phenotypes. *Prenatal diagnosis* is possible by DNA analysis of chorionic villus samples obtained at 11–13wks' gestation. DNA tests are likely to find greater use in the future.

Management *Supportive* for emphysema and liver complications. Quit smoking; consider *augmentation therapy* with human α₁-antitrypsin if FEV₁ <80% of predicted[1] (expensive!) ± *liver transplant* (p231) in decompensated cirrhosis.

Wilson's disease/hepatolenticular degeneration

A rare inherited disorder with toxic accumulation of copper (Cu) in liver and CNS (especially basal ganglia, eg globus pallidus hypodensity ± putamen cavitation). It is treatable, so screen all young patients with cirrhosis. *Genetics:* Autosomal recessive (gene on chromosome 13; codes for a copper transporting ATPase, ATP7B). 27 mutations are known; HIS1069GLU is the commonest.

Signs Children usually present with *liver disease* (hepatitis, cirrhosis, fulminant liver failure); young adults often start with *CNS signs:* Tremor; dysarthria, dysphagia; dyskinesias; dystonias; purposeless stereotyped movements (eg hand clapping); dementia; parkinsonism; micrographia; ataxia/clumsiness. *Affective features:* ▶Ignoring these may cause years of needless misery. Depression/mania; labile emotions; libido↑↓; personality change. *Cognitive/behavioural:* Memory↓; quick to anger; slow to solve problems; IQ↓. *Psychosis:* Delusions; mutism. *Kayser-Fleischer rings:* Cu deposits in iris (Descemet's membrane), pathognomonic but not invariable; may need slit lamp to see). *Also:* Haemolysis; blue lunulae (nails); polyarthritis; hypermobile joints; grey skin; abortions; hypoparathyroidism.

Tests Serum copper and caeruloplasmin usually↓. 24h urinary copper excretion↑ (>100μg/24h, normal <40μg). Liver biopsy: ↑hepatic copper content. Molecular genetic testing can confirm the diagnosis. MRI: basal ganglia degeneration (± fronto-temporal, cerebellar, and brain stem atrophy).

Management *Chelation:* Lifelong penicillamine (500mg/6–8h for 1yr, maintenance: 0.75–1g/d). SE: nausea, rash, WCC↓, Hb↓, platelets↓ haematuria, nephrosis, lupus. Monitor FBC & urinary Cu (and protein) excretion. Say 'report sore throat, T°↑, or bruising at once' in case WCC↓↓. Stop if WCC < 2.5×10⁹/L or platelets falling (or < 120×10⁹/L). *Alternative:* Trientine dihydrochloride 600mg/ 8–12h PO pc (SE: rash; sideroblastic anaemia). *Liver transplant* (p231) if *severe liver disease.* Screen siblings as asymptomatic homozygotes need treatment.

Prognosis Pre-cirrhotic liver disease is reversible. Neurological damage less so. Death occurs from liver failure, variceal haemorrhage (p226), or infection.

---

1 120mg/kg IV every 2wks is conveniently self-given via SC intravenous injection port systems. [@12728289]

Primary biliary cirrhosis (PBC)

Interlobular bile ducts are damaged by chronic granulomatous inflammation causing progressive cholestasis, cirrhosis, and portal hypertension. *Cause:* ?autoimmune. ♀:♂ ≈ 9 : 1. *Prevalence:* ≤4/100,00. *Peak presentation:* ~50yrs old.

Clinical features Often asymptomatic and diagnosed after finding ↑alk phos on routine LFT. Lethargy and pruritus may occur, and can precede jaundice by months to years. Signs: jaundice; skin pigmentation; xanthelasma (p706); xanthomata; hepatomegaly; and splenomegaly.
Complications: Osteoporosis is common. Malabsorption of fat-soluble vitamins (A, D, K) results in osteomalacia and coagulopathy. Other complications: portal hypertension; ascites; variceal haemorrhage; hepatic encephalopathy; HCC (p242).

Tests *Blood tests:* ↑Alk phos, ↑γGT, and mildly ↑AST and ALT; late disease: ↑bilirubin, ↓albumin, ↑PT. 98% are antimitochondrial antibody (AMA) M₂ subtype +ve (highly specific). Other autoantibodies (p421) may occur in low titres. Immunoglobulins are↑ (especially IgM). TSH and cholesterol may be↑.
Radiology: Ultrasound & ERCP (p229) to exclude extrahepatic cholestasis.
Liver biopsy: Granulomas around the bile ducts, progressing to cirrhosis.

Treatment *Symptomatic:* Pruritus: try colestyramine 4g/6–24h PO. Diarrhoea: codeine phosphate, eg 30mg/8h PO. Osteoporosis prevention: p698.

Specific: Fat-soluble vitamin prophylaxis: vitamin A, D, and K. Consider *ursodeoxycholic acid* (UDCA), 13–15mg/kg/d to all patients.[1] It is said to slow disease progression◆ and may obviate the need for *Liver transplantation* (p231), which is the last recourse for patients with end-stage disease (eg bilirubin > 100μmol/L) or intractable pruritus. Recurrence in the graft may occur₆₄ but appears not to influence graft success.

Prognosis Once jaundice develops, survival is <2yrs. In one study, at 2yrs post-transplant, predicted survival without transplant was 55% and actual survival was 79%. At 7yrs, these figures were 22% and 68%, respectively.₆₅

Primary sclerosing cholangitis (PSC)

A disorder of unknown cause characterized by inflammation, fibrosis, and strictures of intra- and extrahepatic bile ducts. Immunological mechanisms are implicated. Associations: UC (in ~80%); HLA-A1, B8, & DR3.

Clinical features Chronic biliary obstruction and secondary biliary cirrhosis lead to liver failure and death (or transplantation) over ~10yrs.
Symptoms: Patients may be asymptomatic and diagnosed incidentally after finding alk phos↑ on LFT; or else symptoms may fluctuate, eg: jaundice; pruritus; abdominal pain; fatigue. *Signs:* Jaundice; hepatomegaly; portal hypertension.
Complications: Bacterial cholangitis; cholangiocarcinoma (10–30%); ↑risk of colorectal cancer. 30% of patients in some series have an overlap syndrome with type 1 AIH (p240).[2]

Tests *Blood:* ↑Alk phos initially followed by ↑bilirubin; hypergammaglobulinaemia; AMA negative, but ANA, SMA, & ANCA may be +ve, see p421. *ERCP* shows multiple strictures of the biliary tree (characteristic 'beaded' appearance). *Liver biopsy* shows a fibrous, obliterative cholangitis.

Management *Drugs:* Some types respond to corticosteroids; colestyramine (=cholestyramine) 4g/6–24h PO for pruritus. Ursodeoxycholic acid improves cholestasis but has no histological effect. Antibiotics for bacterial cholangitis.

Endoscopic stenting helps symptomatic dominant strictures. *Liver transplantation* (p231) is indicated in end-stage disease. Recurrence occurs in 20%; 5yr graft survival is >60%.

---

1 C Levy 2003 *Curr Treat Options Gastroenterol* **6** 93 (Advice from the Mayo clinic).
2 Do anti-mitochondrial, anti-nuclear, anti-smooth muscle, anti-liver kidney microsomal type 1, anti-liver cytosol type 1, perinuclear anti-neutrophil nuclear, & anti-soluble liver antigen antibodies. [@12765484]

Disease associations

Primary biliary cirrhosis (PBC)
- Thyroid disease
- Rheumatoid arthritis
- Sjögren's syndrome (70%)
- Keratoconjunctivitis sicca
- Systemic sclerosis (p420)
- Renal tubular acidosis
- Membranous glomerulonephritis

Primary sclerosing cholangitis (PSC)
- Ulcerative colitis (3% of those with UC have PSC; 80% of those with PSC have UC)
- Crohn's disease (much rarer); HIV infection

Autoimmune hepatitis (AIH)

An inflammatory liver disease of unknown cause[1] characterized by suppressor T-cell defects with autoantibodies directed against hepatocyte surface antigens. Two types are distinguished by the presence of circulating autoantibodies:

Type I   Affects adults or children
            Anti-nuclear antibodies (ANA) and/or
            Anti-smooth muscle antibodies (SMA) +ve in 80%.

Type II   Affects children
            Anti-liver/kidney microsomal type 1 (LKM1) antibodies.

Clinical features Predominantly affects young and middle-aged women. 25% present with acute hepatitis and features of an autoimmune disease, eg fever, malaise, urticarial rash, polyarthritis, pleurisy, or glomerulonephritis. The remainder present insidiously or are asymptomatic and diagnosed incidentally with signs of chronic liver disease (p232). Amenorrhoea is common.

Associations

Pernicious anaemia	Autoimmune haemolysis	Ulcerative colitis
Diabetes	Glomerulonephritis	HLA A1, B8, & DR3 haplotype
Autoimmune thyroiditis	PSC (p238)	

Tests Abnormal LFT (AST↑), hypergammaglobulinaemia (especially IgG), +ve autoantibodies (ANA, SMA, or LKM1). Other autoantibodies, eg anti-soluble liver antigen (SLA) and antimeasles virus may be seen. Anaemia, WCC↓, and platelets↓ indicate hypersplenism. Liver biopsy (p228) shows mononuclear infiltrate of portal and periportal areas + piecemeal necrosis, fibrosis, or cirrhosis. ERCP (p229) helps exclude PSC if alk phos disproportionately ↑.

Diagnosis depends on excluding other diseases as there is no pathognomonic sign or lab test. There is genuine overlap with PBC (p238). Diagnostic criteria exist but are not fully validated (eg the IAHG system). They cannot be universally relied on. International Autoimmune
Hepatitis Group 1999

Management *Prednisolone* 30mg/24h PO for 1 month; ↓by 5mg a month to a maintenance dose of 5–10mg/24h PO. Corticosteroids can sometimes be stopped after 2yrs but relapse occurs in 50–86%. *Azathioprine* (50–100mg/d PO) may be used as a steroid sparing agent. Remission is achievable in 80% of patients within 3yrs. *10- and 20-yr survival rates:* >80%.

Non-standard proposed therapies to avoid steroid side-effects: ciclosporin, budesonide, tacrolimus, mycophenolate mofetil, ursodeoxycholic acid, methotrexate, cyclophosphamide, mercaptopurine, and free radical scavengers.[2]

Liver transplantation (p231) is indicated for decompensated cirrhosis, but recurrence may occur. It is effective (actuarial 10yr survival is 75%).

1 Hepatotropic viruses (eg measles, herpesviruses) and some drugs appear to trigger AIH in genetically predisposed individuals exposed to a hepatotoxic *milieu intérieur*. Viral interferon can inactivate cytochrome P-450 enzymes (∴ ↓ metabolism of ex- or endogenous hepatotoxins). Putative examples of exogenous agents: monosodium glutamate (MSG; E621) and aspartame (E951), which, if regularly consumed in excess, may promote formation of salt bridges between amino acids. These compounds then act as autoantigens causing CD4 T-helper cell activation. J Prandota 2003 *Am J Pharm* **10** 51
2 J Medina 2003 *Aliment Pharmacol Ther* **17** 1

Liver tumours

The commonest liver tumours are secondary (metastatic) tumours eg from breast, bronchus, or the gastrointestinal tract. Primary hepatic tumours are much less common and may be benign or malignant.

Symptoms Fever, malaise, anorexia, weight↓, RUQ pain (∵ liver capsule stretch). Jaundice is late (except with cholangiocarcinoma). Benign tumours are often asymptomatic. Tumours may rupture causing intraperitoneal haemorrhage.

Signs Hepatomegaly (smooth, or hard and irregular, eg metastases, cirrhosis, HCC). Look for signs of chronic liver disease (p53) and evidence of decompensation (jaundice, ascites). Feel for an abdominal mass. Listen for an arterial bruit over the liver (HCC).

Tests *Blood:* FBC, clotting, LFT, hepatitis serology, α-fetoprotein (↑ in 80% of HCC). *Imaging:* Ultrasound or CT to identify lesions and guide diagnostic biopsies. MRI is better for distinguishing benign from malignant lesions. ERCP (p229) and biopsy should be performed for suspected cholangiocarcinoma.

Biopsy under ultrasound or CT guidance may achieve a histological diagnosis; exercise care if potentially resectable, as seeding along biopsy tract may occur.

Other investigations for metastases (eg CXR, mammography, endoscopy, colonoscopy, CT, marrow biopsy) are tailored according to the suspected primary.

Liver metastases signify advanced disease. Treatment and prognosis vary with the type and extent of primary tumour. Chemotherapy may be effective (eg for lymphomas, germ cell tumours). Small, solitary metastases may be amenable to resection. In most, treatment is palliative. Prognosis: <6 months.

Hepatocellular carcinoma (HCC) A malignant tumour of hepatocytes, accounting for 90% of primary liver cancers. Rare in the West (2–3% of cancers), it is common in China and sub-Saharan Africa (40% of cancers).

Causes: Viral hepatitis (persistent HCV or HBV, especially if $>2.3 \times 10^4$ virions/mL)[1]; cirrhosis (alcohol, haemochromatosis, PBC); aflatoxin; parasites (*Clonorchis sinensis*); drugs (anabolic & contraceptive steroids).

Management: Surgical resection of solitary tumours <3cm diameter gives a 3yr survival rate of 59% (baseline 3-yr survival rate is 13%). Chemotherapy, selective tumour embolization, and transplantation are disappointing.

Prognosis: Often <6 months. 95% 5yr mortality. Fibrolamellar HCC, which occurs in children/young adults, has a better prognosis (60% 5yr survival).

Prevention is the key. ►Ensure HBV vaccination (see BOX) ►Do not reuse needles ►Reduce exposure to aflatoxins (anti-humidity measures such as sundrying to ↓spread of this common fungal contaminant in stored maize); this is especially important for those who harbour HBV (risk is highly synergistic).[2]

Cholangiocarcinoma (=Biliary tree malignancy; ~10% of liver primaries.) *Causes:* Flukes (*Clonorchis*, p618) in the East; PSC (p238); congenital biliary cysts; biliary–enteric drainage surgery;⁷¹ N-nitroso toxins.⁷²

The patient: Fever, abdominal pain (±ascites), malaise, bilirubin↑; alk phos↑↑.

Pathology: Usually slow-growing. Most are distal extrahepatic or perihilar.⁷³

Management: 70% are non-resectable.⁷⁴ Of those that are, 76% recur. *Surgery:* eg major hepatectomy + extrahepatic bile duct excision + caudate lobe resection. *Post-op problems:* liver failure (15%), bile leak (17%), GI bleeding (6%); wound infection (6.5%).⁷⁵ *Palliative stenting* of an obstructed extrahepatic biliary tree, percutaneously or via ERCP (p229), improves quality of life. *Prognosis:* ~5 months.

Benign tumours *Haemangiomas* are the commonest benign liver tumours. They are often an incidental finding on ultrasound or CT scan and do not require treatment. Biopsy should be avoided! *Adenomas* are common. *Causes:* anabolic steroids, the Pill; pregnancy. Only treat if symptomatic.

1 Tang B 2004 *J Med Virol* **72** 35 (2.3 × 10⁴ virions/mL by PCR is a low level, so almost all are at risk).
2 Hill A 2003 *BMJ* **i** 995. Aflatoxin binds fatally to guanine in DNA. Genetic crop manipulation may help.

Primary liver tumours

Malignant	Benign
HCC	Cysts
Cholangiocarcinoma	Haemangioma
Angiosarcoma	Adenoma
Hepatoblastoma	Focal nodular hyperplasia
Fibrosarcoma	Fibroma
Leiomyosarcoma	Leiomyoma

Origin of secondary liver tumours

Common in males	Common in females	Less common (either sex)
Stomach	Breast	Pancreas
Lung	Colon	Leukaemia
Colon	Stomach	Lymphoma
	Uterus	Carcinoid tumours

Preventing of hepatitis B, hepatitis B-associated cirrhosis, chronic hepatitis, and hepatic neoplasia

Use hepatitis B vaccine, Engerix B®, 1mL into deltoid; repeat at 1 & 6 months (child: 0.5mL × 3 into the anterolateral thigh). *Indications:* Everyone (WHO advice, even in areas of 'low' endemicity). This strategy is expensive, but not as expensive as trying to rely on the ultimately unsuccessful strategy of vaccinating at-risk groups—health workers (eg GPs, dentists, nurses, etc.), IV drug users, sexual adventurers[1] (homo- or heterosexual), those on haemodialysis, and the sexual partners of known hepatitis B_e antigen+ve carriers. The immunocompromised and others may need further doses. Serology helps time boosters and finds poor or non-responders (correlates with older age, smoking, and ♂ sex). ►*Know your own antibody level!*

Anti-HBs   *Actions and comments:* (UK advice: USA advice is different)

>1000iu/L   Good level of immunity; retest in ~4yrs.

100–1000   Good level of immunity; if level approaches 100, retest in 1yr.

<100   Inadequate; give booster dose and retest.

<10   Non-responder; give booster and retest; if <10, get consent to check hepatitis B status: HBsAg +ve means chronic infection; anti-HB core +ve represents past infection and immunity.

NB: Protective immunity begins about 6wks after the 1st immunizing dose, so it is inappropriate if exposure is recent; here, specific anti-hepatitis B immunoglobulin is the best option if not already immunized.

---

1 Male prostitutes and immigrant prostitutes are new high-risk groups—Huo T 2004 *J Med Virol* **72** 45

Ulcerative colitis (UC)

UC is a relapsing and remitting inflammatory disorder of the colonic mucosa. It may affect just the rectum (proctitis) or extend proximally to involve part or all of the colon (pancolitis). It 'never' spreads proximally to the ileocaecal valve (except for 'backwash ileitis'). *Pathology:* Hyperaemic/haemorrhagic granular colonic mucosa ± 'pseudopolyps' formed by inflammation. Punctate ulcers may extend deep into the lamina propria. *Histology:* See *biopsy,* below. *Cause:* Unknown[1]; there is some genetic susceptibility. *Incidence:* 4–11/100,000 in the developed world. Most present age 15–30yrs. UC is twice as common in non-smokers (the opposite is true for Crohn's disease).

Symptoms Gradual onset of diarrhoea ± blood & mucus. Crampy abdominal discomfort is common; bowel frequency is related to severity of disease (see below). Systemic symptoms are common during attacks, eg fever, malaise, anorexia, weight loss. Urgency and tenesmus occur with rectal disease.

Signs May be none: in acute, severe UC: fever, tachycardia, and a tender, distended abdomen. *Extra-intestinal signs* Clubbing, aphthous oral ulcers, erythema nodosum (PLATE 18), pyoderma gangrenosum, conjunctivitis, episcleritis, iritis, large joint arthritis, sacroiliitis, ankylosing spondylitis, fatty liver, PSC (p238), cholangiocarcinoma—and, very rarely, renal stones, osteomalacia, nutritional deficiencies, and systemic amyloidosis. 7/8

Tests *Blood:* FBC, ESR, CRP, U&E, LFT, and blood cultures. *Stool MC+S and CDT* (p246) to exclude infectious diarrhoea (*Cl. difficile, Salmonella, Shigella, Campylobacter, E. coli, amoebae*). *Abdominal x-ray:* No faecal shadows; mucosal thickening/islands; colonic dilatation (toxic dilatation >6cm); perforation. *Sigmoidoscopy:* Inflamed, friable mucosa. *Rectal biopsy:* Inflammatory infiltrate; goblet cell depletion; glandular distortion; mucosal ulcers; crypt abscesses. *Barium enema:* Loss of haustra; granular mucosa; shortened colon. ▶*Never do a barium enema during an acute severe attack.* Colonoscopy shows disease extent, and allows biopsies to be taken.

Assessing severity

	Mild	Moderate	Severe
Motions/day:	<4	4–6	>6
Rectal bleeding:	Small	Moderate	Large
Temperature at 6AM (p38):	apyrexial	37.1–37.8°C	>37.8°C
Pulse rate (beats/min):	<70	70–90	>90
Haemoglobin:	>11g/dL	10.5–11g/dL	<10.5g/dL
ESR:	<30mm/h		>30mm/h

Complications Perforation and bleeding are 2 serious dangers, also:
- 'Toxic' dilatation of colon (mucosal islands, colonic diameter >6cm).
- Colonic cancer: risk ≈ 15% with pancolitis for 20yrs; 2–4-yearly surveillance colonoscopy may be used, but proving this saves lives is difficult. 7/9

Management *Mild UC:* If <4 motions/d and the patient is well, give prednisolone (eg 20mg/d PO or PR) + mesalazine, eg Pentasa® (500mg as a modified-release 500mg tabs, up to 2g/12h) or Asacol MR® (=400mg tabs; in an acute attack 2tabs/8h; maintenance: 1 tab/8h). 8/0 This may be combined with twice-daily steroid foams (Colifoam®) PR, or prednisolone 20mg retention enemas (Predsol®). If symptoms improve, ↓steroids gradually. If no improvement after 2wks, treat as moderate UC.

Moderate UC: If 4–6 motions/d, but otherwise well, give oral prednisolone 40mg/d for 1wk, then 30mg/d for 1wk, then 20mg for 4 more weeks + sulfasalazine 1g/12h PO + twice-daily steroid enemas.[2] If improving, ↓steroids gradually. If no improvement after 2wks, treat as a severe UC.

---

1 UC & Crohn's *may* involve adhesin-expressing strains of *E. coli* capable of inducing interleukin-8 production and transepithelial migration of WBCs—see Betis F 2003 *Infect Immun* **71** 1774 & *OTM* 2.613
2 Budesonide (Entocort) enemas, 1 nocte, may have fewer SEs ∴ ↓suppression of plasma cortisol. [@7696452]

Severe UC: If systemically unwell and passing >6 motions daily, admit for:
- Nil by mouth and IV hydration (eg 1L of 0.9% saline + 2L dextrose-saline/24h, + 20mmol K⁺/L; less if elderly).
- Hydrocortisone 100mg/6h IV.
- Rectal steroids, eg hydrocortisone 100mg in 100mL 0.9% saline/12h PR.
- Monitor T°, pulse, and BP—and record stool frequency/character.
- Twice-daily exam: document distension, bowel sounds and tenderness.
- Daily FBC, ESR, CRP, U&E ± abdominal x-ray.
- Consider the need for blood transfusion (if Hb < 10g/dL) and parenteral nutrition (if severely malnourished). Give IM vitamins (p254).
- If improving in 5d, transfer to oral prednisolone (40mg/24h) with a 5-ASA (below, eg sulfasalazine 1g/12h) to maintain remission. Sulfasalazine is a combination of 5-aminosalicylic acid (5-ASA) and sulfapyridine (which carries the 5-ASA to the colon).

Topical therapies: Proctitis may respond to *suppositories* (prednisolone 5mg or mesalazine, eg Asacol® 250mg/8h PR or Pentasa® 1g at bedtime).

- Procto-sigmoiditis may respond to *foams* (20mg Predfoam®/12–24h or 5-ASA, eg Asacol® 1g/d PR); disposable applicators aid accurate delivery.
- *Retention enemas* (eg 20mg Predsol®) may be needed in left-sided colitis.

Meta-analyses favour topical 5-ASAs over topical steroids.

Indications for surgery: Typically perforation or massive haemorrhage—or:
- 'Toxic' dilatation of colon (mucosal islands, colonic diameter >6cm).
- Failure to respond to drugs. 85% of those with stool frequency >8/d (or stool frequency 3–8/d and CRP >45) on day 3 will need colectomy. *Procedures:* Proctocolectomy + terminal ileostomy (it may be possible to retain the ileocecal valve, and hence reduce liquid loss);[1] colectomy with later ileo-anal pouch. Total surgical mortality: 2–7%; with perforation, 50%.

Novel therapies: Ciclosporin (=cyclosporin) can benefit patients with steroid refractory UC, although there are reservations about its long-term efficacy. Typical dose: 2–4mg/kg IV. SE: eg nephrotoxicity; K⁺↑; BP↑ (do U&E, LFT and BP often; stop if raised and get expert help). A small trial showed *tacrolimus* may be superior to ciclosporin (=cyclosporin) in maintaining remission. A monoclonal anti-TNF antibody, *infliximab* (p247) may give rapid control and tissue healing in some inflammatory bowel diseases, but randomized trials in UC do not support its use.

Maintaining remission All 5-ASAs (sulfasalazine, mesalazine, and olsalazine) ↓relapse rate from 80% to 20% at 1yr. Maintenance is continued for life. *Sulfasalazine* (1g/12h PO) remains 1st-line if a cheap drug is essential. SEs relate to sulfapyridine intolerance—headache, nausea, anorexia, and malaise. Other allergic/toxic SEs: fever, rash, haemolysis, hepatitis, pancreatitis, paradoxical worsening of colitis, and reversible oligospemia. Monitor FBC. Newer *5-ASAs* deliver the active ingredient (sulfasalazine) but minimize SEs (dyspepsia, nausea ± headache can occur; olsalazine may cause secretory diarrhoea). Rare hypersensitivity reactions: worsening colitis, pancreatitis, pericarditis, nephritis. Examples: *mesalazine* (400–500mg/8h PO) or *olsalazine* (500mg/12h PO)—indicated in sulfasalazine intolerance and young men (less effect on sperm).

Azathioprine (2–2.5mg/kg/d PO) is indicated as a steroid-sparing agent in those with steroid side-effects or those who relapse quickly when steroids are reduced. Treatment should be continued for several months, during which FBC should be monitored every 4–6wks.

1 Nio Y 2004 *Dig Surg.* [@14639037]

Crohn's disease

Crohn's disease is a chronic inflammatory GI disease characterized by trans-mural granulomatous inflammation. It may affect any part of the gut, but favours the terminal ileum and proximal colon. Unlike UC, there is unaffected bowel between areas of active disease (skip lesions).

Cause: Unknown.[1] Mutations of the NOD2/CARD15 gene ↑risk. *Prevalence:* 100/100,000. Smoking ↑risk 3–4-fold. *Associations:* High sugar, low-fibre diet; infective agents (anaerobes); mucins; altered cell-mediated immunity.

Symptoms & signs Diarrhoea, abdominal pain, and weight loss are common. Fever, malaise, anorexia occur with active disease. Look for: Aphthous ulceration; abdominal tenderness; right iliac fossa mass; perianal abscesses/fistulae/skin tags; anal/rectal strictures.

Extra-intestinal signs: Clubbing, erythema nodosum (PLATE 18), pyoderma gangrenosum, conjunctivitis, episcleritis, iritis, large joint arthritis, sacroiliitis, ankylosing spondylitis, fatty liver, primary sclerosing cholangitis, cholangio-carcinoma (rare), renal stones, osteo-malacia, malnutrition, amyloidosis.

Complications Small intestinal obstruction; toxic dilatation (colonic diame-ter >6cm); abscess formation (abdominal, pelvic, or ischiorectal); fistulae, eg colo-vesical (bladder), colo-vaginal, perianal, entero-cutaneous; perforation; rectal haemorrhage; colonic carcinoma.

Tests *Blood:* FBC, ESR, CRP, U&E, LFT, blood culture. Serum iron, B₁₂, and red cell folate if anaemia. *Markers of activity:* Hb↓; ↑ESR; ↑CRP; ↑WCC; ↓albumin.
Stool microscopy/culture & Clostridium difficile toxin (CDT) to exclude infectious diarrhoea (*Cl. difficile, Salmonella, Shigella, Campylobacter, E. coli*).

Sigmoidoscopy and rectal biopsy should be performed even when the mucosa is macroscopically normal (20% have microscopic granulomas).

Small bowel enema: To detect ileal disease (strictures, proximal dilatation, inflammatory mass or fistula). *Barium enema:* This may show 'cobblestoning', 'rose thorn' ulcers, colonic strictures with rectal sparing.

Colonoscopy is indicated if barium enema is equivocal to assess the extent of disease and enable multiple biopsies to be taken.

Management Severity is harder to assess than in UC. Severe symptoms (fever; pulse↑; ↑ESR; ↑CRP; ↑WCC; ↓albumin) merit admission.

Mild attacks: Patients are symptomatic but systemically well. Prednisolone 30mg/d PO for 1wk, then 20mg/d for 1 month. See in clinic every 2–4wks. If symptoms resolve, reduce steroids by 5mg every 2–4wks. Stop steroids only when all parameters have returned to normal.

Severe attacks: Admit for IV steroids, nil by mouth, and IV hydration (eg 1L 0.9% saline + 2L dextrose-saline/24h, + 20mmol K⁺/L, less if elderly). Then:
- Hydrocortisone 100mg/6h IV.
- Treat rectal disease, if present, with rectal steroids twice daily (hydrocorti-sone 100mg in 100mL 0.9% saline/12h PR).
- Metronidazole 400mg/8h PO, or 500mg/8h IV, helps, especially in perianal disease or superadded infection. SE: alcohol intolerance; irreversible neu-ropathy.
- Monitor T°, pulse, BP, and record stool frequency/character.
- Physical examination twice daily.
- Daily FBC, ESR, CRP, U&E, and plain abdominal x-ray.
- Consider need for transfusion (if Hb <10g/dL) and parenteral nutrition.
- If improving after 5d, transfer on to oral prednisolone (40mg/24h).
- If no response (or deterioration) during IV therapy, seek surgical advice.

---

1 *Environmental agents:* Gatti A 2004 *Biomaterials* **25** 385. *Genetics:* colonic involvement is associated with increased CARD15 gene expression in macrophages and intestinal epithelial cells. Berrebi D 2003 *Gut* **52** 840. E. coli adhesins (p244) may also be important.

Additional therapies in Crohn's disease

Azathioprine (2–2.5mg/kg/d PO) is a steroid-sparing agent, eg for those with steroid side-effects or if relapsing rapidly after dose reduction. It takes 6–10wks to work.

Sulfasalazine: 1g/12h PO and other 5-ASAs (p245) are minimally helpful in active Crohn's. They may be reserved for maintenance, eg in preventing the common problem of relapse after resection (Asacol® 2 × 400mg/8h PO has prevented some recurrence, particularly if this dose produces high mucosal levels of 5-ASA).⁸⁶

Elemental diets: (eg E028®)⁸⁷ are as good as steroids in active disease, but are unpalatable and relapse is more common.

Methotrexate: A Cochrane review finds good evidence from a single large randomized trial on which to recommend 25mg IM weekly for induction of remission and complete withdrawal from steroids in patients with refractory Crohn's disease. NNT ≈ 5. There is no evidence on lower doses.[1]

Surgery: 50–80% of patients need ≥1 operation in their life. *Indications for surgery:* Usually failure to respond to drugs—or:
• Intestinal obstruction from strictures
• Intestinal perforation
• Local complications (fistulae, abscesses).

Surgery is never curative: the aim is limited resection of the worst areas. Bypass and pouch surgery is *not* done in Crohn's (∴ ↑risk of recurrence).

Infliximab: This is an anti-tumour necrosis factor monoclonal antibody. It can ↓ Crohn's disease activity. It activates complement, and causes cytotoxicity to CD4+ T-cells, so clearing cells driving the immune response. A single dose of infliximab is given by IVI over 2h on a day ward under expert guidance. NNT ≈ 3–4 (p30). Response may be short-lived. It may be repeated at 8wks. *CI:* Sepsis, LFT↑ >3-fold above top end of normal, concurrent ciclosporin (=cyclosporin) or tacrolimus. *SE:* Rash; ?↑ risk of malignancy.⁸⁸

Cost per qaly: (see p14) £6700 (higher in fistulizing Crohn's).⁸⁹

---

1 Feagan B 2003 *Cochrane Database Syst Rev* CD003459. Adverse effects were not severe.

Irritable bowel syndrome (IBS)

IBS is used to describe a heterogeneous group of abdominal symptoms for which no organic cause can be found. Most are probably due to disorders of intestinal motility.

Clinical features Patients are usually 20–40yrs old and females are more frequently affected than males. *Symptoms:* Central or lower abdominal pain (relieved by defecation); abdominal bloating; altered bowel habit (constipation alternating with diarrhoea); tenesmus; mucus PR. Less commonly: nausea, dyspareunia; pain in the back, thigh, or chest; urinary frequency; depression. Symptoms are chronic (>6 months), and exacerbated by stress, menstruation, or gastroenteritis. *Signs:* Examination is often unremarkable although generalized abdominal tenderness is common. Insufflation of air during sigmoidoscopy may reproduce the pain.

Markers of organic disease: (ie it may well not be IBS) Age >40yrs; history <6 months; anorexia; weight↓; waking at night with pain/diarrhoea; mouth ulcers; rectal bleeding; abnormal investigations. Management: see BOX.

Carcinoma of the pancreas

Epidemiology: Accounts for ≤2% of all malignancy; ~6500 deaths/yr (UK). Incidence is rising (UK). *Typical patient:* Male >60yrs old. *Risk factors:* Smoking, alcohol, diabetes. *Pathology:* Most are ductal adenocarcinoma (metastasize early; present late). 60% arise in the pancreas head, 15% the tail, and 25% in the body. A minority arise from the Ampulla of Vater (ampullary tumour) or pancreatic islet cells (insulinoma, gastrinoma, glucagonomas, somatostatinomas, VIPomas); these have a better prognosis.

Symptoms & signs Tumours in the head of the pancreas present with painless obstructive jaundice. Tumours in the body and tail present with epigastric pain, which typically radiates to the back and may be relieved by sitting forward. Either may cause anorexia, weight loss, diabetes or acute pancreatitis. Rarer features: thrombophlebitis migrans; marantic endocarditis; hypercalcaemia; Cushing's syndrome; ascites (peritoneal metastases); portal hypertension (splenic vein thrombosis); nephrotic syndrome (renal vein metastases). *Signs:* Jaundice + palpable gall bladder (Courvoisier's 'law': painless jaundice + palpable GB implies a diagnosis other than gallstones); epigastric mass; hepatomegaly; splenomegaly; lymphadenopathy; ascites.

Tests *Blood:* Cholestatic jaundice. CA 19–9 (p704) is ↑ in pancreatic cancer but is non-specific. *Imaging:* Ultrasound or CT scan show a pancreatic mass ± dilated biliary tree ± hepatic metastases. Staging CT or endoscopic ultrasound before stent placement in potential surgical candidates. ERCP (p229) delineates the biliary tree anatomy and localizes the site of obstruction. MRI is helpful: sensitivity 84%, specificity 97% vs 70% and 94% for ERCP (p229). *Histology:* Obtainable by ultrasound- or CT-guided percutaneous biopsy.

Treatment Most ductal carcinomas present with metastatic disease; <10% are suitable for radical surgery. *Surgery:* Consider pancreatoduodenectomy (Whipple's, p251) if fit and the tumour <3cm with no metastases. Post-op morbidity is high (mortality <5% in experienced hands). *Post-op chemotherapy* delays disease progression.[1] *Palliation of jaundice:* Endoscopic (ERCP, p229) or percutaneous stent insertion. Rarely, palliative bypass surgery is indicated for duodenal obstruction or unsuccessful ERCP. *Pain relief:* Disabling pain may be relieved by opiates or radiotherapy. Coeliac plexus infiltration with alcohol may be done at the time of palliative surgery or percutaneously.

Prognosis Dismal. Mean survival <6 months. 5yr survival rate: <2%. Overall 5yr survival after Whipples' procedure 5–14%. Patients with the rarer ampullary or islet cell tumours have a much better prognosis.

1 J Dunn *Chirurg* 2003 **74** 191. Older studies used 5-FU 500mg/m², doxorubicin 40mg/m², mitomycin C 6mg/m² every 3wks for 6 cycles. [@8471327]

Management of IBS

The 1st step is to exclude other diagnoses, so:

- If young, with a classic history, FBC, ESR, LFT, coeliac serology (p252), and urinalysis ± sigmoidoscopy with rectal biopsy is sufficient investigation.
- If the patient is aged ≥45yrs or has *any* marker or organic disease, request colonoscopy (barium enema if unavailable).
- If diarrhoea is prominent, do: LFT; stool culture; B12/folate; antiendomysial ab (p252); TSH; consider referral ± ba follow-through ± rectal biopsy.
- Further investigation should be guided by symptoms and include:

  1 Upper GI endoscopy (dyspepsia, reflux)
  2 Duodenal biopsy (coeliac disease), eg if aniendomysial antibodies +ve.
  3 Giardia tests p606 (it often triggers IBS; anti-parasitic R may not help)[92]
  4 Small bowel radiology (Crohn's disease)
  5 ERCP (p229, chronic pancreatitis)
  6 Transit studies and anorectal physiological studies—rarely used.

Refer if: (1) equivocal diagnosis (2) changing symptoms in 'known IBS' (3) *to surgeon* if rectal mucosal prolapse (4) *to dietitian* if food intolerances (5) *to psychiatrists* if stress/depression is pronounced (6) *to gynaecologist* if cyclical pain (endometriosis, OHCS p52) or if difficult pelvic infection, p588.

Treatment Rarely 100% successful so be pragmatic. Careful explanation and reassurance are vital. *Make a good relationship with your patient.*

1 *Food intolerance:* Try exclusion diets (difficult; may lead to obsessions).
2 *Constipation:* See p220; ↑Fibre intake gradually (can paradoxically worsen flatulence/bloating). Fybogel® (ispaghula) or Celevac® (methylcellulose; start with 3–6 tabs night and morning with >300mL fluid) have non-fermentable fibre—and are better than lactulose which ferments (↑gas production is hard to distinguish from bloating).[93]
3 *Diarrhoea:* Bulking agent ± loperamide 2mg after each loose stool; max 16mg/d; SE: Colic, nausea, dizziness, constipation, bloating, ileus.
4 *Colic and bloating:* Antispasmodics may help (eg mebeverine 135mg/8h PO; alverine citrate 60–120mg/8h PO; dicycloverine 10–20mg/8h PO).
5 *Dyspeptic symptoms:* May respond to metoclopramide or antacids.
6 *Psychological R:* Emphasize positive aspects and prognosis: in 50% symptoms go or improve after 1yr; <5% worsen. Symptoms are still troublesome in the rest at 5yrs. *Tricyclic antidepressants* (low dose) are often helpful, eg amitriptyline 10–50mg at night (SE: constipation, dry mouth, etc., OHCS p340). *Psychotherapy* (OHCS p368), *cognitive-behavioural therapy* (OHCS p370), and *gut-focused hypnotherapy*[1] all have roles. Explain that all forms of stress (sexual, physical, or verbal abuse) perpetuate IBS.

The future: Much interest is being expressed in modulating the 'brain–gut' axis by neurotransmitter manipulation. *Visceral hypersensitivity:* Those with IBS have lower visceral pain thresholds than others, and since 5HT antagonists increase pain tolerance, highly selective 5HT₃-receptor antagonists (eg alosetron) are under trial.[94] *Meta-analyses:* Alosetron 1mg/12h PO can ↓symptoms in non-constipated IBS female patients. SE: 25% get constipated. Some on alosetron have developed ischaemic colitis—which could represent a serious side-effect which is why alosetron has had a chequered history. It is not available in the UK. (Efficacy of alosetron is even more unclear in males.)[95]

---

1 12wks of hypnosis helps abnormal sensory perception: 2003 *Aliment Pharmacol Ther* **17** 635. ► Do not think of hypnosis as dubious; it is the neatest way to influence the brain-gut axis, reducing doctor dependency and stopping patients from being patients (passive recipients of suffering). Benefits appear to last ≥5yrs. Gonsalkorale WM *Gut* 2003 **52** 1623

Nutritional disorders Images: www2.msstate.edu/~shbyrd/Disorders.html

Scurvy This is due to lack of vitamin C in the diet. ▶*Is the patient poor, pregnant, or on an odd diet? Signs:* (1) Listlessness, anorexia, cachexia (p66). (2) Gingivitis, loose teeth, and foul-smelling breath (halitosis). (3) Bleeding from gums, nose, hair follicles, or into joints, bladder, gut.
Diagnosis: No test is completely satisfactory. WBC ascorbic acid↓.
Treatment: Dietary education; ascorbic acid 250mg/24h PO.

Beriberi There is heart failure with general oedema (wet beriberi) or neuropathies (dry beriberi) due to lack of vitamin B_1 (thiamine). For treatment and diagnostic tests, see Wernicke's encephalopathy (p738).

Pellagra (Lack of nicotinic acid). *Classical triad:* diarrhoea, dementia, dermatitis (± neuropathy, depression, insomnia, tremor, rigidity, ataxia, fits). It may occur in carcinoid syndrome and anti-TB treatment. It is endemic in China and Africa. *Treatment:* Education, electrolyte replacement, nicotinamide 100mg/4h PO (OTM 1.1045). Look for other vitamin deficiencies.

Xerophthalmia This vitamin A deficiency is a major cause of blindness in the Tropics. Conjunctivae become dry and develop oval or triangular spots (Bitôt's spots). Corneas become cloudy and soft. See *OHCS* p512. Give vitamin A 200,000 iu stat PO, repeat in 24h and a week later (halve dose if <1yr old; quarter if <6 months old); get special help if pregnant; vitamin A embryopathy must be avoided. Re-educate, and monitor diet.

Lathyrism This is an acute spastic paralysis occurring in lathyrus pea eaters (due to a toxin). *Typical patient:* 14yr old African ♂. *Treatment:* Unsatisfactory.

Carcinoid tumours

A diverse group of tumours of argentaffin cell origin, by definition capable of producing 5HT. Common site: appendix (25%) or rectum. They also occur elsewhere in the GI tract, ovary, testis, and bronchi. Tumours may be benign but 80% >2cm across will metastasize. *Symptoms & signs:* Initially few. GI tumours can cause appendicitis, intussusception, or obstruction. Hepatic metastases may cause RUQ pain. Carcinoid tumours may secrete ACTH (∴ Cushing's syndrome; 10% are part of MEN-1 syndrome (p309) and 10% occur with other neuroendocrine tumours. Carcinoid *syndrome* occurs in 10%.

Carcinoid syndrome usually implies hepatic involvement. *Signs:* Paroxysmal flushing (± migrating weals), D&V, abdominal pain, ± CCF (tricuspid incompetence and pulmonary stenosis). *CNS effects:* Many, eg *enhanced* ability to learn new stimulus–response associations. *Carcinoid crisis:* When a tumour outgrows its blood supply, mediators flood out; this is life threatening.

Diagnosis 24h urine 5-hydroxyindoleacetic acid↑ (5HIAA, a 5HT metabolite; levels change with drugs and diet: discuss with lab). If liver metastases are not found, try to find the primary (CXR; chest/pelvis MRI/CT), as curative resection is possible. *New tests:* Plasma chromogranin A (reflects tumour mass); ^{111}Indium octreotide scintigraphy (octreoscan); positron emission tomography (PET).

Treatment *Carcinoid syndrome:* Octreotide (somatostatin analogue) blocks release of tumour mediators and counters peripheral effects. Effects lessen over time. Other options: loperamide or cyproheptadine for diarrhoea; ketanserin (experimental $5HT_2$ antagonist) for flushing; interferon-α. *Tumour therapy:* Surgical debulking (eg enucleating) or embolization of hepatic metastases can ↓symptoms. These must be done with octreotide cover to avoid precipitating a massive carcinoid crisis. Crisis is treated with high-dose octreotide and careful management of fluid balance (central line needed). *Median survival:* 5–8yrs; 38 months if metastases are present, but may be *much* longer (~20 yrs); so beware of giving up too easily, even if metastases are present.

Food mountains, the pellagra paradox, and the sorrow that weeping cannot symbolize[1]

'The sweet smell is a great sorrow on the land. Men who can graft the trees and make the seed fertile and big can find no way to let the hungry people eat their produce ... The works of the roots of the vines, of the trees, must be destroyed to keep up the price ...

There is a crime here that goes beyond denunciation. There is a sorrow here that weeping cannot symbolize. There is a failure here that topples all our success. The fertile earth, the straight tree rows, the sturdy trunks, and the ripe fruit. And children dying of pellagra must die because a profit cannot be taken from an orange. And coroners must fill in the certificates—died of malnutrition—because the food must rot, must be forced to rot.

The people come with nets to fish for potatoes in the river, and the guards hold them back; they come in rattling cars to get the dumped oranges, but the kerosene is sprayed. And they stand still and watch the potatoes float by, listen to the screaming pigs being killed in a ditch and covered with quicklime, watch the mountains of oranges slop down to a putrefying ooze; and in the eyes of the people there is a failure; and in the eyes of the hungry there is a growing wrath. In the souls of the people the grapes of wrath are filling and growing heavy, growing heavy for the vintage.'

How do John Steinbeck's grapes grow in our 21st century soil? Too well; a double harvest, it turns out, as not only is much of the world starving, amid plenty (for those who can pay) but there is a new 'sorrow in our land that weeping cannot symbolize': pathological self-denial—voluntary *self-starvation*, again amid plenty, in pursuit of the body-beautiful according to images laid down by media gods. If gastroenterologists had one wish it might not be the ending of all their diseases, but that human-kind stand in a right-relationship with Steinbeck's fertile earth, his straight trees, his sturdy trunks, and his ripe fruit.

Whipple's procedure

(a) Areas of reflection of different parts

(b) Post-operation

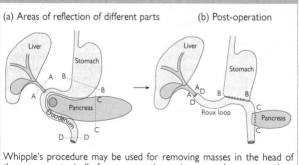

Whipple's procedure may be used for removing masses in the head of the pancreas—typically from pancreatic carcinoma, or less commonly, a carcinoid tumour. [102]

---

1 J Steinbeck *The Grapes of Wrath*, ch 25 http://www.trecc.com/tom/r01.htm

Gastrointestinal malabsorption

Symptoms Diarrhoea; ↓weight; steatorrhoea (fatty stools, hard to flush away). *Deficiency signs:* Anaemia (↓Fe, B₁₂, folate); bleeding (↓vit K); oedema (↓protein). *Common UK causes:* Coeliac disease, Crohn's, chronic pancreatitis. *Others:* ↓Bile: 1° biliary cirrhosis; ileal resection; biliary obstruction; colestyramine. *Pancreatic insufficiency:* Chronic pancreatitis; pancreas cancer; cystic fibrosis. *Small bowel mucosa:* Coeliac and Whipple's diseases (p740); tropical sprue; radiation enteritis; small bowel resection; brush border enzyme deficiencies (eg lactase insufficiency); drugs (metformin, neomycin, alcohol); amyloid (p668). *Bacterial overgrowth:* Spontaneous (especially in elderly); in jejunal diverticula; post-op blind loops. Try metronidazole 400mg/8h PO or oxytetracycline 250mg/8h. *Infection:* Giardiasis; diphyllobothriasis (B₁₂ malabsorption); strongyloidiasis. *Intestinal hurry:* Post-gastrectomy dumping; post-vagotomy; gastrojejunostomy.

Tests FBC (MCV↓, macrocytosis); ↓Ca²⁺(↓vit D due to fat malabsorption); ↓Fe; ↓folate; ↑PT (↓vitamin K); coeliac serology (below). *Stool:* Sudan stain for fat globules; stool microscopy for infestation. *Ba follow-through:* Diverticula; Crohn's; radiation enteritis. *Breath hydrogen analysis:* (bacterial overgrowth). Take samples of end-expired air; give glucose; take more samples at ½h intervals. If there is overgrowth there is ↑exhaled hydrogen. *Small bowel biopsy:* Use endoscopy. *ERCP* (p229) biliary obstruction; chronic pancreatitis.

Tropical malabsorption *Typical causes:* Giardia intestinalis, Cryptosporidium parvum, Isospora belli, Cyclospora cayetanensis, and the microsporidia. *Tropical sprue:* Villous atrophy and malabsorption occurring in the Far and Middle East and Caribbean (it is rarer in Africa[103])—the cause is unknown. Tetracycline 250mg/6h PO + folic acid 15mg/24h PO + optimum nutrition may help. [104]

Coeliac disease is a T-cell mediated autoimmune disease of the small bowel in which prolamin (alcohol-soluble proteins in wheat, barley, rye ± oats) intolerance causes villous atrophy and malabsorption.[1] *Associations:* HLA DQ2 in 95%; the rest are DQ8; autoimmune disease; dermatitis herpetiformis. *Presentation:* Steatorrhoea/offensive stools; other abdominal pain; bloating; nausea/vomiting; aphthous ulcers; angular stomatitis; weight↓; fatigue; weakness; iron-deficiency anaemia; osteomalacia; poor growth (children). One-third are asymptomatic. Occurs at any age (peaks in infancy and 50–60yrs, ♀:♂ > 1). *Diagnosis:* Antibodies: (α-gliadin, transglutaminase, anti-endomysial—an IgA antibody; 95% specific, unless the patient is IgA-deficient). Duodenal biopsy done at endoscopy (p228—as good as jejunal biopsy if ≥4 taken): villous atrophy, reversing on gluten-free diet (along with ↓symptoms and antibodies). *Treatment:* Lifelong gluten-free diet (ie no prolamins). Rice, maize, soya, potatoes, oats (≤50g/d), and sugar are OK. Gluten-free biscuits, flour, bread, & pasta are prescribable. Verify diet by endomysial antibody tests. *Complications:* Anaemia; 2° lactose-intolerance; GI T-cell lymphoma (rare; suspect if worsening despite diet); malignancy (gastric, oesophageal, bladder, breast, brain); myopathies; neuropathies; hyposplenism; osteoporosis.

Chronic pancreatitis Epigastric pain 'bores' through to back (eg relieved by sitting forward or hot water bottles on epigastrium/back: look for *erythema ab igne*'s dusky greyness here); bloating; steatorrhoea; ↓weight; diabetes. *Causes:* Alcohol; rarely: familial; cystic fibrosis; haemochromatosis; pancreatic duct obstruction (stones or pancreatic cancer); hyperparathyroidism. *Tests: Ultrasound* (dilated biliary tree; stones); if normal consider CT/ERCP, p229; *plain film:* speckled pancreatic calcification; glucose↑; breath tests (above). [105] *Drugs:* • Give analgesia (± coeliac-plexus block). • Lipase, eg Creon®. • Fat-soluble vitamins (eg Multivite®). *Diet:* Low fat (+ no alcohol) may help. Medium-chain triglycerides (MCT oil®) may be tried (no lipase needed for absorption, but diarrhoea may be worsened). *Surgery:* For unremitting pain; narcotic abuse (beware of this); weight↓: pancreatectomy or pancreaticojejunostomy.

1 Hyphal wall protein 1 (HWP1) of *Candida albicans* could be one trigger. HWP1 has amino acid seq-uences identical to coeliac disease-related α gliadin T-cell epitopes—M Jansen 2003 *Lancet* **361** 2152 (An epitope is a small part of a macromolecule that is recognized by an antibody.)

Alcoholism

An alcoholic is one whose repeated drinking leads to harm in his work or social life. ▶Denial is a leading feature of alcoholism, so be sure to question relatives. Screening tests: MCV↑; gamma-GT↑. (Note that alcohol can do you good in low doses, eg <21U/wk in men, see p208.)

CAGE questions Ever felt you ought to **c**ut down on your drinking? Have people **a**nnoyed you by criticizing your drinking? Ever felt bad or **g**uilty about your drinking? Ever had an **e**ye-opener to steady nerves in the morning? CAGE is quite good at detecting alcohol abuse and dependence (sensitivity, 43–94%; specificity, 70–97%). See also 'TWEAK' questions, p69.

Organs affected by alcohol • The liver: (Normal in 50% of alcoholics.)
Fatty liver: Acute and reversible, but may progress to cirrhosis if drinking continues (also seen in obesity, DM, and with amiodarone). *Cirrhosis* (p232): 5yr survival is 48% if drinking continues (if not, 77%). *Hepatitis:* TPR↑, anorexia, D&V, tender hepatomegaly ± jaundice, bleeding, ascites, WCC↑, INR↓, AST↑, MCV↑, urea↑ (HRS). 80% progress to cirrhosis (hepatic failure in 10%). *Biopsy:* Mallory bodies ± neutrophil infiltrate. R: see BOX.

- **CNS:** Poor memory/cognition: ▶multiple high-potency vitamins IM may reverse it; cortical atrophy; retrobulbar neuropathy; fits; falls; wide-based gait neuropathy; Korsakoff's ± Wernicke's encephalopathy, p728–p738.
- **Gut:** Obesity, diarrhoea; gastric erosions; peptic ulcers; varices (p226); pancreatitis (acute and chronic).
- **Blood:** MCV↑; anaemia from: marrow depression, GI bleeds, alcoholism-associated folate deficiency; haemolysis; sideroblastic anaemia.
- **Heart:** Arrhythmia; BP↑ cardiomyopathy; sudden death in binge drinkers.

Withdrawal signs Pulse↑; BP↓; tremor; fits; hallucinations (*delirium tremens*)—may be visual or tactile, eg of animals crawling all over one.

Alcohol contraindications Driving; hepatitis; cirrhosis; peptic ulcer; drugs (eg antihistamines); carcinoid; pregnancy (fetal alcohol syndrome—IQ ↓, short palpebral fissure, absent filtrum, and small eyes).

Management *Alcohol withdrawal:* Admit; do BP + TPR/4h. Beware BP↓. For the 1st 3d give generous chlordiazepoxide, eg 10–50mg/6h PO, weaning over 7–14d; alternative: diazepam; the once-preferred chlormethiazole (=clormethiazole) readily causes addiction + respiratory depression (it is said●); phenothiazines are problematic too. • Vitamins may be needed (p738).

Prevention (OHCS p454): Alcohol-free beers; low-risk drinking, eg ≤20U/wk if ♂; ≤15U/wk if ♀—there are no absolutes (risk is a continuum; higher limits are controversial). *1U ≈ 9g ethanol ≈1 spirits measure ≈1 glass wine ≈ ½ pint beer.*

Treating established alcoholics may be rewarding, particularly if they really want to change. If so, *group therapy* or self-help (eg 'Alcoholics Anonymous') may be useful. Encourage the will to change. Think about graceful ways of declining a drink, eg 'I'm seeing what it's like to go without for a bit.' Suggest not buying him- or herself a drink when it is his/her turn. Suggest: 'Don't lift your glass to your lips until after the slowest drinker in your group takes a drink. Sip, don't gulp.' Give follow-up and encouragement.

Relapse: 50% will relapse in the months following initiation of treatment: *anxiety, insomnia, and craving* may be intense, and is mitigated by *acamprosate* (p335); CI: pregnancy, severe liver failure, creatinine >120μmol/L; SE: D&V, libido ↑ or ↓; dose example: 666mg/8h PO if >60kg and <65yrs old.[1]

Reducing pleasure that alcohol brings (and ↓craving): *naltrexone* 50mg/24h PO can halve relapse rates. SE: vomiting, drowsiness, dizziness, cramps, arthralgia. CI: liver failure. It is costly. Confer with experts if drugs are to be used.

1 It has also been used in adolescents. Niederhofer H 2003 *Eur Child Adolesc Psychiatry* **12** 144

Patterns of lab tests in alcoholic and other liver disease

	AST Aspartate aminotransferase	ALT Alanine aminotransferase	MCV Mean cell volume
Alcoholic liver disease	↑↑ *(twice as high as ALT)*	↑	↑↑
Hepatitis C (HCV)	↑ or ↔*	↑↑ *(higher than AST)*	↔
Non-alcoholic fatty liver disease	↑	↑↑	↑ or ↔

*In HCV, AST:ALT ratio is typically <1; ratio may reverse if cirrhosis develops.☐₁₀₇ GGT may be ↑↑ in alcoholic liver disease, but is rather non-specific.

Managing alcoholic hepatitis

- Stop alcohol consumption (for withdrawal symptoms, if chlordiazepoxide by the oral route is impossible, try lorazepam IM).
- High-dose B vitamins IV as Pabrinex®—1 pair of ampoules in 50mL 0.9% saline IVI over ½h; see *Data sheet*—have resuscitation equipment to hand.
- Optimize nutrition (35–40kcal/kg/d non-protein energy) + 1.5g/kg/d of protein (use ideal body weight for calculations eg if malnourished). This prevents encephalopathy, sepsis, and some deaths.
- Daily weight; LFT; U&E; INR. If creatinine↑, get help with this HRS, ie renal failure where the underlying pathology is hepatic. Na⁺↓ is common, but water restriction may make matters worse. See p231.
- Culture ascites fluid—appropriate antibiotics in the light of sensitivities.
- Prednisolone 40mg/d for 5d tapered off over 3wks *may* help.◆[1]

1 Perhaps only if encephalopathy is present; see *Drug Ther Bul* 2003 **41** (July) 49

Renal medicine[1]

Contents

Relevant pages in other chapters: Symptoms and signs: Frequency (p72); loin pain (p76); oedema (p78); oliguria (p78); polyuria (p80).

Surgery: Renal and urological malignancies (p498).

Emergencies: Management of acute renal failure: p824.

Also: Vasculitis (p424); polyarteritis nodosa (p425); urinary retention (p496); incontinence (p500); urological cancers (p498); genitourinary TB (p564); immunosuppressives (p674); biochemistry of renal function (p684); electrolyte physiology (p688); sodium (p688 & p690); potassium (p692); calcium (p694); urate and the kidney (p686); osteomalacia (p700); catheters (p746). *In OHCS:* Gynaecological urology (*OHCS* p70); bacteriuria and pyelonephritis in pregnancy (*OHCS* p160); obstetric causes of acute tubular necrosis (*OHCS* p160); chronic renal disease in pregnancy (*OHCS* p160); UTI in children (*OHCS* p188); urethral valves (*OHCS* p220); horseshoe kidney (*OHCS* p220); ectopic kidney (*OHCS* p220); hypospadias (*OHCS* p220); Wilms' nephroblastoma (*OHCS* p220); acute and chronic renal failure in children (*OHCS* p280); nephritis and nephrosis in children (*OHCS* p282); Potter's syndrome (*OHCS* p120).

Web links for calculating creatinine clearance (CrCl) from serum creatinine (SCr), sex, and ideal body weight (IBW; muscle bulk is important). www.globalrph.com/crcl.htm. It is based on the Cockcroft & Gault equation:

$$CrCl \approx (140 - age) \times IBW/(SCr \times 72) \qquad (\times 0.85 \text{ for females}).$$

Ideal body weight in (kg) $\approx$ 50kg + 2.3kg for each inch of height over 5ft. ♀: IBW $\approx$ 45.5kg + 2.3kg for each inch over 5ft. *Units:* SCr (μmol/L)/88.4 = SCr (mg/dL). The above web calculator deals with both units. *Example:* A 20yr old man with a serum creatinine of 200μmol/L might have a CrCl of 80mL/min (100mL/min is normal); in a little old lady the creatinine clearance for a serum creatinine of 200μmol/L might be <15mL/min (and dialysis may be needed).

---

[1] We thank Dr Patrick Carr who is our Specialist Reader for this chapter.

R **enal disease** typically presents with one or more of rather a short list of clinical syndromes—listed from 1 to 7 below. One underlying pathology may have a variety of clinical presentations.

1 *Proteinuria and nephrotic syndrome:* Normal protein excretion is <150mg/d. In certain circumstances, this may rise to ~300mg/d—eg orthostatic proteinuria (related to posture); during fever, or after exercise. *Proteinuria* (excessive protein excretion) is a sign of glomerular or tubular disease. *Nephrotic syndrome* is the triad of proteinuria (>3g/d, see p270), hypoalbuminaemia (albumin <30g/L) and oedema.

2 *Haematuria and nephritic syndrome:* Haematuria (blood in the urine) may arise from anywhere in the renal tract. It may be *macroscopic* (visible to the naked eye), *microscopic*, or detected as *haemoglobinuria* (haemoglobin in the urine). *Nephritic syndrome* comprises haematuria and proteinuria. It is usually associated with hypertension, pulmonary and peripheral oedema, oliguria (urine output <400mL/d), and a rising plasma urea and creatinine. The question of who to refer haematuria patients to (urologist or nephrologist) is answered on p258.

3 *Oliguria and polyuria:* Oliguria is a urine output of <400mL/d. It is a normal response to hot climates and fluid restriction. *Abnormal causes:* renal perfusion↓, renal parenchymal disease, renal tract obstruction. *Polyuria* is the excretion of larger than normal volumes of urine, usually from high fluid intake. Pathological causes include diabetes mellitus, diabetes insipidus (p326), disorders of the renal medulla (resulting in failure to concentrate the urine), and supraventricular tachycardia.

4 *Renal pain and dysuria: Renal pain* is usually a dull constant pain felt in the loin. It is usually due to renal obstruction (look for swelling or tenderness), acute pyelonephritis, acute nephritic syndrome, polycystic kidneys, or renal infarction. *Renal (ureteric) colic* is severe loin pain which waxes and wanes, is often associated with fever and vomiting, and may radiate to the abdomen, groin, or upper thigh. It is usually caused by a renal calculus, clot, or sloughed papilla. Urinary *frequency & dysuria* (pain on passing urine) are symptoms of cystitis.

5 *Acute renal failure (ARF)* is significant decline in renal function occurring over hours or days, detected by a rising urea and creatinine, with or without oliguria. ARF usually occurs secondary to primary circulatory dysfunction (hypotension, hypovolaemia, sepsis) or urinary obstruction. Less commonly it is due to primary renal disease.

6 *Chronic renal failure (CRF)* is defined as the irreversible, substantial, long-standing loss of renal function. It is classified according to glomerular filtration rate (GFR) into 4 categories: mild (30–50mL/min), moderate (10–29mL/min); severe (<10mL/min) and end-stage (<5mL/min). There is poor correlation between symptoms and signs of CRF. Progression may be so insidious that patients attribute symptoms to age or other illnesses. End-stage renal failure is a degree of renal failure that, without renal replacement therapy, would result in death. In the UK, NICE suggests referral to a nephrologist if serum creatinine is >150μmol/L in diabetes and >200 in heart failure.

7 *Silence:* Serious renal failure may not present with any symptoms. This is why we do U&Es before surgery and other major interventions. *Microalbuminuria* is a silent harbinger of serious renal (and cardiovascular risk). It is described on p288. In one study, 30% of those with type 2 diabetes mellitus died within ~5yrs of developing micro-albuminuria.

Urine

Examine *fresh* urine (MSU) whenever you suspect renal disease. **Dipsticks:**

- *Haematuria:* Renal causes: IgA nephropathy (commonish; p268); glomerulonephritis (p268); interstitial nephritis; polycystic kidney; papillary necrosis; medullary sponge kidney; infections (cystitis, pyelonephritis, TB, schistosomiasis); calculi; neoplasia; trauma; vasculitis (p424); vascular malformation. *Extrarenal:* Calculi; infection (cystitis, prostatitis, urethritis); neoplasia (bladder, prostate, urethra); vasculitis; hypertension; sickle-cell disease; trauma; cyclophosphamide. *Coagulation disorders:* Haemophilia etc.; anticoagulants. *Tests:* Urine MC&S, 24h urine collection (protein, creatinine clearance); FBC, ESR, CRP, U&E. *Others:* Clotting, Hb electrophoresis; AXR (renal stones) renal ultrasound, ± renal biopsy. ▶*Management plan:* Usually refer 1st to a urologist, and do ultrasound. Only refer initially to renal physician if risk of urothelial malignancy is low and risk of glomerulonephritis is not negligible (eg <40yrs old, creatinine↑; BP↑; proteinuria; systemic symptoms; family history of renal disease). [?] Not all women with recurrent UTI + haematuria need cystoscopy, but have a good reason *not* to do cystoscopy (Reynard's rule). [?] *False +ve dipstix haematuria:* Free Hb; myoglobin; eating beetroot; porphyria; alkaptonuria; rifampicin, phenindione, phenolphthalein.

- *Proteinuria:* Normal protein excretion is <150mg/d (may rise to 300mg/d in fever, or with exercise). *Renal causes:* UTI; orthostatic proteinuria; glomerulonephritis; haemolytic-uraemic syndrome; SLE; multiple myeloma; amyloidosis. *Extrarenal causes:* fever; exercise; pregnancy; ↑BP; DM; CCF; vaginal mucus; recent ejaculation. *Tests:* BP; urine MC&S; 24h urine collection (protein excretion, creatinine clearance); renal ultrasound, serum complement. If abnormal, consider renal biopsy. *Microalbuminuria:* (Albumin excretion 25–250mg/24h.) *Causes:* DM; ↑BP; SLE; minimal change glomerulonephritis.

- *Other substances—Glucose:* Low renal threshold (eg chronic renal failure); DM; pregnancy; sepsis; renal tubular damage. *Ketones:* Starvation; ketoacidosis. *Leucocytes:* UTI; vaginal discharge. *Nitrites:* UTI; high-protein meal. *Bilirubin:* Obstructive jaundice. *Urobilinogen:* Pre-hepatic jaundice. *Specific gravity:* Normal range: 1.000–1.030 (useful when assessing degree of proteinuria/haematuria). *pH:* Normal range: 4.5–8 (acid–base balance: p682).

Microscopy Put a drop of fresh urine (MSU or suprapubic aspirate) on a microscope slide, cover with a coverslip and examine under low (×100) and high (×400) power for leucocytes, RBCs, bacteria, crystals, and casts. If renal disease is suspected, a centrifuged urine should be examined.

Leucocytes: >10/mm^3 in an unspun urine specimen is abnormal. Causes: cystitis; urethritis; prostatitis; pyelonephritis; TB; renal calculi; glomerulonephritis; appendicitis; [?] interstitial nephritis; analgesic nephropathy; chemical cystitis.

Red cells: >2/mm^3 in unspun urine is abnormal. *Causes:* See haematuria.

Casts are cylindrical bodies formed in the lumen of distal tubules.

Finely granular and hyaline casts (clear, colourless) are found in: normal concentrated urine, fever, after exercise, or with loop diuretics.

Densely granular casts: GN, diabetic nephropathy, amyloid, or interstitial nephritis.

Fatty casts: Moderate to heavy proteinuria. Don't mistake fat globules for RBCs.

Red cell casts are a diagnostic marvel, as they *prove* that haematuria is glomerular, allowing you to start an interesting dialogue with a nephrologist: 'is there vasculitis (p424), glomerulonephritis (GN), or malignant hypertension?'

White cell casts occur in pyelonephritis and proliferative glomerulonephritis.

Epithelial cell casts occur in acute tubular necrosis or glomerulonephritis.

Crystals are common in old or cold urine and may not signify pathology. Cystine crystals are diagnostic of cystinuria. Oxalate crystals in fresh urine may indicate an increased liability to form calculi.

24h urine for Na$^+$, K$^+$, Ca^{2+}, urea, creatinine ± protein excretion. Take blood simultaneously for creatinine to calculate creatinine clearance (p685).

Urine microscopy

CRYSTALS

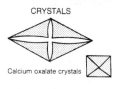

Calcium oxalate crystals

Uric acid crystals

Phosphate crystals

Triple phosphate

Cystine

Tyrosine rods

EPITHELIAL CELLS

Renal tubular epithelial cell

Vaginal squamous epithelial cell

Bladder epithelial cells

Renal papillary epithelial cell

OTHER CELLS

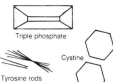

Red blood cells

White (pus) cells (With rods)

Budding yeast

Motile trichomonad

CASTS

Hyaline cast

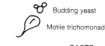

Red cell cast

Granular cast

White cell cast

Finely granular cast

Principle source: M Longmore *An Atlas of Bedside Microscopy* RCGP

259

▶When you find red cells, consider their morphology to understand where in the GU tract they come from. If >10% of RBCs are dysmorphic G1 cells, suspect glomerular bleeding, and look hard for red cell casts. G1 cells have doughnut shapes, target configurations, and membrane protrusions or blebs. Acanthocyturia ≈ RBCs with spicules.
G1 cell images (stained urine cytology): www.uninet.edu/cin2003/conf/nguyen/nguyen.html

Urinary tract imaging

Abdominal x-ray Look at kidneys, path of the ureters, and bladder.
Any abnormal calcification?—related to which of these 3 processes?
1 Calculi (only 80% of stones are visible on plain films: see CT below).
2 Dystrophic calcification, eg in carcinomas or TB (uncommon).
3 Nephrocalcinosis (parenchymal, rare).

Ultrasound (US) is the usual initial image in renal medicine. It shows:
- Renal size—*small* in chronic renal failure, *large* in renal masses, benign cysts,[1] hypertrophy if other kidney missing, polycystic kidney disease, and rarities such as amyloidosis (p668).
- Hydronephrosis, which may indicate renal obstruction or reflux.
- Perinephric collections (trauma, post-renal biopsy).
- Transplanted kidneys (collections, obstruction, perfusion).
- Bladder residual volume.
- Prostate: trans-rectal ultrasound enables US-guided biopsy of focal lesions.
  NB: Prostate size does not correlate with symptoms.

Advantages: Fast; cheap; independent of renal function; no IV contrast or radiation risk. *Disadvantages:* intraluminal masses such as transitional cell carcinomas (TCC) in the upper tracts may not be seen; not a functional study; only suggests obstruction when there is dilatation of the collecting system (~5% of obstructed kidneys have non-dilated systems).

Computer tomography (CT) has revolutionized diagnosis of renal colic. Non-contrast scans are 97% sensitive for calculi, and show many other pathologies. CT has a similar radiation dose to IVU. CT allows detailed characterization of: masses (solid or cystic, contrast enhancement, calcification, local/distant extension, renal vein involvement); renal trauma (2 kidneys, haemorrhage, devascularization, laceration, urine leak); retroperitoneal lesions. CT with IV contrast reveals kidney function.

Intravenous urogram/pyelogram (IVU = IVP) A study for defining anatomy (especially pelvi-calyceal), and for detecting pathology distorting the collecting system. It yields limited functional information. Abdominal films are taken before and after IV contrast, which is filtered by the kidney, reaching the renal tubules at ~1min (nephrogram phase). Later images show contrast in the system (pyelogram), ureters, and bladder. SE: flushing; nausea; rash; contrast nephropathy (caution: if the patient has pre-existing renal failure, DM, or myeloma, check your local policy before requesting a contrast examination).

Retrograde pyelography is good at showing anatomy of the pelvi-calyceal systems and ureters, and detecting pathology such as transitional cell carcinoma (TCC). Contrast is injected via a ureteric catheter.

Percutaneous nephrostomy The renal pelvis is punctured with imaging guidance. Diagnostic images are obtained following contrast injection. A nephrostomy tube may then be placed to allow drainage.

Renal arteriography Still the final arbiter of renal artery stenosis. Therapeutic indications include angioplasty and stenting and selective embolization (bleeding tumour, trauma, or AV malformations).

Magnetic resonance imaging (MRI) offers improved soft tissue resolution; it may be used to clarify equivocal CT findings. Magnetic resonance angiography (MRA) is useful in imaging renal artery stenosis.

Radionuclide imaging Scans quantify each kidney's contribution to renal function, and can detect renal scarring. Radiolabelled metal chelators, eg ^{51}Cr-EDTA (ethylene diamine tetra acetic acid) or ^{99}Tc^{m}DTPA (diethylene triamine penta-acetic acid) can also measure glomerular filtration rate.

---

1 Cysts may be inherited, developmental, or acquired—eg polycystic kidney disease, medullary sponge kidney, multicystic dysplastic kidney, medullary cystic disease, tuberous sclerosis, renal sinus cysts, von Hippel-Lindau's disease. [@9377514]   *We thank Prof Peter Scally for preparing this page.*

Renal biopsy

Most acute renal failure is due to pre-renal causes or acute tubular necrosis, and recovery of renal function typically occurs over the course of a few weeks. Renal biopsy should only be performed if knowing histology will influence management. Once chronic renal failure is established, the kidneys are small, may be hard to biopsy, and the results usually unhelpful.

Indications for renal biopsy:
• What is the cause of this acute renal failure (p272)?
• Investigating glomerulonephritis. Is persistent haematuria from IgA nephropathy, thin basement membrane disease, or hereditary nephropathy?
• What is the cause of this heavy proteinuria (eg >1g/d, when you know that amyloid and DM are not the causes).
• Renal dysfunction post-transplantation: is the cause rejection, drug toxicity, or recurrence of renal disease?

Pre-procedure: Check FBC, coagulation profile, and bleeding time. Obtain written informed consent. Ultrasound (if only 1 kidney, risk is magnified).

Procedure: Biopsy is done under ultrasound guidance with the patient lying in the prone position and the breath held. Samples should be sent to histology for routine stains, immunofluorescence, and electron microscopy. A clear indication on the request form of why the test has been done, eg exclude amyloidosis, will help in the selection of special stains, immunofluorescence and use of electron microscopy.

Post procedure: Bed rest for 12–24h. Monitor pulse, BP, symptoms, and urine colour. Bleeding is the main complication.

Urinary tract infection (UTI)

Definitions *Bacteriuria:* Bacteria in the urine; may be asymptomatic (covert) or symptomatic. *UTI:* The presence of a pure growth of >10^8 colony forming units/L (fresh MSU). UTI sites: bladder (*cystitis*); prostate (*prostatitis*); or kidney (*pyelonephritis*). Up to one-third of women with symptoms do not have bacteriuria; a condition known as *abacterial cystitis* or the *urethral syndrome*. *Classification:* UTIs may be classified as *uncomplicated* (normal renal tract and function) or *complicated* (male patients, abnormal renal tract, impaired renal function, impaired host defences, virulent organism). A *recurrent UTI* is a further infection with a new organism. A *relapse* is a further infection with the same organism. For urethritis, see p588.

Risk factors ♀ sex; sexual intercourse; diaphragm contraceptive; vaginal spermicide; DM; immunosuppression; pregnancy; menopause; urinary tract obstruction (p266); renal stones, instrumentation, or malformation.

Organisms *E. coli* is the commonest (>70% in the community but ≤41% in hospital). Others include *Staphylococcus saprophyticus, Enterococcus faecalis, Proteus mirabilis, Klebsiella* species, *Enterobacter* species, *Acinetobacter* species, *Pseudomonas aeruginosa,* and *Serratia marascens.*

Symptoms *Cystitis:* Frequency; dysuria; urgency; strangury; haematuria; suprapubic pain. *Acute pyelonephritis:* Fever; rigors; vomiting; loin pain and tenderness; oliguria (if acute renal failure). *Prostatitis:* Flu-like symptoms; low backache; few urinary symptoms; swollen, tender prostate.

Signs Fever; abdominal or loin tenderness; renal mass; distended bladder; enlarged prostate. **NB:** see also *vaginal discharge,* p588.

Tests *MSU:* Either microscope MSUs yourself (p259), or dip-test for proteinuria, leucocytes, nitrites (p258), and RBCs. If symptomatic, send a fresh MSU to the lab if any are +ve, or, according to some labs, if ≥2 tests are +ve, but these rules are designed to help the lab, not your patient (ie to reduce workload). Send a lab MSU anyway if the patient is a child (OHCS p188) or pregnant, or ill. A pure growth of >10^8 colony-forming units (CFU)/L is diagnostic. If <10^8 CFU/L and pyuria (eg >20 WBCs/mm^3), the result may still be significant. Cultured organisms are tested for sensitivity to a range of antibiotics.

Blood tests: FBC, U&E, CRP, blood cultures, if systemically unwell.

Ultrasound or IVU/cystoscopy: Consider for: UTI in infants, children, or men; recurrent UTI; pyelonephritis; haematuria; unusual organism; persistent fever; persistent haematuria. *Ultrasound or IVU?* Ultrasound may miss stones, papillary necrosis, small carcinomas, and clubbed calyces. But it avoids contrast agents and radiation, so do it first.

Treatment *Advice:* Drink plenty; urinate often; double voiding (going again after 5min); post-intercourse voiding; wipe front to back after micturition.♀ *Antibiotics:* ►*Know your local pattern of resistance:* increasingly, options are narrowing dangerously (eg nalidixic acid only). *Until the organism is known (MSU):*

Cystitis: Trimethoprim 200mg/12h PO (3d). Alternative: cephalexin 1g/12h. Longer courses (10–14d) may be needed in complicated UTI (see above).

Acute pyelonephritis: Cefalosporin, eg cefuroxime 1.5g/8h IV or 250mg/12h PO.

Prostatitis: Ciprofloxacin 500mg/12h PO for ~4wks. *Pregnancy:* Get expert help.

Prevention: Antibiotic prophylaxis, either continuous or post-coital, decreases infection rates in women with recurrent UTIs. Self-treatment with a single antibiotic dose as symptoms start is an option. Effects of cranberry juice have not been fully assessed, but this long-established alternative remedy may inhibit adherence of *E. coli* to bladder cells.♠ One randomized study over 6 months in 153 elderly women drinking 300mL/d of cranberry (or placebo) juice found that bacteriuria was more common in the placebo group (28% vs 15%). Other studies are equivocal.

Causes of sterile pyuria

►*Always remember renal TB* (do 3 early morning urines). Other causes:
- Inadequately treated UTI
- Appendicitis
- Calculi; prostatitis
- Bladder tumour
- Papillary necrosis from DM or analgesic excess
- UTI with fastidious culture requirement
- Interstitial nephritis, polycystic kidney
- Chemical cystitis eg from cytotoxics

What is the predictive value of urinary symptoms and dipsticks for diagnosing UTI?

In one study of 343 women, the pre-test probability of having UTI if urinary symptoms are present was ~0.5. Positive likelihood ratios (LRs) for UTI were: painful voiding (1.31), urgency (1.29), urinary frequency (1.16), and strangury/urinary tenesmus (1.16). Probability of UTI is lessened by presence of genital discomfort, dyspareunia, vaginal discharge, and perineal discomfort.

Nitrites on dipstick increase the probability of UTI 5-fold, moderate pyuria increases it by >1.5-fold, and the presence of both does so by >7-fold.[1]

1 Llobera J 2003 *Fam Practice* **20** 103 http://fampract.oupjournals.org/cgi/content/abstract/20/2/103

Renal calculi (nephrolithiasis)

Renal stones (calculi) consist mainly of crystal aggregates. Stones form in the collecting ducts and may be deposited anywhere from renal pelvis to urethra.

Epidemiology *Prevalence:* 0.2%. Lifetime incidence: up to 12%. *Peak age:* 20–50yrs. ♂:♀ ≈ 4 : 1. *Risk factors:* Dehydration, UTI, hypercalcaemia; hypercalciuria, ↑dietary oxalate/hyperoxaluria, small intestinal disease or resection, cystinuria, renal tubular acidosis, beryllium or cadmium exposure, drugs (triamterine), genetic factors.

Types of stone Calcium oxalate (39.4%), calcium oxalate/phosphate (13.8%), triple phosphate (15.4%), calcium phosphate (13.2%), uric acid (8%), cystine (2.8%), mixed stones (6.4%).

Clinical features Renal stones may be asymptomatic or present with a variety of symptoms. *Pain:* Stones in the kidney cause loin pain. Stones in the ureter cause renal (ureteric) colic. This classically radiates from the loin to the groin and is associated with nausea and vomiting. Bladder or urethral stones may cause pain on micturition, strangury or interruption of urine flow. *Infection* may be acute, chronic, or recurrent. It may present with cystitis (frequency, dysuria), pyelonephritis (fever, rigors, loin pain, nausea, vomiting), or pyonephrosis (infected hydronephrosis). *Other:* haematuria; proteinuria; sterile pyuria; calculus anuria.

Tests *Blood:* U&E, Ca^{2+}, PO_4^{3-}, total protein, albumin, bicarbonate, urate. *MSU:* MC&S, protein, pH (normal range 4.5–8). *24h urine:* creatinine, Ca^{2+}, urate, oxalate. *Imaging:* Abdominal 'KUB' film (kidneys + ureters + bladder). Look along the line of the ureters for calcification: 80% of renal stones are visible (97% on CT). Renal ultrasound excludes hydronephrosis or hydroureter. CT and ultrasound are replacing IVUs as the image of choice for stones. The latter may show a filling defect or ↓renal function on the side of a calculus.

Management Stones not causing obstruction between attacks of renal colic may be managed conservatively. Advise to increase fluid intake and sieve the urine to catch the stone for biochemical analysis. Note that stones often take ≥30d to pass. *Ureteric stones* <5mm in diameter usually pass spontaneously and their progress can be monitored on serial abdominal films. They may need to be fragmented or removed endoscopically from below. *Pelviceal stones* <5mm do not need treatment unless causing obstruction or infection. Stones <2cm in diameter are suitable for lithotripsy. Stones 2–4cm in diameter with a normal collecting system are also suitable for lithotripsy, provided that measures are taken to prevent obstruction. *Renal colic:* Give IV fluids if unable to tolerate oral fluids, analgesia: eg diclofenac suppository 100mg (single-dose) or morphine 5–10mg IV and metoclopramide 10mg IV and antibiotics (eg cefuroxime 1.5g/8h IV) if evidence of infection. ►*Seek urological help urgently if evidence of obstruction.* Procedures include retrograde stent insertion, nephrostomy, and antegrade pyelography (p260). These may be combined with lithotripsy. Open surgery is rarely needed.

Prevention Drink plenty of fluid, especially in summer or tropics (keep urine output >3L/24h). It may be necessary to drink enough at night to cause voiding 2–3 times per night. *Calcium stones:* ↓calcium intake (dairy products); avoid vitamin D supplements. *Oxalate stones:* ↓oxalate intake (less tea, chocolate, nuts, strawberries, rhubarb, spinach, beans, beetroot); ↓vitamin C intake (citrus fruits). *Triple phosphate stones:* antibiotics. *Uric acid stones:* urinary alkalinization (to maintain pH >6); allopurinol (100–300mg/24h PO). *Cystine stones:* vigorous hydration, D-penicillamine, urinary alkalinization (eg with sodium bicarbonate 5–10g/24h PO in water).

Questions to address when confronted by a stone

- *What is its composition?* In order of frequency, the likely answer is:
  - Calcium oxalate stones: these are spiky   (radiopaque)
  - Calcium phosphate stones are smooth and may be big   (radiopaque)
  - Triple phosphate staghorn stone: big; horny   (radiopaque)
  - Urate; xanthine (smooth, brown, and soft)   (radiolucent)
  - Cystine stones are yellow and crystalline   (semi-opaque)

- *Why has he or she got this stone now?*
  - *'What do you eat?'* Chocolate, tea, rhubarb, spinach ↑oxalate levels.
  - *'Is it summer?'* Seasonal variations in calcium and oxalate levels are thought to be mediated by vitamin D synthesis *via* sunlight on skin.
  - *'What's your job?'* Can he/she drink freely? ►Is there dehydration?
  - *'Do you have any predisposing illnesses/drugs?'* In order of likelihood:
    1. Hypercalciuria/hypercalcaemia (p696, eg hyperparathyroidism, sarcoidosis, neoplasia, Addison's, Cushing's, T_3↑, Li^+, vit D excess)
    2. Medullary sponge kidney[1]
    3. UTI (predisposes to calcium phosphate and staghorn calculi)
    4. Cystinuria
    5. Renal tubular acidosis
    6. Primary or secondary hyperoxaluria
    7. Nephrocalcinosis
    8. Gout and a raised plasma urate
    9. Alkali loss from gut, eg with ileostomy (risk of uric acid stones↑)
    10. Aminoacidurias
    11. Syndromes: *Sjögren's; Lesch-Nyhan* (IQ↓, motor delay, head banging)

- *Is there a family history?* X-linked nephrolithiasis, or Dent's disease: low molecular weight proteinuria, hypercalciuria, nephrocalcinosis?

►Is there infection above the stone? Fever? Loin tender? Pyuria?

---

1 Medullary sponge kidney is a benign typically asymptomatic developmental anomaly of the kidney mostly seen in adult females. *Complications/associations:* UTIs, nephrolithiasis, haematuria and hypercalciuria, hyperparathyroidism (if present, look for genetic markers of MEN type 2A). [@11957291]

Urinary tract obstruction

▶*Urinary tract obstruction is common, often reversible, and should be considered in any patient with impaired renal function.* It may occur anywhere from the renal calyces[1] to the urethral meatus. It may be *partial* or *complete*, *unilateral* or *bilateral*. Obstructing lesions are *luminal* (stones, blood clot, sloughed papilla, renal, ureteric, or bladder tumour), *mural* (eg congenital or acquired stricture, neuromuscular dysfunction, schistosomiasis), or *extra-mural* (abdominal or pelvic mass/tumour, retroperitoneal fibrosis). Unilateral obstruction may be clinically silent (ie normal urine output), if the other kidney is functioning. Bilateral obstruction, or obstruction associated with infection, carry a poor prognosis unless urgently treated.

Clinical features *Acute upper tract obstruction:* Pain in the flank, radiating to groin. There may be superimposed infection ± loin tenderness, or a big kidney.

Chronic upper tract obstruction: Flank pain, renal failure, superimposed infection. Polyuria may occur owing to impaired urinary concentration.

Acute lower tract obstruction: Acute urinary retention typically presents with severe suprapubic pain, often preceded by symptoms of bladder outflow obstruction. Examination: distended, palpable bladder.

Chronic lower tract obstruction: Symptoms: urinary frequency, hesitancy, poor stream, terminal dribbling, overflow incontinence. *Signs:* distended, palpable bladder; big prostate on PR. *Complications:* UTI, acute urinary retention.

Tests *Blood:* U&E, creatinine. *Urine:* MSU; pH (may be ↑ from acidification defect ∵ distal nephron damage). *Ultrasound* (p260) is the image of choice. If there is obstruction, the next test is *antegrade or retrograde ureterograms* (p260): it offers a therapeutic option of drainage. *Radionuclide imaging* enables functional assessment of obstruction. *CT and MRI* also have a role.

Treatment ▶*Drainage is urgent if there might be infection above an obstruction.*

Upper tract obstruction: Nephrostomy for acute obstruction; ureteric stent or pyeloplasty for chronic obstruction.

Lower tract obstruction: urethral or suprapubic catheter. Treat the underlying cause if possible. Beware of a large diuresis after relief of obstruction; a temporary salt-losing nephropathy may occur resulting in the loss of several litres of fluid a day. Monitor weight, fluid balance, and U&E closely.

Peri-aortitis (retroperitoneal fibrosis et *al*)

Peri-aortitis includes idiopathic retroperitoneal fibrosis, inflammatory aneurysms of the abdominal aorta, and perianeurysmal retroperitoneal fibrosis. In this autoimmune condition, inflammation consists of B-cell and CD4(+) T-cell associated vasculitis with fibrinoid necrosis of aortic vasa vasorum and small and medium retroperitoneal vessels. In retroperitoneal fibrosis, the ureters get embedded in dense, fibrous tissue resulting in progressive obstruction.

Associations: Drugs (eg β-blockers, bromocriptine, methysergide); carcinoid tumours; atheroma; mediastinal fibrosis; thyroiditis[2]; ankylosing spondylitis.

Typical patient: Middle-aged ♂ with backache, BP↑, palpable kidney ± oedema.

Tests: Blood: anaemia; uraemia; ↑ESR; ↑CRP; ANA & ANCA +ve, p421. *Imaging:*
• *Ultrasound/IVU:* dilated ureters (hydronephrosis) + medial deviation of ureters.
• *CT/MRI:* peri-aortic mass (this allows biopsy, which confirms the diagnosis).
• *Magnetic resonance angiography* may show iliac vein thrombosis.

Treatment: Retrograde stent placement to relieve obstruction + steroids ± surgery. Laparoscopic ureterolysis is possible.

---

1 Pelvi-uretic junction (PUJ) obstruction is a kind of high obstruction (hereditary or from crossing vessels, seen on spiral CT) or a functional abnormality; stenting or nephrostomy may cure.
2 Vaglio A 2003 *Am J Med* **114** 454 [@12727578] and [@12477237]

Problems of ureteric stenting (depend on site)

Common	Rare
Trigonal irritation	Obstruction
Haematuria	Kinking
Fever	Infection
Infection	Ureteric rupture
Tissue inflammation	Stent misplacement
Encrustation	Stent migration (especially if made of silicone)
Biofilm formation	Tissue hyperplasia

Glomerulonephritis (GN)

Abbreviations: ANA = antinuclear antibody; ASOT = anti-streptolysin O titre; BM = basement membrane (glomerular); EM = electron microscope; ESRF = end-stage renal failure; HCV = hepatitis C virus; IF = immunofluorescence.

Cardinal features Haematuria (may be microscopic, ± red cell casts, p258) and/or proteinuria. Patients may be asymptomatic or present with haematuria, proteinuria, nephrotic syndrome, nephritic syndrome, renal failure, or hypertension. Diagnosis is usually made on renal histology, interpreted in the light of clinical, biochemical, and immunological features. The classification of glomerulonephritis is complex; the most useful one is based in histology.

Tests *Blood:* FBC; U&E; LFT; ESR; CRP; immunoglobulins; serum electrophoresis; complement (C3, C4); autoantibodies: ANA, ANCA (p421), anti-dsDNA (*double stranded DNA*), anti-GBM (*glomerular basement membrane*); blood culture; ASOT; HBsAg; anti-HCV (p576). *Spun urine:* To prove glomerular bleeding, ask a good microscopist about RBC casts (p259), dysmorphic G1 RBCs and acanthocyturia (≥5% of RBCs, p628). *MSU:* MC&S. *24h urine* for protein excretion/creatinine clearance. *CXR; renal ultrasound; renal biopsy (p261).*

Management ▶*Refer to a nephrologist for management.* Keep BP ≤130/80.

IgA nephropathy (Berger's disease) Commonest cause of GN worldwide—eg accounting for ~50% of recurrent haematuria, 40% of asymptomatic, and 10% of acute nephritic pictures. *Typical patient:* Young ♂ with episodic macroscopic haematuria, precipitated by infections (eg pharyngitis). Recovery is usually rapid between attacks. Presentation with nephrotic syndrome or renal failure is rarer. Studies with hepatitis B virus show there is probably a cellular mechanism induced by infection of glomeruli, as well as a humoral mechanism from immune complex deposition. *Diagnosis:* Renal biopsy: mesangial proliferation with +ve immunofluorescence (IF) for IgA and C3. *Prognosis:* 20% of adults develop end-stage renal failure (ESRF) over ~20yrs.

Henoch–Schönlein purpura (HSP) can be regarded as a systemic variant of IgA nephropathy. *Clinical features:* Flitting polyarthritis of the large joints; purpuric rash on the extensor surfaces; abdominal symptoms; GN. *Diagnosis:* Usually clinical. May be confirmed by finding positive IF for IgA and C3 in skin lesions or renal biopsy (identical to IgA nephropathy). *Prognosis:* 50% remission; 15–20% impaired renal function; 3–5% renal failure.

Thin basement membrane nephropathy (Autosomal dominant) There is persistent microscopic haematuria ± minor proteinuria, with normal BP and renal function. *Diagnosis:* Positive family history. Renal biopsy: ↓width of glomerular capillary BM. *Prognosis:* Benign.

Minimal change glomerulonephritis (MCGN) Commonest cause of nephrotic syndrome in children (76%—and 25% of nephrotic adults). *Associations:* Hodgkin's lymphoma; various drugs. *Clinical features:* Nephrotic syndrome; BP↑; renal impairment; especial vulnerability to renal effects of NSAIDs. *Diagnosis:* Selective proteinuria (especially in children). Renal biopsy shows fusion of podocytes on electron microscopy (EM). *Treatment:* Corticosteroids induce remission in >90% of children and 80% of adults (slower response). *Indications for immunosuppression:* (cyclophosphamide, ciclosporin (=cylosporin)): early/frequent relapses; steroid SEs/dependence. *Prognosis:* 1% progress to ESRF.

Focal segmental glomerulosclerosis can be similar to MCGN as only some glomeruli have segmental sclerosis. It may be primary (idiopathic) or secondary (reflux or IgA nephropathy, diffuse proliferative GN, Alport's syndrome, vasculitis (p424), sickle-cell disease, HIV, heroin use). *Clinical features:* Nephrotic syndrome; proteinuria; haematuria; ↓renal function; BP↑. *Renal biopsy:* Segmental areas of glomerular sclerosis, hyalinization of glomerular capillaries and positive IF for IgM and C3. *Treatment:* Poor response to corticosteroids (10–30%). Cyclophosphamide or ciclosporin (=cylosporin) may be used in steroid-resistant cases. *Prognosis:* 30–50% progress to ESRF.

Mesangiocapillary GN Accounts 8% of children and 14% of adults with nephrotic syndrome. *Diagnosis:* Biopsy shows large glomeruli with mesangial proliferation and 'double' BM. 2 histological types: type I (subendothelial deposits) type II (intramembranous deposits). ↓serum C3 and C3 nephritic factor are found in some patients (type II more than type I). *Associations:* Type I: SLE; post-strep; endocarditis; visceral abscess; shunt nephritis; HBV; HCV; leprosy; schistosomiasis; filariasis; mixed cryoglobulinaemia; sickle-cell disease; carcinoma; α_1-antitrypsin deficiency. *Type II:* candidiasis; partial lipodystropy. *Both:* complement deficiency. *Treatment:* None is of proven benefit. *Prognosis:* 50% develop ESRF.

Membranous nephropathy Accounts for 20–30% of nephrotic syndrome in adults; 2–5% in children. *Associations:* Malignancy; drugs (gold, penicillamine, captopril); autoimmune (RA; SLE; thyroid disease); infections (HBV; syphilis; leprosy; filiariasis). *Signs:* Nephrotic syndrome; proteinuria; haematuria; BP↑; renal impairment. 5–10% have renal vein thrombosis. *Diagnosis:* Renal biopsy shows thickened BM, IF +ve for IgG & C3 and subepithelial deposits on EM. *Treatment:* If renal function deteriorates, consider corticosteroids and chlorambucil (Ponticelli regimen). *Prognosis:* Untreated, 15% complete remission, 9% ESRF at 2–5yrs and 41% at 15yrs.

Proliferative GN is classified histologically: focal proliferative; diffuse proliferative; endocapillary proliferative; extracapillary proliferative; mesangial proliferative. The chief cause is post-streptococcal GN. *Clinical features:* Haematuria; proteinuria; nephritic syndrome; nephrotic syndrome; renal failure (rare). *Renal biopsy:* Hypercellularity, mesangial proliferation, inflammatory cell infiltrate, positive IF for IgG and C3 and subepithelial deposits on EM. *Serology:* ↑ASOT; ↓C3. *Treatment:* Antibiotics, diuretics, and antihypertensives as necessary. *Prognosis:* Good.

Rapidly progressive GN (RPGN) ESRF develops over weeks or months. *Causes:*
• Primary systemic vasculitis (see p424—eg Wegener's granulomatosis, polyarteritis, Churg–Strauss syndrome (p425) polyarteritis nodosa, giant cell arteritis, Takayasu's arteritis).
• Antiglomerular basement membrane (GBM) disease (Goodpasture's, p724).
• Systemic disorders: SLE, mixed cryoglobulinaemia; Henoch–Schönlein purpura; relapsing polychondritis, Behçet's disease, rheumatoid arthritis.
• Primary GN (IgA nephropathy, mesangiocapillary GN, membranous GN).
• Infection: (post-streptococcal, IE/SBE, visceral abscess, shunt nephritis).
• Malignancy (carcinoma, lymphoma).
• Drugs (penicillamine, hydralazine, rifampicin).

Clinical features: Symptoms and signs of renal failure. There may be loin pain, haematuria, and systemic symptoms (fever, malaise, myalgia, weight loss).

Renal biopsy: Focal necrotizing GN with crescent formation (crescentic GN).

Lung function tests: Gas transfer (KCO, p170) for pulmonary haemorrhage.

Treatment: High-dose corticosteroids; cyclophosphamide ± plasma exchange/ renal transplantation. *Prognosis:* Poor if initial serum creatinine >600µmol/L.

The nephrotic syndrome

▶*When there is oedema, check an MSU for protein to avoid missing this diagnosis.*

Definition Nephrotic syndrome is the combination of proteinuria (>3g/24h), hypoalbuminaemia (albumin <30g/L), and oedema. It is thought to be due to protein loss resulting in ↓albumin, hence ↓plasma oncotic pressure. However, patients may have a normal or ↑plasma volume suggesting there is no simple relation between renin concentration and salt retention in many patients.[14]

Causes Minimal change GN (glomerulonephritis, p268; commonest in children and young adults); focal segmental glomerulosclerosis; membranous GN; (commonest in middle-aged/elderly); mesangiocapillary GN; proliferative GN; DM; amyloidosis; SLE; Henoch–Schönlein purpura (HSP).

Clinical features *Symptoms* Ask about acute or chronic infections, drugs, allergies, systemic symptoms (vasculitis, p424; malignancy).

Signs: Facial swelling/peripheral oedema (anasarca[1]); xanthelasma; xanthomata; hypertension; pleural effusions; hepatomegaly; ascites.

Complications
• ↑Susceptibility to infection (peritonitis, pneumococcus, eg in children).
• Thromboembolism in 10–40% (DVT, PE, renal vein thrombosis; CNS vessels).
• Hyperlipidaemia.
• Loss of low molecular weight binding proteins in urine.
• Acute renal failure.

Tests *Urine:* Dipstick (haematuria, proteinuria); microscopy (RBCs, casts); culture/sensitivity; 24h collection (protein excretion, creatinine clearance). *Blood:* FBC; U&E; LFT; ESR; CRP; cholesterol; immunoglobulins; serum electrophoresis; complement (C3, C4); autoantibodies (ANA, ANCA, anti-dsDNA, anti-GBM, p268 & p421); HBV serology. *Imaging:* CXR; renal ultrasound. *Renal biopsy:* Do in all adults (and steroid non-responding children, or if unusual features).

Treatment
• Monitor U&E, BP, fluid balance, weight.
• Fluid restriction (1–1.5L/d), salt-restriction (~50mmol/d).
• Diet: avoid excess protein: aim for ≤1g/kg/24h of mainly 1ˢᵗ class protein.[15]
• Diuretics, eg frusemide (=furosemide) eg 80–250mg PO ± metolazone or spironolactone. *Aim for loss of 1kg/d.* Occasionally, to promote diuresis, you may need very high doses of frusemide (eg 250–500mg IV) ± IV salt-poor albumin (rarely used now: evidence of benefit is poor).[16]
• Treat hypertension with conventional regimens (p142).
• In those with chronic nephrotic syndrome, consider drugs to reduce proteinuria, eg ACE-i or ciclosporin (also reduce GFR).
• Prompt treatment of infections. Consider prophylactic penicillin in children and pneumococcal vaccines, p172 (during remission).
• Prophylactic heparin 5000U/12h SC if immobile; warfarin for symptomatic thrombosis. Treatment of asymptomatic thrombosis is controversial.[17]
• Hyperlipidaemia usually improves with resolution of nephrotic syndrome. If prolonged, consider treatment with a statin (p114).

Renal vein thrombosis Clinical prevalence: 6–8% of nephrotics with membranous GN; 1–3% of those with other forms of GN. Radiological prevalence: 10–45% of patients with membranous GN; 10% other causes. *Clinical features:* Loin pain (eg acute) haematuria, proteinuria, renal enlargement and deteriorating renal function. Often asymptomatic and diagnosed incidentally. 35% have coincident PE. *Diagnosis:*[18] Doppler ultrasound, renal angiography (venous phase), spiral CT, or MRI. *Treatment:* Anticoagulate with warfarin for 3–6 months (or until albumin >25g/L). Streptokinase may be used to lyse acute thromboses, but its benefits are unproven.

---

1 ↑Fluid in organs and cavities with severe oedema (+tissue hardening). Anasarca is also seen in: CCF, liver failure, protein-losing enteropathy, fetal hydrops, capillary leak syndrome with monoclonal gammopathy.

Acute renal failure (ARF): Diagnosis

Definition A significant deterioration in renal function occurring over hours or days. Clinically, there may be no symptoms or signs, but oliguria (urine volume <400mL/24h) is common. Biochemically, ARF is detected by rising plasma urea and creatinine. ARF may arise as an isolated problem; more commonly it occurs in the setting of circulatory disturbance, eg severe illness, sepsis, trauma, or surgery—or in the context of nephrotoxic drugs.

Causes *Pre-renal failure* (renal hypoperfusion) and *acute tubular necrosis* (ATN) account for >80% of cases. ATN is usually associated with shock, nephrotoxins (aminoglycosides, amphotericin B, tetracyclines, NSAIDs, ACE-i), rhabdomyolysis, and urinary abnormalities suggestive of tubular dysfunction (see below). Complete recovery of renal function usually occurs within days or weeks. *Urinary obstruction* is a less common but potentially treatable cause. *Rare causes:* Vascular (acute cortical necrosis, large or small vessel obstruction); glomerulonephritis; vasculitis; interstitial nephritis; haematological (myeloma, haemolytic uraemic syndrome, thrombotic thrombocytopenic purpura, p282); hepatorenal syndrome (p472).

Assessment ▶Make sure you know about the renal effects of *all* drugs taken.
1 *Is the renal failure acute or chronic?* Suspect chronic renal failure if:

- History of chronic ill-health or signs of chronic renal failure;
- Previously abnormal blood tests (GP records, laboratory results);
- Small kidneys on ultrasound.

The *presence* of anaemia, $Ca^{2+}\downarrow$ or $PO_4^{3-}\uparrow$ may not help to distinguish ARF from CRF, as these can occur within days, but their *absence* suggests ARF.

2 *Is there urinary tract obstruction?* Obstruction should always be considered as a cause of ARF because it is reversible and prompt treatment prevents permanent renal damage. Obstruction should be suspected in patients with a single functioning kidney, or in those with history of renal stones, anuria, prostatism, or previous pelvic/retroperitoneal surgery. Examine for a palpable bladder, pelvic or abdominal masses, or an enlarged prostate.

3 *Is there a rare cause of ARF?*—eg glomerulonephritis, etc.—see above. These are usually associated with abnormal urinary sediment and warrant urgent renal referral for consideration of a renal biopsy and treatment.

Tests • *Urine:* Dipstick for leucocytes; nitrite; blood; protein; glucose; ketones; specific gravity. *Microscopy* for RBC, WBC; crystals; casts. *Culture* and *sensitivity. Chemistry:* U&E; creatinine; osmolarity; Bence Jones protein. • *Blood tests:* U&E—▶▶beware $K^+\uparrow$; FBC; LFT; clotting; CK; ESR; CRP; ABG; blood cultures. When the cause of ARF is uncertain, consider: serum immunoglobulins; electrophoresis; complement levels (C3/C4); autoantibodies (ANA; ANCA; anti-dsDNA; anti-GBM—p268 & p421) & ASOT. • *CXR:* Pulmonary oedema? • *ECG:* Signs of hyperkalaemia? • *Renal ultrasound:* Renal size or obstruction?

Distinguishing pre-renal failure and ATN

	Pre-renal	ATN
Urine Na (mmol/L)	<20	>40
Urine osmolarity (mosm/L)	>500	<350
Urine/plasma urea	>8	<3
Urine/plasma creatinine	>40	<20
Fractional Na excretion (%)	<1	>2

These indices are of limited clinical use as intermediate values are common, they may be influenced by diuretics and pre-existing tubular disease and 'typical' values do not predict renal prognosis.

Acute renal failure (ARF): Management

►*Enlist specialist help*. While awaiting this, make sure that fresh U&E and urine microscopy results are to hand. Treat the treatable:

• If shock is the cause (↓intravascular volume, *below*), use protocol on p779.
• Urgent US scan (today); you *must* check for a palpable bladder; but absence of this sign does not rule out obstruction. If it *is* palpable, insert a catheter.
• Stop nephrotoxic drugs—eg gentamicin; vancomycin; amphotericin—*any* drug may be nephrotoxic: peripheral eosinophilia is suggestive (unreliable).
• Any sign of a vasculitic cause? Nosebleeds? Rash? Haematuria? ESR↑? CRP↑.
• Find and treat precipitating/exacerbating factors: sepsis/UTI; CCF; BP↑↑.

NB: Assessing signs of ↓intravascular volume can be difficult: look for ↓BP; ↑pulse; urine volume↓; invisible JVP. When in doubt, insert a CVP line to measure the venous pressure. Signs of fluid overloaded: gallop rhythm, ↑BP, ↑JVP, basal crepitations, peripheral oedema.

Monitoring Check pulse, BP, CVP, & urine output hourly. Daily fluid balance + weight chart. Match input to losses (urine, vomit, diarrhoea, drains) + 500mL for insensible losses (more if T°↑).

• Correct volume depletion with intravenous fluid—colloid, saline, or blood (only if plasma ↑K⁺ is not a problem) as appropriate.
• If the patient is septic, take appropriate cultures and treat empirically with antibiotics (p548). Remove any potential sources of sepsis when no longer required, eg IV or urinary catheters.
• Re-check about any nephrotoxic drugs; adjust doses of renally excreted drugs.
• Nutrition is vital: aim for normal calorie intake (more if catabolism↑↑, eg burns; sepsis) and protein ~0.5/kg/d. If oral intake is poor, consider nasogastric nutrition early (parenteral if NGT impossible, p468).

Treat complications *Hyperkalaemia* may cause arrhythmias or cardiac arrest. *ECG changes:* Tall 'tented' T waves; small or absent P wave; increased P–R interval; widened QRS complex; 'sine wave' pattern; asystole. ECG p693. R:

▸▸Intravenous calcium, eg 10mL 10% calcium gluconate IV via a big vein over 1min, repeated as necessary until ECG improves. This is cardioprotective.
▸▸Intravenous insulin + glucose, eg 10U Actrapid® insulin + 50mL of 50% glucose IV over 10min. Insulin stimulates the intracellular uptake of K⁺, lowering serum K⁺ by 1–2mmol/L over 30–60min.
▸▸Consider calcium resonium, eg 15mg/6h PO or PR to bind K⁺ in the gut. SE: constipation.
▸▸Haemodialysis or haemofiltration is usually required if anuric.

Pulmonary oedema (p786). In summary:

▸▸Sit up and give high-flow oxygen by face mask.
▸▸Venous vasodilator, eg morphine 2.5mg IV (+metoclopramide 10mg IV).
▸▸Intravenous diuretic, eg frusemide (=furosemide) 250mg IV over 1 hour.
▸▸If no response, urgent haemodialysis or haemofiltration is necessary.
▸▸Consider continuous positive airways pressure ventilation (CPAP) therapy.
▸▸Consider venesection (100–200mL) if the patient is *in extremis*.
▸▸Intravenous nitrates also have a role (p786).

Bleeding: Impaired haemostasis may be compounded by the precipitating cause. In patients with ARF who are actively bleeding, give:

• Fresh frozen plasma & platelets as needed—if there are clotting problems.
• Blood transfusion to maintain Hb > 10g/dL and haematocrit > 30%.
• Desmopressin (p644) to ↑factor VIII activity, normalizing bleeding time.

Indications for dialysis: • Persistent hyperkalaemia (K⁺ > 7mmol/L) • Severe or worsening metabolic acidosis (pH < 7.2 or base excess <–10) • Refractory pulmonary oedema • Uraemic encephalopathy • Uraemic pericarditis.

Prognosis Worse is oliguric. Mortality depends on cause: burns (80%); trauma/surgery (60%); medical illness (30%); obstetric/poisoning (10%).

Chronic renal failure (CRF)

Definitions The substantial, irreversible, and usually long-standing loss of renal function. CRF can be classified as mild (GFR 30–50mL/min), moderate (GFR 10–29mL/min), severe (GFR <10mL/min), or end-stage (GFR < 5mL/min). End stage renal failure (ESRF) is the degree of renal failure that, without renal replacement therapy, would lead to death.

Causes *Common:* Prostatic hypertrophy; glomerulonephritis; pyelonephritis; interstitial nephritis; DM; BP↑; cystic disease, analgesic nephropathy, renal vascular disease, nephrolithiasis. *Rare:* myeloma, amyloidosis, SLE, scleroderma, vasculitis (p424), haemolytic uraemic syndrome, nephrocalcinosis, gout, renal tumour, cystinosis, oxalosis, Alport's syndrome, Fabry's disease.

History Ask about: past UTI; known hypertension; DM. Any family history of renal disease? Take a careful drug history. Any fatigue, weakness, dyspnoea, pleuritic pain, ankle swelling, restless legs, anorexia, vomiting, pruritus, concentration↓, bone pain, impotence/infertility, or menorrhagia?

Signs: Pallor; yellow skin pigmentation; brown nails; purpura; bruising; excoriation; BP↑; cardiomegaly; pericarditis; pleural effusion; pulmonary or peripheral oedema; retinopathy; proximal myopathy; peripheral neuropathy. Late presentations: arrhythmias; encephalopathy; seizures; coma.

Tests • *Blood:* Hb↓ (normochromic, normocytic); ESR; U&E (↑urea, ↑creatinine); glucose (DM); ↓Ca^{2+}, ↑PO_4^{3-}; ↑alk phos (renal osteodystrophy); ↑PTH (hyperparathyroidism, p308); urate↑. • *Urine:* MC&S; 24h urinary protein; creatinine clearance. • *Renal ultrasound* to exclude obstruction and look at renal size (usually small; normal or large in DM, polycystic kidney disease, amyloidosis, myeloma, systemic sclerosis, and asymmetric in renal vascular disease). Consider IVU or DTPA scan. CXR: Cardiomegaly, pleural/pericardial effusions or pulmonary oedema. *Bone x-rays* may show renal osteodystrophy. • *Renal biopsy* should be considered in patients with normal-sized kidneys.

276

Treatment ▶*Refer early to a nephrologist.* Treat reversible causes: relieve obstruction, stop nephrotoxic drugs, treat hypercalcaemia.

- *Hypertension:* Even a small BP drop may save significant renal function.[19] ACE-i can ↓rate of loss of function even if BP is normal, eg if there is proteinuria (>3g/d). Aim for BP of <130/80 (especially if >3g proteinuria/d).
- *Hyperlipidaemia:* This may contribute to renal damage, and increases the risk of cardiovascular disease. Treat with statins (p706).
- *Oedema:* This may require high doses of loop diuretics, eg frusemide (=furosemide) 250mg–2g/d + metolazone 5–10mg/d (max 80mg/d).
- *Anaemia:* If other causes are excluded, eg iron deficiency, chronic infection, etc. (p626), consider erythropoietin to maintain Hb >11g/dL.
- *Renal bone disease (osteodystrophy):* Treat as soon as ↑PTH. ↓Dietary PO_4^{3-} (less milk, cheese, eggs); phosphate binders (eg Calcichew®)[1]; vitamin D analogues (alfacalcidol = 1α-hydroxycholecalciferol)[2] and Ca^{2+} supplements to ↓risk bone disease, and risk of hyperparathyroidism (2° & 3°, p308).
- *Dietary advice:* Match dietary and fluid intake with excretory capacity. Protein restriction is rarely necessary. Na^+ restriction may help to control BP and prevent oedema. K^+ restriction is only required in hyperkalaemia and acidosis; treat with HCO_3^- supplements.
- *Preparing for dialysis:* Create vascular access, eg arterio–venous fistula 2–3 months before haemodialysis needed. Insert a Tenchkoff catheter 2–3wks before starting peritoneal dialysis. Refer for transplantation, if appropriate.

---

1 Aluminium-containing agents are efficient but potentially toxic. Ca^{2+}-containing agents risk hypercalcaemia and soft tissue calcification. Polyuronic acid derivatives are still under development. [@12656655]
2 Alfacalcidol & 1,25-(OH)2D3 (=1,25-dihydroxycholecalciferol = calcitriol) may be ↓parathyroid hormone, but potent effects on intestinal Ca^{2+} and phosphorus absorption and bone mineral mobilization often leads to PO_4^{3-}↑ and Ca^{2+}↑ (with harmful vascular effects)—so new vitamin D analogues retaining suppressive action on PTH and gland growth, but having less calcaemic and phosphataemic activity are under development, eg 9-nor-1,25-(OH)2D2 and 1,alpha(OH)D2. Teng M 2003 *NEJM* **349** 446 [@12753273]

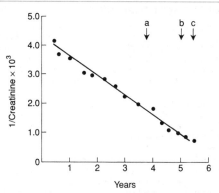

Plot of reciprocal plasma creatinine (µmol/L) against time in a patient with adult polycystic disease. The letters represent life events: (a) work promotion, (b) arterio-venous fistula, and (c) haemodialysis.

Some patients with CRF lose renal function at a constant rate. Creatinine is produced at a fairly constant rate and rises on a hyperbolic curve as renal function declines, so the reciprocal creatinine plot is a straight line, parallel to the fall in GFR. This is used to monitor renal function and to predict need for dialysis—but there is much individual variation in progression, so the plot has limited application.[20] Rapid decline in renal function greater than that expected may be due to: infection, dehydration, uncontrolled ↑BP, metabolic disturbance (eg Ca^{2+} ↑), obstruction, nephrotoxins (eg drugs). Investigation and treatment at this point may delay ESRF.

Background decline is sometimes retardable by using ACE-i with A2A (angiotensin-II blockers). In the COOPERATE randomized prospective trial (over 3yrs) the NNT was ~9 for preventing one case of ESRF (or a doubling of plasma creatinine) by adding losartan (100mg/d)[1] to trandolapril (3mg/d)—ie 11% progressed rather than 23% on ACE-i alone.[21]

Prescribing in renal failure

Relate dose modification to creatinine clearance, and the extent to which a drug is renally excreted. This is significant for aminoglycosides (gentamicin, p710), cefalosporins, and a few other antibiotics (p543–9), lithium, opiates, and digoxin. ►Never prescribe in renal failure before checking how its administration should be altered. Loading doses should not be changed. If the patient is on dialysis (peritoneal or haemodialysis), dose modification depends on how well it is eliminated by dialysis. Consult the drug's *Data Sheet* or an expert. Dosing should be timed around dialysis sessions.

Nephrotoxic drugs: Reduce the dose (the dose adjustment factor, DAF, reflects the fraction excrete unchanged in the urine—(F). DAF = $1/(F(kf-1) + 1)$, where the kf is the relative kidney function = creatinine clearance/120. The usual dose (but not the loading dose) should be *divided* by the DAF. In only a few drugs is F big enough to be important, as below.

Aminoglycosides	0.9	Cefalosporins	1.0
Lithium	1.0	Sulfamethoxazole	0.3–0.5
Digoxin	0.75	Procainamide	0.6
Ethambutol	0.7	Tetracycline	0.4–0.6

1 Get expert advice. ↑Dose *slowly.* SE: BP↓↓ (esp if hypovolaemia); diarrhoea; odd taste; cough; myalgia; migraine; LFT↑; vasculitis. Monitor U&E. Cautions: aortic or mitral stenosis; cardiomyopathy.

Renal replacement therapy

The most widely accepted criterion is creatinine clearance estimated by the Cockcroft–Gault formula (p256) of ~10mL/min (±2).[22] *Early psychological preparation is vital.* Medical preparation involves hepatitis B vaccination and creating an arteriovenous fistula (p289) if haemodialysis is planned option. Choice of haemo- vs peritoneal dialysis depends on medical, social,[1] and psychological factors. **NB:** Kidney function is only partly replaced by dialysis.

Haemodialysis (HD) Blood flows on one side of a semi-permeable membrane while dialysis fluid flows in the opposite direction on the other side. Solute transfer occurs by diffusion. Ultrafiltration is the removal of excess fluid by creating –ve transmembrane pressure. *Problems:* • Disequilibration syndrome • BP↓ • Infection • Vascular access (poor flow, infection, thrombosis, stenosis, bleeding, aneurysm, vascular steal syndrome, ischaemia).

Haemofiltration Blood is filtered across a haemofilter (highly permeable synthetic membrane) allowing removal of waste products by a process of convection (not diffusion). The ultrafiltrate is substituted with an equal volume of replacement fluid. *Advantages:* Less haemodynamic instability; no exposure to dialysis fluid. *Disadvantage:* More expensive than haemodialysis.

Peritoneal dialysis is simple to perform, requires less complex equipment than haemodialysis and is easier at home. It is useful in children, the elderly, and in those with cardiovascular disease or DM. Peritoneal dialysis fluid is introduced into the peritoneal cavity *via* a Tenchkoff catheter and uraemic solutes diffuse into it across the peritoneal membrane. Ultrafiltration may be achieved by adding osmotic agents, eg glucose to the dialysis fluid.

Continuous ambulatory peritoneal dialysis (CAPD) uses the smallest daily volume of dialysate fluid to prevent uraemia. 2L bags are changed 3–5 times a day to produce, with ultrafiltration, a total dialysate of 10L.

Automated peritoneal dialysis uses a cycler machine to enhance solute and fluid removal. Techniques include continuous cyclic peritoneal dialysis (CCPD), intermittent peritoneal dialysis (IPD), night intermittent peritoneal dialysis (NIPD), and tidal intermittent peritoneal dialysis (TIPD). *Problems:* • Peritonitis (60% staphylococci, 20% Gram –ve organisms, <5% fungi) • Exit-site infection • Catheter malfunction • Loss of ultrafiltration • Obesity • Hernias • Back pain • Hyperlidaemia. It is less efficient than haemodialysis and less suitable for larger patients.

Complications of dialysis *Cardiovascular disease,* eg ischaemic heart disease, cardiac failure, cerebrovascular disease is more common in dialysis patients and a major cause of mortality. *Hypertension* persists in 25–30% of patients on haemodialysis. *Anaemia* is common and treated with erythropoietin (and haematinic supplements if deficient). *Bleeding tendency* is due to platelet dysfunction. Acute bleeding is treated with desmopressin and transfusion, as necessary. *Renal bone disease* is treated with alfacalcidol *et al.* (p276), Ca^{2+} supplements, and phosphate binders. *Infections* may be related to UTI or non-sterility during peritoneal dialysis or vascular access procedures. *$β_2$-microglobulin amyloidosis* may cause carpal tunnel syndrome, arthralgia, and fractures. *Acquired renal cysts* occur years after dialysis and may present with haematuria or malignant transformation. *Malignancy* is more common in dialysis patients; some tumours are related to the cause of renal failure, eg urothelial tumours in analgesic nephropathy. *Aluminium toxicity* is now rare.

Stopping dialysis Dialysis can exert a big toll on quality of life, and it may all become too much for patients, eg if very old[23] or there is co-morbidity (eg psychiatric or mobility issues).[1] 8–20% of deaths in dialysis patients are due to its withdrawal.[24] ►*Good palliation allows a good death and mitigates discomfort caused by uraemia:* • Respiratory distress: morphine • Myoclonic jerks: clonazepam • Hallucinations: haloperidol ± midazolam • Secretions: hyoscine. *Doses:* p438. Good communication in the renal team, well-rehearsed protocols, and advance directives (living wills) help the big ethical dilemma.[25]

This is the treatment of choice for end stage renal failure (ESRF). Each patient requires careful medical assessment and consideration of the advantages and disadvantages of dialysis vs transplantation.[1]

Assessment *Note the following:* Pre-existing cardiovascular disease. CMV, zoster, HBV, etc. cause severe disease while immunocompromised. Previous TB may reactivate so isoniazid chemoprophylaxis is given.
• ABO blood group tissue typing for HLA is also required.
• Make sure that a urological assessment is made, where indicated.

Contraindications Active infection; HIV; cancer; severe heart disease.

Types of graft *Living related donor* (LRD) grafts offer the advantages of an optimally timed surgical procedure, HLA haplotype matching, and improved graft survival. *Live unrelated donation* is an option which is becoming commonplace. But this is not legal in the UK, unless done under the complex rules of ULTRA (www.doh.gov.uk/ultra), the unrelated live transplant regulatory authority; expect these rules to change as >6000 are waiting in the UK, often in vain, for a transplant, and altruistic people need to be allowed to realize their own destinies. Consent is problematic, but see p231. *Cadaveric grafts* are obtained from a brainstem dead donor and should ideally be transplanted within 24–36h. Grafts are inserted into an iliac fossa.

Immunosuppressants (Start pre-op.) *Ciclosporin* (=cyclosporin) is the main drug ± *azathioprine/prednisolone*, p674. Doses are slowly reduced over the 1st year. *Others:* tacrolimus (FK506); mycophenylate; anti-T-cell antibodies.

Complications Bleeding; thrombosis; infection; urinary leaks; oliguria.

Acute rejection: (3–6 months post-op) This is characterized by rising serum creatinine ± fever and graft pain. Graft biopsy shows an immune cell infiltrate and tubular damage. R: high-dose corticosteroids. Resistant cases require antithymocyte globulin (ATG) or monoclonal OKT3 antibody.

Chronic rejection: (>6 months) Presents with a gradual rise in serum creatinine and proteinuria. Graft biopsy shows vascular changes, fibrosis, and tubular atrophy. It is not responsive to ↑immunosuppression.

Ciclosporin nephrotoxicity: Afferent arteriole vasoconstriction causes ↓renal blood flow and GFR. There is also chronic tubular atrophy and fibrosis.

Infection: Typically common community infections or those related to ↓T-cell immunity (∵ immunosuppression), eg skin infections (fungi, warts, HSV, zoster) and opportunists (TB, fungi, *Pneumocystis carinii* pneumonia, CMV).

Malignancy: Immunosuppression causes ↑risk of neoplasia ± infection with viruses of malignant potential (EBV, HBV, HHV-8, p726). Typical tumours are squamous cancers, lymphoma (EBV-related), and anogenital ca.

Atheromatous vascular disease: This is commoner in transplant patients than in the general population and is a leading cause of death.

Hypertension: This occurs in >50% of transplant patients and may be due to diseased native kidneys, immunosuppressant drugs or dysfunction in the graft. Management is along standard lines (p142).

Prognosis 1yr graft survival: HLA identical 95%; 1 mismatch 90–95%; complete mismatch 75–80%. Average half-life of cadaveric grafts is 8yrs; 20yrs for HLA-identical living related donor grafts. Risk of neoplasia is ↑ × 5 from immunosuppression, eg skin cancers; lymphomas (eg anaplastic T-cell).

---

1 *Home haemodialysis* gets over some problems with dialysis. Consider in all needing dialysis if: • Willing to learn • Stable on dialysis • No complications • Space for the equipment • No precluding concomitant disease • Good vascular access • There is a carer to assist (get their *informed* consent).

Interstitial nephritides and nephrotoxins

Analgesic nephropathy is associated with the prolonged, heavy ingestion of compound anti-pyretic analgesics. The incidence of analgesic nephropathy has fallen since the withdrawal of phenacetin. *Signs:* Urinary abnormalities (proteinuria, haematuria, casts, RBC, sterile pyuria); UTI; acute pyelonephritis; renal colic; renal obstruction; chronic renal failure; hypertension. *Diagnosis* is based on a history of excess analgesic use, and demonstrating the characteristic renal lesion. *Tests:* IVU shows cortical scarring and clubbed calyces. Retrograde pyelography shows papillary necrosis. Biopsy shows chronic interstitial nephritis or capillary sclerosis. *Treatment:* Stop analgesics; antibiotics for infection; drainage for obstruction; dialysis or transplantation for ESRF.

Interstitial nephritis is an important cause of both acute and chronic renal failure. *Acute interstitial nephritis: Typical cause:* penicillin, frusemide (=furosemide), NSAIDs, or infection (staphylococci, streptococci, *Brucella*, *Leptospira*)—or *no* obvious cause. *Clinical features:* fever; arthralgia; rash (especially if drug related); acute or chronic renal failure; eosinophilia; eosinophiluria; rarely an associated uveitis. *Diagnosis:* biopsy: mononuclear cell infiltration of the renal interstitium and tubules. *Treatment:* ARF: see p274; corticosteroids (unproven, but worth trying). CRF: none. *Prognosis:* favourable in ARF; gradual deterioration in CRF. *Chronic interstitial nephritis* may be a slowly evolving form of the acute disease, or caused by analgesic nephropathy (above) or sickle-cell disease.

Urate nephropathy *Acute crystal nephropathy* may occur when insoluble purines deposit within the tubules causing inflammation or blockage of the tubules. It is caused by gross uric acid overproduction (eg treatment of myeloid tumours) or by inherited diseases (eg Lesch–Nyhan syndrome). The renal parenchyma appears bright on ultrasound and typical birefringent crystals are seen in the urine. *Treatment:* good fluid intake. *Chronic urate nephropathy* typically affects middle-aged men with gout. Histologically, there is interstitial fibrosis with associated vascular changes; crystals are rarely found. *Treatment:* allopurinol (↓dose in renal impairment).

Hypercalcaemic nephropathy is caused by malignancy (commonest); hyperparathyroidism; multiple myeloma; sarcoidosis; vitamin D intoxication. *Clinical features:* Nephrogenic diabetes insipidus (polyuria, polydipsia, dehydration, uraemia); symptoms of hypercalcaemia (nausea, vomiting, constipation, lethargy, weakness, confusion, coma); pancreatitis. *Investigations:* Creatinine↑; Ca^{2+}↑; proteinuria; haematuria; pyuria; hypercalciuria. AXR may show renal calculi/nephrocalcinosis. *Treatment:* IV fluids (3–6L 0.9% saline/24h); loop diuretics; IV disodium pamidronate or similar, p437. Steroids may be useful in sarcoidosis or vitamin D intoxication.

Radiation nephritis *Acute radiation nephritis* (within 1yr of radiotherapy) *Signs:* haematuria, proteinuria, BP↑, anaemia. *Chronic radiation nephritis* may occur after acute radiation nephritis or present with hypertension, proteinuria, anaemia, or end stage renal failure (ESRF) 2–5yrs after exposure to radiation. *Treatment:* control BP, renal replacement therapy for ESRF. *Prevention:* exclusion or shielding of renal areas during radiotherapy.

Balkan nephropathy is characterized by interstitial fibrosis and progressive renal impairment. It is endemic in areas along the River Danube. Environmental and genetic factors are thought to be important. Clinical features: coppery-yellow pigmentation of the palms and soles; β_2-microglobinuria; increased incidence of urothelial tumours (rare).

Nephrotoxins

Many agents may be toxic to the kidneys and cause acute renal failure.

Exogenous nephrotoxins include:
• Analgesics, eg paracetamol and NSAIDs
• Antimicrobials (gentamicin, tetracycline, vancomycin, amphotericin, aciclovir)
• Anaesthetic agents (methoxyflurane, enflurane)
• Chemotherapeutic agents (cisplatin)
• ACE-i and A2As (angiotensin II receptor antagonists)
• Radio-contrast media (especially in diabetes and myeloma)
• Organic solvents (ethylene glycol, carbon tetrachloride)—rare
• Insecticides, herbicides, *Amanita* mushrooms, snake venom—all rare
• Immunosuppressants (ciclosporin (=cyclosporin), methotrexate)—rare.

Endogenous nephrotoxins include:
• Pigments (haemoglobin, myoglobin)
• Crystals (urate, phosphate)
• Tumours (immunoglobulin light chains)

Antimicrobials *Aminoglycosides* (eg gentamicin, amikacin, kanamycin, and streptomycin) are well-recognized nephrotoxins. The typical clinical picture is of mild non-oliguric renal failure which occurs 1–2wks into therapy. The risk of nephrotoxicity is increased by old age, renal hypoperfusion, pre-existing renal impairment, high dosage or prolonged treatment, and co-administration of other nephrotoxic drugs. These circum-stances are common in severely ill patients requiring aminoglycosides. Recovery may be slow, delayed, or incomplete. *Others:* Amphotericin B, sulfonamides, tetracycline; vancomycin. Aciclovir causes crystal nephropathy.

Myoglobin Myoglobin (a muscle protein) can appear in the urine if there is muscle injury or necrosis (rhabdomyolysis). *Causes:* Trauma; ischaemia; coma; immobility; excessive exercise; seizures; myositis; metabolic ($K^+\downarrow$, $PO_4^{3-}\downarrow$); drugs (fibrates, statins); toxins (alcohol, ecstasy, snake bite, carbon monoxide); malignant hyperpyrexia; neuroleptic malignant syndrome; inherited muscle disorders. *Clinical features:* These may be absent or non-specific (muscle pain, swelling, or tenderness). *Tests:* Dark urine which is +ve for blood on dipstick but without RBCs on microscopy. Blood tests: $\uparrow$urea; $\uparrow$creatinine; $\uparrow K^+$; $\downarrow Ca^{2+}$; $\downarrow PO_4^{3-}$. $\uparrow$CK; $\uparrow$LDH; $\uparrow$urate. *Treatment:* Large volumes of IV fluids (up to 12L/d), IV mannitol or urinary alkalinization with IV bicarbonate have been used. Haemodialysis or haemofiltration may be required.

281

Renal vascular disease

Hypertension may be a cause or consequence of renal disease. *Essential hypertension* The extent to which renal impairment develops in mild to moderate hypertension remains controversial. Investigations: p140. Treatment: p142. *Accelerated (malignant) hypertension* is characterized by a severe increase in BP, grade III or IV hypertensive retinopathy (p426) and renal failure. Treatment: p140. *Pregnancy-induced hypertension with proteinuria (pre-eclampsia):* Oedema + proteinuria ± glomerular endotheliosis/obliteration + deposition of fibrin and platelets. *Tests:* **h**aemolysis, **e**levated **l**iver enzymes, **l**ow **p**latelet counts (=HELLP). *Treatment: OHCS p96.*

Renal diseases causing hypertension *Common:* Diabetic nephropathy; chronic glomerulonephritis; chronic interstitial nephritis; polycystic kidneys; renovascular disease. *Rare:* Analgesic nephropathy; vasculitis; SLE; systemic sclerosis; obstructive uropathy; amyloidosis; TB; haemolytic uraemic syndrome; TTP (see below); myeloma; post-partum.

Renovascular disease *Causes:* Atherosclerosis (65–75%, age >50yrs, arteriopaths); fibromuscular dysplasia (younger women). *History:* Coexistent cardiovascular, cerebrovascular, or peripheral vascular disease; deterioration in renal function after ACE-i. *Examination:* Abdominal, carotid, or femoral bruits; absent leg pulses; grade III–IV hypertensive retinopathy. *Tests:* Renal angiography ('gold standard'); others: renal vein renin ratio; captopril challenge test (peripheral renin levels after captopril);[27] isotope renography; CT angiography. *Treatment:* Percutaneous transluminal renal angioplasty or surgery.

Thrombotic thrombocytopenic purpura (TTP) overlaps with HUS (below), but differs in that adult females are chiefly affected, diarrhoea is less marked, and mortality is higher. It is a pentad of: (1) Fever (2) Fluctuating CNS signs (microthrombi, eg causing fits, hemiparesis, ↓consciousness, ↓vision) (3) Microangiopathic haemolytic anaemia (4) Thrombocytopenia (5) Renal failure. *Causes:* see HUS (below). *Other features:* purpura; GI or intracerebral bleeds; haematuria; proteinuria; U&E↑. ►*It is a haematological emergency: get expert help.* Plasma exchange may be life-saving. Ventilation may be needed. Fresh frozen plasma (FFP) and platelet IVI may be needed for severe mucosal or CNS bleeding. There is a role for steroids,[28] vincristine (in steroid non-responders)[29] and splenectomy, if needing repeated plasma exchange.[30]

Haemolytic uraemic syndrome (HUS) is characterized by a microangiopathic haemolytic anaemia, thrombocytopenia, and ARF. Commonest cause of ARF in children. *Infection-associated HUS:* E. coli 0157; *Shigella dysenteriae*; *Streptococcus pneumoniae*; coxsackievirus; echovirus; adenovirus. *Sporadic HUS:* Drugs (the Pill, ciclosporin (=cyclosporin), mitomycin C, 5-fluorouracil, ticlopidine); tumours; pregnancy; SLE; HIV.[31] *Pathogenesis (TTP & HUS):* The key feature may be formation of platelet aggregates, stimulated by endothelial damage, causing release of ultra-large multimers of von Willebrand factor (vWf), so activating platelets. *Tests:* ↓Hb; ↓platelets; ↑neutrophils; blood film (fragmented RBC, ie schistocytes; ↑reticulocytes); ↓Na⁺; ↑creatinine; ↑urate; ↑bilirubin; ↑LDH; ↓haptoglobin;[32] haematuria; proteinuria. *R:* Seek expert advice. Treat hypovolaemia and hypertension. Dialysis, steroids, or plasma exchange may be required. *Prognosis:* It may relapse. 80% may need long-term dialysis (depends on underlying cause). Mortality: <5%.

Cholesterol emboli ►*Suspect in any arteriopath with eosinophilia, purpura* (eg of toes) ± ↑urea.[33] *Prevalence:* 0.3% in unselected necropsies. *Risk:* Atheroma; ↑cholesterol; aneurysms; thrombolysis; arterial procedures. Often spontaneous. *Signs:* Livedo reticularis (p422), purpura, GI bleeding, *progressive renal failure*, myalgia, cyanosis; cholesterol clefts seen in renal or colonic biopsies; they induce evolving fibrosis. *Treatment:* Statins are tried (p706); avoid anticoagulants and instrumentations. *Prognosis:* Often progressive and fatal. A few have regained renal function after dialysis.

Diabetes mellitus (type 2) and the kidney

Diabetes is best viewed as vascular disease—with the kidney as one of its chief targets for end-organ damage. The single most important intervention in the long-term care of DM is the control of BP, to protect the heart, the brain, and the kidney. This organ damage is preventable. ▶Everyone with type 2 DM should either be on an ACE-i (p139) or A2As or have 6-monthly tests for microalbuminuria (25–250mg albumin excreted per day). One convenient way to do this test is to look for an early-morning urine (EMU) albumin : creatinine ratio of >3 (using EMUs improves consistency).

Protect the kidney with ACE-i or angiotensin-2 receptor antagonists (A2A = ARB = AIIAs—such as irbesartan 150–300mg/24h PO or losartan 50mg/d PO; increase dose after 1 month to 100mg daily). Microalbuminuria gives early warning of impending renal problems. SEs of ARAs U&E↑ (monitor K^+ & creatinine periodically); flushing; myalgia; headaches; dyspepsia; cough (rare). Usually, ACE-i are first-line and ARAs for ACE-i intolerant individuals. Occasionally they may be combined, but only by specialists.

▶Example of target BP in DM *if no proteinuria:* 140/80 (negotiate with patient; ensure he/she is well informed); *if proteinuric,* aim for 125/75mmHg.

Do targets work? Target-driven, long-term, intense therapy (including prophylactic aspirin) revolving around microalbuminuria and other risk factors can halve risk of macro- and microvascular events (MI etc.). Steno-2 N=180; 2003

Is microalbuminuria reversible? Answer: sometimes—and more likely if:
• Recent onset • Hb_{A1c} <8% • Systolic <115mmHg • Cholesterol <5mmol/L.[1]

1 Perkins B 2003 *NEJM* **348** 2285 *n*=386; Regression of microalbuminuria had a 6yr cumulative incidence of 58%. This could not be linked specifically to use of ACE-i.

Renal tubular disease

Nephrogenic diabetes insipidus is characterized by renal insensitivity to vasopressin resulting in polyuria, hypernatraemia, and uraemia. It may be *primary* (familial X-linked) or *secondary* to a number of causes:
- Drugs (lithium, diuretics)
- Metabolic (hypokalaemia, hypercalcaemia)
- Tubulointerstitial disease (partial obstruction, pyelonephritis, cystic diseases, granulomatous diseases, sickle-cell disease).

Fanconi syndrome A disturbance of renal tubular function resulting in:
- Generalized aminoaciduria
- Phosphaturia
- Glycosuria
- Rickets (children) or osteomalacia (adults)
- Renal tubular acidosis type 2 (proximal).

Inherited causes: Cystinosis; galactosaemia; glycogen storage disease type 1; fructose intolerance; Lowe's syndrome; tyrosinaemia type 1; Wilson's disease.

Acquired causes: Renal (acute tubular necrosis, hypokalaemic nephropathy, myeloma, Sjögren's syndrome, transplant rejection); hyperparathyroidism; kwashiorkor; drugs (out-of-date tetracycline, iphosphamide); heavy metals (lead, mercury, cadmium, uranium).

Idiopathic Fanconi syndrome: Autosomal dominant. Presents in adulthood with rickets, osteomalacia, and progressive renal failure. *Treatment:* calcitriol; K^+, $NaHCO_3$, PO_4^{3-} supplements.

Cystinosis Autosomal recessive inheritance. The severe infantile form presents with failure to thrive, polyuria, polydipsia, rickets, corneal crystals, retinopathy, hypothyroidism, and renal failure. *Treatment:* vigorous hydration; calcitriol; K^+, $NaHCO_3$, and PO_4^{3-} supplements; thyroxine for hypothyroidism; dialysis or transplantation for end stage renal failure (ESRF). Cysteamine reduces leucocyte cystine and slows glomerular deterioration.

Type 1 (distal) renal tubular acidosis is characterized by an inability to generate acid urine in the distal nephron. *Signs:* Hyperventilation; muscle weakness ($\downarrow K^+$); bone pain (rickets or osteomalacia), nephrocalcinosis; renal calculi; recurrent UTI; renal failure (a late, preventable feature). *Diagnosis:* Urinary pH >6; hypokalaemia; hyperchloraemic metabolic acidosis; hypercalciuria; nephrocalcinosis. *Treatment:* Acute: correct hypokalaemia before acidosis. *Chronic:* oral bicarbonate (1–3mmol/kg/d) and K^+ supplements.

Type 2 (proximal) renal tubular acidosis may occur alone but is usually associated with the Fanconi syndrome. It is characterized by a defect in H^+ secretion and thus HCO_3 reabsorption in the proximal tubule resulting in excess HCO_3 in the urine. *Clinical features:* Polyuria; polydipsia; proximal myopathy; osteomalacia; rickets. Nephrocalcinosis and renal calculi are virtually never seen. *Diagnosis:* Hypokalaemia; hyperchloraemic metabolic acidosis. **NB:** an acid urine can occur with severe metabolic acidosis. *Treatment:* High doses of bicarbonate (eg ≥3mmol/kg/d) are required. *Prognosis:* Good.

Type 4 (hyperkalaemic) renal tubular acidosis occurs in diseases associated with hypoaldosteronism or failure of aldosterone action, eg Addison's disease; inborn errors of steroid metabolism; DM; chronic tubulointerstitial disease; drugs (ACE-i, β-blockers, K^+ sparing diuretics, NSAIDs). Mineralocorticoid deficiency $\downarrow H^+$ secretion in the distal nephron resulting in $\downarrow NH_4^+$ excretion. *Signs:* Urinary pH <5.4; $K^+\uparrow$; hyperchloraemic metabolic acidosis. *Treatment:* Fludrocortisone 0.05–0.15mg PO daily, if acidotic or hyperkalaemic.

Hereditary hypokalaemic tubulopathies *Bartter's syndrome:* Ascending limb involved; mutations eg in genes encoding the Na–K–2Cl cotransporter (NKCC2); see p314; *Gitelman syndrome* (distal convoluted tubule; cause: mutations in the distal tubular Na–Cl cotransporter gene, SLC12A3 on 16q13).

Inherited kidney diseases

Adult polycystic kidney disease (APKD/APRD) *Prevalence:* 1 : 1000. *Inheritance:* Autosomal dominant. Genes on chromosomes 16 (PKD1) and 4 (PKD2). *Signs:* Renal enlargement with cysts; abdominal pain; haematuria; UTI; renal calculi; BP↑; renal failure. Extrarenal: liver cysts; intracranial aneurysms; subarachnoid haemorrhage; mitral valve prolapse; abdominal herniae. *Treatment:* Monitor U&E & BP: treating ↑BP is most important. Treat infections; dialysis or transplantation for ESRF; genetic counselling. *Screening* (eg *magnetic resonance angiography*) eg for 1st-degree relatives of those with stroke. If there is no family history, some centres (USA) still use screening.

Infantile polycystic kidney disease (*OHCS* p220). Prevalence 1 : 40,000. Autosomal recessive (chromosome 6). *Signs:* renal cysts; congenital hepatic fibrosis.

Nephronophthisis An inherited medullary cystic disease. The juvenile form (autosomal recessive) accounts for 10–20% of ESRF in children. *Signs:* Polyuria; polydipsia; enuresis; renal impairment; metabolic acidosis; anaemia; growth retardation; ESRF. Extrarenal signs: retinal degeneration; retinitis pigmentosa; skeletal changes; cerebellar ataxia; liver fibrosis. The adult form (autosomal dominant; restricted to the kidney) is rare.

Renal phakomatoses *Tuberous sclerosis:* (*OHCS* p743) A complex disorder with hamartoma formation in skin, brain, eye, kidney, and heart caused by autosomal dominant genes on chromosomes 9 (TSC1) & 16 (TSC2). *Signs:* skin: adenoma sebaceum, angiofibromas, 'ash leaf' hypomelanic macules, sacral plaques of shark-like skin (shagreen patch), periungual fibromas; IQ↓; fits. *von Hippel–Lindau syndrome* (p736) is the chief cause of inherited renal cancers. *Cause:* germline mutations of the VHL tumour-suppressor gene (also inactivated in most sporadic renal cell cancers).[38]

Alport's syndrome (*OHCS* p742) *Prevalence:* 1 : 5000. Inheritance: X-linked dominant, autosomal dominant, or rarely autosomal recessive. Genes code for type IV collagen molecules, eg *COL4A5, COL4A3, COL4A4*.[9] *Pathology:* thickened GBM with splitting of the lamina densa. *Signs:* Progressive haematuric nephritis, sensorineural deafness, and lenticonus (bulging of the lens capsule, seen on slit-lamp examination). *Treatment:* Control BP; supportive management of renal failure; dialysis; transplantation.

Anderson–Fabry disease X-linked recessive; intralysosomal deposits of trihexoside causing burning pain/paraesthesia in the extremities and angiokeratoma corporis diffusum (blue-black telangiectasia in bathing trunk distribution).

Hyperoxaluria *Primary hyperoxaluria* is due to an autosomal recessive inherited enzyme defect (types I and II) or intestinal hyperabsorption (type III). Do 24h urinary oxalate excretion and creatinine clearance (excretion is misleadingly ↓ in renal failure) if unexplained recurrent calcium oxalate stones.[9TM 2.136] *Secondary hyperoxaluria* is due to small intestine disease/resection, poisoning, pyridoxine deficiency or *Aspergillus* infection. *Signs:* Oxalate stones; nephrocalcinosis; renal failure; cardiac conduction defects; cardiomyopathy; subcutaneous calcinosis; peripheral neuropathy; mononeuritis multiplex; retinal changes; synovitis; osteodystrophy. *Treatment:* High fluid intake; restrict dietary oxalate (tea, chocolate, strawberries, rhubarb, beans, beetroot, celery, nuts); pyridoxine (↓urinary oxalate excretion); hepatic ± renal transplantation.

Cystinuria The commonest aminoaciduria. *Clinical features:* Cystine stones; abdominal pain; haematuria; renal obstruction; UTI. *Treatment:* ↑Fluid intake; $NaHCO_3$ supplements (alkalinizes urine); penicillamine (↓cystine excretion).

Hypomagnesaemia *Autosomal dominant*[(11q23)] and *recessive*[(9q12-22.2)] *hypomagnesaemia. Hypomagnesaemia with hypercalciuria + nephrocalcinosis*[1]: Recessive; the gene ('claudin-16'; 3q27) codes a junctional protein regulating paracellular Mg^{2+} transport in Henlé's loop. *Gitelman syndrome:* Recessive (Mg^{2+}↓; p284).

---

1 Nephrocalcinosis is renal calcification (usually medullary; may cause stones ± UTIs). *Associations:* hyperparathyroidism; distal renal tubular acidosis. Cortical calcification may occur in glomerulonephritis.

Genetics: triumphs and disasters

As soon as genetics solves 1 problem, others appear. You might think that the application of science to medicine is an undisputed boon. Petty has provided a compelling counter-example.[40] A man with adult polycystic kidney disease due to an APKD1 mutation is in end-stage renal failure. A transplant from a matched, living, related, unaffected donor is highly desired. There are problems in his family, but he persuades his adult children to have genetic testing to see if there are eligible donors. Each is apparently happy to donate a kidney to his/her father.

A can of worms is opened when 1 son realizes that he is the only child who can offer a good match—and that his brother is carrying the same mutation as his estranged father (there is a 50:50 chance of passing on the APCD gene). The eligible son would rather save his kidney to help his brother than his father. Old animosities resurface, and the family is in turmoil. How will you feel if the father dies of a complication of dialysis, and both his sons feel guilty forever? We should not be too surprised at all this: often in medicine bad comes out of our good intentions. How can we make good come out of bad? By remembering this example, and not doing tests lightly, and by making genetic counselling as professional as possible, so complications can be foreseen and disasters pre-empted. Furthermore, do not have unreasonable expectations about what genetic counselling can do. The number of diseases being found to have a significant genetic component is increasing faster than geneticists can formulate rational guidelines for screening.[1]

1 Hemminki K 2004 Data for clinical counseling & cancer genetics. *Int J Cancer* **108** 109

Renal manifestations of systemic disease

Amyloidosis (p668) Proteinuria; nephrotic syndrome; renal vein thrombosis; progressive renal failure; renal tubular dysfunction. *Diagnosis:* p668. *Treatment* is of the cause—eg rheumatoid arthritis.

Diabetes 30–40% of patients on dialysis have diabetic nephropathy. *Pathology:* Nodular capillary glomerulosclerosis (Kimmelstiel–Wilson lesion). Early on, there is renal hyperperfusion associated with ↑GFR and ↑renal size. *Microalbuminuria* (albumin excretion 25–250mg/d) occurs 5–15yrs post diagnosis and is associated with a normal GFR and a normal but rising BP.

Type 1 DM nephropathy occurs 10–15yrs post diagnosis and is characterized by macroalbuminuria (albumin excretion >200μg/min or >300mg/d), ↓GFR, and ↑BP. Renal failure occurs 15–30yrs post diagnosis (rare after 30yrs); there may be nephrotic range proteinuria (>3g/d).

Type 2 DM ('maturity onset') nephropathy: ▶See p283 (box). >10–30% have nephropathy at diagnosis, and its prevalence increases linearly with time.

Treatment: Good glycaemic control delays onset and progression of microalbuminuria, but has little effect on established proteinuria. Reducing BP reduces microalbuminuria and attenuates loss of GFR. ACE-i ± A2A (p283) reduce microalbuminuria and slow progression to CRF, even if normotensive.

Infection associated nephropathies are common causes of renal disease. *Glomerulonephritis* is associated with hepatitis B (or C, or less commonly, HIV); SBE/IE, shunt nephritis, visceral abscess, septicaemia, typhoid fever, Legionnaire's disease, TB, leprosy, syphilis, malaria, schistosomiasis, and filiariasis.

Vasculitis (p424)—occurs with HBV, post-streptococcal, staphylococcal, or streptococcal septicaemia.

Interstitial nephritis is seen with *E. coli, Staphylococcus aureus, Proteus,* leptospirosis, hantavirus, and schistosomal infections.

Malignancy *Direct effects:* Renal infiltration (leukaemia, lymphoma); obstruction (pelvic tumours); metastases. *Indirect:* Hypercalcaemia; nephrotic syndrome; acute renal failure; amyloidosis; glomerulonephritis. *Treatment associated:* Nephrotoxic drugs; tumour lysis syndrome; radiation nephritis.

Multiple myeloma is characterized by excess production of monoclonal antibody and/or light chains. Bence Jones proteinuria is common. Myeloma kidney is characterized by accumulation of distal nephron casts. Light chain nephropathy is caused by direct toxic effects of light chains on nephrons. *Clinical features:* ARF; CRF; amyloidosis; nephrotic syndrome; tubular dysfunction; hypercalcaemic nephropathy. *Treatment:* Treat ARF (p274) and hypercalcaemia (p280); chemotherapy; dialysis.

Rheumatological diseases *Rheumatoid arthritis (RA)* NSAIDs may cause ↓GFR or interstitial nephritis. Penicillamine and gold may induce membranous nephropathy. Amyloidosis occurs in 15% of RA patients. SLE involves the kidney in 40–60% of adults. *Clinical features:* proteinuria; haematuria; ↑BP; renal impairment; ARF. Lupus nephritis shows a wide variety of histological patterns. *Treatment:* corticosteroids; immunosuppressants (p422). *Systemic sclerosis* (p420) involves the kidney in 30% of patients. *Clinical features:* proteinuria; haematuria; ↑BP; renal impairment; 'scleroderma crisis' (ARF + malignant hypertension) *Treatment:* control BP; dialysis; transplantation.

Hyperparathyroidism *Nephrocalcinosis:* Deposition of calcium in the renal medulla (seen on plain x-ray). *Renal stones* from associated hypercalcaemia.

Sarcoidosis may involve the kidney in a number of ways. *Abnormal Ca^{2+} metabolism* may cause hypercalciuria, nephrocalcinosis, or nephrolithiasis. *Interstitial nephritis* may present with CRF or ARF. *Glomerular involvement* usually presents with the nephrotic syndrome and is due to membranous glomerulonephritis, other glomerulopathies, or amyloidosis.

Epilogue: the man in a red canoe who saved a million lives

Mostly we commute to work each day driven by motives we would rather not look at too deeply. But one renal physician used a red canoe to commute each day from his houseboat to the hospital. He could have been a very rich man but instead Belding Scribner gave his invention away, and continued his modest existence. He invented the Scribner shunt—a **U** of teflon connecting an artery to a vein, and allowing haemodialysis to be something which could be repeated as often as needed. Before Scribner, glass tubes had to be painfully inserted into blood vessels, which would be damaged by the procedure and haemodialysis could only be done for a few cycles. Clyde Shields was his first patient with chronic renal failure to receive the shunt—on 9 March 1960, and said that his first treatment 'took so much of the waste I'd stored up out of me that it was just like turning on the light from darkness'.[1] Scribner took something that was 100% fatal and overnight turned it into a condition with a 90% survival. In so doing he founded a branch of bioethics because not everyone could have the treatment immediately. This is the branch of ethics that is to do with who gets what—ie distributive justice. In Scribner's day, this was decided by the famous 'Life and Death Committee' which had the unenviable job of choosing who would survive by placing people in order precedence.

Scribner has said that his inventions sprang from his empathy for patients, including himself. 'I was a sickly child' he said, and at various times he needed a heart-lung machine, a new hip, and donated corneas. He was the sort of man whose patients would inspire him to worry away at their problems during the day—and then to awake at night with a brilliant solution.

On 19 June 2003, his canoe was found afloat but empty—and like those ancient Indian burial canoes found at Wiskam which have been polished to an unimaginable lustre by the action of the shifting sands around the Island of the Dead, so we polish and cherish the image of this man who gave everything away.

1 J Lenzer 2003 *BMJ* **ii** 167 and http://seattlepi.nwsource.com/local/127565_scribner20.html For a video of Professor Scribner paddling his canoe and talking about his invention, see http://www.laskerfoundation.org:8080/ramgen/2002_scribner_uwash.rm

Endocrinology[1]

Contents

Relevant pages in other chapters: Diabetic ketoacidosis (p818); hypoglycaemia (p820); the diabetic patient undergoing surgery (p470); the eye in diabetes (*OHCS* p508); thyroid emergencies (p820); thyroid lumps (p516); Addison's disease, thyroid disease, and surgery (p472); Addisonian crisis and hypopituitary coma (p822); phaeochromocytoma emergencies (p822); hyperlipidaemia (p706); natriuretic peptide (BNP, a hormone originating in the heart, p689).

Endocrinology and pregnancy: Thyroid disease in pregnancy (*OHCS* p157); diabetes in pregnancy (*OHCS* p156).

1 We thank Dr Gordon Caldwell who is our Specialist Reader for this chapter.

The essence of endocrinology—for scientists

- Define a clinical syndrome, and match it to a gland malfunction.
- Measure the gland's output in the peripheral blood. Is release diurnal? What other variabilities are there? Define clinical syndromes associated with too much or too little secretion (*hyper-* and *hypo-*syndromes, respectively; *eu-* means normal, neither ↑ nor ↓, as in *euthyroid*).
- Characterize any internal bioassays which nature is kind enough to provide you with. For example you could regard thyroid-stimulating hormone (TSH) as a convenient bioassay of thyroid gland function: the same is true for HbA$_{1c}$ in diabetes mellitus (DM) (p296).
- Find ways of stimulating the gland (usually if hormone deficiency), or, more typically, find out how to replace the missing hormone.
- Find ways of inhibiting the gland (in hormone excess). Measure intermediate metabolites to further define pathophysiology and guide treatment.
- Find a radiological technique to image the gland.
- Aim to halt disease progression. An example is diet and exercise advice which can reduce progression of 'impaired fasting glucose (IFG)' to frank diabetes by 50%.[†] For other glands, halting progression will depend on understanding autoimmunity, and the interaction of endogenous (genetic) and environmental factors. In the case of thyroid autoimmunity (an archetypal autoimmune disease), it is possible to track interactions between genetic and environmental factors (eg smoking and stress) via expression of immunologically active molecules (HLA class I & II, adhesion molecules, cytokines, CD40, and complement regulatory proteins).[1]

The essence of endocrinology—for those doing exams

'What's wrong with *him*?' your examiner asks, baldly. While you apologise to the patient for this rudeness by asking: 'Is it alright if we speak about you as if you weren't there?' think to yourself that if you were a betting man or woman you would wager that the diagnosis will be endocrinological. In no other discipline are Gestalt impressions so characteristic. To get good at recognizing these condition, spend time in endocrinology out-patients and spend time looking at collections of clinical photographs. In addition, specific cutaneous signs are also important, as follows.

Thyrotoxicosis: Hair loss; pretibial myxoedema (p304); onycholysis (nail separation from the nailbed); bulging eyes (exophthalmos).

Hypothyroidism: Hair loss; eyebrow loss; cold; pale skin; characteristic face. (You might, perhaps *should*, fail your exam if you blurt out 'Toad-like face'.)

Cushing's syndrome: Central obesity and wasted limbs (= 'lemon on sticks'); moon facies; buffalo hump; supraclavicular fat pads ± abdominal striae.

Addison's disease: Hyperpigmentation (face, neck, and back of hands).

Acromegaly: Acral (distal) and soft tissue overgrowth; big jaws (macro-gnathia), hands and feet; the skin is thick; facial features are coarse.

Hyperandrogenism (♀): Hirsutism; temporal balding; acne.

Hypopituitarism: Pale or yellow tinged thinned skin, resulting in fine wrinkling around the eyes and mouth, making the patient look older.

Hypoparathyroidism: Dry, scaly, puffy skin; brittle nails; coarse, sparse hair.

Pseudohypoparathyroidism: Short stature; short neck/fingers; calcifications.

DM signs: (There is no Gestalt picture.) Necrobiosis lipoidica; diabetic dermopathy; acanthosis nigricans (dark patches eg in axillae).[2]

1 A Weetman 2003 Autoimmune thyroid disease: propagation and progression *Eur J Endo* **148** 1-9
2 S Jabbour 2003 Skin manifestations of endocrine disorders; guide for dermatologists. [@12688837]

Type 1 diabetes mellitus (DM)

Essence Diabetes results from a lack (or diminished effectiveness) of endogenous insulin. The hyperglycaemia for which diabetes is so famous is just one aspect of a far-reaching metabolic derangement which typically leads to serious vascular events (stroke, MI, retinopathy, and limb ischaemia). Type 1 and type 2 DM (p294) are different entities, with different causes, and natural histories. Type 1 DM (formerly called insulin-dependent diabetes mellitus, IDDM) is usually of juvenile onset but may occur at *any* age, and is characterized by insulin deficiency. Patients *always* need insulin, and are prone to ketoacidosis and weight loss. It is associated with other autoimmune diseases (HLA DR3 & DR4; +ve islet cell antibodies at diagnosis). Concordance is >30% in identical twins. 4 genes are important—one (6q) determines islet sensitivity to damage (eg from viruses or cross-reactivity from cows' milk-induced antibodies).

Presentation *Acute:* Ketoacidosis (p818)—unwell, hyperventilation, ketones on breath, weight loss, polyuria and polydipsia, fatigue. *Subacute:* History as above but longer and in addition lethargy, infection (pruritus vulvae, boils).

Diagnosis Mainly clinical with venous fasting plasma glucose ≥ 7mmol/L. Plasma HCO_3^- and arterial pH may be low, ketones may be present in urine.

Treatment Insulin (see BOX). Education on adjusting insulin dose in the light of exercise & calorie intake to achieve normoglycaemia is vital. Give anti-smoking, foot-care (p298), & pre-conception advice (*OHCS* p94). If pregnant, share care with an interested obstetrician (*OHCS* p156). *Monitor:* BP; Hb$_{A1c}$; creatinine; fundi, p296. There is a need for renal protection eg with ACE-i if microalbuminuria is present (p288).

Dose adjustment for normal eating (DAFNE): One way to optimize control is to use the principles of adult education (eg explicit learning objectives; group learning) in multi-disciplinary teams (specialist diabetic nurses; podiatrists) to fully engage people in self-management. The aim is to promote autonomy and independence (not passive dependency). The randomized DAFNE study found that training in flexible, intensive insulin dosing improved glycaemic control as well as well-being/quality of life.[?] It is resource-intensive.

Insulin dosing during intercurrent illnesses (eg influenza)
• Illness often increases insulin requirements despite reduced food intake.
• Maintain calorie intake using milk or soft drinks containing sugar.
• Check blood glucose ≥ 4 times a day: ↑insulin doses if glucose rising. Patients may need to seek advice from a specialist diabetes nurse or GP.
• Admit if the patient is thirsty, polyuric, dehydrated, or ketotic.
• Admit early if a child or pregnant.

If vomiting, admit—and treat with IV fluids and insulin. Same regimen may be needed during any serious illness. Sliding scales of insulin: see p470.

Managing type 1 diabetes

The aim is to optimize glycaemic control, without risking dangerous hypoglycaemia. 5 other areas need addressing. (1) Maintain renal function (see p288 for the kidney in DM); this will usually mean giving an ACE-i or AT-2 blocker (p288). (2) Control of blood pressure. (3) Prevent eye complications by regular screening (eg retinal photography). (4) Prepare for pregnancy (check contraception if pregnancy not wanted). See *OHCS* p156 for diabetes in pregnancy. (5) Emotional and psychological factors which may be perpetuating unhealthy lifestyles.

Insulin Strength: 100U/mL. There are many types, falling into 6 groups.

1 Ultra-fast acting, eg Humalog® and Novorapid®; inject at start of meal (or immediately after).
2 Soluble insulin eg Humulin S® or Actrapid: inject 15–30min before meals.
3 Intermediate Humulin I® or Insulatard®.
4 Long-acting ('lente'), eg Ultratard®.
5 Long-acting analogue, eg Lantus/insulin glargine, see below.
6 Pre-mixed insulins, eg with ultra-fast component (eg Humalog® Mix 25); or with soluble insulin (eg Humulin® M3 or Mixtard® 30).

Some commonly used insulin regimens

▶Design the insulin regimen to suit your patient's lifestyle (not *vice versa*).

• Twice daily premixed insulins by pen injector—useful in type 2 DM or type 1 with regular lifestyle.
• Before meals ultra-fast or soluble insulin with bedtime intermediate- or long-acting analogue: useful in type 1 DM for achieving a flexible lifestyle (eg skipping meals).
• Once daily before bed intermediate- or long-acting analogue—good initial insulin regimen when switching from tablets in type 2 DM.
• Begin with at least a total daily dose of 1 unit of insulin for every unit of body mass index in adults.
• NB: *Insulin glargine* is a long-acting recombinant human insulin analogue used once daily at bedtime in type 1 or 2 DM; however, not recommended for routine use in type 2 DM (see BNF; NICE guidance). Molecular modification has made an insulin that is soluble at acid pH, but precipitates in subcutaneous tissue and is slowly released from a depot. Given once daily, insulin glargine has comparable efficacy to that of insulins used twice daily. Its rate of hypoglycaemia is ≤ to that of standard insulins, and there is evidence of less nocturnal hypoglycemia. It may be combined with ultra-short acting insulins given at the times of meals. In type 2 DM, if oral agents are failing, it can be added only if a bd dosing is problematic (NICE guidance).
• ▶Strict plasma glucose control *does* reduce renal, CNS, & retinal damage.

Type 2 diabetes mellitus (DM)

Type 2 DM appears to be prevalent at 'epidemic' levels in many places (part of the increase is due to better diagnosis and improved longevity). In areas of Australia, 7% of people over 25yrs old have DM (mostly type 2). Higher prevalence occurs in Asians, men, and the old (18% in men over 80 in Liverpool). Avoid the terms *non-insulin-dependent DM (NIDDM)* and *maturity-onset DM*: most *are* over 40yrs, but teenagers are increasingly getting type 2 DM.

Cause ↓Insulin secretion and insulin resistance associated with obesity ('diabesity'), exercise lack, and calorie excess. ≥80% concordance in identical twins.[1]

Typical natural history *A preliminary phase* of impaired glucose tolerance (IGT) or IFG, see below. (►This a unique window of opportunity for lifestyle intervention.) *A symptomatic phase*: Thirst, polyuria, weight loss. *A phase of complications*: Infections, neuropathy (eg foot ulcers), retinopathy, or arterial disease (eg MI or claudication).

Diagnosis/tests/monitoring *Blood*: Fasting venous glucose↑ (>7mmol/L, unless already on insulin); HbA$_{1c}$↑ (≥6.5%; monitor eg 2–4 times/yr). Random blood glucose tests are unreliable, but if >11.1mmol/L and symptomatic, this is diagnostic. *Urine*: Microalbuminuria (eg annually; defines renal risks, p288); urine analysis. MSU if ill. *Fundoscopy* (p296). *BP*: Keep systolic <140mmHg. *Lipids*: p706. *Foot exam*: Take off shoes and socks at each visit, to assess circulation, sensation, and skin quality; warn not to go barefoot.

Diagnostic criteria If no diabetic symptoms, do not base a diagnosis on 1 glucose value alone. If there is any doubt, use the 2h value in an oral glucose tolerance test (OGTT): look for a level >11.1mmol/L. *How to do a 2h OGTT:*
- Fast overnight and give 75g of glucose in 300mL water to drink.
- Measure venous plasma glucose before and 2h after the drink.

NB: Severe hyperglycaemia in acute infection, trauma, or circulatory or other stress may be transitory: delay *formal* diagnosis (but not management).

Plasma HbA$_{1c}$ values: If >7%, DM is likely (*specificity 99.6%; sensitivity 99%*), and risk of microvascular complications occurs.

Screening for glycosuria: This is easy but ~1% of the population have low renal threshold for glucose; the sensitivity is only 32% (specificity: 99%).

Impaired glucose regulation *not amounting to diabetes* This state lies between *normal glucose homeostasis* and *diabetes*. *Impaired glucose tolerance (IGT)*: Fasting plasma glucose <7mmol/L and OGTT 2h glucose ≥7.8mmol/L but <11.1mmol/L. *Impaired fasting glucose (IFG)*: Fasting glucose levels > normal range, but below the diagnostic level for DM, ie fasting plasma glucose ≥6.1mmol/L but <7mmol/L. Diabetes UK (British Diabetic Association) recommends all those with IFG should have an OGTT to exclude DM.

IFG and IGT denote different abnormalities of glucose regulation (fasting and post-prandial). There may be lower risk of progression to DM in IFG than IGT. Both are managed with lifestyle advice (eg exercise & diet, p91), and regular review. NB: Giving those with heart failure and IFG ACE-i drugs can prevent progression to DM (3% vs 48% over 3yrs).

Gestational diabetes: This term now includes both gestational impaired glucose tolerance (GIGT) and gestational diabetes mellitus (GDM). Use the same diagnostic values as IGT and diabetes above. As glucose tolerance changes during pregnancy, the gestation at which the diagnosis was made needs to be stated. ≥6wks post-partum, do a further 75g OGTT whether she still has diabetes or IGT/IFG. Regardless of the 6wk post-pregnancy result, these women are at ↑risk of later diabetes. See *OHCS* p156.

---

1 Diabetes may be secondary to eg drugs (steroids and thiazides); pancreatic disease (pancreatitis, surgery in which >90% pancreas is removed, haemochromatosis, cystic fibrosis, pancreatic cancer); endocrine disease (Cushing's disease, acromegaly, phaeochromocytoma, thyrotoxicosis); others (acanthosis nigricans, congenital lipodystrophy with insulin receptor antibodies, and glycogen storage diseases).

Managing type 2 diabetes

▶*Patient motivation and education are central.* Aim to avoid complications—hypoglycaemia as well as the long-term effects of hyperglycaemia. Tight BP control (eg systolic ≤140mmHg) is most important for preventing macrovascular disease and mortality. So do a *global* assessment of risk: glucose, BP, left ventricular hypertrophy, cholesterol,[1] and smoking. Don't treat DM in isolation. In the UK, a *National Service Framework (NSF)* governs the delivery of care, setting aims, and prioritizing quality initiatives.

Educate and negotiate on drugs, diet, and the benefits of these issues:
- Specialist *nurse/dieticians, chiropodists, diabetic associations/patient's groups*.
- *Regular* follow-up and *regular* exercise (↓insulin resistance & ↓risk of MI).
- Legal obligations to inform their *driving licence authority* (p162).
- *Diet:* p208—saturated fats↓, sugar↓, starch-carbohydrate↑, moderate protein; don't prohibit coffee (may ↑ insulin sensitivity). If creatinine↑ or microalbuminuria (p288), restrict protein, and give ACE-i (p139) or AT-2 blocker (p283). If diet and exercise do not control glycaemia, use drugs.

Oral hypoglycaemics Start with *metformin* (a biguanide). This helps maintain weight loss (if achieved!) and ↑ insulin sensitivity. SE: anorexia; D&V; B_{12} absorption↓; *not* hypoglycaemia. Avoid if creatinine ≥150µmol/L. *Dose:* 0.5–1g/8h PO pc. Stop if tissue hypoxia (eg MI; sepsis) and 48h before GA and for 3d after contrast medium containing iodine (do U&E).

Next add in a sulfonylurea to ↑insulin secretion (some authorities, but not NICE, say a glitazone[2] is more appropriate as the 2nd add-in drug).
Tolbutamide: Short-acting (hypoglycaemia is rare); 0.5–1.5g in 2–3 doses.
Gliclazide: Medium-acting; 40–160mg PO as a single dose, max 160mg/12h.
Glibenclamide: Long-acting; 2.5–15mg/24h PO at breakfast (rarely used).
Glitazones *Rosiglitazone* 4mg/24h. CI: LFT↑. SE: headache, diarrhoea, dyspepsia, fluid retention (caution in CCF); do LFT every 2 months for 1yr; stop if ALT up >3-fold; alternative: *pioglitazone* 15–30mg/24h. Glitazones ↓insulin resistance. Use if metformin + sulfonylurea combination is problematic: the glitazone replaces whichever is contraindicated or not tolerated.

Other agents *Acarbose* (an α-glucosidase inhibitor) decreases breakdown of starch to sugar. Use as an add-on drug, eg 50mg chewed at start of each meal, start with a once daily dose; max 200mg/8h. SE: wind (can be terrible; less if *slow* dose build-up), abdominal distension/pain, diarrhoea. *Nateglinide:* ↑β-cell insulin release by binding to sulfonylurea receptors. 120mg 30min a.c. Alternative: *Repaglinide.* They may be no better than metformin/glibenclamide at lowering Hb_{A1c}. They target post-prandial hyperglycaemia ($t_{½}$ is short—metformin works mostly on fasting glucose); they may have a role in those with irregular mealtimes if glycaemic control is poor.

Other considerations ACE-i (p139; many good effects, not just BP↓); aspirin + statins (p706; ?for all with DM) to ↓overall risk. Exercise also helps.

Causes of insulin resistance

Syndrome X (central obesity, arteriopathy, glucose↑, and hyperinsulinaemia + BP↑)	Obesity; acromegaly Werner's syn, *OHCS* p758 Renal failure (all types)	Polycystic ovary, p316 Asians[3], pregnancy TB drugs; cystic fibrosis

Mechanisms: ● Obesity may cause insulin resistance by ↑ rate of release of non-esterified fatty acids causing post-receptor defects in insulin's action. ● Mutation of genes encoding insulin receptors. ● Circulating autoantibodies to the extracellular domain of the insulin receptor. R for *syndrome X:* Exercise more; weight↓; statins; hypotensives, hypoglycaemics (eg glitazones).

295

---

1 As DM has so many vascular events, give a statin (p706) if LDL >3mmol/L **or** BP >140. Even consider a statin *whatever* the pre-treatment cholesterol; discuss with your patient. L Lindholm 2003 *Lancet* **361** 2000
2 Glitazones *may* preserve β-cells and control glycaemia for longer than secretagogues or biguanides.
3 Especially Indians (Gujaratis; Punjabis), Sri Lankans, Pakistanis, Bangladeshis.▶Have a lower threshold for diagnosing obesity (BMI >23) and for vigorous intervention in this group. *BMJ* 2003 **327** 1059

Helping people with established diabetes

▶*Focus on education and lifestyle advice.* Promote exercise (to ↑insulin sensitivity), healthy eating (p208) and weight reduction—p208; NICE comments that drugs such as orlistat have a role here if weight loss of >2.5kg has been achieved by lifestyle advice and BMI >28kg/m². ▶*Find out what problems are being experienced* (glycaemic control and morale). ▶*Pre-empt complications.*

Assess those modifiable risk factors important in DM BP: Aim for systolic <140mmHg; *smoking; cholesterol* (p706). *Glycaemic control:* (1) Glycated (glycosylated) haemoglobin (= HbA₁c)—levels relate to mean glucose level over previous 8 wks (ie RBC half-life). The target HbA₁c must be set individually. Tight control is especially vital in pregnancy (OHCS p156) and if there are microvascular complications. In other patients it may occasionally be sensible to opt for less tight control. NB: The 2003 UK prospective diabetes study (UKPDS; N=2489) shows that in type 2 DM, HbA₁c levels remain stubbornly high, despite intensive therapy, (making recent UK HbA₁c targets of ≤7.4% seem impossible). Complications increase with increasing HbA₁c. NB: *fructosamine* (glycated plasma protein) levels reflect control over 2–3 wks: useful in pregnancy to assess shorter term control, and in haemoglobinopathies which interfere with HbA₁c tests. (2) History of hypoglycaemic attacks (and whether symptomatic). (3) Home fingerstick glucose records may be useful.

Look for complications Check injection sites for infection/fat necrosis, then:

• *Vascular disease:* Commonest cause of death. Look for evidence of cerebrovascular, cardiovascular, and peripheral vascular disease. MI is 3–5 times more common in DM and is more likely to be 'silent' (ie without classic symptoms). Stroke is at least twice as common. Women are at high risk—DM removes the cardiovascular advantage conferred by female gender. Reduce other risk factors (see p91). NB: ACE-i also slows progression of renal disease (p283). Treat lipid disorders (p706)—statins, eg simvastatin 40mg nocte, are 1st-line. Good glycaemic control also helps. Fibrates may be useful for ↑triglycerides and ↓HDL. An aspirin a day may ↓risk of MI in diabetics as in non-diabetics (no significant risk to the eye).

• *Kidneys* (p283): Microalbuminuria (p288) reflects early renal disease, and indicates ↑risk for macrovascular disease. Control BP with ACE-i: see p139.

• *Diabetic retinopathy:* (Dilate pupils with 0.5% tropicamide.) Blindness is not *common* and is usually preventable. *Arrange regular fundoscopy for all patients,* including retinal photography, if possible. Refer if maculopathy or pre-proliferative changes or any uncertainty at or around the macula (the most sacred retinal site and the only place capable of 6/6 vision). ▶Presymptomatic screening enables laser photocoagulation to be used. For images of DM retinopathy, see OHCS p508 and its associated colour plates.
Background: Microaneurysms (dots), microhaemorrhages (blots), and hard exudates. Refer to specialist if near the macula. See PLATE 13.
Pre-proliferative retinopathy: Cotton-wool spots (infarcts); microhaemorrhages.
Proliferative retinopathy: New vessels form. Needs *urgent* referral.
Maculopathy: More common in type 2 DM. Suspect if visual acuity↓.
Pathogenesis: Capillary endothelial change→vascular leak → microaneurysms → capillary occlusion→hypoxia + ischaemia→new vessel formation. High retinal blood flow caused by hyperglycaemia (& BP↑ & pregnancy) triggers this, causing capillary pericyte damage. Microvascular occlusion causes *cotton-wool spots* (± *blot haemorrhages* at interfaces with perfused retina). *New vessels* form on disc or ischaemic areas, proliferate, bleed, fibrose, and can detach the retina. Aspirin (2mg/kg/d) may prevent it; there is no evidence of ↑bleeding.[1] *Cataracts:* May be juvenile 'snowflake' form, or 'senile'—which occur earlier in diabetic subjects. Osmotic changes in the lens induced in acute hyperglycaemia reverse after normoglycaemia (so wait before buying glasses).

• *Rubeosis iridis:* New vessels on iris: occurs late and may lead to glaucoma.

• *Metabolic complications:* p818. *Diabetic feet:* p298. *Neuropathy:* p298.

Starting insulin in those with type 2 DM

This is frequently required when control with oral agents is suboptimal (eg HbA~1c~ >7.5–8.0% on maximum oral therapy). The patient must be blood glucose self-testing. Transfer is supervised by a diabetes nurse specialist and dietician. Insulin (p293) may be given initially once or twice a day. Continue metformin to limit weight gain. NICE has commented that long-acting insulin glargine (p293) is not normally needed in this context, unless there is recurrent symptomatic hypoglycaemia or it is necessary to avoid twice daily insulin doses (eg if assistance is needed to inject).

Controlling BP in those with diabetes—3 typical scenarios

1 BP <145/80 and no microalbuminuria and 10yr coronary event risk (CER10, p22) ≤15%, simply check BP every 6 months, or more often.
2 BP ≥ 140/80 and <160/100 and CER10 >15%, but no microalbuminuria, start an antihypertensive (NICE recommends ACE-i, A2A, β-blocker, or a thiazide). Target BP <140/80. For doses and discussion, see p142.
3 BP ≥ 140/80 and microalbuminuria *is* present (urine albumin:creatine ratio ≥ 2.5mg/mmol in men or ≥ 3.5 in women): ensure ACE-i or A2A are part of the approach (unless CI, p139); target BP: <135/75. (NICE guidelines)

▶Aspirin prophylaxis (75mg/d PO) is indicated eg if CER10 >15%.[1]

297

---

1 Aspirin is known to ↓ leucocyte adhesion in diabetic retinal capillaries. It ↓expression of integrins on the surface of leucocytes and it ↓nitric oxide synthetase (eNOS) levels and ↓production of the vasoactive cytokine, tumour necrosis factor, known to be raised in diabetic retinopathy. *BMJ* 2003 **327** 1060

Diabetic neuropathy and diabetic foot care

▶*Amputation is preventable: good care saves legs.* Examine feet regularly. Distinguish between ischaemia (eg critical toes ± absent dorsalis pedis pulses) and peripheral neuropathy (injury/infection over pressure points, eg the metatarsal heads). In practice, many have ischaemia *and* neuropathy.

Symptoms Numbness, tingling, and burning, often worse at night.

Signs Sensation↓ (especially vibration) in 'stocking' distribution; absent ankle jerks; deformity (pes cavus, claw toes, loss of transverse arch, rocker-bottom sole). Neuropathy is patchy, so examine all areas. If the foot pulses cannot be felt, consider Doppler pressure measurement.

Any evidence of neuropathy or vascular disease puts the patient at high risk of foot ulceration. Educate (daily foot inspection, comfortable shoes—ie very soft leather, increased depth, cushioning insoles, weight-distributing cradles, extra cushioning—no barefoot walking, no corn-plasters). Regular chiropody. Treat fungal infections (p612).

Foot ulceration: Usually painless, punched-out ulcer in an area of thick callous ± superadded infection, pus, oedema, erythema, crepitus, odour.

Assess degree of: (1) Neuropathy (clinical). (2) Ischaemia (clinical and Dopplers; consider angiography—even elderly patients may benefit from angioplasty). (3) Bony deformity, eg Charcot joint (clinical, x-ray). (4) Infection (do swabs, blood culture, x-ray; probe ulcer to assess depth).

Management: Regular chiropody (remove dead tissue). Relieve high-pressure areas with bedrest ± therapeutic shoes (Pressure Relief Walkers® and similar shoes may be as good as total contact casts); metatarsal head surgery may be needed. In ischaemia, shoes must be wide-fitting with deep toe boxes to protect vulnerable forefoot margins and toes. If there is cellulitis, admission is mandatory for IV antibiotics: start with benzylpenicillin 600mg/6h IV and flucloxacillin 500mg/6h IV ± metronidazole 500mg/8h IV, refined when microbiology results are known. Get surgical help. Ensure normoglycaemia.

Absolute indications for surgery

- Abscess or deep infection
- Spreading anaerobic infection
- Severe ischaemia—gangrene/rest pain
- Suppurative arthritis

The degree of peripheral vascular disease, patient's general health, and patient request will determine whether local excision and drainage, vascular reconstruction, and/or amputation (and how much) is appropriate.

Types of neuropathy in diabetes

Motor & sensory neuropathy: Symmetric sensory polyneuropathy—distal numbness ('glove and stocking anaesthesia'), tingling, and visceral pain, eg worse at night. *Batting order of drugs to try:* aspirin/paracetamol → tricyclic (amitriptyline 10–25mg nocte; gradually ↑; max 150mg) → gabapentin. *Alternatives:* carbamazepine (p380); lamotrigine; 0.075% capsaicin cream (a counter-irritant). Decompression may help.

Mononeuritis multiplex—especially III & VI cranial nerves. Treatment is difficult. If sudden and severe, immunosuppression with corticosteroids, IV immunoglobulins, and ciclosporin (=cyclosporin) has been tried.

Amyotrophy—painful wasting of quadriceps and other pelvifemoral muscles. Use electrophysiology to show eg lumbosacral radiculopathy, plexopathy, or proximal crural neuropathy. Natural course: variable with gradual but often incomplete improvement. IV immunoglobulins have been used.

Autonomic neuropathy: (biology: p390) Excessive postural BP drop; ↓cerebrovascular autoregulation; urine retention; erectile dysfunction (ED); diarrhoea at night. The latter may respond to long-term codeine phosphate (the lowest dose to control symptoms, eg 15mg/8h PO). Gastroparesis (early satiety, postprandial bloating, nausea/vomiting) is diagnosed by gastric scintigraphy with a ^{99}technetium-labelled low-fat meal. It may respond to antiemetics. Postural hypotension may respond to fludrocortisone 100–300µg/24h PO (SE: oedema).

Preventing loss of limbs: primary or secondary prevention?

Traditionally prevention has involved foot care advice in diabetic clinics (eg 'don't go bare-foot …'), and maintaining good glycaemic and BP control.[1] But despite this, the sight of a diabetic patient minus 1 limb is not rare: whenever we see such patients we should redouble our commitment to primary prevention—ie stopping those at risk from ever getting diabetes. In one randomized prospective study of those with impaired glucose tolerance (IGT) and other risk factors, after 3 yrs, the incidence of diabetes per 100 person-years was 5 in those receiving simple exercise and diet advice, 8 in a group given metformin, and 11 in the placebo group. Advice and metformin decreased incidence of diabetes by 58% (NNT ≈ 7) and 31% (NNT ≈ 14), respectively, compared with placebo.

1 HbA_{1c} ≤ 7.4% and BP ≤ 145/85 are current UK primary care targets (GPs get a quality payment if 70% of their diabetics achieve this level; for non-diabetic hypertensives, the target BP is ≤150/90mmHg).

Hypoglycaemia

►This is the commonest endocrine emergency. Prompt diagnosis and treatment is essential. See p820 for emergency management.

Definition Plasma glucose <2.5mmol/L. Threshold for symptoms varies.

Symptoms *Autonomic*—Sweating; hunger; tremor.

Neuroglycopenic—Drowsiness; seizures; rarely focal symptoms, eg transient hemiplegia, coma. Mutism, mannerisms, personality change, restlessness, and incoherence may lead to misdiagnosis of hysteria or psychosis. Two types:

1 Fasting hypoglycaemia (requires full investigation if documented).
Causes: By far the commonest cause is insulin or sulfonylurea treatment in a known diabetic. In the non-diabetic subject with fasting hypoglycaemia, the following mnemonic is useful: **EXPLAIN**.

Exogenous drugs, eg *insulin* or *oral hypoglycaemics* (p283). Does he have access to these (diabetic in the family)? Body-builders sometimes misuse insulin to improve stamina. *Alcohol*, eg alcoholic on binge with no food. Also: *aminoglutethimide; 4-quinolones; pentamidine; quinine sulfate*.
Pituitary insufficiency.
Liver failure plus some rare inherited enzyme defects.
Addison's disease.
Islet cell tumours (insulinoma, see below) and immune hypoglycaemia (eg anti-insulin receptor antibodies in Hodgkin's disease).
Non-pancreatic neoplasms (especially retroperitoneal fibrosarcomas and haemangiopericytomas).

Diagnosis and investigations
- Document hypoglycaemia by taking finger-prick (on filter-paper at home for later analysis) during attack, or lab glucose if in hospital.
- Exclude liver failure and malaria.
- Admit for 72h fast. Do glucose, insulin, & C-peptide if symptomatic.

Interpreting results
- Hypoglycaemia with high or normal insulin and no elevated ketones. *Causes:* insulinoma; sulfonylurea administration; insulin administration (no detectable C-peptide); insulin autoantibodies.
- Insulin low or undetectable, no excess ketones. *Causes:* Non-pancreatic neoplasm; anti-insulin receptor antibodies.
- Insulin↓, ketones↑. *Causes:* Alcohol; pituitary or adrenal failure.

2 Post-prandial hypoglycaemia May occur eg after gastric surgery ('dumping', p530), and in type 2 diabetes. *Investigation:* Prolonged OGTT (5h, p294).

Treatment ►►See p820. Treat with oral sugar, and a long-acting starch (eg toast); if coma, glucose 25–50g IV (via a large vein with a 0.9% saline flush to prevent phlebitis) or glucagon 0.5–1mg SC/IV/IM (± a repeat after 20min; *follow with carbohydrate*). If episodes are often, advise many small high-starch meals. If post-prandial glucose↓, give slowly absorbed carbohydrate (high fibre). In diabetics, prevent further episodes, by rationalizing insulin therapy (p293).

Insulinoma MEN-1 associated (p309), usually benign islet cell tumour. *Screening test:* Hypoglycaemia + plasma insulin↑ during a long fast. *Suppressive tests:* Give IV insulin and measure C-peptide. Normally exogenous insulin suppresses C-peptide, but this does not occur in insulinoma. *Arterial stimulation[1] with venous sampling (ASVS):* Hyperinsulinaemia as measured eg via splenic or superior mesenteric artery stimulation. *Imaging:* CT/MRI ± endoscopic pancreatic US (all fallible, so don't waste too much time before proceeding to intra-operative visualization ± intra-operative ultrasound). *Treatment:* Surgery.

---

1 With IV 10% calcium gluconate, eg 0.2mL/kg; higher doses may be needed. Test details: www.endocrinesurgeon.co.uk/atoz/calcium%20infusion%20test.html. Get expert help.

Thyroid function tests (TFTs)

Thyroid hormone abnormalities are usually due to a problem with the thyroid gland itself. Primary abnormalities of TSH and thyrotrophin-releasing hormone (TRH) are very rare.

Physiology The hypothalamus secretes TRH, a tripeptide, which stimulates production of TSH, a glycoprotein, from the anterior pituitary. TSH ↑production and release of thyroxine (T4) and triiodothyronine (T3) from the thyroid, which exert –ve feedback on TSH production. The thyroid produces mainly T4, which is 5-fold less active than T3. 85% of T3 is formed from peripheral conversion of T4. Most T3 and T4 in plasma is protein bound, mainly to thyroxine-binding globulin (TBG). The *unbound* portion is the active part. T3 and T4 ↑cell metabolism, via nuclear receptors, and are thus vital for growth and mental development. They also enhance catecholamine effects.

Basic tests • *Hyperthyroidism suspected:* Ask for T3, T4, and TSH. A minority will have elevation of only one thyroid hormone, but all will have ↓TSH (except for the rare phenomenon of a TSH-secreting pituitary adenoma).

• *Hypothyroidism suspected or monitoring replacement treatment:* Ask for only T4, and TSH. Measuring T3 does not add any extra information.

Interpretation of tests

• *If ↑TSH and ↓T4:* Primary hypothyroidism is confirmed.

• *If ↑TSH and normal T4:* Confirmation of compensated or subclinical hypothyroidism (2nd BOX on p307). Treatment depends on clinical state.

• *If ↑TSH and ↑T4:* Consider concordance/compliance problems with T4 replacement, TSH secreting tumour, or thyroid hormone resistance.

• *If ↓TSH and ↑T4 or ↑T3:* Thyrotoxicosis confirmed.

• *If ↓TSH and T4 and T3 normal:* Subclinical thyrotoxicosis, identify cause.

• *If ↓TSH and ↓T4 and ↓T3:* Consider pituitary disease or sick euthyroidism.

• *If normal TSH and T4 abnormal:* Consider hormone-binding problems, eg pregnancy; ↑thyroid-binding globulin; amiodarone; pituitary TSH tumour.

Sick euthyroidism In any systemic illness, TFTs may become deranged. The typical pattern is for 'everything to be low'. Consequently, routine testing of thyroid function in such patients should not be performed.

Special tests *Free T4 & free T3* are useful when a false low or high T4 or T3 is suspected. If unavailable, consider: free thyroxine index which is an estimate of free T4 derived from measuring unoccupied thyroxine-binding sites on TBG. Occasionally, low TSH may be due to non-thyroidal illness: if free T4 >25pmol/L, then there probably really is thyroid disease. *Other tests of thyroid anatomy/pathology:* Consider an *isotope scan* if:

• There is an area of *thyroid enlargement*.

• *Hyperthyroid* but *no thyroid enlargement* (diffuse uptake? solitary nodule?).

• If *hyperthyroid* with one *nodule* (solitary nodule or multinodular?).

• To determine extent of *retrosternal goitre*; to find ectopic thyroid tissue.

• To detect thyroid metastases (whole-body CT).

• Subacute thyroiditis: very low uptake.

Interpretation: The main question is: has the enlarged area increased (hot), or decreased (cold), or the same (neutral) uptake of pertechnetate as the remaining thyroid? 20% of 'cold' nodules are malignant. Few neutral and almost no hot nodules are malignant.

Ultrasound: This distinguishes cystic (usually, but not always, benign) from solid (possibly malignant) 'cold' nodules.

Thyroid autoantibodies: Antithyroid globulin; antithyroid microsomal. Raised in Hashimoto's and some cases of Graves' disease—if positive there is increased risk of hypothyroidism later.

Thyroid-stimulating immunoglobulins: Against TSH receptor. May be raised in Graves' disease. *Serum thyroglobulin:* Useful in monitoring the treatment of carcinoma, and in detection of factitious (self-medicated) hyperthyroidism.

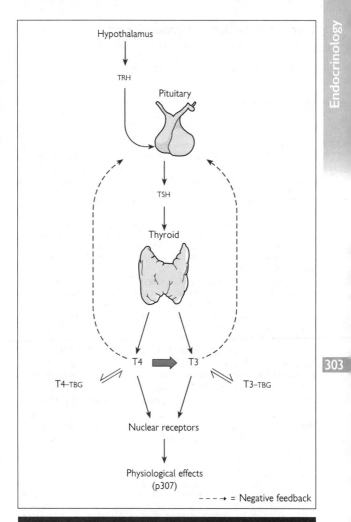

T4–TBG

T3–TBG

- - - → = Negative feedback

The role of scans in monitoring thyroid malignancy

Imaging is most important in following-up differentiated thyroid cancer (DTC) and medullary thyroid cancer (MTC). DTC may be followed with serum thyroidglobulin and ^{131}I whole body scintigraphy when serum thyroglobulin level is ↑. When ^{131}I scintigrams are –ve, thallium scintigraphy (^{201}Tl) may best identify site of recurrent DTC.[39] Alternative radioisotopes, ultrasound, and CT also help localize DTC metastases. MTC recurrences and metastases are more difficult to image. Selective venous catheterization is the most sensitive and specific method for detecting areas of recurrent MTC. High-resolution ultrasound, CT, MRI, and scintigraphy are all used.[40]

Hyperthyroidism (thyrotoxicosis)

Symptoms Weight↓ despite increased appetite, heat intolerance, sweating, diarrhoea, tremor, irritability, frenetic activity, emotional lability, psychosis, itch, oligomenorrhoea. Infertility may be the presenting problem.

Signs Pulse↑, AF, warm peripheries, fine tremor, goitre ± nodules, palmar erythema, hair thinning, lid lag (eyelid lags behind eye's descent as patient watches your finger descend slowly). If BP↑, consider phaeochromocytoma.
Additional signs in Graves' disease: Bulging eyes (exophthalmos, p305); thyroid bruit; ophthalmoplegia; vitiligo; pretibial 'myxoedema' (oedematous swellings above lateral malleoli: the term *myxoedema* is confusing here); thyroid acropachy (an extreme manifestation of autoimmune thyroid disease, with clubbing, painful finger & toe swelling, and periosteal reaction in limb bones).

Tests TSH↓; free T4 and free T3 ↑ (p302). Thyroid scan if subacute thyroiditis suspected or to identify solitary nodules/diffuse multinodular goitre; thyroid autoantibodies. If ophthalmopathy, test visual fields, acuity, and eye movements. Can the lids close fully? If not, there is risk of keratopathy (get help).

Causes *Graves' disease:* Common between 30 and 50 yrs. Genetic influence. ♀ : ♂ ≈ 9 : 1. There are TSH-receptor antibodies (react with orbital autoantigens.) Diffuse thyroid enlargement. Look for associated normochromic normocytic anaemia, ESR↑, Ca^{2+}↑, LFT↑—and type 1 DM and pernicious anaemia. Patients are often hyperthyroid but may be, or become, hypo- or euthyroid.

Toxic adenoma: There is a nodule producing T3 and T4. On scanning, the nodule is 'hot' (p302), and the rest of the gland is suppressed.

Toxic multinodular goitre: This is a common cause of thyrotoxicosis in the elderly, eg in iodine-deficient areas. Treat the thyrotoxicosis, and follow with radioiodine or surgery as indicated. In compressive symptoms, risk of malignancy, or cosmetic deformity develops, surgery may also be indicated.

Self-medication: This is detected by ↑T4, ↓T3, and ↓thyroglobulin.

Subacute (de Quervain's) thyroiditis: Self-limiting, painful goitre. ESR↑. On scans, no radioiodine uptake. *Cause:* ?viral infection in the genetically predisposed.

Follicular carcinoma of thyroid: There may be hyperfunctioning metastases.

Choriocarcinoma; struma ovarii: (Ovarian teratoma containing thyroid tissue).

Drugs: Amiodarone; lithium (↓T4 is commoner); Li^+ may also mask hyperthyroidism by causing cellular unresponsiveness (∴ danger on stopping Li^+).

Exogenous iodine: Contrast media; disinfectants; food contamination.

Treatment

1 **Drugs:** Immediate symptom control: *propranolol* 40mg/6h PO. Thyroid suppression with *carbimazole* eg 15–40mg/24h PO for 4wks, gradually reducing according to TFTs every 1–2 months. Maintain on ~15mg/24h for 12–18 months then withdraw. >50% relapse; warn to get advice if rashes, sore throat, or fevers occur, as 0.03% on carbimazole get agranulocytosis; other SE: rash, headache, alopecia, pruritus, jaundice. Alternative: *propylthiouracil*.

2 **Partial thyroidectomy:** Carries risk of damage to recurrent laryngeal nerves and parathyroids. Patients may be hypo- or hyperthyroid after surgery.

3 **Radioiodine (^{131}I):** This can be repeated until euthyroid but most patients ultimately become hypothyroid. Caution in active Graves' disease. No longer contraindicated in younger women.

4 **In pregnancy and infancy:** Get expert help. See OHCS p157.

Complications *Heart failure* (thyrotoxic cardiomyopathy); *angina; atrial fibrillation* (p130,—seen in ~25%—manage by controlling hyperthyroidism; warfarinize if no contraindication, p648, as 40% have or get emboli). Also: *Osteoporosis; gynaecomastia;* ►► *thyroid storm*, p820; *ophthalmopathy,* see BOX.

Thyroid eye disease

Thyroid eye disease is a clinical diagnosis which may be made in the presence or absence of thyroid autoantibodies. It occurs when there is retro-orbital inflammation and lymphocyte infiltration resulting in swelling of the contents of the orbit. At the time of presentation, the patient may be euthyroid, hypothyroid, or hyperthyroid.

Symptoms Diplopia, eye discomfort, or protrusion ± decreased acuity. ►Decreasing acuity or loss of colour vision may mean optic nerve compression: *Seek expert advice immediately as decompression may be needed.* Nerve damage does not necessarily go hand-in-hand with protrusion. Indeed, if the eye cannot protrude for anatomical reasons, optic nerve compression is all the more likely—a paradox!

Signs Exophthalmos—appearance of protruding eye; proptosis—eyes protrude beyond the orbit (look from above in the same plane as the forehead); conjunctival oedema; corneal ulceration; papilloedema; loss of colour vision. Ophthalmoplegia (especially of upward gaze) also occurs due to muscle swelling and fibrosis.

Tests Rose Bengal drops may stain the upper cornea, indicating superior limbic keratitis, while CT/MRI of the orbits will reveal enlarged eye muscles.

Management Control hyperthyroidism; steroids if ophthalmoplegia or gross oedema. Avoid hypothyroidism. *Get an eye surgeon's help* (eg in papilloedema, vision↓). Stopping smoking may ↓complications. Viscotears® plus Lacrilube® gel at night, for lubrication as often as needed. Lids can be stitched together at the outer corners (lateral tarsorraphy) or may be taped shut. Medical decompression may be achieved with high-dose systemic steroids. Lid retraction may be reduced by guanethidine eyedrops but these are rarely tolerated for long. Surgical decompression uses space in the ethmoidal, sphenoidal, and maxillary sinuses, via a medioinferior approach. Orbital radiotherapy is increasingly used at an early stage, but cytotoxic drugs, and plasmapheresis (p670) are unreliable. Diplopia may be managed with a Fresnel prism stuck to 1 lens of a spectacle, so allowing for reasonably easy changing as the exophthalmos changes.

Eye disease may pre-date other signs of Graves' disease, and does not always respond to treatment of thyroid status. Furthermore, it may develop for the first time following treatment of hyperthyroidism.

Hypothyroidism (myxoedema)

This is common and easy to treat. ►As it is insidious, both the patient and the doctor may not realize anything is wrong, so be alert to subtle and non-specific symptoms, particularly in women over 40yrs old.

Symptoms Tiredness, lethargy, weight↑, constipation, dislike of cold, menorrhagia, hoarse voice, depression, poor cognition/dementia, myalgia.

Signs Bradycardia, dry skin and hair, goitre, slowly relaxing reflexes, CCF, non-pitting oedema (eg eyelids, hands, feet) ± 'toad-like face', pericardial effusion, peripheral neuropathy, cerebellar ataxia.

Diagnosis T4↓, TSH (↑in thyroid failure, slightly ↓ or normal in rare secondary hypothyroidism due to TSH lack from the pituitary, p318). Cholesterol and triglyceride may be↑. Normochromic macrocytic anaemia. CK, AST, and LDH may be↑ due to abnormal muscle membranes. See also p302.

Causes of primary hypothyroidism

Spontaneous primary atrophic hypothyroidism: Common, autoimmune disease which is essentially Hashimoto's without the goitre and is associated with type I diabetes, Addison's disease, or pernicious anaemia. ♀:♂ ≈ 6:1.

Post-thyroidectomy or radioiodine treatment.

Drug-induced: Antithyroid drugs; amiodarone; lithium; iodine.

Subacute thyroiditis: Temporary hypothyroidism after hyperthyroid phase.

Iodine deficiency: Poor diet. *Genetic:* eg with deafness (Pendred's syndrome).

Dyshormonogenesis: Autosomal recessive eg from peroxidase deficiency. Look for ↑radioiodine gland uptake displaced by potassium perchlorate.

Rare associations: Cystic fibrosis, primary biliary cirrhosis, POEMs syndrome (**p**olyneuropathy, **o**rganomegaly, **e**ndocrinopathy, **M**-protein band from a plasmacytoma + **s**kin pigmentation/tethering).

Screen for hypothyroidism if:
- Hyperprolactinaemia
- Post-partum thyroiditis
- Infertility
- Obesity
- Hypothermia
- If neck irradiated
- Cholesterol↑
- Dementia
- Autoimmunity
- Congenital hypothyroidism
- On amiodarone or Li⁺
- Depression ± ↓cognition
- Type 1 DM and pregnant
- Turner's syndrome

Treatment *If healthy and young:* Thyroxine (T4 = levothyroxine), ~100µg/24h PO; review at 12wks. Adjust dose by clinical state and to normalize but not suppress TSH. Then check TSH yearly, at least at first. Osteoporosis is a theoretical risk of overtreating. *If elderly:* Start with 25µg/24h; ↑dose, eg every 4wks (►thyroxine may precipitate angina). Thyroxine's $t_{1/2}$ is ~7d, so any change in dosage will take ~4wks to be assessed accurately by TSH (NB: TSH itself has a $t_{1/2}$ of only ~1h). *If ischaemic heart disease:* Give propranolol 40mg/6h PO and start with 25µg/24h of thyroxine as above. *If diagnosis is in question and T4 already given:* Stop T4; recheck TSH in 6wks.

Causes of goitre + hypothyroidism *Hashimoto's thyroiditis:* Autoimmune disease in which there is lymphocyte and plasma cell infiltration. Usually in women aged 60–70yrs. Often euthyroid. Autoantibody titres high. Treat as above if hypothyroid or to reduce goitre if TSH high. *Drugs:* As above.

The effects of amiodarone on the thyroid are complex and variable. It commonly causes a rise in free T4, and a fall in free T3, but clinically the patient may remain euthyroid. 2% of patients have clinically significant changes—which may be hyperthyroidism or hypothyroidism. Be guided more by clinical state than tests. Seek expert help. Note that $t_{1/2}$ is long (40–100d), so problems persist after withdrawal.

Secondary hypothyroidism (from pituitary failure, p318) is very rare.

Thyroid disease in pregnancy and neonates See *OHCS* p157.

Why are symptoms of hypothyroidism so many, so various, and so subtle?

Almost all our cell nuclei have receptors showing a high affinity for T3: that known as TRα-1 is abundant in muscle and fat; TRα-2 is abundant in brain; and TRβ-1 is abundant in brain, liver, and kidney. These receptors, via their influence on various enzymes, affect the following processes:
- The metabolism of substrates, vitamins, and minerals.
- Modulation of all other hormones and their target-tissue responses.
- Stimulation of O_2 consumption and generation of metabolic heat.
- Regulation of protein synthesis, and carbohydrate and lipid metabolism.
- Stimulation of demand for co-enzymes and related vitamins.

Subclinical hypothyroidism[56]

Features TSH↑ but T4 and T3 ↔, and no obvious symptoms. The context may be follow-up after partial thyroidectomy or ^{131}I, or just a 'routine test' (~10% of those >55yrs old have TSH 3.5–20 mU/L). The risk of progression to frank hypothyroidism is ~2%, but increases as TSH↑. However, this risk doubles if thyroid autoantibodies are present, and is ~10% in men.

Management
- Check thyroid autoantibodies.
- Recheck the history: if any non-specific features (eg depression), discuss benefits of treating (p306) with the patient: they may simply feel better, without realizing that they were not functioning optimally.
- One approach to management is to treat (with thyroxine) those patients with a TSH > 10, or those with positive thyroid autoantibodies, previous Graves' disease, or other organ-specific autoimmunity (type 1 DM, myasthenia, pernicious anaemia, vitiligo).[57] If the patient does not fall into any of these categories, monitor TSH annually.
- Risks from well-managed treatment of subclinical hypothyroidism are small (↑risk of atrial fibrillation and osteoporosis only if over-treated).[58]

Parathyroid hormone & hyperparathyroidism

Parathyroid hormone (PTH) is a peptide which causes ↑Ca^{2+} and ↓PO_4^{3-} reabsorption in the kidney, ↑osteoclast activity, and ↑1,25dihydroxy vitamin D_3 production in the kidney. The overall effect is to ↑Ca^{2+} and ↓PO_4^{3-} in plasma.

Primary hyperparathyroidism (1HPT) Causes: ~80% solitary adenoma, ~15% hyperplasia, ~4% multiple adenomas, ~1.5% primary neoplasia.

Presentation: Often asymptomatic ↑Ca^{2+} or BP↑ on routine tests; osteopenia/osteoporosis (bone pain ± fractures), abdominal pain, renal stones, mood↓, pancreatitis, ulcers (duodenal : gastric ≈ 7 : 1; but gastrinomas common if MEN1).

Other presentations relate to ↑Ca^{2+} and effects of ↑PTH on the skeleton:
- Confusion
- Dehydration
- Mobility↓
- Thirst, nocturia, anorexia (∵ Ca^{2+}↑)
- Stiff joints
- Myopathy

Thirst may be severe. Hyperparathyroidism must pass through your mind whenever a patient says 'I always take a jug of water to bed'.

Associations with multiple endocrine neoplasia (MEN): See BOX.

Blood tests: Ca^{2+}↑, PO_4^{3-}↓ (unless renal failure), alk phos↑, PTH↑, or ↔ creatinine, 24h urine for Ca^{2+}. *DEXA bone scan* (p698). Any evidence of bone reabsorption, ie *osteitis fibrosa et cystica* (brown tumours) and subperiosteal resorption (*hand x-ray*)? Also consider: CXR; *skull x-ray* ('pepper-pot skull'); *pelvic x-ray*.

Treatment Surgical excision[1] prevents fractures and gastric ulcers. Also consider for: brown tumours; osteoporosis; renal calculi; pancreatitis. Pre-op ultrasound can locate the source of PTH. If this fails, try an MIBI scan, before surgical exploration. (MIBI = methoxy-isobutyl isonitrile.) Do plasma Ca^{2+} daily for ≥14d' post-op (danger is Ca^{2+}↓). Mild symptoms may not merit surgery—advise ↑fluid intake to stop stones forming; review every 6 months. *Post-op recurrence:* Seen in ~8% of patients over 10yrs (in one big series).

Secondary hyperparathyroidism (2HPT) (PTH↑ as appropriate for a low Ca^{2+}). Ectopic/metastatic calcification may be a feature (para-articular sites, heart valves, and anterior thigh, and major arteries[2]). *Causes:* chronic renal failure; dietary lack of vit D. *R:* Phosphate binders; vit D analogues; ?calcimimetics[3]—see renal osteodystrophy (bone disease), p276.

Tertiary hyperparathyroidism (3HPT) occurs after prolonged secondary hyperparathyroidism, if 1 or more glands act autonomously (eg with adenoma formation), causing Ca^{2+}↑ from ↑↑ secretion of PTH unlimited by feedback control. It is chiefly seen in chronic renal failure or after renal transplants (in 2%). It may be possible to limit resection to just the adenomatous glands.

Malignant hyperparathyroidism Parathyroid-related protein (PTHrP) produced eg by lung cancers, mimics PTH, resulting in Ca^{2+}↑ (∵ low PTH).

Hypoparathyroidism

Primary hypoparathyroidism PTH secretion↓ due to gland failure, eg removal during neck surgery. *Blood tests:* Ca^{2+}↓, PO_4^{3-}↑ or ↔, alk phos ↔. *Signs and symptoms:* Features of hypocalcaemia (p694). *Associations:* Pernicious anaemia; Addison's; hypothyroidism; hypogonadism. Treatment is with alfacalcidol (p694). Lifelong follow-up required.

Pseudohypoparathyroidism (failure of target cell response to PTH). *Signs:* Round face, short metacarpals and metatarsals. Basal ganglia calcification. Plasma ↑PTH, alk phos normal or ↑. *Treatment:* As for 1° hypoparathyroidism.

Pseudopseudohypoparathyroidism The morphological features of pseudohypoparathyroidism, but with normal biochemistry. The cause is genetic.

---

1 Eg total parathyroidectomy + autotransplantation of 1 gland to a forearm (removable if hyperparathyroidism recurs); without autotransplantation, alfacalcidol or similar (p276) is needed.
2 Other causes: neoplasia, trauma, paraplegia, atheroma, amyloid, CREST (p420); SLE, nephrocalcinosis, chondrocalcinosis, TB, sarcoid, parasites, pseudohypoparathyroidism, myositis ossificans progressiva.
3 Calcimimetics are under development (eg cinacalcet) to amplify sensitivity of extracellular Ca^{2+} sensing receptors (CaR) to extracellular Ca^{2+}, so suppressing PTH with resultant fall in Ca^{2+}. [@12940896]

Autosomal dominant (pre)malignant paraendocrinopathies/ Multiple endocrine neoplasia (MEN)

MEN syndromes are an extraordinary group of genetic tumour syndromes comprising:[67] • MEN1 & 2 • *Neurofibromatosis*, p402, eg with duodenal somatostatinomas + phaeochromocytomas + medullary thyroid cancer (*MTC*) • *Von Hippel Lindau syndrome* (p736) • *Peutz-Jeghers' syndrome* (p732, eg polyposis + endocrine tumours)[68] • *Carney complex*—adrenal hyperplasia + pituitary adenomas + skin & heart myxomas (any chamber) + mucosal lentigos + schwannomas + testicular tumours.[69]

MEN type-1 (=MEN1): Parathyroid hyperplasia (± superimposed clonal tumour growth) + pituitary adenoma + pancreatic tumours—gastrinomas (p740), islet cell tumours (p300), or VIPomas (rare, p218). The MEN1 gene is a tumour suppressor gene; menin, its protein, alters transcription activation.[70] Many cases are sporadic: here typical presentation is in the 3rd–5th decades.

MEN2a: MTC + pheochromocytoma + parathyroid hyperplasia (rarer than with MEN1).[71,72] ►Tests for mutations in the *ret* proto-oncogene are revolutionizing MEN2 treatment by enabling thyroidectomy before neoplasia occurs.[73] **NB:** *ret* mutations rarely contribute to sporadic parathyroid tumours.

MEN2b (= MEN3 = MEN-III)[74] is like MEN2a but has neuro-cutaneous signs (mucosal neuroma 'bumps' eg on: lips, cheeks, tongue, glottis, lids, with visible corneal nerves),[75] and a Marfanoid appearance (p730)—but *without* any hyperparathyroidism.[76] Additional signs: slipped upper femoral epiphyses, and delayed puberty. MEN2b is caused by a mis-sense mutation in the *ret* gene giving rise to a single amino acid substitution (Met918 by Thr).[77]

Adrenal cortex & Cushing's syndrome PLATE 15

Physiology The adrenal cortex produces: *glucocorticoids* (eg cortisol), which affect carbohydrate, lipid, and protein metabolism, and *mineralocorticoids* (eg aldosterone, p688). Corticotrophin-releasing factor (CRF) from the hypothalamus stimulates secretion of ACTH from the pituitary, which in turn stimulates cortisol, and androgen production by the adrenal cortex. Cortisol is excreted as urinary free cortisol and as various 17-oxogenic steroids.

Cushing's syndrome Chronic glucocorticoid excess. 90% are ACTH-dependent; of these 90% are pituitary in origin. 90% of pituitary causes are microadenomas (defined as lesions <1 cm in size) and MRI only detects 70% of them.

ACTH-dependent causes:
- *Cushing's disease:* Adrenal hyperplasia due to excess ACTH from pituitary tumour. Commoner in women. Peak age: 30–50yrs.
- *Iatrogenic:* ACTH administration.
- *Ectopic ACTH production:* Especially small cell lung cancer and carcinoid tumours. Typical features include pigmentation, weight loss, metabolic alkalosis, and hyperglycaemia. Classic features of Cushing's are often absent.
- *Ectopic CRF production* (rare).

ACTH-independent causes:
- *Iatrogenic:* Pharmacological doses of steroids (common).
- *Adrenal adenoma and carcinoma (~20%):* Carcinoma may be associated with abdominal pain and virilization in women.
- *Carney complex:* Cardiac myxoma, freckles, etc., p309. • Alcohol.

The patient *Symptoms:* Weight↑; irregular menses; amenorrhoea; hirsutism♀; impotence♂; depression; weakness; fractures. *Signs:* Tissue wasting; myopathy; thin skin; purple abdominal striae; bruising; osteoporosis; water retention; neck (*buffalo hump*; supraclavicular fat pad); predisposition to infection; ↓wound healing; hirsutism; hypertension; hyperglycaemia (30%).

Tests See BOX. First, confirm the diagnosis, and localize the source on the basis of laboratory testing (below). Then use imaging studies to confirm the likely source. *Note:* adrenal 'incidentalomas' occur on 1% or more of CTs, so identification of an adrenal mass does *not* prove adrenal source of cortisol excess (pituitary incidentalomas are not infrequent either). Abdominal CT if adrenal source is suspected; pituitary MRI (and consider petrosal sinus sampling) if a pituitary source (Cushing's disease) is suspected (p320).

Treatment Depends on the cause.
- Iatrogenic: remove source if possible.
- Surgery: for adrenal adenomas (usually curative) and carcinomas (rarely curative). Radiotherapy and medical treatment follow for carcinoma.
- Cushing's disease: selective removal of pituitary adenoma via a transsphenoidal or very rarely trans-frontal approach. Bilateral adrenalectomy if the source cannot be located, or recurrence post-surgery (but this may be complicated by *Nelson's syndrome* with development of enlarging pituitary tumour and hyperpigmentation). Radiotherapy is used in children and to prevent Nelson's syndrome.
- Ectopic ACTH production may be treated by surgery if the tumour can be located and has not spread. Medical treatment may be required.
- Medical treatment, eg metyrapone, aminoglutethimide, or ketoconazole to ↓plasma cortisol. Adrenolytic agents are also available. Do not expect osteoporosis to fully reverse after drug treatment, but it may after surgery.

Prognosis In 1 study, the easiest variety to diagnose and treat was the adrenal adenoma; adrenal carcinoma was typically incurable. Ectopic ACTH syndrome was amenable to ketoconazole or complete resection of the offending tumour or bilateral adrenalectomy. 44% of pituitary-dependent Cushing's responded to trans-sphenoidal microadenoma resection (recurrence is a problem even after many years).

Assessment of suspected Cushing's syndrome: *screening tests*

- The best screening test is the *overnight dexamethasone suppression test*. Give dexamethasone 1mg PO at midnight; check serum cortisol before, and at 8AM. If level suppresses to <50nmol/L, then it is probably not Cushing's. False negative rate: <2%; false +ve rate: 12.5%.
- *24h urinary free cortisol* (normal: <280nmol/24 h) is an alternative.

NB: False positives ('pseudocushing's') are seen in depression, obesity, alcohol excess, and inducers of liver enzymes which ↑ the rate of dexamethasone metabolism (eg phenytoin, phenobarbital, and rifampicin).

Further tests (False +ves may occur, as above)
- *The 48h dexamethasone suppression test:* Give dexamethasone 0.5mg/6h PO for 2d. Measure cortisol at 0 and 48h (do the last test 6h after the last dexamethasone dose).
- *Circadian rhythm of cortisol secretion:* Requires hospital admission. Normal rhythm (cortisol *lowest* at midnight, *highest* early in the morning) is lost in Cushing's syndrome. Stress, illness, and venepuncture may interfere with the normal rhythm, making interpretation difficult.

Localization tests (where is the lesion?)—If the above are positive.
Plasma ACTH:
- If undetectable, adrenal tumour likely. CT/MRI of adrenal glands. May need to resort to adrenal vein sampling, and *adrenal scintigraphy* (radio-labelled cholesterol derivative).
- If detectable, distinguish pituitary causes from ectopic ACTH production with high-dose dexamethasone suppression test or CRH test.

High-dose dexamethasone suppression test:
  - Give dexamethasone 2mg/6h PO for 2d.
  - Measure plasma and urinary cortisol at 0 and 48h.
  - Complete or partial suppression if Cushing's disease.

CRH test:
  - 100µg ovine corticotrophin releasing hormone IV.
  - Follow cortisol for 120min.
  - Cortisol rises with pituitary disease but not with ectopic ACTH production.

If both tests indicate that cortisol responds to manipulation, image the pituitary (CT/MRI). If not, hunt for the source of ectopic ACTH production.
Plasma sampling from inferior petrosal sinus May help distinguish Cushing's disease from ectopic ACTH production and in lateralizing a pituitary adenoma, if the above tests are discrepant.

Addison's disease (adrenal insufficiency)

Primary adrenocortical insufficiency is rare (incidence ~0.8/100,000). Its signs are capricious; as diagnosis may only be made at necropsy, it is called *the unforgiving master of non-specificity and disguise.* You may diagnose a viral infection or anorexia nervosa in error (K+ is ↓ in the latter but ↑ in Addison's). *Think of Addison's in all those with unexplained abdominal symptoms.*
▶▶Anyone on prednisone for long enough to suppress the pituitary–adrenal axis or who has overwhelming sepsis, or is on anticoagulants, or has metastatic cancer may suddenly develop adrenal insufficiency with deadly hypovolaemic shock, hyperkalemia, hyponatraemia, and hypoglycemia. ▶▶See p822.

Causes 80% autoimmune in UK (↑adrenal antibodies[1] ± associated Graves', Hashimoto's, DM, pernicious anaemia, hypoparathyroidism, vitiligo, coeliac disease). *Others:* TB; metastases (Addison's only if >90% of adrenal tissue lost); lymphoma; HIV (CMV, *Mycobacterium avium*, etc., p581); adrenal bleeding (Waterhouse–Friederichsen, ▶▶p738; SLE; antiphospholipid syndrome).

Symptoms • Fatigue • Abdominal pain • Myalgia • Depression • Anorexia • Weight↓ • D&V (or nausea) • Arthralgia • Psychosis • Weakness • Dizziness • Constipation • Cramps • Self-esteem↓[2] • 'Viral illness' • Fainting • Cold intolerance • Headaches • Confusion

Signs Hyperpigmentation (palmar creases, buccal mucosa); vitiligo; postural hypotension. ▶▶ *Signs of critical deterioration (p822):* Pulse↑; T°↑; shock; coma.

Tests—*General:* K+↑; Na+↓; glucose↓; uraemia; mild acidosis; Ca²⁺↑; eosinophilia; neutropenia; lymphocytosis; Hb↓; LFT↑. *ECG:* PR and QT interval↑.

Specific: Short ACTH stimulation test (Synacthen® test): Do plasma cortisol before and ½h after tetracosactide (=Synacthen®) 250µg IM. Exclude Addison's if initial cortisol >140nmol/L, and 2nd cortisol >500nmol/L. Steroid drugs may interfere with this assay: check with local lab. *ACTH:* In Addison's disease ACTH >300ng/L (inappropriately high). Low in secondary causes.

Plasma renin activity and aldosterone: To assess mineralocorticoid status.

21-Hydroxylase adrenal autoantibodies: In APS-2[1] these may be positive.

AXR (plain abdominal films)/CXR: Any signs of past TB, eg calcification? Have a low threshold for further TB tests (especially if autoantibodies -ve), eg adrenal CT.

Treatment Replace steroids: *hydrocortisone* 20mg in morning, 10mg at bedtime PO. Mineralocorticoid replacement may be needed if postural hypotension, Na+↓, K+↑, or plasma renin↑. If necessary give *fludrocortisone* PO 50µg every 2nd day to 0.15mg daily. Adjust on clinical grounds.

If there is poor clinical response to treatment, suspect an associated autoimmune disease as above (check thyroid; do Coeliac serology, etc.)

Warn against abruptly stopping steroids. Patients should have syringes at home (+ in-date IM hydrocortisone in case vomiting prevents oral intake). Emphasize that prescribing doctors/dentists must know of steroid use (give *steroid card*; advise wearing a bracelet declaring steroid use). Double steroids in febrile illness, injury, or severe stress. For dentistry, double morning hydrocortisone. If vomiting, replace hydrocortisone with hydrocortisone sodium succinate 100mg IM, and get medical help; IV fluids if dehydrated.

Follow-up Yearly (include BP and U&E); watch for other autoimmune disease.

Prognosis Good, if associated diseases (TB; autoimmunity) do not intrude.

Other causes of primary hypoadrenalism *Late-onset congenital adrenal hyperplasia:* Due to 21-hydroxylase deficiency, causing ↑urinary androgens.

1 *Autoimmune polyendocrine syndromes (APS)—APS-1:* Candidiasis + hypoparathyroidism + Addison's ± amenorrhoea. Cause: mutations of AIRE (AutoImmuneREgulator) gene on chromosome 21. [@12817789] *APS-2:* Addison's disease + autoimmune thyroid diseases ± type 1 DM. HLA DR3/DR4-associated. *APS-3:* Autoimmune thyroid disease + autoimmune diseases (excluding Addison's & hypoparathyroidism). **2** *Dehydroepiandrosterone (DHEA)* and DHEA sulfate are adrenal steroid precursors and centrally acting neurosteroids. Glucocorticoid and mineralocorticoid replacement do not correct its lack. When DHEA is given, features such as self-esteem improve. Hunt P 2000 *J Clin Endocrinol Metab* **85** 4650

Hyperaldosteronism

Primary hyperaldosteronism is excess production of aldosterone, independent of the renin-angiotensin system. Consider this when the following features are present: hypertension, hypokalaemia, alkalosis in someone not on diuretics. Sodium tends to be mildly raised or normal.

Causes: >50% due to unilateral adrenocortical adenoma (*Conn's syndrome*). Also: bilateral adrenocortical hyperplasia; adrenal carcinoma (rare); glucocorticoid-remediable aldosteronism (GRA). In GRA, the ACTH regulatory element of the 11β-hydroxylase gene fuses to the aldosterone synthase gene, increasing aldosterone production, and bringing it under the control of ACTH.

Tests: (see BOX) U&E (when not on diuretics, hypotensives, steroids, K^+, or laxatives for 4 wks): do not rely on a low K^+ (>20% are normokalaemic). ↑Aldosterone and ↓renin—normal or high renin excludes the diagnosis. The differential diagnosis relies on assessing the effect of posture on renin, aldosterone, and cortisol (measure at 9AM lying, and at noon standing). If ↓cortisol and ↓aldosterone on standing: ACTH-dependent, ie—Conn's or GRA. If ↓cortisol and ↑aldosterone: angiotensin II-dependent—ie hyperplasia. Do abdo CT/MRI for primary hyperaldosteronism to localize tumour. Seek expert assistance. For GRA (suspect particularly if family history of early hypertension), genetic testing is available. NB: Renal artery stenosis is a more common cause of refractory ↑BP and ↓K^+. evaluate with renal Dopplers, captopril renogram, or angiography (the gold standard).

Treatment: *Conn's:* Surgery (eg laparoscopic); spironolactone up to 300mg per 24h PO for 4wks pre-op. *Hyperplasia:* Spironolactone or amiloride. If GRA is suspected: dexamethasone 1mg/24h PO for 4wks, normalizes biochemistry but not always BP. If BP still↑, give spironolactone; stop dexamethasone.

Secondary hyperaldosteronism Due to a high renin (eg from renal artery stenosis, accelerated hypertension, diuretics, CCF, hepatic failure).

Bartter's syndrome This is a major cause of congenital (recessive) salt wasting—via a Cl⁻ leak in the loop of Henle. Presents in childhood with failure to thrive, polyuria, and polydipsia. BP is *normal* and there is no oedema. Look for hypokalaemia, hypochloraemic metabolic alkalosis, and ↑urinary K^+ and Cl⁻. Plasma renin↑. *Treatments:* K^+ replacement, NSAIDs, amiloride, captopril.

Phaeochromocytoma

This is a rare catecholamine-producing tumour, and a dangerous but treatable cause of hypertension (in <1%). 90% are in the adrenal medulla—unilateral (90%). Inheritance is sometimes as an autosomal dominant.

Associations Sporadic in 84%; others have MEN2a (p309), neurofibromatosis, von Hippel–Lindau syndrome, or Carney complex (p309).

Malignancy 46% have either malignant disease or tumours with some malignant features. Tumours outside the medulla may be in paraganglia (= phaeochrome bodies, ie collections of adrenaline-secreting chromaffin cells)—typically by the aortic bifurcation (called the organ of Zuckerkandl).

The patient Episodic hypertension, anxiety, chest tightness, etc.—see BOX.

Tests Glycosuria during attacks in 30%. Screening: 24h urine collection for 4-OH-3-methoxymandelate (HMMA, VMA) or total (or free) metadrenalines. Full investigation: consult specialist centre: consider meta-iodobenzylguanidine (MIBG) scan or clonidine suppression test, and abdominal CT/MRI.

Treatment Surgery; careful BP control for 2wks pre-op: α-blocker (phenoxybenzamine *before* cardioselective β-blocker). ►Consult anaesthetist. *Post-op:* 24h urine as above; monitor BP (risk of BP↓↓). ►►Emergency ℞: p822.

Follow-up Lifelong, as post-op recurrence may take decades to emerge.

Hypertension: a common context for hyperaldosteronism tests

Think of Conn's in these contexts: hypertension associated with hypo-kalaemia <3.5mmol/L refractory hypertension: severe hypertension occurring before 40yrs of age, especially in women. The aldosterone/renin ratio (ARR) may be a good screening test here. If ratio ≥800 (aldosterone pmol/L): Plasma renin activity (pmol/ml/hr) or aldosterone >1000 further investigation is required ie CT/MRI adrenals. CT only has a specificity of 58% and a positive predictive value of 72%. Adenoma and hyperplasia must then be distinguished, using either NP-59 scintigraphy or adrenal venous sampling.

Adrenal scintigraphy with ^{131}I-labelled 6-β-iodomethylnorcholesterol (NP-59) is a demanding and complex procedure, but it can provide crucial information about adrenal functional status, and guide appropriate management of those with biochemically proven disease—but it does not completely obviate the need for adrenal vein sampling.[25]

The clinical features of phaeochromocytoma

Phaeochromocytomas are rare and present with vague *episodic* features, eg:

- Chest tightness
- 'Spots before the eyes'
- Pins and needles
- Hemianopia
- Pulsatile scotomas

- Skin mottling
- Weight loss
- Dyspnoea
- Purpura
- Sweating

- Abdominal pain
- Tremor
- Cold feet
- Vomiting
- Faints (postural BP drop)

- Palpitations
- Pallor
- Claudication
- Flushing

Symptoms are precipitated by stretching, sneezing, stress, sex, smoking, surgery, or parturition—or by agents such as cheese, alcohol, or the tricyclic you so kindly prescribed, thinking that the patient's bizarre symptoms were only explicable by psychopathology, such as depression.

These crises may last minutes to days. Suddenly patients feel 'as if about to die'—and then get better, or go on to stroke or cardiovascular collapse. On examination, there may be no signs, or hypertension (± signs of cardiomyopathy or heart failure), thyroid swelling (episodic), glycosuria during attacks, or terminal haematuria from a bladder phaeochromocytoma.

Hirsutism, virilism, gynaecomastia, impotence

Hirsutism is common (10% of women) and usually benign. It implies increased hair growth in women, in the male pattern. *If menstruation is normal,* there is almost certainly no increased testosterone production. *If menstruation is abnormal,* the cause is usually *polycystic ovary syndrome* (Stein–Leventhal syndrome): bilateral polycystic ovaries; secondary oligo-menorrhoea; infertility; obesity; hirsutism. The cause is androgen hyper secretion. *Tests:* Ultrasound; ↑plasma LH:FSH ratio, and less consistently, ↑testosterone and ↑oestradiol (see *OHCS* p13 for management). Metformin can restore regular cycles and fertility in some patients. Another cause of hirsutism with irregular menses is *late-onset congenital adrenal hyperplasia*—deficiency of the 21-hydroxylase enzyme in the adrenal gland. See *OHCS* p222. Ovarian tumours are a rare cause, *OHCS* p42.

Management: ▶Be supportive. Explain that she is not turning into a man.
- Depilation with wax or creams, or electrolysis (which is expensive, and time-consuming, but *does* work).
- 1 : 10 hydrogen peroxide to bleach the area.
- Shave regularly.
- Oestrogens help by increasing serum sex hormone-binding globulin—but always combine with a progesterone (= 'the Pill') to prevent excess risk of uterine neoplasia or cyproterone acetate (an anti-androgen and progesto-gen), up to 100mg on days 1–11, with oestrogen on days 1–21. Cypro-terone is also present in the oral contraceptive Dianette®.
- Clomifene (=clomiphene) for infertility (a fertility expert should prescribe).

Virilism is rare. It is characterized by: amenorrhoea; clitoromegaly; deep voice; temporal hair recession; hirsutism. This condition needs further inves-tigation for androgen-secreting adrenal and ovarian tumours.

Gynaecomastia implies an abnormal amount of breast tissue in males (it may occur in normal puberty). It is due to an increase in the oestrogen/androgen ratio. It is seen in syndromes of androgen deficiency (eg Kline-felter's, Kallman's). It may result from liver disease or testicular tumours (oestrogens↑) or accompany hyperthyroidism. The chief causes are drugs: oestrogens; spironolactone; cimetidine; digoxin; testosterone; marijuana.

Erectile dysfunction (ED, impotence—ie inability of an adult male to sustain adequate erection for penetration.) It is common in old age. Psychological causes are common and are more likely if ED occurs only in some situations, if there is a clear stress to account for its onset, and (perhaps) if early morning 'incidental' erections occur (these persist at the onset of organic disease). Psychological causes may exacerbate organic causes. The major organic causes are *smoking*, *alcohol*, and *diabetes*. Other organic causes are as follows.

Drug causes: Antihypertensives (including diuretics and β-blockers), major tranquillizers, alcohol, oestrogens, antidepressants, cimetidine.

Organic causes: Hyperthyroidism, hypogonadism, MS, autonomic neuropathy, atheroma, bladder-neck surgery, prolactin↑, cirrhosis, cancer.

Tests: U&E; LFT; glucose; TFT; LH; FSH; cholesterol; testosterone (eg if libido↓). Nocturnal tumescence studies are not usually needed. Doppler may show ↓blood flow, but is rarely needed as vascular reconstruction is difficult.

Treatment: ● Treat causes. ● Counselling ● Specific interventions. Vacuum aids, implants and intracavernosal injections have largely been supplanted by *oral phosphodiesterase (PDE5) inhibitors* acting by ↑ cyclic guanosine mono-phosphate (GMP). Erection is not automatic (depends on erotic stimuli).
● Sildenafil (Viagra®) 25–100mg ½–1h pre-sex. SE: headache (16%); flushing (10%); dyspepsia (7%); nasal congestion (4%); transient blue/green tingeing of vision via inhibition of retinal PDE6. CI: See BOX. ● Tadalafil (Cialis®; has long $t_{1/2}$) 10–20mg 30min to 12h pre-sex. Don't use > once daily and not every day. SE: headache, dyspepsia, myalgia; ?no visual SEs. ● Vardenafil.

Contraindications to sildenafil/Viagra® and other oral ED agents

Concurrent use of nitrates   Marked renal or hepatic impairment
BP↑↑ or <90/50mmHg; arrhythmias   Stroke in last 6 months
Myocardial infarction <90d ago   Bleeding disorders
Degenerative retinal disorders, eg   Active peptic ulceration
   retinitis pigmentosa (for sildenafil)   Unstable angina

Other cautions
Angina (especially angina during intercourse)
Peyronie's disease
Risk of priapism (sickle-cell anaemia, myeloma, leukaemia)
Concurrent complex antihypertensive regimens
Dyspnoea on minimal effort (sexual activity may be unsupportable)

Use in men with severe coronary disease has been a question, but in one careful study, no adverse cardiovascular effects were detected in men with severe coronary artery disease.

Interactions: Macrolides, anti-HIV drugs, theophylline, ketoconazole, rifampicin, phenytoin, carbamazepine, phenobarbital, grapefruit juice (↑bioavailability).

When does a lifestyle malcontent become a disease?

'When should health providers pay for erectile treatment?' In the UK, the NHS will pay (write 'SLS'/selected list substances on the prescription) if ED is causing severe distress,[1] or there has been:

- Prostatectomy
- Prostate cancer
- Dialysis or a renal transplant
- Spinal cord or pelvic injury
- Radical pelvic surgery[2]
- Diabetes mellitus

- Multiple sclerosis
- Parkinson's disease
- Spina bifida
- Single gene neurological disease
- Poliomyelitis and its after-effects

It is easy to taunt politicians who produce these rather arbitrary-looking criteria by recourse to clever counter-examples, but they really need our support because they are making rationing (which is an inescapable fact of clinical life) *overt, open, available to scrutiny,* and *rational modification.* All too often rationing is covert, and no source takes responsibility for it.

---

1 Criteria include marked disruption to relationships or mood, as judged by any prescriber with purchaser-certified special skill in this area, usually a GP specialist or staff at clinics for ED.
2 Success for reversing ED post-op is only 43% vs 85% in those with neurological conditions.

Hypopituitarism

The 6 anterior pituitary hormones commonly measured are: adrenocortico-trophic hormone (ACTH), growth hormone (GH), follicle-stimulating hormone (FSH), luteinizing hormone (LH), thyroid-stimulating hormone (TSH), and prolactin (PRL). There may be complete loss of anterior pituitary function or selective loss of one hormonal axis, so presentation is very variable.

Causes • Hypophysectomy • Trauma • Pituitary irradiation or adenoma (non-functional or functional with hyposecretion of other hormones, eg acromegaly, prolactinoma, or rarely Cushing's). *Rarer causes:*
• Craniopharyngioma, p320 • Sphenoid meningioma • Abscesses • TB
• Peripituitary glioma • Haemochromatosis • Sheehan's syndrome[1] • Trauma

Features of: *Corticotrophin lack:* Insidious onset afternoon tiredness; dizziness; nausea; pallor; weight↓; postural BP↓; collapse; Na⁺↓, etc., p312.
Gonadotrophin lack: Few, scant, or no menses (oligomenorrhoea; amenorrhoea); fertility↓; libido↓; osteoporosis; breast atrophy; dyspareunia.
Androgen lack: Erectile dysfunction; libido↓; muscle bulk↓; hypogonadism (loss of all hair; small testes; ejaculate volume↓; spermatogenesis↓).
GH lack: Central obesity; atherosclerosis; dry wrinkly skin; strength↓; balance↓; well-being↓; exercise ability↓; cardiac output↓; osteoporosis; glucose↑.
Thyroid lack: Constipated; weight↑; mood↓; dry skin; p306.

Tests (The triple stimulation test is now rarely done.) T4 and TSH reliably diagnoses TSH deficiency. Testosterone, LH, and FSH in men, and a menstrual history + LH and FSH in women are as reliable as the GNRH test. The short Synacthen® test provides sufficient information concerning ACTH deficiency.
• Basal T4, TSH, LH, FSH, prolactin, testosterone. U&E (Na⁺ ∴ dilution), Hb↓ (normochromic, normocytic). *Thyroid deficiency:* T4↓ *but* TSH normal or↓.
• MRI scan; assessment of visual fields.
• *Short Synacthen® test:* (p312—for ACTH deficiency) is nearly as reliable as the insulin tolerance test (ITT), which is now a rarely done 2ⁿᵈ-line gold standard (only do in metabolic units under close supervision).
• *Insulin tolerance test (ITT): CI:* epilepsy, heart disease, adrenal failure. The test involves giving insulin IV, and assessing its effect on cortisol and GH. It is done in morning (water only taken from 22:00h the night before). Have 50% glucose and hydrocortisone to hand and IV line open. Be alert throughout to hypoglycaemia. Consult lab first. *Interpretation:* Glucose must fall below 2.2mmol/L and the patient should become symptomatic. Normal values are: GH >20mU/L, and a peak cortisol >550mmol/L.
• *Arginine + growth hormone releasing hormone test (ARG + GHRH test):* An alternative to the ITT for measuring need for GH; it may have fewer SEs.[2]

Treatment *Hydrocortisone* for secondary adrenal failure (p312). *Thyroxine* if hypothyroid (p306, but TSH useless for monitoring). ♂: 3-weekly *testosterone enanthate* 250mg IM or *transdermal Andropatch®*; apply to clean, dry, unbroken skin on back, upper arm, thigh, or abdomen for 24h (do not use the same site within 7d). ♀: *(pre-menopausal) Oestrogen* (eg as contraceptive steroid pill). Some patients need *growth hormone.* NB: GH has acquired a 'smart drug' status via inappropriate internet advertisements extolling its muscle and potency-enhancing and supposed anti-ageing attributes. SE: prostate hyperplasia; insulin-like growth factor↑ (IGF-1 may ↑risk of cancer, but unproven). If you think your patient might need GH (eg it is known to improve recovery and walking distance after hip surgery), ►ask an endocrinologist first.

Other causes of hypogonadism Trauma, post-orchitis (mumps, brucellosis, leprosy), chemotherapy/irradiation, cirrhosis, alcohol (toxic to Leydig cells), cystic fibrosis, haemochromatosis, syndromes (OHCS p752 eg.): Kleinfelter's (commonest), Laurence-Moon–Biedl, dystrophia myotonica, Prader–Willi, Kallman's (with anosmia + colour blindness; X-linked recessive).

---

1 Sheehan's syndrome (Simmonds' disease) is pituitary necrosis after post-partum haemorrhage.
2 W Kiess 2003 *Clin Endocrinol* **58** 456. Another alternative is a **py**ri**do**stigmine + GHRH (PD + GHRH) test.

NICE guidelines on giving somatropin (GH) in those >25yrs old

Somatotropin is produced by DNA technology; it has the same sequence as human GH. It should only be used in GH deficiency, and if:

1 Peak GH response is <9mU/L (3ng/mL) during an ITT (or equivalent).
2 There is impaired quality of life (QoL), as measured by QoL-AGHDA questionnaires (assessment of hormone deficiency in adults score ≥ 11 points).[1]
3 The person is already receiving treatment for other pituitary hormone deficiencies, as required.

NB: Achieving adult bone mass is a valid indication for somatropin in adults <25yrs old who fulfil criteria 1 but not 2. (Maximum GH secretion is during adolescence; then secretion normally falls by ~14% per decade.)

Self-injection 0.2–0.3mg/d (=0.6–0.9IU); needs ↓ with age; dose titration (1st 3 months of therapy) is done by an endocrinologist. SE: Headache; myalgia; BP↑; carpal tunnel syndrome; fluid retention; ICP↑ (rare). CI: Pregnancy; lactation; major trauma; post-op; malignancy; respiratory failure.

Somatropin should be stopped after 9 months if QoL-AGHDA does not improve by 7 points or more.[1] Using GH in children: See OHCS p184.

1 Improvement in QoL scores during GH replacement has to be viewed with skepticism. This can be dispelled only by randomized trials. Barkan A 2003 J Clin Endocrinol 86 1905

Pituitary tumours

Pituitary tumours (almost always benign adenomas) account for 10% of intracranial tumours. ►Symptoms are caused by local pressure, hormone secretion, or hypopituitarism (p318). There are 3 histological types.

1 *Chromophobe*—70%. Some are non-secretory, but cause hypopituitarism. Local pressure effect in 30%. Half produce prolactin (PRL); a few produce ACTH or GH.

2 *Acidophil*—15%. Secrete GH or PRL. Local pressure effect in 10%.

3 *Basophil*—15%. Secrete ACTH. Local pressure effect rare.

Classification by hormone secreted (may be revealed by immunohistology)

PRL only	35%	ACTH	7%
GH only	20%	LH/FSH/TSH	$\geq 1\%$[1]
PRL and GH	7%	No obvious hormone	30%[2]

Features of local pressure effects Headache; visual field defects (bilateral hemianopia, initially of superior quadrants); palsy of cranial nerves III, IV, VI. Rarely, diabetes insipidus (DI) (p326); which is more likely to result from hypothalamic disease, disturbance of temperature, sleep, and appetite, and erosion through floor of sella leading to CSF rhinorrhoea.

Investigations Pituitary MRI (defines intra- and supra-sellar extension); accurate assessment of visual fields; prolactin, baseline TFTs, short synacthen test, LH/FSH, testosterone, and glucose tolerance test if acromegaly suspected. Water deprivation test if DI is suspected (p326).

Treatment Start hormone replacement as needed, in light of the above.

Surgery: If intrasellar tumour, remove by trans-sphenoidal approach. Suprasellar extension may need a transfrontal approach. *Pre-op:* Check with anaesthetist/surgeon—eg hydrocortisone sodium succinate 100mg IM with pre-med; then every 4h for 72h; then hydrocortisone 20mg PO each morning. *Post-op:* Retest pituitary function (p318) after a few weeks to assess replacement needs.

Medical: Dopamine agonists (p322) are the best treatment for most prolactin-secreting tumours (lowers PRL and can shrink tumour: monitor by MRI). Surgery is not indicated routinely for these. It may also work for some GH-secreting tumours (p322) and also 'non-functional tumours' (some making α-subunit); use higher doses, eg bromocriptine 20–40 mg PO daily.

Radiotherapy: Post-op if complete removal of tumour has not been possible.

Pituitary apoplexy Sudden tumour enlargement due to haemorrhage may cause compression of vessels and neural tissue at the skull base with coma and death without preceding symptoms. Suspect if sudden onset of headache in someone with a known tumour, or if there is sudden headache and loss of consciousness (ie may present like subarachnoid haemorrhage). ΔΔ: Frontal sinusitis, eg when presentation is with fontal tenderness ± periorbital oedema. *Treatment:* Urgent surgery with steroid cover.

Craniopharyngioma Not strictly a pituitary tumour: it originates from Rathke's pouch so is situated between pituitary and the 3rd ventricle floor. 50% present with local pressure effects in children, eg with: headache (50%), vomiting (30%), visual disturbances (20%), polyuria; polydipsia (17%), delayed puberty (20%), short stature (14%), precocious puberty (3%). DI is common. *Tests:* CT/MRI (calcification in 50%). *Treatment:* Surgery; irradiation; test pituitary function (above).

---

1 2003 data show that new(ish) sensitive methods of TSH measurement lead to improved recognition. TSH-secreting tumours are now more frequently found at microadenoma stage, medially located, and *without* associated hypersecretions. In these tumours, somatostatin analogues (p324) are very helpful.
2 Many produce alpha-subunit which may serve as a tumour marker.

Hyperprolactinaemia

This is the most common biochemical disturbance of the pituitary. It tends to present early in women (amenorrhoea) but late in men.

Causes of raised basal plasma prolactin (>390mU/L) Prolactin is secreted from the anterior pituitary and release is inhibited by dopamine produced in the hypothalamus. Therefore, hyperprolactinaemia may result from either excess production, eg prolactinoma, or because of disinhibition, eg compression of the pituitary stalk, reducing local dopamine levels; or due to administration of a dopamine antagonist. A prolactin of 1000–5000mU/L could result from either, but >5000 is likely to be due to an adenoma, with macroadenomas having the highest levels, eg 10,000–100,000.

Physiological: Pregnancy; breast-feeding; stress; sleep.

Drugs and other chemicals (most common cause): Phenothiazines; metoclopramide; haloperidol; α-methyldopa; oestrogens.

Diseases: Prolactinoma, pituitary adenomas, pituitary stalk section, hypothalamic disease, chronic renal failure; hypothyroidism; sarcoidosis.

Symptoms ♀: Libido↓, weight↑, apathy, dry vagina, amenorrhoea; infertility, galactorrhoea. ♂: Impotence, reduced facial hair, galactorrhoea. Osteoporosis and local pressure effects (p320) are also modes of presentation.

Tests Basal plasma prolactin: non-stressful venepuncture between 09.00 and 16.00h. CT/MRI scan of the pituitary fossa if prolactin >1000mU/L.

Management A reasonable approach is as follows:

Microprolactinomas: A tumour <10mm diameter on MRI (~25% of the population have asymptomatic microprolactinomas). Trans-sphenoidal surgery has a high success rate, and a relatively low incidence of side-effects, but is not used in all centres. After surgery, prolactin concentrations are normalized, menstruation starts, and galactorrhoea eliminated in most patients. There is a small but significant recurrence rate.

Alternatively, dopamine agonists such as bromocriptine may be used (1.25mg PO at 22.00 with food; increase weekly by 1.25–2.5mg/d until ~2.5mg/12h). Rarely, patients may require >10mg daily. Follow PRL. Bromocriptine should be stopped in pregnancy—teratogenicity is reported. PRL will rise during pregnancy, there is no need to follow it. If headache or visual loss, check fields and consider neuroimaging. Other SE: pulmonary, pericardial, and retroperitoneal fibrosis; see BNF; watch for cough and dyspnoea.

Macroprolactinomas: A tumour >10mm diameter in association with a prolactin of >3600mU/L is likely to be a macroprolactinoma. If prolactin <3600, then it is probably a non-secretory tumour causing stalk compression and disinhibition of prolactin release. Macroprolactinomas may be treated with bromocriptine, but if there are visual symptoms, pressure effects, or if pregnancy is contemplated (~25% of macroadenomas will expand during pregnancy), then surgery is generally indicated. Usually, a trans-sphenoidal approach is used. Follow-up with serial PRL and MRI. Bromocriptine, and in some cases radiation therapy, may be required post-op because complete surgical resection is uncommon. Pre-op assessment is often difficult: familiarize yourself with case-histories to show complexities of this aspect of endocrinology.[1]

Dopamine agonists Bromocriptine is the established drug, but newer drugs, eg cabergoline (taken weekly) and quinagolide (once daily) are now replacing it (cabergoline *may* be 1st-line therapy). With macroprolactinomas, some centres continue treatment with bromocriptine during pregnancy.

---

1 E Harms 2003 *Dtsch Med Wochenschr* **128** 667. A 46yr-old lady had galactorrhoea for 7yrs, and a ↑prolactin (3133mU/L) and intact pituitary function with no eye signs. MRI showed a 1.9cm pituitary tumour with extrasella extension. Is selective trans-sphenoidal adenomectomy needed for a presumed non-functioning macroadenoma with functional hyperprolactinaemia, or should there be a dopamine-agonist trial? *One possible answer:* try drugs, and monitor MRI if initial prolactin ≥ 2000 mU/L.

Acromegaly

This rare disease is due to hypersecretion of GH from a pituitary tumour. It usually presents between the ages of 30 and 50yrs old.

Prevalence 5 per million.

Clinical features

- *Excessive soft tissue growth:* Coarse, oily skin, large tongue (macroglossia), prominent supraorbital ridge, prognathism, ride-spaced teeth, ↑shoe size, thick spade-like hands, deepening voice, arthralgia, kyphosis, proximal muscle weakness, paraesthesiae—due to carpal tunnel syndrome (p391), progressive heart failure, goitre. Sleep apnoea. Sweating and headache.
- *Features of a pituitary tumour:* Hypopituitarism ± local mass effect (p318).
- *Psychological effects:* Not all patients notice body changes (you may need to study old photos), but take time to ascertain the patient's reaction to their changing body, tactfully ask about associated loss of initiative, decreased spontaneity, mood swings, low self-esteem, body image distortion, disruption in interpersonal relations, social withdrawal, and anxiety.
- *Metabolic effects, eg insulin resistance:* GH acts at several levels to block insulin, including inhibiting phosphorylation of the insulin receptor.

Complications DM; BP↑; left ventricular hypertrophy/cardiomyopathy; colon cancer; ●¯ hyperthyroidism in 4–26% (TSH-dependent or independent).

Investigations

- Isolated GH measurement may show ↑secretion, but levels vary with the time of day and other factors, so random measurements are not diagnostic.
- The definitive test is the OGTT with GH measurement—as described on p294. Collect samples for GH and glucose at: 0, 30, 60, 90, 120, 150min. *Interpretation of OGTT:* normally GH is suppressed, in acromegaly there is no suppression, and levels may rise. False positives: anorexia nervosa, poorly controlled DM, hypothyroidism, Cushing's.
- Serum insulin-like growth factor-1 (IGF-1) is used for screening for acromegaly in some centres. Levels correlate with GH secretion over the past 24h, and so are ↑ if excessive GH secretion, or in pregnancy, or puberty.
- MRI (or CT) scan of pituitary fossa.
- Test pituitary function (p318)—hypopituitarism?
- ECG. Echocardiogram. Visual fields and acuity. Skin thickness.
- Obtain old photos; request a new photo of full face, torso, hands on chest.

Treatment *Trans-sphenoidal surgery:* Usually the treatment of choice. In 60% GH secretion reduces to <10mU/L. 6wks after surgery readmit for OGTT with GH measurement, and full pituitary function testing (p318). If GH fails to suppress below 2.0mU/L, irradiation or medical treatment is needed. Steroids should be stopped before these tests and triple stimulation test may have a role, on day 4 only if no signs of steroid deficiency (postural hypotension, fever, nausea, anorexia). *Yearly follow-up:* (OGTT + GH measurement; T4; PRL; visual fields; x-rays—see above; photos; cardiovascular assessment/ECG).

External irradiation: For older patients or failed surgery. Follow-up as for surgery.

Medical: Somatostatin analogues such as *octreotide* (Sandostatin LAR®, given monthly IM), and *lanreotide* (Somatuline LA®) have displaced dopamine agonists as 1ˢᵗ-line in somatotroph (GH) adenomas (SE: gallstones). Follow-up shows that some cardiac complications resolve after lanreotide (eg LV mass, ventricular filling, and ventricular arrhythmic profile). Monitor glucose tolerance as effects on insulin resistance are unpredictable.

Diabetes insipidus (DI)

This is due to impaired water resorption by the kidney because of reduced ADH secretion from the posterior pituitary (cranial DI), or impaired response of the kidney to ADH (nephrogenic DI).

Symptoms Polyuria; dilute urine; polydipsia; dehydration if not drinking.

Causes of cranial DI Head injury Hypophysectomy Histiocytosis Metastases Sarcoidosis Pituitary tumour Craniopharyngioma Vascular lesion Meningitis Inherited (autosomal dominant)

Idiopathic DI (50%) is often self-limiting, and MRI may show infundibuloneurohypophysitis (known to be lymphocytic, and possibly autoimmune).

Causes of nephrogenic DI Low potassium, high calcium, drugs (lithium, demeclocycline), pyelonephritis, hydronephrosis, pregnancy (rare as a primary cause; due to placental production of vasopressinase; can exacerbate underlying DI from any cause), inherited.

Investigations U&E, Ca^{2+}, plasma, and urine osmolalities.

Plasma osmolality should be high, and urine low. Serum sodium may be high. In psychogenic polydipsia, plasma osmolality is often low.

The water deprivation test will confirm the diagnosis.

The water deprivation test (If 1st morning urine osmolality >600mosmol/kg, DI is excluded.) Stop drugs (eg carbamazepine) before the test.
- Light breakfast, no tea, no coffee, no smoking.
- Weigh at 0, 4, 6, 7, 8h. Stop if >3% body weight lost.
- Supervise carefully to stop patient drinking.
- Empty bladder, then no drinks and only dry food for 8h. Collect urine hourly, measure volume. Measure osmolality at 1, 4, 7, 8h. Stop test if osmolality >600mosmol/kg (DI is excluded).
- Venous sample for osmolality at: 0.5, 3.5, 6.5, 7.5h.
- If plasma osmolality >300mosmol/kg, and urine osmolality <600, give desmopressin 20µg intranasally (or 1µg IM) at 8h. Urine should concentrate within 1h. If plasma osmolality does not rise, do *not* administer desmopressin as hyponatraemia may result.
- Water can be drunk after 8h. Measure urine osmolality at 8, 9, 10, 11, 12h.

Interpreting water deprivation tests: Check if plasma osmolality is >290mosmol/kg to ensure the test has given adequate stimulus for ADH release. *Normal* response is for urine osmolality to be >600mosmol/kg. In *psychogenic polydipsia*, urine is also concentrated (>400mosmol/kg), but rather less than in the normal response. In DI, urine is abnormally dilute (<400mosmol/kg). However, in *cranial* DI, urine osmolality increases >50% after desmopressin, whereas in *nephrogenic* DI, it increases <45% after desmopressin.

Treatment *Cranial DI:* Find the cause. Test pituitary function (p318). Give desmopressin 10–20µg/12–24h intranasally (smallest dose that controls polyuria: higher doses ↑risk of hyponatraemia). An oral formulation is being assessed (DDAVP; there may be fewer problems with water intoxication).

Nephrogenic: Treat the cause. Avoiding high-protein meals and salt may help polyuria. If it persists, try bendrofluazide (=bendroflumethiazide) 5mg PO/24h.

▶▶**Emergency management** *The diagnosis must be made*—eg suitable cause, ↑urine output, urine osmolality↓ (~150mosmol/kg), despite dehydration.
- Do urgent plasma U&E.
- Rehydrate; keep up with output. 5% dextrose, 2L in the 1st hour. If severe hypernatraemia, do not lower Na^+ rapidly, use 0.9% or 0.45% saline.
- Desmopressin 1µg IM (lasts 12–24h).
- In nephrogenic DI, indomethacin 75mg/24h PO can lower urine volume and plasma Na^+.

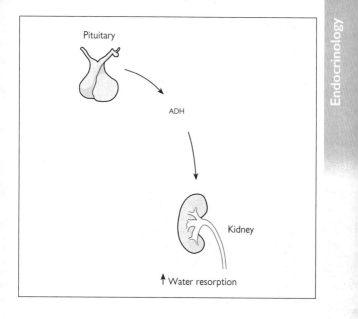

Neurology[1]

Contents

Relevant pages elsewhere: CNS exam/cranial nerve lesions (p55–p57); mental state (p60); psychiatry (p15 & *OHCS* ch 4); nystagmus (p56); facial pain (p72); LP (p752); headache emergencies (p768); coma (p774); coma scale (p776); meningitis (p808); cerebral abscess (p810); status epilepticus (p812); head injury (p814); ↑ICP (p816).

[1] We thank Dr Robert Clifford-Jones who is our Specialist Reader for this chapter.

We dedicate this page to those carers who find themselves responsible for a friend or relative who has a chronic neurological illness, eg stroke, Parkinson's disease, Alzheimer's disease, or motor neurone disease. As a thought-experiment, try spending a morning imagining that you are such a carer—eg trying to expunge the smell of soiled sheets from your clothes, while awaiting a visit from a neighbour, who said he would 'sit with him' so you can catch the bus into town, and, like a guilty hedonist, play truant from your role as nurse for a few sanity-giving hours of normal life. You wait. No one comes. You stop bothering about the smell on your clothes, and turn towards your husband, about to say something, but when your eyes meet his, you realize he does not recognize you—and you keep your thoughts to yourself. Knuckles whiten as you grasp his collar to lift him forward on the commode, and you seem to hear a mocking voice over your shoulder saying: '… so I see we're getting angry with him today, are we?' The ceaseless round from mouth to anus, from bed to chair, from twilight to twilight, continues, *ad infinitum*.

It is all we can do to spend *2 minutes* on this thought-experiment, let alone a morning—or the rest of our lives. We need to be aware of the strategies we adopt to avoid involvement with the naked truth of the shattered lives, which like a tragic subplot, stand behind the farce of morning surgery or out-patients in which we hear ourselves forever saying in plummy complacency: 'And how are *you* today Mrs Salt—your husband, I know… marvellous how you manage. You are a real support to each other. Let me know if I can do anything.' We pretend to be busy, we ensure that we *are* busy, we surround ourselves with students, with white coats, and a miasma of technical expertise—we surround ourselves with *anything* to ensure that there is no chink through which Mrs Salt can shine her rays of darkness. Poor Mrs Salt. Poor us—to be frightened of the darkness, panicking at the thought that we might not have anything to offer, or that we might be called to offer up our equanimity as a sacrifice to Mrs Salt. How dare one little grain upset our carefully contrived universe?

Respite care, medical charities, meals on wheels, laundry services, physiotherapy, transport, day care centres, clubs for carers, visits from district nurses or from a nurse specializing in chronic diseases will go some way to mitigate Mrs Salt's problems. As ever, the way forward is by taking time to listen. Carers' needs evolve. First there is uncertainty, and the need for help in handling this. Next comes the moment of diagnosis with the numbness, denial, and anger that may follow. Then there may be a time of adjusting to reality, characterized by either a frenzied searching for information and advice, or a careful titration by the carer of how much information he or she can handle at any one time. Issues of driving, mobility, finance, sex, and employment are likely to occur throughout the illness, and advice will need to be constantly tailored to suit individual circumstances. But the best thing you can ever offer is the unwritten contract that, come what may, you will be there, available, often ineffectual, but incapable of being alienated by whatever the carer may disclose to you.

The chief questions of bedside neurology

Is there a focal lesion?—or one of the following?

- A general insult, eg trauma, encephalitis, or poisoning, or post-ictal state.
- A lesion of a specific type of nerve cell, eg MND; dementia; subacute combined degeneration of the cord (B$_{12}$↓, p634).
- A disorder of function, eg migraine or epilepsy.
- Medically unexplained symptoms (may have a psychological/psychiatric cause).

A key feature in determining if a focal lesion is present is lack of symmetry—eg one pupil dilated, or an upgoing plantar response.

Where is the lesion? Localization of the site of the lesion depends on recognizing the patterns of cognitive, cranial nerve, motor, and sensory deficits which occur following lesions at different sites in the nervous system. Cognitive, cranial nerve, and motor deficits should be analysed first, and then sensory examination used to confirm the site of the lesion.

Patterns of motor deficits Weakness can arise from lesions of the cortex, corona radiata, internal capsule, brainstem, cord, peripheral nerves, neuro-muscular junction, or muscle. Is the pattern upper or lower motor neurone (UMN or LMN; see BOXES)? *Cortical lesions* may show an unexpected pattern of weakness involving all movements of a hand or foot, with normal or ↓tone—but ↑reflexes more proximally in the arm or leg will suggest an upper rather than lower motor neurone lesion. *Internal capsule* and *corticospinal pathway* brainstem lesions cause contralateral hemiplegia with a pyramidal distribution of weakness (1st BOX). If the hemiplegia occurs with epilepsy, ↓cognition, or homonymous hemianopia (p333), the lesion is in a cerebral hemisphere. A cranial nerve palsy (III–XII) contralateral to a hemiplegia implicates the brainstem on the side of the cranial nerve palsy. *Cord lesions* causing paraplegia (both legs) or quadriparesis/tetraplegia (all limbs) are suggested by finding a motor and reflex level (ie muscles are unaffected *above* the lesion, show LMN signs *at* the level of the lesion, and UMN signs *below* the lesion). *Peripheral neuropathies*: (p390) Most cause a distal pattern of weakness (eg foot-drop or weak hand). Involvement of a single nerve (mono-neuropathy) occurs with trauma or entrapment (carpal tunnel, p391); involvement of several nerves (mononeuritis multiplex) is seen eg in DM.

Sensory deficits Information about the site of a lesion is obtained chiefly from the distribution of the sensory loss, although the range of sensory modalities involved (pain, T°, touch, vibration, and joint position sense) may add information, as pain and T° sensations travel along small fibres in peripheral nerves and spinothalamic tracts in the cord and brainstem—and are distinct from joint position and vibration sense. (The latter travel in fast fibres in the dorsal columns of the cord.) Distal sensory loss suggests a neuropathy and may involve all sensory modalities or be more selective, depending on the pattern of nerve fibre size involved in the peripheral nerve. Individual nerve lesions are identified by their anatomical territories which are usually more sharply defined than those of root lesions (dermatomes, p338), which often show considerable overlap. The hallmark of a cord lesion is a sensory level—ie an area of decreased or absent sensation below the lesion (eg the legs) with normal sensation above this level (eg in abdomen, trunk, and arms). Lateralized cord lesions give a Brown-Séquard syndrome (p720) with dorsal column loss on the side of the lesion and spinothalamic loss in the other legs. Cervical cord lesions (eg syringomyelia, p404 or cord tumours) may cause selective loss of pain and T° sensation with sparing of joint position sense and vibration (dissociated sensory loss). Lateral brainstem lesions show both dissociated and crossed sensory loss with pain and T° loss on the side of the face ipsilateral to the lesion, and contralateral arm and leg sensory loss. Lesions above the brainstem give a contralateral pattern of generalized sensory loss. In cortical lesions, sensory loss is confined to more subtle and discriminating sensory functions (2-point discrimination and stereognosis).

UMN lesions (upper motor neurone)

These are caused by damage to motor pathways anywhere from the motor nerve cells in the precental gyrus of the frontal cortex, through the internal capsule, brainstem, and spinal cord—to the anterior horn cells at the appropriate level in the cord. Typical characteristics are the so-called 'pyramidal'[1] distribution of preferential weakness involving physiological extensors of the upper limb (shoulder abduction; elbow, wrist, and finger extension; and the small muscles of the hand) and the flexors of the lower limb (hip flexion, knee flexion, and ankle dorsiflexion and everters). There is little muscle wasting and *loss of skilled fine finger movements* may be greater than expected from the overall grade of weakness. *Increased tone*, (spasticity) develops in stronger muscles (eg arm flexors and leg extensors). It is manifest as resistance to passive movement that can suddenly be over-come (clasp-knife feel). There is *hyperreflexia*: reflexes are brisk; *plantars are upgoing* (+ve Babinski sign) ± *clonus* (elicited by rapidly dorsiflexing the foot; ≤3 rhythmic, downward beats of the foot are normal; more suggest an UMN lesion) ± a positive *Hoffman's reflex*—passive flicking of a finger (examiner rapidly flexes a DIP joint) causes neighbouring digits to flex. NB: UMN weakness affects *muscle groups* not individual muscles.

LMN lesions (lower motor neurone)

These are caused by damage anywhere from anterior horn cells in the cord, nerve roots, plexi, or peripheral nerves. The distribution of weakness corresponds to those muscles supplied by the involved cord segment, nerve root, part of plexus, or peripheral nerve. See p336. A combination of anatomical knowledge, good muscle testing technique, and experience is needed to distinguish, eg a radial nerve palsy from a C7 root lesion, or a common peroneal nerve palsy from an L5 root lesion (p337).[2] The relevant muscles show *wasting* ± spontaneous involuntary twitching (*fasciculation*)—and feel soft and floppy, providing little resistance to passive stretch (*hypotonia/ flaccidity*). *Reflexes are reduced* or absent, the *plantars remain flexor*. The chief differential is weakness from primary muscle disease—here there is symmetrical loss, reflexes are lost later than in neuropathies, and there is no sensory loss. Myasthenia gravis (MG) causes weakness worsening with use of the affected muscles (↑fatigue); there is little wasting, normal reflexes, and no sensory loss—see p400.

Reflexes and spinal cord level: p55. Spinal roots for each muscle: p336.

Muscle weakness grading (MRC classification)

Grade 0 no muscle contraction Grade 3 active movement against gravity
Grade 1 flicker of contraction Grade 4 active movement against resistance
Grade 2 some active movement   Grade 5 normal power (allowing for age)

Grade 4 covers a big range: 4–, 4, and 4+ denote movement against slight, moderate, and stronger resistance; avoid fudging descriptions—'strength 4/5 throughout' suggests a mild quadriparesis or myopathy. It is better to document 'poor effort' and the maximum grade for each muscle tested.

---

1 *Pyramidal neurons* have basal dendrites and an apical dendrite pointing towards the dorsal cortical border. They are a distinctive cortical feature and are specialized in their dendritic morphology, projection patterns, and localization within the 6 cortical layers. '*Extrapyramidal*' denotes CNS motor phenomena relating to the basal ganglia. Pyramidal lesions result in paresis and spasticity, but extra-pyramidal lesions cause abnormality in initiation and maintenance of movement—negative symptoms include bradykinesia/akinesia (slow/absent movement) and loss of postural reflexes; positive symptoms are tremor, rigidity, and involuntary movements (p352, eg chorea, athetosis, ballismus, and dystonia). **2** The booklet *Aids to the Examination of the Peripheral Nervous System* is invaluable here. ISBN 0-7020-2512-7

Cerebral artery territories

A basic knowledge of the anatomy of the blood supply of the brain is helpful in the diagnosis and management of cerebrovascular disease (p354–362). It is important to be able to identify the area of brain that correlates with a patient's symptoms and identify the affected artery.

Cerebral blood supply The brain is supplied by the 2 internal carotid arteries and the basilar artery (formed by the joining of the 2 vertebral arteries). These 3 vessels feed into an anastomotic ring at the base of the brain called the circle of Willis (below). This arrangement may lessen the effects of occlusion of a feeder vessel proximal to the anastomosis by allowing supply from unaffected vessels. The anatomy of the circle of Willis is, however, highly variable and in many people it cannot provide much protection from ischaemia due to carotid, vertebral, or basilar artery occlusion. Anastomotic supply from other vessels in the neck may mitigate occlusions of feeder vessels—occlusion of the internal carotid in the neck, eg may not cause infarction if flow from the external carotid artery enters the circle of Willis via its anastomosis with the ophthalmic artery.

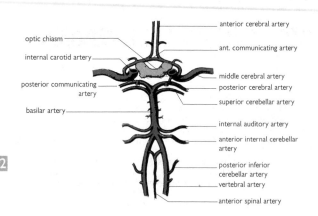

optic chiasm
internal carotid artery
posterior communicating artery
basilar artery

anterior cerebral artery
ant. communicating artery
middle cerebral artery
posterior cerebral artery
superior cerebellar artery
internal auditory artery
anterior internal cerebellar artery
posterior inferior cerebellar artery
vertebral artery
anterior spinal artery

Diagram of the circle of Willis at the base of the brain; see also CT on p363.

Willis and neurology Thomas Willis (1621–75) is one of those happy Oxford heroes belonging to Christ Church College who hold a bogus DM degree—awarded in 1646 for his Royalist sympathies. He had a busy life inventing terms such as 'neurology' and 'reflex'. Not only has his name been given to his famous circle, but he was the first to describe myasthenia gravis, whooping cough, the sweet taste of diabetic urine. He was the first person (few have followed him) who knew the course of the spinal accessory nerve, which he discovered. He is unusual among Oxford neurologists in that, at various times, he developed the practice of giving his lunch away to the poor. He also developed the practice of iatrochemistry: a theory of medicine according to which all morbid conditions of the body can be explained by disturbances in the fermentations and effervescences of its humours.

Arteries and CNS territories

Carotid artery Internal carotid artery occlusion may, at worst, cause total (and usually fatal) infarction of the anterior two-thirds of the ipsi-lateral hemisphere and basal ganglia (lenticulostriate arteries). More often, the picture is similar to a middle cerebral artery occlusion (below).

The cerebral arteries 3 pairs of arteries leave the circle of Willis to supply the cerebral hemispheres; the anterior, middle, and posterior cerebral arteries. The anterior and middle cerebrals are branches of the carotid arteries; the basilar artery divides into the 2 posterior cerebral arteries. These arteries are essentially end arteries (there is no significant anastomosis between them), and ischaemia due to occlusion of any one of them may be reduced, if not prevented, by retrograde supply from meningeal vessels.

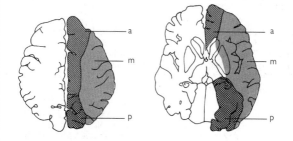

Anterior cerebral artery: ('a' above) Supplies the frontal and medial part of the cerebral hemispheres. Occlusion may cause a weak, numb contralateral leg ± similar, if milder, arm symptoms. The face is spared. Bilateral infarction is associated with an akinetic mute state due to damage to the cingulate gyri (also a rare cause of paraplegia).

Middle cerebral artery: ('m') Supplies the lateral (external) part of each hemisphere. Occlusion may cause: contralateral hemiplegia, hemisensory loss mainly of face and arm; contralateral homonymous hemianopia due to involvement of the optic radiation, cognitive change including dysphasia if the dominant hemisphere is affected, and visuo-spatial disturbance (eg cannot dress; gets lost) with non-dominant lesions.

Posterior cerebral artery: ('p') Supplies the occipital lobe. Occlusion causes contralateral homonymous hemianopia.

Vertebrobasilar circulation Supplies the cerebellum, brainstem, occipital lobes. *Occlusion may cause:* hemianopia; cortical blindness; diplopia; vertigo; nystagmus; hemi- or quadriplegia; unilateral or bilateral sensory symptoms; cerebellar symptoms; hiccups; dysarthria; dysphasia; and coma. Infarctions of the brainstem can produce various syndromes, eg *Lateral medullary syndrome* (occlusion of 1 vertebral artery or the posterior inferior cerebellar artery). It is due to infarction of the lateral medulla and the inferior surface of the cerebellum causing vertigo with vomiting, dysphagia, nystagmus ipsilateral ataxia, and paralysis of the soft palate, ipsilateral Horner's syndrome, and a crossed pattern sensory loss (analgesia to pinprick on ipsilateral face and contralateral trunk and limbs).

Subclavian steal syndrome: Subclavian artery stenosis proximal to the vertebral artery may cause blood to be *stolen* by retrograde flow down this vertebral artery down into the arm, causing brainstem ischaemia after exertion. Suspect if the BP in each arm differs by >20mmHg.

Drugs and the nervous system

The brain is a gland that secretes both thoughts and molecules: both products are modulated by neurotransmitter systems. *Some target sites for drugs:*

1 Precursor of the transmitter (eg L-dopa).
2 Interference with the storage of transmitter in vesicles within the pre-synaptic neurone (eg tetrabenazine).
3 Binding to the post-synaptic receptor site (bromocriptine).
4 Binding to receptor-modulating site (benzodiazepines).
5 Interference with the breakdown of neurotransmitter within the synaptic cleft (monoamine oxidase inhibitors—MAOIs).
6 Reduce *reuptake* of transmitter from synaptic cleft into *pre-synaptic* cell (*selective serotonin reuptake inhibitors*, SSRIs, eg fluoxetine, *OHCS* p340).
7 Binding to pre-synaptic 'autoreceptors'—involved in feedback loops, often reducing neurotransmitter release.

The proven neurotransmitters include:

Amino acids Glutamate and aspartate act as excitatory transmitters on NMDA and non-NMDA receptors—relevant in epilepsy and ischaemic brain damage. Gamma-aminobutyric acid (GABA) is primarily inhibitory. *Drugs enhancing GABA activity are used in:* Epilepsy (phenobarbital, benzodiazepines, vigabatrin); spasticity (baclofen, benzodiazepines).

Peptides Opioids and substance P.

Histamine and **Purines** (such as ATP) Clinical relevance is not clear.

Dopamine (DA) *Drugs enhancing DA activity:* Parkinson's; hyperprolactinaemia; acromegaly. SE: vomiting; BP↓; chorea; dystonia; hallucinations and delusions. *Drugs ↓ DA activity are used in:* schizophrenia (*OHCS* p360, D_2 blockers); delusions; chorea; tics; nausea; vertigo. SE: parkinsonism; dystonias; akathisia.

Serotonin (5-hydroxytryptamine; 5HT) There are many types of receptors, eg: $5HT_{1-4}$. $5HT_1$ has 5 subtypes ($5HT_{1A-E}$). *Agonists:* Lithium$_{1A}$; sumatriptan$_{1D}$. *Partial agonists:* Buspirone$_{1A}$; LSD$_{1A}$; *Antagonists:* Ondansetron$_3$; pizotifen$_{1\&2}$; methysergide$_{1\&2}$; clozapine$_{2C}$—known as low D_2–high $5HT_2$, while risperidone is high D_2–high $5HT_2$ (low D_2 means <60% D_2 occupancy at conventional doses; traditional antipsychotics are just high D_2, ie 60–80%). *Reuptake inhibitors:* Fluoxetine, sertraline, venlafaxine. Ecstasy ↑nerve terminal 5HT release.

Adrenaline (epinephrine) and **non-adrenaline (norepinephrine)** 4 receptor types: α1, α2, β1, β2. Norepinephrine is more specific for α-receptors but both transmitters affect all receptors. In the periphery: α-receptor stimulation leads to arteriolar vasoconstriction and pupillary dilatation; β1 stimulation to increase in pulse and myocardial contractility; β2 stimulation to bronchodilatation, uterine relaxation, and arteriolar vasodilatation.
Drugs enhancing adrenergic activity are used in: Asthma (β2); anaphylaxis (adrenaline); heart failure (dobutamine); depression (MAOIs and tricyclics, the latter may act by increasing synaptic norepinephrine in the CNS).
Drugs reducing adrenergic activity are used in: Angina, ↑BP, arrhythmias, thyrotoxicosis/anxiety (β1); ↑BP from phaeochromocytoma (α).

Acetylcholine (Muscarinic and nicotinic receptors) *Centrally acting anticholinergic drugs are used in:* Parkinsonism, dystonias, motion sickness. Central toxic effects (especially in the elderly): confusion, delusions.
Peripheral antimuscarinic drugs are used in: Asthma (ipratropium); incontinence; to dry secretions pre-op; to dilate pupils; to ↑ heart rate (atropine).
Peripheral cholinergic agonists used in: Glaucoma (pilocarpine); myasthenia (anticholinesterases). SE: sweating, hypersalivation, colic.

Neurotransmitters and CNS drugs

The table below contains some of the drugs most commonly used to modify the activity of central nervous system transmitters. When prescribing for the CNS, it is important to bear in mind (1) that the drug (or a metabolite) must be able to pass through the blood–brain barrier to have an effect (2) the consequences of any sedative effect (3) short- and long-term side-effects (eg tardive dyskinesia with neuroleptic drugs).

Drugs ↑ activity (eg agonists)	Drugs ↓ activity (eg antagonists)
Dopamine	
L-dopa; pergolide; apomorphine	Major tranquillizers
Bromocriptine (D_2-agonist)	Benzisoxazoles (D_2-blocker)
Selegiline (MAO-B inhibitor)	eg risperidone
Amantadine	Some antiemetics
Non-adrenaline & adrenaline less (= norepinephrine & epinephrine)	
Salbutamol (β_2)	Propranolol (β)
Adrenaline (= epinephrine)	Atenolol (β_1)
?Tricyclic antidepressants	Clonidine (α_2-agonist)
MAOI	Phentolamine (α)
5HT	
LSD and other hallucinogens	Pizotifen
Sumatriptan	Benzisoxazoles ($5HT_2$-blockers)
Some tricyclic antidepressants	eg risperidone
eg trazodone	Clozapine (OHCS p360
Buspirone; lithium	$5HT_{2A}$ antagonist)
Fluoxetine (OHCS p340)	Mianserin; ondansetron
Acetylcholine	
carbachol	Atropine; Scopolamine
pilocarpine	Ipratropium
Anticholinesterases	Benzhexol (= trihexyphenidyl)
eg pyridostigmine	Orphenadrine; Procyclidine
GABA (inhibits other transmitters)	
Baclofen (GABA B)	Alcohol abuse[1]: acute effects block
Benzodiazepines	N-methyl-D-aspartate (NMDA) recep-
Valproate	tors; with chronic use, numbers of
Barbiturates	NMDA receptors rise, mediating alcohol
Acamprosate (used in alcohol	withdrawal effects (anxiety, craving)
addiction; derived from taurine)	
Glutamate[1] (an excitatory amino acid)	
	Lamotrigine (used in epilepsy)
	Topiramate (used in epilepsy et al.)[1]
	Acamprosate (↓craving in alcoholics)
	Memantine (Alzheimer's, p376)

335

New drugs are often aimed at multiple neurotransmitters, eg *risperidone* (blocks D_2, $5HT_2$, α_1 and α_2 adrenoceptors, OHCS p360). The smoking-cessation drug *bupropion* (= *amfebutamone*) is said to act via ↑dopamine in the mesolimbic system (mediates dependence) *and* via noradrenergic effects in the locus ceruleus (mediates symptoms of nicotine withdrawal).

---

1 Alcoholics have more glutamate binding sites—so facilitating dopamine neurotransmission in the midbrain—pathways, which, in the ventral tegmental area mediate alcohol's rewarding effects—including craving. Topiramate facilitates GABA function and antagonizes glutamate activity at kainate receptors—and has been found to ↓ cravings in alcoholism. Johnson B 2003 *Lancet* 1677

Testing peripheral nerves

Nerve root	Muscle	Test—by asking the patient to:
C3, 4	Trapezius	Shrug shoulder (via accessory nerve).
C5, 6, 7	Serratus anterior	Push arm forward against resistance; look for winging of the scapula, if weak.
C**5**, 6	Pectoralis major (p major) clavicular head	Adduct arm from above horizontal, and push it forward.
C6, **7**, 8	P major sternocostal head	Adduct arm below horizontal.
C**5**, 6	Supraspinatus	Abduct arm the first 15°.
C**5**, 6	Infraspinatus	Externally rotate arm, elbow at side.
C6, **7**, 8	Latissimus dorsi	Adduct arm from horizontal position.
C5, 6	Biceps	Flex supinated forearm.
C**5**, 6	Deltoid	Abduct arm between 15° and 90°.

Radial nerve

C6, **7**, 8	Triceps	Extend elbow against resistance.
C5, **6**	Brachioradialis	Flex elbow with forearm half way between pronation and supination.
C5, **6**	Extensor carpi radialis longus	Extend wrist to radial side with fingers extended.
C6, 7	Supinator	Arm by side, resist hand pronation.
C**7**, 8	Extensor digitorum	Keep fingers extended at MCP joint.
C**7**, 8	Extensor carpi ulnaris	Extend wrist to ulnar side.
C**7**, 8	Abductor pollicis longus	Abduct thumb at 90° to palm.
C**7**, 8	Extensor pollicis brevis	Extend thumb at MCP joint.
C**7**, 8	Extensor pollicis longus	Resist thumb flexion at IP joint.

Median nerve

C6, 7	Pronator teres	Keep arm pronated against resistance.
C6, 7	Flexor carpi radialis	Flex wrist towards radial side.
C7, **8**, T1	Flexor digitorum superficialis	Resist extension at PIP joint (with proximal phalanx fixed by the examiner).
C7, **8**	Flexor digitorum profundus I & II	Resist extension at index DIP joint of index finger.
C7, **8**, T1	Flexor pollicis longus	Resist thumb extension at interphalangeal joint (fix proximal phalanx).
C8, **T1**	Abductor pollicis brevis	Abduct thumb (nail at 90° to palm).
C8, **T1**	Opponens pollicis	Thumb touches base of 5th finger-tip (nail parallel to palm).
C8, **T1**	1st lumbrical/Interosseus (median & ulnar nerves)	Extend PIP joint against resistance with MCP joint held hyperextended.

Ulnar nerve

C7, **8**, T1	Flexor carpi ulnaris	Flex wrist to ulnar side; observe tendon.
C7, C**8**	Flexor digitorum profundus III and IV	Resist extension of distal phalanx of 5th finger while you fix its middle phalanx.
C8, **T1**	Dorsal interossei	Finger abduction: cannot cross the middle over the index finger (tests index finger adduction too).
C8, **T1**	Palmar interossei	Finger adduction: pull apart a sheet of paper held between middle and ring finger DIP joints of both hands; the paper moves on the weaker side.[1]
C8, **T1**	Adductor pollicis	Adduct thumb (nail at 90° to palm).
C8, **T1**	Abductor digiti minimi	Abduct little finger.
C8, **T1**	Flexor digiti minimi	Flex the little finger at MCP joint.

1 Also, metacarpophalangeal joint flexion may be more on the affected side as flexor tendons are recruited—the basis of Froment's paper sign. Wartenberg's sign is persistent little finger abduction.

Lower limb

Nerve root	*Muscle*	*Activity to test:*
L4, 5, S1	Gluteus medius & minimus (superior gluteal nerve)	Internal rotation at hip, hip abduction.
L5, S1, 2	Gluteus maximus (inferior gluteal nerve)	Extension at hip (lie prone).
L2, **3**, 4	Adductors (obturator nerve)	Adduct leg against resistance.

Femoral nerve

L**1, 2**, 3	Iliopsoas (also supplied via L1, 3, & 3 spinal nerves)	Flex hip against resistance with knee flexed and lower leg supported: patient lies on back.
L2, **3, 4**	Quadriceps femoris	Extend at the knee against resistance. Start with the knee flexed.

Obturator nerve

L2, **3**, 4	Hip adductors	Adduct the leg against resistance.

Inferior gluteal nerve

L**5**, S1, S2	Gluteus maximus	Hip extension ('bury heal into the couch')—with knee in extension.

Superficial gluteal nerve

L**4, 5**, S1	Gluteus medius & minimus	Abduction and internal hip rotation with leg flexed at hip and knee.

Sciatic (and common peroneal*) and sciatic (and tibial**) nerves

*L**4**, 5	Tibialis anterior	Dorsiflex ankle.
*L**5**, S1	Extensor digitorum longus	Dorsiflex toes against resistance.
*L**5**, S1	Extensor hallucis longus	Dorsiflex hallux against resistance.
*L5, S1	Peroneus longus & brevis	Evert foot against resistance.
*L5, S1	Extensor digitorum brevis	Dorsiflex proximal phalanges of toes.
L5, **S1, 2	Hamstrings	Flex the knee against resistance.
L4**, 5	Tibialis posterior	Invert the plantarflexed foot.
**S1, 2	Gastrocnemius	Plantarflex ankle or stand on tiptoe.
L5, **S1, 2	Flexor digitorum longus	Flex terminal joints of the toes.
**S1, 2	Small muscles of foot	Make the sole of the foot into a cup.

337

Quick screening test for muscle power

Shoulder	Abduction	C5	*Hip*	Flexion	L1–L2
	Adduction	C5–C7		Adduction	L2–3
Elbow	Flexion	C5–C6		Extension	L5–S1
	Extension	C7	*Knee*	Flexion	L5–S1
Wrist	Flexion	C7–8		Extension	L3–L4
	Extension	C7	*Ankle*	Dorsiflexion	L4
Fingers	Flexion	C8		Eversion	L5–S1
	Extension	C7		Plantarflexion	S1–S2
	Abduction	T1	*Toe*	Big toe extension	L5

Remember to test proximal muscle power: ask the patient to sit from lying, to pull you towards himself, and to rise from squatting. ►Also, observe walking (easy to forget, even if the complaint is of walking difficulty!).

NB: Root numbers in bold indicate that that root is more important than its neighbour. ►Sources vary in ascribing particular nerve roots to muscles—and there is some biological variation in individuals. The above is a reasonable compromise, based on MRC/*Brain* 2001 guidelines: ISBN 0-7020-2512-7. ►We don't react to nerve damage according to simple anatomy; eg ulnar neuropathy may initiate dystonic flexion or tremor of 4th & 5th digits by inducing a central motor disorder. [@8622720] [@2153273]

Dermatomes

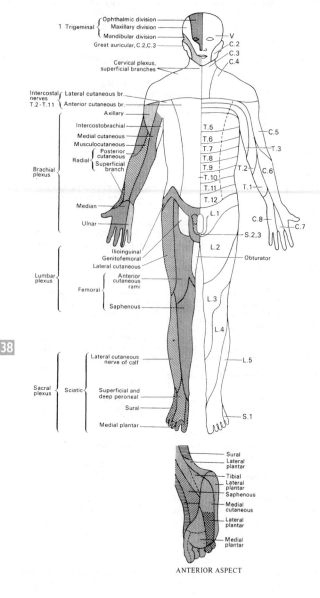

T Trigeminal
- Ophthalmic division
- Maxillary division
- Mandibular division
- Great auricular, C.2, C.3

Cervical plexus, superficial branches

V
C.2
C.3
C.4

Intercostal nerves T.2 - T.11
- Lateral cutaneous br.
- Anterior cutaneous br.
- Axillary

Brachial plexus
- Intercostobrachial
- Medial cutaneous
- Musculocutaneous
- Radial
  - Posterior cutaneous
  - Superficial branch
- Median
- Ulnar

T.5
T.6
T.7
T.8
T.9
T.10
T.11
T.12

C.5
T.3
T.2
C.6
T.1
C.8
C.7

L.1
S.2,3
L.2
Obturator

Lumbar plexus
- Ilioinguinal
- Genitofemoral
- Lateral cutaneous
- Femoral
  - Anterior cutaneous rami
  - Saphenous

L.3
L.4
L.5

Sacral plexus — Sciatic
- Lateral cutaneous nerve of calf
- Superficial and deep peroneal
- Sural
- Medial plantar

S.1

- Sural
- Lateral plantar
- Tibial
- Lateral plantar
- Saphenous
- Medial cutaneous
- Lateral plantar
- Medial plantar

ANTERIOR ASPECT

338

Dermatomes

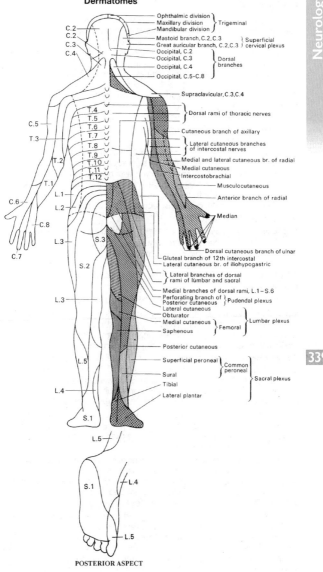

Ophthalmic division
Maxillary division } Trigeminal
Mandibular division
C.2
C.2
Mastoid branch. C.2,C.3 } Superficial
C.3
Great auricular branch. C.2,C.3 } cervical plexus
C.4
Occipital, C.2
Occipital, C.3 } Dorsal
Occipital, C.4 } branches
Occipital, C.5–C.8

Supraclavicular, C.3, C.4

C.5
T.3
Dorsal rami of thoracic nerves
T.4
T.5
T.6
Cutaneous branch of axillary
T.7
T.8
Lateral cutaneous branches
T.9
of intercostal nerves
T.2
T.10
Medial and lateral cutaneous br. of radial
T.11
Medial cutaneous
T.12
Intercostobrachial
T.1
L.1
Musculocutaneous
L.2
Anterior branch of radial

C.6
Median
C.8
C.7
L.3
S.3
Dorsal cutaneous branch of ulnar
Gluteal branch of 12th intercostal
Lateral cutaneous br. of iliohypogastric
S.2
Lateral branches of dorsal
rami of lumbar and sacral
Medial branches of dorsal rami, L.1–S.6
Perforating branch of } Pudendal plexus
Posterior cutaneous }
L.3
Lateral cutaneous
Obturator
Medial cutaneous } Femoral
Saphenous } Lumbar plexus

Posterior cutaneous

L.5
Superficial peroneal } Common
peroneal } Sacral plexus
Sural
L.4
Tibial
Lateral plantar

S.1

L.5

L.5
L.4
S.1
L.5

POSTERIOR ASPECT

Headache

Every day, *thousands* of patients visit doctors complaining of headache; these consultations are rewarding as the chief skill is in interpreting the history, not in *taking* it, so much as in *allowing* it to unfold. Let patients tell you about all the headache's associations, or even *who* their headache is. Stress/tension headache is the usual cause of bilateral, non-pulsatile headache (± scalp muscle tenderness, but without vomiting or sensitivity to head movement,). Here, stress relief, eg massage or antidepressants, may have more to offer than a neurologist. But some headaches are disabling and treatable (migraine, cluster headache), while others are sinister, eg space-occupying lesions, meningitis, subarachnoid haemorrhage (SAH), and giant cell arteritis. These are the headaches you must recognize:

Acute single episode

Meningitis	p368, eg fever, photophobia, stiff neck, rash, coma
Encephalitis	p369, eg fever, odd behaviour, fits or consciousness↓
Tropical illness	p554, eg malaria, +ve travel history, 'flu-like illness
Subarachnoid	p362, haemorrhage → *sudden* headache ± stiff neck
Sinusitis	p554, in OHCS, eg tender face + coryza + post-nasal drip
Head injury	p814, cuts/bruises, consciousness↓; lucid interval, amnesia

Acute recurrent attacks

Migraine	p342, any pre-attack aura? Visual aura? Vomiting? Sensitivity to light, noise, or movement
Cluster headache	p341, typically nightly pain in 1 eye for ~8wks then OK for the next few months—then intermittently repeated
Glaucoma	p427, red eye; sees haloes, fixed big oval pupil; acuity↓

Subacute onset

Giant cell arteritis p424; tender scalp; >50yrs old; acuity↓ (late); ESR↑

Chronic headache (pain for >15d/month for longer than 3 months.[1])

Tension headache 'a tight band round my head'; stress at work/home, mood↓
Chronically ↑ICP eg worse on waking, focal signs, BP↑, pulse↓
Medication misuse p341; medication misuse headache eg from analgesic overuse

Acute single episode *Meningitis, encephalitis, subarachnoid haemorrhage*
If the headache is acute, severe, felt over most of the head and accompanied by meningeal irritation (neck stiffness) ± drowsiness you *must* think of meningitis (p368), encephalitis (p369), or a subarachnoid (p362). Admit immediately for urgent LP (after CT if ↑ICP possible, eg focal signs).

After head injury headache is common after minor trauma. It may be at the site of trauma or be more generalized. It lasts ~2wks and is often resistant to analgesia. Bear in mind subdural or extradural haemorrhage (p366). Sinister signs are drowsiness, focal signs.

Sinusitis: Presents with dull, constant, aching pain over the affected frontal or maxillary sinus, with tender overlying skin ± post-nasal drip. Ethmoid or sphenoid sinus pain is felt deep in the midline at the root of the nose. Pain is worsened by bending over. Often accompanied by coryza (p572), the pain lasts only 1–2wks. Confirm by imaging (eg CT).

Acute glaucoma: Mostly elderly, long-sighted people. Constant, aching pain develops rapidly around 1 eye and radiates to the forehead. *Symptoms:* Markedly reduced vision in affected eye, nausea, and vomiting. *Signs:* Red, congested eye; cloudy cornea; dilated, non-responsive pupil. Attacks may be precipitated by sitting in the dark, eg the cinema, dilating eye-drops or emotional upset. Seek expert help immediately. If delay in treatment of >1h is likely, start IV acetazolamide (500mg over several minutes).

---

[1] International Headache Society revised classification. R Peatfield 2004 *BMJ* **328** 119

Attacks of headache—Cluster headache (CH = migrainous neuralgia): One theory (among many) is that this is caused by superficial temporal artery smooth muscle hyperreactivity to 5HT. There are related hypothalamic grey matter abnormalities. An autosomal dominant gene also has a role.[1] Onset: any age; ♂: ♀ ≥ 5 : 1, commoner in smokers. Pain occurs once or twice every 24h, each episode lasting 15–160min. Clusters typically last 4–12wks and are followed by pain-free periods of months or even 1–2yrs before another cluster begins. Sometimes there are no remissions. *Symptoms:* Rapid onset severe pain around 1 eye which may become watery and bloodshot with lid swelling, lacrimation, facial flushing, and rhinorrhoea. Miosis ± ptosis (20% attacks), remaining permanent in 5%. Pain is strictly unilateral and almost always affects the same side. *The father in extremis:* '…I am careful not to wake the children as I make my way down the stairs. If they were to witness my nightly cluster ritual, they would never see me the same way again. Their father, fearless protector, diligent provider, crawling about in tears, beating his head on the hard wood floor. The pain is so intense I want to scream, but I never do. I go down 3 flights of stairs where I can't be heard, and drop to my knees. I place my hands on the back of my neck, and lock my fingers together. I bind my head between my arms and squeeze as hard as I can in an attempt to crush my skull. I begin to roll around, banging my head on the floor, pressing my left eye with full force of my palm. I search for the telephone that has always been my weapon of choice for creating a diversion, and I beat my left temple with the hand piece. I create a rhythm as I strike my skull, cursing the demon with each blow…'[2] *Treatment:*

- *Acute attack:* 100% O_2 (7–15L/min for 20min) often helps—or *sumatriptan* SC 6mg at attack's onset.
- *Preventives:* verapamil; lithium; steroids; methysergide (SE retroperitoneal fibrosis).

Trigeminal neuralgia: Paroxysms of intense, stabbing pain, lasting seconds, in the trigeminal nerve distribution eg from anomalous intracranial vessels compressing the trigeminal root. It is unilateral, affecting the mandibular and maxillary divisions most often. The face may screw up with pain (hence *tic douloureux*). Pain may recur many times day and night and can often be triggered by touching the skin of the affected area, by washing, shaving, eating, or talking. Typical patient: a man over 50yrs. *Drugs to try:* Carbamazepine (start at 100mg/12h PO; max 400mg/6h; lamotrigine; phenytoin 200–400mg/24h PO; or gabapentin. If drugs fail, surgery may be necessary. This may be directed at the peripheral nerve, the trigeminal ganglion or the nerve root. *Microvascular decompression:* Anomalous vessels are separated from the trigeminal root. *Facial pain differential diagnosis:* See p72.

Headaches of subacute onset Giant cell arteritis: See p424. *Exclude in all >50yrs old presenting with a headache that has lasted a few weeks.* Look for tender, thickened, pulseless temporal arteries + ESR >40mm/h. *Ask about:* Jaw claudication during eating. Prompt diagnosis and steroids avoid blindness.

Chronic headache Tension headache: See above.

Raised intracranial pressure: Headache is a complaint of ~50% patients. Although variable in nature, headaches are characteristically present on waking or may awaken the patient. They are generally not severe and are worsened lying down. If accompanied by other signs of ↑ICP, such as vomiting, papilloedema, epilepsy, progressive focal neurology, or mental change, admit the patient urgently for diagnostic imaging. *LP is contraindicated.* Any space-occupying lesion (neoplasm, abscess, subdural haematoma) may present in this way, as may benign intracranial hypertension.

Medication misuse headache: Culprits are mixed analgesics containing codeine (self-R), or prescribed opiates, ergotamine and triptans. It is a common reason for episodic headaches becoming daily headache. The culprit must be withdrawn, and a preventive added (eg tricyclics, valproate, gabapentin).

341

1 Ekbom K 2003 *Headache* **43** 307   **2** http://www.clusterheadaches.com

Migraine

Migraine causes much misery and costs the UK economy £200 million a year in lost production. Its prevalence is 8%. $\female : \male \approx 2 : 1$.

Symptoms *Classically:* • Visual (or other) aura lasting 15–30min followed within 1h by unilateral, throbbing headache. *Other patterns:* • Aura with no headache • Episodic (often premenstrual) severe headaches, often unilateral, with nausea, vomiting ± photophobia/phonophobia but no aura; may have allodynia—all stimuli produce pain—'I can't brush my hair, wear earrings or glasses, or shave because it's so painful'[6]— (known as *common migraine*).

Aura Visual chaos (cascading, distortion, 'melting' and jumbling of print lines, dots, spots, zig-zag fortification spectra); hemianopia, hemiparesis, dysphasia, dysarthria, ataxia (basilar migraine). Mood or appetite change (↑/↓) or ↑sensory awareness (eg to sound) may occur hours before the aura. Duration of aura is ≤1h, and typically before headache. *Sensory auras:* eg paraesthesiae spreading from fingers to face, or *speech auras:* (8% of auras; eg dysphasia; dysarthria; paraphasia, eg phoneme substitution). *Criteria for diagnosis if no aura:* ≥5 headaches lasting 4–72h with either nausea/vomiting or photophobia/phonophobia *and* ≥2 of these 4 features: • Unilateral • Pulsating • Interferes with normal life • Aggravated by climbing stairs or other routine activity.

Pathogenesis[1] Cerebral oligaemia leading to the aura followed by cerebral and extracranial hyperaemia leading to the headache. The underlying cause of the vascular abnormalities may be dysfunction in the sensory modulation of craniovascular afferents. Attacks are associated with changes in plasma 5HT.

Triggers—eg CHOCOLATE or: Cheese, oral contraceptives, caffeine (or its withdrawal), alcohol, anxiety, travel, or exercise. In ~50%, no trigger is found, and in only a few does avoiding triggers prevent *all* attacks.

Differential Cluster or tension headache, cervical spondylosis; ↑BP; intracranial pathology, sinusitis/otitis media, caries. TIAs may mimic migraine aura. Migraine is rarely a sign of other pathology: don't look too hard for antiphospholipid syndrome, arterio–venous malformations, or microemboli.

Prophylaxis (eg if frequency > twice a month). If one drug does not work after 3 months, try another. Most (>65%) will achieve ↓in attack frequency of 50%.
- Pizotifen 0.5–1mg/8h PO; or 1–3mg PO at night (5HT antagonist). SE: drowsy, weight↑; ↑effects of alcohol; ↑glaucoma risk. Or propranolol 40–120mg/12h PO or amitriptyline 25–75mg nocte; SE: drowsiness, dry mouth, blurred vision.
- 2ⁿᵈ-line: valproate 400–600mg/12h. Verapamil and SSRIs are used but evidence is poor. Gabapentin and topiramate show promise in recent trials.

Treating attacks Low doses may fail as peristalsis is often slow, so try *dispersible* high-dose aspirin 900mg/6h PO pc, or paracetamol 1g/6h PO 10min after metoclopramide solution (5mg PO, ≤15mg/d; beware extrapyramidal SEs) or domperidone. Alternatives: NSAIDs, eg ketoprofen 100mg stat PO,[2] or
- Sumatriptan is a 5HT1B/D *agonist*, constricting cranial arteries. Some trials say that it may be no better than simple analgesia + metoclopramide; others say that the SC form may be best of all (try PO 1ˢᵗ). Rare SEs: arrhythmias or angina ± MI, even if no pre-existing risk. CI: past MI/IHD, coronary spasm, uncontrolled ↑BP, recent lithium, SSRIs or ergot use. Use of newer triptans is controversial.[3]
- Ergotamine (a 5HT agonist, constricting cranial arteries) 1mg PO as the headache begins, repeat at 30min, up to 3mg in a day, and 6mg in a week; or, better, as a *Cafergot®* suppository (2mg ergotamine + 100mg caffeine) to maximum of 2 in 24h; then ≥4 days without. Emphasize dangers of ergotamine (gangrene, permanent vascular damage). CI: the Pill (*OHCS* p64); peripheral vascular disease; ischaemic heart disease; pregnancy; breast-feeding; hemiplegic migraine; Raynaud's; liver or renal impairment; BP↑.

1 P Goadsby *NEJM* 2002 **346** 257   2 M Dib 2003 *Headache* **43** 299
3 Of the oral triptans, rizatriptan is said to have the greatest *early* efficacy. Rizatriptan and zolmitriptan are available as rapidly dissolving wafers. Almotriptan has a response rate similar to oral sumatriptan and may have fewer SEs. [@12739316]

Migraine questions

1 **What is going on in migraine?** Traditionally, the theory has been that there is a vascular problem (constriction during aura, with dilatation causing pain), but MRIs during attacks show that episodic cerebral oedema, dilatation of intracerebral vessels, and ↓water diffusion do not respect vascular territories—so the primary event may be neurological.[1]

2 **Is migraine due to a hyperexcitable brain?** Magnetic studies have shown resting (interictum) hyperexcitability at least in the visual cortex, suggesting a failure of inhibitory circuits. Cortical hyperexcitability may relate to imbalance between neuronal inhibition (mediated by GABA, p335) and excitation (mediated by excitatory amino acids). Putative causes of this include ↓cerebral Mg^{2+} levels, mitochondrial abnormalities, dysfunctions related to ↑nitric oxide, and calcium channelopathy.

3 **Are there any options when standard prophylaxis fails?** Hyperexcitability *may* be reducible by anticonvulsants such as lamotrigine (SE: 'flu-like symptoms, drowsiness, diplopia, confusion, aggression), gabapentin (SE: weight↑, ataxia, vision↓), topiramate (SE: memory and language problems, ataxia, nystagmus), tiagabine (SE: diarrhoea, depression, poor concentration), levetiracetam (SE: somnolence; ataxia, mood swings). Patients will ask about these, and it is necessary to explain that there are side-effects, and the treatment is experimental only. They are also expensive.

4 **For those not wanting drugs, do alternative therapies help?**
- Some people find warm or cold packs to the head helps abort attacks.
- Spinal manipulation receive some support from randomized studies.
- Riboflavin and magnesium may have a role.
- Rebreathing into paper bag (raising P_aCO_2) may abort some attacks.

Migraine, stroke, and the Pill *(combined oral contraception, COC)* Incidence of migraine + Pill-related ischaemic stroke is 8 : 100,000 if aged 20; and 80 : 100,000 in those aged 40yrs. Low-dose COCs only should be used. Those with migraine with aura are known to be at especial risk, precluding use of combined Pills in these women (but no problem with progesterone only or non-hormonal contraception). Risk is further augmented by: • Smoking • Age >35yrs • BP↑ • Obesity (body mass index >30) • Diabetes mellitus • Hyperlipidaemia • Family history of arteriopathy when aged <45yrs. Warn women with migraine to stop Pills at once if they develop aura or worsening migraine—see *OHCS* p65.

343

---

1 D Butteriss 2003 *J Neuroradiol* (serial MRIs in hemiplegic migraine, done in Newcastle, UK)

Blackouts

History It is vital to establish exactly what patients mean by 'blackout'. Do they mean loss of consciousness (LOC)? a fall to the ground without loss of consciousness? a clouding of vision, diplopia, or vertigo? Take a detailed history from the patient *and* a witness (see BOX).

Vasovagal syncope Provoked by emotion, pain, fear or standing too long and due to reflex bradycardia ± peripheral vasodilatation. Onset is over seconds (*not* instantaneous), and is often preceded by nausea, pallor, sweating, and closing in of visual fields (pre-syncope). It cannot occur if lying down. The patient falls to the ground, being unconscious for ~2min. Incontinence of urine is rare. Brief jerking of the limbs is uncommon, but there is no tonic → clonic sequence. After an attack there is no prolonged confusion or amnesia.

Situation syncope *Cough syncope:* Weakness + LOC after a paroxysm of coughing. *Effort syncope:* Syncope on exercise; cardiac origin, eg aortic stenosis, HOCM. *Micturition syncope:* Mostly men, at night. *Carotid sinus syncope:* Carotid sinus hypersensitivity (on head-turning or shaving the neck).

Epilepsy presenting as blackout is most likely to be *grand mal* (LOC) or complex partial (impairment of consciousness). See p378. Attacks vary with the type of seizure, but some features suggest epilepsy as a cause of blackout: attacks when asleep or lying down; aura; identifiable precipitants, eg TV; altered breathing; cyanosis; typical movements; urinary and faecal incontinence; tongue-biting, particularly the side of the tongue, is virtually diagnostic; post-attack drowsiness or coma; amnesia; residual paralysis for <24h.

Stokes–Adams attacks Transient arrhythmias (eg bradycardia due to complete heart block) causing ↓cardiac output and LOC. The patient falls to the ground (often with *no* warning except palpitation), pale, with a slow or absent pulse. Recovery is in seconds, the patient flushes, the pulse speeds up, and consciousness is regained. Injury is a feature of these intermittent arrhythmias. A few clonic jerks may occur if an attack is prolonged. Attacks may happen several times a day and in any posture.

Other causes *Hypoglycaemia:* Tremor, hunger, and perspiration herald light-headedness or LOC; rare in non-diabetics. *Orthostatic hypotension:* Unsteadiness or LOC on standing from lying in those with inadequate vasomotor reflexes: the elderly; autonomic neuropathy (p390); antihypertensive medication; overdiuresis; multi-system atrophy (MSA). ►TIAs rarely cause blackouts.

Drop attacks Sudden weakness of the legs causes the patient, usually an older woman, to fall to the ground. There is no warning, no LOC and no confusion afterwards. The condition is benign, resolving spontaneously after a number of attacks. Drop attacks also occur in hydrocephalus; these patients, however, may not be able to get up for hours.

Other causes *Anxiety:* Hyperventilation, tremor, sweating, tachycardia, paraesthesiae, light-headedness, and no LOC suggest a panic attack. *Factitious blackouts* (Münchausen's, p730). *Choking:* If a large piece of food blocks the larynx, the patient may collapse, turn blue, and be unable to speak. Do the Heimlich manoeuvre immediately to eject the food.

Examination Cardiovascular, neurological. BP lying and standing.

Tests Investigate fully unless clearly syncopal. ECG,[1] 24h (or longer) ECG: (arrhythmia, long Q–T, eg Romano–Ward, p94); U&E, FBC, glucose. Perhaps EEG, sleep EEG, echocardiogram, CT/MRI; HUT.[2] P_aCO_2↓ in attacks suggests hyperventilation as the cause. ►*While the cause is being elucidated, advise against driving.*

---

1 Consider elevating V1-V3 leads from the 4th to the 2nd intercostal space to reveal saddle-shaped ST elevation, the telltale sign of **Brugada syndrome** (p719) [@10809492]—an autosomal SCN5A channelopathy predisposing to VT eg in young men. ECG image: www.smw.ch/images/coupoeil/128-49-184-01.tif
2 Head-up tilt (HUT) tests distinguish vasodepressor from cardio-inhibitory syncope. HUT is +ve if symptoms are associated with a BP drop >30mmHg (vasodepressor; consider β-blockers to counter ↑sympathetic activity)—or bradycardia (cardio-inhibitory; consider pacing). [@9532822]

Taking a history of blackouts

If a series of attacks, ask a witness: During a typical attack…
- Does the patient lose consciousness?
- Does the patient injure himself?
- Does the patient move? Floppy or stiff (suggests epilepsy)? NB: not everything that twitches is epilepsy.
- Is there incontinence? (irrelevant if urine, but faeces suggests epilepsy).
- Is the complexion changed? (White or red suggests arrhythmia, but may occur in temporal lobe epilepsy.)
- Does the patient bite his tongue? (suggests epilepsy).
- What is the patient's pulse like? (abnormalities suggest a CVS cause).
- Are there associated symptoms (palpitations, chest pain, dyspnoea)?
- How long does the attack last?
- Is the patient sleepy before an attack (narcolepsy, p724).

Before the attack:
- Is there any warning?—eg typical epileptic aura or pre-syncope (above)
- In what circumstances do attacks occur? (if watching TV, it is epilepsy)
- Can the patient prevent attacks?

After the attack:
- How much does the patient remember about the attack afterwards?
- Muscle pain afterwards suggests a tonic/clonic seizure
- Is the patient confused or sleepy (post-ictal; narcolepsy)?

Background to attacks: Getting more frequent? Is anyone else in the family getting them? Sudden arrhythmic death[1] may leave no cardiac trace at *post mortem*, or there may be hereditary cardiomyopathy.

▶Witnesses often give conflicting accounts: the most reliable may not be the one with the most medical knowledge. He or she may know what you expect to hear, and furnish you with extra (imagined) material.

Dizziness and vertigo

Complaints of 'dizzy spells' are very common and are used by patients to describe many different sensations. The key to making a diagnosis is to find out exactly what the patient means by 'dizzy' and then decide whether or not this represents vertigo.

Does the patient have vertigo? *Definition:* An illusion of movement, often rotatory, of the patient or his surroundings. In practice, straightforward 'spinning' is rare—the floor may tilt, sink, or rise or '…I veer sideways on walking as if pulled to one side by a magnet'. Vertigo is always worsened by movement. *Associated symptoms:* Difficulty walking or standing; relief on lying or sitting still; nausea; vomiting; pallor; sweating. Attacks may even cause patients to fall suddenly to the ground. Associated hearing loss or tinnitus implies labyrinth or 8th nerve involvement. *What is not vertigo:* Faintness may be described as dizziness but is often due to anxiety with associated palpitations, tremor, and sweating. Anaemia can cause light-headedness as can orthostatic hypotension or effort in an emphysematous patient. But in all of these there is no illusion of movement or typical associated symptoms. Loss of consciousness during attacks should prompt thoughts of epilepsy or syncope rather than vertigo.

Causes Disorders of the labyrinth, vestibular nerve, vestibular nuclei, or their central connections are responsible for practically all vertigo. Only rarely are other structures implicated (see BOX).

Labyrinthine vertigo *Benign positional vertigo:* Displacement of the otoconia (otoliths) from the maculae (the receptor for sensing acceleration in the semicircular canals). Otoconia then settle on the lowest part of the labyrinth. This is curable by the Epley manoeuvre which repositions the particles. *OHCS* p546. *Ménière's disease:* Recurrent, spontaneous attacks of vertigo, hearing loss, tinnitus, and a sense of aural fullness caused by endolymphatic hydrops. Vertigo is severe and rotational, lasts 20min to hours and is often accompanied by nausea and vomiting. Hearing loss is sensorineural, affects primarily low frequencies, fluctuates and is progressive; often to complete deafness of the affected ear. Drop attacks may rarely feature (no loss of consciousness or vertigo, but sudden falling to one side). Acute attacks—bed rest and reassurance. An antihistamine (eg cyclizine) is useful if prolonged. Consider surgery or pharmacological ablation of the vestibular organ in very severe disease. *Ototoxicity:* (eg aminoglycosides) may also cause vertigo and deafness.

Vestibular nerve Damage in the petrous temporal bone or cerebellopontine angle often involves the auditory nerve, causing deafness or tinnitus. Causes: trauma and vestibular schwannomas (acoustic neuromas).

Acoustic neuromas usually present with hearing loss, vertigo coming only later. With progression, ipsilateral cranial nerves V, VI, IX, and X may be affected (also ipsilateral cerebellar signs). Paradoxically, there is rarely VII nerve involvement pre-operatively. Signs of ↑ICP occur late, and indicate a large tumour.

Vestibular neuronitis: Abrupt onset of severe vertigo, nausea, and vomiting, with prostration and immobility. No deafness or tinnitus. May be from a virus in the young, or a vascular lesion in the elderly. Severe vertigo subsides in days, complete recovery takes 3–4wks. Reassure. Sedate.

Herpes zoster: Herpetic eruption of the external auditory meatus; facial palsy ± deafness, tinnitus, and vertigo (Ramsay Hunt syndrome).

Brainstem Infarction of the brainstem (vertebrobasilar circulation) may produce marked vertigo but other lesions may also be responsible (see BOX). Vertigo is protracted as are the associated nausea, vomiting, and nystagmus. It is exceptional for vertigo to be the only symptom of brainstem disease; multiple cranial nerve palsies and sensory and motor tract defects are commonly also seen. Hearing is spared.

Causes of vertigo

Vestibular end-organs and vestibular nerve
Ménière's disease
Vestibular neuronitis (acute labyrinthitis)
Benign positional vertigo (*OHCS* p546)
Motion sickness
Trauma
Ototoxicity (aminoglycosides)
Herpes zoster oticus (Ramsay Hunt syndrome, *OHCS* p756)

Brainstem, cerebellum, and cerebello-pontine angle
MS
Infarction/TIA
Haemorrhage
Migraine (very rarely)
Vestibular schwannoma (acoustic neuroma)

Cerebral cortex
Vertiginous epilepsy

Alcohol intoxication

Cervical vertigo (controversial—neck symptoms are more commonly a result of a patient keeping the neck stiff to avoid exacerbating vertigo).

Deafness

(►See *OHCS* p542 for management)

Simple hearing tests To establish deafness, the examiner should whisper a number increasingly loudly in one ear while blocking the other ear with a finger. The patient is asked to repeat the number. Make sure that failure is not from misunderstanding.

Rinne's test Place the base of a vibrating 256 (or 512) Hz tuning fork on the mastoid process. Then move the fork so that the prongs are 4cm from the external acoustic meatus. The energy in the fork will be lessening, but the sound will appear louder if air conduction (AC) is better than bone conduction (BC). AC is normally better than BC. If not, then it is either conductive deafness or a false negative due to sensorineural deafness with 'hearing' of sound in the other ear. Distinguish from Weber's test (below). If there is hearing loss and AC is better than BC, this suggests sensorineural deafness, ie a cause central to the oval window—eg presbyacusis (from ageing or excess noise) or ototoxic drugs, or post-meningitis.

Weber's test Place a vibrating tuning fork in the middle of the forehead. Ask which side the patient localizes the sound to—or is it heard in the middle? In unilateral sensorineural deafness, the sound is located to the good side. In conduction deafness, the sound is located to the bad side (as if the sensitivity of the nerve has been turned up to allow for poor AC). Neither of these tests is completely reliable.

Conductive deafness Usually due to wax (remove it under direct vision or by syringing with warm water after prior softening with drops, eg olive oil). Also: otosclerosis, otitis media, glue ear (*OHCS* p538).

Causes of sensorineural deafness Presbyacusis (senile deafness), Ménière's disease (*OHCS* p546, causing paroxsmal vertigo, deafness ± tinnitus due to dilatation of the endolymphatic sac). *Other*: Meningitis; acute labyrinthitis; head injury; acoustic neuroma; MS; Paget's disease; excessive noise; aminoglycosides; frusemide (=furosemide); lead; several rare congenital syndromes (*OHCS* p540); maternal infections during pregnancy.

Tinnitus

(See *OHCS* p544)

This is ringing or buzzing in the ears. It is a common phenomenon.

Causes Unknown; hearing loss (20%); wax; viral; presbyacusis; noise (eg gunfire); head injury; suppurative otitis media; post-stapedectomy; Ménière's; head injury; anaemia; BP↑ (found in up to 16%, but it may not be causative). *Drugs*: Aspirin; loop diuretics; aminoglycosides (eg gentamicin). *Psychological associations*: Redundancy, divorce, retirement. ►Investigate unilateral tinnitus fully to exclude a vestibular schwannoma (acoustic neuroma, p346).

Causes of pulsatile tinnitus: (eg audible with stethoscope; do MRI) Carotid artery stenosis/dissection; AV fistulae; glomus jugulare tumours, *OHCS* p544.

Treatment *Psychological support* is very important (eg from a hearing therapist). Exclude serious causes; reassure that tinnitus does not mean madness or serious disease and that it often improves in time. Cognitive therapy is recommended. Randomize trial support specific use of 'tinnitus coping training'.[1] Patient support groups can help greatly.

Drugs are disappointing. Avoid tranquillizers, particularly if depressed (use tricyclic antidepressants here, eg amitriptyline or nortriptyline). Hypnotics at night may be helpful. Carbamazepine has been disappointing; if Ménière's disease is the cause, betahistine will help only a proportion.

Masking may give relief. White noise (like an off-tuned radio) is given via a noise generator worn like a post-aural hearing aid. Hearing aids may help by amplifying desirable sounds. Section of the cochlear nerve relieves disabling tinnitus in 25% of patients (but at the expense of deafness).

---

1 B Kroner-Herwig 2003 *J Psychosom Res* **54** 381. Management of chronic tinnitus. Comparison of an outpatient cognitive-behavioral group training to minimal-contact interventions.

Weak legs and cord compression

Cord compression typically presents with weak legs. There are many causes of weak legs (see BOX) but only 5 cardinal questions: *Was the onset gradual or sudden? At what rate is the weakness progressing? Are the legs spastic or flaccid? Is there sensory loss,[1] in particular a sensory level (a strong indicator of spinal cord disease)? Is there loss of sphincter control (bowels, bladder)?*

Progressive weakness *Rapidly progressing cord compression is an emergency.* Hours make a difference: untreated, irreversible loss of power and sensation below the lesion's level, and a neurogenic bladder and bowel may ensue.

Symptoms: Spinal or root pain[1] may precede leg weakness and sensory loss. Arm weakness is often less severe (suggests a cervical cord lesion). Bladder and anal sphincter involvement happens late and manifests as hesitancy, frequency, and, later, as painless retention. *Signs:* Look for a motor, reflex, and sensory level, with normal findings *above* the level of the lesion, LMN signs *at* the level of the lesion (p331, especially in cervical cord compression, see p396) and UMN signs *below* the level; remember that tone and reflexes are ↓ in acute cord compression—'spinal shock' after trauma, *OHCS* p726.

Causes Secondary malignancy (breast, lung, prostate) in the spine is commonest. Rarer: Infection (epidural abscess), cervical disc prolapse, haematoma (warfarin), intrinsic cord tumour, atlanto–axial subluxation.

Differential diagnosis Transverse myelitis; MS; carcinomatous meningitis; Guillain–Barré (p726); cord infarction, eg due to vasculitis (PAN, syphilis), spinal artery thrombosis, trauma, dissecting aortic aneurysm.

Tests Do not delay imaging at any cost. Speed of imaging should parallel the rate of clinical progression. Spinal x-rays can be helpful, but MRI is the definitive image. Biopsy or surgical exploration may be needed to identify the nature of any mass. *Screening blood tests:* FBC, ESR, B$_{12}$, folate, syphilis serology, U&E, LFT, PSA. Do a CXR (lung malignancy, lung secondaries, TB).

Treatment If malignancy, give dexamethasone IV 4mg/6h while considering more specific therapy, eg radiotherapy or chemotherapy ± decompressive laminectomy; which is most appropriate depends on the type of tumour, the patient's quality of life and the likely prognosis. Epidural abscesses must be surgically decompressed and antibiotics given.

Cauda equina and conus medullaris lesions The big difference between these lesions and those high up in the cord is that leg weakness is flaccid and areflexic, not spastic and hyperreflexic. *Causes:* as above plus canal stenosis; lumbosacral nerve lesions. *Clinical features:* Conus medullaris lesions show early urinary retention and constipation, back pain, sacral sensory disturbance, erectile dysfunction ± leg weakness. Cauda equina lesions feature back pain and radicular pain down the legs; asymmetrical, atrophic, areflexic paralysis of the legs; sensory loss in a root distribution and ↓sphincter power.

Management of the paralysed patient Irrespective of the cause, paralysed patients need especial care. Avoid pressure sores by frequent inspection of weight-bearing areas and turning. Avoid thrombosis in a weak or paralysed limb by frequent passive movement and pressure stockings ± low molecular weight heparin (p648). Bladder care is important (catheterization is only one option) and control of incontinence should not be at the expense of fluid intake (*OHCS* p730). Bowel evacuation may be manual or aided by suppositories. Increasing dietary fibre intake may help. Exercise of unaffected or partially paralysed limbs is important to avoid unnecessary loss of function.

---

1 *Nerve root sensations* may be sharp or dull (like angina if T3–T4 affected) or 'warm glows', or 'as if icy bandages were wrapped round my leg' or rubbed with sandpaper, or sprayed with hot water. *Dorsal column damage* may cause hypersensitivity or vibratory feelings, as if on the deck of a ship under full power, or the limbs may feel twice their normal size.
Spinothalamic symptoms may be 'as if my bones burned, and the flesh was torn away'.

Other causes of leg weakness

- *Chronic spastic paraparesis* MS; intrinsic cord tumours (astrocytomas; ependymomas; haemangioblastomas;[16] metastases, eg from melanoma, lung tumours, etc.[17]) syringomyelia; MND; subacute combined degeneration of the cord (B$_{12}$ deficiency, p634); syphilis; rare non-neoplastic lesions—eg histiocytosis X; schistosomiasis; other parasites (any eosinophilia?).[18]
- *Chronic flaccid paraparesis* Tabes dorsalis; peripheral neuropathies (p392); myopathies (rare; arms are usually involved too, see p398).
- *Unilateral foot drop* DM; stroke; prolapsed disc; MS; common peroneal nerve palsy.
- *Weak legs with no sensory loss* MND; parasaggital meningioma (the rare exception to the 'rule' that weak legs mean cord or more distal problems).
- *Absent knee jerks and extensor plantars* ('MAST'): **m**otor neurone disease, Friedreich's **a**taxia; **s**ubacute combined degeneration of the cord (but knee jerks more often brisk); **t**aboparesis (syphilis, p601).

Specific gait disorders

(Even the best professionals have to employ extraordinary tactics simply to *describe* gaits accurately,[1] never mind *diagnose* them accurately.)
- *Spastic:* Stiff, circumduction of legs ± scuffing of the foot.
- *Extrapyramidal:* Flexed posture, shuffling feet, slow to start, postural instability. *Example:* Parkinson's disease festinating gait.
- *Apraxic:* Pathognomonic 'glueing-to-the-floor' on attempting to walk[19,20] or a wide-based unsteady gait with a tendency to fall. Causes: normal pressure hydrocephalus; multi-infarct states.
- *Ataxic:* Wide-based; falls; cannot walk heel-to-toe. May be caused by cerebellar lesions (eg MS; posterior fossa tumours; alcohol; phenytoin toxicity)—or by proprioceptive sensory loss (eg sensory neuropathies; subacute combined degeneration of the cord).
- *Myopathic:* Waddle (hip girdle weakness). Cannot climb steps.
- *Psychogenic:* Often a bizarre gait not conforming to any pattern of organic gait disturbance. Suspect if there is profound gait disturbance with inability even to stand, without any signs when examined on the couch ('astasia abasia')—but this may occur with midline cerebellar lesions, normal pressure hydrocephalus, and other rare tumours.[20] Video analysis reveals 6 signs of psychogenicity, seen in 97% of patients in one study:[21]
  1 Fluctuations in response to suggestion or distraction.
  2 Excessive hesitation of locomotion incompatible with CNS disease.
  3 'Psychogenic' Romberg test with building-up of sway amplitudes.
  4 Uneconomic postures wasting muscular energy.
  5 'Walking on ice' gait, ie small cautious steps, with ankle joints fixed.
  6 Sudden buckling of the knees, usually without falls.

Tests Spinal x-rays. MRI; FBC, ESR, syphilis serology, serum B$_{12}$, U&E, LFT, PSA (prostate cancer), serum electrophoresis (myeloma); CXR (TB, Ca bronchus); LP (p752); EMG; muscle biopsy; sural nerve biopsy.

351

---

1 *Unda her brella mid piddle med puddle she ninnygoes nannygoes nancing by.* James Joyce *Finnegans Wake.*

Dyskinesia (abnormal involuntary movements)

Tremor *Rest tremor* is rhythmic, present at rest, and abolished on voluntary movement. It occurs in Parkinsonism (p382, with rigidity/bradykinesis). *Intention tremor* is an irregular, large-amplitude shaking worse on reaching out for something. It is typical of cerebellar disease, eg MS. *Postural tremor* is absent at rest, present on maintained posture (eg arms outstretched) and may persist (but is not exaggerated) on movement. *Causes:* Benign essential tremor (autosomal dominant; helped by alcohol); thyrotoxicosis; anxiety; β-agonists (eg salbutamol). Surgery/deep brain stimulation (DBS)[1] helps some tremors.

Chorea, athetosis, and hemiballismus *Chorea:* Non-rhythmic, jerky, purposeless movements which flit from one part of the body to another. Causes are Huntington's and Sydenham's chorea (choreoathetoid movements)—a rare complication of strep infection. The anatomical basis of chorea is uncertain but it is thought of as the pharmacological mirror image of Parkinson's disease (L-dopa worsens chorea). *Hemiballismus:* Large-amplitude, flinging hemichorea (affects proximal muscles) contralateral to a vascular lesion of the subthalamic nucleus (often elderly diabetics). Recovers spontaneously over months. *Athetosis:* Slow, sinuous, confluent, purposeless movements (esp. digits, hands, face, tongue), often difficult to distinguish from chorea. Commonest cause is cerebral palsy (*OHCS* p202). Most other patterns once described as 'athetoid' may now be better characterized as one of the dystonias.

Tics Brief, repeated, stereotyped movements which patients are able to suppress for a while. Tics are common in children, but usually resolve. In *Gilles de la Tourette's syndrome* (p724), multiple motor and vocal tics occur. Consider psychological support, clonazepam or clonidine if tics are severe (haloperidol is more effective but risk of tardive dyskinesia).

Myoclonus Sudden involuntary focal or general jerks arising from cord, brainstem, or cerebral cortex, seen in neurodegenerative disease (eg lysosomal storage enzyme defects), CJD (p720), and myoclonic epilepsies (infantile spasms). *Benign essential myoclonus:* General myoclonus begins in childhood as muscle twitches (eg autosomal dominant and has no other consequences). *Asterixis:* Jerking of outstretched hands (metabolic flap) from loss of extensor tone. *R:* Myoclonus may respond to valproate, clonazepam, or piracetam.

Dystonia Prolonged muscle contraction causing abnormal posture or repetitive movements due to many causes. *Idiopathic torsion dystonia (ITD)*, the commonest, starts in adulthood as a focal dystonia (eg *spasmodic torticollis:* the head is pulled to one side and held there by a contracting sternomastoid). It is worse in conditions of mental or emotional stress. Look for the 'geste antagonistique' (a manual act which controls the deviation of the head, eg a touch of a finger to a jaw). There are no other CNS signs or any secondary cause (eg Wilson's disease). Those <40yrs old need a trial of L-dopa to rule out *dopa-responsive dystonia* (rare). A few ITD patients respond to high-dose trihexyphenidyl (=benzhexol, an anticholinergic). *Blepharospasm* (*OHCS* p522, involuntary contraction of orbicularis oculi) and *writer's cramp*[2] are other focal dystonias. *Acute dystonia* may occur in young men starting neuroleptics (head pulled back, eyes drawn upward, trismus). Use anticholinergics (benzatropine 1–2mg IV). Disabling focal dystonias *may* respond to botulinum toxin injected into the muscle (*OHCS* p522) but there may be SEs. The role of DBS is uncertain.[1]

Tardive dyskinesia Involuntary chewing and grimacing movements due to long-term neuroleptics (eg metoclopramide & prochlorperazine). *Treatment:* Withdraw neuroleptic and wait 3–6 months. The dyskinesia may fail to resolve or even worsen. If so, consider tetrabenazine 25–50mg/8h PO.

---

1 A Lozano 2004 Pallidal stimulation for dystonia *Adv Neurol* 2004 **94** 301. Deep brain stimulation is an experimental technique to alter the net output of the basal ganglia (notably the globus pallidus), which is regulated by the balance of driving and inhibitory circuitry. Any abnormal activity in the outflow nucleus, the globus pallidus interna, is relayed to motor areas of thalamus and brainstem, so these targets also malfunction, so producing the motor defects characterizing parkinsonism and some dystonias.

2 When trying to write, the pen is driven into the paper. Look for hand and forearm spasm ± dystonic arm posture ± focal tremor/myoclonus ± dominant hand muscle hypertrophy. [@10789003] *EMG* may correlate with the two chief physiological events: ↓reciprocal inhibition of wrist flexor motor neurons at rest, and ↑co-contraction of antagonist muscles of the forearm during voluntary activity. [@8749993] *EEG*: abnormal motor command (sensorimotor region β rhythm). [@10762156]. **R:** β-blockers & valproate often fail. Breath-holding or arm cooling may work, as may botulinum & EMG biofeedback. [@10789003]

Stroke: clinical features and investigations

Strokes result from ischaemic infarction or bleeding into part of the brain, manifest by rapid onset (over minutes) of focal CNS signs and symptoms. It is the major neurological disease of our times.

Incidence: 1.5/1000/yr, rising with age to 10/1000/yr at 75yrs. ♂/♀ > 1 : 1.

Causes: • Thrombosis-in-situ
- Heart emboli (AF; IE; MI)
- Atherothromboembolism (eg from carotids)
- CNS bleed (BP↑; trauma; aneurysm rupture).

Rare causes: Sudden BP drop by ≥40mmHg; vasculitis (p424); venous sinus thrombosis (p364). *In young patients suspect:* Thrombophilia (p672); vasculitis; subarachnoid haemorrhage; venous-sinus thrombosis (p364); carotid artery dissection (spontaneous or from neck trauma or fibromuscular dysplasia). ►Do not hesitate to get a neurology, cardiology, or haematology opinion.

Risk factors BP↑, smoking, DM; heart disease (valvular, ischaemic, AF), peripheral vascular disease, past TIA, ↑PCV, carotid bruit, the Pill in smokers, lipids↑ (p706, statins ↓stroke risk by ~17%) excess alcohol; clotting↑ (eg ↑plasma fibrinogen, ↓antithrombin III, see p672).

Signs Sudden onset, or a step-wise progression over hours (even days) is typical. In theory, focal signs relate to distribution of the affected artery (p333), but collateral supplies cloud the issue. *Cerebral hemisphere infarcts* (50%) may cause: contralateral hemiplegia which is initially flaccid (floppy limb, falls like a dead weight when lifted), then becomes spastic (UMN); contralateral sensory loss; homonymous hemianopia; dysphasia. *Brainstem infarction* (25%): wide range of effects which include quadriplegia, disturbances of gaze and vision, locked-in syndrome (aware, but unable to respond). *Lacunar infarcts* (25%): small infarcts around basal ganglia, internal capsule, thalamus, and pons.[2] May cause pure motor, pure sensory, mixed motor and sensory signs, or ataxia; intact cognition/consciousness.

Tests Prompt investigation to confirm diagnosis and avoid further strokes but consider whether results will affect management. Look for:

- *Hypertension:* Look for retinopathy (p426) and a big heart on CXR. **NB:** acutely raised BP is common in early stroke. In general, don't treat (p356).
- *Cardiac source of emboli: Atrial fibrillation (AF):* (p130) Emboli from the left atrium may have caused the stroke. Look for a big left atrium (CXR; echo). *Post-MI:* Mural thrombus is best seen by echocardiography. In stroke from AF or mural thrombus do CT to exclude a haemorrhagic stroke, then start aspirin; wait before commencing full anticoagulation to avoid bleeds into infarcts. *SBE/IE:* (p152) 20% of those with endocarditis present with CNS signs due to septic emboli from valves. Treat as endocarditis; ask a cardiologist's opinion.
- *Carotid artery stenosis:* In carotid territory (p333) stroke/TIA, 2 randomized trials show clear benefit of carotid surgery,[3] so expert bodies affirm that ≥80% stenoses (on Doppler) merit angiography ± surgery—in fit patients.
- *Hypoglycaemia, hyperglycaemia,* and *hyperlipidaemia.*
- *Giant cell arteritis* (p424) eg if ESR↑, or story of headache or tender scalp (not necessarily temporal). Give steroids promptly (p424).
- *Syphilis:* Look for active, untreated disease (p601).
- *Thrombocytopenia* and other bleeding disorders. • *Polycythaemia* (p664).

Tests to exclude preventable causes

Pulse and BP	FBC, platelets	Sickling tests, eg in Blacks
CXR + CT of head	ESR	Blood glucose
ECG	U&E	Syphilis serology if relevant
Carotid doppler	Lipids	Endocarditis tests (p152)

Then consider echocardiography, carotid angiography, and clotting tests.

---

1 TS Eliot reads *The Waste Land:* http://town.hall.org/Archives/radio/IMS/HarperAudio/011894_harp_ITH.html
2 Pontine stroke causes quadriplegia & small pupils ± coma; prognosis: poor. S Tisch 2004. [@14530640]
3 Stenting *may* be an alternative to carotid endarterectomy. S McKevitt *Cerebrovasc Dis* 2004. [@14530635]

Cardiac causes of stroke

Cardioembolic causes are the source of stroke in >30% of patients in population studies. These may recur, unless you prevent them.

►So examine the heart with as much attention as you examine the brain.
- Atrial fibrillation (AF) increases risk of stroke five-fold (up to 5%/yr). This risk rises with age, duration of AF, hypertension, and heart failure—and if the AF follows rheumatic fever. Left ventricular dilatation, left atrial enlargement with stasis, and mitral valve disease particularly risk stroke; this risk can be largely reduced by anticoagulation (to 1.5%/yr).

  Aspirin may be preferable for those at low risk of stroke (<65yrs old, no concurrent vascular risk factors, no history of cerebral events), or for those with high risk of haemorrhage. It is less effective than warfarin, but safer. An alternative for those at high risk of stroke who cannot take warfarin or aspirin, is dipyridamole. *Discuss risks and benefits with the patient*: stroke rate in the elderly is 4.6%/yr for those on aspirin vs 4.3% on warfarin. Aim for an INR of 2.5–3.5 (stroke risk is twice as much for those with an INR of 1.7 as opposed to 2). Adding aspirin to warfarin does not confer additional protection.
- External cardioversion is complicated in 1–3% by peripheral emboli: pharmacological cardioversion may carry similar risks.
- Prosthetic valves risk major emboli; anticoagulate (INR 3.5–4.5, p649).
- Acute myocardial infarct with large left ventricular wall motion abnormalities on echocardiography predispose to left ventricular thrombus. Emboli arise in 10% of these patients in the next 6–12 months; risk being reduced by two-thirds by warfarin anticoagulation.
- Paradoxical systemic emboli via the venous circulation in those with patent foramen ovale, atrial and ventricular septal defects can occur.
- Cardiac surgery, eg bypass graft, carries particular risk (0.9–5.2%).

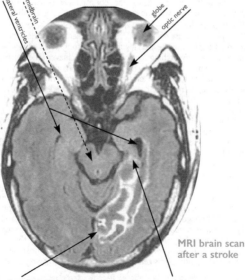

MRI brain scan after a stroke

Area of infarction between the arrows in the territory of the posterior cerebral artery

Stroke: management and prevention

Imaging p405) CT/MRI should now be the rule and is especially important if:
- Unexpected deterioration after the first 24h.
- If unusual features, or diagnosis remains unclear—eg onset slow or not known. Consider especially cerebral tumour and subdural haematoma.
- To distinguish between haemorrhage and ischaemic infarction (do scan within a few days of stroke, eg if considering later anticoagulation).
- Cerebellar stroke—cerebellar haematomas may need urgent surgery.

Differential diagnosis CNS tumour; subdural bleed (p366); Todd's palsy (p736); migraine; hypoglycaemia. Consider drug overdose if comatose. Ischaemic and haemorrhagic stroke are *not* reliably distinguishable clinically but pointers to haemorrhagic stroke are: meningism, severe headache, and coma within hours. Pointers to ischaemic stroke: carotid bruit, AF, past TIA.

Management (See p354 & p358.) Explain what has happened. ►*Communicate fully with patient, relatives and carers* about difficult decisions, eg deciding on the kindest level of intervention (list below) taking into account quality of life, coexisting conditions, and prognosis. Admission to stroke units for nursing/physio saves lives, and is a great motivator. • Unless there is strong suspicion of CNS bleeding, acute aspirin (300mg/24h PO) has a worthwhile effect.
- Nil by mouth if swallowing is a problem (try water on a teaspoon first).
- Maintain hydration, taking care not to overhydrate (cerebral oedema).
- Turn regularly and keep dry (consider catheter) to stop bed sores.
- Monitor BP; but treating even very high levels may harm (unless there is encephalopathy, or aortic dissection): even a 20% fall may impair cerebral perfusion, as autoregulation is impaired.
- If cerebellar haemorrhage possible, immediate referral for evacuation may be needed (familiarize yourself with local current management).

Mortality 20% at 1 month, 5–10%/yr thereafter. **Full recovery** 40%. Drowsiness suggests a poorer prognosis.

Sequelae Pneumonia; depression; contractures; constipation; bed sores; 'I'm a prisoner in my own body'; stress in spouse (eg ± alcoholism); see p329.

Prevention *Primary (ie before a stroke):* Control risk factors (p354: BP, smoking, DM, lipids); exercise helps (HDL↑; glucose tolerance↑). *Help quit smoking:* ►p91. In middle-aged men (especially if ↑BP), quitting ↓risk of stroke, with benefits seen in ≤5yrs. (Switching to pipes or cigars achieves little; former heavy smokers retain some excess risk.) *Lifelong anticoagulants* for those with rheumatic or prosthetic heart valves on left side. Consider warfarin in chronic non-rheumatic AF especially if there are risk factors for vascular disease. Prevention post-TIA (p360). *Secondary (ie preventing further strokes):* Control risk factors. Several large studies suggest considerable advantages from lowering BP and cholesterol (even if not particularly raised). Aspirin (p360) or warfarin if an embolic stroke, or in chronic AF (p130). NB: Combining aspirin with twice-daily modified-release dipyridamole or use of clopidogrel in place of aspirin offers only marginal benefit (?reserve for those in whom risk of further stroke is highest).

The future for ischaemic stroke Some randomized trials suggest rapid assessment of 'brain attacks' (like 'heart attacks') and thrombolysis with alteplase (t-PA) *within 3h of onset of symptoms* decreases risk of adverse outcome by 12%.[1] CI: • Major infarct on CT • Mild deficits • Recent surgery • Past CNS haemorrhage • Recent arterial puncture at a non-compressible site • Anticoagulants or PTT >15s • Platelets <100 × 10^9/L • BP↑.
Thrombolysis cannot be recommended yet in the UK, because the risk of harm has not been fully quantified for NHS patients outside the controlled environment of trials. The position may be different in hospitals which already have CNS thrombolysis teams with a dedicated imaging service on 24h call.

---

1 Although USA doctors may be sued for *not* giving thrombolyis in acute stroke, Cochrane meta-analyses are unconvinced: in the most favourable trial, the placebo group had worse strokes.☞ Despite a favourable re-analysis of the data it remains true that unreasonable data assumptions may have been made. BMJ 2003 i 1234

Summary of emergency management of stroke

Fully appraise yourself of local guidelines—and follow them. In addition:
▸▸Maintain a patent airway
▸▸Ensure hydration
▸▸Prevent hypoxia
▸▸Prevent asphyxia
▸▸Diagnose and treat any fevers
▸▸Treat any hyperglycaemia or hypoglycaemia meticulously
▸▸Meticulous nursing to optimize nutrition and prevent pressure sores.

Rehabilitation after stroke (see p354 for acute stroke)

▶*Good care requires attention to detail.* Principles are of those of *any* chronic disease (p524) and are best realized by specialist rehab or community teams (↓morbidity and institutionalization). *Special points in the early management:*

- Watch the patient swallow a small volume of water; if signs of aspiration (a cough or voice change) make *nil by mouth* for some days; use IV fluids, then semi-solids (eg jelly; avoid soups and crumbly food). Avoid early NG tube feeds (needed only in the few with established chronic swallowing problems). Speech therapists skilled in swallowing difficulties are invaluable here.
- Avoid damaging patients' shoulders through careless lifting.
- Ensure good bladder and bowel care through frequent toileting. Avoid early catheterization which may prevent return to continence.
- Position the patient to minimize spasticity. Get prompt physiotherapy.
- In pseudo-emotionalism (sobbing unprovoked by sorrow, from failure of cortical inhibition of the limbic system), tricyclics or fluoxetine may help.
- Measure time taken to sit up, and to transfer from lying to sitting in a chair; this is a good way to monitor progress with physio/occupational therapy.

Tests: Asking to point to a named part of the body tests *perceptual function.* Copying matchstick patterns tests *spatial ability.*
Dressing or drawing a clock face tests for *apraxia* (p58).
Picking out and naming easy objects from a pile tests for agnosia (acuity OK, but cannot mime use; guesses are way-out, semantically, and phonetically).

Neurorehabilitation takes a functional approach building on what patients can do—with speech- and physiotherapy. Making it fun is an important route to motivation, eg swimming (a hemiplegic arm may be supported on a special float) and video games (which ↑recovery by aiding coordination). The aim is to promote cerebral reorganization. To this end, constraint of the good arm has been found to be helpful (*constraint-induced movement therapy*).

After the stroke: thinking about end-of-life decisions '... And thus the native hue of resolution is sicklied o'er with the pale cast of thought'[1]— the more we think on these issues, the more we tie ourselves in knots, and we risk hanging not just our patients, but also ourselves with all the loose ends engendered by too much philosophy. The following precepts are intended (rather optimistically) to cut through these snares, not to reveal some deep, hidden truth, but to provide a workable framework at the bedside.

- If the patient's views are known, comply with them, except perhaps where doing so entails an illegal act, or one that clearly harms others.
- No person has authority to impose his or her own views on end-of-life decisions. You cannot tell a nurse to stop feeding someone, and expect her to obey you. Consensus is the only practical way forward. Try to get the opinion of more than one relative, and more than one shift of nurses (eg at changeover time). Let everyone have their say. You may learn new and important facts about your patient, which make decisions easier—or harder.
- If consensus is impossible, recourse to the Courts is one option: but remember that judges have no especial skill in this area.

Beware guidelines giving doctors especial powers (such as the BMA guidelines). Doctors may be the worst decision-makers because their closeness to life and death may make them tolerant of ending life—eg if the bed could be used for 'something better'. Even if this is not the case, if society thinks it is the case, then doctors are in an untenable position. Doctors do have a role, though, in facilitating consensus, and documenting it.

Success is often impossible (there are too many grey areas), but if you can stumble from one ambiguity to another without being disheartened, then that is good enough. Your patients will respect your honesty.

---

1 *Hamlet* ACT III, scene 1; William Shakespeare.

Assessing handicap, disability, and independence in daily life

Handicap entails inability to carry out social functions. 'A disadvantage for a given individual, resulting from an impairment or disability, that limits or prevents the fulfillment of a role.' Two people with the same *impairment* (eg paralyzed arm) may have different *disabilities* (one can dress, the other cannot). Disabilities are likely to determine quality of future life. Treatment is often best aimed at reducing disability, not curing disease. For example, Velcro® fasteners in place of buttons may enable a person to dress.

A person with a severe hearing impairment may seem to you to have no disability if they can lip-read. But ask yourself (and your patients, when you get to know them) about the price they pay for rising above their disabilities. Lip-reading, for example, is exhausting, requiring 100% vigilance to make sense of transitory and incomplete visual clues.

Barthel's index of activities of daily living (BAI)

Bowels	0	Incontinent (or needs to be given enemas)
	1	Occasional accidents (once a week)
	2	Continent
Bladder	0	Incontinent, or catheter inserted but unable to manage it
	1	Occasional accidents (up to once per 24 h)
	2	Continent (for more than seven days)
Grooming	0	Needs help with personal care: face, hair, teeth, shaving
	1	Independent (implements provided)
Toilet use	0	Dependent
	1	Needs some help but can do some things alone
	2	Independent (on and off, wiping, dressing)
Feeding	0	Unable
	1	Needs help in cutting, spreading butter, etc.
	2	Independent (food provided within reach)
Transfer	0	Unable to get from bed to commode: the vital transfer to prevent the need for 24-hour nursing care
	1	Major help needed (physical, 1–2 people), can sit
	2	Minor help needed (verbal or physical)
	3	Independent
Mobility	0	Immobile
	1	Wheelchair-independent, including corners, etc.
	2	Walks with help of one person (verbal or physical)
	3	Independent
Dressing	0	Dependent
	1	Needs help but can do about half unaided
	2	Independent (including buttons, zips, laces, etc.)
Stairs	0	Unable
	1	Needs help (verbal, physical, carrying aid)
	2	Independent up and down
Bathing	0	Dependent
	1	Independent (bath: must get in and out unsupervised and wash self; shower: unsupervised/unaided)

The aim is to establish the degree of independence from any help.

Barthel's paradox The more we contemplate Barthel's eulogy of independence, the more we see it as a mirage reflecting a greater truth about human affairs: ►there is no such thing as independence[1]—only interdependence, and in fostering this interdependence lies our true vocation.

---

1 *No man is an Island*, intire of it selfe; every man is a peece of the Continent, a part of the maine; if a Clod bee washed away by the Sea, Europe is the lesse, as well as if a promontorie were, as well as if a Mannor of thy friends or of thine owne were. Any man's death diminishes me, because I am involved in mankinde; And therefore never send to know for whom the bell tolls: It tolls for thee.

John Donne 1572–1631 (meditation XVII) *Selected Prose*, page 101, OUP

Transient ischaemic attack (TIA)

The sudden onset of focal CNS signs or symptoms due to temporary occlusion, usually by emboli, of part of the cerebral circulation is termed a TIA if symptoms fully resolve within 24h (TIAs are often much shorter). They are the harbingers of stroke and MI. If they are recognized for what they are, and preventive measures are prompt, a disastrous stroke may be averted.

Symptoms Attacks may be single or many. Symptoms may be the same or different on each occasions. *Carotid territory ischaemia (p333):* Contralateral weakness/numbness; dysphasia; dysarthria; homonymous hemianopia; amaurosis fugax (one eye's vision is blotted out 'like a curtain descending over my field of view'). *Vertebrobasilar territory:* Hemiparesis; hemisensory loss; bilateral weakness or sensory loss; diplopia; homonymous hemianopia in cortical blindness; vertigo; deafness; tinnitus; vomiting; dysarthria; ataxia.

Signs *(No CNS signs 24h after an attack):* Listen for carotid bruits (p66); their absence does not rule out a carotid source of emboli. NB: tight stenoses often have *no* bruit. Listen for cardiac murmurs suggesting valve disease and identify AF. Fundoscopy during a TIA may reveal retinal artery emboli.

Causes *Atherothromboembolism* from the carotid is the chief cause. Emboli from the heart (AF, mural thrombus post-MI, valvular disease, prosthetic valves); involvement of more than one cerebral artery territory is suggestive. *Hyperviscosity* (p670), eg polycythaemia, sickle-cell anaemia, WCC↑↑ (leukostasis; may need urgent chemotherapy), myeloma and *vasculitis*, eg giant cell arteritis, PAN, SLE, syphilis (and many others) are rarer causes.

Differential diagnosis of brief focal CNS symptoms: *Migraine* (symptoms spread and intensify over minutes, often with visual scintillations before headache); *focal epilepsy* (symptoms spread over seconds and often include twitching and jerking). Sometimes the problem lies in the peripheral nerves. Rare mimics of TIAs: *Malignant hypertension; hypoglycaemia; MS; intracranial lesions; phaeochromocytoma; somatization* (p529).

Tests Aim to find the cause and define vascular risk: FBC, ESR, U&E, glucose, lipids, CXR, ECG, carotid Doppler ± angiography, MRI/CT (any existing infarcts?) ± cardiac echo (rarely shows cardiac cause if no suggestive signs).

Treatment Begin after the first attack—don't wait for another; it could be a stroke. Control risk factors for stroke (p354, eg smoking, BP, lipids, etc.) and MI (p91, and risk equation, p22), the commonest mode of death after TIA. *Reversible risk factors:* Hypertension (cautiously lower; aim for <140/85mmHg, p142); hyperlipidaemia (p706); help to stop smoking (OHCS p452).

- Give an antiplatelet drug: aspirin if no peptic ulcer (~75[1] mg/d for life; probably ↓non-fatal strokes and MI by 25%, and vascular death by 15%).
- Consider oral anticoagulation in AF, mitral stenosis, recent major septal MI, or if there is any other cardiac source of embolism.
- Consider carotid endarterectomy in TIA with carotid distribution if patient is a good operative risk[2] and ≥75% stenosis at the origin of the internal carotid artery. For benefit to outweigh risk, the team's perioperative stroke/mortality rate must be <5%. Intra-operative transcranial Doppler can monitor middle cerebral artery flow. A patch may be used to reduce the chance of restenosis. Do *not* stop aspirin beforehand.

50–70% stenoses *may* benefit from surgery *only in the best hands;* NNT = 15.

Prognosis The risk of stroke and MI is ~7% per year each (the risk of stroke is 12% in the first year and up to 10% subsequently if carotid stenosis is ≥70%). Mortality is ~3 times that of a TIA-free matched population.

---

1 There is *no* dose–response relation for doses between 50 and 1500mg/d: E Johnson 2000 *E-BM* **5** 9
2 *Who risks death/CVA from endarterectomy?* ♀ sex, >75yrs, systolic BP↑, contralateral artery occluded; stenosis of ipsilateral carotid syphon/external carotid; wide-territory TIAs vs just amaurosis fugax.

Subarachnoid haemorrhage (SAH)

Spontaneous bleeding into the subarachnoid space is often a catastrophic event. Incidence: 8/100,000/yr; typical age: 35–65. *Causes:* Rupture of saccular aneurysms are the common cause (80%) with arterio-venous malformations accounting for 15%. No cause is found in <15%. *Associations:* Smoking; BP↑; alcohol misuse; bleeding disorders; mycotic aneurysm post-SBE/IE. Lack of oestrogen (post-menopausal ♀) has been cited. ♀ : ♂ > 1. *Genetics:* Close relatives of those with SAH have a 3–5-fold increase in risk of SAH.

Berry aneurysms Common sites: junction of the posterior communicating with the internal carotid (or of the anterior communicating with the anterior cerebral) or bifurcation of the middle cerebral artery. 15% are multiple. Some are hereditary. Skin biopsy may show Type 3 collagen deficiency and identify relatives at risk. *Associations:* Polycystic kidneys, coarctation of the aorta, Ehlers–Danlos syndrome (hypermobile joints + ↑skin elasticity, OHCS p746).

Clinical features *Symptoms:* Sudden (within a few seconds) devastating headache '*I thought I'd been kicked in the head*', often occipital. Vomiting, collapse (± seizures), and coma frequently follow. Coma/drowsiness may last for days. *Signs:* Neck stiffness (Kernig's +ve) takes 6h to develop; retinal and subhyaloid haemorrhage. Focal neurology *at presentation* may suggest site of aneurysm (eg pupil changes indicating a IIIrd-nerve palsy with a posterior communicating artery aneurysm) or intracerebral haematoma. Later deficits suggest ischaemia from vasospasm, or rebleeding, or hydrocephalus.

Differential In primary care, only 25% of those with severe, sudden 'thunderclap' headache have SAH. In most, no cause is found; the remainder have meningitis, migraine, intracerebral bleeds, or cerebral venous thrombosis.

Sentinel headache SAH patients may earlier have experienced a sentinel headache, perhaps due to a small warning leak from the offending aneurysm (~6%), but the picture is clouded by recall-bias. As corrective surgery is more successful in the least symptomatic, be suspicious of any *sudden* headache, particularly if associated with neck or back pain.

Tests CT (early) shows subarachnoid or ventricular blood but misses 2% of small bleeds. If a –ve scan shows no mass lesion, intracerebral haematoma or hydrocephalus (all contraindications), do an LP, >12h after the onset of headache. The CSF in SAH is uniformly bloody in the early stages of SAH and xanthochromic (yellow) after a few hours. The supernatant from spun CSF is looked at photometrically in the lab to find breakdown products of Hb. Finding bilirubin confirms SAH, and shows that the LP was not a 'bloody tap' (don't rely on there being fewer CSF RBCs in each successive bottle).

Management ▶Get a neurosurgical opinion (immediately if ↓level of consciousness, progressive focal deficit, or cerebellar haematoma suspected).
- Bed rest + chart of BP, pupils, coma level. ?Repeat CT if deteriorating.
- Re-examine CNS often. Prevent the need for straining with stool softeners.
- *Surgery:* Clipping the aneurysm can stop rebleeds and is best in those with few or no symptoms (≤ Grade II). SE: post-craniotomy epilepsy. If surgery is likely, do prompt angiography. Consider evacuation. Guglielmi coils are an alternative with less mortality (1% vs 3.8%, but they don't work in ≥25%).
- *Medical:* Cautiously control *severe* hypertension; analgesia for headache; bed rest ± sedation for ~4wks. Keep properly hydrated (running 'dry' out of respect for ICP↑, worsens vasospasm). *Vasospasm:* Nimodipine (60mg/4h PO for 3wks, or 1mg/h IVI) is a Ca^{2+} antagonist that improves outcome (give to all if blood pressure allows).

Rebleeding is a common mode of death in those who have had a subarachnoid. Rebleeding occurs in 30%, often in the first few days.

Vascular spasm follows a bleed, often causing ischaemia ± permanent CNS deficit. If this happens, surgery is not helpful at the time but may be so later.

Mortality in subarachnoid haemorrhage

Grade:	Signs:	Mortality: (%)
I	None	0
II	Neck stiffness and cranial nerve palsies	11
III	Drowsiness	37
IV	Drowsy with hemiplegia	71
V	Prolonged coma	100

Almost all the mortality occurs in the 1st month. Of those who survive the 1st month, 90% survive a year or more.

Unruptured aneurysms: 'the time-bomb in my head'

Usually, risks of preventive surgery outweigh any benefits, except perhaps in young patients (more years at risk, and surgery is twice as hazardous if >45yrs old) who have aneurysms >7mm in diameter, especially if located at the junction of the internal carotid and the posterior communicating cerebral artery, or at the rostral basilar artery bifurcation, and especially if there is uncontrolled hypertension or a past history of bleeds. Recent data (2003) from the International Study of Unruptured Intracranial Aneurysms (ISUIA) show that relative risks of rupture for an aneurysm 7–12mm across is 3.3; if the diameter is >12mm, the relative risk is 17 times that for aneurysms <7mm across.

In other patients, bear in mind the old adage: 'if it ain't broke; don't fix it'.

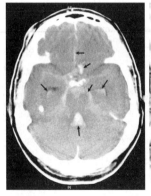 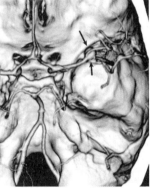

Blood from a ruptured aneurysm occupies the interhemispheric fissure (top arrow), a crescentic intracerebral area presumably near the aneurysm (2nd arrow), the basal cisterns, the lateral ventricles (temporal horns), and the 4th ventricle (bottom arrow).

CT images can be manipulated to show only high-density structures such as bones and arteries containing contrast. Here is a middle cerebral artery aneurysm.

We thank Professor Peter Scally for these CT images and the commentaries on them.

Intracranial venous thrombosis

Isolated sagittal sinus thrombosis (47% of patients) *Presentation:* Headache, vomiting, seizures, papilloedema (one cause of benign intracranial hypertension). If venous infarction supervenes, focal neurology will be seen, eg hemiplegia. Sagittal sinus thrombosis is usually accompanied by thrombosis of other sinuses, eg *lateral sinus thrombosis* (35%—eg with VI and VII cranial nerve palsies, fits, field defect, ear pain), *cavernous sinus thrombosis* (central retinal vein thrombosis, grossly oedematous eyelids, chemosis), *sigmoid sinus thrombosis* (cerebellar signs, lower cranial nerve palsies), *inferior petrosal sinus* (V and VI cranial nerve palsies—Gradenigo's syndrome).

Cortical vein thrombosis This may cause venous infarcts (± focal signs), encephalopathy, seizures, and headache (eg thunderclap headache, ie sudden and severe, ± an ominous snapping). It usually coexists with sinus thromboses, but may be an isolated event.

Predisposing factors In 30%, no cause is found. Previously reports were dominated by postpartum cases, but it is now believed that ♂ : ♀ ≈ 1:1.

Systemic diseases	*Infections*	*Drugs*
Dehydration; diabetes	Meningitis	The Pill
Neoplasms; heart failure	Cerebral abscess	Androgens
Renal/haematological disease	Septicaemia	Antifibrinolytics
Crohn's/UC (p244 & p246)	Fungal infections	
Hyperviscosity (p670)	Otitis media	*Pregnancy/postpartum*
Behçet's disease (p718)		
Activated protein C resistance (p672)		

Differential diagnosis (See subarachnoid differential diagnosis list on p362.) Thunderclap headaches also occur in dissection of a carotid or vertebral artery, as well as in *benign thunderclap headache*.

Emergency investigations in undiagnosed thunderclap headache
- Check that there are no signs of meningitis (p368).
- Do an emergency MRI or CT scan. If CT normal, do LP. Measure the opening CSF pressure.
- If high, and the headache is persisting, and no subarachnoid bleed, suspect cerebral vein thrombosis if predisposing factors. Get neuroimaging help. MRI angiography is the gold standard. **NB:** CT may be normal at first—then at ~1wk develops the delta sign, where a transversely cut sinus shows a contrast filling defect (dark). This may also be an early sign. CSF may be normal, or show RBCs and bilirubin↑—with ↑opening pressure.

Management Seek expert help, eg in interpreting MRI ± MRI angiography. One small randomized study shows that heparin saves lives and improves outcome in survivors. This may be important even in those with haemorrhagic venous infarction.

Prognosis Variable.

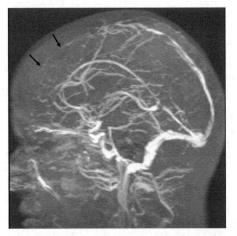

This magnetic resonance venogram (MRV) could look normal at first glance as the hardest thing to see in imaging is often that which is not there. Much of the superior sagittal sinus (SSS) is not demonstrated because it is filled with clot—an SSS thrombosis. The arrows point to where it should be seen. Posteriorly, the irregularity of the vessel indicates non-occlusive clot.

We thank Professor Peter Scally for the image and the commentary.

Subdural haemorrhage

▶Consider this very treatable condition in all whose conscious level fluctuates, and also in those having an 'evolving stroke'—especially if on anticoagulants. Bleeding is from bridging veins between cortex and venous sinuses (vulnerable to deceleration injury), resulting in accumulating haematoma between dura and arachnoid. This gradually raises ICP, shifting midline structures away from the side of the clot and, if untreated, eventual tentorial herniation and coning.

Most subdurals are secondary to trauma but they can occur without. *The trauma may have been so minor or have happened so long ago that it is not recalled.* The elderly are particularly susceptible, as brain shrinkage makes bridging veins more vulnerable. Others at risk are those prone to falls (epileptics, alcoholics) and those on long-term anticoagulation.

Symptoms Development of a subdural haemorrhage may be insidious so be alerted by a fluctuating level of consciousness (present in 35%). Typical complaints are of physical and intellectual slowing, sleepiness, headache, personality change, and unsteadiness.

Signs ↑ICP (p816). Localizing neurological symptoms (eg unequal pupils, hemiparesis) occur late and often long after the injury (63 days average).

CT Shows clot ± midline shift (but beware bilateral isodense clots). Look for crescent-shaped collection of blood over 1 hemisphere. The sickle-shape differentiates subdural blood from extradural haemorrhage.

Differential Evolving stroke, cerebral tumour, dementia.

Treatment Evacuation via burr holes usually leads to full recovery.

▶▶Extradural (epidural) haemorrhage

▶Suspect this if, after head injury, conscious level falls or is slow to improve. Extradural bleeds are commonly due to a fractured temporal or parietal bone causing laceration of the middle meningeal artery and vein, typically after trauma to a temple just lateral to the eye. Any tear in a dural venous sinus will also result in an extradural bleed. Blood accumulates between bone and dura.

Symptoms and signs Look out for a deterioration of consciousness after any head injury that initially produced no loss of consciousness or after initial drowsiness post-injury seems to have resolved. This 'lucid interval' pattern is typical of extradural bleeds. It may last a few hours to a few days before a bleed declares itself by a deteriorating level of consciousness caused by a rising ICP. Increasingly severe headache, vomiting, confusion, and fits can follow, accompanied by a hemiparesis with brisk reflexes and an upgoing plantar. If bleeding continues, the ipsilateral pupil dilates, and coma deepens, a bilateral spastic paraparesis develops, and breathing becomes deep and irregular. Death follows a period of coma and is due to respiratory arrest. Bradycardia and raised blood pressure are late signs.

Tests CT shows a haematoma which is often lens-shaped (biconvex; the blood forms a more rounded shape because the tough dural attachments to the skull tend to keep it more localized). Skull x-ray may be normal or show fracture lines crossing the course of the middle meningeal vessels. Skull fracture after trauma greatly increases the risk of an extradural haemorrhage, and should lead to prompt CT. ▶Lumbar puncture is contraindicated.

Management ▶▶Stabilize and transfer promptly (with skilled medical and nursing escorts) to a neurosurgical unit for clot evacuation (± ligation of the bleeding vessel). Care of the airway in an unconscious patient, and measures to ↓ICP often mandate intubation and ventilation (+ mannitol IVI, p816).

Prognosis Excellent if diagnosis and operation early. Poor if coma, bilateral spastic paresis, or decerebrate rigidity are present pre-op.

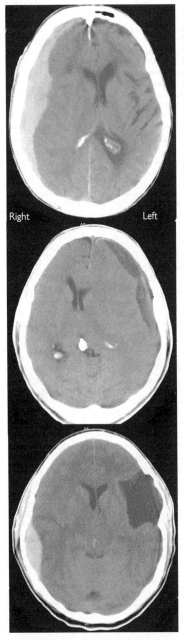

Right   Left

CT images

Figure 1. This image explains the cause as well as the pathology. On the patient's left, the cerebral sulci are prominent and prior to this adverse event would have been even larger. The brain had shrunk within the skull as a result of atherosclerosis, and poor perfusion, leaving large subarachnoid spaces. A simple, quick rotation of the head would have been enough to tear one of the bridging veins, causing this *acute subdural haematoma*.

Figure 2. This fluid collection is of low attenuation compared to the brain, except for a small area of increased attenuation. It is an *acute on chronic subdural haematoma*. But there is more! Look at the shift of midline structures across under the falx cerebri, subfalcine herniation. It is not just caused by the subdural. The left hemisphere is swollen as a result of the compression of the bridging veins in the subdural space, shifting the ventricles and calcified pineal across to the right.

Figure 3. The blood (high attenuation, fusiform or biconvex collection) on the right side is limited anteriorly by the coronal suture and posteriorly by the lambdoid suture. This is therefore an *extradural haematoma*. The low attenuation CSF density collection on the left is causing scalloping of the overlying bone. It is in the typical location of an arachnoid cyst; an incidental finding of a congenital abnormality.

We thank Professor Peter Scally for the images and commentary.

367

Meningitis

Meningitis is inflammation of the meninges caused by bacteria, viruses, fungi, or parasites. ▸▸Bacterial meningitis is a killer, and kills *quickly*. Emergency ℞: p370. Look for rapid onset (<48h) of these signs:

• *Meningeal signs:* Headache; photophobia; stiff neck; Kernig's sign +ve (pain and resistance on passive knee extension with hips fully flexed). Brudzinski's sign +ve (hips flex on bending head forward); opisthotonus.
• *Signs of ↑ICP:* Headache; irritability; drowsiness; vomiting; fits; papilloedema; ↓consciousness/coma; irregular respiration; ↓pulse; ↑BP (late sign).
• *Septic signs:* Malaise; T°↑; arthritis; odd behaviour; rash (any, petechiae suggest meningococcus); DIC (bleeding); slow capillary refill; ↓BP; ↑pulse; tachypnoea.

Tests (follow algorithm, p370) Do not delay treatment for tests. *Lumbar puncture* is critical to diagnosis. Do at once provided no signs of ↑ICP (↓consciousness, *very* bad headache, frequent fits) or focal neurology, in which case do CT first to rule out a mass lesion or hydrocephalus. Send 3 bottles of CSF for Gram stain, Ziehl–Nielsen stain (TB), cytology, virology, glucose, protein, culture ± india ink for cryptococcus. CSF may be normal early on (p752 & p369), so repeat LP if symptoms and signs persist. *CSF in meningitis:* See BOX. Neutrophils > 1180 × 10⁶/L predict bacterial meningitis with >99% certainty. Gram stains of CSF are +ve in 60–90% of bacterial meningitis (~40% if antibiotics have already been given). *Other tests:* Blood cultures; blood glucose (compare to CSF); FBC; U&E; CXR (lung abscess?); culture urine, nasal swabs & stool (virology); skull x-ray if recent head injury. Skin scraping of petechiae for meningococcus may be tried. Where available, PCR ± bacterial antigen tests offer a route to rapid diagnosis.

Risk factors *Place:* Overcrowded closed communities, schools, day centres.
Head injury: Especially basal skull fracture or cranial or spinal surgery.
Septic site: Distant (pneumonia) or near (sinusitis; mastoiditis; otitis media).
Host factors: Complement or antibody deficiency, *OHCS* p201; old or young.
Immunosuppression: Carcinoma; AIDS; no effective spleen; sickle-cell disease; hypogammaglobulinaemia; DM. *Foreign body:* CSF shunts.

Aseptic meningitis CSF has cells but is Gram-stain –ve and no bacteria are cultured on standard media. *Infective:* Virus (echovirus, mumps, coxsackie, herpes simplex/zoster, HIV, measles, 'flu); partly treated bacterial meningitis; fungi; atypical TB; syphilis; Lyme disease; leptospirosis; *Listeria; Brucella.* Parasites: eg rat lungworms (*Angiostrongylus cantonensis*, via raw snail eating); do CSF eosinophil count. *Non-infective:* See below.

Non-infective meningitis Meningeal inflammation can be caused by meningeal infiltration by malignant cells (leukaemia, lymphoma, other tumours); chemical meningitis (intrathecal drugs, contaminants); drugs (NSAIDs, trimethoprim); sarcoidosis; SLE; Behçet's disease.

Differential diagnosis Any acute infection (eg malaria); local infection causing neck stiffness, eg cervical nodes; tetanus (CSF normal in all these). Encephalitis (see BOX); subarachnoid haemorrhage (p362, blood in CSF).

Prognosis and sequelae Acute bacterial meningitis has a mortality of 70–100% untreated; *Neisseria meningitidis* meningitis has an overall mortality in the West of ~15%. Survivors are at risk of permanent neurological deficits including mental retardation, sensorineural deafness (up to 40% although many do recover), and cranial nerve palsies. Viral meningitis is self-limiting, has a good prognosis, and no long-term sequelae.

Recurrent meningitis Is there access to the subarachnoid space *via* occult spina bifida or skull fracture, or one of the above risk factors, or an associated disease, eg SLE, sarcoid, Behçet's (p718), or benign recurrent aseptic Mollaret's meningitis (PCR suggests it may be from herpes simplex)?

Typical CSF in meningitis (There are no hard-and-fast rules)

	Pyogenic	Tuberculous	Viral ('aseptic')
Appearance	Often turbid	Often fibrin web	Usually clear
Predominant cell[1]	Polymorphs	Mononuclear	Mononuclear
Cell count/mm³	Eg 90–1000+	10–1000	50–1000
Glucose[†]	<½ plasma	<½ plasma	>½ plasma
Protein (g/L)	>1.5	1–5	<1
Organisms	In smear and culture	Often absent in smear	Not in smear or culture

[†] Hypoglycorrhachia (↓CSF glucose) also occurs in *parasitic meningitis*; request CSF eosinophil count.

Meningoencephalitis and encephalitis

▶▶ *Herpes simplex encephalitis needs urgent treatment with aciclovir (p568).*

Encephalitis is inflammation of brain parenchyma and is distinguished from meningitis by the relative involvement of meninges and brain. There is usually some degree of inflammation of the parenchyma in meningitis and of the meninges in encephalitis.

Cause Viruses (herpes simplex, commonly; also Japanese B encephalitis, HIV, coxsackie virus, echo virus, rabies, west Nile virus. Think also of *Listeria* (p591), CMV, and toxoplasmosis (p574) if immunocompromised. Measles may cause subacute sclerosing panencephalitis (SSPE[2]) and rubella progressive rubella panencephalitis. *Others:* Borrelia burgdorferi et al. (p600) and Staphylococcus aureus (p590) and other bacteria originating from pus elsewhere (eg frontal sinus; SBE/IE) may reach the brain where they may cause abscesses.

Signs Meningism, consciousness↓, convulsions ± focal CNS or psychiatric features, eg temporal lobe fits, amnesia, or odd behaviours.

Diagnosis is made from:
• Knowledge of local epidemics and of the patient's immunocompetence.
• Unreliable clinical signs (eg temporal lobe signs ± temporal lobe swelling seen on CT or MRI ± periodic complexes on EEG in HSV encephalitis).
• Associated infection (eg mumps).
• CSF microscopy (above; cell count↑; glucose usually ↔).
• Demonstration of virus in CSF, eg serology or PCR (quickest).
• Throat swabs, or stool or CSF culture (the latter rarely contributes much).

Management Get expert help early and admit to ITU for supportive care. In an ill patient, it may be necessary to treat blind with drugs covering all treatable causes of encephalitis. Most important is to realize that any acute encephalitis could be due to HSV and should therefore be treated immediately with aciclovir. Ceftriaxone, benzylpenicillin + thiamine (in case of *Wernicke's* encephalopathy p738) are other reasonable empirical treatments to use until the agent responsible is identified (this may never happen).

369

1 ≤5 lymphocytes/mm³ may be normal, so long as there are no neutrophils. Normal protein: 0.15–0.45g/L. Normal CSF glucose: 2.8–4.2mmol/L (↓by: bacterial, fungal, mumps, carcinomatous meningitis, partially treated bacterial meningitis, herpes encephalitis, hypoglycaemia, sarcoid, CNS vasculitides). The predominant cell type may be lymphocytes in TB, listerial, and cryptococcal meningitis. ▶Normal opening pressure: 7–18cmCSF; in meningitis it may be >40 (typically 14–30cmCSF).

2 SSPE presents ~6yrs after the original infection with personality change, dementia, myoclonic fits, and ataxia, eventually leading to death. Progressive rubella panencephalitis is similar. Post-infectious encephalomyelitis (acute disseminated encephalomyelitis) may occur after measles, zoster, rubella, mumps, mycoplasma or 'flu virus infection, or post-vaccinations www.txt.co.uk/sum.cfm?2. It typically presents with convulsions, coma, fever, urinary retention, or pareses ~2wks after the initial infection. Involuntary movements, cranial nerve lesions, nystagmus, and ataxia are also common. MRI shows demyelination.

▶▶Meningitis treatment

If you suspect meningitis and are outside hospital, *nothing* must delay blind therapy with IV/IM benzylpenicillin 1.2g while awaiting transport. In hospital: ABCs; secure airway; give high-flow O_2. Ask a nurse to draw up cefotaxime 2g[1]

Do septicaemic or meningitic features predominate?

Septicaemic signs to fore, eg ↓capillary refill time (occurs before BP↓); rash

Do not attempt LP
2g cefotaxime IV
Call critical care team for review
    Signs of shock?

Yes → Volume resus
Take to ITU for IVI of inotropes or vasopressors
Aim for systolic BP of >80mmHg and urine flow >30mL/h

No → Careful monitoring
Repeat review

Meningitic features predominate (neck stiffness; photophobia)

Assess carefully before any LP
If signs of ICP↑, BP↓, or respiratory failure, call critical care team
If uncertain ask for urgent senior review

Monitor and stabilize circulation
If no shock, or ICP↑ signs, do LP

2g cefotaxime IV immediately post-LP
If signs of ↑ICP, take to ITU; no LP; 2g cefotaxime IV; nurse at 30°; have low threshold for intubation/ventilation
NB: CT scans do not rule out ICP↑.

Subsequent therapy Cefotaxime 2–4g/8h IVI (eg for 10d); ↓dose in renal failure; see p545 and *datasheet* (SPC). Isolate for 1st 24h. If response to the above is poor, get help. Consider pre-emptive intubation and ventilation ± inotropic/vasopressor support (p788). When you have the time, notify the consultant in community disease control (CCDC). For novel biological agents for meningo-coccaemia, see p739. Rifampicin may be needed to eliminate nasal carriage.

Which antibiotic—when the organism is known? See below + p543 for doses (alternatives in brackets).

Pneumococcus: Cefotaxime (ceftriaxone) ± vancomycin for 10–14d.
Meningococcus: Benzylpenicillin + rifampicin for 2d before discharge (cefotaxime, ceftriaxone).
Haemophilus influenzae: Cefotaxime (ceftriaxone, chloramphenicol; up to >50% may be chloramphenicol-resistant); give rifampicin (20mg/kg/12h PO if >3 months old; max 600mg) for 4d pre-discharge in Type b infection.
Escherichia coli: Cefotaxime (ceftriaxone).
Staph. aureus: Flucloxacillin (p543); for resistant staphs, see MRSA (p590).
Listeria monocytogenes: Gentamicin (p710) + ampicillin (p591) for 10–14d.
Mycobacterium tuberculosis: Rifampicin, ethambutol, isoniazid, *and* pyrazinamide.
Cryptococcus neoformans: Amphotericin B + flucytosine (p612).

Complications Look out for complications: cerebral oedema; cranial nerve lesions; deafness; cerebral venous sinus thrombosis (p364).

Meningococcal prophylaxis Talk to your CCDC. Offer prophylaxis to:
• Household/nursery contacts (ie within droplet range).
• Those who have kissed the patient's mouth.
• Yourself (rarely necessary). Give rifampicin (600mg/12h PO for 2d; children >1yr 10mg/kg/12h; <1yr 5mg/kg/12h) or ciprofloxacin (500mg PO, 1 dose). Neither is guaranteed in pregnancy, but a short course is unlikely to harm and is recommended. *Meningitis vaccination:* See p558.

---

1 Or ceftriaxone. Also give ampicillin 2g/6h IV if >50yrs to cover listeria; amend in the light of blood culture/LP results. Vancomycin ± rifampicin may be needed in some populations. There *may* be a role for dexamethasone 0.15mg/kg/6h IV from just before 1st antibiotic dose. This algorithm is after that of the British Infection Society (2003). It assumes no immunocompromise; if this is possible, get help.

Most frequent organisms in community-acquired meningitis

Vaccination (p558) is successfully reducing haemophilus and meningococcal type C infections: so patterns in the community are changing.

Neonates:
   E. coli
   β-haemolytic streptococci
   L. monocytogenes

Children <14 years:
   H. influenzae if <4yrs and unvaccinated
   Meningococcus (N. meningitidis)
   Streptococcus pneumoniae
   TB (endemic areas)

Adults and older children:
   Meningococcus
   Pneumococcus (Strep. pneumoniae)

Elderly and immunocompromised:
   Pneumococcus
   L. monocytogenes
   TB
   Gram-negative organisms
   Cryptococcus

Hospital acquired (nosocomial) and post-traumatic meningitis

(May often be multi-drug resistant)
   Klebsiella pneumoniae
   E. coli
   Pseudomonas aeruginosa
   Staph. aureus

Meningitis in special situations

Patients with CSF shunts are at especial risk of meningitis (eg staphylococcal), as are those patients having spinal procedures (eg spinal anaesthetics) where *Pseudomonas* species may be the culprit.

Delirium (acute confusional state)

▶Common in hospitalized patients (5-15% patients in general medical or surgical wards) so consider any unexplained behaviour change in a hospital patient as possible delirium and look for an organic cause. There are 7 signs:

1 *Consciousness* is impaired (onset over hours or days). Impaired consciousness is difficult to describe, but when you talk to the patient you have the sense that they are not with you. This has been described more formally as a mild impairment of thinking, attention, and concentration—or more simply as a mild global impairment of cognitive processes associated with a reduced awareness. Conscious level fluctuates throughout the day with confusion typically worsening in the late afternoon and at night.

2 *Disorientation* in time (does not know time, day, or year) and place (often more marked) is the rule.

3 *Behaviour:* Inactivity, quietness, reduced speech, and perseveration (repetition of words) or else hyperactivity, noisiness, and disruptive irritability.

4 *Thinking:* Slow and muddled, commonly with ideas of reference or delusions (eg accusing staff of plotting against them).

5 *Perception:* Disturbed, often with illusions and visual hallucinations (unlike in schizophrenia, where auditory modality dominates) or tactile.

6 *Mood:* Lability, anxiety, perplexity, fear, agitation, or depression.

7 *Memory:* Impaired. Later, patients may be amnesic for the episode.

This is precised and deepened by Conrad's formulation 'The wastes of his weary brain were haunted by shadowy images now—images of wealth and fame... Sometimes he was contemptibly childish. He desired to have kings meet him at railway-stations on his return from some ghastly Nowhere... "Close the shutter". said Kurtz suddenly "I can't bear to look at this." I did so. There was a silence. "Oh, but I will wring your heart yet!" he cried at the invisible wilderness.' 64

Causes (Pain and other psychological states are important co-factors.)
• Infection/contagion (as in Kurtz, above): pneumonia, UTI, wounds; IV lines.
• Drugs: opiates, anticonvulsants, L-dopa, sedatives, recreational, post-GA.
• Alcohol withdrawal (2–5d post-admission; raised LFTs with raised MCV; history of alcohol abuse), also drug withdrawal.
• Metabolic: hypoglycaemia, uraemia, liver failure, U&E imbalance, anaemia.
• Hypoxia: respiratory or cardiac failure.
• Vascular: stroke, myocardial infarction.
• Intracranial infection: encephalitis, meningitis.
• Raised intracranial pressure/space occupying lesions.
• Epilepsy: status epilepticus (see BOX), post-ictal states.
• Trauma, head injury: especially subdural haematoma.
• Nutritional: thiamine, nicotinic acid, or B_{12} deficiency.

Differential diagnosis If agitated, consider anxiety (check conscious level). If delusions or hallucinations, consider primary mental illness (eg schizophrenia) but remember that in hospitalized, ill patients with no psychiatric history, mental illness is rare and delirium is common.

Management After identifying and treating the underlying cause, aim to:

1 Reduce distress and prevent accidents.

2 Nurse in a *moderately lit*, quiet room, ideally with the *same* staff in attendance (minimizes confusion) where the patient can be watched closely. Repeated reassurance and orientation to time and place can help.

3 Minimize medication (especially sedatives). If agitated and disruptive, however, some sedation may be necessary. Use a major tranquillizer—haloperidol 0.5–2mg IM/PO, p15—or chlorpromazine 50–100mg IM/PO (but not in the elderly, in whom it is liable to cause cardiac side-effects and hypotension). Wait 20min to judge effect—further doses can be given if needed. Benzodiazepines may be used for night-time sedation. NB: In alcohol withdrawal do *not* use chlorpromazine, use diazepam instead (p254).

Non-convulsive status epilepticus (NCSE) as a cause of confusion

NCSE is under-diagnosed, and may manifest itself as confusion, impaired cognition/memory, odd behaviour, dreamy derealization,[1][65] aggression, or psychosis ± abnormalities of eye movement, eyelid myoclonus or odd postures. It may or may not occur in the context of classic seizures or ischaemic brain injury (eg subarachnoid haemorrhage).[66] Other causes and associations: drugs (eg antidepressants), infections (eg, arboviruses; HIV; syphilis), neoplasia, dementias, sudden changes in calcium levels,[67] renal failure (eg with cephalosporin therapy or peritoneal dialysis). *Diagnosis:* EEG (eg prolonged 3-per-second spike-wave complexes). Subsequent MRI may show focal oedema (eg in the hippocampus). *Treatment:* Valproate, etho-suximide, or IV benzodiazepines may be indicated (get expert help).[68]

1 The external world is unfamiliar and unreal, and its objects, anchored neither in space nor time, float as in a more or less lucid dream. *Depersonalization* and *derealization* are part of the *dissociative states* (an example of a disorder of consciousness). Dissociation is a mechanism of the mind that separates streams of memories or thoughts from normal consciousness. These mental fragments may then resurface and peruse a life of their own. Causes: Migraine, epilepsy, head injury, stress, and, of course, prolonged sleeplessness (which is why all doctors instinctively understand this odd syndrome).

Dementia

▶Assume confusion is due to acute illness until proved otherwise (p372).

Dementia, which has many causes, entails *impaired cognition with intact consciousness* (unlike delirium). The key is a good history: ask spouse, relatives, or friends about *progressively* impaired cognition/memory (autobiographical[1]; political etc.). Get *objective* evidence. Histories usually go back months or years. There is increasing forgetfulness, and normal tasks of daily living are done with increasing incompetence, eg going to buy sausages 6 times in a day, and then being baffled as to why there is a great mound of sausages in the kitchen. Sometimes the patient appears to have changed personality, eg ↑apathy, uncharacteristically rude or depressed—or with slow, repetitious speech, or literalness. For objective evidence, do tests of cognitive functioning (p59).

Epidemiology Rare below 55yrs of age. 5–10% prevalence above 65yrs. 20% prevalence above 80yrs, and 70% of those over 100yrs.

Commonest causes *Alzheimer's disease (AD)*—see p376. *Vascular dementia:* ~25% of all dementias. It represents the cumulative effects of many small strokes. Look for evidence of vascular pathology (BP↑; past strokes; focal CNS signs). Onset is sometimes sudden, and deterioration is often stepwise.

Lewy body dementia: Characterized by Lewy bodies[2] in brainstem *and* neocortex, *fluctuating* cognitive loss, alertness and attention; parkinsonism (p382); detailed visual hallucinations; falls; loss of consciousness/syncope. It is the 3rd commonest dementia (15–25%) after AD and vascular causes. Older neuroleptics in these patients *often* cause neuropsychiatric SEs. Rivastigmine *may* help.

Fronto-temporal dementia: (Frontal and temporal atrophy) without Alzheimer histology (p376). *Signs:* Behavioural/personality change; early preservation of episodic memory & spatial orientation; disinhibition; hyperorality, stereotyped behaviour, and emotional unconcern. The disinhibition is not *always* bad.[3]

Ameliorable causes T4↓; B₁₂/folate↓; thiamine↓ (eg alcohol); syphilis; some cerebral tumours (eg parasagittal meningioma); subdural haematoma; CNS cysticercosis (p616); normal pressure hydrocephalus (dilatation of ventricles without signs of ↑pressure, ?due to obstructed CSF flow from subarachnoid space; CSF shunts help; it is suggested by incontinence early-on ± gait apraxia).

374

Rarer causes: Alcohol/drug abuse; pellagra (p250), Huntington's (p726); CJD (p720); Parkinson's (p382); Pick's disease; HIV; cryptococcosis (p612); SSPE (p369); progressive leukencephalopathy.

Tests ▶Ensure no treatable cause is missed. FBC, ESR; U&E; Ca²⁺; LFT; TSH; autoantibodies; folate/B₁₂ (treat low-normals); syphilis serology; CT/MRI (any structural pathology?). Consider EEG; CSF; functional imaging (PET; SPECT, ie single photon emission CT; cost ≈ \$74,400 to \$1.9 million per QALY). Metabolic, genetic, and HIV testing after appropriate counselling, as indicated.

Management Neuropsychiatric referral: are specific drugs indicated? (p377)
- Nominate a key worker; make a *care management plan*; get support from social services ± Alzheimer's Society, p377. Ensure access to benefits (p377).
- Carer stress is inevitable (p329), causing ↑morbidity *and* mortality (↑ by 45%): ameliorate this by practical steps and unswerving loyalty (p329).
- GPs have a central role in 'couple focused planning', which acknowledges that needs combine in ways which are not simply additive.
- ▶Give any specific treatment (eg if TSH↑ or B₁₂/folate↓ or equivocal), and treat concurrent illnesses (these may contribute significantly to confusion).

---

1 Autobiographical and political memory are held in different areas: S Black 2004 *Neuropsychologia* **42** 25
2 Lewy bodies are eosinophilic intracytoplasmic neuronal inclusion bodies; there is overlap between Lewy body dementia and Alzheimer's and Parkinson's (PD), making treatment hard as L-dopa can precipitate delusions, and antipsychotic drugs worsen PD. Donepezil may help all 3. [@11981238]
3 An artist who had been constrained by over-adherence to one school of art had a fascinating blossoming of creativity and emotional insight with the arrival of fronto-temporal dementia. *Neurology* 2003 1707. This poses the question of what counts as a disease. If you can answer this question unequivocally perhaps you are over-endowed, fronto-temporally? Let some ambiguity in!

Alzheimer's disease (AD)

This leading cause of dementia is *the* big neuropsychiatric disorder of our times, dominating not just psychogeriatric wards, but the lives of countless children and spouses who have given up work, friends, and all accustomed ways of life to support relatives through the last long years. Their lives can be tormented—'*I am chained to a corpse*' (p329) or transformed, depending on how gently patients exit into their '*worlds of preoccupied emptiness*'. *Mean survival:* 7yrs from onset. Suspect Alzheimer's in adults with enduring,[1] acquired deficits of visual-spatial skill ('he gets lost easily'), memory, and cognition, eg tested by mental test scores + other neuropsychometric tests (p59). Onset may be from 40yrs (earlier, in Down's syndrome, so notions of 'senile' and 'pre-senile' dementia are blurred, and irrelevant). *Cause:* Accumulation β-amyloid peptide, a degradation product of amyloid precursor protein, resulting in progressive neuronal damage, neurofibrillary tangles, ↑numbers of senile plaques, and loss of the neurotransmitter acetylcholine from damage to an ascending forebrain projection (nucleus basalis of Meynert; connects with cortex). AD shares some pathological processes with vascular dementias.

Memory loss is not like loss of land with a rising tide: the last memories to be sunk in the sea of forgetfulness are not earliest or latest, but the deepest, the most personal, and the most bizarre: prime ministers come and go, but, for dementing British patients of a certain age, the last name retained is that of Mrs Thatcher. When this name sinks into oblivion ('*fame's eternal dumping ground*'), often long after that of sovereigns, deities, spouses, and children, one may safely say that the waters have covered the sea.

Risk factors *Defective genes* on chromosomes 1, 14, 19, 21; the apoE4 variant brings forward age of onset. *Insulin resistance* (p295) *may* be important. ◆

Diagnosis is often haphazard, as the exact form of dementia used not to influence outcome, provided B_{12} and TSH were normal. This view is hard to justify now that *specific* treatments are available for Alzheimer's. Specialist input with imaging is the ideal (this helps rule out fronto-temporal dementias, Lewy body, vascular dementias, and Pick's disease).

Presentation Memory/cognition↓; behavioural change (eg aggression, wandering, disinhibition); hallucinations; delusions; apathy; depression; irritability; euphoria. There is no standard natural history. Cognitive impairment is progressive, but behavioural/psychotic symptoms may go after a few months or years. Towards the end, often but by no means invariably, patients become sedentary, taking little interest in anything. Parkinsonism (p382), wasting, mutism, incontinence ± seizures may occur.

Theoretical issues *Potential strategies* (*indicates randomized trial evidence)
- *Prevent breakdown of acetylcholine*,* eg anticholinesterases, etc. (see BOX).
- *Prevent overstimulation of NMDA receptors* by glutamate; memantine (see BOX) is an NMDA antagonist. (NMDA = N-methyl-D-aspartate, p335.)
- *Stimulating nicotinic receptors* may be protective (smoking is *not* a solution!).
- *Preventing neurotoxicity from homocysteine* by ensuring good B_{12} intake (p374).
- *NSAIDs* to ↓production of β-amyloid. NB: NSAIDs don't stop progression of AD.*[2]
- *Some anti-oxidants* may be protective, eg ginkgo biloba or vit C with D.[3]
- ↓*Arteriopathy* (AD risk rises with BP↑) and *normalize pulse pressure* (PP=70–84); if PP > 84mmHg (reflects arterial stiffness) risk of AD is ↑; if PP < 70 (reflects poor perfusion) risk of AD is also raised. *Statins** (p707) may prevent AD eg by ↓brain cholesterol synthesis (∴ less amyloid plaque formation).
- *Cognitively stimulating hobbies* may help: a 1-point rise in cognitive activity score can ↓risk of AD by 33%. NB: *HRT* (OHCS p18) was thought to protect, but the WHIMS* trial found ↑risk of AD (2% vs 1% on placebo). *JAMA 2003 N=4532*

---

1 NB: 'Enduring' need not mean unfluctuating: self-knowledge may come and go, allowing occasional poetic insight, as in Iris Murdoch's poignant self-diagnosis—'I am sailing into the dark'.
2 JAMA 2003 2819. Neither naproxen nor rofecoxib prevents progression of AD. N = 351.
3 P Zandi 2004 *Arch Neurol* **61** 82 (cross-sectional prospective study).

Practical issues in managing Alzheimer's dementia

- *Exclude treatable dementias* (B$_{12}$, folate, syphilis serology, T4, ?HIV); *is this depression masquerading as dementia?* Antidepressant trials may be needed.
- *Treat concurrent illnesses* (many can make dementia worse). In most people, the dementia remains and will progress. Involve relatives and relevant agencies. UK Alzheimer's Disease Society: 0151 298 2444.
- *Avoid drugs that may ↓cognition* (neuroleptics, sedatives, tricyclics, p15).
- In the last stages, feeding by gastrostomy tube has been considered beneficial, but is now thought to be no better than feeding by hand.

- In many countries there is *special help* made available for those looking after demented relatives at home—eg in the UK:

Laundry services for soiled linen	Attendance allowance
'Orange badge' giving priority parking	Respite care in hospital
Carers' groups for mutual support	Council tax rebate (forms
Help from occupational therapist, district	from local council office)
nurses & community psychiatric nurses	Day care/lunch clubs

►See *Living with neurological disease*, p329. *Drugs* which ↑acetylcholine availability for synaptic transmission (by inhibiting the enzyme for its break-down, eg rivastigmine)—or donepezil[1] may delay need for institutional care, but not necessarily its duration. Liaise with a psychogeriatrician. NICE (www.nice.org.uk) asserts that *donepezil, rivastigmine,*[2] and *galanta-mine*[3] should be available for those with mild and moderate AD whose MMSE (p59) score is >12 if expert guidance and a suitable carer is available—and an increase in MMSE and functioning is seen after 2–4 months on a maintenance dose. ►*In general, when you have to choose between interventions of similar or unknown benefit, choose low-technology over high-technology.* The high-technology option can always be added later, but if the fundamentals of care (such as respite admission to give relatives a break) are ignored even the most vigorously pursued high-technology options may fail to produce real benefit.

Antiglutamatergic treatment: Randomized trials show that the NMDA antagonist *memantine* helps moderate-to-severe Alzheimer's disease.[4] Its role is, as yet, ill-defined (*SE:* hallucinations, confusion, hypertonia).

377

1 Wynn Z 2004 [@14564129] Donepezil, dose: eg 5mg/24h PO nocte; ↑ to 10mg nocte after 1 month; cholinergic SEs: D&V, cramps, incontinence—also headaches, dizziness, heart block, psychiatric disturbance, LFT↑.

2 Rivastigmine is a dual acetylcholinesterase/butyrylcholinesterase (AChE/BuChE) inhibitor, and may be better than AChE-selective inhibitors (donepezil; galantamine) vis-à-vis improving apathy, anxiety, depression, hallucinations, and delusions (it also works in a wider range of dementias). [@12139365]

Pre-R orbitofrontal signs (agitation; disinhibition; aberrant motor activity, p387) may predict good response to donepezil, while pre-R hallucinations predict response to rivastigmine. [@ 11261510] [@12094826]

3 Galantamine (=galanthamine; Reminyl®) was originally isolated from daffodils. It is a specific, competitive, and reversible acetylcholinesterase inhibitor, and also an allosteric modulator at nicotinic cholinergic receptor sites potentiating cholinergic nicotinic neurotransmission. See Cochrane. CD001747

4 NMDA. Reisberg B 2003 *NEJM* **348** 1333. N = 252; dose = 20mg memantine daily for 28wks.

Epilepsy: diagnosis

Epilepsy is a recurrent tendency to spontaneous, intermittent, abnormal electrical activity in part of the brain, manifest as *seizures*.[1] These may take many forms: for a given patient they tend to be stereotyped. *Convulsions* are the motor signs of electrical discharges. Many of us would have seizures in abnormal metabolic circumstances—eg $Na^+\downarrow$, hypoxia (reflex anoxic seizures in faints): we would not normally be said to have epilepsy. In deciding if an event is epileptic, don't pay *too* much attention to associated incontinence and abnormal movement (not everything that twitches is epilepsy): but biting the side of the tongue is very suggestive. Prevalence of active epilepsy is ~1%.

The patient There may (rarely) be a *prodrome* lasting hours or days preceding the seizure. It is not part of the seizure itself: the patient or others notice a change in mood or behaviour. An *aura*, which is part of the seizure, may precede its other manifestations. The aura may be a strange feeling in the gut, or a sensation or an experience such as *déjà vu* (disturbing sense of familiarity), or strange smells or flashing lights. It implies a partial seizure (a focal event), often, but not necessarily, temporal lobe epilepsy (TLE). After a partial seizure involving the motor cortex (Jacksonian convulsion) there may be temporary weakness of the affected limb(s) (Todd's palsy). After a generalized seizure, patients may feel awful with headache, myalgia, confusion, and a sore tongue.

Diagnosis Decide first: is this epilepsy? (p344 for $\triangle\triangle$) A detailed description from a witness of 'the fit' is vital. Try hard not to diagnose epilepsy in error—therapy has significant side-effects, the diagnosis is stigmatizing and has implications for employment, insurance, and driving. Decide next what type of seizure it is. The attack's *onset* is the key concern here: partial or generalized? If the seizure begins with focal features, it is a partial seizure, however rapidly it is generalized. Ask next: what if anything brings it on (eg flickering light (TV) or alcohol)? Can this be avoided? TV-induced seizures—almost always generalized—rarely require drugs. Then decide what the best drug is. Start at low dose. Gradually (eg over 8wks) build up until fits are controlled. Persist until drug at maximum dose before considering a change of therapy (p380).

Types

378

1 *Partial seizures:* Features are referable to a part of one hemisphere suggesting structural disease.
  - *Elementary symptoms* (consciousness unimpaired, eg focal motor seizures).
  - *Complex symptoms* (consciousness impaired, eg olfactory aura preceding automatism). Usually TLE.
  - *Partial seizure with secondary generalization:* Evidence of electrical disturbance starting focally, then spreading widely, causing a secondary generalized seizure.

2 *Primary generalized seizures:* No features referable to only one hemisphere.
  - *Absences (petit mal):* Brief (≤10s) pauses, eg suddenly stops talking in mid-sentence, then carries on where left off. Presents in childhood.
  - *Tonic-clonic* (classical *grand mal*). Sudden onset, loss of consciousness, limbs stiffen (tonic) then jerk (clonic); may have one without the other; drowsy after.
  - *Myoclonic jerk* (eg thrown suddenly to ground, or a violently disobedient limb: a patient described it as *my flying-saucer epilepsy*, as crockery which happened to be in the hand would take off).
  - *Atonic* (becomes flaccid).
  - *Akinetic.* Note also *infantile spasms* (OHCS p266).

Causes Often none is found. *Physical:* Trauma, space occupying lesions, stroke, BP↑↑, tuberous sclerosis, SLE, PAN, sarcoid, vascular malformations. *Metabolic:* Alcohol or benzodiazepine withdrawal; glucose ↑ or ↓, $P_aO_2\downarrow$ (eg in brady-arrhythmias), uraemia, $Na^{2+}\uparrow$ or ↓, $Ca^{2+}\uparrow$, liver disease, drugs (eg phenothiazines, tricyclics, cocaine). *Infection:* Encephalitis, syphilis, cysticercosis, HIV.

---

1 ↑Membrane excitation (epileptogenicity) may be related to disorders of synaptic transmission, K^+ channelopathies, or α-subunit mutations (eg SCN2A; SCN1A) of voltage-gated Na^+ channel. *Lancet* 2003 1238

Evaluation of an adult who has just had a first-ever seizure

▶▶For status epilepticus, see p812.

- Obtain as much history as possible from patient and witnesses. Try to form an opinion as to whether the witness is reliable. In the heat of the moment many witnesses may report twitching when none in fact took place (perhaps they want to please you by seeming to be observant and they 'helpfully' fill in the gaps in reality—so, *beware*).
- You must attempt to establish a cause. Adult-onset seizures particularly with focal features are often 'symptomatic', ie secondary to another structural pathology (or cardiac, metabolic, or drug-related problem).
- Clues from the history may point to an obvious illness or other toxic/metabolic cause for the seizure. If not, then these tests may help:
- U&E/LFT, glucose, • Ca^{2+}, PO_4^{3-} • FBC; INR/PTT • Serum & urine toxic screens.
- Blood levels of medications. • Consider LP if CT shows no ↑ICP.
- Imaging: Don't assume that if one CT scan is normal, there is no structural lesion. If epilepsy worsens, consider MRI/MRI angiography to find small areas of cortical dysgenesis, tumours, vascular malformations, and cavernomas (these surgically correctable sporadic or multiple congenital malformations present with fits ± haemorrhage).
- Emergency EEG only if concerned about non-convulsive status (p812; in children, EEG identifies 3-per-second spike-and-wave epilepsy).
- Admission for ~24h is indicated (in <10%) for investigations and observation (eg for intractable seizures or to substantiate ideas of pseudo-seizures, p380). Urgent treatment may be needed if seizures recur.
- You must give advice against driving and document your discussion.

Ideally, all those having a 1st-ever seizure should be seen promptly by a neurologist (NICE advice).

Epilepsy: management   ▶*Status:* p812; *children:* OHCS p266

▶*Involve patients in all decisions.* Compliance depends on communication and doctor–patient concordance issues (p3). Living with epilepsy creates many problems (eg inability to drive, or operate machinery) and fears (eg of sudden death), and drug issues. A problem is that UK neurologists have little time to explore these issues as each could have 1500 people with epilepsy on their books. Each general practice will only have ~50 patients, but GPs may have no special interest in epilepsy. One option is a yearly visit to a GP- or hospital-based *epilepsy nurse*, to monitor drugs, address employment, leisure, and reproductive issues; and, after a few seizure-free years, to see if drugs can be carefully withdrawn (see BOX). These nurses are skilful: respect their role!

Investigating first seizures See p379.

Therapy Treat with 1 drug (with 1 doctor in charge) only. Slowly build up doses (over 2–3 months) until seizures are controlled, or toxic effects are manifest, or maximum drug dosage reached. Beware drug interactions (consult formulary). Most specialists would not recommend treatment after 1 fit but would start treatment after 2. ▶Discuss options with the patient. If your patient has only 1 fit every 2yrs, he or she may accept the risk (particularly if there is no need to drive or operate machinery) rather than have to take drugs every day.

Generalized: Try sodium valproate as first-line, then lamotrigine (see BOX). Also use valproate, and ethosuximide for absence seizures.

Partial with or without secondary generalization: Carbamazepine is first-line, then try sodium valproate.

Commonly used drugs *Carbamazepine:* Start with 100mg/12h PO; maximum dose: 800–1000g/12h. A slow-release form is available, which is useful if intermittent side-effects experienced when dose peaks. Toxic effects: rash, nausea, diplopia, dizziness, fluid retention, hyponatraemia, blood dyscrasias.

Sodium valproate: Start with 300mg/12h PO PC, max 30mg/kg (or 3g) daily. The BNF suggests LFT & INR during the first 6 months of therapy (but most hepatic failure is in those <3yrs old on multi-drug regimens). Toxic effects: sedation, tremor, weight↑, hair thinning, ankle swelling, hyperammonaemia (causing encephalopathy), liver failure. Drug levels are not helpful.

Phenytoin: Although an effective and well-tried anticonvulsant, it is no longer 1st line for generalized or partial epilepsy owing to toxicity: nystagmus, diplopia, tremor, dysarthria, ataxia. SEs: intellect↓, depression, poor drive, polyneuropathy, acne, coarsening of facial features, gum hypertrophy, blood dyscrasias. Furthermore, dosage is difficult, and may require monitoring (p711).

Other drugs Phenobarbital; benzodiazepines; newer agents (see BOX).

Changing drugs *Indications:* On inappropriate drug; side-effects unacceptable; treatment failure. *Method:* Begin new drug at its starting dose. At the same time, withdraw the old drug, eg over 6wks (sooner if toxicity: get help). Slowly ↑ new drug to middle of its therapeutic range.

When it all goes wrong *Sudden unexpected death in epilepsy (SUDEP)* is more common in uncontrolled epilepsy and in youth, and may be related to nocturnal seizure-associated apnoea. Those with epilepsy have a mortality rate 3-fold that of controls. Over 700 epilepsy-related deaths are recorded per year in the UK; up to 17% are SUDEPs. For help with families of those with SUDEP, contact '*Epilepsy Bereaved*',ᵁᴷ 01235 772852.

Uncontrolled epilepsy

Review diagnosis. Ask a neurologist to help. Is the diagnosis of epilepsy correct? (bear in mind non-epileptic attack disorder). If it is epilepsy, is the patient on the appropriate drug for the seizure type, and has the top dose been prescribed and taken? Has an evolving underlying structural or metabolic abnormality been excluded? A low grade glioma may not show up on initial MRI. Aim to use 1 drug only. If seizures are not controlled, switch to the 2nd most appropriate drug. Only consider maintenance on 2 drugs if all appropriate drugs have been tried singly at their top dose.

Newer drugs NICE asserts that these are 2nd-line, ie if valproate and carbamazepine are contraindicated or problematic, eg: poor seizure control; fertile women; or drug interactions. They are costly, eg £100/month VS £12.

Lamotrigine is licensed as monotherapy and as an add-on for secondary generalized epilepsy. It is also useful in primary generalized epilepsy. *Monotherapy dose:* 25mg/24h PO for 14d, ↑ to 50mg daily for a further 14d, then increase by no more than 50–100mg every 7–14d; usual maintenance as monotherapy, 50–100mg/12h. (500mg daily may be needed.) ▶Halve monotherapy doses if already on valproate; double if on carbamazepine or phenytoin. *SE:* Rash (may be serious; typically occurs in 1st 8wks, especially if valproate co-prescribed; warn patients to see a doctor at once if rash or 'flu symptoms associated with hypersensitivity develop; do FBC; U&E; LFT; INR). *Other SEs:* fever; malaise; 'flu symptoms; drowsiness; LFT↑; photosensitivity; diplopia; vision↓; vomiting; aggression; tremor; agitation. Interactions (see BNF): anticonvulsants (as above); antimalarials; antidepressants.

Gabapentin is a weak anticonvulsant (a clearer indication is pain syndromes).

Topiramate and *levetiracetam* are powerful new anticonvulsants for secondary generalized seizures. Their exact role is to be defined.

Vigabatrin: Only use this agent in infantile spasms, owing to unacceptably high incidence of visual field defect side-effects.

Non-epileptic attack disorder (pseudo or psychogenic seizures) These are not infrequent: suspect this if there are uncontrollable symptoms, no learning disabilities, and CNS exam, CT, MRI, and EEG are normal.

381

Stopping anticonvulsants

Most patients are seizure-free within a few years of starting drugs. More than 60% remain so when drugs are withdrawn. After assessing risks and benefits for the individual patient (eg the need to drive), withdrawal may be tried, if the patient meets these criteria: normal CNS examination, normal IQ, normal EEG prior to withdrawal, seizure-free for >2yrs, and no juvenile myoclonic epilepsy. In one study (N = 459), over 5yrs 52% remained seizure-free, compared with 67% continuing their medication.

▶Discuss risks and benefits with patients. Informed choices are vital.

One way[1] to withdraw drugs in adults is to ↓the dose by 10% every 2–4wks (for carbamazepine, lamotrigine, phenytoin, valproate, and vigabatrin) and by 10% every 4–8wks for phenobarbital (=phenobarbitone), benzodiazepines, and ethosuximide. Alternative (MRC regimen): ↓ every 4wks by:

Phenobarbital	30mg	Valproate	200mg
Phenytoin	50mg	Primidone	125mg
Carbamazepine	100mg	Ethosuximide	250mg

Driving and jobs (p162). *Epilepsy in pregnancy* (OHCS p161).

1 *Drug Ther Bul* 2003 41 (June) 41

Parkinson's disease (PD) and parkinsonism

Parkinsonism is a syndrome of *tremor, rigidity, bradykinesis (slowness)*, and loss of postural reflexes. *Prevalence:* 1 : 200 if >65yrs old.

Tremor: 4–6Hz (cycles per sec). It is most marked at rest and coarser than cerebellar tremor. It is typically a 'pill rolling' of thumb over fingers.

Rigidity: ↑Resistance to passive stretch of muscles throughout range of movement (*lead-pipe*); tone may be broken-up by tremor (*cogwheel rigidity*). Unlike in spasticity, rigidity is present equally in flexors and extensors.

Bradykinesis: Slowness of movement initiation with progressive reduction in speed and amplitude of repetitive actions; also monotonous speech (± dysarthria). Expressionless face. Dribbling. Short shuffling steps with flexed trunk as if forever a step behind one's centre of gravity (*festinant gait*). Feet as if frozen to the ground. Peristalsis↓. Blink rate↓. Fidgeting↓. Micrographia.

Parkinson's disease is one cause of parkinsonism (due to degeneration of substantia nigra dopaminergic neurones; the pathological hallmark is Lewy bodies in this area, p374). Degeneration may be related to mitochondrial DNA dysfunction.⁜ Symptoms usually start between 50 and 70yrs old.

Management: ▶Get help (neurologist, physiotherapist, and specialist nurse).

1 Forge a therapeutic and humanizing alliance between the specialists, the patient, and his or her carer: in the end, this is the only way to confront what is an incurable disease; see p329. Respite care is much valued by carers.

2 Assess disability and cognition regularly and objectively (eg time how long to walk 10 metres; can he/she dress alone, and turn over in bed?).

3 Start drugs when PD is seriously interfering with life (not too soon, as L-dopa's effects wear off with time; explain this to patients, and let them choose). Use the lowest dose giving symptom relief, without troublesome SEs. *Dopaminergic drugs* (see BOX) eg L-dopa: Start at 50mg/12h PO (after food, to avoid nausea/vomiting). Increase dose to 100mg/8h, then slowly ↑ to 800mg/24h (in divided doses). Give enough peripheral dopa-decarboxylase inhibitor (≥25mg/100mg L-dopa). Balance improved mobility with L-dopa's SEs—eg nausea and unwanted movements—seen after ~2yrs' treatment (± orthostatic hypotension, arrhythmias, and psychiatric disturbance).

4 Episodes of multidisciplinary rehabilitation improve mobility and morale. ⁜

5 Over years, drugs may get less effective with switching between times of exaggerated involuntary movement and of immobility ('on–off'); *slow-release L-dopa* (BOX) aims to help this (evidence is poor); once it occurs, it may be irreversible: there is evidence that early use of dopaminergic agonists (eg ropinirole, see BOX) may reduce this, and allow lower doses of L-dopa.

6 Anticholinergics/antimuscarinics (see BOX) help motor symptoms. *CI:* Urinary retention, angle-closure glaucoma, GI obstruction, prostatism. *SE:* Dry mouth, dizziness, vision↓, urinary retention, pulse↑, anxiety, confusion, excitement, agitation, hallucinations, insomnia, memory↓.

7 Modafinil (100–200mg bd *before* noon; *CI:* BP↑) helps *daytime sleepiness.*⁜ *Psychosis & dementia* often complicate PD; get further help, p374. Older antipsychotics worsen PD, but consider rivastigmine or atypical neuroleptics.⁜

8 Assess for depression (seen in ~50%); antidepressants may worsen PD; nortriptyline (25mg/8h) may be least problematic here; mirtazapine is an antidepressant which may ↓tremor (≤30mg nocte; SE: BP↓; LFT↑; WCC↓).

Treatment of drug-induced parkinsonism It may be unwise to reduce or stop the culprit drug (eg in schizophrenia where relapse could spell catastrophe), so try adding in an antimuscarinic (eg procyclidine 2.5mg/8h PO).

Causes of parkinsonism Neurodegeneration; *neuroleptics* (eg metoclopramide, prochlorperazine, haloperidol); *arteriosclerosis*. Rarely *postencephalitis; supranuclear palsy* (Steele–Richardson–Olszewski syndrome with absent vertical gaze, both upward and downward, and dementia); *multisystem atrophy* (MSA) *(formerly Shy-Drager syndrome)* (orthostatic BP↓, atonic bladder); *carbon monoxide poisoning; Wilson's disease; communicating hydrocephalus.*

Drugs combining L-dopa and dopa-decarboxylase inhibitors

Trade name	L-dopa content (mg)	Benserazide (mg)	Carbidopa (mg)
Madopar 62.5®	50	12.5	
Madopar 125®	100	25	
Madopar CR® controlled release	100	25	
Madopar 250®	200	50	
Sinemet 62.5®*	50		12.5
Sinemet 110®*	100		10
Sinemet 275®*	250		25
Sinemet Plus®	100		25
Half Sinemet CR®	100		25
Sinemet CR®	200		50

*The proportion of carbidopa may be suboptimal.

Generics: Madopar® is co-beneldopa (1 part benserazide to 4 parts levodopa). Sinemet® is co-careldopa (carbidopa with levodopa). Doses are expressed as co-careldopa *x/y*, where *x* and *y* are strengths in mg of carbidopa and levodopa, respectively; eg Sinemet 275® = co-careldopa 25/250 = 25mg carbidopa + 250mg levodopa.

Older dopamine agonists *Pergolide:* Start at 50μg/24h PO for 2d. Increase by 100–150μg every 3rd day over the next 12d. Further increases of 250μg every 3rd day may be tried. Usual maintenance dose: 1mg/8h. Tablets are 50μg (white), 250μg (green), and 1mg (pink). During titration, the dose of L-dopa may be decreased cautiously.

Bromocriptine: Week 1: 1.25mg at night PO with food. *Week 2:* 2.5mg at night. *Week 3:* 2.5mg/12h. *Week 4:* 2.5mg/8h. Increase by 2.5mg/d at weekly intervals. Max dose = 5 × 2.5mg/8h. SE (both drugs): Hallucinations, BP↓, constipation, confusion, drowsiness, retroperitoneal fibrosis.

Subcutaneous apomorphine (an injectable D_1 and D_2 dopamine agonist) may help patients with severe on-off effects. Injections or continuous infusion may be required. Liaise with a special PD centre.

New dopamine agonists Ropinirole and pramipexole are better tolerated than older agonists and are easier to titrate up to the best dose. They are now often used as initial therapy in younger patients to ↓risk of dyskinesias (and at all ages as an adjunct to L-dopa). *Ropinirole dose:* eg 250μg/8h PO increased by small weekly increments to 3mg/8h if needed; tabs are 250μg, 1mg, 2mg, & 5mg. SE: drowsiness; nausea; hallucinations in 17%. *Entacapone:* This decreases peripheral L-dopa metabolism by catechol-O-methyltransferase (COMT) inhibition. It may lessen the 'off' time in those with wearing off effects. SE: red-brown urine, dyskinesia, nausea, vomiting, orthostatic hypotension, sleep disorders, hallucinations, dry mouth, Hb↓, LFT↑.

Anticholinergics *Benzhexol* (=*trihexyphenidyl*): 1mg daily, gradually ↑ to 5mg/8h PO (max: 20mg/24h); elderly: lower doses. *Orphenadrine:* 50mg/8h PO; max 400 mg daily; elderly: lower doses. They help motor function (as add-ons, or monotherapy); meta-analyses don't strongly support a specific effect on tremor. *Interactions:* phenothiazines; antihistamines; antidepressants.

Non-standard treatments *Neural transplants* and *gene therapy* may be future (problematic) options.[1] *Selegiline* (MAO-B inhibitor) may delay need for L-dopa by a few months, but has serious SEs (BP↑; AF). *Deep brain stimulation* (p352) is experimental; it *may* improve on–off phenomena.[2]

1 J Kordower J 2003 *Ann Neurol* **53** S120. Gene delivery of glial cell line-derived neurotrophic factor for PD.
2 Detante O 2004 *Adv Neurol* 2004 309. High-frequency stimulation of the subthalamic nucleus in PD.

Multiple sclerosis (MS)

This relapsing/remitting disorder consists of plaques of demyelination (and axon loss) at sites throughout the CNS (but not peripheral nerves). Pathogenesis involves focal disruption of the blood–brain barrier and associated immune response and myelin damage as well as neurodegenerative processes.[1]

Epidemiology Commoner in temperate areas, but prevalence is very variable: England 40/100,000; SE Scotland 200/100,000;▩ rarer in Black Africa and Asia. Lifetime UK risk: ~1 : 1000. Adult travellers take their risk with them; children acquire the risk of where they settle. ♀ : ♂ > 1; mean age of onset is 30yrs. There is speculation about the role of EBV.[2] *Poor prognostic signs:* Older males; motor signs at onset; many relapses early on; many MRI lesions.

Presentation is usually monosymptomatic: unilateral optic neuritis (pain on eye movement and rapid deterioration in central vision); numbness or tingling in the limbs; leg weakness or brainstem or cerebellar symptoms such as diplopia or ataxia. Less often there may be more than 1 symptom. Other signs: see BOX. Symptoms may worsen with heat (eg a hot bath) or exercise. *Progression/prognosis:* Early on, relapses (which can be stress induced)▩ may be followed by remission/full recovery. With time, remissions are incomplete, so disability accumulates. Steady progression of disability from the outset also occurs, while some patients experience no progressive disablement at all.

Examination Look carefully for CNS deficits other than the presenting problem. Lhermitte's symptom (paraesthesiae in limbs on flexing neck) may be positive (also in cervical spondylosis or B_{12} deficiency).

Diagnosis This is clinical, requiring demonstration of lesions disseminated in time and space, unattributable to other causes. Isolated CNS deficits are never diagnostic, but may become so if a careful history reveals previous episodes, eg unexplained blindness for a week. *The role of MRI:* See BOX.

Tests None is pathognomonic. *CSF:* up to 50 lymphocytes/mm³, protein ≤1g/L ± oligoclonal bands of IgG on electrophoresis. Delayed visual, auditory, and somatosensory *evoked potentials.* MRI is sensitive but not specific for plaque detection and may exclude other causes, eg cord compression. Correlation of MRI with clinical condition is poor. *Antibodies to myelin oligodendrocyte glycoprotein* (MOG) and *myelin basic protein* (MBP) in those with a single MS-like clinical lesion can predict time to conversion to definite MS.▩

Treatment *Methylprednisolone* 1g/24h IV/PO for 3d shortens relapses; use sparingly (≤ ×2/yr, ∴ steroid SEs). It does not alter the overall prognosis.

Disease-modifying agents: Interferon (INF-1b; INF-1α): Trials show that these can ↓relapses by 30% in active relapsing-remitting MS (RRMS);▩ they also ↓lesion accumulation on MRI.▩ Their power to ↓disability remains controversial, as does benefit in secondary and primary progressive (SP & PP) MS. Licensed for use by neurologists, they are expensive (~£200/wk; £0.8 million/QALY, p14).●▩ SE: 'flu-like symptoms, depression, abortion. CI: depression, LFT↑, pregnancy, uncontrolled epilepsy. The UK DoH, the Association of British Neurologists, and the drug industry have agreed a scheme to make INF more available according to agreed criteria and effectiveness monitoring. Newer agents (role uncertain): *Glatiramer; mitoxantrone* (? for secondary progressive MS).▩ *Palliation:* ►Help to live well with disability (p524). *Spasticity: Baclofen* 5–30mg/8h PO; *diazepam* ≤ 5mg/8h PO; *dantrolene* 25mg/d; ↑ at weekly intervals (max 100mg/6h); *tizanidine* 2mg/24h PO; ↑at intervals of >3d in steps of 1mg/12h (max 8mg/8h). The role for intrathecal baclofen, phenol nerve block, botulinum toxin, and cannabis is uncertain.▩ (N = 630) *Urgency/ Frequency:* Measure post-micturition residual urine. If >100mL teach intermittent self-catheterization. If <100mL, try oxybutynin 2.5mg/8h or tolterodine.

1 P Matthews 2003 *Neurology* **60** 1949 &1157; degeneration is early in primary progressive and relapsing MS.
2 L Levin 2003 *JAMA* **289** 1533. EBV is not a *proven* cause but in 1 study risk ↑ ×30 if anti-EBV antibodies ↑↑. In susceptible people, these antigens might cross-react with myelin. Other evidence of an infective cause includes case-clustering: peak clustering of MS is at age 18yrs—T Riise 1991 *Am J Epi* **113** 932

Clinical features of MS

- Fatigue
- Motor:
  Weakness
  Spasticity
- Altered sensation:
  Numbness; pins & needles
- Pain:
  Trigeminal neuralgia
  Dysaesthesia
- Bladder: eg urge incontinence
- GI: swallowing disorders; constipation
- Sexual dysfunction (impotence)
- Visual defects on exercise (∵ ↑T°, this is Uhthoff's phenomenon)[1]
- Diplopia; nystagmus; optic neuritis
- Cerebellum: ataxia; intention tremor
- Cognition↓; memory↓; dementia.
- Vertigo
- Depression[2] or, rarely, euphoria
- Epilepsy and aphasia are rare.

Proposed McDonald criteria for diagnosing MS 📖 106

Clinical presentation	Additional data needed
2 or more attacks (relapses) with 2 or more objective clinical lesions	None; clinical evidence will do (imaging evidence desirable; must be consistent with MS)
2 or more attacks with 1 objective clinical lesion	Dissemination in space, shown by: • MRI OR • +ve CSF and ≥2 MRI lesions consistent with MS OR • Further attack involving different site
1 attack with 2 or more objective clinical lesions	Dissemination in time, shown by • MRI OR 2nd clinical attack
1 attack with 1 objective clinical lesion (monosymptomatic presentation)	Dissemination in space: • MRI OR +ve CSF if ≥2 MRI lesions consistent with MS • AND dissemination in time shown by MRI or 2nd clinical attack[3]
Insidious neurological progression suggestive of MS (primary progressive MS)	Positive CSF AND Dissemination in space shown by: • MRI evidence of ≥9 T2 brain lesions • or 2 or more cord lesions • or 4–8 brain and 1 cord lesion • or +ve visual evoked potential (VEP) with 4–8 MRI lesions • or +ve VEP + <4 brain lesions + 1 cord lesion • AND Dissemination in time shown by MRI or continued progression for ≥1yr

Attacks: These must last >1h, eg motor weakness etc., see. BOX above.
Time between attacks: 30d. *MRI abnormality:* 3 out of 4:
  1 1 Gadolinum (Gd)-enhancing or 9 T2 hyperintense lesions if no Gd-enhancing lesion
  2 1 or more infratentorial lesions
  3 1 or more juxtacortical lesions
  4 ≥3 periventricular lesions (1 spinal cord lesion = 1 brain lesion)
CSF: Oligoclonal IgG bands in CSF (and not serum) or ↑IgG index.
Evoked potentials: (EP) This counts if delayed but well-preserved waveform.
What provides MRI evidence of dissemination in time? A Gd-enhancing lesion demonstrated in a scan done at least 3 months following onset of clinical attack at a site different from attack, OR
In absence of Gd-enhancing lesions at a 3-month scan, follow-up scan after an additional 3 months showing Gd-lesion or new T2 lesion. 📖 107

385

1 Medline[@7751837] 2 Depression is common and treatable, eg fluoxetine 20mg/24h. Avoid ECT.
3 Prospective studies are needed to optimize MRI criteria. *Neurology* 2003 **60** 27 [@12525713]

Space-occupying lesions

Signs Features of ↑intracranial pressure, evolving focal neurology, seizures, false localizing signs, cognitive or behavioural change, local effects (eg proptosis; epistaxis). *Raised ICP* (p816): Headache (p340), vomiting, papilloedema (only in 50% of tumours), altered consciousness. *Seizures:* Seen in ≤50% of tumours. Suspect in all adult-onset seizures, especially if focal, or with a localizing aura or post-ictal weakness (Todd's palsy, p736). *Evolving focal neurology:* Depends on the site (see BOX for localizing signs). Ask first *where* the mass is then *what* it is. Frontal lobe, non-dominant, and temporal lobe masses present late. *False localizing signs:* These are caused by ↑ICP. VI nerve palsy is commonest (p56) due to its long intracranial course. *Subtle personality change:* Irritability, lack of application to tasks, lack of initiative, socially inappropriate behaviour.

Causes Tumour (primary or secondary), aneurysm, abscess (25% multiple); chronic subdural haematoma, granuloma p199, eg tuberculoma), cyst (eg cysticercosis). *Histology:* 30% secondaries (breast, lung, melanoma; 50% multiple). Primaries include: Astrocytoma, glioblastoma multiforme, oligo-dendroglioma, ependymoma (all <50% 5yr survival), cerebellar haem-angioblastoma (40% 20yr survival); meningioma (♀ : ♂ ≈ 2 : 1).

Differential diagnosis Stroke, head injury, vasculitis (p424), eg SLE, syphilis, PAN, giant cell arteritis, MS, encephalitis, post-ictal (Todd's palsy p736), metabolic, or electrolyte disturbances. Also colloid cyst of the 3rd ventricle and benign intracranial hypertension (see below).

Tests CT; MRI (good for posterior fossa masses). Consider biopsy. Avoid LP (risks coning, ie cerebellar tonsils herniate through the foramen magnum).

Tumour management *Benign:* Complete removal if possible but some may be inaccessible. *Malignant:* Complete removal of gliomas is difficult as resection margins are rarely clear, but surgery does give a tissue diagnosis and allows debulking pre-radiotherapy. If a tumour is inaccessible but causing hydrocephalus, a ventriculo-peritoneal shunt can help. Radiotherapy is used post-op for gliomas or metastases and as sole therapy for some tumours if surgery is impossible. Chemotherapy is used in gliomas (uncertain value). Prophylaxis for epilepsy is important, but frequently fails. Treat headache (eg codeine 60mg/4h PO). Dexamethasone 4mg/8h PO for cerebral oedema. Mannitol if ↑ICP acutely, p816. Meticulous palliative treatment (p438).

Prognosis Complete removal of a benign tumour achieves cure but the prognosis of those with malignant tumours is poor.

Colloid cyst of the third ventricle These congenital cysts declare themselves in adult life with memory loss, headaches (often positional), obtundation (blunting of consciousness), incontinence, dim vision, bilateral paraesthesiae, weak legs, and drop attacks with no LOC. *Tests:* CT scan/MRI. *Treatment:* Excision or ventriculo-peritoneal shunting.

Benign intracranial hypertension (Pseudotumor cerebri) Think of this in those presenting as if with a mass (headache, ↑ICP and papilloedema)—*when none is found.* Typical patients are obese women with blurred vision ± diplo-pia, VI nerve palsy, and an enlarged blind spot, if papilloedema is present (it usually is). Consciousness and cognition are preserved. *Cause:* Often unknown, or secondary to venous sinus thrombosis, or drugs, eg tetracycline, minocycline, nitrofurantoin, vitamin A, isotretinoin, danazol, and somatropin.

Treatment: Acetazolamide, loop diuretics, prednisolone (start at ~40mg/24h PO; more SE than diuretics); advise weight loss. Consider optic nerve sheath fenestration if drugs fail and visual loss is progressing. 📖108

Prognosis: Often self-limiting. Permanent significant visual loss in 10% (ie not so benign). CSF shunting ± optic nerve sheath fenestration can help vision. 📖109

Localizing signs

Temporal lobe Seizures (complex partial ± automatisms); hallucinations (smell, taste, sound, *déjà vu*); complex partial with automatisms; dysphasia; field defect (contralateral upper quadrantanopia); forgetfulness; psychosis; fear/rage; hypersexuality.

Frontal lobe Hemiparesis; seizures (focal motor seizures, eg aversive seizures involving head and eyes); personality changes (indecent; indolent; indiscreet); positive grasp reflex (fingers drawn across palm are grasped) significant only if unilateral; dysphasia (Broca's area p58); loss of smell unilaterally. *Orbitofrontal syndrome:* Lack of empathy; disinhibition; ↓social skills; over-eating; rash actions (mania); over-familiar; unconscious imitation of postures (eg when you put your feet on the desk, or sit on the floor); 'utilization behaviour' (whatever is provided is used, however inappropriately—eg hand the patient spectacles, and he puts them on, hand him another pair, and this goes on his nose too, ditto for a 3rd pair).

Parietal lobe Hemisensory loss; ↓2-point discrimination; astereognosis (↓ability to recognize object in hand by touch alone); sensory inattention; dysphasia (p58); Gerstmann's syndrome (p724; ie left–right disorientation, finger agnosia, dyscalculia, and dysgraphia).

Occipital lobe Contralateral visual field defects (homonymous hemianopia); hallucinations such as palinopsia (persisting or recurring images, once the stimulus has left the field of view).[1]

Cerebellum ('DASHING') **D**ysdiadochokinesis; **a**taxia (truncal); **s**lurred speech; **h**ypotonia; **i**ntention tremor; **n**ystagmus; **g**ait abnormality. *Dysdiadochokinesis* is impaired *rapidly alternating* movements, eg pronation–supination. NB: If the truncal ataxia is worse on eye closure, the lesion is in the dorsal columns, not cerebellum.

Cerebellopontine angle (Usually vestibular schwannoma).
Ipsilateral deafness; nystagmus; reduced corneal reflex, facial weakness; ipsilateral cerebellar signs, papilloedema; and VI nerve palsies.

Corpus callosum (a rare site for lesions)
Usually severe rapid intellectual deterioration with focal signs of adjacent lobes; signs of loss of communication between lobes (eg left hand unable to carry out verbal commands).

Midbrain (eg pineal gland tumours or midbrain infarction)
Failure of up or down gaze; light/near dissociated pupil responses, with convergence retraction nystagmus —upward saccadic retracting pulses from co-contraction of opposing horizontal muscles, precipitated by attempted up-gaze. The eyes retract in their sockets because of contraction of the medial recti, eg while looking at a down-moving target.

---

1 Greek *palin* (again) and *opsia*, vision. Polyopia is seeing multiple images. P Shah *Lancet* 2003 1098

Bell's palsy

An *idiopathic* palsy of the facial nerve (VII) resulting in a unilateral facial weakness or paralysis. Other causes of a facial palsy must be excluded before a diagnosis of Bell's palsy is made (see BOX). Many now suspect that Bell's is a viral neuropathy—HSV-1 has been implicated.

Incidence ~20/100,000/yr; risk ↑ in pregnancy (3-fold) and diabetes (~5-fold).

Symptoms Onset of facial weakness is rapid and may occur with or be preceded by pain below the ear. Weakness worsens for 1–2d before stabilizing, and pain resolves within a few days. Symptoms and signs are unilateral. If bilateral, consider other diagnoses (eg sarcoidosis; Lyme disease).

- Unilateral facial weakness with sagging of the mouth (it is drawn towards the normal side on smiling, producing a grimace).
- Food gets trapped between gum and cheek; drinks and saliva leak out.
- Speech difficulty ∵ adynamic lip (marginal mandibular branch of VII).
- Taste impairment on the anterior part of the tongue.
- Intolerance of loud, high-pitched sound (hyperacusis ∵ paralysis of stapedius).
- Failure of eye closure may cause a watery or dry eye, ectropion (sagging and turning-out of the lower lid), conjunctivitis, or injury from foreign bodies.

Enquire about prodromal pain behind the ear. There is some evidence that if this precedes facial paralysis by more than 4d, prognosis is good.

Ask the patient to wrinkle up the forehead and close the eyes forcefully. Test buccinator by whistling/blowing out the cheeks (*buccina* is Latin for trumpet).

Natural history Those with incomplete paralysis and no axonal degeneration typically recover completely within a few weeks. Those with complete paralysis nearly all fully recover too but ~15% have axonal degeneration (recovery frequently begins only after 3 months, may be incomplete, fail to happen at all, or else be complicated by the formation of aberrant reconnections). These produce synkinesis, eg eye blinking is accompanied by synchronous upturning of the mouth. Misconnection of parasympathetic fibres can produce so-called crocodile tears when eating stimulates unilateral lacrimation. Cutting the tympanic branch of IX solves this problem (rarely needed).

Tests *Electroneurography* at 1–3wks can predict delayed recovery by identifying axonal degeneration but does not influence management.

Serology may show a 4-fold rise in antibody to varicella zoster virus.

MRI ± *LP* help rule out other diagnoses (only needed in atypical presentations).

Management If presentation is within 6d of onset, prednisolone (eg 50mg/24h PO for 5d ± 10mg/day for 5 more days) is given by most to try to prevent weakness becoming paralysis by reducing nerve oedema.[1] Evidence for prednisolone is not universally acknowledged. **NB:** Many 'Bell's cases' are now thought to be due to herpes viruses, and some studies (with flaws) support using antivirals (aciclovir or valaciclovir) with prednisolone. Meta-analyses say that more data are needed with follow-up >12 months.

- Protect the eye with dark glasses and by instilling artificial tears (eg hypromellose) if there is any evidence of drying.
- Encourage regular eyelid closure by pulling down the lid by hand.
- Use tape to close the eyes at night.
- If ectropion is severe, lateral tarsorrhaphy (partial lid-to-lid suturing) can help.
- If recovery fails in the long term (wait >12 months), plastic surgery to help lid closure and to straighten the drooping face can be attempted. In good hands, results may be satisfactory.

---

1 Many neurologists give steroids 'to reduce oedema in the nerve', particularly if seen within 6d of onset. One helpful study—Shafshak T 1994 *J Laryng & Otol* **108** 940 [@7829945] showed that the extra benefit of steroids may be confined to those treated within 24h of onset. Spontaneous recovery is good in any case (85%). NNT = 3. Older randomized studies have been inconclusive, but did not look specifically at early treatment. Meta-analyses also favour steroids (E-BM 1997 **2** 79).

Other causes of a VII nerve palsy[123]

Infection

Ramsay Hunt syndrome (cephalic herpes zoster, *OHCS* p756). This is peripheral facial nerve palsy accompanied by an erythematous vesicular rash on the ear (zoster oticus) or in the mouth. (Famciclovir 500mg/8h PO + prednisolone may be indicated.)[124]

Lyme disease[1]

HIV

Meningitis

Polio

TB

Chronic meningitis (eg fungal)

Brainstem lesions

Brainstem tumour

Stroke

MS

Cerebello-pontine angle lesions

Acoustic neuroma (p346); meningioma

Systemic disease

Diabetes mellitus

Sarcoidosis[1] (facial palsy is the commonest CNS sign of sarcoidosis)[125]

Guillain–Barré syndrome[1]

ENT and other rare causes

Orofacial granulomatosis—recurrent VII palsies

Parotid tumours

Cholesteatoma

Otitis media

Trauma to skull base

Diving—barotrauma + temporal bone pneumocel[126]

Pregnancy/delivery, via intracranial hypotension[127]

---

1 Common causes of a bilateral facial palsy in some countries.

Mononeuropathies

These are lesions of individual, including cranial, nerves. Trauma is the main cause. *Others*: leprosy; DM. If ≥2 peripheral nerves are affected, the term *mononeuritis multiplex* is used (causes: 'WARDS PLC': **W**egener's granulomatosis, **a**myloidosis, **r**heumatoid, **D**M, **s**arcoidosis, **P**AN, **l**eprosy, **c**arcinomatosis).

Median nerve C6–T1 *At the wrist:* (eg lacerations; carpal tunnel syndrome—see BOX) Weakness of abductor pollicis brevis and sensory loss over the radial 3½ fingers and palm. Lesions confined to the anterior interosseous nerve (neuralgic amyotrophy[1]; trauma): weakness of flexion of the distal phalanx of the thumb and index finger. *Proximal lesions* (eg at the elbow) may show combined defects.

Ulnar nerve C7–T1 Vulnerable to elbow trauma; *Signs:* Weakness/wasting of medial (ulnar side) wrist flexors; weakness/wasting of the interossei (cannot cross the fingers in the 'good luck' sign) and medial 2 lumbricals (claw hand); wasting of the hypothenar eminence which abolishes finger abduction and sensory loss over the medial 1½ fingers and the ulnar side of the hand. Flexion of 4th & 5th DIP joints is weak. Treatment: see BOX. With lesions at the wrist (digitorum profundus intact), claw hand is more marked.

Radial nerve C5–T1 This nerve opens the fist. Damaged by compression against the humerus. Test for wrist and finger drop with elbow flexed and arm pronated. Sensory loss: variable; test dorsal aspect of root of thumb.

Sciatic nerve L4–S2 Damaged by pelvic tumours or fractures to pelvis or femur. Lesions affect the hamstrings and all muscles below the knee (foot drop), with loss of sensation below the knee laterally.

Common peroneal nerve L4–S2 Frequently damaged as it winds round the fibular head by trauma or even prolonged sitting cross-legged. Lesions lead to inability to dorsiflex the foot (foot drop), evert the foot, extend the toes—and sensory loss over dorsum of foot.

Tibial nerve S1–3 Lesions lead to an inability to stand on tiptoe (plantarflexion), invert the foot, or flex the toes. Sensory loss over the sole.

Autonomic neuropathy

This may be isolated or part of a generalized sensory motor peripheral neuropathy. *Causes:* DM; amyloidosis; Guillian–Barré. *Signs:* Postural hypotension (faints after standing, eating, exercise, or hot baths), impotence, sweating↓, diarrhoea (especially nocturnal)/constipation, urinary retention, Horner's (p726).

Autonomic function tests Postural drop of ≥30/15mmHg is abnormal.
- A variation of <10bpm with respiration is abnormal (do resting ECG).
- Bladder pressure studies (*cystometry*). • *Pupils:* Instil 0.1% epinephrine (dilates if post-ganglionic sympathetic denervation, not if normal); 2.5% cocaine (dilates if normal; not if sympathetic denervation); 2.5% methacholine (constricts if parasympathetic lesion). These are rarely used.

Primary autonomic failure Occurs alone, as part of MSA (p382) or, rarely, with Parkinson's. Middle-aged/elderly men are most affected. Onset is insidious (symptoms as above) and progression over several years is typical. Extra-pyramidal symptoms (p382) may precede those of autonomic failure in MSA although the condition may be unmasked by a sudden worsening of mild postural hypotension when presumed classical Parkinson's is treated with L-dopa. Patients rarely survive >10yrs after diagnosis of MSA.

Treatment Treat causes; offer compression stockings; advise to stand slowly. Head-up tilt of the bed at night ↑renin release, so decreasing fluid loss and raising standing BP. If post-prandial dizziness, advise eating little and often, and to ↓carbohydrate and alcohol intake. Reserve fluid-retaining drugs (fludrocortisone 0.1mg/24h PO, ↑ as needed) for severe disease.

---

1 Radiculitis (eg of C5 & C6, after an infection or an immunization into deltoid) causes pain then weakness (may involve the diaphragm). It resolves over months. *J Peripher Nerv Syst* 2002 **198** & OTM

Carpal tunnel syndrome: the commonest mononeuropathy

9 tendons and the median nerve compete for space within the wrist. Compression is common, especially in women who have narrower wrists but similar-sized tendons to men. (NB: For similar reasons, the tibial nerve may be compressed: the tarsal tunnel syndrome—causing unilateral burning sole pain, eg on walking or standing.)

The patient: Aching pain in the hand and arm (especially at night), and paraesthesiae in thumb, index, and middle fingers, all relieved by dangling the hand over the edge of the bed and shaking it. There may be sensory loss and weakness of abductor pollicis brevis ± wasting of the thenar eminence. Light touch, 2-point discrimination, and sweating may be impaired.

Associations: Pregnancy, rheumatoid, DM, hypothyroidism, dialysis, trauma.

Tests: Neurophysiology helps by confirming the lesion's site and severity (and likelihood of improvement after surgery). Maximal wrist flexion for 1min (Phalen's test) may elicit symptoms (unreliable!). Tapping over the nerve at the wrist induces tingling (Tinel's test; also rather non-specific).

Treatment: Splinting, local steroid injection (*OHCS* p658) ± decompression surgery; many alternative therapies are tried: meta-analyses are doubtful.[1]

Managing ulnar mononeuropathies from entrapments

The ulnar nerve 'asks for trouble' in at least 5 places around the elbow, beginning proximally at the arcade of Struthers (a musculofascial band ~8cm proximal to the medial epicondyle) and ending distally where it exits the flexor carpi ulnaris muscle in the forearm. Most commonly compression occurs at the epicondylar groove or at the point where the nerve passes between the 2 heads of the flexor carpi ulnaris muscle (true *cubital tunnel syndrome*). Trauma can easily damage the nerve against its bony confines (the medial condyle of the humerus—the 'funny bone'). Normally, the ulnar nerve suffers stretch and compression forces at the elbow that are moderated by its ability to glide in its groove. When normal excursion is restricted, irritation ensues. This may cause a vicious cycle of perineural scarring, consequent loss of excursion, and progressive symptoms—without there being any antecedent trauma.

Rest and avoiding pressure on the nerve helps but if symptoms continue, night-time soft elbow splinting (to prevent flexion to >60°) is warranted, eg for 6 months. For chronic neuropathy associated with weakness, or if splinting fails, a variety of surgical procedures have been tried. For moderately severe neuropathies, decompressions *in situ* may help, but often fail. Medial epicondylectomies are effective in ≤50% (there is a high rate of recurrence). Subcutaneous nerve re-routings (transpositions) may be tried. Intramuscular and submuscular transpositions are more complicated, but the latter may be preferable.

Compressive ulnar neuropathies at the wrist (*Guyon's canal*—between the pisiform and hamate bones) are less common, but they can also result in disability. *Thoracic outlet compression* is another cause of a weak numb hand. Electromyography (EMG) helps define the anatomic site of lesions.

---

1 *Cochrane meta-analysis of 21 carpal tunnel trials:* 7 (but not 2) weeks' ultrasound can help. Compared to placebo, diuretics & NSAIDs gave no benefit. Vit. B6 did not help (N = 50). Those adopting the namaste (prayer) posture in yoga may obviate need for surgery: the forced wrist extension helps (N = 53). Trials of ergonomic keyboards give equivocal results for pain and function. Trials of magnet therapy, laser acupuncture, and exercise showed no benefit. Chiropractic care can increase distress.

Polyneuropathies

Polyneuropathies are generalized disorders of peripheral nerves (including cranial nerves) whose distribution is usually bilaterally symmetrical and widespread—usually a distal pattern of muscle weakness and sensory loss (known as 'glove and stocking anaesthesia'). They may be classified by time course (acute or chronic); by the functions disturbed (motor, sensory, autonomic, mixed); or by the underlying pathology (demyelination, axonal degeneration, or both). Guillain–Barré syndrome (p726), for example, is a subacute, predominantly motor, demyelinating neuropathy, whereas chronic alcohol abuse leads to a chronic, initially sensory then mixed, axonal neuropathy. Causes of polyneuropathies appear in the BOX.

Mostly motor	Mostly sensory
Guillain–Barré syndrome	Diabetes mellitus
Lead poisoning	Uraemia
Charcot–Marie–Tooth syndrome	Leprosy

Symptoms *Sensory neuropathy:* Numbness; 'feels funny'; tingling or burning sensations often affecting the extremities first ('glove and stocking' distribution). There may be difficulty handling small objects such as a needle.

Motor neuropathy: Often progressive (may be rapid) weakness or clumsiness of the hands; difficulty walking (falls; stumbling); respiratory difficulty. Signs are those of a LMN lesion: wasting and weakness most marked in the distal muscles of hands and feet (foot or wrist drop). Reflexes are reduced or absent. Involvement of the respiratory muscles may be shown by a ↓vital capacity.

Cranial nerves: Difficulties swallowing; speaking; double vision.

Autonomic neuropathy: See p390.

Diagnosis The history is vital; make sure you are clear about the illness's time course; the precise nature of the symptoms; any preceding or associated events (eg *Campylobacter* D&V before Guillain–Barré syndrome; weight↓ in cancer; arthralgia from a connective tissue disease); travel; sexual history (infections); alcohol use; medications; and family history. Pain is typical of neuropathies due to DM or alcohol. *Examination:* Do a careful neurological examination looking particularly for lower motor signs (weakness, wasting, reduced or absent reflexes) and sensory loss which should be carefully mapped out for each modality. Do not forget to assess the autonomic system (p390) and cranial nerves (p56). Look also for signs of trauma (eg finger burns) indicating reduced sensation. Scuff marks on shoes suggest foot drop. If there is nerve thickening think of leprosy or Charcot–Marie–Tooth. Examine other systems for clues to the cause, eg signs of alcoholic liver disease.

Tests FBC, ESR, glucose, U&E, LFT, thyroid function tests, B_{12}, protein electrophoresis, ANCA (p421), ANA, CXR, urinalysis, and consider an LP. Consider specific genetic tests for inherited neuropathies (eg Charcot–Marie–Tooth syndrome, p720), lead levels, and antiganglioside antibodies. Nerve conduction studies help by distinguishing demyelinating from axonal neuropathies.

Treatment Treat the cause if possible (eg withdraw precipitating drug). Involve physiotherapists and occupational therapists. Care of the feet and shoe choice is important in sensory neuropathies to minimize trauma and subsequent disability. In Guillain–Barré syndrome (p726) and chronic inflammatory demyelinating polyradiculoneuropathy (CIDP),[1] IV immunoglobulin helps. Steroids and other immunosuppressants may help vasculitic neuropathy.

---

1 CIDP is an autoimmune demyelinating disease of peripheral nerves and their roots causing weakness and sensory loss in the extremities + peripheral nerve enlargement. It is relapsing-remitting or there is step-wise progression. Cranial nerves are typically spared. CSF protein↑.

Causes of polyneuropathies

Inflammatory
Guillain–Barré syndrome, CIDP (see footnote), sarcoidosis

Metabolic
Diabetes mellitus, renal failure, hypothyroidism, hypoglycaemia, mitochondrial disorders

Vasculitides (p424)
Polyarteritis nodosa, rheumatoid arthritis, Wegener's granulomatosis

Malignancy
Paraneoplastic syndromes (especially small cell lung cancer), polycythaemia rubra vera (rare; p664)

Infections
Leprosy, syphilis, Lyme disease (p600), HIV

Vitamin deficiencies and excesses
Lack of B_1, B_6, B_{12} (eg alcoholic), folate; also excess vit B_6 (100mg/d)

Inherited
Refsum's syndrome (p734); Charcot–Marie–Tooth syndrome (p720), porphyria (p708), leukodystrophy (and many more)

Toxins
Lead, arsenic

Drugs
Alcohol, cisplatin, isoniazid, vincristine, nitrofurantoin. Less frequently: metronidazole, phenytoin

Others
Paraproteinaemias, eg multiple myeloma, amyloidosis (p668)

Bulbar palsy

This is palsy of the tongue, muscles of chewing/swallowing, and facial muscles due to loss of function of brainstem motor nuclei. Signs are of a *LMN lesion*; eg flaccid, fasciculating tongue (p56, like a sack of worms); jaw jerk is normal or absent, speech is quiet, hoarse, or nasal.

Causes: MND (below); Guillain–Barré; polio; syringobulbia (p404); brainstem tumours; also as part of *central pontine myelinolysis* (CPM, in malnourished alcoholics or in rapid correction of hyponatraemia). CPM causes progressive and fatal quadriparesis, mutism, dysarthria, and bulbar palsy (but spontaneous resolution can occur—monitor MRI).

Pseudobulbar palsy An *UMN lesion* involving muscles of eating, swallowing, and talking due to bilateral lesions above the midpons. The tongue is spastic, the jaw jerk increased, and speech like Donald Duck. Emotions may be labile (eg giggling during examination). *Causes:* Pseudobulbar palsy is more common than bulbar palsy, and is caused by *strokes* affecting corticobulbar pathways bilaterally, *MS*, and *MND*.

Motor neurone disease (MND)

MND is caused by degeneration of neurones in motor cortex, cranial nerve nuclei, and anterior horn cells. Upper and lower motor neurones may be affected but there is *no* sensory loss or sphincter disturbance—so distinguishing MND from MS and polyneuropathies. MND never affects external ocular movements (cranial nerves III, IV, and VI) which distinguishes it from myasthenia (p400). The cause is unknown, but as MND, like polio, affects anterior horn cells, viruses are suggested. 3 MND patterns:

1. • *Bulbar palsy* This accounts for about 25% of patients.
2. • *Amyotrophic lateral sclerosis (ALS)* (50%) Combined LMN wasting and UMN signs (p331) contribute to weakness. Risk↑ ~2-fold in Gulf war veterans. If familial, suspect copper/zinc superoxide dismutase mutations (SOD1).
3. • *Progressive muscular atrophy* (25%) Anterior horn cell lesion, affecting distal muscles before proximal. Better prognosis than ALS (see above).

394

Prevalence 7/10,000. ♂ : ♀ ≈ 3 : 2. ≤10% are autosomal dominant.

▶Think of MND in those >40 with stumbling (spastic gait, foot-drop), weak grip (door-handles are difficult), or aspiration pneumonia. Look for UMN signs: weakness; spasticity; brisk reflexes; plantars↑; and LMN signs: weakness; wasting; fasciculation of tongue, abdomen, back, thigh. Is speech or swallowing affected? Diagnosis is strongly supported by combinations of progressive UMN and LMN signs with involvement of ≥2 limbs, or a limb and bulbar muscles. Fasciculations are not enough to diagnose an LMN lesion: look for weakness too. MRI of brain and cord helps exclude structural causes; LP helps to exclude inflammatory ones, and neurophysiology can detect subclinical denervation and help exclude motor neuropathies.

Prognosis MND is incurable (eg fatal within 5yrs; median UK age at death is 60yrs). Prognosis is worse with bulbar-onset disease (≤1.5yrs from diagnosis).

Treatment Because of the rapid course of the illness, its rarity, and its frightening nature, a multi-disciplinary approach is best—neurologist, GP, hospice, physio, OT, speech and language therapists, dietician, and social services—with early help from the MND association (tel. 08457 626262).
Antiglutamate drugs: Riluzole (see BOX) prolongs life by ~3 months; it is costly.
Spasticity: As for MS (p384).
Drooling: Propantheline 15–30mg/8h PO; amitriptyline 25–50mg/8h PO.
Dysphagia: Blend food; would he or she like a nasogastric tube, or percutaneous catheter gastrostomy?—or would this prolong death?
Joint pains and distress: Analgesic ladder (p439) NSAIDs etc.; then opioids.
Respiratory failure (± aspiration pneumonia & sleep apnoea): Non-invasive ventilation at home in selected patients may give valuable palliation.

Following in the footprints of free radicals

Post-mortem studies show that changes to proteins and DNA which are signs or 'footprints' of free radical damage are more pronounced in MND brains than in controls. Also, cultured fibroblasts from those with MND show excessive sensitivity to oxidative insults. However, these findings do not explain 2 key MND phenomena:

1 **Why is there predilection for motor neurones?** One answer may be the sheer length and complex cytoarchitecture of motor cells, with their 1 metre axons and high levels of neurofilament proteins, and low levels of Ca^{2+}-buffering proteins (thought to be protective). We note that motor cells with the shortest axons (to the eye's external muscles) are unaffected in MND; this is not true of the tongue which only requires slightly longer axons. Another answer is that it is **not** only motor neurones which are affected: changes are seen in other areas, and we note that specific aphasia-dementia syndromes occur in MND.[1]

2 **Why do some MND brains have excess levels of glutamate?** (Glutamate is the chief excitatory neurotransmitter.) This is thought to be due to decreased activity of the excitatory amino acid transporter (EAAT2), which mops up glutamate—hence the notion that MND is an 'excitotoxic' phenomenon.

Motor cells have high levels of Cu/Zn superoxide dismutase (thought to protect normal motor cells from glutamate toxicity/oxidative stress). But a high level may itself be damaging, given certain genetic or acquired vulnerabilities. Transgenic mice exhibiting high levels of superoxide dismutase do indeed develop an MND phenotype.

These ideas are speculative, but important (perhaps) in understanding and criticizing future therapeutic options. *Riluzole*, for example, is an Na-channel blocker which inhibits glutamate's release. Neurotrophic factors can protect motor neurones and one (*insulin-like growth factor*) has been found which (in one unreplicated trial) slows MND's progression. Effects of free radical manipulation can be unpredictable. The antioxidant *vitamin E* can protect transgenic mice from developing an MND-like picture—but trials in humans are disappointing.

Apoptosis is a hallmark of MND, and genetically induced overexpression of proteins inhibiting cell death via apoptosis (Bcl-2) in transgenic mice can slow motor neurone degeneration.

---

1 Microvacuolation and ubiquitin +ve deposits in parietotemporal cortex—Catani M 2004. [@14560061]

Cervical spondylosis

Cervical spondylosis with compression of the cord (myelopathy) and nerve roots is the leading cause of progressive spastic quadriparesis with sensory loss below the neck: but most people with cervical spondylosis have no impairment—just degeneration of the annulus fibrosus of cervical intervertebral discs ± bony spurs which narrow the spinal canal and intervertebral foramina. As the neck flexes and extends, the cord is damaged as it is dragged over these protruding osteophytes anteriorly and indented by a thickened ligamentum flavum posteriorly.

Symptoms of cord compression

1 Neck pain and stiffness
2 Arm pain (brachialgia)
3 Spastic leg weakness ± ataxia.

Crepitus (palpable creaking), restricted neck movement and neck pain without neurological complaint are very common in people over 50yrs so ask about other symptoms. Arm pain is felt as stabs in the pre- or post-axial borders of the upper limb, or as a constant, dull ache in forearm or wrist. Hands may be weak and clumsy and numbness or paraesthesiae may be experienced in part of the hand or forearm. Weakness which is often more marked in one leg than the other and unsteadiness in walking are typical of myelopathy. The leg feels heavy and stiff and the toe often scrapes the floor. Progression results in bilateral, worsening weakness and reduced walking distance. Numbness and tingling of the feet and ankles are common. Bladder trouble is late (hesitancy or precipitancy); incontinence is uncommon.

Signs: Limited, painful neck movement ± crepitus—be careful! Neck flexion may produce tingling down the spine—a positive Lhermitte's symptom. This does not help decide if cord or roots or both are involved.

Arm: LMN signs at the level of the compressed cord or roots and UMN signs below. Atrophy of hand and forearm muscles may be visible. Sensory loss, especially pain and temperature.

Leg: Spasticity; weakness; brisk reflexes ± plantars extensor. Position and vibration sense↓. Examine cutaneous sensation from below upwards to show any sensory level (often several segments below level of cord compression).

Root compression (radiculopathy) Pain in arms and fingers and diminished reflexes, dermatomal sensory disturbance (numbness, tingling), LMN weakness and eventual wasting of muscles innervated by the affected root. *Typical motor and sensory deficits from individual root involvement:*

C5/C6	Weak biceps & deltoid; ↓supinator & biceps jerks, Numb thumb
C7	Weak triceps & finger extension; ↓triceps jerks; numb middle finger
C8/T1	Weak finger flexors & small muscles of the hand; numb 5th & ring finger
C4/C5	Elbow sensation, supraspinatus.

Tests MRI is the localizing image of choice. The time it takes to walk 30m may be used for monitoring purposes: it is a valid and cheap test.

Differential diagnosis MS, neurofibroma of the nerve root, subacute combined degeneration of the cord (from B_{12} deficiency).

Treatment A firm neck collar restricts anterior–posterior movement of the neck so may relieve pain, but patients dislike them. Don't dismiss those with chronic root pain in the arm as suffering simply from 'wear and tear' spondylosis. Be optimistic: they may improve over months; if not, they *may* benefit considerably from surgical root decompression if there is significant MRI abnormality.[1] Consider this if objective evidence of a root lesion or myelopathy, and especially if the history is short, and myelopathy is progressing. Progression is usually halted and leg weakness may improve. Operative risk is small.

1 Cochrane review on the role of surgery in cervical spondylotic radiculomyelopathy. I Fouyas 2002

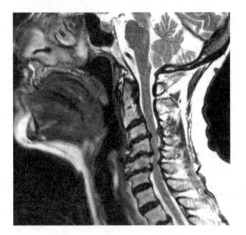

A T2 weighted MR image. The CSF consequently looks bright. The spinal cord is compressed between the osteophytes anteriorly and the ligamentum flavum posteriorly.

We thank Professor Peter Scally for the image and the commentary.

Primary disorders of muscle (myopathies)

Signs and symptoms *Muscle weakness* Rapid onset suggests a toxic, drug, or metabolic cause. *Excess fatigability* (weakness increases with exercise) suggests myasthenia (p400). *Myotonia* (delayed muscular relaxation after contraction, eg on shaking hands) is characteristic of myotonic disorders. Spontaneous *pain* at rest occurs in inflammatory disease as does local tenderness. Pain on exercise suggests ischaemia or metabolic myopathy (eg McArdle's disease). *Oddly firm* muscles (due to infiltrations with fat or connective tissue) suggest pseudohypertrophic muscular dystrophies. Muscle *tumours* are rare; common causes of *lumps* are herniation of muscle through fascia, haematoma, and tendon rupture. *Fasciculation* (spontaneous, irregular, and brief contractions of part of a muscle) suggest anterior horn cell or root disease. Look carefully for evidence of systemic disease. *Tests:* Consider EMG ± muscle biopsy; and investigations relevant to systemic causes (eg TSH, p302). Many genetic disorders of muscle can be detected by DNA analysis, and muscle biopsy is now reserved for when genetic tests are non-diagnostic (eg Duchenne's or myotonic dystrophy). *There are 6 main types:*

1 *Muscular dystrophies* are a group of genetic diseases with progressive degeneration and weakness of specific muscle groups. The primary abnormality may be in the muscle membrane. Secondary effects are marked variation in size of individual fibres and deposition of fat and connective tissue. The commonest is *Duchenne's muscular dystrophy* (pseudohypertrophic; sex-linked recessive—30% from spontaneous mutation) and is (almost always) confined to boys. The Duchenne gene is on the short arm of the X chromosome (X p23), and its product, dystrophin, is absent (or present in only very low levels). Serum creatine kinase is raised >40-fold. It presents at ~4yrs old with increasingly clumsy walking, progressing to difficulty in standing and respiratory failure. Some survive beyond 20yrs. There is no specific treatment. Home ventilation is used. Genetic counselling is vital. *Fascioscapulohumeral muscular dystrophy* (Landouzy–Dejerine) is almost as common. *Inheritance:* Autosomal dominant (4q35). *Typical age of onset:* 12–14yrs. *Early symptoms:* Inability to puff out the cheeks, difficulty raising the arms above the head (eg changing light-bulbs). *Signs:* Weakness of face ('ironed out' expression), shoulders, and upper arms (often asymmetric with deltoids spared) ± foot-drop ± winging of the scapulae (∵ weakness of thoracoscapular muscles) ± scoliosis ± anterior axillary folds ± horizontal clavicles. ≤20% need a wheelchair by 40yrs old.

2 *Myotonic disorders* are characterized by myotonia (tonic spasm of muscle). Muscle histology shows long chains of central nuclei within the fibres. The chief disorder is *Dystrophia myotonica*[1] (autosomal dominant). Typical onset: 25yrs with weakness (hands, legs, sternomastoids) and myotonia. Muscle wasting and weakness in the face gives a long, haggard appearance. Other features: cataract; frontal baldness (men); atrophy of testes or ovaries; cardiomyopathy; mild endocrine abnormalities (eg DM); and mental impairment. Most patients die in middle age of intercurrent illness. Mexiletine may help the myotonia. Genetic counselling is important.

3 *Acquired myopathies of late onset* are often a manifestation of systemic disease. Look carefully for evidence of: carcinoma; thyroid disease (especially hyperthyroidism); Cushing's disease; hypo- and hypercalcaemia.

4 *Inflammatory disorders:* Inclusion-body myositis,[2] polymyositis et al. (p420).

5 *Neuromuscular junction disorders:* Myasthenia gravis (p400).

6 *Toxic myopathies:* Alcohol; statins; steroids; chloroquine; colchicine; procainamide; zidovudine; vincristine; ciclosporin; hypervitaminosis E; cocaine.

---

1 Various channelopathies may cause other myotonias via mutations in genes encoding chloride, sodium, and calcium channels in skeletal muscle. *Curr Treat Options Neurol* 2000 **2** 31
2 Inclusion-body myositis is commoner in old age, often affects mainly distal muscles and is progressive and uninfluenced by steroids. Histologically, ringed vacuoles + intranuclear filamentous inclusions are characteristic—*Semin Neurol* 2003 **23** 199. Small trials of methotrexate preceded by 7d of IV anti-T-lymphocyte immunoglobulin have been conducted with some (small) success—*Neurology* 2003 **61** 260

Myasthenia gravis (MG)

Essence An antibody-mediated, autoimmune disease with too few functioning muscle acetylcholine receptors, leading to muscle weakness. Antiacetylcholine receptor antibodies are detectable in 90% of patients, and cause depletion of functioning postsynaptic receptor sites.

Presentation Can present at any age with increasing muscular fatigue. If <50yrs old, myasthenia is commoner in women, associated with other autoimmune diseases and thymic hyperplasia. Over 50, it is commoner in men, and associated with thymic atrophy or, rarely, a thymic tumour. Muscle groups commonly affected (most likely first): extraocular; bulbar; face; neck; limb girdle; trunk. Look especially for: ptosis; diplopia; 'myasthenic snarl' on smiling. On counting aloud to 50, the voice weakens. Reflexes are normal. Weakness may be exacerbated by pregnancy, $K^+\downarrow$, infection, overtreatment, change of climate, emotion, exercise, gentamicin, opiates, tetracycline, quinine, quinidine, procainamide, β-blockers.

Associations: Thymic tumour; hyperthyroidism; rheumatoid arthritis; SLE.

Tests *Tensilon® test* (only do if resuscitation facilities and atropine are to hand). Prepare 2 syringes, 1 with 10mg edrophonium and one with 0.9% saline. Give 1st 20% of each separately IV as test dose. Ask independent observer to comment on effect of each. Wait 30s before giving rest of each syringe. The test is +ve if edrophonium improves power in ~1min. The test may not be as dramatic as it is stated. Others: *Antiacetylcholine receptor antibody* ↑ in 90% (70% in ocular-confined MG). *Neurophysiology* (decremental response in muscle to repetitive nerve stimulation ± ↑'jitter' in single-fibre studies). *CT of thymus.* **NB:** ptosis improves by >2mm after ice applied to the (shut) affected lid for >2min. This is the basis of a new non-invasive test.

Treatment options

1 Symptomatic control with anticholinesterase eg *pyridostigmine* 60–450mg/24h PO taken through the day; SE: diarrhoea, colic, controllable by propantheline 15mg/8h PO; cholinergic SE: salivation↑; lacrimation; sweats; vomiting; miosis.

2 Immunosuppression with *prednisolone* (single-dose alternate day regimen + osteoporosis prophylaxis); start at 5mg, increase by 5mg/wk up to 1mg/kg on each treatment day; ↓dose on remission (may take months). SE: weakness (hence low starting dose); may be combined with *azathioprine* 2.5mg/kg/d (do FBC & LFT weekly for 8wks, then 3 monthly) or weekly *methotrexate*.

3 *Thymectomy:* Consider if onset before 50yrs old and disease is not easily controlled by anticholinesterases. Expect remission in 25% and worthwhile benefit in a further 50%. Thymectomy is also necessary for thymomas to prevent local invasion (but MG symptoms are often unaffected).

4 *Plasmapheresis* or IV *immunoglobulin* (IVIg) gives ~2–4wks' benefit (useful in crises or pre-thymectomy, eg IVIg 0.4g/kg daily for 5d pre-op).

Prognosis Relapsing or slow progression. If thymoma, 5yr survival is 68%.

Myasthenic syndrome

This typically occurs in association with small cell lung cancer (Eaton–Lambert syndrome) or, less commonly, with other autoimmune disease. Unlike true MG, it: • Affects especially proximal limbs and trunk (rarely the eyes) • Autonomic involvement is common (especially dry mouth) • There is *hypo*-reflexia • Only a slight response to edrophonium • Repeated muscle contraction may lead to *increased* muscle strength and reflexes • It is the presynaptic membrane which is affected (the carcinoma appears to provoke production of antibody to Ca^{2+} channels). Treatment (by experts): 3,4-diaminopyridine.
▶ Do regular CXRs as symptoms may predate lung cancer by ≥4yrs.

Other causes of muscle fatigability Polymyositis; SLE; botulism; Takayasu's disease (fatigability of the extremities). For other myopathies, see p398.

Neurofibromatosis

Type 1 neurofibromatosis (NF1, von Recklinghausen's disease)
Prevalence: 1 in 2500, ♀:♂ ≈ 1:1; no racial predilection. Inheritance is autosomal dominant, the gene is on chromosome 17. Expression of Type 1 neurofibromatosis (NF1) is variable, even within a family.

Signs *Café-au-lait spots* are flat, coffee-coloured patches of skin seen in the 1st year of life (clearest in UV light), increasing in size and number with age. Adults have ≥6, >15mm across. They do *not* predispose to skin cancer.

Freckling occurs in axillae, groin, neck base, and submammary area (♀) and is usually present by age 10.

Dermal neurofibromas appear at puberty and are small, violaceous nodules, gelatinous in texture. They may become papillomatous. They are not painful but may itch. Numbers increase over time.

Nodular neurofibromas arise from nerve trunks. Firm and clearly demarcated, they can give rise to paraesthesiae if pressed.

Lisch nodules are hamartomas on the iris which cannot be seen with the naked eye (use a slit lamp). They develop in early childhood and are harmless. Other signs: short stature and macrocephaly are also seen.

Complications These occur in ~one-third of NF1 patients. Mild learning disabilities are common. *Local effects of neurofibromas:* Nerve roots—compression; gut—bleeds, obstruction; bone—cystic lesions; pseudarthrosis; scoliosis. Hypertension (6%) due to renal artery stenosis or phaeochromocytoma. Plexiform neurofibromas (large, subcutaneous swellings). Malignancy (5% patients with NF1): optic glioma, sarcomatous change in a neurofibroma. Epilepsy risk ↑ (slight). There is a rare association with carcinoid syndrome (p250).

Management By a multi-disciplinary team including clinical geneticist, neurologist, and surgeon, orchestrated by the GP. Yearly measurement of BP and cutaneous survey is advised. Dermal neurofibromas are unsightly, and catch on clothing; if troublesome, lesions can excised, but removal of all lesions is unrealistic. Genetic counselling is important (*OHCS* p212).

Type 2 neurofibromatosis (NF2)
Autosomal dominant inheritance. Much rarer than NF1 with a prevalence of only 1 in 35,000. The gene responsible is on chromosome 22.

Signs *Café-au-lait spots* are fewer than in NF1. *Bilateral vestibular schwannomas* (acoustic neuromas) become symptomatic in the teens or twenties when sensorineural hearing loss is the 1st sign. There may be tinnitus and vertigo. The rate of tumour growth is unpredictable and variable. The tumours are benign but cause problems by pressing on local structures and by ↑ICP. *Juvenile posterior subcapsular lenticular opacity* (a form of cataract) occurs before other manifestations and can be useful in screening those at risk.

Complications Schwannomas of other cranial nerves, spinal nerve roots, or peripheral nerves. Meningiomas (45% NF2) which may be multiple. Glial tumours also but less commonly. Consider NF2 in any young person presenting with one of these tumours in isolation.

Management Hearing tests yearly from puberty with brain MRI only if abnormalities detected. A negative MRI in the late teens is helpful in assessing risk to any offspring. A clear scan at 30yrs (unless a family history of late onset) indicates that the gene has not been inherited. Treatment of vestibular schwannomas is neurosurgical and complicated by hearing loss/deterioration and facial palsy. Mean survival from diagnosis has been reported at 15yrs and best practice is still unclear.

Don't be put off by the excessive amount of detail on this page: you could leave it until later (the details are required to make sense of difficult presentations).

Diagnostic criteria for neurofibromatosis

NF1 (von Recklinghausen's disease)

Diagnosis is made if 2 of the following are found:

1 ≥6 *café-au-lait* macules >5mm (prepubertal) or >15mm (post-pubertal)
2 ≥2 neurofibromas of any type or 1 plexiform
3 Freckling in the axillary or inguinal regions
4 Optic glioma
5 ≥2 Lisch nodules
6 Distinctive osseous lesion typical of NF1, eg sphenoid dysplasia
7 First degree relative with NF1 according to the above criteria

Differential: McCune–Albright syndrome (*OHCS* p754), multiple lentigenes,[1] urticaria pigmentosa (*OHCS* p602).

NF2

Diagnosis is made if either of the following are found:

1 Bilateral vestibular schwannomas seen on MRI or CT
2 First degree relative with NF2 and either:

  (a) Unilateral vestibular schwannoma
  (b) One of the following:

      Neurofibroma
      Meningioma
      Glioma
      Schwannoma
      Juvenile cataract (NF2 type).

Differential: NF1.

---

1 May be part of the LEOPARD syndrome, a complex dermatosis with dominant autosomal transmission; L = lentigines, E = ECG anomalies, O = ocular hypertelorism (eyes wide-spaced), P = pulmonary stenosis, A = anomalies of the genital organs, R = retarded growth, D = deafness. www.txt.co.uk/sum.cfm?11

Syringomyelia

Syrinx was one of those versatile virgins of Arcadia who, on being pursued by Pan to the banks of the river Ladon, turned herself into a reed—from which Pan made his pipes, and, in so doing, she gave her name to all manner of tubular structures, eg syringes—and syrinxes, which are tubular or slit-like cavities which form in or close to the central canal of the cervical spinal cord.

Cause Most commonly associated with base of brain abnormalities (eg the Arnold–Chiari malformation, in which the cerebellum extends through the foramen magnum). Less common associations include basilar invagination,[1] atlanto-axial fusion, localized arachnoiditis, and dural cysts. Pathogenesis is debated but probably involves changes in CSF flow dynamics around the cervical cord and between the spinal and intracranial CSF compartments. Syrinxes can also develop after cord injury or within spinal tumours.

As syrinxes enlarge, they expand into adjacent grey and white matter, compressing decussating spinothalamic fibres anteriorly, the ventral horns which contain anterior horn cells, and the descending corticospinal fibres. Extension into the brainstem is called *syringobulbia*. Sudden development or worsening of signs may occur during coughing or sneezing as acute rises in venous pressure causes extension of the syrinx.

Cardinal signs Wasting and weakness of the hands and arms, with loss of pain and temperature sensation (dissociated sensory loss, p330) over the trunk and arms, eg in a cape distribution (suspended sensory loss)—reflecting early involvement of fibres conveying pain and temperature sensation which decussate anteriorly in the cord, and of cervical anterior horn cells. Sensory loss may lead to painless burns and Charcot's joints.

Other features: *Horner's syndrome* (cervical sympathetics) and *UMN signs in the legs ± body asymmetry*, limb hemihypertrophy, or podomegaly/chiromegaly (unilaterally enlarged hands or feet, perhaps from release of trophic factors via the anterior horn cells). *Eye movement abnormalities* (esp. downbeat nystagmus; also diplopia, oscillopsia,[2] and tunnel vision) are due to associated base of brain (foramen magnum) abnormality. *Charcot's (neuropathic) joints:* On losing sensation, joints are destroyed by too great a range of movement, becoming swollen and mobile. *Causes:* DM (tarsometatarsal, tarsal, ankle), tabes dorsalis (eg knee), paraplegia (eg hips), syringomyelia (eg shoulder), leprosy, spinal osteolysis/cord atrophy (eg systemic sclerosis).

Investigations MRI scan.

Natural history The symptoms may be mild and unchanging for years, but then there may be a rapid deterioration.

Treatment Surgical decompression at the foramen magnum may be tried if there is a Chiari malformation. It aims to promote free flow of CSF through the foramen magnum, preventing syrinx dilatation. These procedures may relieve pain, and prevent progression of symptoms.

Tropical spastic paraplegia/HTLV-1 myelopathy

There is spastic paraplegia, with paraesthesiae, sensory loss, and disorders of micturition which progresses over weeks or months, and becomes disabling. It is typically caused by sexually acquired human T-cell lymphotropic virus type I (HTLV-1) retrovirus infection (endemic in Japan, the Caribbean, Africa, South America, and the Southern USA). HTLV-1 also causes adult T-cell leukaemia—but rarely in the same individual as the myelopathy.

---

1 The top of the odontoid process (part of C2) migrates upwards (congenitally or in rheumatoid arthritis or osteogenesis imperfecta) causing foramen magnum stenosis ± medulla oblongata compression. Consider basilar invagination if the odontoid tip is ≥4mm above McGregor's line (drawn from the upper surface of the posterior edge of the hard palate to the most caudal point of the occipital curve).
2 Oscillopsia (sensation of oscillation of objects viewed) in brainstem disorders not causing nystagmus is attributed to failure of vestibular-ocular reflex to compensate for head movement. [@12131465]

Neuroradiology (CT and MRI)

Computer tomography (CT) works by identifying x-ray attenuation of materials, measured in Hounsfield units (HU), eg bone +1000, water 0, and air –1000HU. You see the x-ray attenuation of an area as a shade of grey. At the extremes, high attenuation is white and low attenuation is black. The attenuation of biological soft tissues is in a narrow range from about +80 for blood and muscle, to 0 for CSF, and down to –100 for fat. IV contrast may be given, demonstrating initially an angiographic effect, the high attenuation contrast in the vessels making them appear white. Later, if there is a defect in the blood–brain barrier, as with neoplasms or infection, contrast will extravasate, giving an enhancing, white7 area in the cerebrum or cerebellum. Some intracranial components do not have a blood–brain barrier and enhance normally: pituitary gland and choroid plexus.

Compared with MRI, CT is good at showing acute haemorrhage and fractures, and is much easier to do in ill or anaesthetized patients—so is valuable in emergencies. Fresh blood is of higher attenuation (∴ whiter) than brain tissue. Attenuation of haematomas declines as Hb breaks down so that a sub-acute subdural haematoma at 2wks may have an attenuation the same as adjacent brain, making it difficult to detect. A chronic subdural haematoma will be of relatively low attenuation.

CT is commonly performed in acute stroke to exclude haemorrhage (eg pre-anticoagulation). The actual area of infarction/ischaemia will not show up for a day or so, and will be low-attenuation cytotoxic oedema (intracellular oedema mainly confined to the grey matter).

Tumours and abscesses can have common features, eg a ring enhancing mass, surrounding vasogenic oedema, and mass effect. Vasogenic oedema is extracellular and spreads through the white matter. Mass effect causes compression of the sulci and ipsilateral ventricle, and may also cause herniation, subfalcine, trans-tentorial, or tonsillar. ▶On p367 there is an image of this.

One indication for CT scan is acute, severe headache. If there is concern about subarachnoid haemorrhage, a non-contrast CT may show acute blood. Even if it does not, it will show if the basal cisterns are normal and therefore lumbar puncture is probably safe.

Magnetic resonance imaging (MRI) An image is made by disturbing a nucleus in a strong magnetic field by using a radiofrequency pulse at the resonant frequency, and detecting the signal as the nucleus (usually hydrogen) returns to equilibrium. *Example image*: p354. The chief image sequences are:

- *T1 weighted images:* give good anatomical detail to which the T2 image can be compared/related. Fat is brightest (signal intensity↑); other tissues are darker to varying degrees. Flowing blood appears black.
- *T2 weighted images:* These provide the best detection of pathology, most pathology having some oedema fluid, therefore appearing white. Fat and fluid appear brightest. ▶For an example of this, see p397.

Advantages of MRI:	*Disadvantages of MRI:*
Non-ionizing radiation	High cost
Shows vasculature without contrast	Claustrophobia (in magnet tunnel for 15–60min—hypnosis, music, or sedation may be needed)
Images can easily be produced in any plane, eg sagittal or coronal (good for spinal cord and blood vessels)	Motion artefact ∵ ↑imaging time
Visualization of posterior fossa and other areas prone to bony artefact on CT, ie cranio–cervical junction	Unhelpful in imaging calcium
High inherent soft tissue contrast	Unsuitable for those with ferromagnetic foreign bodies (pacemakers, CNS vascular clips, cochlear implants, valves, shrapnel, etc.)
Precise staging of malignancy, eg involvement of bone marrow	Difficult in anaesthetized patients

Models of brain functioning

A superficial reading of the foregoing pages might lead one to the conclusion that the structure of the adult brain is fixed, and that a circumscribed lesion will produce reproducible, predictable results (if we remember our neuroanatomy correctly). Furthermore, if a certain phenomenon appears when part of the brain (say area A) is stimulated, and is lost when the same part of the brain is injured, we happily conclude that area A is the centre for laughter, fear, or whatever the phenomenon is. A lesion here, and you will stop laughing for ever, we might think. An area on the hard disk of our mind has been scratched. The grey cells do not regenerate themselves, so the brain carries on as before with this one defect. The more we look at the brain, the more wrong this model becomes.

If our brains were like a computer, the more tasks we did at the same time, the slower we would do any one task. In fact, our performance can improve, the more simultaneous tasks we take on. This is why music helps some of us concentrate. Experiments using functional MRI show that listening to polyphonic music recruits memory circuits, promoting attention, and aids semantic processing, target detection, and some forms of imagery.[1]

Another way in which our brains are not like a computer is that we are born with certain predispositions and expectations. Our hard disk never was blank. Just as the skin on the feet of new-born babies is thicker than other areas (as if feet were made with a pre-knowledge of walking, or somehow expecting walking), so our brains are made expecting a world of stimuli, which need making sense of by reframing sequential events in terms of cause and effect. We cannot help unconsciously imposing cause and effect relationships on events which are purely sequential. This unconscious reframing no doubt has survival value.

The model we have of brain function is important because it influences our attitude to our patients. If we are stuck with a neuroanatomical model, we will be rather pessimistic and guarded in our assessment of how patients may recover after neurological events. If we use a model which is more holistic and reality based, such as the Piaget-type model in which the brain is seen as intrinsically unstable and continually re-creating itself, we will grant our patients more possibilities. Our model of the brain must encompass its ability to set goals for itself, and to be self-actuating. Unstructured optimism is unwarranted, but structured optimism is to some extent a self-fulfilling prognosis. For many medical conditions, the more optimistic we are, and the more we involve our patients in their own care and its planning, the faster and better they will recover. If we combine this with the observed fact that those with an optimistic turn of mind are less likely to suffer stroke,[2] we can reach the conclusion that emotional well-being predicts subsequent functional independence and survival. When this hypothesis is tested directly in a prospective way, the effect of emotional well-being is found to be direct and strong and independent of other factors such as functional status, sociodemographic variables, chronic conditions, body mass index, etc.

So the conclusion is that the brain has an unknown amount of inherent plasticity, and an unknown potential for healing after injury—uninjured areas may take on new functions, and injured parts may function in new ways.[3] The great challenge of neurology is to work to maximize this potential for recovery and re-creation. This demands knowledge of your patient, as well as knowledge of neuroanatomy and neurophysiology. The point is that there is no predefined limit to what is possible.

1 P Janata 2003 *Cogn Affect Behav Neurosci* 2 121
2 G Ostir 2001 *Psychosom Med* 63 210. N = 2478 (6yr prospective population-based cohort study).
3 In early frontotemporal dementia, artistic creativity may blossom—suggesting that language is not required for, and may even inhibit, certain types of visual creativity. B Miller 2003 *Neurology* 60 1707

Rheumatological & related illnesses[1]

Contents

Relevant pages elsewhere: Charcot's joints (p404). Eponymous syndromes: Behçet's disease (p718); Sjögren's syndrome (p734); Wegener's granulomatosis (p738).

Points to note in the rheumatological history

Age, occupation, origin (eg SLE is commoner in Afro-Caribbeans and Asians).

• *Presenting symptoms*

Joints:	Pain; morning stiffness (eg RA)
	Pattern of distribution
	Swelling; loss of function
Extra-articular:	Rashes, photosensitivity (SLE)
	Raynaud's (SLE; CREST, p420; poly- and dermatomyositis)
	Dry eyes or mouth (Sjögren's)
	Diarrhoea/urethritis (Reiter's)
	Red eyes, eg ank. spond., p418
	Nodules or nodes (RA; TB)
	Mouth/genital ulcers (Behçet's)
	Weight loss (eg TB arthritis)

• *Rheumatological and related diseases:* eg Crohn's/UC in ankylosing spondylitis; psoriasis, gonorrhoea, or Reiter's-associated arthritis (p418)
• *Current & past drugs:* Disease modifying drugs, eg gold et al
• *Family history:* Arthritis; psoriasis (psoriatic arthropathy)
• *Social history:* Functioning, eg dressing, writing, walking, domestic, situation social support, home adaptations

Existential approaches to rheumatology patients Like François Verret's productions, rheumatological encounters are often multimedia affairs, with conflicting lines of story and mime, ever-changing charts of painful, disjointed images, puzzling manifestations, disorganized articulations, and absurdly irrelevant facts that may prove crucial in certain undeclared contexts. The diagnosis you arrive at will depend on which layer of this multimedia event you attend to. No single interpretation is universally valid, and in your attempts to lead an authentic life on the wards and in clinics you may frequently need to change your angle of approach. When in doubt (the only valid state of the thinking doctor), ask your patient what is most important.

---

1 *We thank Dr Gavin Clunie who is our Specialist Reader for this chapter.*

Points to note in assessing the locomotor system

This aims to screen for most rheumatological conditions, and to assess motor disability. It is based on the GALS locomotor screen (below).

Essence Ask questions; look; 'feel'; move. If a joint *feels normal* to the patient, *looks normal* to you, and has *full range of movement*, it usually *is* normal.

3 screening questions • Are you free of any muscle pain or stiffness? • Can you dress all right? • Can you manage stairs? If 'Yes' to all 3, muscle and joint problems are unlikely. If 'No' to any, go into detail.

GALS screening examination To be done in light underwear (no corsets).

Spine: Observe from behind: Is muscle bulk OK (buttocks, shoulders)? Is the spine straight? Symmetrical paraspinal muscles? Swellings/ deformities? *Observe from the side:* Normal cervical and lumbar lordosis? Kyphosis? *'Touch your toes, please':* Is lumbar spine flexion normal? *Observe from in front* for the rest of the examination. Ask him to: *'Tilt head towards shoulders'* (without moving the shoulders): is lateral neck flexion normal?

Arms: 'Arms straight': Tests elbow extension. Also tests forearm supination/ pronation. *'Put hands behind head'*—tests functional shoulder movement. *Examine the hands:* See p39. Any deformity, wasting, or swellings? *'Put index finger on thumb'*—tests pincer grip. Assess dexterity.

Legs: Observe legs: Normal quadriceps bulk? Any swelling or deformity or length discrepancy?

Find any knee effusion: With patient supine, do the patella tap test. If there is fluid, consider aspirating and testing it for crystals or infection?

Observe feet: Any deformity? Are arches high or flat? Any callosities? These may indicate an abnormal gait of some chronicity.

Gait: 'Walk over there please': Is the gait smooth? Good arm swing? Stride length OK? Normal heel strike and toe off? Can he turn quickly?

Other manoeuvres

• Palpate for typical fibromyalgia tender points (*OHCS* p675).
• *Squeeze across 2nd–5th metacarpophalangeal joints.* Pain may denote joint or tendon synovitis. Repeat for metatarsophalangeal joints.
• *Passively flex knee and hip to the full extent.* Is movement limited?
• *Internally/externally rotate each hip in flexion.*

The GALS system for quickly recording your findings

<pre>
        G (Gait) ✓
                    Appearance: Movement:
    A (Arms)   ✓   ✓
    L (Legs)   ✓   ✓
    S (Spine)   ✓   ✓

                    A ✓ means normal. If not normal, then put a cross
                    with a note to explain what the exact problem is.
</pre>

Back pain

This is very common, and often self-limiting; *but be alert to sinister causes.*
Key points in the history: (1) Onset: sudden (related to trauma?) or gradual?
(2) Are there motor or sensory symptoms? (3) Is bladder or bowel affected?
Pain worse on movement and relieved by rest is often mechanical. If it is
worse after rest, an inflammatory cause should be considered.

Examination: (1) With the patient standing (straight legs), gauge the extent
and smoothness of lumbar forward/lateral flexion and extension. (2) Neurological deficits: peri-anal sensation; upper and lower motor neurone (UMN &
LMN) signs in legs (p331); (3) Signs of generalized disease suggest malignancy.
Dorsal root irritation causes pain in relevant dermatomes, worsened by coughing and bending forward. *Lasègue's sign* is +ve if straight leg raising on supine
patient is painful in buttock/back/other leg and restricted to <45°. It suggests
lumbar disc prolapse irritating nerve roots (although inter-observer reproducibility is poor for this test, do not assume that there is some gold standard which will reveal all: 20–30% of 'normals' with *no* back pain have *some*
disc protrusion on MRI; in finding out if this is significant, we rely on signs
such as Lasègue's sign). Its sensitivity is ~0.9 and its specificity is 0.26.

Neurosurgical emergencies • *Acute cauda equina compression:* Alternating
or bilateral root pain in legs, saddle anaesthesia (ie bilaterally around anus),
and disturbance of bladder or bowel function • *Acute cord compression:* Bilateral pain, LMN signs at level of compression, UMN and sensory signs below,
spincter disturbance. Causes (same for both types of compression): bony
metastasis (look for missing pedicle on x-ray), myeloma, cord or paraspinal
tumour, TB (p564), abscess. ▶▶Urgent treatment prevents irreversible loss:
laminectomy for disc protrusions; decompression for abscess; radiotherapy
for tumours.

Tests MRI is the best way to illustrate cord compression, myelopathy, spinal
neoplasms, cysts, haemorrhages, and abscesses (myelography, plain x-rays,
and CT are problematic). FBC, ESR (↑in myeloma, infections, tumours), U&E,
PSA, and bone scan 'hot spot' suggest neoplastic diagnoses.

Causes Age determines the most likely causes.
- 15–30yrs: Prolapsed disc, trauma, fractures, ankylosing spondylitis (AS)
(p418), spondylolisthesis (eg L5 shifts forward on S1), pregnancy.
- 30–50yrs: Degenerative spinal disease, prolapsed disc, malignancy (lung,
breast, prostate, thyroid, kidney).
- >50yrs: Degenerative, osteoporosis, Paget's, malignancy, myeloma (request
serum electrophoresis), lumbar canal/lateral recess spinal stenosis.

Rarer causes: Cauda equina tumours, spinal infection (usually staphylococcal,
also *Proteus*; *Escherichia coli*; *S.typhi*; TB). Often no systemic signs of infection.

Treatment Specific causes need specific treatment. Usually no cause is
found, so treat empirically: avoid precipitants; arrange physiotherapy or
manual therapy. Analgesia, and carrying on with life is better than bed rest
(>3 days is rarely justifiable[1]) or physiotherapy. In certain patients there are
roles for disc, epidural or nerve root injections and surgical procedures:
foramenotomy, stabilization, or laminectomy.

Features which may indicate sinister back pain
- Young (<20yrs) or old (>55yrs)
- Violent trauma
- Alternating sciatica
- Bilateral sciatica
- Weak legs
- Weight loss
- PUO; ESR↑ (>25mm/h, p670)
- Taking systemic steroids
- Progressive, continuous, non-mechanical pain
- Systemically unwell; drug abuse; HIV +ve
- Spine movement in *all* directions painful
- Localized bony tenderness
- CNS deficit at more than one root level
- Pain or tenderness of thoracic spine
- Bilateral signs of nerve root tension
- Past history of neoplasia

1 A firm mattress is often recommended, but in fact medium types are better (N=313; *Lancet* 2003 1599).

Arthritis—general points

Features of inflammatory arthritis Pain, stiffness (especially early morning), loss of function, and signs of inflammation at 1 or more joints.

Diagnosis ►Consider septic arthritis in any sudden onset monoarthritis. Features may be less overt if immunodeficient or if underlying joint disease. Aspirate the joint. ►Look for blood, crystals, and pus (polarized light microscopy, culture, Gram stain). Sepsis may destroy a joint within 24h. On microscopy, finding WBCs in the aspirate fluid suggests sepsis or crystal arthritis. If in doubt, treat initially for sepsis, as described below.

Causes—*Monoarthritis*

Septic arthritis (eg *staphs, streps, Gram −ve bacilli, gonococci,* TB)
Psoriatic and reactive arthritides
Trauma (haemarthrosis)
Calcium pyrophosphate dihydrate (CPPD) crystals (p416); gout
Osteoarthritis
Monoarthritic presentation of a polyarticular disease (eg RA)

Polyarthritis (eg >2 swollen painful joints)

Viruses, eg *mumps, rubella, parvovirus B19, EBV, hepatitis B, enteroviruses,* HIV, α-viral arthropathy[1]
Rheumatoid (RA) or osteoarthritis (OA)
Spondyloarthritides
Connective tissue diseases (eg systemic lupus erythematosus, SLE)
Crystal arthropathies (gout, CPPD, p416)
Post-streptococcal reactive arthritis
Sarcoidosis

Assess Extent of joint involvement (include spine), symmetry, disruption of joint anatomy, limitation of movement (by pain or contracture), effusions and peri-articular involvement. See p409 for a full assessment. Associated features: dysuria or genital ulcers, skin or eye involvement, lungs, kidneys, heart, GI (eg mouth ulcers, bloody diarrhoea), and CNS.

Urine: Dipstick urine for blood and protein. If +ve, arrange urgent microscopy (?casts), culture, and Gram stain.

Radiology: Look for erosions, calcification, widening or loss of joint space, changes in underlying bone (eg periarticular osteoporosis, sclerotic areas, osteophytes) of affected joints. Image sacroiliac joints if considering a spondyloarthritis (irregularity of lower third); CXR in RA, SLE, vasculitis, and TB. In septic arthritis, x-rays may be normal, as may be ESR and CRP (if CRP ↑, expect it to fall with treatment).

Joint aspiration: OHCS p656. Microscopy (+culture): any blood, crystals, or pus? Do polarized light microscopy for urate or CPPD crystals (see above & p416).

Blood: Culture if sepsis is possible. FBC, ESR, urate, urea, and creatinine if systemic disease. Rheumatoid factor, antinuclear antibody, and other autoantibodies (p421). In trauma, arthroscopy may help. Consider HIV serology.

Treatment is determined by the cause. If **septic arthritis** is suspected,[2] give good analgesia and flucloxacillin (for staphs—in adults: ½–1g/6h slowly IV) + benzylpenicillin 1.2g/4h IV ± gentamicin (p710) until sensitivities are known. In infants, *Haemophilus* is common, so give cefotaxime too (50mg/kg/12h IV slowly). Look for atypical mycobacteria and fungi if HIV +ve. Ask a microbiologist how long to continue treatment (≥2wks IV, then 3wks PO). Consider aspiration (arthrocentesis), lavage, and debridement—arthroscopic (eg for knee) or open (eg for hip or shoulder, with GA; this allows biopsy—helpful for TB). Ask for orthopaedic advice. If a joint prosthesis is *in situ*, get orthopaedic advice before aspiration. Splint for ≤48h; then give physiotherapy. ►*Ask yourself* 'how did the organism get there?' Is there immunosuppression, or a focus of infection (eg pneumonia, in 50% of those with pneumococcal arthritis)?

---

1 Via mosquitoes: Chikungunya, O'nyong, Mayaro, Ross River, Sindbis, Barmah Forest viruses [@7728877]
2 Rare but serious cause of irreversible loss of joint function. More common in RA and in those with joint prostheses—where infection is particularly difficult to treat; use vancomycin + fusidic acid. ►Get help *Rheum Dis Clin North Am* 2003 **29** 61 *Advances in managing septic arthritis.*

Synovial fluid in health and disease[1]

Aspiration of synovial fluid is used primarily to look for infectious or crystal (gout and CPPD crystal arthropathy, p416).

	Appearance	Viscosity	WBC/mm³	Neutrophils
Normal	Clear, colourless	↑	≤200	None
Non-inflammatory[2]	Clear, straw	↑	≤5000	≤25%
Haemorrhagic[3]	Bloody, xanthochromic	Varies	≤10,000	≤50%
Acutely inflamed[4]	Turbid, yellow	↓		
• Crystal			~14,000	~80%
• Rheumatic fever			~18,000	~50%
• RA			~16,000	Varies
Septic	Turbid, yellow	↓		
• TB			~24,000	~70%
• Gonorrhoeal			~14,000	~60%
• Septic (non-gonococcal)[5]			~65,000	~95%

Palliative care in chronic arthritis

The ideal option is inpatient or home-based rehabilitation with physiotherapy, group exercise programmes, hydrotherapy, swimming, thermal treatments, endurance training, and relaxation strategies. This is known to reduce pain and to increase function (both long- and short-term). See M Weigl 2004 *Ann Rheum Dis* **63** 360.

1 Wallach, Interpretation of Diagnostic Tests: A Synopsis of Laboratory Medicine, 5e, Little, Brown, Boston.
2 Eg degenerative joint disease.
3 Eg tumours, haemophilia, trauma.
4 Eg Reiter's, CPPD crystals (p416), SLE.
5 Includes staphs, streps, and Pseudomonas (eg post-op).

Rheumatoid arthritis (RA)

Typically a persistent, symmetrical, deforming, peripheral arthropathy. Peak onset: 5th decade. ♀:♂ > 2 : 1. Prevalence: 0.5–1% (higher in smokers).[1] Genetics: HLA DR4 linked in caucasians (DRβ1 epitope)

Presentation Typically with swollen, painful, and stiff hands and feet, especially in the morning. This can fluctuate and larger joints become involved. Less common presentations are:

1 Recurring monoarthritis of various joints (*palindromic*—'*was I saw!*'[2]).
2 Persistent monoarthritis (often of 1 knee).
3 Systemic illness (pericarditis, pleurisy, weight↓) with minimal joint problems at first. (Commoner in men.)
4 Vague limb girdle aches.
5 Sudden onset of widespread arthritis.

Signs At first, swollen fingers and MCP joint swelling. Later, digital ulnar deviation and dorsal wrist subluxation. Boutonnière and swan-neck deformities of fingers (see BOX) or Z-deformity of thumbs. Hand extensor tendons may rupture and adjacent muscles waste. Foot changes are similar. Larger joints may be involved. Atlanto-axial joint subluxation may threaten the cord.

Extra-articular Anaemia; nodules; lymphadenopathy; vasculitis; carpal tunnel syndrome; multifocal neuropathies; splenomegaly (5%; but only 1% have Felty's syndrome: leucopenia, lymphadenopathy, weight loss, p722). Eyes: episcleritis; scleritis; keratoconjunctivitis sicca. Other signs: pleurisy, pericarditis. Pulmonary fibrosis. Osteoporosis. Amyloidosis. Associated with increased risk of ischaemic heart disease and lymphomas.

X-rays ↑Soft tissue; juxta-articular osteoporosis; ↓joint space. Later: bony erosions ± subluxation ± complete carpal destruction.

Blood tests ESR↑; HB↓; MCV ↔; WCC↓; platelets↑. *Rheumatoid factor* often –ve at start, becoming +ve in 80% (also +ve in: Sjögren's: 100%; SLE: 30%; mixed connective tissue disease (MCTD): 30%; systemic sclerosis: 30%); ANA +ve in 30%.

Treatment ►Encourage regular exercise, physio- and occupational therapy.
• Household aids and personal aids (orthoses), eg wrist splints.
• Intra-lesional steroids (for joint injection technique, see *OHCS* p656–8).
• Surgery—to relieve pain, improve function, and to prevent disease complications (eg ulna stylectomy; joint replacements).
• Oral drugs: if no contraindication (asthma, active peptic ulcer) start an NSAID: often, NSAIDs, such as ibuprofen 400mg/8h, after food do not control symptoms or are not tolerated (GI bleeds). Consider COX II selective NSAID if needing maximum dose regular NSAID or age >65 (NICE recommendations): rofecoxib (Vioxx® 25mg/24h PO); celecoxib 200mg/12h PO, or etodolac 600mg od. Avoid NSAIDs if on warfarin. Patients who need low dose aspirin ± prednisolone will also need regular proton pump inhibitor such as lansoprazole. One cannot predict which NSAID a patient will respond to: different ones can be tried. Disease-modifying anti-rheumatic drugs (DMARDs) should be considered early (see BOX). Regular monitoring is vital.
• Steroids may ↓joint damage and control difficult symptoms—eg prednisolone 7.5mg/d PO, but place in treatment schema is controversial. One problem is ↓ bone density over long periods. *Osteoporosis prevention:* p698.
• Leflunomide ↓ autoimmune effects (takes months to work). For 1st 6 months, do FBC 2-weekly + monthly LFT, BP, & U&E. Stop if: platelets <150×10⁹/L; WBC <4×10⁹/L, or AST↑ by >3-fold or rashes, etc. ►See BNF.
• Manage cardiovascular risk factors (p91) as atherosclerosis is accelerated.[1]

1 Stolt P 2003 *Ann Rheum Dis* 62 835 & Caplan M 2003 *Lancet* 361 1068.
2 *Palin dromo* is Greek for 'to run to and fro' or 'to recur'. Verbal palindromes read equally well forwards or back, to and fro, as in *Lager, Sir, is regal*. In rheumatological palindromes, arthritis lasting hours or days runs to and fro, visiting and revisiting 3 or more sites, typically knees, wrists, & MCP joints. It may presage RA, SLE, Whipple's, or Behçet's disease. Remissions are (initially) complete, leaving no radiological mark. Patient diaries *might* reflect wrist, ankle, shoulder, and interphalangeal arthritis, tempting obsessive diagnosticians to hope (unreasonably) for a perfectly palindromic week, eg *Was I saw!*

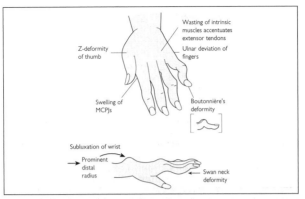

Wasting of intrinsic muscles accentuates extensor tendons

Ulnar deviation of fingers

Z-deformity of thumb

Swelling of MCPJs

Boutonnière's deformity

Subluxation of wrist

Prominent distal radius

Swan neck deformity

Influencing biological events in RA

The chief biological event is inflammation. Monocytes traffic into joints, cytokines are produced, fibroblasts and endothelial cells are activated, and tissue proliferates. Fluid is generated (effusion) and cytokines and cellular processes erode cartilage and bone. Cytokines also produce systemic effects: fatigue, accelerated atherosclerosis, and accelerated bone turnover.

Disease-modifying drugs (DMARDs) Start DMARDs if there is persisting synovitis for >6wks. Sulfasalazine and methotrexate are typical 1st choices and are often used together.

- *Sulfasalazine:* Common SE: nausea, headaches, diarrhoea, marrow↓, sperm count↓, rash, oral ulcers.
- *Methotrexate:* Avoid in liver disease and pregnancy and if alcohol consumption↑; caution if pre-existing lung disease. SE: mucositis, nausea, fatigue/lethargy, pneumonitis (rare; can be life-threatening), AST & ALT↑. Give concurrent folate supplements, eg folic acid 5mg/wk, PO.
- *Ciclosporin:* SE: nausea, tremor, gingival hypertrophy, hypertension, renal impairment/hypertension.
- *Gold:* SE: marrow↓, proteinuria, rash, hepatitis.
- *Azathioprine:* SE: marrow↓, nausea, LFT↑, oncogenic (do TPMT[1] test 1st).
- *Penicillamine:* SE: marrow↓, proteinuria, taste↓, oral ulcers, myasthenia.
- *Hydroxychloroquine:* SE: rash, diarrhoea, rarely retinopathy, tinnitus, headache.

►See *OHCS* p672 for dosages and further details.

Anti-cytokine therapy *Tumour necrosis factor α (TNFα)* is a key cytokine over-produced in RA synovium. Infliximab (chimeric murine/human anti-TNF antibody given IVI every 8wks p247), etanercept (TNFα receptor/Ig Fc fusion protein given 25mg SC twice weekly), and Humira (fully human anti-TNF monoclonal given as 40mg SC every 2wks). Infliximab and etanercept are NICE approved for progressive RA after 2 DMARD failures. *SE:* Rashes, nausea, diarrhoea, and infections (eg reactivation of TB). Neutralizing antibodies can ↓efficacy especially with infliximab; ANA and even SLE-type illness can evolve. Long-term safety issues are opaque (?↑risk of cancer) but responses can be striking compared with other DMARDs.

---

1 TPMT = thiopurine methyltransferase. TPMT alleles associated with ↓activity of TPMT is a cause of withdrawal of azathioprine. TPMT genotyping may allow high doses of AZA in those with normal TPMT alleles to improve immunosuppression. *Rheumatology* 2003 **42** 40

Osteoarthritis (OA)

OA is the commonest joint condition. Women are prone to symptomatic OA ($\female:\male \approx 3:1$). *Mean age at onset:* 50yrs. OA is usually primary, but may be secondary to any joint disease/injury or some diseases (eg haemochromatosis).

Signs & symptoms In single joints, pain on movement, worse at end of day; background pain at rest; stiffness; joint instability. In polyarticular OA with Heberden's nodes ('nodal OA'), the most commonly affected joints are DIP, thumb metacarpophalangeal joints, cervical and lumbar spine, and knee. There may be joint tenderness, derangement, ± bony swelling (eg Heberden's nodes, ie bony lumps at DIP joints), poor range of movement, and some (though usually limited) synovitis.

Imaging/tests *Radiology:* Loss of joint space, subchondral sclerosis and cysts, marginal osteophytes. *CRP* can be elevated slightly.

Treatment Regular paracetamol for pain. If no good, try NSAIDs (see BOX & p414), or low-dose tricyclic for night pain. Reduce weight; walking aids; supportive footwear; physiotherapy ± joint replacement for end-stage OA. Do exercises (eg regular quadriceps exercises in knee OA) and keep active.

Crystal arthropathies PLATE 16

Gout In the acute stage there is severe pain, redness, and swelling of the joint—often the metatarsophalangeal joint of the big toe (podagra). Attacks are due to the deposition of sodium monourate crystals in and around joints and may be precipitated by trauma, surgery, starvation, infection, or diuretics. With long-term hyperuricaemia, after repeated attacks, urate deposits (tophi) are found in peripheries, eg pinna, tendons, joints. 'Secondary' causes: polycythaemia, leukaemia, cytotoxics, renal impairment, long-term alcohol excess. *Diagnosis* depends on finding urate crystals in tissues and synovial fluid (serum urate not always ↑). Synovial fluid microscopy: negatively birefringent crystals; neutrophils (+ingested crystals). X-rays may show only soft-tissue swelling in the early stages. Later, well-defined 'punched out' lesions are seen in juxta-articular bone. There is no sclerotic reaction, and joint spaces are preserved until late. *Prevalence:* ~½–1%. $\male:\female \approx 5:1$.

Treating acute gout: Use a strong NSAID (eg naproxen). If contraindicated (eg peptic ulcer), give colchicine 0.5mg/8–12h, or 0.5mg/2–3h PO until pain goes or D&V occurs or 6mg given. **NB:** in renal impairment, NSAIDs and colchicine are problematic: steroids may be effective, but have their own SE (get expert help). *Preventing attacks:* Avoid prolonged fasts, alcohol excess, and high purine food.[1] Lose weight. Avoid low-dose aspirin (it ↑ serum urate). Consider reducing serum urate with long-term allopurinol, but not until 3wks after an attack. Start with regular NSAID or colchicine cover as introduction of allopurinol may cause gout attack. *Allopurinol dose:* 100–300mg/24h PO PC, adjust in the light of serum urate (typically 200mg/24h; max 300mg/8h). SE: rash, fever, WCC↓. If simple treatment fails, refer to rheumatologists.

Calcium pyrophosphate dihydrate (CPPD) arthropathy Risk factors:
• Dehydration • Intercurrent illness • Hyperparathyroidism • Myxoedema • PO_4^{3-}↓;Mg^{2+}↓ • Osteoarthritis; old age • Haemochromatosis • Acromegaly

Acute CPPD monoarthritis (pseudogout): Similar to gout; affects different joints (mainly wrist or knee). *Chronic CPPD:* Destructive changes like OA, but more severe; affecting eg knees (also wrists, shoulders, hips). Can present as polyarthritis (pseudo-rheumatoid) *Tests:* Polarized light microscopy of joint fluid: crystals are weakly positively birefringent. Associated with soft-tissue calcium deposition on x-ray, eg triangular ligament in wrist or in cartilage (chondrocalcinosis). *Treatment:* NSAIDs help but are rarely sufficient and often contraindicated in the elderly; consider steroids eg triamcinolone IM 60mg or prednisolone EC 20mg/d for 2wks. For chronic disease, consider hydroxychloroquine 200mg/d, upto 200mg/12h PO.

Prescribing NSAIDs: dialogue with patients

Most patients prescribed NSAIDs do not need them all the time, but some patients obediently take them continuously, as prescribed, with not infrequent serious side-effects, such as GI bleeding. *Bleeding is more common in those who know less about their drugs.* So explain that:

- Drugs are for relief of symptoms: *on good days none may be needed.*
- Abdominal pain may be a sign of impending gut problems: stop the tablets, and come back for more advice if symptoms continue.
- Ulcers may occur with no warning: *report black motions (± faints) at once.*
- Don't supplement prescribed NSAIDs with ones bought over the counter (eg ibuprofen): mixing NSAIDs can increase risks 20-fold.
- Smoking and alcohol ↑NSAID risk.

NB: Patients often ask about alternatives to NSAIDs, such as glucosamine (it acts on cartilage—dose example: 500mg/12h with food); it is better tolerated, but is not free of SEs (rash, drowsiness, headache).

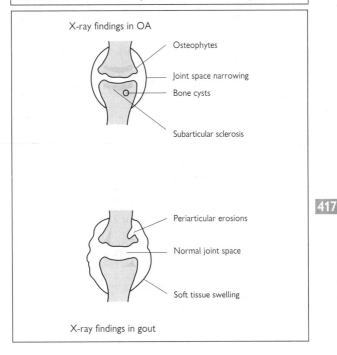

X-ray findings in OA

Osteophytes

Joint space narrowing

Bone cysts

Subarticular sclerosis

Periarticular erosions

Normal joint space

Soft tissue swelling

X-ray findings in gout

1 Less offal; oily fish; roes; anchovies; mussels; crabs; prawns; shrimps; meat/yeast extracts; spinach; chocolate; caffeine, eg in cough-and-cold remedies. Cherries may actually help (↑urate excretion).

Spondyloarthritides

Ankylosing spondylitis (AS) *Prevalence:* 0.25–1%. *Men present earlier.* ♂ : ♀ ≈ 6 : 1 at 16yrs old, and ≈ 2 : 1 at 30yrs old. >95% are HLA B27 +ve.

Symptoms: The typical patient is a young man presenting with low back pain, spinal morning stiffness, progressive loss of spinal movement (spinal ankylosis) who later develops kyphosis, neck hyperextension (question mark posture), and spino-cranial ankylosis. Other features and associations:

- Thoracic excursion decreased
- Chest pain
- Hip involvement
- Knee involvement
- Enthesitides[1] of calcanea, tibial or ischial tuberosities, or plantar fascia
- Crohn's/UC, psoriaform rashes, amyloid
- Carditis; iritis; recurrent sterile urethritis
- Aortic valve disease

Investigations: Diagnosis is clinical, supported by radiology findings (may be normal in early disease). Look for irregularities, erosions, or sclerosis affecting both sides of the lower third of the sacroiliac joints. Later: squaring of the vertebra, 'bamboo spine', erosions of the apophyseal joints, obliteration of the sacroiliac joints (sacroiliitis also occurs in reactive arthritides, Crohn's disease, psoriatic arthropathy, Brucella arthritis). Other tests: FBC (normochromic anaemia); ESR↑; ↑IgA, ↑CRP.

Treatment: Exercise, not rest, for backache; if able to cooperate with intense exercise regimens to maintain posture and mobility. NSAIDs may help pain and stiffness. Sulfasalazine and methotrexate help peripheral arthritis and enthesitis. Efficacy is 'proved' with infliximab (p247; but currently not other anti-TNF therapies). Rarely, spinal osteotomy is useful. Difficult-to-fix osteoporotic spinal fractures can occur (long-term bisphosphonates may prevent this).

Mortality: 1.5-fold higher than expected (eg from secondary amyloidosis or cardiovascular causes).

Enteropathic spondyloarthropathies Inflammatory bowel disease and GI bypass surgery (and possibly Whipple's and Coeliac disease, p740) are associated with spondyloarthritis.

Psoriatic arthritis See *OHCS* p586. Often asymmetrical, involves DIP joints, spine, typically causing dactylitis. X-ray changes can be misinterpreted as OA: entirely enthesopathic subforms exist. Associated with synovitis, acneiform rashes, palmo-plantar pustulosis, hyperostoses and (sterile) osteomyelitis (SAPHO). Responds to NSAIDs, methotrexate, ciclosporin (=cyclosporin), and anti-TNFα therapies (p247).

Reactive arthritides/Reiter's syndrome *Presentation:* Secondary to *Chlamydia trachomatis* urethritis, *Campylobacter jejuni*, *Salmonella*, *Shigella*, and *Yersinia* species. A typical story: a young man with recent non-specific urethritis (NSU, p586)—which may be asymptomatic; it may also follow dysentery (epidemics occur, eg in war). Often large joint, lower limb mono- or oligoarthritis or enthesitis; it may be chronic or relapsing. *Also:* Iritis, keratoderma blenorrhagica (brown, aseptic abscesses on soles and palms and circinate balanitis—painless serpiginous penile rash—(secondary to *C trachomatis*); mouth ulcers; enthesitis (plantar fasciitis, Achilles tendonitis) and aortic incompetence (rare). *Tests:* ESR & CRP ↑ or ↔. Culture stool if diarrhoea, serum for serology. Consider sexual health review. X-rays: periostitis at ligamentous entheses; enthesopathic erosions. *Management:* Rest; splint affected joints; NSAIDs or steroids. Consider sulfasalazine or methotrexate. Treating the original infection (p586 & p588) makes little difference on outcome.

---

1 Enthesitis ≈ painful inflammation/fasciitis where bone meets a joint capsule, ligament, or tendon.

Spondyloarthritides typically hold these features in common

1 Seronegativity (rheumatoid factor –ve).
2 Pathology in spine (spondylo-) and sacroiliac (SI) joints, ie 'axial arthritis'.
3 Asymmetrical large-joint oligoarthritis (ie few joints) or monoarthritis.
4 Inflamed tendon ligament union sites (enthesis), eg plantar fasciis, Achilles tendonitis, costochondritis, or digit tendon sheaths (dactylitis).
5 Extra-articular manifestations eg: uveitis, psoriaform rashes, Crohn's, UC.
6 HLA B27 association (88–96% of those with AS).

Spondyloarthritides show much overlap with one another. They are treated with physio- and occupational therapy, advice on posture, NSAIDs, sulfasalazine, methotrexate, IV bisphosphonates (p437), and infliximab (p415).

Arthritides unassociated with rheumatoid factor (sero –ve)

Lyme disease (p600), Behçet's (p718), leukaemia (p652), pulmonary osteoarthropathy (p182), endocarditis, acromegaly (p324), Wilson's disease (p236), familial Mediterranean fever (p552), sarcoid (p198), haemophilia, sickle-cell (p640), haemochromatosis (p234), and infections, eg from:

Post-streptococcal	*Hepatitis B*	*Rubella*
Parvovirus B19	*& Chl pneumoniae* (p174)	*Ureaplasma;* HIV
Vibrio parahaemolyticus	*Borrelia burgdorferi* (p600)	*Clostridium difficile*

Chronic arthritis in children (ie before 16yrs) takes several forms, and is classified into juvenile idiopathic arthritis (JIA) subforms:

• Systemic arthritis (formerly Still's disease)
• Oligoarthritis (1–4 joints affected in first 6 months)
• Polyarthritis (RhF –ve)
• Polyarthritis (RhF +ve)
• Psoriatic arthritis
• Enthesitis-related arthritis at ligament/tendon insertion into bone.

NB: JIA shares only some features with RA:

JIA shares these in common with RA:	*JIA and RA differ in these ways:*
Both display destructive arthropathy	RA is more likely to run in families
Autoimmune with autoantibodies	RA is more homogeneous than JIA
Both have HLA associations[1]	RA has poorer outcomes than JIA

Children with chronic arthritis need regular ophthalmic review to detect occult uveitis—and regular monitoring of growth and development.

---

1 3 haplotypes (DRB1*08-DQA1*0401-DQB1*0402; DRB1*11-DQA1*05-DQB1*03; & DRB1*1301-DQA1*01-DQB1*06) associate with ↑risk of JIA. DRB1*04-DQA1*03-DQB1*03 has ↓risk. *Rheumatology* 2002 **41** 1183

Autoimmune connective tissue diseases

Essence Included under this heading are: SLE (p422, the group prototype), diffuse/limited cutaneous systemic sclerosis, primary Sjögren's syndrome (p734), idiopathic inflammatory myopathies, MCTD, relapsing polychondritis, and Behçet's disease (p718). They overlap with each other, may affect many organ systems, and often respond to immunosuppressives (p674).[1]

Systemic sclerosis The 2 main forms:

• *Limited cutaneous systemic sclerosis:* (of which *CREST syndrome* is part) calcinosis (subcutaneous tissues), **R**aynaud's, o**e**sophageal and gut dysmotility, **s**clerodactyly, and **t**elangiectasia. 'Limited' to face and limbs distal to elbows or knees. Often associated with anticentromere antibodies and (initially) subclinical pulmonary hypertension.

• *Diffuse cutaneous systemic sclerosis:* 'Diffuse' defines skin involvement. More profound internal organ involvement. Often associated with lung (anti-Topo I [scl70] antibodies), cardiac, and renal changes. *Prognosis:* Often poor.

• *Therapy:* Calcium antagonists, ACE-i and A2R blockers (p288) for Raynaud's. Prostacyclin by IVI is being evaluated. Consider cyclophosphamide for lung disease. Meticulous BP control (ACE-i) if any renal crisis. Endothelin-1 receptor blockade (bosentan) if pulmonary hypertension and renal crisis.

Mixed connective tissue disease (MCTD) combines features of SLE, systemic sclerosis, and polymyositis. Renal & CNS signs are rare. Anti-RNP (ribonuclear protein) antibody is present (without other types of ANA).

Relapsing polychondritis attacks the pinna, nasal septum ± larynx (∴ stridor). *Association:* Aortic valve disease; arthritis; vasculitis. *R:* Steroids.

Polymyositis and dermatomyositis

Both conditions cause symmetrical, proximal muscle weakness from muscle inflammation. Associated with malignancy (in 9–23%). Dysphagia, dysphonia (problems with the mechanics, not the idea, of speech production, ie phonation), facial oedema, or respiratory weakness may develop.

Skin signs Macular rash (if over back & shoulder the *shawl sign* is +ve). 25% have a lilac-purple (*heliotrope rash*) on cheeks, eyelids and light-exposed areas, ± nail-fold erythema (*dilated capillary loops*), and roughened red papules over extensor surfaces of phalanges (*Gottron's papules*—pathognomonic if CK↑ + muscle weakness). Also *mechanic's hands* (rough, cracked skin on the lateral and palmar surfaces of the fingers and hands, with irregular 'dirty' lines—particularly in the antisynthetase syndrome [anti-Jo1].

Systemic signs Fevers, Raynaud's; lung involvement (20%); polyarthritis/ arthralgia (40%); calcifications; retinitis (like cotton-wool patches); myocardial involvement (myocarditis; arrhythmias); dysphagia and gut dysmotility.

Diagnosis Muscle enzymes (ALT & CK) ↑ in plasma; electromyography (EMG): shows fibrillation potentials; muscle biopsy. *Autoantibody (ab) associations:* Myositis-specific: anti-Mi-2, anti-Jo1 (look for lung fibrosis too). *Overlap syndromes:* Scleroderma with dermatomyositis (eg anti-PM-Scl +ve) or polymyositis/alveolitis (eg anti-Jo1 +ve). ∆∆: Subacute weakness from: inclusion-body myositis; muscular dystrophies; SLE myositis; polymyalgia; systemic sclerosis; endocrine/metabolic myopathies; rhabdomyolysis (p281).

Management Investigate extensively for malignancy; get expert help; rest and prednisolone help (start with 1mg/kg/24h PO). Immunosuppressives (p674) and cytotoxics are also used early, eg azathioprine, methotrexate, cyclophosphamide, or ciclosporin (=cyclosporin). High-dose immune globulin has a role. Doses vary: eg, 0.4g/kg/d for 5d each month, or 1g/kg daily for 2d each month (eg for 4 months). Dapsone can help skin disease.

A more aggressive form with prominent vasculitis occurs in children.

Plasma autoantibodies: disease associations

Antinuclear antibody (ANA)	+ve in (%)	Smooth muscle antibody (SMA)	+ve in (%)
SLE	95	Chronic active hepatitis	40–90
RA	32	Primary biliary cirrhosis	30–70
JIA (p419)	76	Idiopathic cirrhosis	25–30
Chronic active hepatitis	75	Viral infections	80
Sjögren's syndrome	68	(low titres)	
Systemic sclerosis	64	'Normal' controls	3–12
'Normal' controls[2]	0–2	(↑ with age: 20% at 70yrs)	

Gastric parietal cell antibody		Mitochondrial autoantibodies, AMA	
Pernicious anaemia (adults)	>90%	Primary biliary cirrhosis	60–94%
Atrophic gastritis:		Chronic active hepatitis	25–60%
Females	60%	Idiopathic cirrhosis	25–30%
Males	15–20%	'Normal' controls	0.8%
Autoimmune thyroid disease	33%		
'Normal' controls	2–16%		

Antibody to reticulin	
Coeliac disease	37%
Crohn's disease	24%
Dermatitis herpetiformis	17–22%
'Normal' controls	0–5%

Thyroid antibodies	Microsomal (%)	Thyroglobulin (%)
Hashimoto's thyroiditis	70–91	75–95
Graves' disease	50–80	33–75
Myxoedema	40–65	50–81
Thyrotoxicosis	37–54	40–75
Juvenile lymphocytic thyroiditis	91	72
Pernicious anaemia	55	
'Normal' controls (50% in older women)	10–13	6–10

Rheumatoid factor	+ve in (%)		
RA	70–80	Juvenile arthropathy	see p419
Sjögren's syndrome	≤100	Infective endocarditis	≤50
Felty's syndrome	≤100	SLE	≤40
Systemic sclerosis	30	'Normal' controls	5–10

It is associated with viral hepatitis, infectious mononucleosis, TB & leprosy.

ANCA-associated vasculitis: (No complement consumption or immune complex deposition.) Signs relate eg to respiratory tract or kidney. 2 types:

• *Classical antineutrophil cytoplasmic antibody (cANCA): Target:* serine protease 3: +ve in Wegener's disease (p738) in >90% of patients.

• *Perinuclear antineutrophil cytoplasmic antibody (pANCA): Target:* myeloperoxidase; +ve in ~80% pauci-immune crescentic GN (p268) and systemic vasculitides, eg microscopic polyangiitis (a vasculitis of kidney ± lung, pANCA +ve in ~75%).

NB: Churg–Strauss (p425) may be associated with p- and cANCA.

1 These and ill-defined/incomplete *autoimmune syndromes* (Raynaud's phenomenon, cold agglutinin disease, thyroiditis, nephrotic syndrome; vasculitis) are associated with ↑risk of lymphoma/CLL.
Undifferentiated connective tissue disease (UCTD) is diagnosed on the basis of signs suggesting a connective tissue disease and the presence of autoantibodies such as ANA, anti-dsDNA, -Sm, -RNP, -SSA, -SSB, -Scl-70, -centromere, -Jo1, -PM-Scl [@12846049].
2 The concept of normal is opaque here as autoantibodies are often present (eg in 88%) up to a decade before overt signs of illness occur—Arbuckle M 2003 *NEJM* **349** 1526

Systemic lupus erythematosus (SLE)

SLE is a non-organ-specific, autoimmune disease in which autoantibodies are produced against a variety of autoantigens (eg ANA). Immunopathology results in polyclonal B-cell secretion of pathogenic autoantibodies and subsequent formation of immune complexes which deposit in sites such as the kidneys. ♀ : ♂ ≈ 9 : 1. *Prevalence:* ~0.2%. **Common in:** Pregnancy; Afro-Caribbeans; Asians—and if HLA B8, DR2 or DR3 +ve. ~10% of relatives of SLE patients are affected. It is a remitting and relapsing illness, with peak age at diagnosis being 30–40yrs (in UK). *Clinical features:* See BOX. In addition: T°↑ (77%); splenomegaly; lymphadenopathy; alopecia (in 70%) recurrent abortion; retinal exudates; pulmonary oedema; fibrosing alveolitis; myalgia (50%); anorexia (40%); myositis; migraine (40%); ESR↑ (CRP often ↔: think of SLE whenever someone has a multisystem disorder and ESR↑ but CRP↔). OTM 3.87

Immuno-genetics 95% are ANA +ve. High titre of antibodies directed against double-stranded DNA is almost exclusive to SLE. Its absence does not exclude it. 40% are Rh factor +ve. 11% have false +ve syphilis serology from IgG anticardiolipin antibodies. Antibodies to Ro (SS-A), La (SS-B), and U1 ribonuclear protein help define overlap syndromes (eg with Sjögren's, p734).

Monitoring activity *3 best tests:* (1) ESR (2) Complement: C3↓, C4↓; C3d↑ (denotes degradation products of C3, hence it moves in the opposite way) (3) Double-stranded (anti-ds) DNA antibody titres. OTM 3.86 *Others:* BP, urinalysis, U&E, FBC.

Drug lupus This is caused by isoniazid, hydralazine (if >50mg/24h in slow acetylators), procainamide, chlorpromazine, minocycline. Lung and skin signs prevail over renal and CNS signs. It remits if the drug is stopped. Sulfonamides and the Pill may exacerbate idiopathic SLE.

Antiphospholipid syndrome SLE may occur with arterial or venous thromboses, livedo rash, stroke, adrenal haemorrhage, migraine, miscarriages, myelitis, myocardial infarct, multi-infarct dementia, and cardiolipin antibodies. *Presentation:* Abdominal pain (55%); BP↓ (54%); fever (40%); nausea (31%); weakness (31%), altered mental status (19%). Venous thrombi occur more often if lupus anticoagulant is +ve, and arterial thrombi if IgG or IgM antiphospholipid antibody +ve. R: Long-term warfarin (INR ≈ 3) may be used.

Treatment Refer to a rheumatologist. NSAIDs. Sun-block creams (OHCS p595).

- *Hydroxychloroquine* if joint or skin symptoms are uncontrolled by NSAIDs, ≤3.25mg/kg/12h PO (max 200mg/12h). SE: irreversible retinopathy—annual ophthalmic referral[1] is recommended (?needed only after ~6yrs of R).
- *High-dose prednisolone* is kept for severe episodes of SLE (~1mg/kg/24h PO for 6wks or pulse IV methylprednisolone), may be combined with other immunosuppressive agents (eg cyclophosphamide), or 'steroid-sparing agents', eg azathioprine, methotrexate, or mycophenolate.
- *Low-dose steroids* may be of value in chronic disease.
- *Cyclophosphamide* is indicated for some nephritides. Dose example: 0.5–3mg/kg/d PO; intermittent pulses of 20mg/kg/month IV—give fewer SE. Its role in CNS disease is unclear.
- *Azathioprine* 1–2.5mg/kg/d PO can be a 'steroid-sparer' SE: lymphoma.
- *Renal transplantation* may be needed; nephritis recurs in ~50%, on biopsy, but is a rare cause of graft failure (graft survival 87% at 1yr and 60% at 5yrs).

The future Agents which interfere with T-cell–B-cell collaboration, such as CTLA4-Ig and anti-CD154 monoclonal antibodies are theoretically attractive, but randomized trials are absent or disappointing. Recently immunotherapy with anti-CD20 antibody (rituximab, p660) has shown promise.

---

1 Do visual acuity, colour vision, visual fields, fundoscopy ± electroretinography ± fluorescein angiography, if ≥5yrs of treatment is needed, or a change in vision occurs.

Revised criteria for diagnosing SLE

1 *Malar rash (butterfly rash):* Fixed erythema, flat or raised, over the malar eminences, tending to spare the nasolabial folds.

2 *Discoid rash:* Erythematous raised patches with adherent keratotic scaling and follicular plugging ± atrophic scarring. Think of it as a 3-stage rash affecting ears, cheeks, scalp, forehead, and chest: erythema → pigmented hyperkeratotic oedematous papules → atrophic depressed lesions.

3 *Photosensitivity* on exposed skin representing unusual reaction to light.

4 *Oral ulcers:* Oral or nasopharyngeal ulceration.

5 *Arthritis:* Non-erosive arthritis involving 2 or more peripheral joints, characterized by tenderness, swelling, or effusion. Joint involvement is seen in 90% of patients. Deforming arthropathy may occur due to capsular laxity (Jaccoud's arthropathy). Aseptic bone necrosis also occurs.

6 *Serositis:* (a) Pleuritis (pleuritic pain or rub—80% of all patients have lung function abnormalities; 40% have dyspnoea) pleural effusion OR (b) Pericarditis (ECG or pericardial rub or evidence of pericardial effusion).

7 *Renal disorders:* (a) Persistent proteinuria >0.5g/d (or >3+ on dipstix) OR (b) *Cellular casts*—may be red cell, granular, or mixed.

8 *CNS disorders:* (a) Seizures, in the absence of causative drugs or known metabolic imbalance, eg uraemia, ketoacidosis, or U&E↑ OR *Psychosis* in the absence of causative drugs/metabolic derangements, as above.

9 *Haematological disorders:* (a) *Haemolytic anaemia* with reticulocytosis OR (b) *Leukopenia*, ie WCC <4 ×10^9/L on ≥2 occasions OR (c) *Lymphopenia*, ie <1.500 ×10^9/L on ≥2 occasions OR (d) *Thrombocytopenia*, ie platelets <100 ×10^9/L in the absence of a drug effect.

10 *Immunological disorders:* (a) *Anti-DNA* antibody to native DNA in abnormal titre OR (b) *Anti-Sm* antibody to Sm nuclear antigen OR (c) Antiphospholipid antibody +ve based on:

   (1) an abnormal serum level of IgG or IgM anticardiolipin antibodies,
   (2) positive result for lupus anticoagulant using a standard method, or
   (3) false positive serological test for syphilis +ve for >6 months and confirmed by *Treponema pallidum* immobilization or fluorescent treponemal antibody absorption tests.

11 *Antinuclear antibody:* Positive in 95%.

Diagnose SLE in the appropriate clinical setting if ≥4 out of the 11 criteria are present, serially or simultaneously.

Vasculitis

Vasculitis, defined as any inflammatory disorder of blood vessels (typically non-infectious), can affect vessels of any organ. It may be occlusive (necrotizing, as in SLE) or non-occlusive, as in Henoch–Schönlein purpura (p726). It can occur *de novo*, eg polyarteritis (see BOX), Churg–Strauss, Behçet's, Giant cell arteritis (GCA), Takayasu's, and Wegener's (Chapter 18), or be from drugs or infection (syphilis is an endarteritis obliterans)—or be mediated by complement activation induced by immune complexes in autoimmunity (eg SLE, RA). ► *Consider vasculitis as a diagnosis for any unidentified multisystem disorder.* Organ involvement can be from acute vasculitis or end-organ damage resulting from recurrent vasculitis. *Features seen in many vasculitides:*

- General: fever; malaise; weight↓; arthralgia; myalgia; ESR↑.
- Skin: purpura; ulcers; livedo reticularis; nailbed infarcts; digital gangrene.
- Eyes: episcleritis; ulceration; visual loss.
- ENT: epistaxis; nasal crusting; stridor; deafness.
- Pulmonary: haemoptysis; dyspnoea.
- Cardiac: loss of pulses; heart failure; myocardial infarction; angina.
- GI: abdominal pain (any viscus may infarct); malabsorption because of chronic ischaemia.
- Renal: BP↑ haematuria; proteinuria; casts; acute/chronic renal failure.
- Neurological: mononeuritis multiplex; sensorimotor neuropathy; fits; hemiplegia; chorea; psychoses; confusion; cognition↓; mood↑↓; odd behaviour.

Diagnosis: This is based on clinical findings, supported by histological and occasionally angiographic findings. ANCA may be +ve (p421).

Treatment: Treat hypertension meticulously. Refer to experts. Use high-dose prednisolone, and cyclophosphamide if major organ involvement.

Polymyalgia rheumatica (PMR)

Common in those over 70yrs who have symmetrical aching and morning stiffness in shoulders and proximal limb muscles for >1 month ± mild polyarthritis, tenosynovitis (eg carpal tunnel syndrome, p391 occurs in 10%), depression, fatigue, fever, weight↓, and anorexia. It may come on suddenly, or over 1 month. It overlaps with GCA. ♀:♂ ≈ 2:1 *Tests:* ESR usually 40mm/h; CK usually ↔; alk phos↑. *Differential diagnosis:* Recent onset RA; hypothyroidism, primary muscle disease, occult malignancy or infection, neck lesions, bilateral subacromial impingement lesions (*OHCS* p612), spinal stenosis (*OHCS* p622). *Treatment:* Prednisolone 15–20mg/24h PO; ↓dose slowly, eg by 1mg/month (in the light of symptoms & ESR). Most need steroids for ≥2yrs. Preventing osteoporosis is essential (p698).

Giant cell (cranial/temporal) arteritis (GCA)

GCA is associated with polymyalgia in 25% of people. Common in the elderly, it is rare under 55yrs. *Symptoms:* Headache, scalp and temporal artery tenderness (eg on combing hair), jaw claudication, amaurosis fugax, or sudden blindness in one eye. *Tests:* ESR↑, CRP↑, platelets↑, alk phos↑, HB↓. ►If you suspect GCA, do an ESR, start prednisolone 40–60mg/24h PO *immediately*. Some advocate higher doses (?IV) if visual symptoms (ask an ophthalmologist). Osteoporosis prophylaxis essential. Get temporal artery biopsy in the next few days. Skip lesions occur, so don't be put off by a –ve biopsy. NB: the immediate risk is blindness, but longer term, the main cause of death and morbidity in GCA is steroid treatment! Reduce prednisolone after 5–7d in the light of symptoms and ESR; ↑dose if symptoms recur. Typical course: 2yrs, then complete remission.

Polyarteritis nodosa (PAN)

PAN is a necrotizing vasculitis that causes aneurysms of medium-sized arteries.[1] ♂ : ♀ ≈ 2 : 1. Sometimes PAN is associated with HBsAg.

Signs and symptoms:

- General features: Fevers, abdominal pain, malaise, weight↓, arthralgia.
- Renal: (75%) Main cause of death. Hypertension, haematuria, proteinuria, renal failure, intrarenal aneurysms, vasculitis.
- Vascular: BP↑; vasculitis; erectile dysfunction.
- Cardiac: (80%) Second biggest cause of death. Coronary arteritis and consequent infarction. ↑BP and heart failure. Pericarditis. In Kawasaki disease (childhood PAN variant, *OHCS* p750) coronary aneurysms occur.
- Pulmonary: Pulmonary infiltrates and asthma occur in vasculitis (some say that lung involvement is incompatible with PAN, calling it then Churg—Strauss syndrome).
- CNS: (70%) Mononeuritis multiplex, sensorimotor polyneuropathy, seizures, hemiplegia, psychoses.
- GI: (70%) Abdominal pain (any viscus may infarct), malabsorption because of chronic ischaemia.
- Skin: Urticaria, purpura, infarcts, livedo reticularis,[2] nodules.
- Blood: WCC↑; eosinophilia (in 30%), anaemia, ESR↑, CRP↑.

Diagnosis: This is most often made from clinical features in combination with renal or mesenteric angiography. ANCA (p421) is classically negative.

Treatment: Treat hypertension meticulously. Refer to experts. Use high-dose prednisolone, and then cyclophosphamide.

---

1 The term **microscopic polyangiitis** (MPA) denotes small vessel vasculitis (capillaritis ± venulitis). ANCA (p421) associated pauci-immune segmental and crescentic glomerulonephritis are leading signs—as in other small vessel vasculitides (Wegener's & Churg-Strauss). J Barlow 2003 *Cur Op Neph* **12** 267

2 Stasis in skin venules, eg induced by cold, causes immune complex deposition and pink-blue mottling (cutis marmorata). If this becomes irreversible, it is called livedo reticularis.

Rheumatological and other systemic conditions causing eye signs

The eye plays host to many diseases: the more you look, the more you'll see, and the more you'll enjoy medicine, for the eye is beautiful, and its signs are legion.

Granulomatous disorders Syphilis, TB, sarcoidosis, leprosy, brucellosis, and toxoplasmosis all inflame the eye; either front chamber (anterior uveitis/iritis) or back chamber (posterior uveitis/ choroiditis). Refer to an ophthalmologist. In sarcoid there may be cranial nerve palsies.

Collagen diseases cause inflammation of the eye coat (episcleritis/scleritis). Conjunctivitis is found in Reiter's; episcleritis in PAN and SLE; uveitis in AS and Reiter's (p418). Scleritis in RA and Wegener's is potentially damaging to the eye. Refer patients with eye pain immediately. In dermatomyositis, there is orbital oedema with retinopathy showing cotton-wool spots (micro-infarcts).

Keratoconjunctivitis sicca (Sjögren's syndrome, p734.) There is reduced tear formation (<10mm in 5min on Schirmer filter paper test), producing a gritty feeling in the eyes. Decreased salivation also gives a dry mouth (xerostomia). It is associated with collagen diseases. Treatment is with artificial tears (tears naturale, or hypromellose drops).

Vascular retinopathy (p141) may be *arteriopathic* (arteriovenous nipping: arteries nip veins where they cross) or *hypertensive*—with arteriolar vasoconstriction and leakage (hard exudates, macular oedema, haemorrhages, and, rarely, papilloedema). Thickened arterial walls are shiny ('silver wiring'). Narrowed arterioles lead to localized infarction of the superficial retina, seen as cotton-wool spots and flame haemorrhages. Leaks from these appear as hard exudates ± macular oedema/papilloedema (rare). The grading of hypertensive retinopathy from I to IV is considered obsolescent by some, partly because changes due to arteriopathy and those due to hypertension are confused, and also because some grades exist in normotensive, non-diabetic people.

Emboli passing through the retina produce *amaurosis fugax* (p360; any carotid bruits?). *Retinal haemorrhages* are common in leukaemia; comma-shaped conjunctival haemorrhages and retinal new vessel formation may occur in sickle-cell disease; optic atrophy in pernicious anaemia. Note also Roth spots (retinal infarcts) in endocarditis (p152).

Retinal vein occlusion is caused by BP↑, age, or hyperviscosity (p670). Suspect in any acute fall in acuity. If it is the central vein, the fundus is like a stormy sunset (those angry red clouds are haemorrhages). In branch vein occlusion, changes are confined to a wedge of retina. Get expert help.

Metabolic disease Diabetes: p296. Hyperthyroid exophthalmos: p305. Lens opacities: hypoparathyroidism. Conjunctival and corneal calcification may occur in hypercalcaemia, including hyperparathyroidism. In gout, conjunctival deposits of monosodium urate may give sore eyes.

Systemic infections Septicaemia may seed to the internal eye causing infection in the vitreous (endophthalmitis). Syphilis can cause chorioretinitis or iritis; congenital syphilis causes a pigmented retinopathy.

AIDS and HIV (See p580.) Those who are HIV+ve may develop CMV retinitis, characterized by cotton-wool retinal spots with flame haemorrhages ('pizza pie' fundus, signifying superficial retinal infarction). This may be asymptomatic but can cause sudden visual loss. If it is present, it implies full-blown AIDS + a CD4 count <100 × 10⁶/L. Cotton-wool spots on their own indicate HIV retinopathy and may occur before the full HIV picture.

Candidiasis of the vitreous is found mostly in IV drug abusers and is hard to treat. Kaposi's sarcoma may affect the lids or conjunctiva.

Differential diagnosis of 'red-eye'

	Conjunctiva	Iris	Pupil	Cornea	Anterior chamber	Intraocular pressure	Appearance
Acute glaucoma	Both ciliary and conjunctival vessels injected Entire eye is red	Injected	Dilated, fixed, oval	Steamy, hazy	Very shallow	Very high	
Iritis	Redness most marked around cornea Colour does not blanch on pressure	Injected	Small, fixed	Normal	Turgid	Normal	
Conjunctivitis	Conjunctival vessels injected, greatest toward fornices Blanch on pressure Mobile over sclera	Normal	Normal	Normal	Normal	Normal	
Subconjunctival haemorrhage	Bright red sclera with white rim around limbus	Normal	Normal	Normal	Normal	Normal	

After RD Judge, GD Zuidema, FT Fitzgerald Clinical diagnosis 5 ed. Little Brown, Boston.

Skin manifestations of systemic diseases

Erythema nodosum (PLATE 18) Painful, red, raised lesions on shin fronts (± thighs/arms). *Causes*: sarcoidosis; drugs (sulfonamides, the Pill, dapsone); bacteria (streptococci, *Mycobacterium*—TB, leprosy); *Less common*: Crohn's; UC; BCG vaccination; leptospirosis; *Yersinia*; various viruses and fungi.

Erythema multiforme (PLATE 17) 'Target' lesions (symmetrical ± central blister, on palms/soles, limbs, and elsewhere). Often with mouth, genital, and eye ulcers and fever (= Stevens–Johnson syndrome). Associated with: drugs (barbiturates; sulfonamides); infections (herpes; Mycoplasma; orf, p540); collagen disorders. 50% are idiopathic. Get expert help in severe disease.

Erythema chronicum migrans Presents as small papule which develops into a spreading large erythematous ring, with central fading. It lasts from 48h to 3 months. May be multiple. *Cause*: Lyme disease (p600).

Erythema marginatum Pink coalescent rings on trunk which come and go. It is seen in rheumatic fever (or rarely other causes, eg drugs).

Pyoderma gangrenosum Recurring nodulo-pustular ulcers, ~10cm wide, with tender red/blue overhanging necrotic edge, healing with cribriform scars. (on leg, abdomen, or face). *Associations*: UC; Crohn's; autoimmune hepatitis; neoplasia; Wegener's; myeloma. ♀:♂ > 1:1. *Treatment*: Get help. Saline toilet, high-dose oral or intralesional steroids ± ciclosporin (=cyclosporin) ± topical antibiotic.

Vitiligo *Vitellus* is Latin for *spotted calf*: typically white patches ± hyperpigmented borders. Sunlight makes them itch. *Associations*: Autoimmunity: Graves', Addison's, Hashimoto's, DM, alopecia areata, hypoparathyroidism, premature ovarian failure. Treat by camouflage cosmetics and sunscreens (± steroid creams ± dermabrasion). UK vitiligo society: 020 7840 0855.

Specific diseases and their skin manifestations

Diabetes mellitus Infections; ulcers; *necrobiosis lipoidica* (shiny area on shin with yellowish skin ± telangiectasia); *granuloma annulare* (OHCS p578).

Gluten-sensitive enteropathy (coeliac disease) *Dermatitis herpetiformis* (itchy blisters, eg in groups on knees, elbows, and scalp). The itch (which can drive patients to suicide) responds to dapsone 100–200mg/24h PO within 48h—and this may be used as a diagnostic test. The maintenance dose may be as little as 50mg/wk. In 30% this will need to be continued, despite having a gluten-free diet. SE (dose related): haemolysis, hepatitis, agranulocytosis. CI: G6PD-deficiency. Risk of lymphoma↑ (with coeliac disease *and* dermatitis herpetiformis)—so surveillance is needed.

Malabsorption Dry pigmented skin, easy bruising, hair loss, leuconychia.

Hyperthyroidism *Pretibial myxoedema* (red oedematous swellings above lateral malleoli, progressing to thickened oedema of legs and feet), *thyroid acropachy* (clubbing + subperiosteal new bone in phalanges).

Other endocrine diseases See p291.

Neoplasia *Acanthosis nigricans*: Pigmented, rough thickening of axillary or groin, skin with warty lesions, associated especially with stomach cancer. *Dermatomyositis* (p420). *Skin metastases*. *Acquired icthyosis*: Dry scaly skin associated with lymphoma. *Thrombophlebitis migrans*: Successive crops of tender nodules affecting blood vessels throughout the body, associated with pancreatic cancer (especially body and tail tumours).

Crohn's Perianal/vulval ulcers; erythema nodosum; pyoderma gangrenosum.

Liver disease Palmar erythema; spider naevi; gynaecomastia; decrease in pubic hair; jaundice; bruising; scratch marks.

Dermatomyositis Gottron's papules; shawl sign; lilac rash on lids (p420).

Skin diagnoses not to be missed

Malignant melanoma ♀ : ♂ ≈ 1.5 : 1. UK incidence: 3500/yr. 800 deaths (up ≥80% in last 20yrs). Sunlight is a major cause, particularly in the early years. Diagnosis can be tricky, but most have ≥1 major component on the Glasgow checklist: ⬚ They may occur in pre-existing moles. ►When in doubt, refer.

Major	Minor	Less helpful signs
• Change in size	• Inflammation, crusting, or bleeding	• Asymmetry
• Change in shape	• Sensory change	• Irregular colour
• Change in colour	• Diameter >7mm (unless growth is in the vertical plane: beware)	• Elevation
		• Irregular border

Neighbouring 'satellite' lesions may occur. If smooth, well-demarcated, and regular, it is unlikely to be a melanoma. Treatment: *OHCS* p584.

Squamous cell cancer This usually presents as an ulcerated lesion, with hard, raised edges. They may begin in solar keratoses (below), or be found on the lips of smokers or in long-standing gravitational leg ulcers. Metastases are rare, but local destruction may be extensive. *Treatment:* Total excision. **NB:** the condition may be confused with a keratoacanthoma—a fast-growing, benign, self-limiting papule plugged with keratin.

Basal cell carcinoma (rodent ulcer) Typically, pearly nodule with rolled telangiectatic edge usually on the face. Metastases are very rare. It is locally destructive epithelioma (if left untreated). Lesions on trunk can appear as red scaly plaques with raised smooth edge. *Cause:* UV exposure. *Treatment:* Excision is best; radiotherapy can be used for larger lesions in the elderly. Cryotherapy ± curettage can be used in non-critical sites.

Bowen's disease Slow-growing red scaly plaque, eg on lower legs. *Histology:* Full-thickness dysplasia (carcinoma-*in-situ*). Infrequently progresses to squamous cell cancer. Penile Bowen's disease is called Queyrat's erythroplasia. *Treatment:* Cryotherapy; topical 5-flurouracil as above; photodynamic therapy. For a few dozen images, see www.txt.co.uk/full.cfm?1118.

Actinic keratoses appear on sun-exposed skin as crumbly, yellow-white crusts. Malignant change may occur. Treatment: cautery; cryotherapy; twice-daily 5% 5-fluorouracil (5-FU) cream (with this sequence of events: erythema → vesiculation → erosion → ulceration → necrosis → healing epithelialization). Healthy skin is unharmed. Treatment is usually for 4wks, but may be prolonged. There is no significant systemic absorption if the area treated is <500cm². Avoid in pregnancy. The hands should be washed after applying the cream. Alternative: diclofenac gel (3%; Solaraze®, use thinly bd for ≤90d).

Secondary carcinoma The most common metastases to skin are from breast, kidney, and lung. The lesion is usually a firm nodule, most often on the scalp. See acanthosis nigricans (p428).

Mycosis fungoides is a lymphoma (cutaneous T-cell lymphoma, as in Sézary syndrome) which is usually confined to skin. It causes itchy, red plaques.

Leukoplakia This appears as white patches (which may fissure) on oral or genital mucosa (where it may itch). Frank carcinomatous change may occur.

Leprosy Suspect in any anaesthetic hypopigmented lesion (p598).

Syphilis Any genital ulcer is syphilis until proved otherwise. Secondary syphilis: papular rash—including, unusually, on the palms[1] (p601).

Others Kaposi's sarcoma (p726); Paget's disease of the breast (p732).

---

1 *Other causes:* Stevens–Johnson synd.; hand, foot & mouth disease; also palmar erythema of liver disease.

Oncology[1]

Contents

Relevant pages in other chapters: Leukaemias and lymphomas (p650–60); myeloma (p666); immunosuppressive drugs (p674); pain (p454); dying at home (OHCS p442); facing death (p7)

For specific cancers, see the relevant chapter, eg *Surgery*, p444.

Communication

This chapter starts with communication because this is the first step in overcoming or coming to terms with cancer. As a thought experiment, consult yourself on how you would feel on receiving a diagnosis of cancer. Shocked, numb, frantic, panicky, emotionless, resigned ('I knew all along...')? All these and other emotions are likely to be manifest in your patients. Some doctors instinctively turn away from 'undisciplined squads of emotions' and try to stop them taking over consultations. A more positive approach is to try to use these emotions to benefit and motivate your patient—through listening to, and addressing, their worst fears. ►*Include your patient in all decision-making processes.* Many patients (not just the young and well informed) will appreciate this—and the giving of information and the sharing of decisions is known to reduce treatment morbidity. So, even when this is physically exhausting (the same ground may need covering many times) it is definitely worth spending this time. A huge amount is forgotten or fails to register the first time, so videos and written information are important. Be sure to ask, in an open way, about use of alternative therapies. This is often a sign of undisclosed fear of recurrence. Ask about this and by good communication and the promoting of autonomy, your patient's fear-driven wish to try dangerous or untried therapies may be trumped by a spirit of rational optimism.

1 *We thank Dr P Hoskins, who is our Specialist Reader for this chapter.*

Looking after people with cancer

No rules guarantee success, but there is no doubt that getting to know your patient, making an agreed management plan, and seeking out the right expert for each stage of treatment *all* need to be central activities in oncology. These issues centre around communication, and the personal attributes of the doctor as a physician. There is nothing unique about oncology here—but in oncology these issues are highly focused. Remember, it is never too early to start palliative care (*with* other treatments).

Psychological support Examples include:
- Allowing the patient to express anger, fear—or any negative feeling (anger can anaesthetize pain).
- Counselling, eg with a breast cancer nurse (mastectomy preparation).
- Biofeedback and relaxation therapy can ↓side-effects of chemotherapy.
- Cognitive and behavioural therapy reduces psychological morbidity associated with cancer treatments. See OHCS p370.
- Group therapy (OHCS p372) reduces pain, mood disturbance, and the frequency of maladaptive coping strategies.
- Meta-analyses have suggested that psychological support can have some effect on improving outcome measures such as survival.

Streamlining care pathways Care pathways map patient journeys in a health system: symptoms felt → GP appointment → referral → hospital appointment → consultant clinic → imaging → 1st treatment (surgery, etc). Each arrow represents a possibility for fatal delay. 48h access to GPs, GP referral under the 2wk rule (hospital must see within 2wks—this inevitably makes other equally or more deserving patients wait longer) and e-booking (like on-line airline seat reservations) are unreliable ways of speeding up the crucial arrow pointing to 1st treatment. The only way to do this is to increase capacity (beds, nurses, doctors, equipment, and theatres).

Hints on breaking bad news
1 Choose a quiet place where you will not be disturbed. This may be impossible—but at least give it some thought.
2 Find out what the patient already knows or surmises (often a great deal). Surmises are not static and change rapidly, so that when you try to verify what your patient is telling you by going over the same ground again, you may get quite a different impression—both may be valid.
3 Find out how much the person wants to know. You can be surprisingly direct about this. 'Are you the sort of person who, if anything were amiss, would want to know all the details?'
4 Give some warning—eg 'there is some bad news for us to address'.
5 Share information about diagnosis, treatments, and prognosis. Specifically list supporting people (eg nurses) and institutions (eg hospices). Try asking 'Is there anything else you want me to explain?' Don't hesitate to go over the same ground repeatedly. Allow denial: don't force the pace.
6 'Cancer' has negative connotations for many people. Address this, and explain that ~50% of cancers are cured in the developed world.
7 Listen to any concerns raised; encourage the airing of feelings.
8 Summarize and make a plan. Offer availability.
9 Follow through. The most important thing is to leave the patient with the strong impression that, come what may, you are with them whatever, and that this unwritten contract will not be broken.

Don't imagine that a single blueprint will do for everyone. ►Be prepared to use *whatever* the patient gives you. This requires close observation of verbal and non-verbal cues. Practise in low-key interactions with patients—so when great difficulties arise, you have a better chance of helping. Because humans are very complex, we all frequently fail. Don't be put off: keep trying, and, afterwards, recap with a colleague, so you keep learning.

Oncology and genetics

A number of gene mutations, which predispose to cancer, have been identified: a list of the more common ones appears in the BOX.

Familial breast/ovarian cancer Most breast and ovarian cancer is sporadic, but ~5% are due to germline mutation in either BRCA1 (17q) or BRCA2 (13q). Both genes function as tumour suppressors. Carrying a BRCA1 mutation confers a lifetime risk of developing breast cancer of 70–80%, and ovarian cancer of 30–40%. Mutations in BRCA2 are much less likely to cause ovarian cancer, but may cause male breast cancer in some families. The incidence of mutations varies according to the population sampled. In families with ≥4 cases of breast cancer collected by the Breast Cancer Linkage Consortium, the disease was linked to BRCA1 in 52% of families and BRCA2 in 32%. Individuals from families in which a mutation has not been detected can be given risk estimation based on number of individuals affected and age of onset of cancer. There is no consensus on efficacy of mammographic and ovarian ultrasound screening with analysis of CA125 and CEA serum markers in individuals at moderate risk. There is debate about cost–benefits of screening and risks of radiation exposure from regular mammography. Those at high risk of developing breast or ovarian cancer may opt for prophylactic mastectomy and oophorectomy both of which lower, but do not completely remove, the risk of developing cancer derived from those sites. Drugs have an uncertain role in prevention in high-risk patients; anastrozole is under trial (IBIS-II).[9]

Familial colorectal cancer ~20% of those with colorectal cancer have a family history of the disease. Personal risk of colorectal cancer is proportionate to the degree of family history: the relative risk (RR) is about: ×2 for people with any family history; ×5 if 2 affected 1st degree relatives; and ×3 for an affected 1st degree relative aged <45yrs at diagnosis. On the basis of empirical risk estimation, some people may be recommended colonoscopic surveillance, but weigh against the dangers of long-term, invasive screening for each at-risk individual. Hereditary non-polyposis colorectal cancer (HNPCC) is a syndrome of familial aggregation of colorectal (mainly), endometrial, ovarian, gastric, upper urinary tract, small intestinal, pancreatic, and other cancers. Many HNPCC families have mutations in 1 of 5 DNA mismatch repair genes. Lifetime risk of colorectal cancer for relatives who carry a mutation is 60%, and women with a mutation have a 40% lifetime risk of endometrial cancer. Surveillance for HNPCC families is 2-yearly with colonoscopy ± gynaecological surveillance—or even prophylactic surgery. These mutations account for ~2% of all UK colorectal cancers.

Familial adenomatous polyposis is due to germline mutations in the APC gene. Offspring are at 50% of risk of being a gene carrier, and gene penetrance approaches 100% for colorectal cancer by 50yrs old. *Peutz-Jeghers' syndrome* has a 10–20% lifetime risk of colorectal cancer, and has been shown to be due to germline mutations in STK11, a serine threonine kinase (locus: 19p14).

Familial prostate cancer ~5% of those with prostate cancer have a family history: the genetic basis is multifactorial. There is a modestly elevated life time risk of prostate cancer for male carriers of BRCA1 and BRCA2 mutations, although the molecular basis of this remains to be elucidated. Mutations in BRCA1/BRCA2 or in the genes on chromosomes 1 and X do not account for all family clusters of prostate cancer and so it is clear that other genes must be involved. In 1 twin study, 42% of the risk was found to be genetic.[10]

Genetic tests can also tell if chemotherapy is likely to work: chemotherapy fails in 17% of colon cancer patients—ie those with certain mutations.[1]

---

1 Shown by the microsatellite instability status being 'high-frequency'. Microsatellites are stretches of DNA in which a short section is repeated several times. 5-FU chemotherapy only improves survival in microsatellite stable or low-frequency microsatellite unstable tumours. S Gallinger 2003 *NEJM* **249** 209

Examples of cancers with a familial predisposition

Cancer/syndrome	Gene	Chromosome	
Breast and ovarian cancers	BRCA1	17q	(OPPOSITE)
	BRCA2	13q	
HNPCC	MSH2	2p	(OPPOSITE)
	MLH1	3p	
	PMS2	7p	
Familial polyposis (colorectum)	APC	5q	
von Hippel–Lindau (kidney, CNS)	VHL	3p	(p309)
Carney complex	PRKAR1A	17q	(p309)
Multiple endocrine neoplasia Type I (pituitary, pancreas, thyroid)	MEN1	11q	(p309)
Multiple endocrine neoplasia Type 2	RET	10q	(p309)
Basal cell naevus syndrome (CNS, skin)	PTCH	9q	
Retinoblastoma (eye, bone)	Rb	13q	(OHCS p485)
Li–Fraumeni syndrome (multiple)	TP53	17p	(OHCS p752)
Neurofibromatosis Type I (CNS; rare)	NF1	17q	(p402)
Neurofibromatosis Type 2 (common) (meningiomas, auditory neuromas)	NF2	22	(p402)
Familial melanoma	INK4A	9p	

Oncological emergencies

▶A patient who becomes acutely unwell can often be made more comfortable with simple measures, but some problems require specific treatment.

Febrile neutropenic patients See p650.

Spinal cord compression Requires urgent and efficient treatment to preserve neurological function. A high index of suspicion is essential. *Causes:* Typically extradural metastases. Others: extension of tumour from a vertebral body, direct extension of the tumour, or crush fracture. *Signs & symptoms:* Back pain with a root distribution, weakness and sensory loss (a level may be found), bowel and bladder dysfunction. *Tests:* Urgent MRI. *Management:* Dexamethasone 8–16mg IV then 4mg/6h PO. Discuss with neurosurgeon and clinical oncologist immediately.

Superior vena cava (SVC) obstruction with airway compromise SVC obstruction is not an emergency unless there is tracheal compression with airway compromise: usually there is time to plan optimal treatment, and this is to be preferred, rather than rushing into therapy which may not be beneficial. *Causes:* Typically lung cancer; rarely from causes of mediastinal enlargement (eg germ cell tumour); lymphadenopathy (lymphoma); thymus malignancy; thrombotic disorders (eg Behçet's or nephrotic syndromes); thrombus around an IV central line; hamartoma; ovarian hyperstimulation (OHCS p75); fibrotic bands (lung fibrosis after chemotherapy). *Signs & symptoms:* Dyspnoea; orthopnoea; swollen face & arm; cough; plethora/cyanosis; headache; engorged veins. *Pemberton's test:* On lifting the arms over the head for >1min, there is ↑facial plethora/cyanosis, JVP↑ (non-pulsatile), and inspiratory stridor. *Tests:* Sputum cytology, CXR, CT, venography. *Management:* Get a tissue diagnosis if possible, but bronchoscopy may be hazardous. Give dexamethasone 4mg/6h PO. Consider balloon venoplasty and SVC stenting, eg prior to radical or palliative chemo- or radiotherapy (depending on tumour type).

Hypercalcaemia Affects 10–20% of patients with cancer, and 40% of those with myeloma. *Causes:* Lytic bone metastases, production of osteoclast activating factor or PTH-like hormones by the tumour. *Symptoms:* Lethargy, anorexia, nausea, polydipsia, polyuria, constipation, dehydration, confusion, weakness. Most obvious with serum Ca^{2+} >3mmol/L. *Management:* Rehydrate with 3–4L of 0.9% saline IV over 24h. Avoid diuretics. Give bisphosphonate IV (consider maintenance therapy, IV or PO). Best treatment is control of underlying malignancy. In resistant hypercalcaemia, consider calcitonin.

Raised intracranial pressure Due to either a primary CNS tumour or metastatic disease. *Signs & symptoms:* Headache (often worse in the morning), nausea, vomiting, papilloedema, fits, focal neurological signs. *Tests:* Urgent CT is important to diagnose an expanding mass, cystic degeneration, haemorrhage within a tumour, cerebral oedema, or hydrocephalus due to tumour or blocked shunt since the management of these scenarios can be very different. *Management:* Dexamethasone 4mg/6h PO, radiotherapy, and surgery as appropriate depending on cause.

Tumour lysis syndrome Rapid cell death on starting chemotherapy for rapidly proliferating leukaemia, lymphoma, myeloma, and some germ cell tumours can result in a rise in serum urate, K^+, and phosphate, precipitating renal failure. Prevention is with good hydration and *allopurinol* 24h *before* chemotherapy; dose example if renal function OK: 300mg/12h PO. If creatinine >100μmol/L: 100mg alternate days. Haemodialysis may be needed in renal failure. More potent uricolytic agents: recombinant urate oxidase (*rasburicase*) 200μg/kg/d IVI for 5–7d; SE: fever; D&V; headache; rash; bronchospasm; haemolysis. It may interfere with uric acid tests; see *datasheet*.

Inappropriate ADH secretion p690; **febrile neutropenic regimen** p650.

Treating hypercalcaemia with bisphosphonates

Ensure adequate hydration (eg with 0.9% saline IVI). Zoledronic acid and pamidronate are 2 options.

Disodium pamidronate

Calcium (mmol/L; corrected)[15]	Single-dose pamidronate (mg)
<3	15–30
3–3.5	30–60
3.5–4	60–90
>4	90

Infuse slowly, eg 30mg in 300mL 0.9% saline over 3h via a largish vein. Max dose: 90mg. Response starts at ~3–5d, peaking at 1wk.

SE: 'Flu symptoms, bone pain, $PO_4^{3-}\downarrow$, bone pain, myalgia, nausea, vomiting, headache, lymphocytopenia, $Mg^{2+}\downarrow$, seizures (rare).

Zoledronic acid is significantly more effective in reducing serum Ca^{2+} than previously used bisphosphonates.[16] Usually, a single dose of 4mg IVI over 2h will normalize plasma Ca^{2+} within a week. A higher dose should be used if corrected Ca^{2+} is >3mmol/L. *SE:* 'Flu symptoms, bone pain, $PO_4^{3-}\downarrow$, confusion, thirst, taste disturbance, nausea, pulse↓, WCC↓, creatinine↑.

Sodium clodronate and *ibandronic acid* are other bisphosphonates.
Corrected calcium in mmol/L = serum Ca^{2+} – [0.02 × serum albumin in g/L] + 0.8.

Symptom control in severe cancer

Pain ▶Do not be miserly with analgesia: aim to *prevent*—or *eliminate* pain.

Types of pain Don't assume that the cancer is the cause (abdominal pain, eg, may be from constipation). Seek the mechanism. Pain caused by nerve infiltration and damage via local pressure may respond to amitriptyline (eg 10–50mg at night) rather than opioids. Bone pain (eg presenting with back pain) may respond to NSAIDs, radiotherapy, or a nerve block.

▶Identify each symptom and type of pain.

Management (1) Pain is affected by mood, morale, and meaning. Explain its origin to both the patient and relatives, and plan rehabilitation goals. (2) Use oral analgesics if possible—aim to prevent pain with regular prophylactic doses (eg 4-hourly); do not wait for pain to recur. (3) Modify the pathological process where possible, eg radiotherapy; hormones; chemotherapy; surgery.

With analgesia, work up the pain ladder until pain is relieved (see BOX). Monitor response carefully. Laxatives (eg co-danthrusate 10mL PO at night) and antiemetics (below) are often needed with analgesics. *Adjuvant analgesics:* (previously termed co-analgesics) NSAIDs, steroids, muscle relaxants, anxiolytic, anti-depressants.

Giving oral morphine: Start with aqueous morphine 5–10mg/4h PO. A double dose at night can be used to promote 8h of sleep. Most patients need no more than 30mg/4h PO. A few need much more. Aim to change to modified-release morphine (eg MST® tablets every 12h), when daily morphine needs are known. In morphine-resistant pain (persisting when 60mg/4h is given), consider adjuvant analgesics, methadone, or ketamine (specialist use only).

Vomiting: Prevent from before the 1st dose of chemotherapy, to avoid anticipatory vomiting before the next dose. Give orally if possible, but if severe vomiting prevents this, give rectally or subcutaneously by syringe driver. *Agents to try:* Cyclizine ≤50mg/8h PO; metoclopramide 10mg/8h PO; ondansetron 4–8mg/8–12h PO/IV; haloperidol 0.5–2mg/24h (max 5mg).

Breathlessness: Consider supplementary O_2 or morphine. Use of relaxation techniques and benzodiazepines can be useful. Assess for pleural or pericardial effusion. If there is significant pleural effusion, consider thoracocentesis ± pleurodesis. If there is a malignant pericardial effusion, consider pericardiocentesis (p757), pericardiectomy, pleuropericardial windows, external beam radiotherapy, percutaneous balloon pericardiotomy, or pericardial instillation of immunomodulators or sclerosing bleomycin.

Pruritus (itching): See p76.

Venepuncture problems: Repeated venepuncture with the attendant risk of painful extravasation and phlebitis may be avoided by insertion of skin tunnelled catheter (eg a Hickman line)—a single or multilumen line—into a major central vein (eg subclavian or internal jugular). It is inserted using a strict aseptic technique. Patients can look after their own lines at home, and give their own drugs. Problems include: infection, blockage (flush with 0.9% saline or dilute heparin, eg every week), axillary, subclavian, or superior vena cava thrombosis/obstruction, and line slippage. Even more convenient portable delivery devices are available, allowing drugs to be given at a preset time, without the patient's intervention.

The analgesic ladder[18] [19]

(See p454 for NNT)

Rung 1 *Non-opioid* Aspirin; paracetamol; NSAID

Rung 2 *Weak opioid* Codeine; dihydrocodeine; dextropropoxyphene; tramadol; oxycodone (some place this on rung 3)

Rung 3 *Strong opioid* Morphine; diamorphine; hydromorphine; fentanyl ± adjuvant analgesics.

If 1 drug fails to relieve pain, move up ladder; do not try other drugs at the same level. In new, severe pain, rung 2 may be omitted.[20]

Syringe drivers deliver opioids, haloperidol, cyclizine and metoclopramide and hyoscine, giving 24h cover. If you have no syringe driver, consider suppositories (below) or *fentanyl transdermal patches:* If not previously exposed to morphine, start with one low-strength patch (25µg/h). Remove after 72h, and place a new patch at a different site. 25, 50, 75, and 100µg/h patches are made. $t_{1/2} \approx 17h$. See BNF.

Suppositories can also be used if unable to tolerate oral route. For pain: try oxycodone 30mg suppositories (eg 30mg/8h ≈ 30mg morphine). Agitation: try diazepam 10mg/8h suppositories.

Other agents and procedures to know about (alphabetically listed)
- Bisacodyl tablets (5mg), 1–2 at night, help opioid-induced constipation.
- C(h)olestyramine 4g/6h PO (1h after other drugs) helps itch in jaundice.
- Enemas, eg arachis oil, may help resistant constipation.
- H_2-antagonists (eg cimetidine 400mg/12h PO) help gastric irritation— eg associated with gastric carcinoma.
- Haloperidol 0.5–5mg/24h PO helps agitation, nightmares, hallucinations, and vomiting.
- Hydrogen peroxide 6% cleans an unpleasant-feeling coated tongue.
- Hyoscine hydrobromide 0.4–0.6mg/8h SC or 0.3mg sublingual: vomiting from upper GI obstruction or noisy bronchial rattles.
- Nerve blocks may lastingly relieve pleural or other resistant pains.
- Low-residue diets may be needed for post-radiotherapy diarrhoea.
- Metronidazole 400mg/8h PO mitigates anaerobic odours from tumours; so do charcoal dressings (Actisorb®).
- Movicol® sachets 2–4/12h for 48h to shift resistant constipation with overflow.
- Naproxen 250mg/8h with food: fevers caused by malignancy or bone pain from metastases (consider splinting joints if this fails).
- Pineapple chunks release proteolytic enzymes when chewed, eg for a coated tongue. (Sucking ice or butter also helps the latter.)
- Spironolactone 100mg bd PO + bumetanide 1mg/24h PO for ascites.
- Steroids: dexamethasone: give 8mg IV stat to relieve symptoms of superior vena cava or bronchial obstruction—or lymphangitis carcinomatosa. Tablets are 2mg (≈15mg prednisolone). 4mg/12–24h PO may stimulate appetite, or reduce ICP headache, or induce (in some patients) a satisfactory sense of euphoria.
- Table fans ± supplemental humidified O_2 helps hypoxic dyspnoea.
- Thoracocentesis (±bleomycin pleurodesis) in pleural effusion.

Cancer therapy

Cancer affects 30% of the population: 20% die from cancer. Management requires a multidisciplinary team and communication is vital (p432). Most patients wish to have some part in decision making at the various stages of their treatment, and to be informed of their options. Patients are becoming better informed through self-help groups and access to the Internet. Most patients undergo a variety of treatments during the treatment of their cancer and your job may be to orchestrate these.

Surgery In many cases a tissue diagnosis of cancer is made with either a biopsy or formal operation to remove the primary tumour. Although it is sometimes the only treatment required in early tumours of the GI tract, soft tissue sarcomas, and gynaecological tumours, it is often the case that best results follow the combination of surgery and chemotherapy. Surgery also has a role in palliating advanced disease.

Radiotherapy Uses ionizing radiation to kill tumour cells. See p442.

Chemotherapy Cytotoxics should be given under expert guidance by people trained in their administration. Drugs are often given in combination with a variety of intents: *Neoadjuvant*—to shrink tumours to reduce the need for major surgery (eg mastectomy). There is also a rationale which considers early control of micro-metastasis. *Primary therapy*—as the sole treatment for haematological malignancies. *Adjuvant*—to reduce the chance of relapse, eg breast and bowel cancers. *Palliative*—to provide relief from symptomatic metastatic disease and possibly to prolong survival.

Important classes of drugs include:

- Alkylating agents, eg cyclophosphamide, chlorambucil, busulfan.
- Antimetabolites, eg methotrexate, 5-fluorouracil.
- Vinca alkaloids, eg vincristine, vinblastine.
- Antitumour antibiotics, eg actinomycin D, doxorubicin.
- Others, eg etoposide, taxanes, platinum compounds.

Side-effects depend on the types of drugs used. Nausea/vomiting are most feared by patients and are preventable or controllable in most. Alopecia can also have a profound impact on quality of life. Neutropenia is most commonly seen 10–14d after chemotherapy (but can occur within 7d for taxanes) and sepsis requires immediate attention. ▶▶See p650.

Extravasation of a chemotherapeutic agent: Suspect if there is pain, burning or swelling at infusion site. *Management:* Stop the infusion, attempt to aspirate blood from the cannula, and then remove. Take advice. Administer steroids and consider antidotes.[1] Elevate the arm and mark site affected. Review regularly and apply steroid cream. Apply cold pack (unless a vinca alkaloid, in which case a heat compress should be applied). Consider report to National Extravasation Scheme. Early liaison with plastic surgeon may be needed.

Communication ▶*Include the patient in the decision-making process, p432.*

---

1 Some recommend (on scant evidence) topical dimethylsulfoxide (DMSO) and cooling after extravasation of anthracyclines or mitomycin, locally injected hyaluronidase if vinca alkaloids involved, and locally injected sodium thiosulfate (sodium hyposulfite) if chlormethine (mechlorethamine; mustine).

Avoiding pointless procedures in patients with cancer

Surgery is often curative (eg for colorectal cancers), while other surgery restores function, or deals with local recurrence, or reduces tumour bulk. But ambitious surgery is often pointless if the cancer has already spread beyond the organ in question. A key process in planning the right procedure is to interest a radiologist in your problem. This may require more than scrawling a request on an x-ray form. The range of imaging available is constantly changing, and the radiologist may need detailed information to allow best use of the scans available—eg:

Computer tomography (CT): Extensive application in many cancers.

MRI: Allows precise staging in areas occult to CT (eg marrow); see p405.

Bone scan: Helps staging/follow-up of prostate, breast, and lung ca.

Sestamibi scan: Localizing active disease in breast cancer and thyroid (eg if not iodine-avid). Like bone scans, it uses technetium (^{99m}Tc).

Thallium scan: Helps localize viable tissue, eg in brain tumours.

Gallium scan: Helps staging and follow-up in lymphoma.

Octreotide scan: Localizes cancers with somatostatin receptors (eg pancreas, medullary thyroid, neuroblastoma, and carcinoid tumours).

Monoclonal antibodies: (^{99m}Tc-labelled tumour antibodies). Helps staging by detecting tumour antigen, eg in lung, colon, and prostate cancer.

FDG PET: Positron emission tomography (PET) detects high rates of aerobic metabolism, eg in lung, colon, breast, and testis. FDG = 2-[18F]fluoro-2-deoxy-D-glucose.

MIBG scan (^{131}I): Localizing noradrenaline production, eg phaeochromocytoma. MIBG = meta-iodobenzylguanidine.

Radiotherapy

Radiotherapy uses ionizing radiation to produce free radicals which damage DNA. Normal cells are better at repairing this damage than cancer cells, so are able to recover before the next dose (or fraction) of treatment.

Radical treatment is given with curative intent. The total doses given range from 40–70Gy (1Gy = 100cGy = 100rads) in 15–35 daily fractions. Some regimens involving giving several smaller fractions a day with a gap of 6–8h (CHART). Combined chemoradiation is used in some sites, eg anus and oesophagus, to increase response rates.

Palliation aims to relieve symptoms. Doses: 8–30Gy, given in 1, 2, 5, or 10 fractions. Bone pain, haemoptysis, cough, dyspnoea, and bleeding are helped in >50% of patients. *'Will this patient benefit from radiotherapy?'* is a frequently asked question. For a formal example assessing risks and benefits, 🗌. When in doubt, ask an expert (or 2).

Early reactions Occur during, or soon after treatment.

- Tiredness: common after radical treatments; can last weeks to months.
- Skin reactions: These vary from erythema to dry desquamation to moist desquamation to ulceration; on completing treatment, use moisturizers.
- Mucositis: all patients receiving head and neck treatment should have a dental check-up before commencing therapy. Avoid smoking, alcohol, and spicy foods. Antiseptic mouthwashes may help. Aspirin gargle and other soluble analgesics are helpful. Treat oral thrush.
- Nausea and vomiting: occur when stomach, liver, or brain treated. Try a dopamine antagonist 1st. If unsuccessful, try 5HT$_3$ antagonist, p438.
- Diarrhoea: usually after abdominal or pelvic treatments. Maintain good hydration. Avoid high-fibre bulking agents; try loperamide.
- Dysphagia. Thoracic treatments.
- Cystitis. Pelvic treatments. Drink plenty of fluids. NSAIDs, eg diclofenac.
- Bone marrow suppression. More likely after chemotherapy or when large areas are being treated. Usually reversible.

Late reactions Occur months, or years after the treatment.

- CNS: somnolence, 6–12wks after brain radiotherapy. Treat with steroids. Spinal cord myelopathy—progressive weakness. MRI is needed to exclude cord compression. Brachial plexopathy—numb, weak, and painful arm after axillary radiotherapy. Reduced IQ can occur in children receiving brain irradiation if <6yrs old.
- Lung: pneumonitis may occur 6–12wks after thoracic treatment, eg with dry cough ± dyspnoea. Treatment: prednisolone 40mg reducing over 6wks.
- GI: xerostomia—reduced saliva. Treat with pilocarpine 5mg/8h or artificial saliva. Care must be taken with all future dental care as healing is reduced. Benign strictures—of oesophagus or bowel. Treat with dilatation. Fistulae—need surgical intervention.
- GU: urinary frequency—small fibrosed bladder after pelvic treatments. Fertility—pelvic radiotherapy (and cytotoxics) may affect fertility, so ova or sperm storage should be considered. This is a complex area: get expert help. See BOX. In premature female menopause or reduced testosterone—replace hormones. Vaginal stenosis and dyspareunia. Impotence—can occur several years after pelvic radiotherapy.
- Others: panhypopituitarism, following radical treatment involving pituitary fossa. Children need hormones checking regularly as growth hormone may be required. Hypothyroidism—neck treatments, eg for Hodgkin's lymphoma. Cataracts. Secondary cancers, eg sarcomas usually 10 or more years later.

Fertility issues in cancer patients

Plan with patients *before* treatment.

Chemotherapy and radiotherapy often damage germ-cell spermatogonia (∴ impaired spermatogenesis ± sterility in the male), and may hasten oocyte depletion (premature menopause in women). As treatments become more effective and survival improves, there are more survivors in the reproductive years for whom parenting is a top priority.[] There is nothing like the hope of creating new life to sustain patients through the difficult times of radio- and chemotherapy, so make sure this hope is well founded.

Semen cryopreservation from men and older boys with cancer must be offered before therapy. With modern fertility treatment (*OHCS* p57), even poor quality samples can yield successful pregnancies.[] Another option is use of spermatozoa from cryopreserved testicular tissue followed up with intracytoplasmic sperm injection (ICSI). If your patient is a man some years after cancer therapy who is unable to have children, refer him to a specialist. ▶*Do not write him off as infertile*—testicular sperm extraction (TESE) with ICSI can yield normal pregnancies.[]

Cryopreservation of embryos and *ovarian tissue banking* are harder options in women.[] Harvesting and storing ovarian cortical tissue from girls and young women before potentially gonadotoxic therapy is only available in some centres.[] Success depends on the integrity of the uterus, and in some cancers this may have been badly affected by radiotherapy. For ethical issues and the UK Human Embryology Authority, see *OHCS* p57.

Survival—European figures

On average, 40.5% of men and 53.6% of women survive >5yrs after a cancer diagnosis (respectively, in England, 37.1% of men and 50.8% of women).[] These statistics are based on 1.8 million adults and 24,000 children diagnosed between 1990 and 1994 and followed to 1999. (England has probably caught up since then—see the Cancer Plan/Care Pathways, p433.) Early diagnosis, a full range of treatment options, and the money spent by nations on health care all have an impact on survival.[]

Surgery[1]

Contents

Relevant pages in other chapters:

▶See *Gastroenterology* and *Dictionary of symptoms and signs* (p206 & p64).

Urology pages in other chapters: UTI/urine (p258–62); haematuria (p258); prostatism (p80); gynaecological urology (*OHCS* p70); stones (p264); GU obstruction (p266).

1 We thank Mr A Purushotam who is our Specialist Reader for this chapter.
2 ▶▶These are the three conditions where the promptest surgery is essential; ▶ notify the duty surgical registrar or consultant, and theatre, *at once*.

The language of surgery

Incisions have names

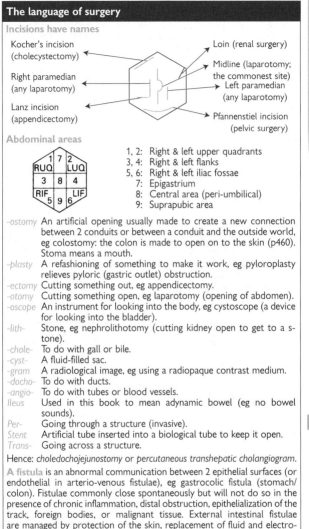

Kocher's incision (cholecystectomy)

Loin (renal surgery)

Midline (laparotomy; the commonest site)

Left paramedian (any laparotomy)

Right paramedian (any laparotomy)

Lanz incision (appendicectomy)

Pfannenstiel incision (pelvic surgery)

Abdominal areas

	7	
1 RUQ		2 LUQ
3	8	4
5 RIF	9	6 LIF

1, 2: Right & left upper quadrants
3, 4: Right & left flanks
5, 6: Right & left iliac fossae
7: Epigastrium
8: Central area (peri-umbilical)
9: Suprapubic area

-ostomy An artificial opening usually made to create a new connection between 2 conduits or between a conduit and the outside world, eg the colostomy: the colon is made to open on to the skin (p460). Stoma means a mouth.

-plasty A refashioning of something to make it work, eg pyloroplasty relieves pyloric (gastric outlet) obstruction.

-ectomy Cutting something out, eg appendicectomy.

-otomy Cutting something open, eg laparotomy (opening of abdomen).

-oscope An instrument for looking into the body, eg cystoscope (a device for looking into the bladder).

-lith- Stone, eg nephrolithotomy (cutting kidney open to get to a stone).

-chole- To do with gall or bile.

-cyst- A fluid-filled sac.

-gram A radiological image, eg using a radiopaque contrast medium.

-docho- To do with ducts.

-angio- To do with tubes or blood vessels.

Ileus Used in this book to mean adynamic bowel (eg no bowel sounds).

Per- Going through a structure (invasive).

Stent Artificial tube inserted into a biological tube to keep it open.

Trans- Going across a structure.

Hence: *choledochojejunostomy* or *percutaneous transhepatic cholangiogram*.

A **fistula** is an abnormal communication between 2 epithelial surfaces (or endothelial in arterio-venous fistulae), eg gastrocolic fistula (stomach/colon). Fistulae commonly close spontaneously but will not do so in the presence of chronic inflammation, distal obstruction, epithelialization of the track, foreign bodies, or malignant tissue. External intestinal fistulae are managed by protection of the skin, replacement of fluid and electrolytes, parenteral nutrition and, if this fails, operation.

A **sinus** is a blind-ending track, typically lined by epithelial or granulation tissue, which opens on to an epithelial surface.

An **ulcer** (p486) is an abnormal break in an epithelial surface.

An **abscess** is a cavity containing pus. For different types, consult the *index*. Remember the aphorism: *if there is pus about, let it out*—and remember that all such aphorisms also have their limitations.

445

Pre-operative care

Aims ▶*To ensure that, as far as possible, any fears are addressed and the patient understands the nature, aims, and expected outcome of surgery.*

- Ensure that the right patient gets the right surgery. Have the symptoms and signs changed? If so, inform the surgeon.
- Get informed consent (see BOX); explain the 'op' and reasons for it (diagrams help); outline serious/commoner (>1%) complications; leave time for questions. If you find ambivalence or any problem, eg confusion, get help.
- In the UK, those >16yrs can give valid consent. Those <16yrs can give consent for a medical decision provided they understand what it involves. *If <18yrs and refusing life-saving surgery*, talk to the parents and your senior; the law is unclear. You may need to contact the duty judge in the High Court.
- Assess/balance risks of anaesthesia, and maximize fitness. Is he a smoker? Optimizing oxygenation/perfusion *before* major surgery improves outcome.
- Check anaesthesia/analgesia type with anaesthetist. *Aim to allay anxiety and pain.*

Pre-op checks Assess cardiorespiratory system, exercise tolerance, existing illnesses, drugs, and allergies. Is the neck unstable (eg arthritis complicating intubation)? Assess past history of: myocardial infarction, diabetes, asthma, hypertension, rheumatic fever, epilepsy, jaundice. Assess any specific risks, eg is the patient pregnant? Is the neck/jaw immobile (intubation risk)? Has there been previous anaesthesia? Were there any complications (eg nausea, deep vein thrombosis, DVT)? ▶Is DVT/PE prophylaxis needed (p456)? ▶If patient for 'unilateral' surgery, mark the correct arm/leg/kidney.

Family history May be relevant eg in malignant hyperpyrexia (p450); dystrophia myotonica (p398); porphyria; cholinesterase problems; sickle-cell disease.

Drugs Any drug/plaster/antiseptic allergies? ▶Inform the anaesthetist about *all* drugs even if 'over-the-counter'. For *diabetes*, see p470.
Antibiotics: Tetracycline and neomycin *et al.* may ↑neuromuscular blockade.
Anticoagulants: Tell the surgeon. Avoid epidural, spinal, and regional blocks.
Anticonvulsants: Give as usual pre-op. Post-op, give drugs IV (or by NGT) until able to take orally. Valproate: give usual dose IV. Phenytoin: give IV slowly (<50mg/min; monitor ECG). IM phenytoin absorption is unreliable.
β-blockers: Continue up to and including the day of surgery as this precludes a labile cardiovascular response.
Contraceptive steroids: See BNF. Stop 4wks before major (or leg) surgery, and ensure alternative contraception is used.
Digoxin: Continue up to and including morning of surgery. Check for toxicity (ECG; plasma level); do plasma K⁺ and Ca²⁺ (suxamethonium ↑K⁺ and can lead to ventricular arrhythmias in the fully digitalized).
Diuretics: Beware hypokalaemia, dehydration. Do U&E (and bicarbonate).
HRT: There may be some increased risk of DVT/PE. *Steroids:* See p472.
Levodopa: Possible arrhythmias when patient under GA.
Lithium: Get expert help; it may potentiate neuromuscular blockade and cause arrhythmias. See OHCS p354.
MAOI: Get expert help as interaction with opiates and anaesthetics may cause hypotensive/hypertensive crises.
Eye-drops: β-blockers get absorbed; anticholinesterases ↑[suxamethonium].
Tricyclics: These enhance adrenaline (epinephrine) and arrhythmias.

Preparation ▶Fast the patient—and nil by mouth for ≥2h pre-op.
- Is any bowel or skin preparation needed, or prophylactic antibiotics (p448)?
- Start DVT prophylaxis as indicated, eg graduated compression stockings (not if poor foot pulses) + heparin 5000U SC pre-op, then every 12h SC until ambulant. Low molecular weight heparin: p194.
- Write up the pre-med (p450); book any pre-, intra-, or post-operative x-rays or frozen sections. Book post-operative physiotherapy.
- If needed, catheterize and insert a Ryle's tube (p743) before induction.

Pre-operative examination and tests

▶*Careful planning is the key to preventing perioperative death.* A good thought exercise is to imagine yourself at the next surgical *Mortality Meeting* and ask 'If I were looking back at the pre-op period, knowing that this patient had died, would I still consider that surgery was indicated?' The UK National Confidential Enquiry into Perioperative Deaths (NCEPOD) has found that 'too many' operations are performed on moribund patients.

It is the anaesthetist's duty to assess suitability for anaesthesia. The ward doctor assists with a good history and examination, and should also reassure, inform, and get written consent from the patient (remembering to consent for further procedures that may become necessary during the operation eg orchidectomy in orchidopexy procedures).

Be alert to chronic lung disease, BP↑, arrhythmias, and murmurs (endocarditis prophylaxis needed?—see p154).

Tests ▶Be guided by the history and examination, and local protocols.

- U&E, FBC, and ward tests for blood glucose in most patients. If Hb <10g/dL tell anaesthetist. Investigate/treat as appropriate. U&E are particularly important if the patient is starved, diabetic, on diuretics, a burns patient, has hepatic or renal diseases, has an ileus, or is parenterally fed.
- Crossmatching: group and save for mastectomy, cholecystectomy. Crossmatch 2 units for Caesarean section; four units for a gastrectomy, and >6 units for abdominal aortic aneurysm (AAA) surgery.
- Specific blood tests: LFT in jaundice, malignancy, or alcohol abuse.
 Amylase in acute abdominal pain. Blood glucose if diabetic (p470).
 Drug levels as appropriate (eg digoxin, lithium).
 Clotting studies in liver disease, DIC (p650), massive blood loss, patients already on sodium valproate, warfarin, or heparin.
 HIV, HBsAg in high risk patients—after appropriate counselling.
 Sickle test in those from Africa, West Indies, or Mediterranean—and others whose origins are in malarial areas (including most of India).
 Thyroid function tests in those with thyroid disease.
- CXR: if known cardiorespiratory disease, pathology or symptoms, possible lung metastases, or >65yrs old.
- ECG: if >55yrs old or poor exercise tolerance, or history of myocardial ischaemia, hypertension, rheumatic fever, or other heart disease.
- Lateral cervical spine x-ray: if history of rheumatoid arthritis, ankylosing spondylitis or Down's syndrome, to warn about difficult intubations.

American Society of Anesthesiologists (ASA) classification
1 Normally healthy.
2 Mild systemic disease.
3 Severe systemic disease that limits activity; not incapacitating.
4 Incapacitating systemic disease which poses a threat to life.
5 Moribund. Not expected to survive 24h even with operation.

You will see a space for an ASA number on most anaesthetic charts. It is a health index *at the time of surgery*. The prefix **E** is used in emergencies.

447

Obtaining informed consent

This is complex: UK law implies that we are either fully competent or 'incompetent' but things are not so clear-cut, so ...
- Use only words the patient understands.
- Ensure that he believes your facts and can retain the pros and cons long enough to inform his decision. See p231 for difficult areas, eg transplantation. Fact sheets for individual operations are often helpful.
- Make sure his choice is free from pressure from others.

Prophylactic antibiotics in gut surgery

Meta-analyses show that a single dose given just before surgery is as beneficial as more prolonged regimens in colorectal surgery. Metronidazole *alone* is probably suboptimal. There is no evidence that 3rd generation cefalosporins are better than cheaper, older cefalosporins (p544).

Wound infections These occur in 20–60% of those undergoing GI surgery. Sepsis may lead to haemorrhage, wound dehiscence, and initiate a fatal chain of events. Prophylaxis substantially reduces infection rates. *Rules for success:*

• Give the antibiotic just before (eg 1h) surgery; often it can be stopped after 24h.
• Give it IV or IM (or as a suppository for metronidazole).
• Use antibiotics which will kill anaerobes and coliforms.
• Consider use of perioperative supplemental oxygen. This is a practical method of reducing the incidence of surgical-wound infections.

Antibiotic regimens There is usually a local preference; examples:
Biliary surgery: Broad-spectrum penicillin (eg ampicillin 500mg IV/8h for 3 doses) or cefalosporin (eg cefuroxime 1.5g/8h, 1–3 doses IV/IM).
Appendicectomy: A 1–3-dose regimen of metronidazole suppositories 1g/8h, + cefuroxime 1.5g/8h IV or gentamicin IV (p710).
Colorectal surgery: Cefuroxime 1.5g/8h + metronidazole 500mg/8h, 1–3 doses IV.
Vascular surgery: Co-amoxiclav 1.2g IV on induction; if penicillin-allergic, cefuroxime 1.5g IV/IM + metronidazole 500mg IV. Single stat doses are best.

Bowel preparation in colorectal surgery

Bowel preparation is often used before colorectal surgery to minimize the risk of post-operative infectious complications. Preparation may involve 'low-residue' diets, restriction to free fluids 24h pre-op, and laxatives/washouts.

Laxatives or washouts may be needed if a primary anastomosis is to be formed, or to allow visualization of the bowel eg at colonoscopy (p228). Usually no laxatives are needed for right-sided operations (eg right hemicolectomy); the patient is just put on a 'low-residue' diet for a few days pre-op. For left-sided operations and rectal operations (eg left hemicolectomy, anterior resection), laxatives are usually used. ►Check with the surgeon what preparation he prefers. *Example:* 1 sachet of Picolax® (10mg sodium picosulfate with magnesium citrate) given on the morning before surgery and a 2nd sachet during the afternoon before surgery; use with care if any risk of perforation. Washouts (if used) should be continued until evacuation is clear.

There is some controversy about whether mechanical bowel preparation is of any real benefit other than for visualization. Some studies have suggested that it does not significantly reduce post-operative infectious complications.

Sutures

Sutures (stitches) are central to the art of surgery. The range of types available may appear confusing. Generally, they are absorbable or non-absorbable and their structure may be divided into monofilament, twisted, or braided. Examples of absorbable sutures are catgut, polydioxanone (PDS), polyglactin (Vicryl®), and polyglycolic acid (Dexon®). Non-absorbable sutures include silk, nylon, and prolene. Monofilament sutures are quite slippery but minimize infection and produce less reaction. Braided sutures have plaited strands and provide secure knots, but they may allow infection to occur between their strands. Twisted sutures have 2 twisted strands and similar qualities to braided sutures.

The time of suture removal depends on the site and the general state of the patient. Face and neck sutures tend to be removed after 5d (may be earlier in children), scalp and back of neck after 5d, and abdominal incisions after 5–10d. In patients with poor wound healing, eg on steroids, with malignancy, infection, or cachexia (p66), the sutures may need 14d or longer.

Anaesthesia

Before anaesthesia, explain to the patient what will happen and where he will wake up, otherwise the recovery room or ITU will be frightening. Explain that he may feel ill on waking. The premedication aims to allay anxiety and to make the anaesthesia itself easier to conduct. Typical regimens might include:

- *Anxiolytics:* Benzodiazepines eg temazepam 10–20mg PO. In children, midazolam 0.5mg/kg rectally 30min prior to procedure is effective.
- *Analgesics:* See p454. The patient should not be in pain prior to surgery. Opioids, local anaesthetic blocks and non-steroidal anti-inflammatory drugs (NSAIDs) (beware bleeding risk) are all used. In children or anxious adults, local anaesthetic cream (eg Emla® Amitop®) may be used on a few sites for the anaesthetist's IVI.
- *Antiemetics:* 5-HT$_3$ antagonists (eg ondansetron 4mg IV/IM)are the most effective agents; others (eg metoclopramide 10mg PO/IM/IV) are also used.
- *Antacids:* Ranitidine 50–100mg IV in patients at particular risk of aspiration.
- *Antisialogues:* Glycopyrronium (200–400µg in adults, 4–8µg/kg in children; given IV/IM 30–60min before induction) is sometimes used to decrease secretions that may cause respiratory obstruction in smaller airways.
- *Antibiotics:* See p448.

Give oral premedication 1–2h before surgery (1h if IM route used).

The side-effects of anaesthetic agents

Hyoscine, atropine: Tachycardia, urinary retention, glaucoma.

Opioids: Respiratory depression, cough reflex↓, vomiting, constipation.

Thiopentone (=thiopental; for rapid induction of anaesthesia): Laryngospasm.

Propofol: Respiratory depression, cardiac depression, pain on injection.

Volatile agents eg isoflurane: Nausea, vomiting, cardiac depression, respiratory depression, vasodilation, hepatotoxicity (see BNF).

The complications of anaesthesia are due to loss of:

Pain sensation: Urinary retention, diathermy burns.

Consciousness: Cannot communicate 'wrong leg/kidney'. NB: in some patients (eg 0.15%) *retained* consciousness is the problem. Awareness under GA sounds like a contradiction of terms, but remember that anaesthesia is a process rather than an event. Such awareness can lead to ill-defined, delayed neuroses and post-traumatic stress disorder (OHCS p347).

Muscle power: Corneal abrasion, no respiration, no cough (leads to pneumonia and atelectasis—partial lung collapse causing shunting ± impaired gas exchange: it starts minutes after induction, and may be related to the use of 100% O$_2$, supine position, surgery and age as well as to loss of power). Cannot phonate (speak) and is unable to impart vital information—eg 'I am in pain …' when paralysed and in pain, and unable to communicate.

Local anaesthesia If unfit/unwilling to undergo general anaesthesia, local nerve blocks or spinal blocks (contraindication: anticoagulation) using long-acting local anaesthetics (eg bupivacaine) may be indicated.

Drugs complicating anaesthesia ▶Inform anaesthetist. See p446 for lists of specific drugs, and actions to take.

Malignant hyperpyrexia This is a rare complication, precipitated by eg halothane or suxamethonium, exhibiting autosomal dominant inheritance. There is a rapid rise in temperature (>1°C every 30min); masseter spasm may also be an early sign. Complications include hypoxaemia, hypercarbia, hyperkalaemia, metabolic acidosis, and arrhythmias. ▶Get expert help immediately. It may respond to prompt treatment with dantrolene. Give 1mg/kg every 5min IV—up to 10mg/kg in total (OHCS p772).

Principles and practical conduct of anaesthesia

▶The general principles of anaesthesia centre on the triad of *hypnosis*, *analgesia*, and *muscle relaxation*.

The conduct of anasthesia typically involves:

- *Induction:* either *intravenous* (eg propofol 1.5–2.5mg/kg IV at a rate of 20–40mg every 10s; thiopentone is an alternative) or, if airway obstruction or difficult IV access, *gaseous* (eg sevoflurane or nitrous oxide, mixed in O_2).
- *Airway control:* either using a face mask, an oro-pharyngeal (Guedel) airway or by intubation. The latter usually requires muscle relaxation with a depolarizing/non-depolarizing neuromuscular blocker (*OHCS* p767).
- *Maintenance of anaesthesia:* either a volatile agent added to N_2O/O_2 mixture, or high-dose opiates with mechanical ventilation, or IV infusion anaesthesia (eg propofol 4–12mg/kg/h IVI).
- *End of anaesthesia:* Change inspired gases to 100% oxygen only, then discontinue any anaesthetic infusions and reverse muscle paralysis. Once spontaneously breathing, place patient in recovery position and give oxygen by face mask.

For further details, see the chapter titled *Anaesthesia* in *OHCS* (p760).

Some post-operative complications

Pyrexia Mild pyrexia in the first 24h is typically from atelectasis (needs prompt physio, not antibiotics), or tissue damage or necrosis but ↑temperature post-op should stimulate an infection screen. Check the chest for pneumonia, the wound for infection, and the abdomen for signs of peritonism (eg anastomotic leakage) or UTI. Examine sites of IV cannulae and check for signs of meningism and endocarditis. Check the legs for DVT. Send blood for FBC, U&E, CRP, and culture. Dipstick the urine. Consider MSU, CXR, and abdominal ultrasound/CT depending on clinical findings.

Confusion This may manifest as agitation, disorientation, and attempts to leave hospital especially at night. Gently reassure the patient in well-lit surroundings. See p372 for a full work-up: the common causes are:

- Hypoxia (pneumonia, atelectasis, LVF, PE)
- Infection (see above)
- Drugs (opiates, sedatives, and many others)
- Alcohol withdrawal
- Urinary retention; MI or stroke
- Liver/renal failure

Occasionally, sedation is necessary to examine the patient; consider midazolam (see p757; antidote: flumazenil) or haloperidol 0.5–2mg IM. Reassure relatives that post-op confusion is common and reversible.

Shortness of breath or hypoxia Any previous lung disease?
Sit up and give oxygen, monitoring peripheral O_2 saturation by pulse oximetry (p168). Examine for evidence of:

- Pneumonia/pulmonary collapse/aspiration
- LVF (MI or fluid overload)
- Pulmonary embolism (p194)
- Pneumothorax (p194; due to CVP line or intercostal anaesthetic block).

Do FBC, arterial blood gases, CXR, and ECG. Manage according to findings.

BP↓ If severe, tilt bed head down and give O_2. Check pulse rate and measure BP yourself; compare it with that prior to surgery. Post-op ↓BP is commonly due to hypovolaemia resulting from inadequate fluid input so check fluid chart and replace losses, usually with colloid initially. Monitor urine output; consider catheterization. A CVP line may be useful to monitor fluid resuscitation. Hypovolaemia may also be caused by haemorrhage so review wounds and abdomen. If severe, return to theatre for haemostasis. Beware cardiogenic causes and look for evidence of MI and PE. Consider sepsis and anaphylaxis. Management: p778.

Urine output↓ (oliguria) Aim for output of >30mL/h in adults (½mL/kg/h). Anuria means a blocked or malsited catheter (and never, we hope, an impending lawsuit: both ureters tied). Flush or replace catheter. *Oliguria is usually due to inadequate replacement of lost fluid.* Treat by increasing fluid input. Acute renal failure may follow shock, nephrotoxic drugs, transfusion, or trauma.

- Review fluid chart and examine for signs of volume depletion.
- Urinary retention is also common, so examine for a palpable bladder.
- Establish normovolaemia (a CVP line may help here, normal is 0–5cm H_2O relative to sternal angle); you may need 1L/h IVI for 2–3h.
- Catheterize bladder (for accurate monitoring); check U&E.
- If intrinsic renal failure is suspected, refer to a nephrologist early.

Nausea/vomiting Any mechanical obstruction, paralytic ileus, or emetic drugs (opiates, digoxin, anaesthetics)? Consider AXR, NGT, and antiemetic.

Other post-op complications Pain (p454), DVT (p456), pulmonary embolus (p194; massive PE: p802), wound dehiscence (p458), complications in post-gastric surgery (p530), other complications of specific operations (p458).

Post-operative bleeding

- Primary haemorrhage: ie continuous bleeding, starting during surgery. Replace blood loss. If severe, return to theatre for adequate haemostasis. Treat shock vigorously (p778).
- Reactive haemorrhage: haemostasis appears secure until BP rises and bleeding starts. Replace blood and re-explore wound.
- Secondary haemorrhage occurs 1 week or 2 post-op and is the result of infection.

Surgical drains in the post-operative period

The decision when to insert and remove drains may seem to be one of the great surgical enigmas—but there are basically 2 types to get a grip on. Most are inserted to drain the area of surgery and are often put on gentle suction. These are removed when they stop draining. The other type of drain is used to protect sites where leakage may occur in the post-operative period such as bowel anastomoses. These form a tract and are removed after about 1wk.

'Shortening a drain' means withdrawing it (eg by 2cm/d). This allows the tract to seal up, bit by bit.

Discharging patients after day-case surgery

▶After day-case surgery, don't discharge until 'LEAP-FROG' is established:

Lucid, not vomiting, and cough reflex established.

Easy breathing; easy urination.

Ambulant without fainting.

Pain relief + post-op drugs dispensed + given. Does he understand doses?

Follow-up arranged.

Rhythm, pulse rate, and BP checked one last time. Is trend satisfactory?

Operation site checked and explained to patient.

GP letter sent with patient or carer. He *must* know what has happened.

The control of pain

We humans are the most exquisite devices ever made for the experiencing of pain: the richer our inner lives, the greater the varieties of pain there are for us to feel—and the more resources we will have for mitigating pain. If you can connect with your patient's inner life you may make a real difference. *Never forget how painful pain is*—nor how fear magnifies pain. Try not to let these sensations, so often interposed between your patient and his recovery, be invisible to you as he or she bravely puts up with them.[1]

Guidelines for success Review & chart each pain carefully and individually.

- Identify and treat the underlying pathology wherever possible.
- Give regular doses rather than on an *as required* basis.
- Choose the best route: oral, PR, IM, epidural, SC, inhalation, or IV.
- Explanation and reassurance contribute greatly to analgesia.
- Allow the patient to be in charge. This promotes well-being, and does not lead to overuse. Patient-controlled continuous parenteral morphine delivery systems are useful.

Non-narcotic (simple) analgesia Paracetamol: 0.5–1.0g/4h PO (up to 4g daily). Caution in liver impairment. NSAIDs, eg ibuprofen 400mg/8h PO or diclofenac 75mg/12h PO, or 100mg PR/IM stat; these are good for musculoskeletal pain and renal colic. CI: peptic ulcer, clotting disorder, anticoagulants. Cautions: asthma, renal or hepatic impairment, pregnancy, and the elderly. Aspirin is contraindicated in children due to the risk of Reye's syndrome (*OHCS* p756).

Opioid drugs for severe pain *Morphine* (eg 10–15mg/2–4h) *or diamorphine* (5–10mg/2–4h PO, SC, or slow IV, but you may need much more) are best. NB: These are 'controlled' drugs. For terminal care, see p438.

Side-effects of opioids: These include nausea (so give with an antiemetic, eg prochlorperazine 12.5mg/6h IM), respiratory depression, constipation, cough suppression, urinary retention, BP↓, and sedation (do not use in hepatic failure or head injury). Dependency is rarely a problem. Naloxone may be needed to reverse the effects of excess opioids (p830).

How effective are standard analgesics? Pain is subjective, but its measurement by patients is surprisingly consistent and reproducible. The table below gives 'number needed to treat' (NNT, p30), ie the number of patients who need to receive the drug for one to achieve at least 50% pain relief over 4–6h (the range is 95% confidence intervals).

Codeine[60mg]	11–48	Paracetamol[1000mg]	3–4
Tramadol[50mg]	6–13	Paracetamol[1000mg]/codeine[60mg]	2–3
Aspirin[650mg]/codeine[60mg]	4–7	Diclofenac[50mg]	2–3
Paracetamol[650mg]/proproxyphene[100mg]	4–6	Ibuprofen[400mg]	2–3

Epidural analgesia Opioids and anaesthetics are given into the epidural space by infusion or as boluses. Ask the advice of the Pain Service (if available). SE: thought to be less as drug more localized: watch for respiratory depression; local anaesthetic-induced autonomic blockade (BP↓).

Adjuvant treatments Eg radiotherapy for bone cancer pain; anticonvulsants, antidepressants or steroids for nerve pain, antispasmodics, eg hyoscine (Buscopan® 10–20mg/8h) for intestinal, renal, or bladder colic. If brief pain relief is needed (eg for changing dressings or exploring wounds), try inhaled nitrous oxide (with 50% O_2—as Entonox®) with an 'on demand' valve. Transcutaneous electrical nerve stimulation (TENS), local heat, local or regional anaesthesia, and neurosurgical procedures (eg excision of neuroma) may be tried but can prove disappointing. Treat conditions that exacerbate pain (eg constipation, depression, anxiety).

---

1 Compare with Proust's '*egg of pain* ... this structure ... interposed between the face of a woman and the eyes of her lover which encases it and conceals it as a mantel of snow conceals a fountain ...' Marcel Proust 1925 *Remembrance of Things Past* **11**; *Albertine Disparue* 30, Chatto

Why is controlling post-operative pain so important?

- Psychological reasons: pain control is a humanitarian undertaking.
- Social reasons: pain relief makes surgery less feared by society.
- Biological reasons: there is evidence for the following sequence: pain → autonomic activation → increased adrenergic activity → arteriolar vaso-constriction → reduced wound perfusion → decreased tissue oxygenation → delayed wound healing → serious or mortal consequences.

Deep vein thrombosis (DVT)

DVTs occur in ~20% of surgical patients, and many non-surgical patients. 65% of below-knee DVTs are asymptomatic; these rarely embolize to the lung.

Risk Age↑, pregnancy, synthetic oestrogen, surgery (especially pelvic/orthopaedic), past DVT, malignancy, obesity, immobility, thrombophilia (p672).

Signs • Calf warmth/tenderness/swelling • Mild fever • Pitting oedema Homans' sign (↑resistance/pain on forced foot dorsiflexion) should never be performed as it may dislodge thrombus.

Differential diagnoses Cellulitis (may coexist); ruptured Baker's cyst (both may coexist).

Tests *D-dimer blood tests* are sensitive but not specific for DVT. They are also raised in infection, pregnancy, malignancy and post-op. A –ve result, combined with a low pretest clinical probability score (see BOX) is sufficient to exclude DVT. If D-dimer↑, or the patient has a high/intermediate pretest clinical probability score, do *compression ultrasound*. If this is –ve, a repeat ultrasound may be performed at 1wk to catch early but propagating DVTs. *Venography* is rarely necessary. Do *thrombophilia tests* (p672) if there are no predisposing factors, in recurrent DVT, or if there is a family history of DVT.

Prevention • Stop the Pill 4wks pre-op. • Mobilize early. • Heparin 5000U/12h SC; low molecular weight heparin (LMWH, eg enoxaparin 20mg/24h SC for 7d, starting 2h pre-op, or dalteparin) may be better (less bleeding, no monitoring needed). • Support hosiery (CI: ischaemia). • Intermittent pneumatic pressure, until 16h post-op. • Newer drugs, eg fondaparinux, *may* be better than LMWH.

Treatment Meta-analyses have shown LMWH (eg enoxaparin 1.5mg/kg/24h SC) to be superior to unfractionated heparin (dose guided by APTT, p648), but extensive ileofemoral thrombi may still require unfractionated heparin as such patients were excluded from the trials. Start warfarin simultaneously, stopping heparin when INR is 2–3; treat for 3 months (6 months if no cause is found; lifelong in recurrent DVT or thrombophilia) *Inferior vena caval filters* may be used in active bleeding, or when anticoagulants fails, to minimize risk of pulmonary embolus. *Preventing post-phlebitic change*: thrombolytic therapy (to reduce damage to venous valves) and graduated compression stockings have both been tried, but neither has been conclusively shown to be beneficial.

Swollen legs

Bilateral oedema implies systemic disease with ↑venous pressure (right heart failure) or ↓intravascular oncotic pressure (any cause of albumin↓, so test the urine for protein). It is *dependent* (distributed by gravity), which is why legs are affected early, but severe oedema extends above the legs. In the bed-bound, fluid moves to the new dependent area, causing a sacral pad. The exception is the local increase in venous pressure occurring in IVC obstruction: the swelling neither extends above the legs nor redistributes. Causes: • Right heart failure (p136) • Albumin↓ (p702) • Venous insufficiency: *acute*, eg prolonged sitting, or *chronic*, with haemosiderin-pigmented, itchy, eczematous skin ± ulcers. • Vasodilators, eg nifedipine • Pelvic mass (p64). • Pregnancy—if BP↑ + proteinuria, diagnose pre-eclampsia (OHCS p96): find an obstetrician urgently. *In all the above, both legs need not be affected to the same extent.*

Unilateral oedema: Pain ± redness implies DVT or inflammation, eg cellulitis or insect bites (any blisters?). Bone or muscle may be to blame, eg trauma (check sensation and pulses: a compartment syndrome with ischaemic necrosis needs prompt fasciotomy); tumours; or necrotizing fasciitis, p486.

Impaired mobility suggests trauma, arthritis, or a Baker's cyst (p718).

Non-pitting oedema is oedema you cannot indent: see p78.

Treatment Treat the cause. Giving diuretics to everyone is not an answer. Ameliorate dependent oedema by elevating the legs (ankles higher than hips—do not just use foot stools); raise the foot of the bed. Graduated support stockings may help (CI: ischaemia).

Pretest clinical probability scoring for DVT[1]

In patients with symptoms in both legs, the more symptomatic leg is used.

Clinical feature	Score
Active cancer (treatment within last 6 months or palliative)	1 point
Paralysis, paresis, or recent plaster immobilization of leg	1 point
Major surgery or recently bedridden for >3d in last 4wks	1 point
Local tenderness along distribution of deep venous system	1 point
Entire leg swollen	1 point
Calf swelling >3cm compared to asymptomatic leg (measured 10cm below tibial tuberosity)	1 point
Pitting oedema (greater in the symptomatic leg)	1 point
Collateral superficial veins (non-varicose)	1 point
Alternative diagnosis as likely or more likely than that of DVT	−2 points

3 or more points: high probability; *1-2 points:* intermediate probability; *0 or less points:* low pretest probability of DVT.

Air travel and DVT

In 1954, Homans first reported an association between air travel and venous thromboembolism. Recently, the supposed risk of DVT and subsequent pulmonary emboli associated with air travel (the so-called 'economy-class syndrome') has been the subject of much public scrutiny. Factors such as dehydration, immobilization, decreased oxygen tension, and prolonged pressure on the popliteal veins resulting from long periods in confined aircraft seats have all been suggested to be contributory factors.[21] While the evidence linking air travel to an increased risk of DVT is still largely circumstantial, the following facts may help answer questions from your patients, family, and friends:

- The risk of developing a DVT from a long distance flight has been estimated at 0.1–0.4/1000 for the general population.[22]
- There is an increased risk of pulmonary embolus associated with long distance air travel.[23]
- Compression stockings may decrease the risk of DVT, though they may also cause superficial thrombophlebitis.
- The role of prophylactic aspirin is still under investigation.
- Measures to minimize risk of DVT include leg exercises, increased water intake, and refraining from alcohol or caffeine during the flight.

9 questions to ask those with swollen legs

- Is it *both* legs?
- Any trauma?
- Any pain?
- Is she pregnant?
- Any pitting?
- Any skin changes?
- Is she mobile?
- Past diseases/on drugs?
- Any oedema elsewhere?

1 PS Wells 1997 *Lancet* **350** 1795–8

Specific post-operative complications

Laparotomy In the elderly, or the malnourished, the wound may break down from a few days to a few weeks post-op, particularly if infection or haematoma is present, or there has been major surgery in a patient already compromised, eg by cancer, or because this is a 2nd laparotomy.

The warning sign of wound dehiscence is a pink serous discharge. It should always be assumed that the defect involves the whole of the wound. Serious wound dehiscence may lead to a 'burst abdomen' with evisceration of bowel (mortality 15–30%). If you are on the ward when this happens, put the guts back into the abdomen, and place a sterile dressing over the wound. Call your senior. Allay anxiety, give parenteral pain control, set up IVI, and return patient to theatre.

Incisional hernia is a common (15%) problem, reparable by mesh insertion.

Biliary surgery After exploration of the common bile duct (CBD), a T-tube is usually left in the bile duct draining freely to the exterior. A T-tube cholangiogram is performed at 8–10d and if there are no retained stones, the tube may be pulled out.

Retained stones may be removed by ERCP (p229), further surgery, or instillation of stone-dissolving agents (via T-tube to dissolve the stone). If there is distal obstruction in the CBD, fistula formation may occur with a chronic leak of bile. Other complications of biliary surgery are CBD stricture; cholangitis; bleeding into the biliary tree (haemobilia) which may lead to biliary colic, jaundice, and haematemesis; pancreatitis; and leak of bile causing biliary peritonitis. If jaundiced, it is important to maintain a good urine output as the danger is the hepatorenal syndrome (p472).

Thyroid surgery Recurrent and/or superior laryngeal nerve palsy (hoarseness); hypoparathyroidism (p308), causing hypocalcaemia (p694); hypothyroidism; thyroid storm (p820). Tracheal obstruction due to haematoma in the wound may occur. ▶▶Relieve by immediate removal of stitches or clips; may require urgent surgery.

Prostatectomy See p497.

Haemorrhoidectomy Constipation; infection; stricture; bleeding. 1 week's lactulose + metronidazole (p547) starting pre-op ↓pain, and time off work.

Mastectomy Arm oedema; skin necrosis.

Arterial surgery Bleeding; thrombosis; embolism; graft infection; myocardial infarct. Complications of aortic surgery: gut ischaemia; renal failure; respiratory distress; bleeding into the gut (aorto-enteric fistula); trauma to ureters; and anterior spinal artery (leading to paraplegia).

Colonic surgery Sepsis; ileus; fistulae; anastomotic leaks; obstruction; haemorrhage; trauma to ureters or spleen.

Small bowel surgery *Short gut syndrome* may result from substantial resections of small bowel. Diarrhoea and malabsorption (particularly of fats) lead to a number of metabolic abnormalities including deficiency in vitamins A, D, E, K, and B_{12}, hyperoxaluria (causing renal stones), and bile salt depletion (causing gallstones).

Tracheostomy Stenosis; mediastinitis; surgical emphysema.

Splenectomy Acute gastric dilatation (a serious consequence of failing to use a nasogastric tube, or to check that the one in place is actually working); thrombocytosis; sepsis. ▶Lifetime sepsis risk is partly preventable with pre-op vaccines—ie *Haemophilus* type B, meningococcal, and pneumococcal (p558 & p172) and prophylactic penicillin (p671).

Genitourinary surgery Septicaemia (from instrumentation in the presence of infected urine); urinoma—rupture of a ureter or renal pelvis leading to a mass of extravasated urine.

Gastrectomy See p530.

Stoma care

A stoma is an artificial union made between 2 conduits (eg a choledocho-jejunostomy) or, more commonly, between a conduit and the outside—eg a colostomy, in which faeces are made to pass through a hole in the abdominal wall into an adherent plastic bag, hopefully as 1–2 formed motions per day. (Mouths and anuses are natural stomas.) The physical and psychological aspects of stoma care must not be undervalued. Be alert to any vicious cycle in which a skin reaction leads to leakage → fear of going out into the world → fear of eating → poor skin nutrition → further skin reactions → further leakage → more depression. These cycles can be circumvented by the stoma nurse (below), who is expert in knowing which device to use when—and when to provide a shoulder to cry on.

When choosing the site for a colostomy, avoid areas in scars, the area around the waistline, and creases (so stand the patient up while planning).

The *stoma nurse* is expert in fitting secure, odourless devices. Ensure patients have her phone number for use before and after surgery. Her visits are more useful than any doctor's in explaining what is going to happen, and what the colostomy will be like, and in troubleshooting post-op problems. ►*Early direct self-referral prevents problems.* Without her, a patient may reject his colostomy, never attend to it, or become suicidal.

Pre-op, confirm that he is unsuited to 1 of the newer colostomy prevent-ing operations (eg employing muscle fibres from gracilis muscle).

1 *Loop colostomies:* A loop of colon is exteriorized, opened, and sewn to the skin. A rod under the loop prevents retraction and may be removed after 7d. This is often called a defunctioning colostomy but this is not strictly true as faeces may pass beyond the loop. A loop colostomy is used to pro-tect a distal anastomosis or to relieve distal obstruction. It is often tempo-rary, and more prone to complications than end colostomies.

2 *End colostomy:* The bowel is divided; the proximal end brought out as a stoma. The distal end may be: • resected, eg abdominoperineal excision of the rectum. • closed and left in the abdomen (Hartman's procedure) • exteriorized, forming a 'mucous fistula'.

3 *Double-barreled (Paul-Mikulicz) colostomy:* The colon is brought out as a double-barrel. It may be closed using an enterotome.

Incidence: 50,000 colostomies/yr (UK). Most manage their own colostomies well, and the cost for appliances is ~£1300/yr (allowing for a bag-use rate of 1–3/d). If there is an allergic-type reaction to the adhesive or other part of the device, a change of device may be all that is needed. Contact your local specialist nurse. Avoid most creams which tend to be troublesome if of an oily nature—Comfeel® is an exception.

Ileostomies protrude from the skin and emit fluid motions which contain active enzymes (so skin needs protecting). End ileostomy usually follows proctocolectomy, typically for UC. Loop ileostomy can be used to tempo-rarily protect distal anastomoses.

Total anorectal reconstruction: an alternative to colostomy Total anorectal reconstruction uses gracilis muscle disconnected distally and wound around the anus and induced to contract by a pulse generator implanted in the abdomen, with bowel action triggered by a hand-held radiofrequency controller. We regard it as still rather experimental, but patients will ask about it. Warn them that normal-quality continence cannot be achieved because of lack of sensation of the arrival of stools. Outcomes seem to correlate with surgical experience.

For posterior sagittal anorectoplasty (PSARP), see *OHCS* p218. There is some evidence from non-randomized trials that sphincter saving operations are not associated with poorer disease-free survival compared with abdomino-perineal resection in those with lower-third rectal carcinomas.

Complications of stomas

▶Liaise with the stoma nurse, starting pre-operatively.

Early:

- Haemorrhage at stoma site
- Stoma ischaemia
- High output (especially ileostomies—can lead to $K^+\downarrow$)
- Obstruction secondary to adhesions
- Stoma retraction.

Delayed:

- Obstruction (failure at operation to close lateral space around stoma)
- Dermatitis around stoma site
- Stoma prolapse
- Parastomal hernia
- Fistulae
- Psychological problems.

IV fluids on the surgical ward

Pre-op fluids Avoid rushing dehydrated patients to theatre before adequate resuscitation. Anaesthesia compounds shock by causing vasodilatation and depressing cardiac contractility. Exceptions are exsanguination from a ruptured ectopic pregnancy, major trauma, or a ruptured aortic aneurysm, where blood is lost faster than it can be replaced.

Post-operative fluids A normal requirement is 2–3L/24h which allows for urinary, faecal, and insensible loss.

A standard regimen: (One of many) 2L 5% dextrose with 1L 0.9% saline/24h. Add K^+ post-op (20mmol/L). See p680 for other examples. More K^+ is needed if losses are from the gut (eg diarrhoea, vomiting, intestinal fistula, high output stoma). More saline is appropriate for those at risk of hyponatraemia: ▶See BOX.

When to increase the above regimen:
- Dehydration: this may be by ≥5L if severe. Replace this slowly.
- Shock (all causes, except for cardiogenic shock).
- Operative losses: check operation notes for extent of bleeding in theatre.
- Losses from gut: replace NGT aspirate volume with 0.9% saline.
- Transpiration losses: feverish patients and burns.
- Pancreatitis: there are large pools of sequestered fluid which should be allowed for.
- Losses from surgical drains: check fluid charts and replace significant losses.
- Low urine output (the night after surgery) is almost always due to inadequate infusion of fluid. Check JVP, and review for signs of cardiac failure. Treat by increasing IVI rate unless patient is in heart or renal failure, or profusely bleeding (when blood should be transfused). If in doubt, a fluid challenge may be indicated: 200mL of colloid (eg Gelofusine®) over 30–60 min, with monitoring of urine output. Then you may increase IVI rate eg to 1L/h of 0.9% saline for 2–3h. Only if output does not increase should a diuretic be considered; a CVP line may be needed if estimation of fluid balance is difficult. A normal value is 0–5cm of water relative to the sternal angle.

If not catheterized exclude retention, but otherwise do not catheterize until absolutely necessary.

When to decrease the above regimen: Acute renal failure—give 500mL plus the previous day's output (▶with no K^+). *Heart failure*—halve the volume (1–1.5L/24h).

Guidelines for success (see also p688)
- Be simple. Chart losses and replace them. Know the urine output. Aim for 60mL/h; 30mL/h is the minimum in adults (½mL/kg/h).
- Measure plasma U&E if the patient is ill. Regular U&Es are not needed on young, fit people with good kidneys.
- Start oral fluids as soon as possible.

What fluids to use ▶*Haemorrhagic/hypovolaemic shock* (see p778): Insert 2 large IV cannulae, for fast fluid infusion. Start with crystalloid (eg 0.9% saline) or colloid (eg Gelofusine®) until blood is available. The advantage of crystalloids is that they are cheap—but they do not stay as long in the intravascular compartment as colloids, as they equilibrate with the total extracellular volume (dextrose is useless for resuscitation as it rapidly equilibrates with the enormous intracellular volume). In practice, the best results are achieved by combining crystalloids and colloids. Aim to keep the haematocrit at ~0.3, and urine flowing at >30mL/h. Monitor pulse and BP often.

Septicaemic shock: Use a plasma-like substance (eg Gelofusine®).

Heart or liver failure: Avoid sodium loads: use 5% dextrose.

Excessive vomiting: Use 0.9% saline: replace losses, including K^+.

Hyponatraemia: it matters—and it is preventable[29]

If 5% dextrose is infused post-operatively, the dextrose is quickly used, rendering the fluid hypotonic. This causes hyponatraemia (nausea, head-aches, weakness, cognition↓, coma, death)—especially in those at risk: on excessive doses of thiazide diuretics, females (especially pre-menopausal) and those undergoing physiological stress, which causes inappropriate ADH secretion, hence the low Na^+. In some individuals, only marginally low plasma Na^+ levels cause serious effects (eg ~128mmol/L). Risk of harm is minimized by following these rules:

- Know the pre-op U&E.
- Don't infuse dextrose without saline.
- Do a post-op U&E. Look at the result (Obvious, and so forgettable).
- Don't attribute odd CNS signs to non-existent strokes/TIAs if Na^+↓.
- Don't ignore low sodiums. Get help if you don't know what to do.

Treatment: (▶p690) 0.9% saline IVI; do U&E every 2h; aim to bring Na^+ up to 130mmol/L by 1–2mmol/L per hour. Diuretics eg frusemide (=furosemide) may be useful in acute hyponatraemia, or if the patient is symptomatic. Hypertonic saline (eg 1.8% saline) should only be used in emergencies when the patient has profound neurological symptoms (seizures, coma).

Blood transfusion and blood products

▶Blood should only be given if strictly necessary.

- Know *and* use local procedures to ensure that the right blood gets to the right patient at the right time. See p447 for quantities to request.
- Take blood for crossmatching from only 1 patient at a time. Label immediately. This minimizes risk of wrong labelling of samples.
- When giving blood, monitor TPR and BP every ½h.
- Do not use giving sets which have contained dextrose or Gelofusine®

Group-and-save (G&S) requests Find out your local guidelines for elective surgery. Having crossmatched blood to hand may not be needed if a blood sample is already in the lab, with group determined, with any atypical antibodies (ie G&S).

Whole blood (rarely used) *Indications:* Exchange transfusion; grave exsanguination—use crossmatched blood if possible, but if not, use 'universal donor' group O Rh−ve blood, changing to crossmatched blood as soon as possible. ▶Blood >2d old has no effective platelets.

Red cells (packed to make haematocrit ~70%) Use to correct anaemia or blood loss. 1U ↑Hb by 1–1.5g/dL. In anaemia, transfuse until Hb ~ 8g/dL.

Platelet transfusion (p662) Not usually needed if not bleeding or count is >20 × 10^9/L. If surgery is planned, get advice if <100 × 10^9/L.

Fresh frozen plasma (FFP) Use to correct clotting defects: eg DIC (p650), warfarin overdosage where vitamin K would be too slow, liver disease, thrombotic thrombocytopenic purpura (p282). It is expensive and carries all the risks of blood transfusion. Do not use as a simple volume expander.

Human albumin solution (Plasma protein fraction) is produced as 4.5% or 20% protein solution and is basically albumin to use for protein replacement. Both the solutions have much the same Na^+ content and 20% albumin can be used temporarily in the hypoproteinaemic (eg liver disease; nephrotic) who is fluid overloaded, without giving an excessive salt load.

Others Cryoprecipitate (a source of fibrinogen); coagulation concentrates (self-injected in haemophilia); immunoglobulin (anti-D, OHCS p109).

Complications of transfusion ▶Management of acute reactions: see BOX

- *Early (within 24h):* Acute haemolytic reactions (eg ABO or Rhesus incompatibility), anaphylaxis, bacterial contamination, febrile reactions (eg from HLA antibodies), allergic reactions (eg itch, urticaria, mild fever), fluid overload, transfusion-related acute lung injury (TRALI)—basically ARDS due to anti-leucocyte antibodies in donor plasma.
- *Delayed (after 24h):* Infections (eg viruses: hepatitis B/C, HIV; bacteria; protozoa; prions), iron overload (treatable with desferrioxamine), graft-versus-host disease, post-transfusion purpura—potentially lethal fall in platelet count 5–7d post-transfusion requiring specialist treatment with IV immunoglobulin and platelet transfusions.

Massive blood transfusion This is defined as replacement of an individual's entire blood volume (>10U) within 24h. *Complications:* platelets↓, Ca^{2+}↓, clotting factors↓, K^+↑, hypothermia.

Transfusing patients with heart failure If Hb≤5g/dL with heart failure, transfusion with packed red cells is vital to restore Hb to safe level, eg 6–8g/dL, but must be done with great care. Give each unit over 4h with frusemide (=furosemide, eg 40mg slow IV/PO; do not mix with blood) with alternate units. Check for ↑JVP and basal lung crepitations; consider CVP line. If CCF gets worse, and immediate transfusion is essential, try a 2–3U exchange transfusion, removing blood at same rate as transfused.

▶There is a role for patients having their own blood stored pre-op for later use (*autologous transfusion*). Erythropoietin (EPO) can be used to increase the yield of autologous blood in normal individuals.

Transfusion reactions

A rapid spike of temperature (>40°C) at the start of a bag indicates that the transfusion should be stopped (suggests intravascular haemolysis or bacterial contamination). For a slowly rising temperature (<40°C), slow the IVI—this is most frequently due to antibodies against white cells.

Acute transfusion reactions	Action
Acute haemolytic reaction (eg ABO incompatibility) Agitation, T°↑ (rapid onset), ↓BP, flushing, abdominal/chest pain, oozing venepuncture sites, DIC (p650).	STOP transfusion. Check identity and name on unit; tell haematologist; send unit + FBC, U&E, clotting, cultures, & urine (haemoglobinuria) to lab. Keep IV line open with 0.9% saline. Treat DIC (p650).
Anaphylaxis Bronchospasm, cyanosis, ↓BP, soft tissue swelling.	SLOW or STOP the transfusion. Maintain airway and give oxygen. Contact anaesthetist. ▶▶see p780.
Bacterial contamination T°↑ (rapid onset), ↓BP, and rigors.	STOP the transfusion. Check identity against name on unit; tell haematologist and send unit + FBC, U&E, clotting, cultures & urine to lab. Start broad-spectrum antibiotics.
TRALI (See OPPOSITE) Dyspnoea, cough; CXR 'white out'	STOP the transfusion. Give 100% O₂. Treat as ARDS. ▶▶see p190. Donor should be removed from donor panel.
Non-haemolytic febrile transfusion reaction Shivering and fever usually 30–60min after starting transfusion.	SLOW or STOP the transfusion. Give an antipyretic, eg paracetamol 1g. Monitor closely. If recurrent, use leucocyte-depleted blood or WBC filter.
Allergic reactions Urticaria and itch.	SLOW or STOP the transfusion; give chlorpheniramine (= chlorhenamine) 10mg slow IV/IM. Monitor closely.
Fluid overload Dyspnoea, hypoxia, tachycardia, ↑JVP, and basal crepitations.	SLOW or STOP the transfusion. Give oxygen and a diuretic, eg frusemide (=furosemide) 40mg IV initially. Consider CVP line and exchange transfusion.

Blood transfusion and Jehovah's witnesses

These patients are likely to refuse even vital transfusions on religious grounds.[1] These views must be respected, but complex issues arise if the patient is a child, or (perhaps) an adult who lives a sheltered life, and may not be able to give, or withhold consent in an informed way. When in doubt, apply to the Court. Judges tend to take a narrow view on this,[2] acting as if any immediate benefit to life must trump putative benefits in any life hereafter. How can refusal be informed, it might be argued, if only the physical (and not the metaphysical) consequences of transfusion can be foreseen? Even if metaphysical considerations are put on one side, it is a question whether giving a transfusion against consent could amount to a degrading act or torture, against which the European Convention on Human Rights gives absolute, inalienable protection. ▶Some patients may not want to forsake their principles but would not mind too much being told what to do, thereby not being the means of their child's destruction, while being true to their beliefs. It is possible to hold 2 incompatible beliefs at the same time.[1]

1 Accepting transfusion implies self-expulsion from this church, but it is no longer a disfellowshipping event with active expulsion—D Sharp 2000 *Lancet* **356** 8. See also R Yate 2000 *Lancet* **356** 69
2 V Wason 1998 Court Order (High Court Family Division) Re L (A Minor), June 1–10

Nutritional support in hospital

▶Over 25% of hospital inpatients may be malnourished. Hospitals can become so focused on curing disease that they ignore the foundations of good health. Malnourished patients recover more slowly, and experience more complications, than those well fed.[32]

Why are so many hospital patients malnourished?

1 Increased nutritional requirements (eg sepsis, burns, surgery).
2 Increased nutritional losses (eg malabsorption, output from stoma).
3 Decreased intake (eg dysphagia, sedation, coma).
4 Effect of treatment (eg nausea, diarrhoea).
5 Enforced starvation (eg prolonged periods *nil by mouth*).
6 Missing meals through being whisked off, eg for investigations.
7 Difficulty with feeding and no one available to give enough help.
8 Unappetizing food: 'They feed me stuff I wouldn't give my cat'.

Identifying the malnourished patient

History: Recent weight change; recent reduced intake; diet change (eg recent change in consistency of food); nausea, vomiting, pain, diarrhoea which might have led to reduced intake.

Examination: Examine for state of hydration (p688): dehydration can go hand-in-hand with malnutrition, and overhydration can mask the appearance of malnutrition. Evidence of malnutrition: skin hanging off muscles (eg over biceps); no fat between fold of skin; hair rough and wiry; pressure sores; sores at corner of mouth. Calculate the body mass index (p208); BMI< 19kg/m² suggests malnourishment.

Investigations: Generally unhelpful. Low albumin suggestive, but is affected by many things other than nutrition.

Prevention of malnutrition
Assess nutrition state and weight on admission, and eg weekly thereafter. Identify those at risk (see above). Ensure that investigations and the like don't interfere substantially with meals. Provide appetizing food to the patient when he wants to eat it.

Calorie needs
Most patients are well-nourished with 2000–2500kCal (20–40kCal/kg) and 7–14g nitrogen every 24h. Even catabolic patients rarely need more than 2500kCal. Very high calorie diets (eg 4000kCal/24h) can lead to fatty liver. If patient requires nutritional support, seek help from dietician.

Approximate energy contents
Glucose 4kCal/g; fat 10kCal/g. (To convert kCal to kJ multiply by 4.2.)

Enteral nutrition (ie nutrition given into gastrointestinal tract)

If at all possible give nutrition by mouth. An all-fluid diet can meet requirements (but get advice from dietician). If danger of choking (eg after stroke), consider semi-solid diet before abandoning food by mouth.

Tube feeding: This is giving liquid nutrition *via* a tube, eg placed endoscopically, radiologically, or surgically (directly into stomach, ie gastrostomy). Use nutritionally complete, commercially prepared feeds. Standard feeds (eg Nutrison standard®, Osmolite®) normally contain 1kCal/mL and 4–6g protein per 100mL. Most people's requirements are met in 2L/24h. Specialist advice from dietician is essential. Nausea and vomiting is less of a problem if feed given continuously with pump, but may have disadvantages compared with intermittent nutrition.

Guidelines for success
• Use fine-bore NG feeding tube when possible.
• Check position of nasogastric tube before starting feeding.
• Build up feeds gradually to avoid diarrhoea and distension.
• Weigh weekly, check blood glucose and plasma electrolytes (including phosphate, zinc, and magnesium, if previously malnourished).
• Close liaison with a dietician is essential.

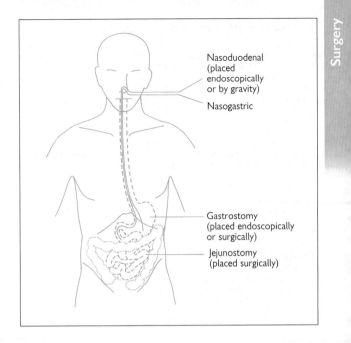

Parenteral (intravenous) nutrition

Do not undertake parenteral feeding lightly: it has risks. Specialist advice is vital. Only consider it if the patient is likely to become malnourished without it. This normally means that the gastrointestinal tract is not functioning (eg bowel obstruction), and is unlikely to function for at least 7d. Parenteral feeding may supplement other forms of nutrition (eg in active Crohn's disease when insufficient nutrition can be absorbed in the gut) or be used alone (total parenteral nutrition—TPN). Even if there is GI disease (eg pancreatitis), studies show that enteral nutrition is safer, cheaper, and at least as efficacious.

Administration Nutrition is normally given through a central venous line as this usually lasts longer than if given into a peripheral vein. A peripherally inserted central catheter (PICC line) is another option. Insert under strictly sterile conditions and check its position on x-ray.

Requirements There are many different regimens for parenteral feeding. Most provide ~2000kCal and 10–14g nitrogen in 2–3L; this usually meets a patient's daily requirements of 20–40kCal/kg and 0.2g nitrogen/kg. ~50% of calories are provided by fat and 50% by carbohydrate. Regimens comprise vitamins, minerals, trace elements, and electrolytes; these will normally be included by the pharmacist.

Complications[1]

Sepsis: (Eg *Staphylococcus epidermidis* and *Staphylococcus aureus*; *Candida*; *Pseudomonas*; infective endocarditis.) Look for spiking pyrexia and examine wound at tube insertion point. If central venous line related sepsis is suspected, the safest course of action is always to remove the line. Do not attempt to salvage a line when *S. aureus* or *Candida* infection has been identified. Antimicrobial-impregnated central lines decrease the incidence of line-related infections.

Thrombosis: Central vein thrombosis may occur, resulting in pulmonary embolus or superior vena caval obstruction (p436). Heparin in the nutrient solution may be useful for prophylaxis in high-risk patients.

Metabolic imbalance: Electrolyte abnormalities (including K^+, calcium, phosphate, zinc, magnesium); plasma glucose; deficiency syndromes.

Mechanical: Pneumothorax; embolism of IVI tip.

Guidelines for success
- Liaise closely with nutrition team and pharmacist.
- Meticulous sterility. Do not use central venous lines for uses other than nutrition. Remove the line if you suspect infection. Culture its tip.
- Review fluid balance at least twice daily, and requirements for energy and electrolytes daily.
- Check weight, fluid balance, and urine glucose daily throughout period of parenteral nutrition. Check plasma glucose, creatinine and electrolytes (including calcium and phosphate), and full blood count daily until stable and then 3 times a week. Check LFT and lipid clearance three times a week until stable and then weekly. Check zinc and magnesium weekly throughout.
- Do not rush. Achieve the maintenance regimen in small steps.

---

1 For more information on complications of central lines, see DC McGee 2003 *NEJM* **348** 1123
For children, see Brit. Assoc for Parenteral and Enteral Nutrition 2000 *Guidelines* ISBN 1-899-467-408

Diabetic patients on surgical wards

Insulin-dependent diabetes mellitus (eg Type 1 diabetes mellitus)
- Patients are often well informed about their diabetes; involve them fully when managing their diabetic care.
- Stress or intercurrent illness increases basal insulin needs (see p292).
- Always try to put the patient first on the list (surgery, endoscopy, bronchoscopy, etc.). Inform the surgeon and anaesthetist early.
- Stop all long–acting insulin the night before. Get IV access *before* you need it urgently. If surgery is in the morning, stop all SC morning insulin. If surgery is in the afternoon, have the usual short-acting insulin in the morning at breakfast. No medium- or long-acting insulin.
- Check blood glucose hourly. Aim for 7–11mmol/L during surgery.
- Check U&E pre-op. Start an IVI of 1L of 5% dextrose with 20mmol KCl/8h. Dextrose saline can be given if Na⁺ low, but do not give *only* saline; dextrose may need constant infusion to maintain blood glucose.
- Start an infusion pump with 50U short-acting insulin (eg Actrapid®) in 50mL 0.9% saline. Give according to sliding scale below adjusted in the light of blood glucose.
- Post-op, continue IV insulin and dextrose until patient tolerating food. Fingerprick glucose check every 2h. Switch to usual SC regimen.

Practical hints:
- Some centres prefer to control blood sugar with a glucose-potassium-insulin (GKI) infusion—see BOX.
- If the patient is having minor surgery, and thus will definitely be able to eat post-op, IV insulin may not be necessary. Some advocate giving the patient a small glucose drink early on the morning of surgery, and delaying their morning insulin dose and breakfast till after the procedure.
- If in doubt, check with the anaesthetist.

Non-insulin-dependent diabetes mellitus (≈Type 2 diabetes)
- These patients are usually controlled on oral hypoglycaemics (p295). If diabetes poorly controlled (eg fasting glucose >10mmol/L), treat as for Type 1 diabetes.
- Do not give long-acting sulphonylureas (eg glibenclamide) on the morning of surgery, as they can cause prolonged hypoglycaemia on fasting.
- Beware lactic acidosis in patients on biguanides (eg metformin).
- If the patient can eat post-operatively, simply omit tablets on the morning of surgery and give post-op with a meal.
- If the patient is having major surgery with restrictions to eating post-op, check fasting glucose on the morning of surgery and start IV or SC insulin given according to sliding scale. Post-op, consult the diabetic team as the patient may need a phase of insulin to supplement their oral hypoglycaemics.

Diet-controlled diabetes Usually no problem, though patient may temporarily become insulin dependent post-op. Monitor fingerprick glucose before meals and bedtime. Avoid giving 5% dextrose IVI as a fluid replacement as blood glucose will rise.

IV Insulin sliding scale (This is only a guide; values are in mmol/L.)

Fingerprick glucose	IV soluble insulin[1]	Alternative SC insulin[2]
<2 ►►See p820	None (50% glucose IV)	None (50% glucose IV)
2–5	No insulin	No insulin
5–10	1u/h	2u/h (rough guide only)
10–15	2u/h	5u/h
15–20	3u/h	7u/h
>20	6u/h: get urgent diabetologist review if >20mmol/L	

[1] Check glucose hourly and adjust insulin accordingly.
[2] ► Only use SC route if IV route is problematic as it is associated with much variability; check finger prick glucose every 2–4h if NBM—or pre-meals if using SC insulin to supplement other hypoglycaemics.

GKI infusions (glucose, K⁺ & insulin)

▶A problem when giving IV insulin and IV dextrose simultaneously through separate intravenous lines is that if one cannula becomes blocked, the patient may become hypo- or hyperglycaemic. If the glucose and insulin are given through the same cannula, however, and the 3-way converter becomes blocked, the syringe driver may retrogradely fill the infusion set with insulin. When the cannula is subsequently resited and the infusion restarted, the patient will receive this large accumulated dose of insulin. This has caused lethal hypoglycaemia, so some centres now use GKI infusions instead of sliding scales.

- A 500mL bag of 5% dextrose ± KCl is given over 6h, with a short-acting insulin (eg Actrapid®) added according to blood glucose:

Blood glucose (mmol/L)	Insulin dose (units/bag)	Serum K⁺ (mmol/L)	KCl to be added (mmol/bag)
<4	None	<3	20
4–6	5	3–5	10
6–10	10	>5	None
10–20	15		
>20	20		

- Check blood glucose every 3h. If levels too high or low, start a new 500mL bag of 5% dextrose with the correct insulin dose.
- Check U&E daily.

GKI infusions are useful when close monitoring of blood glucose is not possible, but may not be suitable in poorly controlled diabetes.

NB: regimens vary and sometimes more insulin will be required; eg if shocked, severely ill, or if on steroids or sympathomimetics, 2–4 times as much insulin may be needed. See BNF section 6.1.

Jaundiced patients undergoing surgery

Patients with obstructive jaundice are particularly prone to developing renal failure after surgery (the hepatorenal syndrome). This may be from the toxic effect of bilirubin on the kidney. In practice this means that a good urine output must be maintained in such patients around the time of surgery.

Pre-operative preparation Avoid morphine in the premedication.
- Insert IV line and run in 1L of 0.9% saline over 30–60min following pre-med (unless the patient has heart failure), to produce a moderate diuresis peri-operatively. A loop diuretic (eg frusemide (=furosemide)) may be needed to ensure a diuresis. Pre-op mannitol is no longer routine in jaundiced patients.
- Insert a urinary catheter.
- A 'renal' dose dopamine (2–5µg/kg/min) IVI *may* be indicated: remember there may be side-effects from any central line used, and from the drug:
  - Sepsis (immune dysfunction) – Arrhythmias – Gut and myocardial perfusion↓
  - Diuresis when hypovolaemic – Catabolism↑ – Gastric motility decreased
  - Pulmonary hypertension – Impaired hypoxic ventilatory responses
- Check clotting, and consider giving prophylactic vitamin K (p644) even if clotting function is normal.

During surgery
- Measure urine output hourly.
- Give 0.9% saline IV to match the urine output.

For 48h after surgery
- Measure urine output every 2h; measure urea and electrolytes daily.
- Give 0.9% saline at rate to match urine output and fluid lost through NGT; and give 2L of dextrose–saline every 24h.
- Give furosemide if urine output is poor despite adequate hydration.
- Give 20mmol of K⁺/L of fluid after 24h post-op if urine output good.

Surgery in those on steroids or anticoagulants

Steroids Patients may need extra steroid cover to cope with the stress of surgery. The amount of extra cover needed depends on the extent of the surgery and the pre-op dose of steroids. *Major surgery:* Typically give hydrocortisone 50–100mg IV with the pre-med and then every 8h IV/IM for 3d. Then return to previous medication. *Minor surgery:* Prepare as for major surgery except that hydrocortisone is given for 24h only. The major risk with adrenal insufficiency is hypotension, so if this is encountered without an obvious cause, it may be worthwhile giving a dose of 50mg hydrocortisone IV.

Those on stable long-term anticoagulants Contact your lab, and inform the surgeon and anaesthetist. Very minor surgery has been undertaken without stopping warfarin (check INR). In major surgery, drugs may be stopped for 2–5d pre-op. The risks and benefits are individual to each patient, so exact rules are impossible. Discuss these issues when arranging consent. Vitamin K or FFP may be needed in emergency surgery. One elective option is conversion to heparin (stop 6h prior to surgery, and monitor APTT perioperatively): unfractionated heparin's short $t_{1/2}$ allows swift reversal with protamine (p648). ►*Monitor clotting meticulously.*

Thyroid disease and surgery

Thyroid surgery for hyperthyroidism If severe, give carbimazole until euthyroid (p304). Arrange operation date and 10–14d before this, start aqueous iodine oral solution (Lugol's solution), 0.1–0.3mL/8h PO well diluted with milk or water. Continue until surgery.

Mild hyperthyroidism Start propranolol 80mg/8h PO and Lugol's solution as above at the 1ˢᵗ consultation. Stop Lugol's solution on the day of surgery but continue propranolol for 5d post-op.

Surgery in the obese

It has long been believed that obesity increases the risk of post-operative complications. Obesity has been shown to increase risks of cardiac and spinal surgery. Indeed, 50 years ago obesity was considered a contraindication to elective surgery.

A recent study has suggested, however, that obesity in itself may not be a risk factor for most complications. Overall incidence of complications after elective general surgery did not differ significantly between obese and non-obese patients, though only 1.7% of the 6336 patients in the trial had a BMI >40kg/m^2. The only post-operative complication found to have an increased incidence in the obese was wound infection after open surgery. Overall it would seem that the practice of forcing patients to lose weight prior to elective general surgery may be inappropriate.[1]

473

1 D Dindo 2003 Lancet 361 2032

The acute abdomen (X-RAY PLATE 1)

Someone who becomes acutely ill and in whom symptoms and signs are chiefly related to the abdomen has an acute abdomen. Prompt laparotomy is sometimes essential: *repeated examination is the key to making the decision.*

Clinical syndromes that usually require laparotomy

1 *Rupture of an organ* (Spleen, aorta, ectopic pregnancy) Shock (eg faints or BP↓ by ≥20mmHg on standing) is a leading sign. Abdominal swelling may be seen. Any history of trauma? Peritonism may be surprisingly mild. *Delayed* rupture of the spleen may occur weeks after trauma.

2 *Peritonitis* (Perforation of peptic ulcer, diverticulum, appendix, bowel, or gall bladder) Signs: prostration, shock, lying still, +ve cough test (p52), tenderness (± rebound/percussion pain, p82), board-like abdominal rigidity, guarding, and no bowel sounds. Erect CXR may show gas under the diaphragm (X-RAY PLATE 1). NB: *acute pancreatitis* (p478) causes these signs, but does *not* require a laparotomy—so always check serum amylase.

Syndromes that may not require a laparotomy

1 *Local peritonitis:* Eg diverticulitis, cholecystitis, salpingitis, and appendicitis. (The latter *will* need surgery.) If abscess formation is suspected (swelling, swinging fever, and WCC↑), arrange a diagnostic ultrasound or CT. Drainage can be percutaneous (ultrasound or CT guided), or by laparotomy. Look for 'a sentinel loop' on the plain AXR (p493).

2 *Colic* is a regularly waxing and waning pain, caused by muscular spasm in a hollow viscus, eg gut, ureter, uterus, or gall bladder (in the latter, pain is often dull and constant). Colic causes restlessness, unlike peritonitis.

Obstruction of the bowel See p492.

Tests U&E; FBC; amylase; LFT; CRP; urinoscopy; laparoscopy may avert open surgery. CT can be helpful *provided it is readily available and causes no delay;* 1 study found that early CT for an acute abdomen increases accuracy of diagnosis, while decreasing length of hospital stay and mortality. [a]

Pre-op care ►Do not rush to theatre. Anaesthesia compounds shock, so resuscitate properly first (p779) unless blood is being lost faster than it can be replaced in ruptured ectopic pregnancy, *OHCS* p24, or a leaking abdominal aneurysm, p480. Put to bed, then:

- Nil by mouth for ≥2h pre-op
- Relieve pain (p454)
- Blood culture
- Consent
- Plain x-ray[1]
- IVI (0.9% saline)
- CXR + ECG if >50yrs
- IV/PR antibiotics[2]
- Treat shock (p778)
- Crossmatch, eg 2U

The medical acute abdomen Irritable bowel syndrome (p248) is the chief cause, [a] so *always* ask about other episodes of pain associated with loose stools, relief by defecation, bloating, and urgency. Other causes:

Myocardial infarction	Pneumonia (p172)	Sickle-cell crisis (p640)
Gastroenteritis or UTI	Tabes (p601)	Phaeochromocytoma (p822)
Diabetes mellitus (p292)	Zoster (p568)	Malaria (p560)
Bornholm disease (p720)	Tuberculosis (p566)	Typhoid fever (p596)
Pneumococcal peritonitis	Porphyria (p708)	Cholera (p596)
Henoch–Schönlein (p726)	Thyroid storm (p820)	*Yersinia enterocolitica* (p593)
Narcotic addiction	PAN (p425)	Lead colic

Computer help Accuracy in diagnosing acute abdomen is ~45%; this is improvable to ~70–80% by using a computer, not because computers are so clever, but because they are so stupid—and rigid: they have no intuition, and they need clear answers to a full set of questions. They allow no escape. You have to take a proper history, and you have to conduct a careful examination. This enforced virtue accounts for most (but not all) of the improved performance when a computer is used.

---

1 Consider erect or decubitus films (but rarely helpful, in fact).
2 Give antibiotics if peritonitis, eg cefuroxime 1.5g/8h IV + metronidazole 500mg/8h IV/PR.

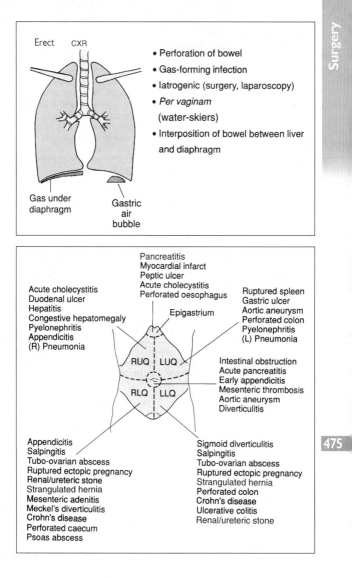

Erect CXR

- Perforation of bowel
- Gas-forming infection
- Iatrogenic (surgery, laparoscopy)
- *Per vaginam*
  (water-skiers)
- Interposition of bowel between liver
  and diaphragm

Gas under diaphragm

Gastric air bubble

Pancreatitis
Myocardial infarct
Peptic ulcer
Acute cholecystitis
Perforated oesophagus

Acute cholecystitis
Duodenal ulcer
Hepatitis
Congestive hepatomegaly
Pyelonephritis
Appendicitis
(R) Pneumonia

Epigastrium

Ruptured spleen
Gastric ulcer
Aortic aneurysm
Perforated colon
Pyelonephritis
(L) Pneumonia

RUQ | LUQ

RLQ | LLQ

Intestinal obstruction
Acute pancreatitis
Early appendicitis
Mesenteric thrombosis
Aortic aneurysm
Diverticulitis

Appendicitis
Salpingitis
Tubo-ovarian abscess
Ruptured ectopic pregnancy
Renal/ureteric stone
Strangulated hernia
Mesenteric adenitis
Meckel's diverticulitis
Crohn's disease
Perforated caecum
Psoas abscess

Sigmoid diverticulitis
Salpingitis
Tubo-ovarian abscess
Ruptured ectopic pregnancy
Strangulated hernia
Perforated colon
Crohn's disease
Ulcerative colitis
Renal/ureteric stone

Acute appendicitis

This is the most common surgical emergency (lifetime incidence: 6%).

Pathogenesis Gut organisms invade the appendix wall after lumen obstruction by lymphoid hyperplasia, faecolith, or filarial worms—or there may be impaired ability to prevent invasion, brought about by improved hygiene (so less exposure to gut pathogens). This 'hygiene hypothesis' explains the rise in appendicitis rates in the early 1900s and its later decline (as pathogen exposure dwindles further).

Symptoms As inflammation begins, there is central abdominal colic. Once peritoneum becomes inflamed, the pain shifts to the right iliac fossa and becomes more constant. Anorexia is almost invariable but vomiting rarely prominent. Constipation is usual. Diarrhoea may occur.

Signs	Lying still	Signs in the right iliac fossa:
Tachycardia	Foetor ± flushed	Tenderness, guarding (p72)
Fever 37.5–38.5°C	Coughing hurts	Rebound tenderness (p82)
Furred tongue	Shallow breaths	PR painful on right

Special tests: Rovsing's sign (pain more in the RIF than the LIF when the LIF is pressed). In women, do a vaginal examination: does she have salpingitis (+ve cervical excitation, OHCS p50)? CT (if diagnosis unclear: reduces -ve appendicectomy rate, but may cause fatal delay).[1]

Variations in the clinical picture ● The infant with watery diarrhoea and vomiting: appendicitis *may* be a complication of simple gastroenteritis.
● The boy with vague abdominal pain who will not eat his favourite food.
● The shocked, confused octogenarian who is not in pain.

Hints
● Don't rely on tests, eg WCC; CRP; urinoscopy; CT (may cause fatal delay).
● If the child is anxious, use his hand to press his belly.
● Do not ignore right-sided tenderness on rectal examination: it may be the only sign of appendicitis.
● Expect your diagnosis (both of 'appendicitis' and 'not appendicitis') to be wrong half the time. This means that those who seem not to have appendicitis should be re-examined often. Laparoscopy may be helpful.

Differential diagnosis	Cholecystitis	Crohn's disease
Ectopic pregnancy	Diverticulitis	Perforated ulcer
Mesenteric adenitis	Salpingitis	Food poisoning
Cystitis	Period pains	Meckel's diverticulitis

Treatment Prompt appendicectomy. Metronidazole 1g/8h + cefuroxime 1.5g/8h, 1 to 3 doses IV starting 1h pre-op,[2] reduces wound infections. Laparoscopic appendicectomy reduces recovery time and incidence of wound infections, but increases risk of intra-abdominal abscesses.

Complications Perforation (does not appear to cause later infertility in girls); appendix mass; appendix abscess.

An appendix mass may result when an inflamed appendix becomes covered with omentum. US/CT may help with the diagnosis. Some advocate early surgery, but initial management is usually conservative—NBM and antibiotics (eg cefuroxime 1.5g/8h IV and metronidazole 500mg/8h IV). Mark out the size of the mass and proceed to drainage if the mass develops into an abscess (see below). If the mass resolves some perform an interval (ie delayed) appendicectomy. Exclude colonic tumour unless too young for this to be a consideration.

An appendix abscess may result if an appendix mass fails to resolve. Signs of abscess formation include enlargement of the mass or if the patient gets more toxic (pain↑; temperature↑; pulse↑; WCC↑). Treatment usually involves drainage, either surgical or percutaneous (under radiological guidance). Antibiotics alone may bring about resolution, eg in >90% of children.

1 For a review of diagnosing suspected appendicitis, see EK Paulson 2003 *NEJM* **348** 236–42
2 More SE and resistance problems if >1 dose; *Drug Ther Bul* 2004 9

Appendicitis in pregnancy

Appendicitis occurs in ~1/1000 pregnancies. It is not commoner, but mortality is higher, especially from 20wks gestation. Perforation is commoner (15–20%), and increases fetal mortality from ~1.5% (for simple appendicitis) to ~30%. As pregnancy progresses, the appendix migrates, so pain is often less well localized, and signs of peritonism less obvious. ►Prompt assessment is vital; laparotomy should be performed by an experienced surgeon (*OHCS* p135).

Acute pancreatitis

►This unpredictable disease (overall mortality 10–15%) is usually managed on surgical wards, but because surgery is often not involved, it is easy to think that there is no acute problem: *there is*—due to self-perpetuating pancreatic inflammation (and of other retroperitoneal tissues). Litres of extracellular fluid are trapped in the gut, peritoneum, and retroperitoneum. There may be rapid progress from a phase of mild oedema to one of necrotizing pancreatitis. In fulminating cases, the pancreas is replaced by black fluid. Death may be from shock, renal failure, sepsis, or respiratory failure, with contributory factors being protease-induced activation of complement, kinin, and the fibrinolytic and coagulation cascades.

Causes 'GET SMASHED': Gallstones, Ethanol, Trauma, Steroids, Mumps, Autoimmune (PAN), Scorpion venom, Hyperlipidaemia (↑Ca^{2+}, hypothermia), ERCP, (also emboli), Drugs (eg azathioprine, asparaginase, mercaptopurine, pentamidine, didanosine, ?diuretics); also pregnancy. Often none found.

Symptoms Gradual or sudden severe *epigastric* or *central abdominal pain* (radiates to back); vomiting is prominent. Sitting forward may relieve pain.

Signs (may be mild in serious disease!) Tachycardia, fever, jaundice, shock, ileus, rigid abdomen ± local/generalized tenderness and periumbilical discolouration (Cullen's sign or, at the flanks, Grey Turner's sign).

Tests Serum amylase >1000U/mL (lesser rises in cholecystitis, mesenteric infarction, GI perforation, renal failure; *amylase may be normal even in severe pancreatitis as amylase starts to fall within the 1st 24–48h*). Serum lipase is more sensitive and specific for pancreatitis, and may eventually replace amylase measurement. Blood gases. Abdominal films: no psoas shadow (retroperitoneal fluid↑), 'sentinel loop' of proximal jejunum (solitary air-filled dilatation). Erect CXR helps exclude other causes that may cause perforation. CT helps assess severity. Ultrasound (if gallstones, AST↑ too). ERCP. *Differential diagnosis:* Any acute abdomen (p474), myocardial infarct.

Management Obtain expert help. Nil by mouth (may need NGT).
1 Set up IVI and give plasma expanders (eg Gelofusine®) and 0.9% saline until vital signs are satisfactory and urine flows at >30mL/h. If shocked or elderly, consider CVP. Insert a urinary catheter.
2 Analgesia: pethidine 75–100mg/4h IM, or morphine (a better analgesic, but *may* cause Oddi's sphincter to contract more) + prochlorperazine.
3 Hourly pulse, BP, and urine flow; daily FBC, U&E, Ca^{2+}, glucose, amylase, blood gas. Repeat ultrasound may show peripancreatic fluid.
4 If worsening, take to ITU. O_2 if P_aO_2↓. In suspected abscess formation or pancreatic necrosis (on contrast-enhanced CT), consider parenteral nutrition ± laparotomy & debridement. Antibiotics may help in *severe* disease.
5 ERCP + gallstone removal may be needed if there is progressive jaundice.

Prognosis (See BOX) C-reactive protein can be a helpful marker. Some patients suffer *recurrent oedematous pancreatitis* so often that near-total pancreatectomy is contemplated. Evidence is accumulating that 'oxidant' stress is important here, but initial clinical trials of free radical scavengers have been disappointing.

Complications—*Early:* Shock, ARDS (p190), *renal failure*, DIC, Ca^{2+}↓, (10mL of 10% calcium gluconate IV slowly is, rarely, necessary; albumin replacement has also been tried), *glucose*↑ (transient; 5% need insulin). *Later* (>1wk): *Pancreatic necrosis, pseudocyst* (fluid in lesser sac, eg at ≥6wks), with fever, a mass, and persistent ↑amylase/LFTs. It may resolve or need drainage, externally, or into the stomach (may be laparoscopically). *Abscesses* need draining. *Bleeding* is from elastase eroding a major vessel (eg splenic artery); embolization of the artery may be life-saving. *Thrombosis* may occur in the splenic and gastroduodenal arteries, or in the colic branches of the superior mesenteric artery (SMA), causing bowel necrosis.

Modified Glasgow criteria for predicting severity of pancreatitis

▶3 or more positive factors detected within 48h of onset suggest severe pancreatitis, and should prompt transfer to ITU.
Mnemonic: PANCREAS

- P_aO_2 <8kPa
- Age >55yrs
- Neutrophils: WBC >15 x 10^9/L
- Calcium <2mmol/L
- Renal function: Urea >16mmol/L
- Enzymes: LDH >600iu/L; AST >200iu/L
- Albumin <32g/L (serum)
- Sugar: blood glucose >10mmol/L.

These criteria have been validated for pancreatitis caused by gallstones and alcohol; Ranson's criteria are valid for alcohol-induced pancreatitis only.

Aneurysms and dissections of arteries

'True' aneurysms are abnormal dilatations of arteries. They should be distinguished from 'false' aneurysms, which are collections of blood around a vessel wall eg following trauma.

Aneurysms may be fusiform or sac-like (eg Berry aneurysms in the circle of Willis). Common sites: aorta, iliac, femoral, and popliteal arteries. Atheroma is the usual cause; also connective tissue disorders (eg Marfan's, Ehlers–Danlos), and infections (eg endocarditis, or tertiary syphilis).

Complications from aneurysms: rupture; thrombosis; embolism; pressure on other structures; infection.

Thoracic aorta dissection Blood splits aortic media with sudden tearing chest pain (±radiation to back). As dissection unfolds, branches of the aorta occlude leading sequentially to hemiplegia (carotid), unequal arm pulses and BP, paraplegia (anterior spinal artery), and anuria (renal arteries). Aortic incompetence and inferior MI may develop if dissection moves proximally. ▶▶*All patients with ascending aorta dissections should be considered for surgery:* get cardiological advice. • Crossmatch 10U blood; do ECG & CXR (expanded mediastinum is rare). • CT/MRI or transoesophageal echocardiography (TOE). Take to ITU; hypotensives: keep systolic at ~100–110mmHg: labetolol (p142) or esmolol (p129; $t_{\frac{1}{2}}$ is ultra-short) by IVI is helpful here. Perioperative mortality: ≤12%.

Ruptured abdominal aortic aneurysm (AAA) Death rates/year from ruptured AAAs rise with age: 125/million in those aged 55–59; 2728/million if over 85yrs.

Signs & symptoms: Intermittent or continuous abdominal pain (radiates to back, iliac fossae, or groins), collapse, and an *expansile* abdominal mass (ie the mass expands and contracts: swellings that are pulsatile merely transmit the pulse, eg nodes overlying arteries). The main differential diagnosis is pancreatitis. If in doubt, assume a ruptured aneurysm.

Management: ▶Summon a vascular surgeon and an experienced anaesthetist. Warn theatre. Put up several large IVIs. Treat shock with ORh−ve blood (if desperate), but keep systolic BP ≤100mmHg (but note: *raised* BP is common early on). Do an ECG, and take blood for amylase, Hb, crossmatch (10–40U may eventually be needed). Take the patient straight to theatre. Do not waste time doing x-rays: fatal delay may result, though CT can be helpful in a stable patient with an uncertain diagnosis. Catheterize the bladder. Give prophylactic antibiotics eg ampicillin + flucloxacillin—both 500mg IV. Surgery involves clamping the aorta above the leak, and inserting a Dacron® graft (eg 'tube graft' or, if significant iliac aneurysm also, a 'trouser graft' with each 'leg' attached to an iliac artery). Mortality—treated: 21–70%; untreated: 100%.

Unruptured AAA[1] Prevalence: 3% of those >50yrs. Often symptomless, they *may* cause abdominal/back pain. They may be discovered incidentally on abdominal examination (this misses ~⅓ of even quite big aneurysms). Trials suggest that aneurysms <5.5cm across might safely be monitored by regular examination and ultrasound/CT. Risk of rupture below this size is <1%/yr, compared with ~25%/yr for aneurysms >6cm across. Aneurysms larger than this, rapidly expanding (>1cm/yr) or symptomatic should be considered for elective surgery. It should be noted that ~75% of aneurysms monitored in this way will eventually need repair. Elective operative mortality is ~5%. Studies show that age >80yrs is NOT a reason to decline surgery.

Big operations can sometimes be avoided by inserting stented grafts via the femoral artery. When successfully positioned, such stents can lead to shorter hospital stays and fewer transfusions than with conventional surgery. Many patients are not suitable for such stents, however, because of the anatomy of their aneurysms. There is also a risk that the stent will leak.[1]

1 Further reading: PT O'Gara 2003 *Circulation* **107** e43

Population screening for AAAs

A number of recent studies have looked at the screening of asymptomatic patients in 'at-risk' groups for AAA. A multi-centre study showed that ultrasound screening of 65–74yr old men decreases mortality related to AAA. The cost per life-year gained was £28,400 after 4yrs, and is expected to drop to a quarter of this figure after 10yrs.[1]

One aspect of screening for AAA that is easily overlooked is the ~5% elective operative mortality associated with surgery. This makes informed consent (the Rees' rules, *OHCS* p430), a key issue in developing ultrasound-based screening of 'healthy' people.

1 Multi-centre aneurysm screening study (MASS) 2002 *BMJ* **325** 1135–8

Diverticular disease

A *diverticulum* is an outpouching of the wall of the gut. The term *diverticulosis* means that diverticula are present, whereas *diverticular disease* implies they are symptomatic. *Diverticulitis* refers to inflammation within a diverticulum. Although diverticula may be congenital or acquired and can occur in any part of the gut, by far the most important type are acquired colonic diverticula, to which this page refers.

Pathology Most occur in the sigmoid colon with 95% of complications at this site but right-sided diverticula do occur. Lack of dietary fibre is thought to lead to high intraluminal pressures which force the mucosa to herniate through the muscle layers of the gut. One-third of the population in the Western world has diverticulosis by the age of 60yrs.

Diagnosis *PR examination* (may reveal a pelvic abscess, or colorectal cancer, the chief competing diagnosis), *sigmoidoscopy, barium enema, colonoscopy.* CT may be more useful than ultrasound, and plain films may only be useful in showing vesical fistulae.

Complications of diverticulosis

1 *Painful diverticular disease:* There may be altered bowel habit; pain—usually colicky, left-sided, and relieved by defecation; nausea and flatulence. *A high-fibre diet* (wholemeal bread, fruit and vegetables, see p208) is usually prescribed. *Antispasmodics*, such as mebeverine, 135mg/8h PO may help. *Surgical resection* is occasionally resorted to.

2 *Diverticulitis*—with features above + pyrexia, WCC↑, ESR↑, and a tender colon, and there may be localized or generalized peritonism. Treatment: bed rest, NBM, IV fluids, and antibiotics: see BOX.

3 *Perforation:* There is ileus, peritonitis ± shock. *Mortality:* 40%. Manage as for an acute abdomen (p474). At laparotomy, a Hartman's procedure may be used (temporary colostomy + partial colectomy). It is sometimes possible to do colon lavage via the appendix stump, then immediate anastomosis (so avoiding repeat surgery to close the colostomy).

4 *Haemorrhage* is usually sudden and painless. It is a common cause of big rectal bleeds. Bleeding usually stops with bed rest. Transfusion may be needed. Embolization or colonic resection may be necessary after locating bleeding points by angiography or colonoscopy (here diathermy ± local epinephrine injections *may* obviate the need for surgery).

5 *Fistulae:* Colon–small bowel, or colon–vaginal, or colon–bladder (pneumaturia ± intractible UTIs). Treatment is surgical, eg colonic resection.

6 *Abscesses* eg with swinging fever, leucocytosis, and localizing signs eg boggy rectal mass (pelvic abscess—drain rectally). If no localizing signs, remember the aphorism: *pus somewhere, pus nowhere = pus under the diaphragm.* A subphrenic abscess is a horrible way to die, so do an *urgent* ultrasound. Antibiotics ± ultrasound-guided drainage may be needed.

7 *Post-infective strictures* may form in the sigmoid colon.

Angiodysplasia

Angiodysplasia refers to submucosal arteriovenous malformations that typically present as fresh PR bleeding in the elderly. The underlying aetiology is unknown. *Pathology:* 70–90% of lesions occur in the right colon, though angiodysplasia can affect anywhere in the gastrointestinal tract. *Diagnosis:* PR examination, barium enema, colonoscopy may exclude competing diagnoses; [99mTc] radionucleotide imaging is useful to identify lesions during active bleeding. Mesenteric angiography is particularly helpful in diagnosing angiodysplasia, and allows therapeutic embolization during active bleeding. CT angiography offers a non-invasive alternative. *Treatment:* Options include embolization, endoscopic laser/electrocoagulation, and surgical resection of the affected bowel.

Managing diverticulitis[1]

▶Beware diverticulitis in immunocompromised patients (eg on steroids) who often have few symptoms, and may present late.

- Mild attacks can be treated at home with bowel rest (fluids only) + co-amoxiclav (p543, or metronidazole 400mg/8h PO, or ciprofloxacin).
- If oral fluids cannot be tolerated or pain cannot be controlled, admit to hospital for bed rest, NBM, IV fluids and antibiotics eg cefuroxime 1.5g/8h IV with metronidazole 500mg/8h IV/PR, until the results of cultures are available. Avoid morphine as this aggravates colonic spasm. Most settle on this regimen but there may be abscess formation (necessitating drainage) or perforation. The latter requires peritoneal lavage and formation of a proximal colostomy. The perforation may be resected at the 1st operation or later. Mortality following perforation approaches 40%.

Surgery: The need for surgery is reflected by the degree of infective complications, which may be classified thus:

Stage 1: small confined pericolonic abscesses: *surgery rarely needed.*

Stage 2: larger abscesses: *may resolve without surgery.*

Stage 3: generalized suppurative peritonitis: *surgery required.*

Stage 4: faecal peritonitis: *surgery required.*

- For severe or recurrent diverticulitis: ~20% will require surgery.
- Elective sigmoid resection after medical management can be a 1-stage (eg laparoscopic) procedure.
- Emergency colonic resection is usually a 2-stage procedure (initially resection of diseased segment and end colostomy and oversewing of stump—Hartman's procedure; later closure of colostomy).

---

1 For a review on acute diverticulitis, see LB Ferzoco 1998 *NEJM* **338** 1521

Gallstones

Bile contains cholesterol, bile pigments (from broken down Hb), and phospholipids. If the concentrations of these vary, different kinds of stones may be formed. *Pigment stones:* Small, friable, and irregular. Causes: haemolysis. *Cholesterol stones:* Large, often solitary. Causes: female sex, age, obesity. *Mixed stones:* Faceted (calcium salts, pigment, & cholesterol). *Gallstone prevalence:* 8% of those over 40yrs. 90% remain asymptomatic. *Risk factors for stones becoming symptomatic:* smoking; parity. Stones may cause acute or chronic cholecystitis, biliary colic, pancreatitis, or obstructive jaundice (p222).

Acute cholecystitis follows stone impaction in the neck of the gall bladder (GB), which may cause continuous epigastric or RUQ pain, vomiting, fever, local peritonism, or a GB mass. The main difference from biliary colic is the inflammatory component (local peritonism, fever, WCC↑). If the stone moves to the CBD, jaundice may occur.

Murphy's sign: Lay 2 fingers over the RUQ. Ask the patient to breathe in. This causes pain and arrest of inspiration as an inflamed GB impinges on your fingers. It is only +ve if the same test in the LUQ does not cause pain. *Tests:* WCC, ultrasound (thickened GB wall, pericholecystic fluid, and stones), HIDA cholescintigraphy (useful if diagnosis uncertain after ultrasound). Gallstones are only radio-opaque on plain abdominal films in ~10% of cases.

Treatment: NBM, pain relief, IVI, and antibiotics (eg cefuroxime 1.5g/8h IV). In suitable candidates, do cholecystectomy (laparoscopic if no question of GB perforation) within 72h; early surgery is associated with fewer complications and lower conversion rates to open cholecystectomy. *Mortality:* <1%. If delayed, relapse occurs in 18%. Otherwise, operate after 6–12wks. In elderly or high-risk patients unsuitable for surgery, percutaneous cholecystostomy may be useful; cholecystectomy can still be performed at a later date. Cholecystostomy is also the treatment of choice for acalculous cholecystitis.

Chronic cholecystitis Stones cause chronic inflammation ± colic. Vague abdominal discomfort, distension, nausea, flatulence, and intolerance of fats may also be caused by reflux, ulcers, irritable bowel syndrome, relapsing pancreatitis, or tumour (stomach, pancreas, colon, GB).

Ultrasound is used to image stones, and to assess common bile duct (CBD) diameter. MRCP (p229) is increasingly being used to check for stones in the CBD.

Treatment: Cholecystectomy (eg laparoscopic). If ultrasound shows a dilated CBD with stones, ERCP (p229) with sphincterotomy is used to remove stones, usually prior to surgery. No comparative trials favour lithotripsy.

Biliary colic RUQ pain (radiates to back) ± jaundice. *Treatment:* Pain control: morphine[1], eg 5–10mg IM/4h + antiemetic. Elective cholecystectomy. *Differential diagnosis* can be hard as the above may overlap. Urinoscopy, CXR, and ECG help exclude other diseases. *Other presentations:*

- *Obstructive jaundice with CBD stones*—ERCP with sphincterotomy then cholecystectomy may be needed, or open surgery with CBD exploration (if there is no obstruction/cholangitis, a stone-trapping basket on the end of a choledochoscope introduced through the cystic duct at laparoscopy can be done as part of laparoscopic cholecystectomy).
- *Cholangitis* (bile duct infection) causing RUQ pain, jaundice, and rigors. Treat with eg cefuroxime 1.5g/8h IV and metronidazole 500mg/8h PR.
- *Gallstone ileus:* A stone perforates the GB, entering the duodenum; it may then obstruct the terminal ileum. X-ray: air in CBD, small bowel fluid levels, and a stone. Duodenal obstruction is rarer (Bouveret's syndrome).
- *Pancreatitis* • *Empyema:* The obstructed GB fills with pus.
- *Silent stones:* Some advise elective surgery. Dissolution of cholesterol stones by oral ursodeoxycholic acid is expensive, and often causes diarrhoea.

---

1 Morphine is a better analgesic than pethidine, but may cause more Oddi sphincter contraction, p478.

Complications of gallstones

1 In the gall bladder
  Biliary colic
  Acute and chronic cholecystitis
  Empyema
  Mucocele
  Carcinoma
2 In the bile ducts
  Obstructive jaundice
  Pancreatitis
  Cholangitis
3 In the gut
  Gallstone ileus

Diseases having biliary complications

Causes of cholecystitis and biliary symptoms, other than gallstones, are
rare, eg:
- Infections:
  - Typhoid   - Brucellosis   - Ascariasis
  - Cryptosporidiosis, p556   - Opisthorchiasis
- Complications of parenteral nutrition
- Polyarteritis nodosa (p425)
- Hormonal: release of cholecystokinin
- Structural abnormality of the cystic duct
- High pressure spincter of Oddi.

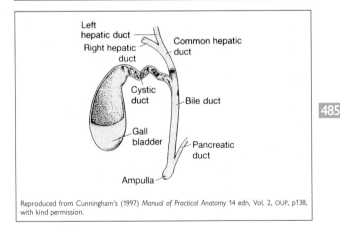

Reproduced from Cunningham's (1997) *Manual of Practical Anatomy* 14 edn, Vol. 2, OUP, p138,
with kind permission.

Gangrene and necrotizing fasciitis

Gangrene is death of tissue from poor vascular supply. Tissues are black and may slough. If tissue death and infection occur together, *wet gangrene* exists. *Dry gangrene* means death with *no* infection. Note a line of demarcation between living and dead tissue. Take cultures; look out for group A streptococci (a cause of Fournier's- or Meleney's-type gangrene, a rapidly progressive necrotizing fasciitis or myositis). ▶*In any atypical cellulitis, get prompt surgical help*. Radical debridement (eg preserving a skin flap) ± amputation is needed, always covered by antibiotics, including eg 5 days of IV benzylpenicillin 600mg/6h starting 1h pre-op, to prevent gas gangrene (± clindamycin 0.6–1.2g/6h IVI/IM). Get the help of a plastic surgeon. Remember TB in any necrotizing infection.

Gas gangrene is a *Clostridium perfringens* myositis. Risk factors: diabetes, trauma, malignancy. Toxaemia, delirium, and haemolytic jaundice occur early. There is oedema, crepitus (usually), and bubbly brown pus. *Treatment:* Remove all dead tissue (eg amputation); benzylpenicillin. Hyperbaric O_2, clindamycin (900mg/6h) & metronidazole have a role.

Skin ulcers

Ulcers are abnormal breaks in an epithelial surface. *Causes of skin ulcers:* Venous disease, peripheral arterial disease, neuropathy, diabetes (ulcers can be neuropathic and/or ischaemic), vasculitis, infection (eg TB, esp. *Mycobacteria ulcerans*, the cause of Buruli ulcer), malignancy (eg squamous or basal cell carcinoma, p430), sickle-cell anaemia, pyoderma gangrenosum (p428), trauma. *The history:* ask about number, pain, and trauma; is the history long or short? Is the patient taking steroids? Is the patient a bit odd? (remember self-induced ulcers: *dermatitis artefacta*). Has a biopsy been taken? *Examination:* note features such as *site*, *surface area, edge, base, discharge, lymphadenopathy, sensation*, and *healing*.

Site Above the medial malleolus is the favourite place for *gravitational ulcers* (mostly related to superficial venous disease, but may reflect venous hypertension via damage to the valves of the deep venous system, eg 2° to DVT). Venous hypertension leads to the development of superficial varicosities and skin changes (lipodermatosclerosis = induration, pigmentation, and inflammation of the skin of the lower leg). Minimal trauma to the leg leads to ulceration which often takes many months to heal.

Ulcers on the sacrum or greater trochanter suggests *pressure sores* (OHCS p597), particularly if the patient is bed-bound with suboptimal nutrition.

Surface area Draw a map of the area to quantify and time any healing.

Shape Oval, *circular* (cigarette burns), *serpiginous* (granuloma inguinale, p586); *scrofuloderma* (*tuberculosis colliquativa cutis*).

Edge Eroded ≈ active and spreading; shelved/sloping ≈ healing; punched-out ≈ syphilis; rolled/everted ≈ malignant.

Base Any muscle, bone, or tendon destruction (malignancy; pressure sores)?

Discharge Culture before starting any antibiotics (which usually don't work). A watery discharge is said to favour TB; bleeding ≈ malignancy.

Associated lymphadenopathy This suggests infection or malignancy.

Sensation Decreased sensation around the ulcer implies neuropathy.

Position in phases of extension/healing Healing is heralded by granulation, scar formation, and epithelialization. Inflamed margins ≈ extension.

▶Managing ulcers is often difficult. Treat the cause. Optimize nutrition. Are there adverse risk factors (drug addiction, or risk factors for arteriopathy, eg smoking etc)? Get expert nursing care. Consider referral to community nurse, varicose leg ulcer clinic: 'Charing-cross' 4-layer compression bandaging may help (if arterial pulses OK: ankle : brachial pressure index should be greater than 0.8) and is better than standard bandages.

Ischaemia of the gut

►AF with abdominal pain should suggest the idea of bowel ischaemia.

Acute small bowel ischaemia[63] This may follow superior mesenteric artery (SMA) embolism or thrombosis, low flow states or mesenteric vein thrombosis. Embolism is now uncommon and thrombosis is the commonest cause of acute ischaemia. Low flow states usually reflect poor cardiac output but there may be other factors such as DIC. Venous thrombosis is uncommon and tends to affect smaller lengths of bowel.

A classical clinical triad: Acute severe abdominal pain; no abdominal signs; and rapid hypovolaemia (causing shock). Pain tends to be constant and central, or around the right iliac fossa. The degree of illness is often out of proportion to the clinical signs. *Tests:* There may be Hb↑ (due to plasma loss), WCC↑, modestly raised plasma amylase, and a persistent metabolic acidosis. Early on the abdominal x-ray shows a 'gasless' abdomen. Arteriography helps but many diagnoses are made at laparotomy. CT/MR angiography may provide a non-invasive alternative to conventional arteriography. *Treatment:* Fluid replacement, antibiotics (gentamicin + metronidazole, p547) and, usually, heparin. If arteriography is performed, thrombolytics may be infused locally via the catheter. At surgery dead bowel must be removed. Revascularization may be attempted on potentially viable bowel but is difficult and often needs a second laparotomy. *Prognosis:* Poor (<20% survive).

Chronic intestinal ischaemia This relative rarity is classified into *small bowel* or *colonic* ischaemia. *Small bowel ischaemia* may be acute or chronic and is typically due to SMA disease. Less common causes of ischaemia include vasculitis (p424), trauma, radiotherapy, and strangulation, eg hernias. It presents quite a different picture to acute ischaemia, with severe, colicky postprandial abdominal pain ('gut claudication') with PR bleeding ± ↓weight (food hurts). It is difficult to diagnose but, following angiography, surgery may be helpful.

Colonic ischaemia usually follows low flow in the inferior mesenteric artery territory. *Presentation:* Lower left-sided abdominal pain and bloody diarrhoea. There may be pyrexia, tachycardia, blood per rectum, and a leucocytosis. Usually this 'ischaemic colitis' resolves, but it may progress to gangrenous ischaemic colitis. *Tests:* Barium enema may show 'thumb-printing' indentation of the barium due to submucosal swelling. Symptoms may be mild and result in stricture formation. *Treatment:* This is usually conservative with fluid replacement and antibiotics. Most recover but strictures are common.

Gangrenous ischaemic colitis This may follow ischaemic colitis and is signalled by more severe pain, peritonitis, and hypovolaemic shock. After resuscitation, necrotic bowel should be resected and a colostomy formed.

Volvulus (rotation) of the stomach

If the stomach twists, the classical triad of gastro-oesophageal obstruction may occur: vomiting (then non-productive retching), pain, and failed attempts to pass an NG tube. Regurgitation of saliva also occurs. Dysphagia and noisy gastric peristalsis (relieved by lying down) may occur in chronic volvulus.

Risk factors *Congenital:* Paraoesophageal hernia, congenital bands, bowel malformations, pyloric stenosis. *Acquired:* Gastric/oesophageal surgery.

Tests Look for gastric dilatation and a double fluid level on erect films.

Treatment If acutely unwell, arrange prompt resuscitation and laparotomy. In organoaxial volvulus, rotation is typically 180° left to right, about a line joining the relatively fixed pylorus and oesophagus. Mesenteroaxial rotation is at right angles to this line (and is from right to left). Laparoscopic management may be possible.[64]

Arterial supply of the colon

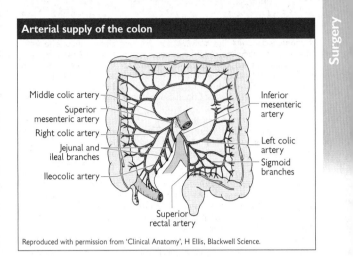

Middle colic artery
Superior mesenteric artery
Right colic artery
Jejunal and ileal branches
Ileocolic artery
Inferior mesenteric artery
Left colic artery
Sigmoid branches
Superior rectal artery

Reproduced with permission from 'Clinical Anatomy', H Ellis, Blackwell Science.

Limb embolism and ischaemia

Chronic ischaemia This is 'always' due to atherosclerosis. Its chief feature is intermittent claudication (from the Latin, meaning *to limp*). Cramping pain is felt in the calf, thigh, or buttock after walking for a fairly fixed distance (the *claudication distance*). *Ulceration, gangrene,* and foot pain *at rest*, eg burning pain at night relieved by hanging legs over side of bed are cardinal features of critical ischaemia. Buttock claudication ± impotence imply Leriche's syndrome (p728).

Signs: Absent pulses; cold, white leg(s); atrophic skin; punched out ulcers (often painful); postural colour change. *Tests:* Exclude DM, arteritis (ESR/CRP). Do FBC (anaemia, infection); U&E (renal disease); lipids (dyslipidaemia); syphilis serology; ECG (cardiac ischaemia). Do clotting and group & save if planning arteriography. *Ankle—brachial pressure index (Doppler):* Normal ≈ 1. Claudication ≈ 0.9–0.6. Rest pain ≈ 0.3–0.6. Impending gangrene ≤0.3 or ankle systolic pressure <50mmHg. Do *arteriography, digital subtraction arteriography* or *colour duplex imaging* to assess the extent and location of stenoses and the quality of distal vessels ('*run off*'). If *only* distal obliterative disease is seen, and little proximal atheroma, suspect arteritis, previous embolus, or diabetes mellitus.

Management: Many claudicants improve with *conservative treatment*, ie quit smoking, ↓weight, more exercise—ideally a supervised exercise programme. Treat diabetes, hypertension (avoid β-blockers), and hyperlipidaemia. Aspirin has a role. Vasodilators rarely help.

Percutaneous transluminal angioplasty is good for short stenoses in big arteries (a balloon is inflated in the narrowed segment). Stents maintain artery patency after angioplasty, and are beneficial for iliac artery disease. If atheromatous disease is extensive but distal run off is good (ie distal arteries filled by collateral vessels), he may be a candidate for *arterial reconstruction* by a bypass graft. Vein grafts are often used but prosthetic grafts are an option. Aspirin helps prosthetic grafts to remain patent; warfarin may be better after vein grafts and in high-risk patients.

Sympathectomy (chemical or surgical) may help relieve rest pain. It may not be appropriate in diabetic patients with peripheral neuropathy.

Amputation may relieve intractable pain and death from sepsis and gangrene. The decision to amputate must be made by the patient, usually against a background of failed alternative strategies. The level of amputation must be high enough to ensure healing of the stump. Rehabilitation should be started early with a view to limb fitting.

Acute ischaemia This may be due to thrombosis *in situ* (eg in ~41%), emboli (38%), graft/angioplasty occlusion (15%), or trauma. There is little difference in presenting signs. Mortality: 22%. Amputation rate: 16%.

Signs/symptoms: 6 Ps—the part is **p**ale, **p**ulseless, **p**ainful, **p**aralysed, **p**araesthetic, and '**p**erishing with cold'. Onset of fixed mottling implies irreversibility. Emboli commonly arise from the heart (infarcts, AF) or an aneurysm (aorta, femoral, or popliteal). ▶The limb may be red, but only when dependent, leading to disastrous misdiagnosis of gout or cellulitis.

Management: ▶This is an emergency and may require urgent open surgery or angioplasty. If diagnosis is in doubt, do urgent arteriography. If the occlusion is embolic, the options are surgical embolectomy (Fogarty catheter) or local thrombolysis, eg t-PA (p645). Anticoagulate with heparin after either procedure. Later, look for the emboli's source: echocardiogram; ultrasound of aorta, popliteal and femoral arteries. Ischaemia following trauma and acute thrombosis may require urgent reconstruction.

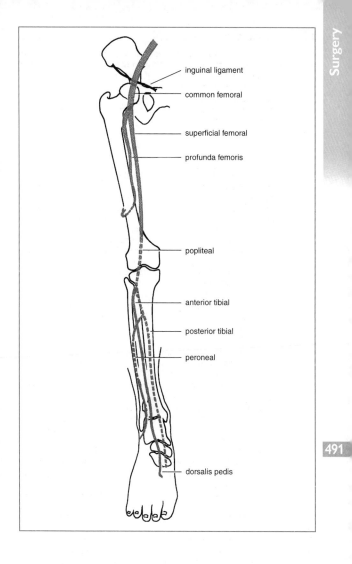

inguinal ligament

common femoral

superficial femoral

profunda femoris

popliteal

anterior tibial

posterior tibial

peroneal

dorsalis pedis

Obstruction of the bowel (X-RAY PLATE 3)

Features of obstruction Anorexia, nausea, vomiting with relief. Colicky abdominal pain with distension. Constipation need not be absolute (ie *no* faeces or flatus passed) if obstruction is high. Active, 'tinkling' bowel sounds. For the features of gastric volvulus, see p488.

On AXR (plain abdominal x-ray) look for abnormal gas patterns (gas in the fundus of stomach and throughout the large bowel is normal). On erect AXR look for horizontal fluid levels.

The key decisions

1 *Is the obstruction of the small or large bowel?* In small bowel obstruction, vomiting occurs earlier, distension is less, pain is higher in the abdomen. *The AXR (see BOX) plays a key role in diagnosis.* In small bowel obstruction, AXR shows central gas shadows and no gas in the large bowel. Small bowel is identified by valvulae conniventes that completely cross the lumen (large bowel haustral folds do *not* cross all the lumen's width).

   In large bowel obstruction, pain is more constant; AXR shows gas proximal to the block (eg in caecum) but not in the rectum. If the ileocaecal valve is competent, pain may be felt over a distended caecum (see below).

2 *Is there ileus* (functional obstruction due to reduced bowel motility) or *mechanical obstruction?* In ileus there is no pain; bowel sounds are absent.

3 *Is the bowel strangulated?* Signs: the patient is more ill than you would expect. There is a sharper and more constant pain than the central colicky pain of the obstruction and it tends to be localized. Peritonism is the cardinal sign. There may be fever and WCC↑.

Causes *Small bowel:* Adhesions, hernias external/internal, intussusception, Crohn's, gallstone ileus, tumour, foreign body (eg smuggled cocaine), TB.
Large bowel: Tumour, sigmoid or caecal volvulus, faeces, diverticulitis.

Management • *General principles:* The site, speed of onset, and completeness of obstruction determine therapy. Strangulation and large bowel obstruction require surgery soon. Paralytic ileus and incomplete small bowel obstruction can be managed conservatively, at least initially.

• *Conservative options:* Pass NGT and give IV fluids to rehydrate and correct electrolyte imbalance, see p462—ie 'drip and suck'.

• *Surgery:* Strangulation requires emergency surgery, as does 'closed loop obstruction'—large bowel obstruction with tenderness over a grossly dilatated caecum (>8cm), which occurs when the ileocaecal valve remains competent despite bowel distension. Usually large volumes of IV fluid must be given. For less urgent large bowel obstruction, there is time for an enema to try to clear the obstruction and to correct fluid imbalance.

Sigmoid volvulus occurs when the bowel twists on the mesentery and can produce severe, rapid strangulated obstruction. There is a characteristic AXR with an 'inverted U' loop of bowel. It tends to occur in the elderly, constipated patient, and is often managed by sigmoidoscopy and insertion of a flatus tube, but sigmoid colectomy is sometimes required. For gastric volvulus, see p488.

Pseudo-obstruction is like mechanical GI obstruction but no cause for obstruction is found. *Predisposing factors:* Malignancy, electrolyte disturbances (eg ↓K⁺), recent surgery. *Presentation:* There is nausea and post-prandial bloating. Acute colonic pseudo-obstruction is called Ogilvie's syndrome (p732). *Treatment:* Manage conservatively. Neostigmine or colonoscopic decompression are sometimes useful in acute cases. Weight loss is a problem in chronic pseudo-obstruction.

▶There is a case for investigating the cause by colonoscopy or water-soluble contrast enema in most instances of suspected mechanical obstruction.

Plain abdominal films (X-RAY PLATE 1 & 3)

These are rarely diagnostic, and are non-contributory in most mild or moderate instances of abdominal pain. They may help in GI obstruction. Gas pattern is best seen on supine images. Occasionally surgeons may prefer erect films to demonstrate fluid levels. Free intraperitoneal gas (signifying perforation) is best seen on erect CXRs when it is subdia-phragmatic (p475). Small bowel is recognized by its central position and valvulae conniventes, which reach from one wall to the other. Large bowel is more peripheral and the folds go only part of the way across the lumen.

Where to look:

1 Gas patterns: *Look for:* An abnormal quantity of gas in the stomach, small intestine, or colon. Normal diameter of the small intestine is 2.5cm, of the colon 5cm. Dilated small intestine occurs with obstruction and paralytic ileus. Dilated large bowel occurs with both these causes but also consider toxic dilatation in someone who is really sick—and, in the elderly, benign hypotonicity.

  Local peritoneal inflammation can cause localized ileus (a sentinel loop of intraluminal gas) and gives a clue to the site of pathology.

Cholecystitis		Pancreatitis
Appendicitis		Diverticulitis

  Gas outside the lumen: You must explain any gas outside the stomach, small intestine, and colon. It could be a pneumoperitoneum, or gas in the urinary tract or biliary tree.

2 Biliary tree and right urinary tract. The ureter passes near the tips of the lumbar transverse processes, crosses the sacro-iliac joint, down to the ischial spine, and turns medially to join the bladder. *Look for:* Calcification in the gall bladder, kidney, or ureter.

3 Left urinary tract: *Look for:* Calcification in the left kidney or ureter.

4 Bones: *Look for:* Scoliosis, degenerative disease, metastatic deposits (osteolytic or osteoblastic), Paget's disease.

5 Soft tissues: *Look for:* Size/position of: liver, spleen, kidneys, bladder.

Don't expect too many answers from the plain abdominal films. Develop and rely on your clinical skills. Remember that at the end of the day the most common diagnosis for abdominal pain is abdominal pain of unknown origin. Think of the major pathologies.

Some paediatric surgical emergencies

Congenital hypertrophic pyloric stenosis ▶See *OHCS* p198. This usually presents not at birth but in the first 3–8wks as projectile vomiting. ♂: ♀ ≈ 4 : 1. The baby is malnourished and always hungry and the diagnosis is made by palpating the pyloric mass in the RUQ during a feed. There may also be visible gastric peristalsis passing from the LUQ. The baby can be severely alkalotic and depleted of water and electrolytes. This needs correcting *before* surgery. Pass an NGT (p743). *Treatment:* Ramstedt's pyloromyotomy which involves incision of the muscle down to the mucosa.

Intussusception The small bowel telescopes, as if it were swallowing itself by invagination. *Presentation:* Patients may be any age (usually 5–12 months) presenting with *episodic* intermittent inconsolable crying, with drawing the legs up (colic) ± bilious vomiting. He may (but need not) pass blood PR (like redcurrant jam or merely flecks: do a PR). A sausage-shaped abdominal mass may be felt. He may become shocked, and moribund. *Tests/Management:* The least invasive approach is ultrasound with reduction by air enema (preferred to barium). Pneumatic reduction, by passing a balloon catheter PR under radiographic control, is another option that is effective in up to 80% of patients. CT may be problematic, and is less available. Plain abdominal films may be reserved for when perforation is suspected. Doppler studies to show bowel viability have been used but are non-standard. If reduction by enema fails, surgical reduction is needed. Any necrotic bowel should be resected.

Pre-op care: ▶▶Resuscitate, crossmatch blood, pass nasogastric tube. NB: children >4yrs present differently: rectal bleeding is less common, and they are more likely to have a long history (>3wks) and some sort of contributing pathology, eg Henoch–Schönlein purpura, cystic fibrosis, Peutz–Jeghers' syndrome[?], ascariasis, nephrotic syndrome or tumours such as lymphomas—in the latter, obstructive symptoms caused by intussusception are the most frequent mode of presentation. Recurrence rate: ~5%.

Torsion of the testis

The aim is to recognize this condition before the cardinal signs and symptoms are fully manifest, as prompt surgery saves testes.

▶If in any doubt, surgery is required.

Symptoms: Sudden onset of pain in one testis, which makes walking uncomfortable. (Pain in the abdomen, nausea, and vomiting are common.)

Signs: Inflammation of one testis—it is tender, hot, and swollen. The testis may lie high and transversely. Torsion may occur at any age but is most common at 11–30yrs.

Tests: Doppler USS (may demonstrate lack of blood flow to testis) and isotope scanning may be useful, but must not delay surgical exploration.

Treatment: ▶Ask consent for possible orchidectomy + *bilateral* fixation (orchidopexy). At surgery expose and untwist the testis. If its colour looks good, return it to the scrotum and fix *both* testes to the scrotum.

Differential diagnosis: The main one is epididymitis but here the patient tends to be older, there may be symptoms of urinary infection, infected urine, and more gradual onset of pain. Also consider tumour, trauma, and an acute hydrocoele. NB: *torsion of the hydatid of Morgagni*—remnants of the Müllerian ducts—occurs a little earlier, and causes less pain (the patient can often walk with no pain, unlike in testicular torsion)—and its tiny blue nodule may be discernible under the scrotum. It is thought to be due to the surge in gonadotrophins which signal the onset of puberty.[?] *Idiopathic scrotal oedema* is a benign condition, and is differentiated from torsion by the absence of pain and tenderness.[?]

Urinary retention & benign prostatic hyperplasia

Retention means not emptying the bladder (·.· obstruction or ↓detrusor power).

Acute retention The bladder is usually tender, containing ~600mL of urine. The cause in men is usually prostatic obstruction, eg precipitated by anticholinergics, 'holding on', constipation, pain, anaesthetics, alcohol, infection (p262). *Questions to detect obstruction:* see p52.

Examine: Abdomen, PR, perineal sensation (cauda equina compression).

Investigations: MSU, U&E, FBC, and prostate-specific antigen (PSA) (p705).[1] Renal ultrasound if renal impairment.

Tricks to aid voiding: Analgesia, privacy on hospital wards, ambulation, standing to void, voiding to the sound of running taps—or in a hot bath.

If the tricks fail: Catheterize (p746) and try a *prostate procedure* (below). After eg 7d, try a *trial without catheter* may work (esp. if <75yrs old or <1L drained or retention was triggered by a passing event, eg general anaesthesia).

Prevention: Finasteride, below, reduces prostate size and retention risk.

Chronic retention is more insidious. Bladder capacity may be >1.5L. Presentation: overflow incontinence, acute on chronic retention, a lower abdominal mass, UTI, or renal failure. Prostatic enlargement is the common cause. Others: pelvic malignancy; rectal surgery; DM; CNS disease eg transverse myelitis/MS; zoster (S2–S4). ►Only catheterize the patient if there is pain, urinary infection, or renal impairment (eg urea >12mmol/L). Institute definitive treatment promptly. Intermittent self-catheterization is sometimes required (p746).

Catheters and catheterization See p746. **Prostate cancer** p498.

Benign prostatic hypertrophy (BPH) is common (24% if aged 40–64; if older, 40%). ↓Urine flow (eg <15mL/s) is associated with frequency, urgency (►p52) and voiding difficulty. *Managing BPH:*

History: severity of symptoms and impact on life. Rectal examination.
Effect on bladder/kidneys: ultrasound (residual volume↑, hydronephrosis).
U&E: renal function.
MSU: rule out infection.
Rule out cancer: PSA[1], transrectal ultrasound ± biopsy. Then consider:

1 *Transurethral resection of the prostate* (TURP, a common operation; ≤14% become impotent). Crossmatch 2U. Consider perioperative antibiotics, eg cefuroxime 1.5g/8h IV, three doses. Beware excessive bleeding post-op and clot retention. ~20% of TURPs need redoing within 10yrs.

2 *Transurethral incision of the prostate* (TUIP) involves less destruction than TURP, and less risk to sexual function, while achieving similar clinical improvement in symptoms. It achieves its effect by relieving pressure on the urethra. It is perhaps the best surgical option for those with small glands <30g—ie ~50% of those operated on in some areas.

3 *Retropubic prostatectomy* is an open operation.

4 *Transurethral laser-induced prostatectomy* (TULIP).

5 *Drugs* may be useful in mild disease, and while awaiting TURP, eg:
  • α-blockers: eg *tamsulosin* 400µg/24h PO; alternatives: alfuzosin, doxazosin, terazosin. These ↓smooth muscle tone (prostate *and* bladder). SE: drowsiness, depression; dizziness; BP↓; dry mouth; ejaculatory failure; extrapyramidal signs; nasal congestion; weight↑. They are the drugs of choice.
  • 5α-reductase inhibitors: *finasteride*[2] (5mg/d PO ↓testosterone's conversion to dihydrotestosterone). It is excreted in semen, so warn to use condoms; ♀: avoid handling crushed pills. SE: impotence; libido↓. Effects on prostate size are limited and slow, so, if α-blockers fail, many try surgery next.

6 *Wait and see* is an option, but risks incontinence, retention, and renal failure.

---

1 Do venepuncture for PSA *before* PR, as PR can ↑total PSA by ~1ng/mL (free PSA ↑by 10%)[@10565747]
2 Finasteride can prevent retention but has odd effects on risk of prostate cancer. The PCPT trial (N= 18882) showed a ↓risk of indolent cancers, but ↑risk of Gleason >7 (p498). P Scardino *NEJM* 2003

Advice for patients concerning transurethral prostatectomy

Pre-op consent issues may centre on risks of the procedure, eg:

- Haematuria/haemorrhage
- Haematospermia
- Hypothermia
- Urethral trauma/stricture
- Post TURP syndrome (T°↓; Na⁺↓)
- Infection; prostatitis
- Impotence ~10%
- Incontinence ≤10%
- Clot retention near strictures
- Retrograde ejaculation (common)

Post-operative advice:

- Avoid driving for 2wks after the operation.
- Avoid sex for 2wks after surgery. Then get back to normal. The amount ejaculated may be reduced (as it flows backwards into the bladder—harmless, but may cloud the urine). It means you may be infertile. Impotence may be a problem after TURP, but do not expect this: in some men, erections improve. Rarely, orgasmic sensations are reduced.
- Expect to pass blood in the urine for the first 2wks. A small amount of blood colours the urine bright red. Do not be alarmed.
- At first you may need to urinate *more* frequently than before. Do not be despondent. In 6wks things should be much better—but the operation cannot be guaranteed to work (8% fail, and lasting incontinence is a problem in 6%; 12% may need repeat TURPs within 8yrs, compared with 1.8% of men undergoing open prostatectomy).
- If feverish, or if urination hurts, take a sample of urine to your doctor.

Urinary tract malignancies

Renal cell carcinoma (hypernephroma, Grawitz tumour) arises from the proximal renal tubular epithelium.

Epidemiology: 90% of renal cancers; mean age 55yrs; ♂:♀ = 2:1.

Clinical features: 50% are incidental findings during abdominal imaging for other symptoms. Haematuria, loin pain, abdominal mass, anorexia, malaise, weight loss, PUO may occur. Rarely, invasion of left renal vein compresses the left testicular vein causing a left varicocoele. Spread may be direct (renal vein), via lymph nodes, or haematogenous (bone, liver, lung).

Tests: Blood: FBC (polycythaemia from erythropoeitin secretion); ESR; U&E; alk phos. *Urine:* RBCs; cytology. *Imaging:* Ultrasound; CT/MRI; renal angiography (if partial nephrectomy or palliative embolization are being considered; angiography can be done by CT); IVU (filling defect in kidney ± calcification); CXR ('cannon ball' metastases).

Treatment: Radical nephrectomy. Metastatic disease is reason to consider immunotherapy with interferon-α or interleukin-2. *Prognosis:* 5yr survival: 45%.

Transitional cell carcinoma (TCC) may arise in the bladder (50%), ureter, or renal pelvis. *Epidemiology:* age >40yrs; ♂:♀ = 4. *Risk factors:* Smoking; drugs (cyclophosphamide, phenacetin); industrial carcinogens (azo-dyes, β-naphthalene). Schistosomiasis is a risk factor for squamous cell carcinoma of the bladder. *Presentation:* Painless haematuria; frequency, urgency, dysuria, or urinary tract obstruction. *Diagnosis:* Urine cytology; IVU; cystoscopy + biopsy; CT/MRI scan. *Treatment:* See *Bladder tumours*, p502. *Prognosis:* Varies with clinical stage/histological grade: 10–80% 5yr survival.

Wilms' tumour (nephroblastoma, *OHCS* p220) is a childhood tumour of primitive renal tubules and mesenchymal cells. It presents with an abdominal mass and haematuria. *Investigations:* Urine cytology; ultrasound; IVU; renal angiography; CT/MRI scan. Avoid biopsy. *Treatment:* Nephrectomy; radiotherapy; chemotherapy. *Prognosis:* 90% 5yr survival.

Prostate cancer is the 2nd commonest malignancy of men. *Incidence:* Rises with age: 80% in men >80yrs (in autopsy studies). *Associations:* ↑testosterone, +ve family history (p434). Most are adenocarcinomas arising in the peripheral prostate. Spread may be local (seminal vesicles, bladder, rectum) via nodes, or haematogenously (sclerotic bony lesions). *Symptoms:* May be asymptomatic or nocturia, hesitancy, poor stream, terminal dribbling, or urinary obstruction. Weight↓ ± bone pain suggests metastases. *Digital rectal exam:* May show a hard, irregular prostate. *Diagnosis:* ↑PSA (p705; normal in 30% of small cancers); transrectal ultrasound and biopsy; bone x-rays; bone scan; CT/MRI. *Staging:* MRI. If contrast-enhancing magnetic nanoparticles are used, sensitivity for detecting affected nodes rises from 35% to 90%.

Treatment: Local disease: Which is better: *radical prostatectomy* (+immediate goserelin if node +ve; a widely used regimen), *radiotherapy* or *watchful waiting* with serial PSA monitoring? One trial (N = 695) found radical prostatectomy improved disease-specific mortality, but not overall survival, when compared with watchful waiting. Radical surgery doubles rates of erectile dysfunction and incontinence. Do transurethral resection for obstruction. Brachytherapy is being assessed for local disease. *Metastatic disease:* hormonal drugs may give benefit for 1–2yrs. Gonadotrophin-releasing analogues, eg 12-weekly goserelin (10.8mg SC as Zoladex LA®) first stimulate, and then inhibit pituitary gonadotrophin output. Alternatives: cyproterone acetate; flutamide; diethylstilboestrol. *Symptomatic treatment:* analgesia; treat hypercalcaemia; radiotherapy for bone metastases or spinal cord compression.

Prognosis: 10% die in 6 months, but 10% live >10yrs. *Screening:* Rectal examination; PSA; transrectal ultrasound. There are problems with all (p705).

Advice to asymptomatic men asking for a PSA test

The prostate lies below the bladder, and surrounds the tube taking urine out. Prostate cancer is common in older men. Many men over 50 (to whom this advice applies) consider a PSA test on their blood to detect prostatic cancer. *Is this a good idea?*

- The test is not very accurate, and we cannot say that those having the test will live longer—even if they do turn out to have prostate cancer. This is because the cancer is often very lazy, so that, in most men with prostate cancer, death is from an unrelated cause.
- The test itself has no side-effects, provided you don't mind giving blood and time. But if the test is falsely positive, you may needlessly have more tests, such as sampling the prostate by the back passage (which may cause bleeding and infection in 1–5% of men).
- Only one in three of those with a high PSA level will have cancer.
- You may also be worried needlessly if later tests put you in the clear.
- Even if a cancer is found, there is nothing we can do to tell you for sure whether it will impinge on your health. Treatment may be recommended—and then you might end up having a bad effect from treatment which was not even needed.
- There is more bad news for those who *do* turn out to have prostate cancer: we do not even know for sure how to treat it! Options are radical surgery to remove the prostate (this treatment may be fatal itself in 0.2–0.5% of patients), radiotherapy, or hormones.
- There is indirect evidence of benefit of screening from the USA where fewer radical prostatectomies reveal cancer-affected lymph nodes than those done before widespread PSA-based screening. Intensive screening and treatment for prostate cancer does not, however, appear to be associated with lower prostate-specific mortality in retrospective studies.

Ultimately, you must decide for yourself what you want.

Prognostic factors in prostate cancer

A number of prognostic factors are used to help determine whether watchful waiting or aggressive therapy should be undertaken in prostate cancer. These include age, pretreatment PSA level, tumour stage (as measured by the TNM system[1]), and tumour grade—as measured by its Gleason score. Gleason grading is from 1 to 5, with 5 being the highest grade, and carrying the poorest prognosis. A pathologist determines the Gleason grade by analysing histology from two separate areas of tumour specimen, and adds them to get the total Gleason score for the tumour, from 2 to 10. Scores from 8 to 10 suggest an aggressive tumour, from 5 to 7 suggest intermediate grade, whereas from 2 to 4 suggest indolent tumour. Patients with high Gleason scores are more likely to be treated aggressively, especially if they are young and/or have higher stage disease.

1 See www.prostateinfo.com/patient/treatment/tnm.asp for the full TNM staging for tumour spread.

Urinary incontinence

▶Think twice before inserting a urinary catheter.
▶Carry out rectal examination to exclude faecal impaction.
▶Is the bladder palpable after voiding (retention with overflow)?

Anyone might 'wet themselves' on a long coach ride (we all would if the journey was long enough). Do not think of people as either dry or incontinent but as incontinent in certain circumstances. Attending to these circumstances is as important as focusing on the physiology.

Incontinence in men Enlargement of the prostate is the major cause of incontinence: urge incontinence (see below) or dribbling may result from the partial retention of urine. TURP may weaken the bladder sphincter and cause incontinence. Troublesome incontinence needs specialist assessment.

Incontinence in women (See also *Voiding difficulty*, OHCS p71.)

1 *Functional incontinence*, ie when physiological factors are relatively unimportant. The patient is 'caught short' and too slow in finding the toilet because of eg immobility or unfamiliar surroundings.

2 *Stress incontinence:* Leakage of urine due to incompetent sphincter. Leakage typically occurs when intra-abdominal pressure rises (eg coughing, laughing). The key to diagnosis is the loss of small (but often frequent) amounts of urine when coughing, etc. Examine for pelvic floor prolapse. Look for cough leak with the patient standing and with full bladder. Stress incontinence is common during pregnancy and following childbirth. It occurs to some degree in about 50% of post-menopausal women. In elderly women, pelvic floor weakness, eg with uterine prolapse or urethrocele (OHCS p54) is the commonest cause.

3 *Urge incontinence* is the most common type seen in hospital practice. The urge to pass urine is quickly followed by uncontrollable complete emptying of the bladder as the detrusor muscle contracts. Large amounts of urine flow down the patient's legs. In the elderly it is usually related to detrusor instability (a urodynamic diagnosis—see BOX) or organic brain damage. Look for evidence of: stroke; Parkinson's; dementia. Other causes: urinary infection; diabetes; diuretics; 'senile' vaginitis; urethritis.

In both sexes incontinence may result from diminished awareness due to confusion or sedation. Occasionally incontinence may be purposeful (eg preventing admission to an old people's home) or due to anger.

Management *Check for:* UTI; diabetes mellitus; diuretic use; faecal impaction. Do U&E. *Stress incontinence:* pelvic floor exercises may help. Intravaginal electrical stimulation may also be effective, but is not acceptable to many women. A ring pessary may help uterine prolapse, eg while awaiting surgical repair (this must be preceded by cystometry and urine flow rate measurement to exclude detrusor instability or sphincter dyssynergia). Surgical options for stress incontinence include Burch colposuspension and sling procedures; a variety of minimal access techniques (eg involving tension-free vaginal tape) have also been tried but remain unproven.

If urge incontinence: examine for spinal cord and CNS signs (including cognitive test, p59); and for vaginitis—treat with estriol 0.1% cream (eg Ovestin®, one applicator dose twice weekly for a few months)—consider cyclical progesterone if prolonged use, if no hysterectomy, to avoid risk of uterine cancer. The patient (or carer) should complete an 'incontinence' chart for 3 days to obtain the pattern of incontinence. Maximize access to toilet; advise on toileting regimen (eg every 4h). The aim is to keep bladder volume below that which triggers emptying. Drugs may help reduce night-time incontinence (see BOX) but are generally disappointing. Consider aids (absorbent pad; Paul's tubing if ♂).

▶Do urodynamic assessment before any surgical intervention.

Managing detrusor instability

Agents for detrusor instability:	Symptoms that they may improve:
Tolterodine 1–2mg/12h PO; SE: dry mouth, eyes, & skin; drowsiness, abdominal pain, urinary retention	Frequency, urgency (alternative: oxy-butynin, but more SEs). Avoid in myasthenia, and if glaucoma or UC are uncontrolled
Imipramine 50mg PO at night	Nocturia, enuresis, coital incontinence
Oestrogens	Post-menopausal urgency, frequency + nocturia may be improved by raising the bladder's sensory threshold
Surgery, eg clam ileocystoplasty	(The bladder is bisected, opened like a clam, and 25cm of ileum is sewn in)
Neuromodulation via transcuta-neous electrical stimulation	(Stimulates afferent nerve fibres to modulate bladder reflexes, suppressing involuntary detrusor contractions)
Hypnosis, psychotherapy, bladder training	(These all require good motivation)

NB: Desmopressin nasal spray 20μg as a night-time dose may have a role in ↓urine production, but not in the elderly (SE: fluid retention, heart failure).

Bladder tumours

What appear as benign papillomata rarely behave in a purely benign way. They are almost certainly indolent transitional cell (urothelial) malignancies. Adenocarcinomas and squamous cell carcinomas are rare in the West (the latter may follow schistosomiasis). UK incidence ≈ 1 : 5000/yr. ♂/♀ ≈ 4 : 1. Histology is important for prognosis: Grade 1—differentiated; Grade 2—intermediate; Grade 3—poorly differentiated. 80% are confined to bladder mucosa, and only ~20% penetrate muscle (increasing mortality to 50% at 5yrs).

Presentation Painless haematuria; recurrent UTIs; voiding irritability.

Associations Smoking; aromatic amines (rubber industry); chronic cystitis; schistosomiasis (↑risk of squamous cell carcinoma); pelvic irradiation.

Tests • Urine: Microscopy/cytology (cancers may cause sterile pyuria).
• IVU may show filling defects ± ureteric involvement.
• Cystoscopy with biopsy is diagnostic.
• Bimanual EUA helps assess spread.
• CT/MRI or lymphangiography may show involved pelvic nodes.

Staging Complex and changing (EUA = examination under anaesthesia)

Tis	Carcinoma-in-situ	Not felt at EUA
Ta	Tumour confined to epithelium	Not felt at EUA
T1	Tumour in mucosa or submucosa	Not felt at EUA
T2	Superficial muscle involved	Rubbery thickening at EUA
T3	Deep muscle involved	EUA: mobile mass
T4	Invasion beyond bladder	EUA: fixed mass

Treatment of transitional cell carcinoma (TCC)

Tis/Ta/T1: (80% of all patients.) Diathermy via cystoscope. Consider intravesical chemotherapeutic agents (eg mitomycin C) for multiple small tumours or high-grade tumours. Immunotherapy with intravesical BCG (p558) is useful in high-grade tumours and carcinoma-in-situ.

T2–3: Radical cystectomy is the 'gold standard'. Radiotherapy gives worse 5yr survival rates than surgery, but preserves the bladder. 'Salvage' cystectomy can be performed if radiotherapy fails, but yields worse results than primary surgery. Post-op chemotherapy (eg M-VAC: methotrexate, vinblastine, adriomycin, and cisplatin) is toxic but effective. Methods to preserve the bladder with transurethral resection/partial cystectomy + systemic chemotherapy have been tried, but long-term results are disappointing. ▶The patient should have all these options explained by a urologist *and* an oncologist.

T4: Usually palliative chemo/radiotherapy. Chronic catheterization and urinary diversions may help to relieve pain.

Cystectomy complications include sexual and urinary malfunction. To avoid a urostoma, a new bladder may be made from the patient's ileum.

Follow up History, examination, and regular cystoscopy: *high-risk tumours:* every 3 months for 2yrs, then every 6 months; *low-risk tumours:* first follow-up cystoscopy after 9 months, then yearly.

Tumour spread Local—to pelvic structures; lymphatic—to iliac and para-aortic nodes; haematogenous—to liver and lungs.

Survival This depends on age at surgery. For example, the 3yr survival after cystectomy for T2 and T3 tumours is 60% if 65–75yrs old, falling to 40% if 75–82yrs old (in whom the operative mortality is 4%). With unilateral pelvic node involvement, only 6% of patients survive 5yrs. The 3yr survival with bilateral or para-aortic node involvement is nil.

Massive bladder haemorrhage may complicate treatment; consider alum solution bladder irrigation (safer than formalin): it is an in-patient procedure.

Is asymptomatic microscopic haematuria significant?[1]

Dipstick tests are often done routinely as part of a new admission. If microscopic haematuria is found, but the patient has no related symptoms, what does this mean? Before rushing into a barrage on investigations, consider:

- One study found incidence of urogenital disease (eg bladder cancer) was no higher in those with asymptomatic microhaematuria than those without.
- Asymptomatic microscopic haematuria is the sole presenting feature in only 4% of bladder cancers, and there is no evidence that these are less advanced than malignancies presenting with macroscopic haematuria.
- When monitoring those with treated bladder cancer for recurrence, microscopic haematuria tests have a sensitivity of only 31% in those with superficial bladder malignancy, in whom detection would be most useful.
- Although 80% of those with flank pain due to a renal stone have microscopic haematuria, so will >50% of those with flank pain but no stone.

The conclusion is not that urine dipstick testing is useless, but that results need should not be interpreted *in isolation*. Take a holistic view. Smokers and those with a +ve family history for urothelial malignancy may be investigated differently from those with no risk factors (eg ultrasound, cystoscopy ± referral to a renal physician in some patients), but in a young fit athlete, the diagnosis is more likely to be exercise-induced haematuria. Wise doctors liaise with their patients. 'Shall we let sleeping dogs lie?' is a reasonable question for *some* patients. Give the facts and let him or her decide, reserving to yourself the right to present the facts in certain ways, depending on your instincts, and those of a trusted colleague. Remember that medicine is for gamblers (p26), and wise gamblers assess the odds against a shifting set of circumstances. When in doubt, there is nothing wrong in selecting a good guideline for your patient, eg that from SIGN.

Scottish intercollegiate guidelines network
www.show.scot.nhs.uk/sign/pdf/sign17.pdf

1 P Malmström 2003 *BMJ* **326** 813

Breast lumps and breast carcinoma

▶All solid lumps need histological or cytological assessment.

History Previous lumps, family history, pain, nipple discharge, change in size related to menstrual cycle, parous state, last period, drugs (eg HRT).

Examination Inspect (arms up and down). Note position, size, consistency, mobility, fixity, and local lymphadenopathy. Any nipple discharge or recent nipple inversion? Is the skin involved (eg dimpling, *peau d'orange*)?

Investigation All lumps should undergo *triple assessment* comprising *clinical examination* (above), *radiology*, and *histology/cytology* (see BOX).

Causes of lumps Fibroadenoma, cyst, cancer, fibroadenosis (focal or diffuse nodularity), periductal mastitis (often secondary to duct ectasia), fat necrosis, galactocoele, abscess, 'non-breast' lumps—eg lipomas, sebaceous cysts.

Causes of discharge Duct ectasia (green/brown/red, often multiple ducts and bilateral), intraduct papilloma/adenoma/carcinoma (bloody discharge, often single duct), lactation. *Management:* diagnose the cause (mammogram, ductogram, microdochectomy/total duct excision); then treat appropriately.

Breast cancer *Risk factors:* Nulliparity, 1st pregnancy >30yrs old, early menarche, late menopause, HRT (esp combined HRT), obesity, BRCA genes (p434), not breast-feeding, past breast ca, the Pill (possibly). *TNM staging:* T1 <2cm. T2 2–5cm. T3 >5cm. T4 Fixity to chest wall or *peau d'orange*. N1 Mobile ipsilateral nodes. N2 Fixed nodes. M1 Distant metastases. *Treating early cancer:* • *Surgery:* Wide local excision (WLE) or mastectomy ± breast reconstruction + axillary nodes sampling or surgical clearance. Local excision followed by radiotherapy gives equal survival, but higher local recurrence rates, than mastectomy. • *Radiotherapy:* For tumours at high risk of local recurrence, post-mastectomy radiotherapy to the chest wall ↑survival & ↓local recurrence in pre-menopausal women receiving adjuvant chemotherapy. Radiotherapy to the breast following WLE ↓local recurrence. Radiotherapy to the axilla is used if lymph node +ve on sampling and complete surgical clearance was not performed. • *Chemotherapy* improves survival (esp. if younger and node +ve), eg an anthracycline (epirubicin is less cardiotoxic than doxorubicin) + 5-FU + cyclophosphamide ± methotrexate. If this fails, vinorelbine or capecitabine with docetaxel (a taxane) may be indicated. NICE 2003 • *Endocrine therapy* aims to ↓oestrogen activity, and is used in all oestrogen receptor (ER) or progesterone receptor (PR) +ve disease (it may also be of slight benefit in ER/PR –ve tumours). The ER blocker tamoxifen is widely used, eg 20mg/d PO for 5yrs post-op (saves 12% of patients: may rarely cause uterine cancer so warn to report vaginal bleeding). Aromatase inhibitors (eg anastrozole) that target oestrogen synthesis can also be used, and may be better tolerated than tamoxifen. In pre-menopausal women with ER+ve tumours, ovarian ablation either via surgery, radiotherapy, or GnRH analogues (p498, eg goserelin) improves recurrence and survival. *Distant disease:* Assess LFT, Ca^{2+}, CXR, skeletal survey, bone scan, liver ultrasound, or CT. DXT (p442) to painful bony lesions. Tamoxifen is 1st choice in ER+ve disease; if successful initially, but then relapse, consider chemotherapy. Tumours +ve for the HER2 protein may respond to the monoclonal antibody trastuzumab.

Preventing breast cancer deaths: • Promoting 'breast awareness' • Mammography (offered every 3yrs to UK women from 50yrs to 70yrs old). 2-view mammograms are used; radiation risk is 'negligible'. Detection rates are 6.4 cancers per 1000 'healthy' women over 50yrs. Screening ↓breast cancer deaths by 25% in this age group. Annual mammograms do not significantly lower mortality (compared to 3-yearly screening). Cost: £40 per woman screened, £6000 per cancer detected; also false +ves may cause needless alarm.

NB: The fall in death rates from 51 to 35 per 100,000 during 1990–2000 is largely attributed to wider use of tamoxifen.

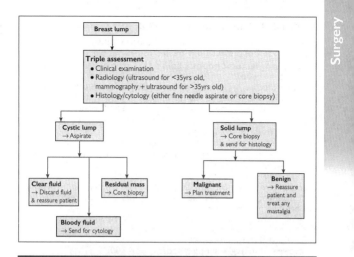

Sentinel node biopsy

▶Sentinel node biopsy may reduce the number of needless axillary clearances in lymph node –ve patients, thus decreasing post-op morbidity. It remains controversial. A typical procedure is as follows:

- A vital blue dye and/or radiocolloid is injected perioperatively into the periareolar area or the area of the primary tumour.
- A small incision is made in the axilla, and a gamma probe/visual inspection is used to identify the sentinel node.
- The sentinel node is biopsied and sent for histology ± immunohistochemistry.

Multi-centre trials suggest that the sentinel node can be identified in 90% of patients. False negative rates of 9–14% are reported, though these drop to <5% as surgeons become more experienced with the technique.[105]

Prognostic factors in breast cancer

▶A variety of prognostic factors are assessed in invasive breast cancer, including tumour size, grade, lymph node status, ER/PR status,[1] and presence of lympho-vascular invasion. The Nottingham Prognostic Index (NPI) is widely used to predict survival and risk of relapse, and thus help select appropriate adjuvant systemic therapy:[106]

NPI = 0.2 x tumour size (cm) + histological grade + nodal status[2]

If treated with surgery alone, 10yr survival rates are: *NPI <2.4:* 95%; *NPI 2.4–3.4:* 85%; *NPI 3.4–4.4:* 70%; *NPI 4.4–5.4:* 50%; *NPI >5.4:* 20%.

---

1 ER/PR = oestrogen receptor/progesterone receptor.
2 Nodal status is scored 1–3: 1 = node –ve; 2 = 1–3 nodes +ve; 3 => 3 nodes +ve for breast cancer. Histological grade is also scored 1–3.

Colorectal adenocarcinoma

This is the 2nd most common cause of cancer deaths in the UK (19,000 deaths/yr). 56% of presentations are in those >70yrs old.

Predisposing factors Neoplastic polyps, UC, Crohn's, familial adenomatous polyposis, and HNPCC (p434), previous cancer, low-fibre diet♠. NSAIDs may be protective. *Genetics:* No close relative affected: colorectal cancer risk is 1:50. One 1st degree relative affected: risk=1:17; if 2 affected, 1:10 (refer when 10yrs younger than the youngest affected relative).

Presentation depends on site: *Left-sided*: Bleeding PR; altered bowel habit; tenesmus; mass PR (60%). *Right*: Weight↓; Hb↓; abdominal pain. *Either*: Abdominal mass; obstruction; perforation; haemorrhage; fistula.

Tests FBC (microcytic anaemia); faecal occult blood (FOB); proctoscopy, sigmoidoscopy, barium enema or colonoscopy (can be done 'virtually' by CT); LFT, CT/MRI; liver ultrasound. CEA may be used to monitor disease and effectiveness of treatment (p704). If polyposis in family, refer for DNA testing once a patient is >15yrs old. Genetic testing may also help determine who will benefit from chemotherapy—see p434.

Staging is by Dukes' classification:

		Treated 5yr survival (%):
A	Confined to bowel wall	~90
B	Extension through bowel wall	~65
C	Involvement of regional lymph nodes	~30
D	Distant metastases	<10

Spread Local, lymphatic, or by blood (liver, lung, bone) or transcoelomic.

Treatment Surgery aims to cure (ideally). Exact technique may ↑survival times by up to 50% (eg in TME[1]): so expert training is vital. *Hemicolectomies: Right* is for caecal tumours, ascending or proximal transverse colon. *Left* is for tumours in the distal transverse colon or descending colon. *Sigmoid colectomy* is for tumours of sigmoid colon.

Anterior resection is for low sigmoid or high rectal tumours. Anastomosis is achieved at the first operation (stapling devices are helpful).

Abdomino-perineal (A-P) resection is for tumours low in the rectum (<~8cm from anal canal): permanent colostomy and removal of rectum and anus (but see p460 for total anorectal reconstruction).

Radiotherapy may be used pre-op in Ca rectum to ↓local recurrence; it *may* ↑survival by 10%. Pre-op radiotherapy ± 5-FU is also used to downstage initially unresectable rectal tumours. Post-op radiotherapy is only used in patients with rectal tumours at high risk of local recurrence.

Chemotherapy: There is good evidence that 5-FU ± folinic acid for 1yr post-op reduces Dukes C mortality by ~25%. The role of chemotherapy in Dukes B tumours is under investigation. Chemotherapy is also used in palliation of metastatic disease; newer agents (eg irinotecan, oxaliplatin) may provide more options. Patients with single-lobe hepatic metastases and no extra-hepatic spread may be suitable for curative surgery with liver resection.

Prognosis 60% are amenable to radical surgery, and 75% of these will be alive at 7yrs (or will have died from non-tumour-related causes).

Polyps are lumps that appear above the mucosa. There are 3 types:

1 *Inflammatory:* Ulcerative colitis, Crohn's, lymphoid hyperplasia.
2 *Hamartomatous:* Juvenile polyps, Peutz–Jeghers' syndrome (p732).
3 *Neoplastic:* Tubular or villous adenomas: malignant potential, esp. if >2cm.

Symptoms of polyps: Passage of blood/mucus PR. They should be biopsied and removed if they show malignant change. Most can be reached by the flexible colonoscope and diathermy can avoid the morbidity of partial colectomy. Check resection margins are clear of tumour.

---

1 TME=total mesorectal excision; entails sharp dissection to yield an intact mesorectal envelope: A Martling 2000 *Lancet* 356 **93**

Location of cancers of the large bowel

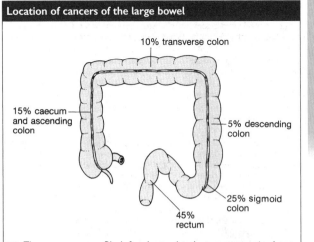

10% transverse colon

15% caecum and ascending colon

5% descending colon

25% sigmoid colon

45% rectum

NB: These are averages: Black females tend to have more proximal neoplasms, while White men tend to have more distal neoplasms.

Examples of clinical scenarios prompting urgent referral (eg by fax) for surgeon's assessment within 2wks if:

• Rectal bleeding and a persistent change in bowel habit for >6wks.
• Persistent rectal bleeding without anal symptoms in those over 45yrs, with no obvious external evidence of benign anal disease.
• Recent onset of looser stools and/or increased frequency of defecation, persisting for >6wks.
• Iron-deficiency anaemia without an obvious cause and Hb <10g/dL.
• An easily palpable abdominal or rectal mass.

Universal adult screening for colorectal cancer

507

►A number of screening methods have been proposed. Evidence from randomized trials is currently only available for FOB screening, however.
• FOB screening every 2yrs with home tests reduces mortality by 15–33%, but false +ve rates are high (up to 10% of those screened) and there are problems with acceptability. The patient has to be on a special diet while 2 out of 3 consecutive stool samples are tested. Sample rehydration improves sensitivity but increases false +ves.
• Sigmoidoscopy can be used to screen for left-sided lesions with 90% sensitivity and 99% specificity within the region of the scope. Case–control studies suggest ~60% reduction in risk of death from colorectal cancer by the finding of a lesion within the reach of the scope. Limitations include acceptability, cost, and not picking up right-sided lesions.
• Colonoscopy examines all the colon and is the most accurate test. It is already used in those at ↑risk of colorectal cancer due to personal or family history, adenoma, or UC/Crohn's. Limitations include perforation problems (2/1000 vs 1/10,000 for sigmoidoscopy), cost, need for sedation, acceptability to patients, and the availability of trained endoscopists.

Carcinoma of the stomach

Incidence of adenocarcinoma at the gastro-oesophageal junction is increasing in the West, though incidence of distal & body gastric carcinoma has fallen sharply. It remains a tumour notable for its gloomy prognosis and non-specific presentation.

Incidence 23/100,000 in the UK, but there are unexplained wide geographical variations, being especially common in Japan. Associations:
- Blood group A
- Atrophic gastritis; pernicious anaemia
- Social class ↓
- H.pylori (p214)
- Adenomatous polyps
- Smoking

Pathology The adenocarcinoma may be polypoid, ulcerating, or leather bottle type (linitis plastica). Some are confined to mucosa and submucosa—so-called 'early' gastric carcinoma.

Presentation *Symptoms:* Often non-specific. Dyspepsia (p70) lasting >1 month in patients aged ≥40–50yrs demands GI investigation. Others: weight ↓, vomiting, dysphagia, anaemia. *Signs* suggesting incurable disease: epigastric mass, hepatomegaly, jaundice, ascites (p518), large left supraclavicular (Virchow's) node (Troissier's sign), acanthosis nigricans (p428). *Spread* is local, lymphatic, blood-borne, and transcoelomic eg to ovaries (Krukenberg tumour).

Tests Gastroscopy + multiple ulcer edge biopsies. ▶Aim to biopsy all gastric ulcers as even malignant ulcers may appear to heal on drug treatment. Endoscopic ultrasound (EUS) and CT/MRI are useful for staging.

Treatment Localized disease may be treated by curative gastrectomy, either D_1 resection (excision of tumour and perigastric nodes) or D_2 resection (basically a D_1 resection extended to include nodes around the coeliac axis). There is controversy about whether D_2 is better than D_1; D_2 resections should only be done in specialist units. For tumours in the distal ⅔, a partial gastrectomy may suffice, but, if more proximal, total gastrectomy may be needed. The role of chemotherapy is under investigation. Endoscopic mucosal resection is used for early tumours confined to the mucosa.

Palliation is often needed for obstruction, pain, or haemorrhage. In metastatic disease, chemotherapy increases quality of life and survival. Judicious use of surgery and radiotherapy may also be helpful.

5yr survival <10% overall, but nearly 20% for patients undergoing radical surgery. The prognosis is much better for 'early' gastric carcinoma.

Carcinoma of the oesophagus

Incidence Australia <5/100,000/yr; UK <9; Brittany >50; Iran >100. *Risk factors:* Diet, alcohol excess, smoking, achalasia, Plummer–Vinson syndrome (p212), obesity, reflux oesophagitis ± Barrett's oesophagus (p718); there is a 44-fold ↑risk of adenocarcinoma if severe reflux for >10 yrs).

Site 20% occur in the upper part, 50% in the middle, and 30% in the lower part. They may be squamous cell or adenocarcinomas (incidence rising).

The Patient Dysphagia, weight ↓, retrosternal chest pain, lymphadenopathy (rare). *Signs from upper ⅓ of oesophagus:* Hoarseness; cough (may be paroxysmal if aspiration pneumonia). *Differential:* See *dysphagia*, p212.

Tests Barium swallow, CXR, oesophagoscopy with biopsy/brushings/EUS, CT/MRI. Staging laparoscopy if significant infra-diaphragmatic component.

Treatment Survival rates are poor with or without treatment. If localized T1/T2 disease radical curative oesophagectomy may be tried. Transhiatal oesophagectomy is associated with less morbidity than transthoracic resection, though the latter *may* be associated with ↑long-term survival. Pre-op chemotherapy (cisplatin + 5-FU) improves survival. Chemoradiotherapy without surgery may be the definitive treatment for proximal squamous cell tumours. Palliative therapy in advanced disease primarily aims to restore swallowing with chemo/radiotherapy, stenting, and laser therapy.

TNM typing in oesophageal cancer

Spread of oesophageal cancer is direct, by submucosal infiltration and local spread—or to nodes, or, later, via the blood.

T_{is} carcinoma-*in-situ*	NX nodes cannot be assessed
T1 invading lamina propria/submucosa	N0 no node spread
T2 invading muscularis propria	N1 regional node metastases
T3 invading adventitia	M0 no distant spread
T4 invasion of adjacent structures	M1 distant metastasis

Lumps

▶Examine the regional lymph nodes as well as the lump. If the lump is a node, examine its area of drainage.

History How long has it been there? Does it hurt? Any other lumps? Is it getting bigger? Ever been abroad? Otherwise well?

Physical exam Remember the 6 Ss: site, size, shape, smoothness, surface, and surroundings. Other questions: does it transilluminate (see below)? Is it fixed to skin or underlying structures? Is it fluctuant? Lumps in certain sites call to mind particular pathologies (see lumps in groin and scrotum p512). Remember to feel if a lump is pulsatile; this may seem to be a minor detail until faced with a surprise on a minor operations list.

Transilluminable lumps After eliminating as much external light as possible, place a bright, thin 'pencil' torch on the lump, from behind, so the light is shining through the lump towards your eye. If the lump glows red it is said to transilluminate. Fluid-filled lumps such as hydrocoeles are good examples of transilluminable swellings.

Lipomas These benign fatty lumps, occurring wherever fat can expand (*not* scalp or palms), have smooth, imprecise margins, and a hint of fluctuance. They only cause symptoms via pressure. Malignant change is very rare (suspect if rapid growth, hardening, or vascularization occurs). Multiple scattered lipomas, which may be painful, occur in Dercum's disease.

Sebaceous cysts These are intradermal, so you cannot draw the skin over them. Look for the characteristic punctum marking blocked sebaceous outflow. Infection is quite common, and foul pus exits through the punctum. *Treatment:* Shelling them out whole can be tricky: learn from an expert.

Causes of lymph node enlargement Infections: glandular fever; brucellosis; TB; HIV; toxoplasmosis; actinomycosis; syphilis. Others: malignancy (carcinoma, lymphoma); sarcoidosis.

Cutaneous abscesses Staphylococci are the most common organisms. *Haemolytic streptococci* are only common in hand infections. Proteus is a common cause of non-staphylococcal axillary abscesses. Below the waist faecal organisms are common (aerobes and anaerobes). *Treatment:* Incision and drainage alone usually cures. *Boils (furuncles)* are abscesses which involve a hair follicle and its associated glands. *A carbuncle* is an area of subcutaneous necrosis which discharges itself on to the surface through multiple sinuses.

Rheumatoid nodules These are collagenous granulomas which appear on the extensor aspects of joints—especially the elbows. They occur in established cases of rheumatoid arthritis.

Ganglia These are degenerative cysts from an adjacent joint or synovial sheath commonly seen on the dorsum of the wrist or hand and dorsum of the foot. They may transilluminate. 50% will disappear spontaneously. Aspiration may be effective, especially when combined with instillation of steroid and hyaluronidase.[20] For the rest, the treatment of choice is excision rather than the traditional blow from your bible (the *Oxford Textbook of Surgery*!).

Fibromas These may occur anywhere in the body, but most commonly they are under the skin. These whitish, benign tumours contain collagen, fibroblasts, and fibrocytes.

Dermoid cysts contain dermal structures; often found in the midline.

Malignant tumours of connective tissue These include the fibrosarcoma, liposarcoma, leiomyosarcoma (smooth muscle), and rhabdomyosarcoma (striated muscle). Sarcomas are staged using a modified TNM system which includes tumour grade. Needle-core (Trucut) biopsies of large tumours precede excision. Any lesion suspected of being a sarcoma should not be simply enucleated in what might wrongly be considered a 'conservative' procedure.

Lumps in the groin and scrotum

▶Any lump within the tunica vaginalis is cancer until proved otherwise. 🔲
▶Acute, tender enlargement of the testis is torsion until proved otherwise.

Diagnosing groin lumps Think of nearby structures: femoral/inguinal hernias, saphena varix (p528—both have cough impulse), nodes, femoral aneurysm, ectopic testis, skin lumps, psoas abscess (may present with back pain, limp, and swinging pyrexia. Diagnose with ultrasound).

Diagnosis of lumps in the scrotum

1 *Can you get above it?* If not, it is an inguinoscrotal hernia (inguinal hernia extending into scrotum, p527).
2 *Is it separate from the testis?*
3 *Is it cystic or solid?* (Does it transilluminate? See p510.)
    Separate and cystic—epididymal cyst.
    Separate and solid—epididymitis (may also be orchitis).
    Testicular and cystic—hydrocoele.
    Testicular and solid—tumour, orchitis, granuloma (p198), gumma (p601).
Ultrasound may help in sorting out testis tumours from other lumps. Do not assume that an injured testis was normal before the injury: this is not a rare mode of tumour presentation; ultrasound may help here.

Epididymal cysts These usually develop in adult life and contain either clear or milky (spermatocoele) fluid. They lie above and behind the testis. Remove if they are symptomatic.

Hydrocoeles (fluid within the tunica vaginalis) may be *primary* (idiopathic—associated with a patent processus vaginalis, which typically resolves during the first year of life) or *secondary*. Primary hydrocoeles are more common, larger, and usually develop in younger men. If secondary, suspect associated testis tumour, trauma, or infection. Hydrocoeles are treated by aspiration (may need repeating) or surgery.

Epididymo-orchitis Causes: *Chlamydia* (eg if <35yrs old; erythromycin may be the best remedy here), *Escherichia coli*, mumps, gonococcal infection, or TB. The area is usually tender. Take a urine sample; look for urethral discharge. A 'first catch' is more likely to show abnormalities than an MSU.

Testis tumours are the commonest malignancies in males aged 15–44.

Varieties: Seminoma (30–40yrs); teratoma (20–30yrs); tumours of Sertoli or Leydig cells. ~10% of malignancies occur in undescended testes, even after orchidopexy. A contralateral tumour is found in 1 in 20 instances.

Typical presentation: Painless testis lump, noticed after trauma or infection.
Risk factors: Undescended testis; infant hernia; infertility. 🔲 *Spread:* Lymphatic: to para-aortic nodes; then to mediastinum. *Haematogenous:* to lungs.
Staging is essential: (1) No evidence of metastasis. (2) Infradiaphragmatic node involvement. (3) Supradiaphragmatic node↑. (4) Lung involvement.
Tests: (To allow staging) CXR, CT, excision biopsy. α-fetoprotein (eg >3iu/mL)[1] and β-human chorionic gonadotrophin (β-HCG) are useful tumour markers and help monitor treatment; check *before* and *during* treatment.
Treatment: Orchidectomy (inguinal incision; occlude the spermatic cord before mobilization to ↓risk of intra-operative spread). Options are constantly being refined (surgery, radiotherapy, chemotherapy). Seminomas are exquisitely radiosensitive. Stage 1 seminomas may be treated by orchidectomy + radiotherapy to give cure rates of ~95%. Do close follow-up to detect relapse. Cure of teratomas, even if metastases are present, is achieved by 3–4 cycles of *bleomycin* + *etoposide* + *cisplatin*. 🔲
5yr survival: This is good (≥70%—more for early disease).
Prevention of late presentation: Self-examination.

---

1 AFP is *not* raised in pure seminoma (*may also be raised in:* hepatitis, cirrhosis, hepatocellular carcinoma, open neural tube defects).

Diagnosis of scrotal masses[1]

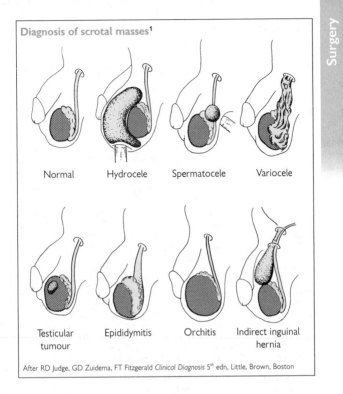

Normal   Hydrocele   Spermatocele   Variocele

Testicular tumour   Epididymitis   Orchitis   Indirect inguinal hernia

After RD Judge, GD Zuidema, FT Fitzgerald *Clinical Diagnosis* 5th edn, Little, Brown, Boston

1 A varicocele is formed by dilated veins in the pampiniform plexus of the spermatic cord, often visible as distended scrotal blood vessels that feel like 'a bag of worms'. They are associated with male subfertility, though varicocele repair (via surgery or embolization) seems to have little effect on subsequent pregnancy rates—see J Evans 2003 *Lancet* **361** 1849

Lumps in the neck

▶Don't biopsy lumps until tumours within the head and neck have been excluded by an ENT surgeon. Culture all biopsied lymph nodes for TB.

Diagnosis First of all ask how long the lump has been present. If <3wks, self-limiting infection is the likely cause and extensive investigation is unwise. Next ask yourself where the lump is. Is it intradermal?— (eg sebaceous cyst with a central punctum). Is it a lipoma (p510)? If the lump is not intradermal, and is not of recent onset, you are about to start a diagnostic hunt over complicated terrain:

Midline lumps: If patient is <20yrs old, the likely diagnosis is a dermoid cyst (ie sequestrations of epidermoid tissue), or, if it moves on protruding the tongue and is below the hyoid, a thyroglossal cyst (fluctuant lump developing in cell rests in thyroid's migration path; treatment: surgery; they are the commonest congenital cervical cystic lump).[124]

In patients >20yrs old, it is probably a thyroid mass, unless it is bony hard, when the diagnosis may be a chondroma.

Submandibular triangle: (Below jaw; above anterior belly of digastric.) If <20yrs, self-limiting lymphadenopathy is likely. If >20, exclude **malignant lymphadenopathy** (eg firm, and non-tender). ▶Is TB likely? If it is not a node, think of submandibular **salivary stone, sialadenitis,** or **tumour.**

Anterior triangle: (Below digastric and in front of sternomastoid.) Nodes are common (see above): examine the areas which they serve (skin, mouth, throat, thyroid; is the spleen enlarged?—this may indicate lymphoma).

Branchial cysts emerge under the anterior border of sternomastoid where the upper third meets the middle third; age <20. They are due to non-disappearance of the cervical sinus (where the 2nd branchial arch grows down over the 3rd and 4th). Lined by squamous epithelium, their fluid contains cholesterol crystals. Treat by excision. **Cystic hygromas** arise from the jugular lymph sac; transilluminate brightly. Treat by surgery or hypertonic saline sclerosant. **Carotid body tumours** (chemodectoma) are very rare, move from side to side but not up and down, and splay out the carotid bifurcation. It is usually firm and occasionally soft and pulsatile. It does not usually cause bruits. It may be bilateral, familial, and malignant (5%). This tumour should be suspected in masses just anterior to the upper third of sternomastoid. Diagnose by digital computer angiography. Treatment: extirpation by vascular surgeon. If the lump is in the supero-posterior area of the anterior triangle, is it a **parotid tumour** (more likely if >40yrs)? **Laryngocoeles** are uncommon causes of anterior triangle lumps: they are painless, and may be made worse by blowing. These cysts are classified as external, internal, or mixed, and may be associated with laryngeal cancer.

Posterior triangle: (Behind sternomastoid, in front of trapezius, above clavicle.) If there are many small lumps, think of **nodes**—TB, viruses such as HIV or EBV (infectious mononucleosis), any chronic infection or, if over 20yrs, consider lymphoma or metastases eg from GI or bronchial or head and neck neoplasia. **Cervical ribs** may intrude into this area.

Tests Ultrasound shows lump consistency. CT defines masses in relation to their anatomical neighbours. Do virology and Mantoux test. CXR may show malignancy or reveal bilateral hilar lymphadenopathy; here you should consider sarcoid. Consider fine-needle aspiration (FNA).

Salivary gland pathology

There are 3 pairs of major salivary glands: parotid, submandibular, and sublingual (also numerous minor glands).

History: lumps; swelling related to food; pain; taste; dry eyes.

Examination: note external swelling; look for secretions; bimanual palpation for stones. Examine VII nerve and regional nodes.

Cytology: This may be ascertained by FNA.

Recurrent unilateral pain and swelling is likely to be due to a stone. 80% are submandibular. The classical story is of pain and swelling on eating—with a red, tender, swollen, but uninfected gland. The stone may be seen on plain x-ray or by sialography. Distal stones are removed via the mouth but deeper stones may require excision of the gland.

Chronic bilateral symptoms may coexist with dry eyes and mouth and auto-immune disease, eg Mikulicz's or Sjögren's syndrome (p730 & p734).

Fixed swellings may be from tumours or sarcoid—or are idiopathic.

Salivary gland tumours: '80% are in the parotid, 80% of these are pleomorphic adenomas, 80% of these are in the superficial lobe.'

▶Any salivary gland swelling must be removed for assessment if present for >1 month. VII nerve palsy signifies malignancy.

Benign or malignant:	*Malignant:*	*Malignant:*
Cystadenolymphoma	Mucoepidermoid	Squamous carcinoma
Pleomorphic adenoma	Acinic cell	Adenocarcinoma
		Adenoid cystic carcinoma

Pleomorphic adenomas often present in middle age and grow slowly. Removed by superficial parotidectomy. Adenolymphomas: usually older men; soft; treat by enucleation. Carcinomas: rapid growth; hard fixed mass; pain; facial palsy. Treatment: surgery + radiotherapy. Surgery complications: (1) Facial palsy—often brief. Have a facial nerve stimulator in theatre to aid identification. (2) Salivary fistula: often close spontaneously. (3) *Frey's syndrome* (gustatory sweating); tympanic neurectomy may help here.

Lumps in the thyroid

PLATE 14

Examination Watch the neck during swallowing water. Stand behind and feel thyroid for size, shape (smooth? one or many nodules?), tenderness, and mobility. Percuss for retrosternal extension. Any nodes? Bruits? If the thyroid is enlarged (goitre), ask these 3 questions:

1 Is the thyroid smooth or nodular?
2 Is the patient euthyroid, thyrotoxic (p304), or hypothyroid (p306)?
   Smooth, non-toxic goitre: Endemic (iodine deficiency); congenital; goitrogens; thyroiditis; physiological; Hashimoto's thyroiditis (an autoimmune disease thought to be due to apoptosis induced by lymphocytes bearing Fas ligands combining with thyrocytes bearing Fas.)
   Smooth, toxic goitre: Graves disease.
3 Any nodules? Many or one? If >4cm across, malignancy is more likely.[25]
   Multi-nodular goitre (PLATE 14): Usually euthyroid but hyperthyroidism may develop. Hypothyroidism and malignancy are rare.

The *single thyroid lump* is a common problem; ~10% will be malignant.
Causes: Cyst, adenoma, discrete nodule in multi-nodular goitre, malignancy. First ask: is he/she thyrotoxic? Do T3 & T4. Then: • *Ultrasound,* to see if the lump is solid or cystic or part of a group of lumps • *Radionucleotide scans* may show malignant lesions as hypofunctioning or 'cold', whereas a hyper-functioning 'hot' lesion suggests adenoma • *FNA*[1] and do cytology on the fluid.
►No clinical/lab test is good enough to tell for sure if follicular neoplasms found on FNA are benign, so such patients are referred for surgery.[26]

What should you do if high-resolution ultrasound shows impalpable nodules?
Such thyroid nodules can usually just be observed[27] provided they are:
• <1cm across (most are; ultrasound can detect lumps <2mm; such 'inciden-talomas' occur in 46% of routine autopsies) and asymptomatic.
• There is no past history of thyroid cancer or radiation.
• No family history of medullary cancer. (If any present, do ultrasound-guided FNA; excise if cytology is malignant.)

Thyroid neoplasia[2] 5 types:
1 *Papillary:* 60%. Often in young; spread to nodes and lung. Treatment: total thyroidectomy (to remove non-obvious tumour) ± node excision + radio-iodine to ablate residual cells may all be needed. Give T4 to suppress TSH. Prognosis is better if young and female.
2 *Follicular:* ≤25%. Middle-aged, spreads early via blood (bone, lungs). Well-differentiated. Treat by total thyroidectomy and T4 suppression and radioiodine (^{131}I) ablation.
3 *Anaplastic:* Rare. ♀ : ♂ ≈ 3 : 1. Elderly, poor response to any treatment. In the absence of unresectable disease, excision + radiotherapy may be tried.
4 *Medullary:* 5%. Sporadic (80%) or part of MEN syndrome (p309). May pro-duce calcitonin. They do not concentrate iodine. Do thyroidectomy + node clearance (do phaeochromocytoma screen pre-op). External beam radiotherapy should be considered to prevent regional recurrence.
5 *Lymphoma:* 5%. ♀:♂ ≈ 3:1. May present with stridor or dysphagia. Do full staging pre-treatment (chemoradiotherapy). Assess histology for mucosa-associated lymphoid tissue (MALT) origin (associated with a good prognosis).

Thyroid surgery *Indications:* Pressure symptoms, hyperthyroidism, carci-noma, cosmetic reasons. Render euthyroid pre-op, by antithyroid drugs and/or propranolol. Check vocal cords by indirect laryngoscopy pre- and post-op.

Complications *Early:* Recurrent laryngeal nerve palsy, haemorrhage (►if compresses airway, instantly remove sutures for evacuation of clot), hypo-parathyroidism (check plasma Ca^{2+} daily, usually transient), thyroid storm (symptoms of severe hyperthyroidism—treat by propranolol PO or IV, antithy-roid drugs, and iodine, p820). *Late complications:* Hypothyroidism.

1 FNA = fine needle aspirate 2 For a review of thyroid carcinoma, see S Sherman 2003 *Lancet* **361** 501–11

Abdominal masses

As with any mass, determine size, site, shape, and surface. Find out if it is pulsatile and if it is mobile. Examine supraclavicular and inguinal nodes. Is the lump ballottable (like bobbing an apple up and down in water)?

Right iliac fossa masses

Appendix mass/abscess	Intussusception	Transplanted kidney
Caecal carcinoma	TB mass	Kidney malformation
Crohn's disease	Amoebic abscess	Tumour in an
Pelvic mass (see below)	Actinomycosis (p591)	undescended testis

Abdominal distension Flatus, fat, fluid, faeces, or fetus? Fluid may be outside the gut (ascites) or sequestered in bowel (obstruction; ileus). To demonstrate ascites elicit signs of a fluid thrill and/or shifting dullness (p53).

Causes of ascites:
Malignancy;[¶] pancreatitis[¶]
Low albumin (eg nephrosis)
Myxoedema; CCF pericarditis
Infections—especially TB

Ascites with portal hypertension:
Cirrhosis
Portal nodes
Budd–Chiari syndrome[¶] (p720)
IVC or portal vein thrombosis

Tests: Aspirate ascitic fluid (paracentesis) for cytology, culture, & protein level (≥30g/L in diseases marked[¶]) with an 21G needle in RIF (p748); ultrasound. Protein level rarely helps diagnostically; it tends to rise with diuretic therapy.

Left upper quadrant mass Is it spleen, stomach, kidney, colon, pancreas, or a rare cause (eg neurofibroma)? Pancreatic cysts may be true (congenital; cystadenomas; retention cysts of chronic pancreatitis; cystic fibrosis); or pseudocysts (fluid in lesser sac from acute pancreatitis).

Splenomegaly Causes are often said to be *infective, haematological, neoplastic*, etc., but grouping by *associated feature* is more useful clinically:

Splenomegaly with fever	*With lymphadenopathy*	*With purpura*
Infection* (malaria, hepatitis,*	Glandular fevers*	Septicaemia; typhus
SBE/IE, EBV*, TB, CMV, HIV)	Leukaemias; lymphoma	DIC; amyloid*
Sarcoid, malignancies*	Sjögren's syndrome	Meningococcaemia
With arthritis Sjögren's	*With ascites*	*With a murmur* SBE/IE
Rheumatoid arthritis; SLE	Carcinoma	Rheumatic fever
Infection, eg Lyme (p600)	Portal hypertension*	Hypereosinophilia
Vasculitis/Behçet's (p424)	(see above)	Amyloid* (p668)
With anaemia Sickle-cell*	*With weight↓ +CNS signs*	*Massive splenomegaly*
Thalassaemia;* POEM (p306)	Cancer, lymphoma, TB	Malaria; myelofibrosis
Leishmaniasis;* leukaemia*	Arsenic poisoning	CML;* leishmaniasis
Pernicious anaemia (p634)	Paraproteinaemia*	Gaucher's syndrome*

See OUP's **Mentor**, for a full list of causes by *any* association; * = causes of hepatosplenomegaly.

Smooth hepatomegaly Hepatitis, CCF, sarcoid, early alcoholic cirrhosis (a small liver is typical later); tricuspid incompetence (pulsatile liver).

Craggy hepatomegaly Secondaries or 1° hepatoma. (Nodular cirrhosis typically causes a small, shrunken liver, not an enlarged craggy one.)

Pelvic masses *Is it truly pelvic?*—Yes, if by palpation you cannot 'get below it'. Causes: fibroids, fetus, bladder, ovarian cyst/malignancies.

Investigating lumps There is much to be said for performing an early CT to save time and money compared with leaving the test to be the last in a long chain of tests. If unavailable, ultrasound is the first test. Others: IVU, liver and spleen isotope scans, Mantoux test (p566). Routine tests: FBC (with film), ESR, U&E, LFT, proteins, Ca^{2+}, CXR, AXR, biopsy tests; a tissue diagnosis may be made using a fine needle guided by ultrasound or CT control. MRI and spiral CT also have a role.

Around the anus

Pruritus ani Itch occurs if the anus is moist or soiled, eg fissures, incontinence, poor hygiene, tight pants, threadworm, fistula, dermatoses, lichen sclerosis, anxiety, contact dermatitis. *Treatment:*

- Careful hygiene
- Moist wipe post-defecation
- Try anaesthetic cream
- No spicy food
- No steroid/antibiotic creams

Fissure-in-ano This is a midline longitudinal split in the squamous lining of the lower anus—often, if chronic, with a mucosal tag at the external aspect—the 'sentinel pile'. 90% are posterior (anterior ones follow parturition), and are perpetuated by internal sphincter spasm. ♂:♀ >1:1.

- Most are due to hard faeces. They make defecation very painful—and spasm may constrict the rectal artery, making healing difficult.
- Rare causes: syphilis, herpes, trauma, Crohn's, anal cancer, psoriasis.
- Examine with a bright light. Do a PR ± sigmoidoscopy. Groin nodes suggest a complicating factor (eg immunosuppression from HIV).
- Try 5% lignocaine (=lidocaine) ointment, extra dietary roughage + good anal toilet. Glyceryl trinitrate ointment (0.2–0.3%) relieves pain and ischaemia caused by chronic fissures and spasm, and can prevent need for surgery, but may cause headache. Trials suggest that botulinum toxin injection is more effective than glyceryl trinitrate.[128] If conservative measures fail, consider day-case *lateral partial internal sphincterotomy; manual anal dilatation* (under GA) is also used, but has fallen out of favour due to ↑ risk of post-op anal incontinence (24.3% vs 4.8% for lateral sphincterotomy).[129]

The perianal haematoma (also called a thrombosed external pile). Both names are wrong because it is a clotted venous saccule. It appears as a 2–4mm 'dark blue berry' under the skin. It may be evacuated via a small incision under local anaesthesia or left alone if present for >1day.

Pilonidal sinus Obstruction of natal cleft hair follicles ~6cm above the anus, with ingrowing of hair, excites a foreign body reaction, and may cause devious secondary tracks which open laterally ± abscesses, with foul-smelling discharge. (Barbers get these sinuses between their fingers.) ♂:♀ ≈ 10:1. *Treatment* is excision of the sinus tract ± primary closure, but is unsatisfactory in 10% of patients. Consider pre-op cefuroxime (eg 1.5g IV + metronidazole 1g IV). Complex tracks can be laid open and packed individually, or skin flaps can be used to cover the defect.

Rectal prolapse The mucosa, or rectum in all its layers, may descend through the anus. This leads to incontinence in 75%. It is due to a lax sphincter and prolonged straining. Treatment: fix rectum to the sacrum (± rectosigmoidectomy with no abdominal wound, as exposure is via amputating the prolapse) or encircle the anus with a Thiersch wire.

Anal ulcers are rare: consider Crohn's disease, anal cancer, TB, syphilis.

Skin tags seldom cause trouble but are easily excised. **Piles** See p522.

Anorectal abscesses are usually caused by gut organisms (rarely staphs or TB). ♂:♀ ≈ 1.8. *Location:* Perianal (~45%), ischiorectal (≤30%), intersphincteric (>20%), supralevator (~5%). Redness and swelling may spread well into the buttock. PR may be too painful. Do incision & drainage, eg under GA (+ fistulotomy if needed, eg in Crohn's disease). *Associations:* DM, Crohn's, malignancy. Don't rely on antibiotics.

Anal cancer *UK incidence:* 300/yr. *Risk* ↑: Syphilis, anal warts (HPV 16, 6, 11, & 18 implicated), anoreceptive homosexuals (often young). *Histology:* Squamous cell (80%); rarely basaloid, melanoma, or adenocarcinoma. *The Patient* may present with bleeding, pain, bowel habit change, pruritus ani, masses, stricture. *Differential diagnosis:* Condyloma acuminata, leucoplakia, lichen sclerosus, Bowen's, or Crohn's disease. *Treatment: Radiotherapy + 5-FU + mitomycin/cisplatin* is usually preferred to *anorectal excision & colostomy,* and 75% of patients retain normal anal function.[130]

Examination of the rectum and anus

Explain what you are about to do. Make sure curtains are pulled and doors are closed. The patient (and passers-by!) will appreciate it. Have the patient on his left side, his knees brought up towards the chest. Use gloves and lubricant. Part the buttocks and inspect the anus. Press your index finger against the side of the anus. Ask the patient to breathe deeply and insert your finger slowly; press with the pad of the finger first then twist and push in the tip. Feel for masses (haemorrhoids are not palpable) or impacted stool. Twist your arm so that the pad of your finger is feeling anteriorly. Feel for the cervix or prostate. Note consistency and size of prostate. Obliteration of its midline sulcus is a sign (unreliable) of prostate cancer. If there is a concern about the spinal cord, ask the patient to squeeze your finger and note the tone. Note stool or blood on the glove and test for occult blood. Wipe anus. Consider proctoscopy (for the anus) or sigmoidoscopy (which mainly inspects the rectum).

Haemorrhoids (piles)

The anus is lined by mainly discontinuous masses of spongy vascular tissue—the anal cushions, which contribute to anal closure. Viewed from the lithotomy position, their positions are at 3, 7, and 11 o'clock. They are attached by smooth muscle and elastic tissue, but are prone to displacement and disruption, either singly or together. The effects of gravity (our erect posture), increased anal tone (?stress), and the effects of straining at stool may make them become both bulky and loose, and so to protrude to form piles (Latin *pila*, meaning a ball). They are vulnerable to trauma and bleed readily from the capillaries of the underlying lamina propria, hence their other name—haemorrhoids (meaning *running blood* in Greek). Because the bleeding is from capillaries, it is bright red. (Piles are *not* varicose veins.)

Classification *1st-degree piles* remain in the rectum. If *2nd-degree,* they prolapse through the anus on defecation but spontaneously reduce. *3rd-degree piles:* As for second-degree but require digital reduction. *4th-degree piles:* These remain persistently prolapsed.

As there are no sensory fibres above the dentate line (squamomucosal junction), piles are not painful unless they thrombose when they protrude and are gripped by the anal sphincter, blocking venous return.

Differential diagnosis Perianal haematoma, fissures, abscess, tumour, proctalgia fugax (idiopathic, intense, stabbing rectal pain). Never ascribe bleeding to piles without adequate examination or investigation.

Causes Constipation with prolonged straining is the key factor. Congestion from a pelvic tumour, pregnancy, CCF, or portal hypertension are important in only a minority of cases.

Pathogenesis There is a vicious circle: vascular cushions protrude through a tight anus, become more congested, so hypertrophying to protrude again more readily. These protrusions may then strangulate.

The patient notices bright red rectal bleeding, often coating stools or dripping into the pan after defecation. There may be mucous discharge and pruritus ani. Severe anaemia may occur. In all rectal bleeding do:

- An abdominal examination to rule out other diseases.
- A rectal examination: prolapsing piles are obvious. Internal haemorrhoids are not palpable.
- Proctoscopy to see the internal haemorrhoids.
- Sigmoidoscopy to identify rectal pathology higher up (you can get no higher up than the rectosigmoid junction).

The best treatment Unknown, as meta-analyses differ. *Infra-red coagulation* applied for 1.5–2s, 3–8 times to localized areas of piles works by coagulating vessels, and tethering mucosa to subcutaneous tissue. Doing all the piles may take a few sessions. *Sclerosants* (2mL of 5% phenol in oil injected into the pile above the dentate line; SE: impotence; prostatitis) or *rubber band ligation* (SE: bleeding; infection); do <3 band-treatments per session; a cheap treatment, but needs skill. Banding produces an ulcer to anchor the mucosa (SE: pain, bleeding, infection). Freezing (cryo) is also used. A high-fibre diet may also help. Soft paraffin soothes.

In all but 4th degree piles, these may obviate need for haemorrhoidectomy (excision of piles ± ligation of vascular pedicles, as day-case surgery, needing ~2wks off work, p458). SE: haemorrhage or stenosis. Stapled haemorrhoidectomy results in a shorter hospital stay and quicker return to normal activity than conventional surgery, provided the surgeon has the technical experience.

Treatment of prolapsed, thrombosed piles is with analgesia, and bed rest. Pain usually resolves in 2–3 wks. Some surgeons advocate early operation.

Hernias

Definition Any structure passing through another so ending up in the wrong place is a *hernia*. Hernias involving bowel are said to be *irreducible* if they cannot be pushed back into the right place. This does not mean that they are either necessarily obstructed or strangulated. Gastrointestinal hernias are *obstructed* if bowel contents cannot pass through them—the classical features of intestinal obstruction soon appear. They are *strangulated* if ischaemia occurs—the patient becomes toxic and requires urgent surgery.

Inguinal hernia The commonest kind, described on p526.

Femoral hernia Bowel enters the femoral canal, presenting as a mass in the upper medial thigh or above the inguinal ligament where it points down the leg, unlike an inguinal hernia which points to the groin. They occur more often in women than men and are likely to be irreducible and to strangulate. *Anatomy:* The *neck* of the hernia is felt below and lateral to the pubic tubercle (inguinal hernias are above and medial to this point). The boundaries of the femoral canal are *anteriorly* and *medially* the inguinal ligament; *laterally* the femoral vein and *posteriorly* the pectineal ligament. The canal contains fat and Cloquet's node. *Treatment:* Surgical repair is recommended.

Paraumbilical hernias These occur just above or below the umbilicus. Risk factors are obesity and ascites. Omentum or bowel herniates through the defect. Surgery involves repair of the rectus sheath.

Epigastric hernias These pass through linea alba above the umbilicus.

Incisional hernias These follow breakdown of muscle closure after previous surgery (seen in 11–20%). If obese, repair is not easy. A randomized trial of repairs favoured mesh over suture techniques.[35]

Spighelian hernias These occur at the lateral edge of the rectus sheath, below and lateral to the umbilicus.

Lumbar hernias These occur through 1 of the lumbar triangles.

Richter's hernia This involves bowel wall only—not lumen.

Obturator hernias These occur through the obturator canal. Typically there is pain along the medial side of the thigh in a thin woman.

Other examples of hernias

- Of the nucleus pulposus into the spinal canal (slipped disc).
- Of the uncus and hippocampal gyrus through the tentorium (tentorial hernia) in space-occupying lesions.
- Of the brainstem and cerebellum through the foramen magnum (Arnold–Chiari malformation).
- Of the stomach through the diaphragm (hiatus hernia, p216).
- Of the terminal (intravesical) portion of the ureter into the bladder, with cystic ballooning between the mucosa and muscle layers. This is a *ureterocele* (*kēlē* is Greek for hernia), and results from stenosis of the ureteral meatus. Causes may be congenital (eg persistence of Chawalla's membrane), or rarely schistosomiasis or phaeochromocytoma. This intra-bladder hernia may cause obstruction ± UTI—or even herniate into the urethra and present as an interlabial mass. Management may involve endoscopic meatotomy or ureterocelectomy ± reimplantation.

Some examples of hernias

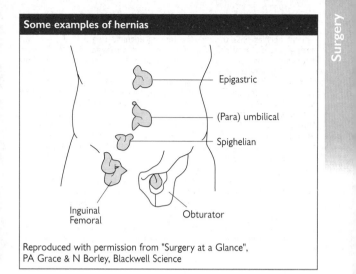

- Epigastric
- (Para) umbilical
- Spighelian
- Inguinal Femoral
- Obturator

Reproduced with permission from "Surgery at a Glance",
PA Grace & N Borley, Blackwell Science

Inguinal hernias

Indirect hernias pass through the internal inguinal ring and, if large, out through the external ring. Direct hernias push their way directly forward through the posterior wall of the inguinal canal, into a defect in the abdominal wall. Predisposing conditions: chronic cough, constipation, urinary obstruction, heavy lifting, ascites, previous abdominal surgery. There are 2 landmarks to identify: *The internal ring* may be defined as being the *inguinal ligament's mid-point*, 1½ cm above the femoral pulse (which crosses the *mid-inguinal point;* distinguishing this from the inguinal ligament's mid-point is probably useful only in finals examinations). *The external ring* is just above and medial to the pubic tubercle (the bony prominence forming the medial attachment of the inguinal ligament). Relations of the inguinal canal are:

Floor: Inguinal ligament.
Roof: Fibres of transversalis and internal oblique.
Front: External oblique aponeurosis + internal oblique for the lateral ⅓.
Back: Laterally, transversalis fascia; medially, conjoint tendon.

It contains the *spermatic cord* (*round ligament* if ♀) & the *ilioinguinal nerve*.

Examining the patient Always look for previous scars, feel the other side and examine the external genitalia. Then ask: • Is the lump visible? If so, ask the patient to reduce it—if he cannot, make sure that it is not a scrotal lump. Ask him to cough. Inguinal hernias appear inferomedial to the external ring. • If no lump is visible, feel for a cough impulse. • If there is no lump, ask the patient to stand and repeat the cough.

Distinguishing direct from indirect hernias This is loved by examiners but is of little clinical use. The best way is to reduce the hernia and occlude the internal ring with two fingers. Ask the patient to cough—if the hernia is restrained, it is indirect, if it pops out, it is direct.

Indirect hernias:	Direct hernias:	Femoral hernias:
Common (80%)	Less common (20%)	More frequent in females
	Reduce easily	Frequently irreducible
Can strangulate	Rarely strangulate	Frequently strangulate

Irreducible hernias You may be called because a long-standing hernia is now irreducible and painful. It is always worth trying to reduce these yourself—to prevent strangulation and bowel necrosis (a grave event, demanding prompt laparotomy). Learn how to do this from an expert—ie one of your patients who has been reducing his hernia for years, then you will be well-equipped to act correctly when the incipient emergency presents. Notice that such patients use the flat of the hand, directing the hernia from below, up towards the contralateral shoulder. Sometimes, as the hernia obstructs, reduction requires perseverance, which may be rewarded by a gurgle from the retreating bowel, and can thus spare unnecessary surgery.

Repairs Advise patients to diet and stop smoking pre-op. Mesh techniques (eg Lichtenstein repair) have replaced older methods such as the 'Shouldice' repair, with its multilayered suture involving both anterior and posterior walls of the inguinal canal. In mesh repairs, a polypropylene mesh reinforces the posterior wall. Recurrence rate is less than with older methods (eg <2% vs 10%). Local anaesthetic techniques and day-case 'ambulatory' surgery may halve the price of surgery. This is important because this is one of the most common operations (>100,000 per year in the UK).

Laparoscopic repair is also possible, and gives similar recurrence rates. There is less post-operative pain and an earlier return to work after a laparoscopic repair, and undiagnosed contralateral hernias can be identified. Laparoscopic repair *may* cost more than conventional surgery (p534).◄

Return to work: we used to advise 4wks' rest and convalescence over 10wks, but with new mesh repairs, if comfortable, return to manual work (& driving) after ≤2wks is OK; explain pre-op.

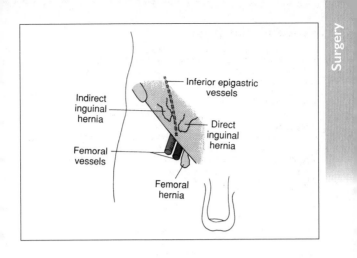

Varicose veins (VVs)

Blood from superficial veins of the leg passes into the deep veins by means of perforator veins (perforating deep fascia) and at the sapheno-femoral and sapheno-popliteal junctions. Valves prevent blood from passing from deep to superficial veins. If they become incompetent (venous hypertension from prolonged standing, occlusion by fetus, ovarian tumour, previous DVT) dilatation (*varicosities*) of the superficial veins occurs. Other risk factors may include genetic predisposition but probably not female sex.[17]

Symptoms 'My legs are ugly'. Note that pain, cramps, tingling, heaviness, and restless legs are often attributed to VVs, but careful studies show these common symptoms are only slightly commoner in those with VVs (63% vs 45%; and early surgery does not prevent later complications).[19]

Signs Oedema; eczema; ulcers; haemosiderin skin staining; haemorrhage; phlebitis. On their own, even in (non-smoking) Pill takers, and even associated with phlebitis, VVs don't cause DVTs (*proximally spreading phlebitis of the long saphenous vein in the thigh may be an exception*).

Method of examination (Start with the patient standing.)

1 Note signs of poor skin nutrition: ulcers usually above the medial malleolus (varicose ulcers, *OHCS* p474) with deposition of haemosiderin causing brown edges, eczema, and thin skin. Inspect the legs from anterior thigh to medial calf (long saphenous vein) and the back of the calf (short saphenous vein). Palpate veins for tenderness (due to phlebitis) and hardness (due to thrombosis).

2 Feel for a *cough impulse* at the sapheno-femoral junction (≈ incompetence). *The percussion test:* tap the top of a vein and feel how far down its length you can feel repercussions (interrupted by competent valves).

3 *Trendelenburg's test* assesses if the sapheno-femoral junction valve is competent: lie the patient down and raise the leg to empty the vein. Place 2 fingers on the sapheno-femoral junction (5cm below and medial to femoral pulse). Ask him to stand keeping the fingers in place. If the varicosities are controlled, they will not rapidly fill. Release the fingers to confirm that they then fill. This shows that there is sapheno-femoral incompetence and the operation of sapheno-femoral disconnection (Trendelenburg's operation) should help. If the varicosities are not controlled, then there must be incompetence at a lower level.

4 *The tourniquet test* is similar to Trendelenburg's test, but instead of controlling varicosities with the fingers, use a tourniquet tied around the thigh at the level of the sapheno-femoral junction. If the varicosities are not controlled, repeat the test with the tourniquet lower down the thigh, until the level at which there is incompetence is identified.

5 *Perthes' test* determines if the deep femoral veins are competent. With the patient standing and veins filled, a tourniquet is placed around the mid-thigh and the patient walks for 5min. If the saphenous veins collapse below the tourniquet, the deep veins are patent and the communicating veins are competent; if unchanged, both saphenous and communicating veins are incompetent; if the veins increase in prominence and pain occurs, the deep veins are occluded.

6 *Doppler ultrasound probes*, to listen to flow in incompetent valves, eg the sapheno-femoral junction, or the short saphenous vein behind the knee (the calf is squeezed, and flow on release lasting over ½–1 second indicates significant reflux). If incompetence is not identified and treated at the time of surgery, varicosities will return.

▶Before surgery, ensure that all varicosities are indelibly marked *on either side* (to avoid tattooing if the incision is made through inked skin).

Saphena varix This is a dilatation (varicosity) in the saphenous vein at its confluence with the femoral vein. It is one of the many causes of a lump in the groin (p512). Because it transmits a cough impulse, it may be mistaken for an inguinal or femoral hernia—but on closer inspection, it may have a bluish tinge to it, and it disappears on lying down.

Treating varicose veins

▶NICE guidelines suggest that the criteria for specialist referral of patients with VVs should be bleeding, pain, ulceration, superficial thrombophlebitis, or 'a severe impact on quality of life'.

- *Patient education:* Avoid prolonged standing; support stockings; lose weight; regular walks (calf muscle action aids venous return).
- *Injection therapy:* especially for varicosities below the knee if there is no gross sapheno-femoral incompetence. Sclerosant (eg ethanolamine) is injected at multiple sites and the vein compressed for a few weeks to avoid thrombosis (intravascular granulation tissue obliterates the lumen). Unsuitable for perforation sites. A novel development of this technique involves mixing the sclerosant with air to form a foam that is injected at a single site, and spreads rapidly throughout the veins. Ultrasound monitoring prevents inadvertent spread of foam into the femoral vein.
- *Surgery:* There are several choices, depending on vein anatomy and surgical preference, eg sapheno-femoral disconnection; multiple avulsions; stripping from groin to upper calf (stripping to the ankle is not needed, and may damage the saphenous nerve). *Post-op:* Bandage legs tightly, and elevate for 24h. Then encourage regular walking eg 3miles/d, taken as many short walks.

When do varicose veins become an illness?

The obvious answer is that they do so when they hurt. But for some patients, this is too simple. Thanks to Albert Camus, we know that 'certain illnesses are desirable: they provide a compensation for a functional disorder which, in their absence, would express itself in a more serious disturbance'. In one study ~50% of those undergoing VV surgery were in emotional turmoil—perhaps many opted for surgery as a displacement activity to confronting deeper problems. ▶We adopt the sickness role when we want sympathy. Somatization is hard to manage: here is one general approach to consider: Give time; don't dismiss these patients as 'just the "worried well"'.

- Explore the factors perpetuating illness behaviour (disordered physiology, misinformation, unhelpful 'coping' behaviour, social stressors).
- Agree a plan that makes sense to the patient's holistic view of himself.
- Treat any underlying depression (drugs & cognitive therapy, *OHCS* p370).

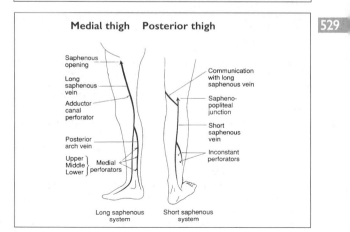

Medial thigh   Posterior thigh

Saphenous opening
Long saphenous vein
Adductor canal perforator
Posterior arch vein
Upper
Middle ⎱ Medial perforators
Lower ⎰

Communication with long saphenous vein
Sapheno-popliteal junction
Short saphenous vein
Inconstant perforators

Long saphenous system   Short saphenous system

Gastric surgery and its aftermath

▶Indications for gastric surgery include gastric carcinomas and peptic ulcers, though medical therapy (p214) has made elective surgery for the latter rare.

Operations for benign gastric ulceration Those near the pylorus may be considered similarly to duodenal ulceration (p532). Away from the pylorus, elective operation is rarely needed as ulcers respond well to medical treatment, stopping smoking, and avoidance of NSAIDs. In patients who are unable to tolerate medical treatment, a laparoscopic highly selective vagotomy (HSV) can be performed.

Emergency surgery is sometimes needed for haemorrhage or perforation. Haemorrhage is usually treated by underrunning the bleeding ulcer base or excision of the ulcer. If the former is done, then a biopsy should be taken to exclude malignancy. Perforation is usually managed by excision of the hole for histology, then closure.

Operations for duodenal ulceration See p532.

Gastric carcinoma (See p508.) Curative surgical options include D_1 resection (removal of tumour and perigastric lymph nodes) and D_2 resection (removal of the D_1 tier of lymph nodes and the next tier out, along the coeliac axis). There is considerable controversy as to which should be performed, as some studies have shown worse morbidity and mortality for D_2 resections performed in Western countries. It is likely that the results reflect the lack of dedicated specialists such as those in Japan, where gastric carcinoma is particularly common. D_2 resections should therefore only be performed in specialist centres.

Partial gastrectomy (the Billroth operations)

Billroth I: Partial gastrectomy with simple re-anastomosis (rejoining).

Billroth II (Polya gastrectomy): Partial gastrectomy. The duodenal stump is oversewn (leaving a blind loop), and anastomosis is achieved by a longitudinal incision further down (into the proximal jejunum).

Physical complications of gastrectomy and peptic ulcer surgery

▶As peptic ulcer surgery is largely obselete, these complications are mainly of historical interest only.

Recurrent ulceration: Symptoms are similar to those experienced pre-operatively but complications are more common and response to medical treatment is poor. Further surgery is difficult.

Abdominal fullness: Feeling of early satiety (perhaps with discomfort and distension) improving with time. Advise to take small, frequent meals.

Dumping syndrome: Fainting and sweating after eating due to food of high osmotic potential being dumped in the jejunum, causes oligaemia from rapid fluid shifts. 'Late dumping' is due to rebound hypoglycaemia and occurs 1–3h after meals. Both tend to improve with time but may be helped by eating less sugar, and more guar and pectin (slows glucose absorption). Acarbose may also help to reduce the early hyperglycemic stimulus to insulin secretion.

Bilious vomiting: This is difficult to treat—but often improves with time.

Diarrhoea: May be disabling after vagotomy. Codeine phosphate may help.

Gastric tumour: A rare complication of any surgery which ↓acid production.

Amylase↑: If abdominal pain too, this may indicate afferent loop obstruction after Billroth II surgery (needs emergency surgery).

Metabolic complications *Weight loss:* Often due to poor calorie intake.

Bacterial overgrowth ± malabsorption (the blind loop syndrome) may occur.

Anaemia: Usually from lack of iron hypochlorhydria and stomach resection. B_{12} levels are frequently low but megaloblastic anaemia is rare.

Osteomalacia: There may be pseudofractures which look like metastases.

Complications of peptic ulcer surgery

	Partial gastrectomy	Vagotomy & pyloroplasty	Highly selective vagotomy
Recurrence	2%	7%	>7%
Dumping	20%	14%	6%
Diarrhoea	1%	4%	<1%
Metabolic	++++	++	0

(These values are approximate and depend on the skill of the surgeon.)

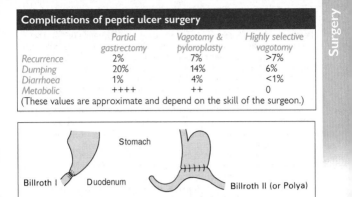

Stomach

Billroth I — Duodenum

Billroth II (or Polya)

Operations for duodenal ulcer

Peptic ulcers usually present as epigastric pain and dyspepsia (p214). There is no reliable method of distinguishing clinically between gastric and duodenal ulcers. Although management of both is usually medical in the 1ˢᵗ instance (with *H. pylori* eradication, p215), surgery still has a role.

Surgery is usually only required for complications such as *haemorrhage*, *perforation*, and *pyloric stenosis*, though may be considered for the few patients who are not responsive/tolerant to medical therapy.

Several types of operation have been tried but, as whenever considering an operation, one must consider efficacy, side-effects, and mortality.

1 **Elective surgery** may be undertaken for patients who are intolerant to or who fail to respond to medical treatment:

   a. *Highly selective vagotomy:* May be useful in patients unable to tolerate medical treatment. The vagus supply is denervated only where it supplies the lower oesophagus and stomach. The nerve of Laterget to the pylorus is left intact; thus, gastric emptying is unaffected. The results of surgery are greatly dependent on the skill of the surgeon.

   b. *Vagotomy and pyloroplasty:* A vagotomy reduces acid production from the stomach body and fundus, and reduces gastrin production from the antrum. However, it interferes with emptying of the pyloric sphincter and so a drainage procedure (eg pyloroplasty) must be added. This operation is now almost obselete, and is only performed in exceptional circumstances.

   c. *Gastrectomy* (p530) is rarely required in the modern management of peptic ulcer disease.

2 **Emergency surgery** may be required for the following complications:

   a. *Haemorrhage* may be controlled endoscopically by adrenaline injection, diathermy, laser coagulation, or heat probe. Operation should be considered for severe haemorrhage or rebleeding, especially in the elderly. At surgery, the bleeding ulcer base is underrun or oversewn.

   b. *Perforation* Most patients undergo surgery, though some advocate an initial conservative approach (NBM, NG tube, IV antibiotics) in patients without generalized peritonitis—this can prevent surgery in up to 50% of such cases. If emergency surgery is required, laparoscopic repair of the hole will usually suffice. *H. pylori* eradication should be commenced post-op (p214).

   c. *Pyloric stenosis* This is a late complication, presenting with vomiting of large amounts of food some hours after meals. (Adult pyloric stenosis is a complication of duodenal ulcers, and has nothing to do with congenital hypertrophic pyloric stenosis.) *Treatment:* Endoscopic balloon dilatation, followed by maximal acid suppression (p214), may be tried in the 1ˢᵗ instance (NB: 5% risk of perforation). If this is unsuccessful, a drainage procedure (eg gastro-enterostomy or pyloroplasty) ± highly selective vagotomy may be performed, often laparoscopically. The operation should be done on the next available list, after correction of the metabolic defect—hypochloraemic, hypokalaemic metabolic alkalosis.

Fundoplication for gastro-oesophageal reflux

The goal This is to re-establish lower oesophageal sphincter tone.

The procedure This involves wrapping the gastric fundus around the lower oesophagus, closing the hiatus, and securing the wrap in the abdomen. There are various types of procedure eg Nissen (360° wrap), Toupet (270° posterior wrap), Watson (anterior hemifundoplication).

Access Now usually performed laparoscopically which, when performed in specialist centres, is at least as effective at controlling reflux as open surgery but with a lower mortality . Wound infections and respiratory complications are also more common in open surgery, and the incidence of dysphagia is similar for the two procedures—but see p534.

Minimally invasive surgery

The term 'keyhole surgery' or minimal access surgery may be preferred, because these procedures can be as invasive as any laparotomy, having just the same set of side-effects—plus some new ones. It is the size of the incision and the use of laparoscopes which marks out this branch of surgery. Laparoscopy has been well established in gynaecology for many years where initially a purely optical telescope, held by the surgeon, was used for visualization. The development of miniaturized video cameras was the impetus to the widespread use of laparoscopy, as it allowed an assistant to have the same view as the surgeon. The surgeon could therefore operate with *both* hands, while his assistant held the laparoscope and retracted the viscera. Laparoscopic cholecystectomy was shown to be possible, and became the method of choice. Laparoscopy is now in widespread use for diagnostic purposes and for other conditions, such as appendicectomy, fundoplication, splenectomy, and adrenalectomy. It is currently under evaluation for hernia repair, colectomy, nephrectomy (in renal transplants), parathyroidectomy, sentinel node biopsy, and perforated peptic ulcer repair.

As a rule of thumb, whatever can be done by laparotomy can also be done with the laparoscope. This does not mean that it *should* be done, but if the patient feels better sooner, has less post-operative pain, and can return to work earlier, and have fewer complications, then these specific techniques will gain ascendency—provided hospitals can afford the equipment.

It is worth noting that advantages do not include time. In upper GI procedures, laparoscopic procedures take longer than open procedures. Also, the patient needs to spend a night in hospital, usually. This has economic implications when comparing laparoscopic inguinal hernia repair with its open alternative done under local anaesthesia (after which the patient can go home the same day). On the other side of the economic equation for hernia repair is that pain >24h post-op is less after laparoscopic procedures, and the patient can return to full employment after a week. In addition, laparoscopic repair allows detection of a previously undiagnosed contralateral hernia. Which method makes economic sense depends on who is doing the calculation; NICE concluded that open hernia repair was cheaper, but their calculations did not include out of hospital costs.◆

Problems with minimal access surgery: for the surgeon

Inspection: Anatomy looks different due to the different surgical approach.
Palpation is impossible during laparoscopic procedures. This may make it hard to locate colon lesions prior to cutting them out. This means that pre-operative tests may need to be more extensive (eg colonoscopy *and* barium enema).
Skill: Here the problem is not just that a new skill has to be learned and taught. Old skills may become attenuated if most cholecystectomies are performed via the laparoscope, and new practitioners may not achieve quite the level of skill in either sphere if they try to do both.

Problems for the patient and his general practitioner

Post-operative complications: What may be quite easily managed on a well-run surgical ward (eg haemorrhage) may prove a challenge for a GP and be terrifying for the patient, who may be all alone after early discharge.

Loss of tell-tale scars: After laparoscopy there may only be a few abdominal stab wounds, so the GP or the patient's future carers have to guess at what has been done. The answer here is to communicate carefully and thoroughly with the patient, so that he or she knows what has been done.

Problems for the hospital Just because minimal access surgery is often cost-effective, it does not follow that hospitals can afford the procedures. Instruments are continuously being refined, and quickly become obsolete—so that many are now produced in disposable single-use form. Because of budgeting boundaries, hospitals cannot use the cash saved, by early return to work or by freeing-up bed use, to pay for capital equipment and extra theatre time that may be required.

Exposing patients to our learning curves? The jury is still out …

All surgeons, indeed all doctors, get better over time (for a while), as they perform new techniques with increasing ease and confidence. Mortality rates inevitably vary. When Wertheim did his first radical hysterectomies, his first dozen patients died—but then someone survived, and he assumed it was a good operation, and pressed ahead. He was a brave man, and thousands of women owe their lives to him. But if he had tried to do this today, he would have been stopped. The UK's General Medical Council (GMC), and other august bodies constantly tell us that we must protect the public by reporting doctors whose patients have low survival rates. The reason for this is partly ethical, and partly an attempt to preserve self-regulation.

The defining feature of any profession lies, the GMC assumes, in self-regulation. To preserve this, we have the toughest professional codes of practice and disciplinary procedures of any group of workers. It is assumed that doctors are loyal to each other out of self-interest, and that this loyalty is bad. This has never been tested formally, and is not evidence-based. We can imagine two clinical worlds: one of constant 'reportings' and recriminatory audits, and another of trust and teamwork. Both are imperfect, but we should not assume that the first world would be better for our patients.

It is easy to say that our patients demand honesty, and so long as we are doing our best, and referring where needed, all will be well. But honesty is opaque at the bedside. We never know the *whole* truth about our past performance. (All our patients with such-and-such a colostomy left hospital alive—but perhaps they all committed suicide later?) Should we tell our patient that this is the first time we have done this sort of operation unsupervised? When patients are sick with fear, they do not, perhaps, want to know everything. We may tell to protect ourselves. We may *not* tell to protect ourselves. Perhaps what we should do is, in the privacy of our own hearts, to appeal to those 12 dead women-of-Wertheim—a jury as infallible as sacrificial—and try to hear their reply. And to those who complain that in doing so we are playing God, it is possible to reply with some humility that, whatever it is, it does not *seem* like play.

▶'It is amazing what little harm doctors do when one considers all the opportunities they have'.   Mark Twain

Infectious diseases (ID)[1]

Contents

---

1 We thank Dr David Chadwick who is our Specialist Reader for this chapter.

UK notifiable diseases[ND]

Inform the Consultant in Communicable Disease Control (CCDC).

Anthrax	Malaria	Rubella
Cholera	Measles	Scarlet fever
Diphtheria	Meningitis (acute)	Smallpox; tetanus
Dysentery (amoebic, typhoid, and paratyphoid)	Meningococcal sepsis	Tuberculosis
	Mumps	Typhus
	Ophthalmia neonatorum	Viral haemorrhagic fevers, eg lassa & yellow fevers
Encephalitis	Plague	
Food poisoning	Poliomyelitis	
Leprosy	Rabies	Viral hepatitis
Leptospirosis	Relapsing fever	Whooping cough

UK HIV reporting is voluntary (and in strict confidence) to the Communicable Disease Surveillance Control, 61 Colindale Ave, London NW9 5EQ (tel: 020 8200 6868 or 020 8965 1118).

Getting the balance right in studying infectious diseases

It is not possible for any ID chapter to be constructed so that it has the right balance throughout the world. Many of our readers come from communities where tetanus and malaria are daily problems—whereas, in UK consulting rooms, chest, GU, and ENT infections are likely to dominate. In Western hospital specialist ID practice, the chief problems are:
- Respiratory tract infections (p172–p180, and *Emergencies*, p800)
- Hospital acquired infections (eg p174 & p565)
- Infections in immunocompromised hosts, eg febrile neutropenia (p650)
- Infections associated with general surgery (p448 & p452)
- Infections in intensive care unit patients (examples on p548 & p613)
- Osteomyelitis (*OHCS* p644) and prosthetic joint infections (*OHCS* p655)
- HIV/AIDS (p578–85)
- Illness in a returning traveller (p554).

But in all areas, the pitfalls are the same: not taking time to find out about your patient—where he has been, what his hobbies are (and his work), and whom he has had contact with. Always have a high index of suspicion for TB, and always remember that ID rarities are often very treatable.
►Two heads are better than one: so when in doubt, get help.

The classification of pathogens

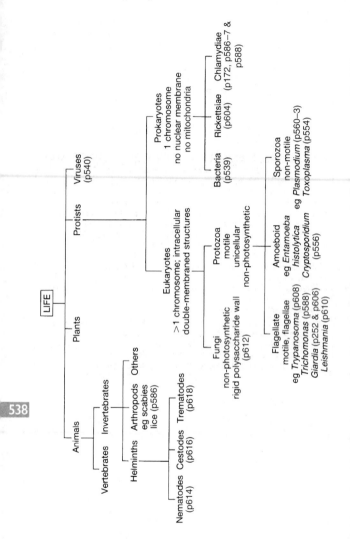

If the classification above seems too conventional, try this method, translated from a Chinese encyclopaedia by Michel Foucault in *The Order of Things*:
'Animals are divided into the following categories: (a) belonging to the Emperor, (b) embalmed, (c) tame, (d) sucking pigs, (e) sirens, (f) fabulous, (g) stray dogs, (h) included in the present classification, (i) frenzied, (j) innumerable, (k) drawn with a very fine camelhair brush, (l) etc, (m) having just broken the water pitcher, (n) that from a long way off look like flies.'

Examples of pathogens from various types of bacteria

This table is not exhaustive; it is simply a guide for the forthcoming pages.

Gram positive cocci

Staphylococci (p590):
  coagulase +ve, eg *Staphylococcus aureus*
  coagulase −ve, eg *Staph. epidermidis*

Streptococci[1] (p590):
  β-haemolytic streptococci
    Streptococcus pyogenes (Lancefield group A)
  α-haemolytic streptococci
    Strep. mitior
    Strep. pneumoniae (pneumococcus)
    Strep. sanguis
  Enterococci (non-haemolytic)[2]:
    Enterococcus mutans
    E. faecalis
  Anaerobic streptococci

Gram positive bacilli (rods)

Aerobes
  Bacillus anthracis (anthrax: p590)
  Corynebacterium diphtheriae (p590)
  Listeria monocytogenes (p591)
  Nocardia species

Anaerobes:
  Clostridium
    Cl. botulinum (botulism: p830)
    Cl. perfringens (gas gangrene: p591)
    Cl. tetani (tetanus: p594)
    Cl. difficile (diarrhoea, p218)
  Actinomyces:
    Actinomyces israeli (p591), *A. naeslundii*
    A. odontolyticus, A. viscosus

Obligate intracellular bacteria:

Chlamydia (p586, p174, *OHCS* p50)
  Chlamydia trachomatis (*OHCS* p512)
  C. psittaci
  C. pneumoniae
Coxiella burnetii (p604)
Bartonella (p604)
Ehrlichia (p604)
Rickettsia (typhus, p605)
Legionella pneumophilia (p174)
Mycoplasma pneumoniae (p174)

Gram negative cocci

Neisseria:
  Neisseria meningitidis (meningitis, septicaemia)
  N. gonorrheae (gonorrhoea, p588)
Moraxella:
  Moraxella catarrhalis (pneumonia, p593)

Gram negative bacilli (rods)

Enterobacteriaceae (p556 & p592):
  Escherichia coli
  Shigella species (p596)
  Salmonella species (p596)
  Citrobacter freundii, C. koseri
  Klebsiella pneumoniae, K. oxytoca
  Enterobacter aerogenes, E. cloacae
  Serratia marascens;
    Proteus mirabilis/vulgaris
  Morganella morganii
  Providencia species
  Yersinia enterocolitica, Y. pestis
  Y. paratuberculosis
  Pseudomonas aeruginosa (p592)
  Haemophilus influenzae (p592)
  Brucella species (p592)
  Bordetella pertussis (p592)
  Pasteurella multocida (p593)
  Vibrio cholerae (p596)
  Campylobacter jejuni (p556)

Anaerobes:
  Bacteroides (wound infections, p448)
  Fusobacterium
  Helicobacter pylori (p214)

Mycobacteria:
  Mycobacterium tuberculosis (TB, p564–8)
  M. bovis
  M. leprae (leprosy, p598)
'Atypical' mycobacteria:
  M. avium intracellulare (p580)
  M. scrofulaceum, M. kansasii
  M. marinum, M. malmoense
  M. ulcerans, M. xenopi, M gordonae
  M. fortuitum, M. chelonae, M. flavescens
  M. smegmatis-phlei
Spirochaetes (p600–3):
  Treponema (syphilis; yaws; pinta)
  Leptospira (Weil's dis; canicola fever)
  Borrelia (relapsing fever; Lyme dis)

---

1 Streps are classified according to haemolytic pattern (α, β-, or non-haemolytic) or by Lancefield antigen (A–G), or by species (eg *Strep. pyogenes*). There is much crossover among these groups; the above is a generalization for the chief pathogens.
2 Clinically, epidemiologically and in terms of treatment, enterococci behave unlike other streps.

Viruses (classification)

DNA viruses

A *Double-stranded DNA*

- Papovavirus   Papilloma virus: human warts
  JC virus: Progressive multifocal leucoencephalopathy, PML

- Adenovirus   >30 serotypes
  10% viral respiratory disease
  7% viral meningitis

- Herpes viruses   Alphaherpesvirus$^\alpha$ (eg neurotropic) beta-$^\beta$ (eg epithe-
  liotropic) & gammaherpesvirus$^\gamma$ (lymphotropic):
  Herpes simplex virus$^\alpha$ (HSV) 1 & HSV 2 (p568)
  Herpes (varicella) zoster virus$^\alpha$ (p568)
  Cytomegalovirus$^\beta$—CMV, also called HHV-5, (p574)
  Herpes virus 6$^\beta$ & 7$^\beta$ (HHV-6 & 7): roseola infantum
  (mild, OHCS p214); also post-transplant, like CMV
  Epstein–Barr virus (EBV) (p570)$^\gamma$
  –infectious mononucleosis (glandular fever)
  –Burkitt's lymphoma; nasopharyngeal carcinoma
  HHV-8$^\gamma$: Kaposi's sarcoma (p726)

- Pox viruses   (1) Variola: smallpox (now officially eradicated)[1]
  (2) Vaccinia, cowpox
  (3) Orf, cutaneous pustules, caught from sheep
  (4) Molluscum contagiosum, pearly umbilicated
  papules, typically seen in children or with HIV.

- Hepatitis B virus (see p576)

B *Single-stranded DNA*

- Erythrovirus   Erythema infectiosum (fifth disease, OHCS p214)
  formerly parvovirus   'slapped cheek' appearance ± aplastic crises

RNA viruses

A *Double-stranded RNA*

- Reovirus   eg rotavirus, infantile gastroenteritis

B *Positive single-stranded RNA*

- Picornavirus   (1) Rhinovirus, common cold, >90 serotypes
  (2) Enterovirus
      (i) Coxsackie A (meningitis, gastroenteritis)
        Coxsackie B (pericarditis, Bornholm disease)
      (ii) Polio virus
      (iii) Echovirus (30% viral meningitis)
      (iv) Hepatitis A virus

- Togavirus   (1) Rubella
  (2) Alphavirus
  (3) Flavivirus (yellow fever, dengue, hepatitis C)

- Coronavirus   eg Urbani SARS-associated coronavirus[2]

C *Negative single-stranded RNA*

- Orthomyxovirus   Influenza A, B, C
- Paramyxovirus   Parainfluenza, mumps, measles, respiratory
  syncitial virus (RSV)
- Arenavirus   Lassa fever, some viral haemorrhagic fevers,
  lymphocytic-choriomeningitis virus (LCM)
- Rhabdovirus   Rabies
- Bunyavirus   Some viral haemorrhagic fevers

D Retrovirus

- HIV-1, HIV-2, (p578)
- HTLV-1, HTLV-2

---

1 Although officially declared eradicated by WHO in 1979, there have been some recent concerns that the virus may fall into the hands of those who would use it as a biological weapon.
2 Severe acute respiratory syndrome (SARS) presents with fever, dry cough, headache, and hypoxaemia. The virus is named after Carolo Urbani, the doctor who discovered, and subsequently died from, SARS.

Travel advice[1]

The majority of travel-related illnesses are not infections, eg accidents, violence, myocardial infarction. Most infections are due to ignorance or indiscretions. ▶*Advice to travellers is more important than vaccination*: eg simple hygiene, malaria prophylaxis, and protective measures. Take time to advise travellers on the benefits of safe sex and the risks of HIV and other STDs. *Malaria* is a big killer; see p562 for prevention. For *cholera* and *traveller's diarrhoea*, see p596 & p556.

Vaccinations: [L = live vaccine]	Doses needed	Gap between doses: 1st & 2nd	2nd & 3rd	Booster interval
Yellow fever[L]	1			10yrs
Typhoid SC (Typhim VI®)	1			3yrs
Tetanus	3	4wks	4wks	10yrs
Polio[L]	3	>4wks	>4wks	10yrs
Rabies pre-exposure	3	7–28d	6–12 months	2–3yrs
Meningococci	1			3yrs
Japanese encephalitis	3	1–2wks	2–4wks	2yrs
Tick encephalitis	3	1–3 months	9–12 months	3yrs
Hepatitis A (Havrix monodose®)	1	6–12 months		10yrs
if 1–15yrs use Havrix Junior®	1	6–12 months		
Hepatitis B	3	1 month	5 months	5yrs
if travelling soon:	3	1wk	3wks	1yr

*If live oral form used, give 3 doses (1 capsule on alternate days, 1h ac, with a cool drink).

If only 1 attendance is possible, all is not lost (make up *en route*): *malaria prophylaxis/advice*: p562. Suggested vaccines: *Africa:* Meningitis, typhoid, diphtheria, tetanus, polio, hepatitis A ± yellow fever. *Asia:* Meningitis (quadrivalent vaccine against meningitis A, C, W135, and Y for Saudi Arabia), typhoid, diphtheria, tetanus, polio, hepatitis A. Consider rabies and encephalitis. *S America:* Typhoid, diphtheria, tetanus, polio, hepatitis A ± yellow fever. *Travel if immunocompromised:* Avoid live[L] vaccines. Hepatitis B vaccine: p243.

Preventing traveller's diarrhoea

Water: If in doubt, boil all water. Chlorination is an alternative but does not kill amoebic cysts. Tablets are available from pharmacies. Filter water before purifying. It is important to distinguish between simple gravity filters and water purifiers (which also attempt to sterilize chemically). Choose a unit which is verified by bodies such as the London School of Hygiene and Tropical Medicine (eg the MASTA *Travel Well Personal Water Purifier*). Make sure that all containers are disinfected. Try to avoid surface water and intermittent tap supplies. In Africa assume that all unbottled water is unsafe. With bottled water, ensure the rim is clean and dry. Avoid ice.

Other water-borne diseases include schistosomiasis (p618).

Food: Hot, well-cooked food is safest. Avoid salads and peel your own fruit. If you cannot wash your hands, discard the part of the food which you are holding (with bananas, careful unzipping obviates this precaution). In those in whom traveller's diarrhoea might be most serious, consider a standby course of ciprofloxacin.

1 R Dawood *Traveller's Health*, OUP. Further information is available from: www.cdc.gov/travel (USA site) or www.doh.gov.uk/traveladvice/index.htm (UK site).

Susceptibility of some bacteria to certain antibiotics

	Penicillin V & G	Ampicillin & Amoxicillin	Flucloxacillin	Ticarcillin, piperacillin, Azlocillin	Cefradine & Cefazolin	Cefuroxime	Ceftriaxone & Cefotaxime	Ceftazidime	Imipenem & Meropenem	Erythromycin	Clindamycin	Tetracyclines	Chloramphenicol	Trimethoprim	Vancomycin & Teicoplanin	Aminoglycosides, eg Gentamicin	Metronidazole	Ciprofloxacin	Co-amoxiclav
Staph. aureus (penicillin-sensitive)	1	2	2	0	2	2	2	2	2R	2R	2R	2R	0	2	2	2	0	2	2
Staph. aureus (penicillin-resistant)	R	R	2	0	2	2	2	2	2R	2R	2R	2R	0	2	2	2	0	2	2
Strep. (group A)	1ᵃ	2	2	2	2	2	2	2	2	2	2	2R	R	2	2	R	0	2	2
Strep. pneumoniae	1	2	2	2	2	2	2	2	2	2	2	2R	R	2	2	R	0	2	2
Enterococcus foecalis	R	1	2	R	R	R	R	R	0	R	R	2R	R	R	2	R	0	R	1
N. meningitidis	1	2	0	2	2	0	0	0	0	R	R	2R	0	R	0	0	0	2	0
Listeria monocytogenes	0	2	0	2	0	0	0	0	2	R	R	2R	2	R	0	2	0	R	0
H. influenzae	R	1R	0	2	1	2	2	2	2	R	R	2R	2	2	R	R	0	2	2
E. coli	R	2R	R	1R	1R	2	2	2	2	R	R	R	1R*	R	R	2	0	2	2
Klebsiella species	R	R	R	1R	1R	2	2	2	2	R	R	R	1R*	R	R	2	0	2	2
Serratia/Enterobacter species	R	R	R	2R	2R	2R	2	R	R	R	R	R	1R*	R	R	2	0	2	2R
Proteus species	R	R	R	1R	2R	2	2	2	2	R	R	R	1R*	R	R	2	0	2	2
Pseudomonas aeruginosa	R	R	R	1R	R	R	R	1R	2	R	R	R	1R*	R	R	1	0	1	R
Bacteroides fragilis	2	R	R	R	R	R	R	R	0	2R	2R	2R	R	R	1	R	1	2	2
Other Bacteroides species	2	R	R	R	R	R	R	R	0	R	R	R	R	R	1	R	1	R	1
Clostridium difficile	0	0	0	0	0	0	0	0	0	0	2R	0	0	0	2	0	1	0	0

Note: 1 = susceptible, 1ˢᵗ choice. 2 = 2ⁿᵈ choice. R = resistance likely. 0 = usually inappropriate. R* = resistance is rare in most areas.

ᵃHigh proportion of isolates from S Europe, S Africa, & USA now show intermediate or high-level resistance.

NB: This table is a guide only, and different populations will exhibit their own (changing) patterns of resistance.

▲ In practice, the best thing is often to talk to a microbiologist.

Antibiotics: penicillins

General advice The most common error is to give antibiotics without knowing the causative organism and then to stop them before the infection is controlled. This may promote the spread of antibiotic resistance (see p590). In general, avoid giving antibiotics until the lab has cultured the organism unless the patient is very ill and in need of immediate treatment (see *Empirical treatment* p548). In which case, culture blood, MSU, sputum, and any other relevant samples before treating.

Antibiotic (*and its uses*):	*Usual adult dose*:	*In renal failure*:
Amoxicillin As ampicillin but better absorbed PO. For IV therapy, use ampicillin.	250–500mg/8h PO 3g/12h in recurrent or severe pneumonia	↓Dose if CC <10 (CC = creatinine clearance, mL/min)
Ampicillin Broader spectrum than penicillin; more active against Gram −ve rods, but β-lactamase sensitive. Amoxicillin is better absorbed PO.	500mg/4–6h IM/IV	↓Dose dose if CC < 10
Benzylpenicillin = penicillin G Most streptococci, meningococcus, gonococcus, syphilis, gas gangrene, anthrax, actinomycosis, and many anaerobes.	300–600mg/6h IV, 2.4g/4h in meningitis. If dose >1.2g, inject at rate <300mg/min	Massive doses may cause Na+↑ & K+↓, and, in renal failure, seizures
Co-amoxiclav Augmentin® = clavulanic acid 125mg + amoxicillin 250mg; use as for ampicillin but β-lactamase resistance confers a much broader spectrum. May cause LFT↑.	1–2 tab/8h PO; Avoid clavulanic acid toxicity (LFT↑) by giving 2nd tab as amoxicillin. IV form: p593	If CC 10–50, give 1–2 tab/12h; if CC <10, 1–2 tab/24h
Flucloxacillin (cloxacillin) For Gram +ve β-lactamase producers (staphylococci).	250–500mg/6h PO/IM; take ½h before food. 0.5–2g/6h IV	Dose unaltered if CC >10
Phenoxymethylpenicillin = penicillin V As for penicillin G but less active. Used as prophylaxis or to complete an IV course.	250–500mg/6h PO; take ½h before food	In severe renal failure, give doses every 12h
Piperacillin Very broad spectrum incl. anaerobes & *Pseudomonas*. Inactive against *Staphs*. Reserve only for those with severe infections. May be used with aminoglycosides (but not in the same IVI).	3–4g/4–6h slowly IV if severe infection. Tazocin® = tazobactam 500mg + piperacillin 4g: dose: 4.5g/8h IV over 3–5min	↓Dose if CC↓: CC 10–50: 4g/6h CC <10: 3–4g/8h
Procaine penicillin (= procaine benzylpenicillin) Depot injection; good for syphilis and gonorrhoea. Only available on a named patient basis in the UK.	Syphilis: 600mg/24h IM for 14d, gonorrhoea: start dose 3.6g if female, 2.5g if male	Dose unaltered
Ticarcillin Very broad spectrum, eg *Pseudomonas, Proteus*. Use with an aminoglycoside. More active than azlocillin or piperacillin.	Timentin® contains 3g ticarcillin + 200mg clavulanic acid; dose: 3.2g/8h IV (/4h in severe infections)	If CC 10–50 dose is 2g/4–8h If CC < 10, dose is 2g/12h

Penicillin side-effects ● Hypersensitivity: rash (ampicillin rashes need not indicate penicillin allergy but 'penicillin-allergic' implies allergy to *all* penicillins); serum sickness (2%); anaphylaxis (<1 : 100,000). ● In huge overdose or intrathecal injection: seizures and coma. ● Diarrhoea (pseudomembranous colitis, p219, is rare). ● U&E imbalance if given IV.

Antibiotics: cephalosporins

Spectrum Most cephalosporins are active against staphylococci (including β-lactamase producers), streptococci (except group D, *Enterococcus faecalis & faecium*), pneumococci, *E. coli*, some *Proteus, Klebsiella, Haemophilus, Salmonella,* and *Shigella*. 2nd generation drugs (cefuroxime, cefamandole) are active against *Neisseria* and *Haemophilus*. 3rd generation drugs (cefotaxime, ceftazidime, ceftriaxone) have better activity against Gram −ve organisms. Ceftazidime has less Gram +ve activity, especially against *Staph. aureus,* and is used in the treatment of *Pseudomonas* infections.

Uses Indications are controversial and vary from place to place. Oral cephalosporins (cefaclor, cefadroxil, cefradine, cefalexin, cefuroxime axetil) may be used in pneumonias, otitis media, skin and soft tissue lesions, and UTIs, but they are not 1st-line agents. They may be used as 2nd-line agents, or to complete a course that was started with an IV cephalosporin. The major use of cephalosporins is parenteral, eg as prophylaxis in surgery (p448) and in post-operative infection. Suspected life-threatening infections, eg severe pneumonia, meningitis, or Gram −ve septicaemia may be treated empirically with a 3rd generation drug. Cephalosporins may also become the drugs of 1st choice in certain situations, such as penicillin sensitivity (NB: 10% cross-sensitivity) or where aminoglycosides are better avoided, but they have no unique role here.

The principal **adverse effect** of the cephalosporins is hypersensitivity. This is seen in <10% of penicillin-sensitive patients. There may be GI upset, reversible changes in liver function tests, eosinophilia, rarely neutropenia, nephrotoxicity, and colitis. There are reports of clotting abnormalities, and there may be false +ve results for glycosuria or the Coombs' test. There is increased risk of nephrotoxicity when first generation cefalosporins are co-administered with frusemide (= furosemide), gentamicin, and vancomycin, but 2nd and 3rd generation drugs are probably safe. Most broad-spectrum cephalosporins potentiate warfarin.

Antibiotic	Adult dose	Notes
		For body surface area calculations see www.bnf.org/BNFExtraFrame.htm
Cefaclor	250mg/8h PO Max: 4g/24h	No dose change in RF
Cefadroxil	500mg–1g/12h PO	In RF give 1g loading dose, then: if CC^M 26–50: 1g/12h if CC^M 11–25: 1g/24h if CC^M 0–10: 1g/36h
Cefalexin	500mg/8h PO Max: 4g/24h PO	↓dose proportionately in RF if CC < 60 if CC <10: 500mg/24h
Cefamandole	500mg–2g/4–8h IM/IV	Similar to cefuroxime In RF give 1–2g loading dose, then: if CC 50–80: 750mg–2g/6h if CC 25–50: 750mg–2g/8h if CC 10–25: 500mg–1.25g/8h if CC 2–10: 500mg–1g/12h if CC <2: 250–750mg/12h
Cefepime[4]	1–3g/12h IVI	Good activity against *Pseudomonas,* enterobacter, other resistant Gram −ve organisms, and *S. aureus.* if CC 10–50: 1–2g/12h if CC ≤10: 1g/24h

Antibiotic	Adult dose	Notes
Cefpirome[4]	1–2g/12h IV over 5min	Broad spectrum, used eg in polymicrobial infection; pyelonephritis; pneumonia. Not for MRSA (p590) or bacteroides. Good against enterobacter.[?] In renal failure, load with 1–2g, then: if CC 20–50: 500mg–1g/12h if CC 5–20: 500mg–1g/24h
Cefixime	Syrup = 100mg/5mL ½–1yr: 3.75mL/d 1–4yrs: 5mL/d 5–10yrs: 10mL/d Adult dose: 200mg/12–24h PO	Active against streptococci, coliforms, *Haemophilus*, *Proteus* and anaerobes, staphylococci, *E. faecalis,* and *Pseudomonas* are resistant. In RF: normal dose if CC >20mL/min
Cefotaxime[3]	1–2g/12h IV/IM Max 4g/8h (gonorrhoea: 500mg stat)	Broad spectrum. For serious infections only (severe pneumonia, meningitis). Unreliable activity against *Pseudomonas*. If CC <10, give 2g/24h max.
Cefoxitin	1–2g/6–8h IV/IM Max 12g/24h Gonorrhoea: 2g stat (deep IM) with probenecid 1g PO	Active against *Bacteroides*, so useful in bowel surgery and pre-operatively. In RF load with 1–2g, then: if CC 10–50: 1–2g/8–12h if CC <10: 2g/24–48h
Cefradine	250–500mg/6h PO or 500mg–1g/12h PO or 500mg–2g/6h IM/IV	Less active than cefuroxime In RF load with 750mg, then give 500mg at frequency dictated by CC: if CC > 20: 500mg/6h if CC 5–20: 250mg/6h if CC < 5: 250mg/50–70h
Ceftazidime[3]	UTI: 500mg–1g/12h Other: 1–2g/8h Max: 1g/8h if elderly Route: IV/IM but avoid IM if dose >1g	Broad spectrum, incl. most *Pseudomonas* For serious infections only. Used in blind treatment of neutropenic sepsis. In RF load with 1g, then: if CC 31–50: 1g/12h if CC 16–30: 1g/24h if CC 6–15: 500mg/24h if CC ≤ 5: 500mg/48h
Ceftriaxone[3]	1–4g daily IM/IV give ≤1g at each IM site with 3.5mL 1% lignocaine (=lidocaine)	Many Gram +ve and –ve infections. Used in meningitis (p370), pre-colonic surgery, and gonorrhoea. No activity against *Listeria*, enterococci, and *Pseudomonas*. Can be used in RF unless CC < 10, then limit dose to 2g/d and check levels
Cefuroxime	250–500mg/12h PO 750mg–1.5g/8h IV/IM; Max IV: 3g/8h In RF ↓dose	Broad spectrum & good Gram –ve activity. Used in: surgical prophylaxis; post-op infections; severe pneumonia. if CC 10–20: 750mg/12h if CC < 10: 750mg/24h

545

RF = renal failure; CC= creatinine clearance; CC^M= CC/1.73m^2 body area; [4]= 4th generation cephalosporin; [3]= 3rd generation cephalosporin

Antibiotics: others

Antibiotic (and uses)	Adult dose	Notes (CC=creatinine clearance, mL/min)
Amikacin See gentamicin.	7.5mg/kg/12h IV; (lower dose in renal failure)	Resistance is less common than with gentamicin.
Azithromycin See clarithromycin, also good against *N. gonorrhoae*.	500mg PO for 3d.	SE: See erythromycin.
Chloramphenicol Rarely used 1ˢᵗ-line. May be used in typhoid fever & *Haemophilus* infection. Also in blind R̥ of meningitis if patient allergic to both penicillins and cephalosporins. Avoid late in lactation & pregnancy.	12.5mg/kg/6h PO or IV; 25mg/kg/6h may be used in septicaemia or meningitis	SE (rare): marrow aplasia (check FBC often), neuritis, GI upset. Avoid long or repeated courses and in liver impairment or if CC <10mL/min. *Interactions:* warfarin, rifampicin, phenytoin, sulfonylureas, phenobarbital.
Ciprofloxacin Used in adult cystic fibrosis, typhoid, *Salmonella*, *Campylobacter*, prostatitis, and serious or resistant infections. Avoid overuse.	250–750mg/12h PO 200–400mg/12h IVI over ≥½h (over 1h, if 400mg used)	A good oral anti-pseudomonal agent. β-lactamase-resistant. Halve dose if CC <10. SE: rashes, D&V, LFT ↑; potentiates theophylline.
Clarithromycin A macrolide, like erythromycin, used for: *S. aureus*, streptococci, *Myco-plasma*, *H. pylori*, *Chlamydia*, MAI (p580).	250–500mg/12h PO for 7–14d. *H. pylori*: 500mg/12h PO for 1wk as triple therapy (p215). MAI may need 12wks (p580)	Halve dose if CC <10. *Interactions:* ergot, warfarin, carbamazepine, theophyllines, zidovudine; never use with terfenadine or pimozide.
Clindamycin Active against Gram+ve cocci including penicillin resistant staph, and anaerobes.	150–300mg/6h PO; max 450mg/6h PO. 0.2–0.9g/ 8h IV or IM (by IVI only, if >600mg used)	Stop if diarrhoea occurs (pseudomembranous colitis, p219). Used in *Staph.* bone/joint infection.
Co-trimoxazole Sulfamethoxazole 400mg + trimethoprim 80mg. 1ˢᵗ choice in *Pneumocystis carinii* (p580–3), toxoplasmosis and nocardia. NB: can act against *S. aureus*.	960mg–1.44g/12h PO/IVI; see *Pneumocystis* (p580)	SE (mostly ∵ sulfonamide, elderly at ↑risk): jaundice; Stevens–Johnson syn; marrow depression; folate↓. If CC 15–30, halve dose frequency after 3d. Avoid if CC <15. CI: G6PD deficiency.
Doxycycline Used in travellers' diarrhoea, *Chlamydia*, leptospirosis, syphilis, & brucellosis.	200mg PO on 1ˢᵗ day then 100mg/24h; max 200mg/d in severe infections	As for tetracycline, but may be used in renal failure.
Erythromycin Macrolide, used in penicillin allergy. Used 1ˢᵗ line in atypical pneumonia, p174.	250–500mg/6h PO (≤4g/d in *Legionella*). 6.25–12.5mg/kg/6h IVI (adult and child)	SE: D&V; phlebitis in IV use. Potentiates warfarin,theophylline, terfenadine, ergotamine, carbamazepine.
Fusidic acid Narrow-spectrum antistaph agent (incl. some MRSA, p590); used in osteomyelitis.	500mg/8h PO 500mg/8h IV over 6h; avoid intravenous route if possible.	Combine with another antistaphylococcal drug. SE: GI upset, reversible changes in LFTs.

Antibiotic (and uses):	Adult dose	Notes
Gentamicin Spectrum-wide but poor against streps & anaerobes, so use with a penicillin and/or metronidazole. Synergy with ampicillin against Enterococcus. For potentially serious Gram –ve infections or prophylaxis in IE.	0.7–1.7mg/kg/8h IV ↓Dose in renal failure (►see p710) *Typical once daily dose:* 160mg/d in *uncomplicated* infection. *Single stat dose for 'simple' infections:* 5mg/kg then no more or review.	►See *nomogram*, p710. In uraemia, give usual loading dose then decrease frequency. Avoid: • Prolonged use • Concurrent frusemide (=furosemide) • In pregnancy or myasthenia gravis. SE: oto- & nephrotoxicity.
Imipenem (+cilastatin) Very broad spectrum: Gram +ve & –ve organisms, anaerobes & aerobes. β-lactam stable.	250–500mg/6h IVI; dose if CC 6–20: 250mg/12h or 3.5mg/kg/d, whichever is less; high doses risk fits. CC <5, dialyse	Avoid in pregnancy and lactation. SE: fits; D&V; myoclonus, eosinophilia, WCC↓, Coombs' +ve; LFTs abnormal.
Linezolid Oxazolidinone used vs MRSA, VISA, & VRE[1]	600mg/12h PO/IV	May cause reversible pancytopenia if R >2wks
Meropenem See imipenem.	0.5–1g/8h IVI, max 2g/8h	Causes fewer fits than imipenem.
Metronidazole Drug of choice vs anaerobes, *Gardnerella, Entamoeba histolytica,* & *Giardia-lamblia;* use PO in pseudo-membranous colitis.	400mg/8h PO. PR dose: 1g/8h for 3d then 1g/12h. IVI dose: 500mg/8h for ≤7d	Disulfiram reaction with alcohol, interacts warfarin, phenytoin, cimetidine; care in liver failure. Breast-feeding and pregnancy: avoid high-dose regimens.
Minocycline Spectrum > tetracycline.	100mg/12h PO	As tetracycline, but more SE (hepatitis, pneumonitis).
Nitrofurantoin UTI.	50mg/6h PO with food	CI: CC <50. SE: fibrosis.
Oxytetracycline	250–500mg/6h PO	See tetracycline.
Rifampicin[UK]= **Rifampin**[US] Mycobacteria, prophylaxis in meningitis contacts.	Dose example: 450–600mg/24h PO before breakfast. See TB, p566	↓Dose in liver disease. Interferes with contraceptive Pill. SE: p566.
Teicoplanin See vancomycin, but not given PO.	IV/IM: 400mg/12h for 3 doses, then 200mg/24h	Longer half-life than vancomycin.
Tetracycline Used in chronic bronchitis; 1st line in *Chlamydia,* Lyme disease, mycoplasma, brucellosis, rickettsia.	250–500mg/6h PO ac 500–1000mg/12h IVI (not if liver disease). IV preparation not available in UK.	Avoid if <12yrs old, in pregnancy, and if CC <50. Absorption ↓by iron, milk, and antacids. SE: photosensitivity, D&V.
Tobramycin As gentamicin; better against *Pseudomonas.*	1mg/kg/8h IVI Dose↓ in renal failure	Less toxic than gentamicin. Once daily dose: 5.1mg/kg/d.
Trimethoprim Used in UTI, COPD. Dose in prophylaxis: 100mg/24h PO.	200mg/12h PO	SE depressed marrow, D&V. CC 10–50: 200mg/18h PO. CC <10: 200mg/24h PO.
Vancomycin PO: pseudomembranous colitis if metronidazole is contraindicated; IV: MRSA & other Gram +ve organisms (not *Erysipelothrix* species).	125mg/6h PO; 500mg/6h IVI over 1h or 1g/12h IVI over 100min; do peak level 2h post-IVI, eg after dose 3; aim for <30mg/L, & <10mg/L before dose 4	In renal failure, get help; nomograms are available, eg ⁸⁄₆ SE: renal and oto-toxicity. Do not overuse (↑risk of multiple resistance, p590).

1 MRSA: p590; VISA: vancomycin-intermediate resistant *S. aureus*; VRE: vanco. resistant enterococci

Empirical 'blind' treatment

History: A detailed history may reveal the source of infection: ask about respiratory, GI and GU symptoms; any travel or possible immunocompromise?

Examination: Look at the temperature chart and examine for localizing signs.

Investigations: If possible, culture all possible sources before treating (blood, sputum, urine, faeces, skin/wound swabs, CSF, aspirates). Also check FBC, ESR, CRP, U&E, LFT, clotting, atypical serology, malaria film, acute phase serum save, serum for virology, CXR, ABG (as clinically indicated). Dipstick the urine.

Treatment: Follow local guidelines. Change to the most appropriate drug once sensitivities are known. Treatment of most infections should not exceed 7d. Intravenous antibiotic therapy should preferably not exceed 48h; review the need and change to PO if possible. If in doubt, ask a microbiologist.

Infection	Treatment (pen. = penicillin, p543)
Urinary tract infection	Trimethoprim 200mg/12h PO
Cellulitis	Co-amoxiclav (or flucloxacillin + pen.)
Wound infection	Await swab results
	Otherwise, flucloxacillin 1g/6h IV
Pneumonia	
Mild community-acquired	Amoxicillin 500mg/8h PO
Possible atypical pneumonia	Erythromycin 500mg/6h PO
Severe community-acquired	Cefuroxime 1.5g/8h IV
	+ erythromycin 1g/6h IV
Hospital-acquired	Cefuroxime 1.5g/8h IV
	or Tazocin® 4.5g/8h IV[1]
Meningitis (p370; p808)	
Meningococcus ⎫	▶▶Benzylpenicillin 2.4g/4–6h slowly IV
Pneumococcus[2] ⎬	(1.2mg IM stat, pre-hospital)
Haemophilus ⎭	and ceftriaxone 2g/12h IV
Listeria	Add ampicillin 2g/4h IVI
If HSV encephalitis possible	Add aciclovir 10mg/kg/8h IVI
Endocarditis (p152)	
Empirical therapy	Benzylpenicillin[2] + gentamicin IV, p710
Strep. viridans	Benzylpenicillin[2] + gentamicin IV
Enterococcus faecalis	Amoxicillin[2] + gentamicin IV
Staph. aureus, Staph. epidermidis	Flucloxacillin[2] + gentamicin IV
Prosthetic valve	Vancomycin + gentamicin + rifampicin
Osteomyelitis/Septic arthritis	Flucloxacillin 1g/6h IV
	then clindamycin PO
Septicaemia	
Urinary tract sepsis	Cefuroxime 1.5g/8h IV + gentamicin IV
	5mg/kg once daily is typical max dose;
	rarely, 7mg/kg is needed, less if obese; p710
Intra-abdominal sepsis	Cefuroxime 1.5g/8h IV
	+ metronidazole 500mg/8h IVI
Meningococcal sepsis	▶▶Ceftriaxone 2g/12h IV
Neutropenic sepsis	Tazocin® 4.5g/8h IV[1] over 3–5min
	+ netilmicin eg 6mg/kg IV once daily
Skin or bone source	Flucloxacillin 1g/6h IV
Unknown cause	Cefuroxime 1.5g/8h IV
	+ gentamicin 5mg/kg IV once daily, p710
	+ metronidazole 500mg/8h IVI

▶All IV does should be given slowly, eg over 5mins.

Prognosis: Poor if very old or young, BP↓, WCC↓, $P_a O_2$↓, DIC, hypothermia.

---

1 Tazocin = piperacillin 4g (p543) + tazobactam 500mg.
2 Use vancomycin if penicillin-allergic, or suspected penicillin resistance eg MRSA.

Using a side-room laboratory

Urine Dipstick analysis should always be performed. If positive for leucocytes, nitrites, blood, or protein, send for MC+S. If positive for glucose or ketones, suspect diabetes. If heavily positive for protein, check 24h collection for protein. Urine microscopy: p258.

Blood Adhere to universal precautions: all specimens could be HBsAg, HCV, or HIV +ve. To make a *thick blood film* (malaria diagnosis), use fresh whole blood: a small blob should be spread out somewhat untidily to cover ~1cm², thinly enough for watch hands to be seen through. The untidiness is helpful to the microscopist because it provides areas of varying thickness, some of which will be ideal for what is often a tricky task. Label and allow to dry. To make a *thin blood film*, put 1 drop of blood near one end of the slide. Take another slide, place its end in the drop of blood, angled at 45°. Push the slide away from you to spread the blood into a thin film (practice makes perfect!). Allow the film to dry, fix in methanol for 5s, then stain as follows.

Leishman's stain: Cover with 10 drops of Leishman's stain. After 30s add 20 drops of water. Leave for 15min. Pick up the slide with forceps (to avoid purple fingers) and rinse in fast-flowing tap water—for 1s only. Allow to dry. Now examine under oil immersion. Note red cell morphology. Do a differential white count. Polymorphs have lobed nuclei. Lymphocytes are small (just larger than red cells) and round, having little cytoplasm. Monocytes are larger than lymphocytes, but similar, with kidney-shaped nuclei. Eosinophils are like polymorphs, but have prominent pink-red cytoplasmic granules. Basophils are rare, and have blue granules. Learn to use a white cell counting chamber—don't expect this to be as accurate as electronic methods.

Field's stain is easy to use and gives good results for malaria, and allows detection of trypanosomes and filaria. Dip the slide in solution A for 5s and solution B for 3s. Dip in tap water for 5s after each staining. Stand to dry. Examine thick films for at least 5min before saying that it is negative. **NB:** ward *serology tests*, eg *ParaSight F®* are available for *P. falciparum*, but cannot replace microscopy as they are not 100% sensitive[1] and parasites are not quantified (needed to plan treatment).

Pus (Gram stain) Make a smear; fix by gentle heat. Flood the slide with cresyl violet for 30s. Wash in running water. Flood with Lugol's iodine for 30s. Wash with running water. Decolourize with acetone for 1–3s until no blue colour runs out. Counterstain for 30s with neutral red or safranin. Wash and dry. Gram +ve organisms appear blue-black; Gram −ve ones look red, but are easier to miss.

549

Near-patient chemistry In one sense this is less taxing than the above tests—the skill lies in the people who made the reagents easy to use. A very real problem is quality control and the black box effect: when you put a strip into a machine, eg to measure cardiac enzymes, you cannot observe the workings of the black box—it simply produces a deceptively accurate-looking figure. Frequent calibration of biochemical equipment is only a partial answer to this. It is only after you have spent a long time trying to get good results from near-patient analysers, and comparing paired samples with the lab, that one really appreciates the reproducibility, and reliability of the formal laboratory. ►Speed of reporting is useless if you cannot trust the results.[2]

Drug abuse and infectious diseases

►Always consider this when there are evasive answers or unexplained findings, especially in younger patients. Ask direct questions: 'Do you use any drugs? Have you ever injected drugs? Does your partner use any drugs? Do you share needles? Have you ever had a HIV test? How do you finance your drugs?' List drugs used, and prescribed drugs, with names of prescriber.

Behavioural clues:
- Temporary resident seen by GP 'Just passing through your area'.
- Demands analgesia/antiemetics. Knows pharmacopoeia well: 'I just need some pethidine for my renal colic/sickle-cell crisis'.
- Erratic behaviour on the ward; unexplained absences; mood swings.
- Unrousable in the mornings; agitation from day 2.
- Heavy smoking; strange smoke smells (cannabis, cocaine, heroin).

Physical clues:
- Acetone or glue smell on breath (solvent abuse).
- Small pupils (opiates), reversed by naloxone.
- Needle tracks on arms, groin, legs, between toes; IV access hard.
- Abscesses and lymphadenopathy in nodes draining injection sites.
- Signs of drug-associated illnesses (eg endocarditis, p152; AIDS, p580, chronic viral hepatitis).

Common and possible presentations in drug abusers

Unconscious (see p774)	Narcotics (naloxone, p830), barbiturates, solvents, benzodiazepines (if in ITU consider flumazenil 0.2mg IV over 15s then 0.1mg/min as needed, to 2mg if on ITU).
Psychosis or agitation	Ecstasy (p831), LSD, amphetamine, anabolic steroids, benzodiazepines. Haloperidol may help (p15).
Asthma or dyspnoea	Is there opiate-induced pulmonary oedema? NB: Asthma may follow the smoking of heroin.
Lung abscess	Right-sided endocarditis (*Staph*) until proved otherwise.
Fever/PUO	Is it endocarditis, eg with no cardinal signs (p152)?
Shivering & headache	After a 'bad hit' (chemical/organism contamination). Do blood cultures; start eg gentamicin (p547 & p710).
Hyperpyrexia	Ecstasy (p831). Beware myoglobinuria, DIC, renal failure.
Abscesses	If over injection site, then often of mixed organisms.
DVT (p456)	Eg on injecting suspended tablets into groin. Is there compression damage (compartment syndrome)? Do CK.
Pneumonia	Pneumococcus, haemophilus, TB, pneumocystis (p580).
Tachyarrhythmia	(If young); cocaine, amphetamines, endocarditis.
Jaundice	Hepatitis B, C, or D; anabolic steroids (cholestasis).
'Glandular fever'	May be presentation of HIV seroconversion illness.
Osteomyelitis	Including spinal. *Staph. aureus*/Gram –ve organisms.
Constipation	If severe, opiate abuse may be the cause.
Blindness	Consider fungal ophthalmitis ± endocarditis.
Runny nose	Opiate withdrawal (+colic/diarrhoea, yawns, lacrimation, dilated pupils, insomnia, piloerection, myalgia, mood↓; can occur in neonates if mother is an opiate abuser); cocaine use.
Neuropathies	(And any odd CNS signs) Consider solvent abuse.
Infarctions	(eg of spinal cord, brain, heart): suspect cocaine use.

General management A non-judgemental approach will produce better cooperation and may avoid self-discharge. Establish firm rules of acceptable ward behaviour. NSAIDs are useful for pain relief. Do not prescribe benzodiazepines or chlormethiazole (=clormethiazole). Methadone may be needed if opiate addicts develop withdrawl symptoms while in hospital.

Commercial sex workers need STD screen, speculum exam (OHCS p2), and cervical cytology as carcinoma-*in-situ* is common (OHCS p35). Screen for hepatitis B (vaccination, p243, use gloves); safe sex and safe injection advice. HIV testing (p578). ►Liaise with community teams. See OHCS p362.

The vocabulary of drug abusers

The first step in helping a drug abuser is to communicate. To understand what he or she is telling you, the following may be helpful.

Amphetamines	Speed; whiz; Billy; pink champagne
Amyl-nitrate	Goldrush; poppers; snappers
Barbiturates	Barbs; idiot pills
Cocaine	Coke; Charlie; uncle; the white; the nice; snow; rock; crack; nuggets; wash; gravel
Dihydrocodeine	DFs
Drug-induced sleep	Gauching; nodding; going on the nod
Drug intoxication	Stoned; off it; bladdered; ripped; wiped out
Heroin (± cocaine)	Smack; the nasty; gear; brown; scag; hit; Harry
Ecstasy (MDMA)	E; X; echo; disco biscuit; love drug; XTC
Febrile reaction	Bad hit
Filter	A bud (usually a cigarette tip, through which drugs are drawn before being injected)
Injecting	Hitting up; jacking up; cranking; having a dig
Subcutaneous	Skin popping
IM	Muscle popping
Subclavian	Pocket shot
Failed	Miss
LSD	Acid; trips; cardboard; tabs
Marijuana	Weed; pot; draw; ganja; grass; resin; Mary; hash
Methadone	Mud
Needles	Spikes; nails
Obtaining drugs	Score (selling drugs = deal)
PCP	Angel dust; KJ; ozone; missile
Physeptone ampoules	Amps
Prostitution	Working the block/square; doing business; on the game; on the batter; flogging one's golly
Prostitute's client	Mush; punter
Shoplifting	Grafting
Smoking cocaine	Bonging
Smoking heroin	Chasing the dragon
Syringes	Works; tools (barrel of a syringe = gun)
Temazepam	Temazies
Tourniquet	Key
Wanted by police	'On me toes'; keeping head down
White heroin	China white
Withdrawing from opiates	Turkeying, clucking
Zopiclone	Zim-zims

Pyrexia of unknown origin (PUO)

Contrary to Gustave Flaubert, most fevers are not caused by plums, melons, April sunshine, etc., but by self-limiting viral infections. Here fever may be caused by the body's immune response to infection resulting in the production of interferons and cytokines. A PUO is defined as a prolonged fever (>3 wks), which resists diagnosis after a week in hospital. Indicators of bacteraemia include confusion, renal failure, neutrophilia, ↓plasma albumin, and ↑CRP (acute phase response, p702).

Causes Infection (23%); multisystem diseases, eg connective tissue diseases (22%); tumours (20%); drug fever (3%); miscellaneous diseases (14%). It is often impossible to reach a diagnosis (25% in this series).

- **Infections** *Abscesses* (lung, liver, subphrenic, perinephric, pelvic); empyema; *bacteria* (*Salmonella, Brucella, Borrelia,* leptospirosis); rheumatic fever; endocarditis (may be culture-negative, eg Q fever); TB (CXR may be normal, culture sputum, urine ± gastric aspirate); other *granulomas* (actinomycosis, toxoplasmosis); *parasites* (eg amoebic liver abscess, malaria, schistosomiasis, trypanosomiasis); fungi and HIV. Asking '*Where have you been*' is vital: find an expert on that area, or else you will miss diagnoses you may have never heard of, eg melioidosis (*Burkholderia* (p621) is the commonest cause of fatal bacteraemic pneumonia in parts of SE Asia).
- **Neoplasms** Especially *lymphomas* (any pattern: the Pel–Ebstein fever, p658, is rare). Occasionally *solid tumours* (GI; renal cell). Patients may not feel hot during fevers. Fever with *leukaemia* is usually infective.
- **Connective tissue disease** Rheumatoid arthritis, polymyalgia rheumatica, Still's disease, giant cell arteritis, SLE, PAN, Kawasaki disease.
- **Others** Drugs (T°↑ may occur months after starting but remits within days of stopping; eosinophilia is a clue); pulmonary embolism; stroke; Crohn's; ulcerative colitis; sarcoid; amyloid; familial Mediterranean fever—recurrent polyserositis (peritonitis, pleurisy) + fevers, abdominal pain, and arthritis; treat with colchicine; cause: gene defect, eg at 16p13.

Examples of intermittent fevers SBE; TB; filarial fever; amyloid; *Brucella*. *Daily fever spikes:* Abscess; malaria; schistosomiasis; *Saddleback fever (eg fever for 7d, then ↔ for 3d):* Colorado tick fever; Borrelia; Leptospira; dengue; Ehrlichia (p604). *Longer periodicity:* Pel–Ebstein (p658). *Remitting* (diurnal variation, not dipping to normal): Amoebiasis; malaria; Salmonella; Kawasaki disease, CMV.

History Note especially sexual history, IV drug abuse, immunosuppressive illness, foreign or distant travel (►see p554), animal (or people) contacts, bites, cuts, surgery, rashes, mild diarrhoea, drugs (including non-prescription), immunization, sweats, weight↓, lumps, and itching.

Examination Remember teeth, rectal/vaginal exams, skin lesions, lymphadenopathy, hepatosplenomegaly (p518), nails, joints, temporal arteries.

Tests *Stage 1(the first days):* FBC, ESR, U&E, LFT, CRP, WBC differential, acute phase serum save, blood cultures (several, from different veins, at various times of day; prolonged culture may be needed for *Brucella*); baseline serum for virology, sputum microscopy and culture (specify for TB), urine dipstick, microscopy, and culture stool for microscopy (ova, cysts, and parasites), CXR.
Stage 2: Repeat history and examination every day. Protein electrophoresis, CT (chest, abdomen). Rheumatoid factor, ANA, antistreptolysin titre, Mantoux, ECG, bone marrow, lumbar puncture. Consider PSA, carcionembryonic antigen, and withholding drugs, one at a time for 48h each. Consider temporal artery biopsy (p424). HIV test counselling.
Stage 3: Follow any leads uncovered. Consider echocardiography, radio-nucleotide scans (eg indium-labelled white cell scan, gallium scan), CT, barium studies, IVU, liver biopsy, exploratory laparotomy. ?Bronchoscopy.
Stage 4: ?Treat for TB, endocarditis, vasculitis, or trial of aspirin/steroids.

New infectious diseases

Many of the diseases which preoccupy consultants in infectious diseases are new—food-borne *E. coli*, waterborne *Cryptosporidium*, airborne Legionnaire's disease, blood-borne hepatitis C, and sexually transmitted HIV have come to the fore only in the last 30yrs. Why have these years been so tumultuous in the ID world? The short answer (at least for some of these) is greed, and our desire to exploit nature. For example, economic drive builds dams (↑breeding grounds for vectors by orders of magnitude) and forces land development, putting people closer to vectors, eg ticks, mosquitoes, and rodents. Intensive farming is also making it easier for infectious agents to jump the species barrier (think of CJD, p720).

For the long answer, turn to the Institute of Medicine's list of 8 reasons:[15]
1 War and famine (threats of bioterrorism add another dimension, threatening re-emergence of once-vanquished diseases such as smallpox).
2 Microbial adaptation and change.
3 Human susceptibility to infection (increased immunocompromise).
4 Climate and weather which lead to changing ecosystems.
5 Human demographics (especially economic development and land use).
6 International travel and commerce.
7 Technology and industry.
8 Breakdown of public health measures with poverty and social inequality.

Travel is a leading cause: West Nile virus, for example, reached New York from its ancestral home in the Middle East on a bird carried by a ship or plane.[16] With SARS, the precise tourists, businessmen, and doctors who have taken the virus from Hong Kong to Hanoi, Singapore, and Toronto have been identified. Similar stories may under-pin the spread of HIV, Hantavirus, Ebola, Nipah, and Hendra viruses.[17]

Can we win? No: we cannot win against infectious diseases. All we can do is live with them. To help us do this in ways which are not too destructive, we need robust public health surveillance institutions, political will, quarantine laws, and above all, openness and cooperation. SARS and its spread underline these facts in a particularly graphic way: as the Chinese and other less-than-open societies have found out, when it comes to reporting infectious diseases, lying means dying.

Diagnosing the tropical traveller

Tropical medicine centres UK: Liverpool 0151 708 9393, London 020 7388 9600, Birmingham 0121 766 6611.

In every ill traveller, consider:

1 *Malaria* (p560 & p562): Presentation: fever, rigors, headaches, dizziness, 'flu-like symptoms, diarrhoea, thrombocytopenia. Complications: anaemia, hyperparasitaemia (>5%), renal failure, pulmonary oedema, cerebral oedema. Diagnosis: serial thick and thin blood films. NB: mosquitoes may stowaway in luggage causing malaria in non-tropical areas.

2 *Typhoid* (p596): Presents with fever, relative bradycardia, abdominal pains, dry cough, constipation, lymphadenopathy, headache, splenomegaly ± rose spots (rare). *Complication:* GI perforation. *Diagnosis:* blood or BM culture.

3 *Dengue fever (DF)* (p602): Presents with fever, headache, myalgia, rash (flushing or petechial), thrombocytopenia, and leucopenia. Diagnosis: serology.

4 *Amoebic liver abscess* (p606): Presents with fever, jaundice, RUQ pain. Do serology and ultrasound. Blood cultures to rule out septicaemia.

▶NB: A visit to the tropics does not preclude the mundane fevers—eg 'flu.

Jaundice Think of viral hepatitis, cholangitis, liver abscess, leptospirosis, typhoid, malaria, dengue fever, yellow fever, haemoglobinopathies.

Hepatosplenomegaly (p518). Viral hepatitis, malaria, *Brucella*, typhoid, leishmaniasis, schistosomiasis, toxoplasmosis.

Gross splenomegaly Malaria, visceral leishmaniasis (kala-azar).

Diarrhoea & vomiting (p556 & p218) *E. coli* (Travellers' diarrhoea) is commonest. Consider *Salmonella*, *Shigella*, *Campylobacter*, *Giardia lamblia*, *Vibrio Cholerae*, etc. (p556). See p218 for general management. If diarrhoea prolonged, consider protozoal infection of small bowel or tropical sprue (p252). In HIV: cryptosporidia, microsporidia, and *Isospora belli* (need special stains).

Respiratory symptoms Common respiratory pathogens (p174), typhoid, *Legionella*, TB, Q fever, histoplasmosis, Löffler's syndrome (p728).

Arthritis Gonococcus; septicaemia; viruses (Ross river, Chikungunya et al p412).

Erythema nodosum (PLATE 18) *Causes:* streps, TB, leprosy, fungi, Crohn's, ulcerative colitis, sarcoidosis, pregnancy, drugs (sulfonamides, the Pill).

Anaemia hookworm, malaria, kala-azar, haemolysis, malabsorption.

Skin lesions scabies (itchy allergic rash + burrows, eg in finger web-spaces; p586 & OHCS p600), orf (pustules), molluscum contagiosum (pearly, punctate, papules), leprosy (p598, anaesthetic, hypopigmented areas), tropical ulcers, typhus ('eschar' = scab), leishmaniasis (ulcers/nodules), onchocerciasis (itchy nodules), myiasis (nodules—larvae of various insects), drug reactions.

Acute abdomen Perforation of a typhoid ulcer, toxic megacolon in amoebic or bacillary dysentery, sickle-cell crisis, ruptured spleen.

Rarities to consider ▶Use local emergency isolation policy.

- *Rabies* (p602) and other CNS viral infections, eg encephalitis (p369).
- *Yellow fever* (p602) Suspect in travellers from Africa.
- *Lassa fever:* Occurs in Nigeria, Sierra Leone, or Liberia. *Signs:* Fever; exudative sore throat; face oedema; collapse. △: PCR/EM; serology. R: Isolate & refer.
- *Marburg and Ebola virus:* Seen in Sudan, Zaire, Kenya. *Signs:* Fever, myalgia, D&V, pleuritic pain, hepatitis, shock, and bleeding tendency. A maculo-papular rash appears on day 5–7 and desquamates in <5d. Patients may bleed from all orifices and gums. △: PCR/EM; serology. R: Isolate & refer.
- *Viruses causing haemorrhage:* Dengue, Marburg, Lassa, Ebola, Crimea-Congo fever, haemorrhagic fever with renal syndrome, yellow fever. ▶See p602.

The details of the travel history (eg areas visited, immunization and prophylaxis taken, any exposure to disease) are very important, even if you cannot interpret them yourself. Seek expert opinion early.

Incubation times for fever in the tropical traveller[1]

▶The incubation times below are typical, but considerable variation occurs.

<14d	14d to 6wks	>6wks
Undifferentiated fever		
Malaria	Malaria	Malaria
Typhoid	Typhoid	Hepatitis B or E
Leptospirosis	Leptospirosis	Kala-azar
Dengue fever	Hepatitis A or E	Lymphatic filariasis
Rickettsiae	Acute schistosomiasis	Schistosomiasis
Acute HIV infection	Acute HIV infection	Amoebic liver abscess
Fever with CNS signs		
Viral and bacterial meningitis and encephalitis	East African trypanosomiasis	Rabies
East African trypanosomiasis	Rabies	
Poliomyelitis		
Fever with chest signs		
Influenza	Tuberculosis	Tuberculosis
Legionellosis	Q fever	
Q fever		
Acute histo-plasmosis		
SARS		
Fever with diarrhoea		
(see p556)		

1 ET Ryan 2002 *NEJM* **347** 505

Gastroenteritis

Ingestion of certain bacteria, viruses, and toxins (bacterial and chemical) is a common cause of diarrhoea and vomiting (p86 & p218). Contaminated food and water are common sources, but often no specific cause is found. Ask about details of food and water taken, cooking method, time till onset of symptoms, and whether fellow-diners were affected. Ask about swimming, canoeing, etc. NB: *Food poisoning is a notifiable disease (p537) in the UK.*

Organism/Source	Incubation	Clinical features	Food
Staph. Aureus	1–6h	D&V, P, hypotension	Meat
Bacillus cereus	1–5h	D&V	Rice
Red beans	1–3h	D&V	
Heavy metals, eg zinc	5min–2h	V, P; with zinc, (delayed fever ± 'flu-like features after exposure at work)	
Scrombotoxin	10–60min	D, flushing, sweating erythema, hot mouth	Fish
Mushrooms	15min–24h	D&V, P, fits, coma, hepatic and renal failure	
Salmonella	12–48h	D&V, P, fever, septicaemia	Meat, eggs, poultry
Cl. perfringens	8–24h	D, P afebrile	Meat
Cl. botulinum	12–36h	V, paralysis	Processed food
Cl. difficile	1–7d	Bloody D, P, toxic megacolon (p219)	
Vibrio parahaemolyticus	12–24h	Profuse D; P, V	Seafood
Vibrio cholerae	2h–5d	See p596	Water*
Campylobacter	2–5d	Bloody D, P, fever	Milk, poultry, water*
Listeria		meningoencephalitis; 'I've got 'flu'; miscarriages	Cheese, pâtés
Small round-structured viruses (SRSV)	36–72h	D&V, fever malaise	Any food
E. coli type 0157	12–72h	Cholera/typhoid-like;* haemolytic-uraemic syn, p282a	
Y. enterocolitica	24–36h	D, P, fever	Milk*
Cryptosporidium[1]	4–12d	D in HIV	Cow→water→man
Giardia lamblia	1–4wks	See p606	Water*
Entamoeba histolytica	1–4wks	See p606	*
Rotavirus	1–7d	D&V, fever, malaise	*
Shigella	2–3d	Bloody D, P, fever	Any food

V = vomiting; **D** = diarrhoea; **P** = abdominal pain.
*May be food- or water-borne.

Tests *Stool microscopy and culture,* if the patient has been abroad, is from an institution or at day care, or an outbreak is suspected. In these circumstances, culture of the food source is also useful.

Prevention Basic hygiene. When abroad, avoid unboiled/unbottled water, ice cubes, salads, and peel own fruit. Eat only freshly prepared hot food or thoroughly rewarmed food.

Management Usually symptomatic. Maintain *oral fluid intake* (±oral rehydration sachets). For severe symptoms (but not in dysentery) give *antiemetic* (eg prochlorperazine 12.5mg/6h IM) and an *antidiarrhoeal* (eg codeine 30mg PO/IM or loperamide 4mg stat then 2mg after each loose stool). *Antibiotics are only indicated if systemically unwell, immunosurpressed or elderly:*
- Cholera: tetracycline reduces transmission.
- *Salmonella:* ciprofloxacin 500mg/12h PO, 200–400mg/12h IVI over 60min.
- *Shigella* and *Campylobacter:* ciprofloxacin 500mg/12h PO.

1 Cryptosporidium is a fungus prevalent in HIV infection, eg related to drinking unboiled water. Self-limiting if CD4 count is ≥100. Quantify oocyst excretion. If ℞ is needed, ask a microbiologist. Various treatments are tried, eg azithromycin with paromomycin 1g/12h PO, but none is of proven value.

Immunization

Active immunization usually stimulates the immune system (humoral and cellular immunity). *Passive immunization* provides pre-formed antibody (non-specific or antigen-specific).

Immunizations The UK DoH schedule (^{L} = live vaccine)

3d	BCG^L (if TB in family in last 6 months). See below.
	Hepatitis B vaccine if mother is HBsAg +ve; p243 & *OHCS* p208.
2 months	DTwP-HiB (diphtheria, tetanus, whole cell pertussis, *Haemophilus influenzae* Type *b*) + meningitis c conjugate (MCC) vaccine + oral Polio^L.
3 months	Repeat DTwP-HiB and Polio^L and MCC.
4 months	Repeat DTwP-HiB and Polio^L and MCC.
	NB: a Hib booster may be needed >1 month after dose 3.
12–18 months	Measles/mumps/rubella^L (MMR$_{II}$® vaccine[1]): 0.5mL SC.
4–5yrs	DTaP (diphtheria, tetanus, and acellular pertussis) and Polio^L booster. MMR$_{II}$® dose 2.
10–14yrs	BCG^L, MMR (any age) ×1 if infant doses missed.
15–18yrs	Polio^L + tetanus + low-dose diphtheria booster. MCC if unvaccinated and aged between 15 and ~24yrs.
Any age	Consider yearly 'flu vaccine (if in 'at risk' category, p572).
Adults	Boosters eg of tetanus and Polio^L. Pneumococcal vaccine.

►*An acute febrile illness is a contraindication to any vaccine.* Give live vaccines either together, or separated by ≥3wks. Caution with live vaccines in patients who are immune-deficient (transplants, cancer chemotherapy, steroids, HIV infection)—seek expert advice.

►*Contraindications to vaccines:* see *OHCS* p208.

►**Bacille Calmette–Guérin (BCG)** Live attenuated anti-TB vaccine (works in up to 80% subjects for ~10yrs, but considerable regional variation in effectiveness). If TB is rife, or if past TB in family in the last 6 months, give BCG intradermally. Make a 7mm blanched weal between the top and middle thirds of the arm (deltoid's insertion) or, for cosmetic reasons, the upper, outer thigh. Expect to feel marked resistance as the injection is given. If, during the injection, propagation of the weal stops, the vaccine is going too deep: re-insert the needle. A swelling appears after 2–6wks, developing into a papule or small ulcer. Avoid air-occluding dressings. SE: pain, local abscess. CI: pyrexia, oral steroids, sepsis, or eczema at vaccination site, immune pareses (eg AIDS and malignancy).

Mantoux test (p566) Offered to those at risk of TB (eg TB contacts, health workers) and those aged 10–13yrs (to identify those needing BCG).

Travel immunization See p541. Take expert advice (*Schools of Tropical Medicine:* London: 020 7636 8636; Liverpool: 0151 708 9393).

►*Advice to travellers is more important than vaccination:* eg simple hygiene, malaria prophylaxis, and protective measures, advice about safe sex.

Immunization in special situations If *splenectomized/hyposplenic (eg sickle cell):* MCC; polyvalent pneumococcal; Hib; annual 'flu vaccine. *Chronic lung, heart, liver or kidney disease, diabetes:* pneumococcal; annual 'flu vaccine.

Other vaccines Hepatitis B (p243); influenza; pneumococcal[2] (p172); meningococcal (Mengivac® = group A & C), for short-term use, eg travel abroad. Leave ≥2wks after routine MCC before giving Mengivac®. Ideally this gap should be >6 months, but children <5yrs may not have responded well to their 1st dose of MCC.

1 There have been reports of associations between MMR vaccination and bowel disease ± autism. These have been dismissed by vaccination committees in many countries.● B Taylor 2002 *BMJ* **324** 393
2 Pneumococcal vaccination may ↓invasive disease in young children: C Whitney 2003 *NEJM* **348** 1737

Malaria^ND: clinical features and diagnosis

▶Always check for malaria in any sick patient from an endemic area.

Plasmodium protozoa, injected by the female *Anopheles* mosquito (~120 sporozoites/bite), multiply in RBCs (>10^8–10^{12} trophozoites per infection) so causing haemolysis, RBC sequestration, and cytokine release. Protective factors: sickle-cell trait, Melanesian ovalocytosis, G6PD deficiency, certain HLA types, eg B53 allele (found in many non-Europeans, enables killing of parasite-infected hepatocytes by cytotoxic T lymphocytes).

Malaria is one of the most common causes of fever and illness in the tropics. *P. falciparum* is estimated to kill 1 million people each year.

P. falciparum malaria *Incubation:* 12d. Most travellers present within 2 months. *Symptoms:* Non-specific flu-like prodrome: headache, malaise, myalgia, and anorexia followed by fever and chills ± faints. Classic periodic fever (peaking every 3rd day, ie tertian) and rigors are unusual initially. *Signs:* Anaemia, jaundice, and hepatosplenomegaly. No rash or lymphadenopathy. *Complications:* Cerebral malaria (p810): fits ± confusion then coma. Focal signs unusual. May have variable tone, extensor posturing; upgoing plantars, dyscon-jugate gaze; teeth-grinding. In children, seizures are common. Mortality: ~20%. *Metabolic (lactic) acidosis* giving laboured deep (Kussmaul's) breathing also major cause of death. *Anaemia* is common due to haemolysis of parasitized and unparasitized RBCs, and may be particularly severe in young children. *Hyperparasitaemia* (>5% of RBCs parasitized). *Hypoglycaemia* occurs in severe malaria (25% of children, 8% of adults), pregnancy, or with quinine therapy. *Acute renal failure* from acute tubular necrosis, sometimes with haemoglobin-uria ('blackwater fever'), and *pulmonary oedema* (ARDS, p190) are important causes of death in adults. Shock may develop in severe malaria (*algid malaria*) from supervening bacterial septicaemia, dehydration or, rarely, splenic rupture. In pregnancy, the risk of death (mother or fetus) is high (*OHCS* p159). Use chemoprophylaxis in pregnant women in endemic areas of transmission.

Benign malaria has a very low mortality. The acute febrile illness is very similar to that of uncomplicated *falciparum* malaria. Incubation periods may be longer: 5–10% of *P. malariae* malaria presents over 1yr after infection. *Complications:* Relapse occurs as parasites lie dormant in the liver (*P. vivax* and *ovale*) or at low levels in the blood (*P. malariae*). Nephrotic syndrome (glomerulonephritis) may occur in chronic *P. malariae* infection.

Diagnosis Serial thin & thick blood films (needs much skill, don't always believe –ve reports, or reports based on thin film examination alone); if *P. falciparum*, what is the level of parasitaemia? Rapid stick tests now available if microscopy cannot be performed or previously treated seriously ill patient: see p549 for ParaSight F® Serology not useful. Other tests: FBC (anaemia, thrombocytopenia), clotting (DIC, p650), glucose (hypoglycaemia), ABG/lactate (lactic acidosis) U&E and creatinine (renal failure), urinalysis (haemo-globinuria, proteinuria, casts), blood culture.

Poor prognostic signs (Severe *falciparum* malaria) Age <3yrs, pregnancy, respiratory distress, fits, coma, absent corneal reflexes, papilloedema, pulmonary oedema, HCO_3 <15mmol/L, plasma or CSF lactate >5mmol/L, glucose <2.2mmol/L, hyperparasitaemia (>5% RBCs or 250,000/μL), Hb <5g/dL, DIC, creatinine >265μmol/L. If ≥20% (or >10^4/μL) of parasites are mature trophozoites or schizonts, the prognosis is poor, even if few parasites seen (reflects critical mass of sequestered RBCs); malaria pigment in >5% of neutrophils.

Pitfalls in malaria

- Failure to take a full travel history, including stop-overs in transit and failure to check if the patient has already received treatment which might make the blood smear negative.
- Delay in treatment while seeking lab confirmation.
- Failure to examine enough blood films before excluding the diagnosis.
- Belief that drugs will work, when the parasite is often one step ahead.
- Not having IV quinine available immediately. (Quinidine is an alternative.)
- Not observing *falciparum* patients closely for the first few days.
- Forgetting that malaria is an important cause of coma, deep jaundice, severe anaemia, and renal failure in the tropics.

Malaria: treatment and prophylaxis

Treatment If species unknown or mixed infection, treat as *P. falciparum*. Nearly all *P. falciparum* is now resistant to chloroquine and in many areas is also resistant to Fansidar® (pyrimethamine + sulfadoxine). If in doubt consider as resistant. Chloroquine is the drug of choice for benign malarias in most parts of the world, but chloroquine-resistant *P. vivax* occurs in Papua New Guinea, Indonesia, some areas of Brazil, Colombia, and Guyana. Never rely on chloroquine if used alone as prophylaxis.

Falciparum malaria: If can swallow and no complications (p560), give 600mg quinine salt/8h PO for 7d, + either tetracycline 250mg/6h, doxycycline 100mg/12h, or clindamycin 300mg/6h for 7d. *Alternatives:* artemether-lumefantrine (eg Riamet®) 4 tabs twice daily (see BNF) OR atovaquone + proguanil (Malarone®) 4 tabs once daily (both for 3d with food). If seriously ill, take to ITU, and give quinine or artesunate or artemether IV: ▶▶p810.

Benign malarias: Give chloroquine PO as 600mg base, 300mg 6h later, then 300mg/24h for 2d. If *P. vivax/ovale,* give primaquine 15mg/24h for 14–21d (22.5mg if Chesson strain from SE Asia/west Pacific) after chloroquine to treat liver stage and prevent relapse. Screen for G6PD deficiency first.

Other treatments: Tepid sponging + paracetamol for fever. Transfuse if severe anaemia. Consider exchange transfusion if patient severely ill. Treat 'algid' malaria as malaria + bacterial shock (p778). Monitor TPR, BP, urine output, blood glucose frequently. Daily parasite count, platelets, U&E, LFT.

Examples of prophylaxis *Prophylaxis does not give full protection.* Risks are very variable; get local advice. Avoid mosquito bites between dusk and dawn: wear long-sleeved clothes, use repellents (DEET), insecticide-treated bed nets.

Except for Malarone®, take drugs from 1wk before travel (to reveal any SE) and continue for 4wks after return. None are required if just visiting cities of East Asia. There is no good protection for parts of SE Asia.

Recommended prophylaxis: *Caribbean, North Africa, and Middle East:* chloroquine ± proguanil. *Latin America, sub-Saharan Africa, SE Asia, and Oceania:* mefloquine, doxycycline, or Malarone® *South Asia:* chloroquine + proguanil. *Indonesia and the forests of Malaysia and Sarawak:* chloroquine + proguanil.
▶If area has poor medical care and traveller not pregnant, also carry standby treatment course (eg Riamet® Malarone®).

Adult prophylactic doses: *Chloroquine (base[1]):* 300mg/wk PO. *Proguanil:* 200mg/24h PO. *Doxycycline:* 100mg/24h PO. *Mefloquine:* 250mg/wk PO for adults if no risk of pregnancy. *Malarone®:* 1 tablet/24h PO starting 1d before travel, and continuing till 7d after return from malarious area.

562 *Antimalarial SE: Chloroquine:* headache, psychosis, retinopathy (chronic use). *Fansidar®:* Stevens–Johnson syn., erythema multiforme, LFT↑, blood dyscrasias. *Primaquine:* Epigastric pain, haemolysis if G6PD-deficient, methaemoglobinaemia. *Mefloquine:* Nausea, dizziness, dysphoria, sleep disturbance, serious neuropsychiatric symptoms, long $t_{1/2}$. Ideally start prophylaxis 3wks prior to travel to reveal any SE. Avoid mefloquine if: • Low risk of chloroquine-resistant malaria, eg 2wk trip to East African coastal resort • Past or family history of epilepsy, psychosis need to perform delicate tasks (eg pilots) • Risk of pregnancy within 3 months of last dose. Interactions: quinidine, halofantrine. *Malarone®:* Abdominal pain, nausea, headache, dizziness.

The future Genetic manipulation of the *Anopheles* mosquito can confer refractoriness to malaria, though how these genes could be spread worldwide is unclear. A number of vaccines targeting pre-erythrocytic, erythrocytic, and mosquito stages of the malaria life cycle are in development, but for the time being, the best hope may be for longer lasting insect nets.

---

1 150mg chloroquine base ≈ 250mg chloroquine phosphate (PO) ≈ 200mg chloroquine sulfate (IV).

Malaria prophylaxis a rough guide in children

Age	Weight (kg) (a better guide than age)	Chloroquine (base) weekly (mg)	Proguanil daily (mg)	Mefloquine weekly (mg)	Doxy* daily (mg)
<12wks	<6	37.5	25	—	—
<1yr	6–9.9	75	50	62.5	—
1–3yrs	10–15.9	112.5	75	62.5	—
4–7yrs	16–24.9	150	100	125	—
8–12yrs	25–44.9	225	150	187.5	—
~Adult	>45	300	200	250	100

*Doxy = doxycycline.

Mycobacterium tuberculosis: clinical features

►TB kills nearly 3 million/yr worldwide. If one includes HIV-related TB, then TB is the leading infectious cause of death worldwide, even though it has been highly treatable for 50yrs. Worldwide prevalence: 2 billion people; UK incidence: 7000/yr. 10% are drug-resistant; more in the USA.

Primary TB Initial infection is usually pulmonary (by droplet spread). A peripheral lesion forms (Ghon focus), and its draining nodes are infected (Ghon complex). There is early distant spread of the bacilli, then an immune response suspends further multiplication at all sites. Primary TB is often asymptomatic, or there is fever, lassitude, sweats, anorexia, cough, sputum, erythema nodosum (PLATE 18), or phlyctenular conjunctivitis (small, multiple, yellow-grey nodules near the limbus). Acid-fast bacilli (AFBs) may be found in sputum. CXR may help. The commonest non-pulmonary *primary* infection is GI, typically affecting the ileocaecal junction and associated lymph nodes.

Post-primary TB Any form of immunocompromise may allow reactivation, eg malignancy; diabetes; steroids; debilitation (esp. HIV or old age). The lung lesions (usually upper lobe) progress and fibrose. Any other site may become the main clinical problem. Tuberculomas contain few AFB, unless they erode into a bronchus, where the favourable environment ensures rapid multiplication, rendering the patient highly contagious (open TB). In the elderly, immunocompromised or Third World children, dissemination of multiple tiny foci throughout the body (including back to the lungs) results in miliary TB.

- *Pulmonary TB:* This may be silent or present with cough, sputum, malaise, weight loss, night sweats, pleurisy, haemoptysis (may be massive), pleural effusion, or superimposed pulmonary infection. *Investigation and treatment:* see p566. An aspergilloma/mycetoma (p180) may form in the cavities.
- *Miliary TB:* Occurs following haematogenous dissemination. Clinical features may be non-specific. CXR shows characteristic reticulonodular shadowing. Look for retinal TB. Biopsy of lung, liver, lymph nodes, or marrow may yield AFB or granulomata.
- *Meningeal TB:* (p368) Subacute onset of meningitic symptoms: fever, headache, nausea, vomiting, neck stiffness, and photophobia. *Treatment:* see OHCS p260.
- *Genitourinary TB:* May cause frequency, dysuria, loin/back pain, haematuria, and, classically, sterile pyuria. Take 3 early morning urine samples (EMU) for AFB. Renal ultrasound may help. Renal TB may spread to bladder, seminal vesicles, epididymis, or fallopian tubes. Endometrial TB: see OHCS p36.
- *Bone TB:* (OHCS p644) Look for vertebral collapse adjacent to a paravertebral abscess (Pott's vertebra). Do x-rays and biopsies (for AFB stains and culture).
- *Skin TB (lupus vulgaris):* Look for jelly-like nodules, eg on face or neck.
- *Peritoneal TB:* This causes abdominal pain and GI upset. Look for AFB in ascites (send a *large* volume to lab); laparotomy may be needed.
- *Acute TB pericarditis:* Think of this as a primary exudative allergic lesion.
- *Chronic pericardial effusion and constrictive pericarditis:* These reflect chronic granulomata. Fibrosis and calcification may be prominent with spread to myocardium. (Giving steroids to these patients for 11wks with their anti-TB drugs reduces need for pericardiectomy.)

Additional points in all those with TB:

►Advise HIV testing.

►Notify consultant in communicable disease control (CCDC) to arrange contact tracing and screening (preferably by a chest physician).

►Explain that prolonged treatment will be necessary.

►Explain that taking the tablets as prescribed is important. Monitoring of blood tests will be needed (LFTs). Explain that directly observed therapy (DOT) may be needed to ensure that the right pills are swallowed.

►Explain the need for respiratory isolation procedures while infectious.

►Check regularly for drug compliance and toxicity.

TB with AIDS and multi-drug resistant (MDR) TB

▶Directly observed treatment strategy (DOTS) prevents MDR-TB. In areas where MDR-TB is common, DOTS-plus (involving the rational use of second-line drugs) may be a solution.◆

TB is a common, serious, but treatable complication of HIV infection (p580). It is estimated that 30–50% of those with AIDS in the developing world also have TB. TB is probably no more infectious when occurring in the context of HIV. Interactions of HIV and TB are as follows:

• Mantoux tests may be negative.
• Increased reactivation of latent TB.
• Presentation may be atypical.
• Previous BCG vaccination does not prevent development of TB.
• Smears may be negative for AFB. Smears that are positive tend to contain few AFB. This makes culture all the more important and is vital to characterize drug resistance.
• Atypical CXR: lobar or bibasal pneumonia, hilar lymphadenopathy.
• Extrapulmonary and disseminated disease is much more common.
• More toxicity from highly-active antiretroviral therapy (HAART, p584) and anti-TB therapy due to drug interactions.
• Antiretroviral therapy reconstitutes CD4 count and immune function, which may lead to a paradoxical worsening of TB symptoms, called the 'immune reconstitution inflammatory response' (IRIS).
• Seek expert help on need for isoniazid prophylaxis in HIV +ve individuals (p566). Lifelong prophylaxis with isoniazid is probably *not* helpful (controversial), but regular clinical monitoring is vital.

▶*Respiratory isolation is essential* when TB patients are near HIV +ve patients. Nosocomial (hospital-acquired) and MDR-TB are now major problems worldwide, affecting both HIV +ve and HIV –ve people. Mortality is ~80% in patient-to-patient spread. Test TB cultures against 1st and 2nd line chemotherapeutic agents; 5+ drugs may be needed in MDR-TB :

First line antitubercular agents:		*Second line antitubercular agents:*	
Isoniazid	Streptomycin	Ofloxacin	Aminosalicylic acid
Rifampicin	Amikacin	Ciprofloxacin	Clarithromycin
Pyrazinamide	Kanamycin	Cycloserine	Azithromycin
Ethambutol	Capreomycin	Ethionamide	

Stopping the spread of MDR-TB Chief goals: *early identification; full treatment; isolation.* Control may be linked to:

• Early isolation of suspected patients. A suspicious CXR or a past history of MDR-TB is enough. Don't wait to prove the diagnosis.
• The ability to obtain Ziehl–Nielsen (ZN)/auramine stains 24h a day.
• Directly observing & confirming that patients take all prescribed drugs.
• Wearing of special masks by staff and the patient if s/he leaves the isolation room (avoid this if possible).
• Sputum induction/expectoration being confined to isolation rooms.
• Doors to isolation rooms having automatic closing devices.
• Providing negative air pressure in isolation rooms.
• Only stop isolation after ≥3 sputum samples are AFB –ve on culture for MDR-TB.
• Frequent tuberculin skin surveillance tests for workers and contacts.

Guidelines on MDR-TB are continually under review. Discuss appropriate treatment with a microbiologist, and refer early to a consultant in infectious diseases. Specific advice is available from the British Thoracic Society and the USA National Institutes of Health.

Tuberculosis[ND]: diagnosis and treatment

Diagnosis In all suspected cases, it is important to obtain the relevant clinical samples (sputum, pleural fluid, pleura, urine, pus, ascites, peritoneum, or CSF) for culture to establish the diagnosis. ▶Get advice on testing contacts.[1]

Microbiology: Send multiple sputum for MC+S for AFB (acid-fast bacillus), pleural aspiration and biopsy if there is an effusion. If sputum negative, bronchoscopy with biopsy and bronchoalveolar lavage may be helpful. Biopsy any suspicious lesions in liver, lymph nodes or bone marrow.

AFB are bacilli that resist acid–alcohol decolourization under auramine or Ziehl–Neelsen (ZN) staining. Cultures undergo prolonged incubation (up to 12wks) on Lowenstein–Jensen medium.

TB PCR: Allows rapid identification of rifampicin (and likely multi-drug) resistance. Occasionally useful for diagnosis in sterile specimens.

Histology: The hallmark is the presence of *caseating granulomata*.

Radiological features: CXR may show *consolidation, cavitation, fibrosis*, and *calcification* in pulmonary TB.

Immunological evidence of TB may be helpful:
- *Tuberculin skin test:* TB antigen is injected intradermally and the cell-mediated response at 48–72h is recorded. A positive test indicates that the patient has immunity. It may indicate previous exposure or BCG. A strong positive test probably means active infection. *False negative tests* occur in immunosuppression, including miliary TB, sarcoid, AIDS, lymphoma.
- *Mantoux test:* Serial dilutions of TB antigen provide 1, 10, and 100 tuberculin units (TU), respectively. The test is +ve if it produces ≥10mm induration, and –ve if <5mm. This test is overrated in diagnosing TB and its use is controversial.
- *Heaf and Tine tests* are used for screening. They consist of a circle of primed needles which inject the tuberculin.
- If active TB is strongly suspected, use 1 TU. If it is positive, infection is likely. Otherwise, interpret in the clinical context.

Treatment of pulmonary TB *Before treatment:* Stress importance of compliance (helps the patient and prevents the spread of resistance). Check FBC, liver, and renal function. Test colour vision (Ishihara chart) and acuity before and during treatment as ethambutol may cause (reversible) ocular toxicity. ▶Patients often forget to take pills, so consider DOT, as follows:
- *Initial phase* (8wks on 3–4 drugs):
  1 Rifampicin 600–900mg (child 15mg/kg) PO 3 times/wk.
  2 Isoniazid 15mg/kg PO 3 times/wk + pyridoxine 10mg/24h.
  3 Pyrazinamide 2.5g PO (2g if <50kg) 3 times/wk (child 50mg/kg).
  4 If resistance possible, add ethambutol 30mg/kg PO 3 times a week, or streptomycin 0.75–1g/24h IM (child 15mg/kg/24h).
  Monitor LFT weekly.
- *Continuation phase* (4 months on 2 drugs) rifampicin and isoniazid at same doses. (2 Rifinah 300® tablets = rifampicin 600mg + isoniazid 300mg). If resistance is a problem, use ethambutol 15mg/kg/24h PO.
- Give pyridoxine throughout treatment.
- Steroids *may* be indicated in meningeal and pericardial disease, p564.

Main side-effects ▶Seek help in renal or hepatic failure, or pregnancy.

Rifampicin: Hepatitis (a small rise of AST is acceptable, stop if bilirubin rises), orange discolouration of urine and tears (contact lens staining), inactivation of the Pill, 'flu-like syndrome with intermittent use.

Isoniazid: Hepatitis, neuropathy, pyridoxine deficit, agranulocytosis.

Ethambutol: Optic neuritis (colour vision is the first to deteriorate).

Pyrazinamide: Hepatitis, arthralgia (gout is a contraindication).

1 Spread the net wider than just household contacts: S Vervner 2004 *Lancet* **363** 212

Chemoprophylaxis for asymptomatic tuberculous infection

Immigrant or contact screening may identify patients with TB without symptoms or radiographic changes. In such patients, chemoprophylaxis may be useful to kill the infective organisms and prevent possible disease progression at a later date. This involves administration of one or two anti-TB drugs for shorter periods than for symptomatic disease (eg rifampicin and isoniazid for 3 months, or isoniazid alone for 6 months). Suitable patients for chemoprophylaxis include adults with documented recent tuberculin conversion, and young immigrants (16–34yrs) who are Heaf grade 3–4 positive without prior BCG vaccination.

►Seek expert advice, or consult the latest British Thoracic Society guidelines (www.brit-thoracic.org.uk).

►In all cases, standard anti-TB therapy should be initiated once any evidence of active disease (clinical or radiographic) is found.

Preventing TB in HIV +ve people

Primary prophylaxis against TB is indicated in some HIV +ve patients. In Africa, about 50% of those with HIV develop TB, and 80% of those with TB are HIV +ve.[1] Isoniazid (eg 300mg/d PO; children 5mg/kg, max 300mg; give with pyri-doxine) is the most common agent used. If there is a known contact with a person infected with isoniazid-resistant TB, rifampicin is an alternative. The duration of prophylaxis has been the subject of debate; 9 months is probably correct for isoniazid, lifelong prophylaxis is probably not helpful. ►Seek expert advice early. If prophylaxis is not used, monitor clinical state and CXR.

Indications for primary prophylaxis:

• If the patient has not had BCG and the Mantoux test is >5mm (Heaf 1–4).
• If BCG vaccinated (>10yrs ago), consider prophylaxis if Mantoux >10mm (Heaf 3–4).
• If there is recent exposure to someone with active TB.

1 WHO 2004; see http://allafrica.com

Herpes infections

Varicella zoster (PLATE 19) Chickenpox (*OHCS* p216) is the primary infection; after infection virus remains dormant in dorsal root ganglia. Reactivation causes shingles. Shingles affects 20% at some time. High-risk groups: elderly or immuno-suppressed. *Clinical features:* Pain in a dermatomal distribution precedes malaise and fever by a few days. Some days later macules, papules, and vesicles develop in the same dermatome. Thoracic dermatomes and the ophthalmic division of trigeminal nerve (ophthalmic shingles, *OHCS* p484) are most vulnerable. If the sacral nerves are affected, urinary retention may occur. Motor nerves are rarely affected. *Ramsay-Hunt syndrome* (zoster of the ear + VIIth nerve palsy, *OHCS* p756). Recurrence suggests immunosuppression. *Investigations* are rarely necessary. Rising antibody titres and culture or electron micro-scopy of vesicle fluid confirm the diagnosis. *Indications for treatment:* Most patients will want treatment (to ↓risk of post-herpetic neuralgia); if seen early, give aciclovir eg 800mg 5 times a day PO for 5–7d. If immunocompromised, give 10mg/kg/8h by slow IVI for 10d. Alternatives: valaciclovir or famciclovir. Control pain with oral analgesic ± low-dose amitriptyline. There is evidence to support a 4wk course of prednisolone to reduce post-herpetic neuralgia. If the conjunctiva is affected, apply 3% aciclovir ointment 5 times a day. Beware iritis. Measure acuity often. Advise to report *any* visual loss at once (*OHCS* p484). SE of aciclovir: renal impairment (check U&E) vomiting, urticaria, encephalopathy. *Complications:* Post-herpetic neuralgia in the affected dermatome can persist for years, and be very hard to treat. Try carbamazepine, phenytoin, amitriptyline, gabapentin, or capsaicin cream (counter-irritant). As a last resort, ablation of the appropriate ganglion may be tried. ▶Refer to a pain clinic.

Herpes simplex virus (HSV) Manifestations of primary infection:

1 *Systemic infection,* eg fever, sore throat, and lymphadenopathy may pass unnoticed. If immunocompromised, it may be life-threatening with fever, lymphadenopathy, pneumonitis, and hepatitis.

2 *Gingivostomatitis:* Ulcers filled with yellow slough appear in the mouth.

3 *Herpetic whitlow:* A breach in the skin allows the virus to enter the finger, causing a vesicle to form. Often affects childrens' nurses.

4 *Traumatic herpes (herpes gladiatorum):* Vesicles develop at any site where HSV is ground into the skin by brute force.

5 *Eczema herpeticum:* HSV infection of eczematous skin; usually children.

6 *Herpes simplex meningitis:* This is uncommon and usually self-limiting (typically HSV II in women during a primary attack).

7 *Genital herpes:* Usually HSV II. ♂: grouped vesicles and papules develop around anus and penis (with pain, fever, and dysuria) ± palms, feet, or throat. ♀: *OHCS* p30. Give analgesia + famciclovir 250mg/8h (500mg if immunocompromised) PO for 5d (recurrences: 125mg/12h PO; 500mg/12h if immunocompromised). Advise condoms even for oral sex. If frequent (≥6/yr) or severe recurrences, continuous aciclovir ≤400mg/12h PO.

8 *HSV keratitis:* Corneal dendritic ulcers. *Avoid steroids.* See *OHCS* p480.

9 *Herpes simplex encephalitis:* Usually HSV I. Spreads centripetally, eg from cranial nerve ganglia, to frontal and temporal lobes. ▶Suspect if fever, fits, headaches, odd behaviour, dysphasia, hemiparesis, or coma or subacute brainstem encephalitis, meningitis, or myelitis. *Diagnosis:* Urgent PCR on CSF sample (CT/MRI and EEG may show temporal lobe changes but are non-specific and unreliable; brain biopsy rarely required). Seek expert help: admit to ITU; careful fluid balance to minimize cerebral oedema (consider mannitol, p816); ▶▶*prompt* aciclovir, eg 10mg/kg/8h IV for 10d, saves lives. Mortality: 19% if treated with aciclovir, 70% if untreated.

Tests: Rising antibody titres in 1° infection; culture; PCR for fast diagnosis.

Recurrent HSV: HSV lying dormant in ganglion cells may be reactivated by illness, immunosuppression, menstruation, or even sunlight. Cold sores (perioral vesicles) are one manifestation. Aciclovir cream may be disappointing.

Infectious mononucleosis (glandular fever)

This is a common disease of young adults which may pass unnoticed or cause acute illness. Spread is thought to be by saliva or droplet. The incubation period is uncertain, but may be 4–5wks. The disease is caused by the Epstein–Barr virus (EBV), which preferentially infects B-lymphocytes. There follows a proliferation of T-cells (the 'atypical' mononuclear cells) which are cytotoxic to EBV-infected cells. The latter are 'immortalized' by EBV infection and can, very rarely, proliferate to form a picture indistinguishable from immunoblastic lymphoma in immunodeficient individuals (whose suppressor T-cells fail to check multiplication of these B-cells).

Symptoms and signs Sore throat, fever, anorexia, malaise, lymphadenopathy, palatal petechiae, splenomegaly, hepatitis, and haemolytic anaemia. Occasionally encephalitis, myocarditis, pericarditis, neuropathy. Rashes may occur, particularly if the patient is given ampicillin (but this does not indicate lifelong ampicillin allergy).

Investigations *Blood film* shows a lymphocytosis (up to 20% of WBC) and atypical lymphocytes (large, irregular nuclei). Such cells may be seen in many viral infections (eg CMV, HIV, parvovirus, dengue fever), toxoplasmosis, leukaemias, lymphomas, drug hypersensitivity, and lead poisoning.

Heterophil antibody tests (eg Monospot® or Paul-Bunnell): Heterophil antibodies develop early and disappear after ~3 months. These antibodies agglutinate sheep red blood cells. They can be absorbed (and thus agglutination is prevented) by ox red cells, but not guinea-pig kidney cells. This pattern distinguishes them from other heterophil antibodies. These antibodies do not react with EBV or its antigens. *False +ve* Monospot® tests may occur in hepatitis, parvovirus infections, lymphoma, leukaemia, rubella, malaria, carcinoma of pancreas, and SLE.

Immunology: EBV-specific IgM implies current infection. IgG shows that the patient has been previously infected.

Differential diagnosis Streptococcal sore throat (may coexist), CMV, viral hepatitis, HIV seroconversion illness, toxoplasmosis, leukaemia, diphtheria.

Treatment Avoid alcohol. Prednisolone PO is recommended (rarely) for severe symptoms or complications (80mg, 45mg, 30mg, 15mg, and 5mg on successive days, then stop). Its use is non-standard. *Ampicillin and amoxicillin should not be given for sore throats as they may cause a severe rash in those with acute EBV infection.*

Complications Depression, tiredness, and lethargy which may persist for months. Also, thrombocytopenia, ruptured spleen, splenic haemorrhage, upper airways obstruction (may need observation on ITU), secondary infection, pneumonitis, aseptic meningitis, Guillain–Barré syndrome, renal failure, lymphoma, and autoimmune haemolytic anaemia. All are rare.

Other EBV-associated diseases EBV is associated with Burkitt's lymphoma (p660) in Africa, and nasopharyngeal carcinoma in Asia. EBV+ve large cell (B-cell) lymphomas occasionally appear in the immunocompromised, eg post-transplantation lymphoproliferative disorder.[1] The EBV genome has also been found in the Reed–Sternberg cell of Hodgkin's lymphoma. Oral hairy leucoplakia (p210) is caused by EBV and may respond to antivirals such as aciclovir and valaciclovir.

---

1 EBV, HHV-6, and HHV-8 (p726) form a group of lymphotropic herpes viruses. EBV may cause tumours if immunosuppression suppresses EBV-specific cytotoxic CD8+ T-cells. R Ganschow 2004 *J Pediatr Gastroenterol* **38** 198 [@14734884]

Influenza

This is the most important viral respiratory infection because of its frequency and complication rate, particularly in the elderly. In pandemics, millions may die, particularly when new strains evolve. The virus (RNA orthomyxovirus) has three types (A, B, C). Only types A and B cause significant morbidity in humans. Subtyping (for type A) is by haemagglutinin (H) and neuraminidase (N) characteristics. Frequent mutations give strains with new antigenic properties. Minor changes (antigenic drift) and especially major changes (antigenic shift) place whole areas at risk. WHO classification specifies: type/host origin/geographic origin/strain no./year of isolation/subtype, eg A/Swine/Taiwan/2/87/ (H3, N2).

Spread is by droplets. *Incubation period:* 1–4d. *Infectivity:* 1d before to 7d after symptoms start. *Immunity:* Those attacked by one strain are immune to that strain only. *Convalescence:* May be slow.

Symptoms Fever, headache, malaise, myalgia, prostration, nausea, vomiting, conjunctivitis/eye pain (even photophobia). Also depression.

Tests *Serology* (paired sera; takes >2wks). *Culture* (1wk, from nasopharyngeal swabs). *PCR:* (eg 36h; sensitivity 94.2%; specificity ~100%).

Complications Bronchitis (20%), pneumonia (esp. *Staph. aureus*), sinusitis, otitis media, encephalitis, pericarditis, Reye's syndrome (coma, LFT↑).

Treatment Bed rest ± aspirin. If severe pneumonia (± 2 dry infections), most authorities recommend rapid transfer to ITU as sepsis and hypoxia may rapidly progress to circulatory collapse and death.

Antivirals: Amantadine 100mg/24h PO for 5d eases symptoms in H2,N2; H3,N2; & H1,N1 outbreaks, but is only effective against type A virus. *Zanamivir* (an inhaled neuraminidase inhibitor) shortens attacks by 24–48h, and is active against influenza types A and B. It is not a universal panacea; consider if complications would be serious (eg cardiovascular or chronic respiratory/renal disease; diabetes; immunosuppression; ≥65yrs old: see BOX and www.nice.org.uk advice). Dose: two blisters (2 × 5mg)/12h for 5d (before any other inhalers); start within 48h of symptom onset. NB: Inhalation is not an ideal route, eg if elderly. SE: bronchospasm; oropharyngeal oedema. *Oseltamivir* eg 75mg/12h PO for 5d is an orally administered alternative.

Prevention • Use whole *trivalent vaccine* (from inactivated viruses), reserving split (fragmented virus) for those <13yrs old. It is prepared from current serotypes and takes <2wks to work. *Indications:* Diabetes; chronic lung, heart or renal disease; immunosuppression; haemoglobinopathies; medical staff; those ≥65yrs old, especially in institutions. The logistics of vaccinating all those in the at-risk groups pose a challenge, particularly in ageing populations. *Dose:* 0.5mL sc (once). In children repeat after 6wks (½ dose if <3yrs old). *SE:* Mild pain or swelling (17%). Fever, headaches, and malaise are reported in 10%. Guillain–Barré and pericarditis are rare. • *Oseltamivir* 75mg/24h PO has been provisionally recommended by NICE for post-exposure prophylaxis in at-risk patients (ie immunocompromised, diabetics, chronic renal or lung disease, significant cardiovascular disease, or age >65yrs) in whom vaccination is either contraindicated, yet to take effect, or not well matched to the circulating strain of virus.

The common cold (coryza)

Rhinoviruses are the main culprits (>80 strains), and cause a self-limiting nasal discharge (which becomes mucopurulent over a few days). *Incubation:* 1–4d. *Complications:* (6% in children) Otitis media, pneumonia, febrile convulsions. *Treatment:* None is usually needed. If nasal obstruction in infants hampers feeding, 0.9% saline nose drops may help. In adults, a careful study has shown that zinc gluconate trihydrate 13.3mg in a candy lozenge, 5× daily, reduced duration by ~50%; SE: nausea, metallic taste.

NICE advice on antivirals for preventing and treating influenza

▶NICE states that 'at risk' individuals are those with any of the following: chronic respiratory diease (asthma, copd), significant cardiovasular disease (excluding patients with hypertension alone), chronic renal impairment, diabetes mellitus, age >65yrs, or patients who are immunocompromised.

Zanamivir (Relenza®): Recommended for *treatment* (eg 10mg/12h for 5d, given as 2 blisters inhaled via a Diskhaler® device) of 'at risk' adults and children aged >12yrs. Zanamivir must only be offered if treatment can be started within 48h of the onset of symptoms. The patient must know, or be correctly taught, how to use the Diskhaler® to deliver the drug.

Oseltamivir (Tamiflu®): Recommended for *treatment* (eg 75mg/12h PO for 5d) of 'at risk' adults, and children aged >1yr.

Recommended for *prophylaxis* (eg 75mg/24h PO for 7d) in 'at risk' patients aged >13yrs who have *both* not been effectively protected by vaccination, *and* have been exposed to someone with an influenza-like illness. This includes those in whom vaccination is contraindicated, and those vaccinated less than 2–3wks previously (it takes this long for immunity to develop). Also recommended for prophylaxis for 'at risk' patients aged >13yrs, who live in a residential care establishment where a resident/staff member has an influenza-like illness, regardless of whether or not the patient has been vaccinated.

NB: *in 'flu epidemics,* the prophylactic dose may be given for up to 6wks.

For both treatment and prophylaxis, oseltamivir should only be offered if the patient was exposed within the last 48h.

Amantadine: Not recommended by NICE for either treatment or prophylaxis of influenza.

For latest updates on these NICE guidelines on the prophylaxis and treatment of influenza, consult the www.nice.org.uk website.

Genetic reassortment and influenza pandemics

Influenza virus can achieve genetic diversity via a process known as reassortment whereby 2 different virus sources shuffle genetic material. (In addition stepwise single mutations can accumulate to produce new strains.) Reassortment is particularly dangerous when one of the viral sources is from an animal source (eg poultry)—of which the human population has had no previous immunological exposure.[1]

1 W Barclay 2004 *BMJ* **328** 238

Toxoplasmosis

The protozoan *Toxoplasma gondii* infects via gut, lung, or broken skin. Cats (the primary host) excrete oocysts, but the ingestion of poorly cooked infected meat by humans may be as important as contact with cat faeces. In humans, the oocysts release trophozoites, which migrate widely, with a predilection for eye, brain, and muscle. Toxoplasmosis occurs worldwide, but is common in the tropics. Infection is lifelong. HIV may reactivate it. NB: rats are also sources of infection.

The Patient ►*In any granulomatous uveitis or necrotizing retinitis, think of toxoplasmosis, especially in the immunosuppressed.* Most infections are asymptomatic: in the UK 50% have been infected by 70yrs. Symptomatic acquired toxoplasmosis resembles infectious mononucleosis, and is usually self-limiting. Eye infection, usually congenital, presents with posterior uveitis, often in the 2nd decade of life, and may cause cataract. In the immunocompromised (eg AIDS), myocarditis, encephalitis, focal neurological signs, stroke or fits may occur.

Tests Acute infection is confirmed by a 4-fold rise in antibody titre over 4wks or specific IgM (unreliable if HIV +ve). The toxoplasma 'dye test' was the first serological test used. Parasite isolation is difficult; lymph node or CNS biopsy may be diagnostic. Cerebral CT may show characteristic multiple ring-shaped contrast-enhancing lesions.

Treatment♦ Often none is needed: seek expert advice. If the eye is involved, or in the immunocompromised, pyrimethamine 25–50mg/8h PO for 5d, then 25–50mg/24h PO for 4wks, + sulfadiazine ≤1g/6h PO *may* be needed. SE: renal stones. ►If pregnant, get expert help. Consider spiramycin ± sampling of fetal cord blood, eg at 21wks for IgM (indicates severe infection). For HIV, see p580.

Congenital toxoplasmosis (*OHCS* p98) May cause abortion, neonatal fits, choroidoretinitis, hydrocephalus, microcephaly, or cerebral calcification. Worse prognosis if early infection.

Cytomegalovirus (CMV)

CMV may be acquired by direct contact, blood transfusion, or organ transplantation. After acute infection, CMV becomes latent but the infection may reactivate at times of stress or immunocompromise. If immunocompetent, primary infection is usually asymptomatic, but acute hepatitis may occur. In transplant recipients or post bone marrow transplantation: fever > pneumonitis > colitis > hepatitis > retinitis. In AIDS: retinitis > colitis > CNS disease. (Here '>' means 'is commoner than'.)

Diagnosis of acute CMV infection is difficult; growth of the virus is slow and there may be prolonged CMV excretion from a distant source of infection. Serology is much more helpful; specific IgM indicates acute infection (unreliable if HIV +ve). CMV PCR (including quantitative tests) of blood/CSF/broncho-alveolar lavage are becoming widely available.

Treat only if serious infection (eg immunocompromised), with ganciclovir 5mg/kg/12h IVI over 1h via a central line. Alternatives: valganciclovir, foscarnet. Immunization is being explored. For CMV in HIV, see p580.

Prevention post-transplantation If seropositive pre-op, ganciclovir, eg 2.5mg/kg/d IV for the first 2 post-op weeks. If seronegative pre-op, valaciclovir 2g/6h PO for 90d reduces the incidence and delays the onset of CMV disease. Use CMV-negative, irradiated blood when transfusing transplant recipients, leukaemics, or HIV patients.

Congenital CMV (*OHCS* p98) Look for: jaundice, hepatosplenomegaly, and purpura. Chronic defects include mental retardation, cerebral palsy, epilepsy, deafness, and eye problems. Treatment: none is established.

T. gondii: a subtle parasite

Oocysts excreted in cat faeces can stay in the soil for months, where rats typically pick them up. They become infected, and, under the direction of *Toxoplasma* in the amygdala, these rats lose their innate fear of cats, and so tend to get eaten—so the parasite ensures its success by facilitating its jump from its intermediate to its definitive host.

In humans, the following CNS effects have been observed:
- Confusion, seizures, and signs of brainstem or spinal cord injury.
- A *latent* phase of toxoplasmosis is well-recognized: less so are subtle personality changes. Loss of fear of cats is *not* reported, but there are changes in willingness to accept group moral standards, in proportional to the latent period's length.
- Meningoencephalitis + localizing signs (fever + headache → drowsiness → coma → death, eg over a few days or weeks). CSF: mild lymphocytic pleocytosis and moderate protein elevation.
- Multifocal myelin loss, and microglial nodules.
- *Pseudotumour cerebri* syndrome: transient intracranial hypertension.
- Space-occupying mass with focal ± intracranial hypertension mimicking a tumour or a brain abscess.
- Multiple mass lesions that can be the cause of hemisensory abnormalities, hemiparesis, cranial nerve palsy, aphasia, and tremors.

In some areas (eg India), toxoplasmosis is the most common HIV-associated CNS opportunistic infection.

Viral hepatitis

Hepatitis A virus (HAV) RNA virus *Spread:* Faecal–oral, often in travellers or institutions. Most infections occur in childhood. *Incubation:* 2–6wks. *Symptoms:* Prodromal symptoms include fever, malaise, anorexia, nausea, arthralgia. Jaundice develops ± hepatomegaly, splenomegaly, and adenopathy. *Tests:* Serum transaminases rise 22–40d after exposure. IgM rises from day 25 and signifies recent infection. IgG remains detectable for life. *Treatment:* Supportive. Avoid alcohol. Rarely, interferon-α for fulminant hepatitis. *Prevention:* Passive immunization with normal human immunoglobulin (0.02mL/kg IM) gives <3 months' immunity to those at risk (travellers, household contacts). Active immunization is with Havrix Monodose®, an inactivated protein derived from HAV. *Dose:* if >16yrs old, 1 IM dose (1mL to deltoid) gives immunity for 1yr (10yrs if further booster is given at 6 months). Use Havrix Monodose Junior® if 1–15yrs old. *Prognosis:* Usually self-limiting. Fulminant hepatitis occurs rarely. Chronic liver disease does not occur.

Hepatitis B virus (HBV) DNA virus. *Spread:* Blood products, IV drug abusers, sexual intercourse, direct contact (African children), vertical transmission (Asia). Risk groups: health workers, Haemophiliacs, haemodialysis, sexually promiscuous, homosexuals, and IV drug users (IVDU). Endemic in the Far East, Africa, and Mediterranean. *Incubation:* 1–6 months. *Clinical features:* Resemble hepatitis A but extrahepatic manifestations are more common, eg arthralgia, urticaria. *Tests:* HBsAg (surface antigen) is present from 1 to 6 months after exposure. HBeAg (e antigen) is present for 1½–3 months after the acute illness and implies high infectivity. The persistence of HBsAg for >6 months defines carrier status and occurs in 5–10% of infections (chronic infection). Antibodies to HBcAg (anti-HBc) imply past infection; antibodies to HBsAg (anti-HBs) alone implies vaccination. HBV PCR allows monitoring of response to therapy. *Vaccination* (▶p243) may be universal in childhood or just for high-risk groups. Passive immunization (specific anti-HBV immunoglobulin) may be given to non-immune contacts after high-risk exposure. *Treatment:* Supportive. Avoid alcohol. Chronic HBV may respond to interferon-α or other antivirals, eg lamivudine, adefovir. Immunize sexual contacts. *Complications:* Fulminant hepatic failure (rare); relapse; prolonged cholestasis; chronic hepatitis (5–10%); cirrhosis; hepatocellular carcinoma (HCC: 10-fold ↑risk if HBsAg +ve, 60-fold ↑risk if both HBsAg and HBeAg +ve); glomerulonephritis; cryoglobulinaemia.

Hepatitis C virus (HCV) RNA flavivirus. *Spread:* Blood, IVDU, sexual, unknown (40%). Early infection often mild/asymptomatic. ~85% develop chronic infection; 20–30% get cirrhosis within 20yrs; a few also get hepatocellular cancer (HCC). *Tests:* LFT (typically AST : ALT <1 until cirrhosis develops, p254), anti-HCV antibodies, recombinant immunoblot assay, HCV-PCR. Liver biopsy if HCV-PCR +ve to assess degree of liver damage and need for R. *Treatment:* Interferon-α + ribavirin is used in chronic infection; peginterferon-α may be superior to IFN-α. Treating acute infection with IFN-α may ↓ progression to chronic disease.◆ *Complications:* Irritability, cirrhosis, HCC.

Hepatitis D virus (HDV) Incomplete RNA virus, exists only with HBV. *Spread:* Coinfection or superinfection with HBV. *Clinical features:* Increased risk of acute hepatic failure and cirrhosis. *Tests:* Anti-HDV antibody. *Treatment:* Interferon-α has limited success in treatment of HDV infection.

Hepatitis E virus (HEV) RNA virus. Similar to HAV. Common in India. High mortality in pregnancy. *Diagnosis:* Serology. No effective treatment/vaccine.

Hepatitis GB Parenterally transmitted. Causes asymptomatic post-transfusion hepatitis. One type (HGB-C) can cause fulminant liver failure.

Differential diagnosis *Acute hepatitis:* Alcohol, drugs, toxins, EBV, CMV, leptospirosis, malaria, Q fever, syphilis, yellow fever. *Chronic hepatitis:* Alcohol, drugs, autoimmune hepatitis (p240), Wilson's disease (p236).

Serological markers of HBV infection

	Incubation	Acute	Carrier	Recovery	Vaccinated
LFTs		↑↑↑	↑	Normal	Normal
HBsAg	+	+	+		
HBeAg	+	+	+/−		
Anti-HBs				+	+
Anti-HBe			+/−		
Anti-HBc IgM		+	+/−		
Anti-HBc IgG		+	+	+	

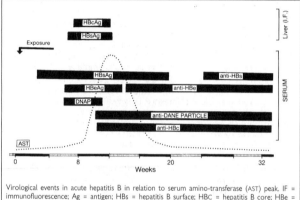

Virological events in acute hepatitis B in relation to serum amino-transferase (AST) peak. IF = immunofluorescence; Ag = antigen; HBs = hepatitis B surface; HBC = hepatitis B core; HBe = hepatitis B e antigen; DNAP = DNA polymerase.

Using ribavirin with peginterferon-α in HCV: *NICE advice 2004*

This combination is indicated in moderate and severe chronic hepatitis C infection if liver biopsy shows necro-inflammation and fibrosis. Efficacy is less if: • HCV genotype G1, 4, 5, or 6 is involved[1] • ↑Viral load • Older patients • Excessive delay before Rx starts • Blacks (vs Caucasians) • Male sex • HIV+ve.

NB: Pegylated interferon has an inert tail retarding its elimination (hence it may be given SC once weekly). Giving these drugs is a specialist role, so the main thing is for non-specialists is to know the contraindications, to prevent inappropriate referral. CI: • Allergy to or past use of interferon • Autoimmune hepatitis • Severe liver dysfunction or decompensated cirrhosis • Age <3yrs • Severe, unstable or uncontrolled heart disease in past 6 months • Past severe psychiatric conditions (esp. depression) • Pregnancy/lactation • Haemoglobinopathies (a CI to ribavirin).

577

1 Interferon-α Rx is either for 24wks (genotype 2 & 3) or 48wks for G1 (commonest in UK) & G4–6.

Human immunodeficiency virus (HIV)

Over 40 million people are HIV positive; over half are in Africa (WHO 2004). HIV-1 (a retrovirus) is responsible for most cases worldwide. HIV-2, a related virus, produces a similar illness, perhaps with a longer latent period.

More than 3 million have acquired immunodeficiency syndrome (AIDS); most are women and children in sub-Saharan Africa. AIDS is one end of a spectrum of disease caused by HIV, and is defined as the presence of one or more AIDS-defining illnesses ± evidence of HIV infection. *UK incidence:* >4400/yr (more heterosexually acquired than homosexually since 1999).

Transmission is by sexual contact (75%, including oral, in ~5%), infected blood or blood products, IV drug abuse or perinatally. In developed countries, the screening of blood donors and sterilizing blood products has greatly reduced the risk. In the developing world, increasing numbers of infected children being born (*OHCS* p98).

Immunology HIV binds, via its gp120 envelope glycoprotein, to CD4 receptors on helper T-lymphocytes, monocytes, macrophages, and neural cells. CD4 +ve cells migrate to the lymphoid tissue where the virus replicates producing billions of new virions. These are released, and in turn infect new CD4 +ve cells. As the infection progresses depletion or impaired function of CD4 +ve cells predisposes to the development of immune dysfunction.

Virology HIV is a double-stranded RNA retrovirus. After entry into the cell, the viral reverse transcriptase enzyme (hence retrovirus) makes a DNA copy of the RNA genome. The viral integrase enzyme then integrates this into the host DNA. The core viral proteins are initially synthesized as large polypeptides, that are cleaved by the viral protease enzyme into the enzymes and building blocks of the virus. The completed virions are then released from the cell by characteristic budding. The number of circulating viruses (viral load) predicts progression to AIDS.

Stages of HIV infection *Acute infection* is often asymptomatic. *Seroconversion* may be accompanied by a transient illness 2–6wks after HIV infection: fever, malaise, myalgia, pharyngitis, maculopapular rash or meningoencephalitis (rare). A period of *asymptomatic infection* follows although one-third of patients will have *persistent generalized lymphadenopathy (PGL)*, defined as nodes >1cm diameter at ≥2 extra-inguinal sites, persisting for 3 months or longer. Later, non-specific constitutional symptoms develop: fever, night sweats, diarrhoea, weight loss. There may also be minor opportunistic infections, eg oral *Candida*, oral hairy leucoplakia, herpes zoster, recurrent herpes simplex, seborrhoeic dermatitis, tinea infections. This collection of symptoms and signs is referred to as the *AIDS-related complex (ARC)* and is regarded as a prodrome to AIDS. *AIDS* is a stage in HIV infection characterized by the presence of an indicator diseases (p580). The CD4 count is usually <200 × 10^6/L.

AIDS prognosis Untreated, death in ~20 months; longer if treated, p584.

Diagnosis is based on detecting anti-HIV antibodies in serum. Acute infection may be detected by the presence of P24 antigen or HIV RNA by PCR and precedes the appearance of IgM and IgG (within 3 months). During the asymptomatic period, there are high titres of IgG to core and envelope proteins. As immunodeficiency develops, IgG titre to core protein falls, and P24 antigenaemia recurs. New rapid diagnostic kits for detecting anti-HIV antibodies have been developed.

Prevention Condoms for *any* sexual contact, or abstinence; blood screening; disposable equipment, and, in the case of infants, perinatal antiretroviral therapy for mother and infant (± Caesarean section), and bottle-feeding (but may ↑overall mortality, if hygiene is poor).

Complications of HIV infection

▶All patients with a new diagnosis of HIV should have a tuberculin test and be tested for toxoplasma, CMV, hepatitis B/C, and syphilis serology, to identify past or current infections that may develop as immunosuppression progresses.

- **Pulmonary** *Pneumocystis carinii* pneumonia is the most common life-threatening opportunistic infection in AIDS (p174). Treatment: high-dose co-trimoxazole IV or pentamidine by slow IVI for 2–3wks. Steroids are beneficial if severe hypoxaemia. Primary prophylaxis (eg co-trimoxazole PO) is indicated while CD4 count <200 × 10⁶/L. Secondary prophylaxis is essential after 1ˢᵗ attack until CD4 count >200 × 10⁶/L. Other pathogens include *pyogenic bacteria* (atypical presentation); *M. tuberculosis* (p566); *M. avium intracellulare* (MAI); *fungi* (*Aspergillus*, cryptococcus, histoplasma); CMV. Also: *Kaposi's sarcoma*, lymphoma, lymphoid interstitial pneumonitis, and non-specific pneumonitis.

- **Gut** Oral pain may be caused by *candidiasis*, HSV or aphthous ulcers, or tumours. *Oral Candida* is treated with nystatin suspension/pastilles or amphotericin lozenges. *Oesophageal* involvement causes dysphagia ± retrosternal discomfort. R: fluconazole, ketoconazole, or itraconazole PO for 1–2wks. Relapse is common. HSV and CMV also cause oesophageal ulceration which may be difficult to differentiate from *Candida* by barium studies. *Anorexia and weight loss* are common in HIV infection. *Deranged LFT and hepatomegaly* are common; causes include drugs, viral hepatitis, AIDS sclerosing cholangitis, or MAI. MAI causes fever, night sweats, malaise, anorexia, weight↓, abdominal pain, diarrhoea, hepatomegaly, and anaemia. *Diagnosis:* blood cultures, biopsies (lymph node, liver, colon, bone marrow). R: ethambutol + clarithromycin + rifabutin/rifampicin (see BOX). *Primary prophylaxis:* eg azithromycin 1200mg weekly, while CD4 <100 × 10⁶/L. *Chronic diarrhoea* may be caused by bacteria (*Salmonella, Shigella, Campylobacter*, atypical mycobacteria, *Cl. difficile*), protozoa (*Cryptosporidium* p556, *Microsporidium, Isospora belli, cyclospora*), or viruses (CMV, adenovirus). *Perianal disease* may be due to recurrent HSV ulceration, perianal warts, squamous cell carcinoma (rare). Kaposi's sarcoma (p726) and lymphomas can also affect the gut.

- **Neurological** *Acute HIV* is associated with transient meningoencephalitis, myelopathy, and peripheral neuropathy. *Chronic HIV* is associated with several CNS syndromes: AIDS-related dementia, HIV-related meningitis, CMV encephalitis, PML, p540[1]), and vacuolar myelopathy. *T. gondii* (p574) is the chief CNS pathogen in AIDS, presenting with focal symptoms/signs. CT/MRI shows ring-shaped contrast enhancing lesions. Treat with pyrimethamine (and folinic acid) + sulfadiazine or clindamycin for 6 months. Lifelong secondary prophylaxis is needed. Primary prophylaxis (eg co-trimoxazole PO) is only indicated in patients with serum antitoxoplasma IgG and CD4 <100 × 10⁶/L. *Cryptococcus neoformans* (p612) causes an insidious meningitis, often without neck stiffness. Diagnosis: India Ink staining and culture of CSF, or detection of cryptococcal antigen in blood/CSF. Treatment: amphotericin + flucytosine IV; fluconazole in milder cases. 20% mortality despite treatment. Secondary prophylaxis with fluconazole is needed until CD4 >150 × 10⁶/L and cryptococcal antigen negative. *Tumours* affecting the CNS include primary cerebral lymphoma, B-cell non-Hodgkin's lymphoma. CSF JC virus PCR is useful in distinguishing lymphoma from PML.

- **Eye** CMV retinitis (acuity↓ ± blindness) may affect 45% of those with AIDS. Fundoscopy shows characteristic 'mozarella pizza' appearance. Treatment: IV ganciclovir or foscarnet. Alternatives: valganciclovir PO, IV cidofovir, or ganciclovir-containing intraocular implants (NB: risk of post-op retinal detachment, 1 implant does not prevent disease in the other eye). Treatment has traditionally been lifelong, but trials suggest that therapy may be stopped in some patients when CD4 >150 × 10⁶/L after HAART (p584).

- **TB** p566 • **Leishmaniasis** p610 • **Kaposi's sarcoma** p726.

---

1 PML is caused by the JC virus (named after the initials of its 1ˢᵗ patient).

Treatment of opportunistic infections in HIV[1]

Infection	Treatment/side-effects
Tuberculosis	This is the most lethal opportunistic infection (WHO 2004); ►see p565.
Pneumocystis carinii	Co-trimoxazole (=trimethoprim 1 part + 5 parts sulfamethoxazole) 120mg/kg/d IVI in 3–4 divided doses for 14d. (SE: nausea, vomiting, fever, rash, myelosuppression) OR
	Pentamidine isetionate 4mg/kg/d by slow IV infusion for 14–21d (SE: hypotension, hyper- or hypoglycaemia, renal failure, hepatitis, myelosuppression, arrhythmias).
	Prednisolone 40–60mg PO daily (reducing dose) if severe hypoxaemia. 2nd line agents: primaquine + clindamycin, trimetrexate + calcium folinate, atovaquone.
	Secondary prophylaxis (eg co-trimoxazole 480mg/24h PO; same dose as primary prophylaxis) essential after 1st attack.
Candidiasis	Local treatment: Nystatin suspension/amphotericin lozenges 4 times/d.
	Systemic treatment: Fluconazole 50–200mg/d PO (SE: nausea, hepatitis) or ketoconazole 200mg/d PO (SE: nausea, hepatitis, rash, platelets↓) or itraconazole 200mg/d PO (SE: CCF, nausea, hepatitis). Amphotericin B (p180) is used in severe systemic infections. Relapse is common.
Toxoplasmosis	Sulfadiazine 1g/6h (or clindamycin 600–1200mg/6h) + pyrimethamine eg 25mg/8h PO + folinic acid 15mg/d. Secondary prophylaxis: halve doses.
Cryptococcal meningitis	Amphotericin B (see BNF for regimens) and flucytosine 25mg/kg/6h IV eg for 4 months or until clinically stable (SE: nausea, vomiting, rash, myelo-suppression, renal impairment). OR, in milder disease fluconazole 800mg on days 1–3, then 400–800mg/d (better tolerated). Secondary prophylaxis: fluconazole 200mg/24h PO.
CMV retinitis	Induction: ganciclovir 5mg/kg/12h IV for 14–21d (SE: myelosuppression) or foscarnet 60mg/kg/8h IV for 2wks, then reduce. SE: renal impairment, U&E imbalance, ulcers). Alternatives: valganciclovir 900mg/12h PO for 3wks, then 900mg/12h PO OR cidofovir: start with 5mg/kg IV once weekly for 2wks (given with probenecid and IV fluids), then reduce to weekly doses. Oral ganciclovir (1g/8h PO with food) is less effective. Maintenance therapy may be discontinued in some patients with CD4 > 150 × 10⁶/L (p580).
MAI[2]	Clarithromycin 500mg/12h + ethambutol 15mg/kg/24h + either rifabutin or rifampicin 450–600mg/d ± ciprofloxacin 500mg/12h, all PO. Secondary prophylaxis is required eg clarithromycin 500mg/12h + ethambutol 15mg/kg/24h; may be discontinued when culture –ve, CD4 >100 × 10⁶/L, and HIV viral load <10,000/mL after HAART (p584).

581

1 For more doses, see GAT^sandford 2003 or the British National Formulary (www.bnf.org).
2 MAI = Mycobacterium avium intracellulare (=MAC, ie M. avium complex, p580).

What every doctor should know about HIV

Preventing HIV spread • Promote *lifelong* safer sex, barrier contraception, and reduction in the number of partners. Videos, followed by interactive discussions, is one way to double the use of condoms. Another way is the *100% condom programme* involving distribution of condoms to brothels, with enforcement programmes enabling monitoring and encouraging condom use at any sex establishment. Such programmes are estimated to have prevented 2 million HIV infections in Thailand.
- Warn everyone about the dangers of sexual tourism/promiscuity.
- Tell drug users not to share needles. Use needle exchange schemes.
- Vigorous control of other STDs can reduce HIV incidence by 40%.
- Strengthen awareness of clinics for STDs.
- Reduce unnecessary blood transfusions.
- Encourage pregnant women to have HIV tests. (Caesarean sections and zidovudine during birth can prevent vertical transmission, *OHCS* p98.)

Occupational exposure and needle-stick injury
(Seroconversion rate: ~0.4% for HIV; 30% for Hepatitis B if HBeAg +ve)
- Wash well; encourage bleeding; do not suck or immerse in bleach.
- Note name, address, and clinical details of 'donor'.
- Report incident to Occupational Health and fill in an accident form.
- Store blood from both parties. If possible ascertain HIV, HBV, and HCV status of both. Immunize (active and passive) against hepatitis B at once, if needed. Counsel (HIV risk <0.5% if 'donor' is HIV +ve) and test recipient at 3, 6, and 8 months (seroconversion may take this long).
- Weigh risks by questioning 'donor'; if HIV+ve, what is the CD4 and viral load count? Before prophylaxis, do a pregnancy test. Get informed consent. Was there a large inoculum? Was injury deep? (Mucous membrane exposure carries very low risk.) Give 4wks of drugs, if possible within 1h of exposure: **Low-risk:** No antiviral medication. **Higher-risk:** Typically *zidovudine* 250mg/12h + *lamivudine* 150mg/12h, and particularly for worst episodes (deep puncture from wide-bore needle causing bleeding), *indinavir* 800mg/8h OR *nelfinavir* 750mg/8h, all PO.

HIV test counselling If in doubt, get help from a genitourinary clinic.
- Determine level of risk (eg unprotected sex; sex overseas).
- Explore benefits of the test (eg anxiety↓; protection of partner; planning the future; avoiding vertical transmission; getting treatment).
- What are the difficulties? Will you tell family and friends? Explain possible effects on: job, mortgage, insurance (in the UK there is no obligation for doctors to disclose HIV status).
- Do post-test counselling (eg to re-emphasize ways to ↓risk exposure).
- *Counselling throughout HIV illness:* A key issue when a person is dying from HIV is making a will. Legal help may be needed on housing, employment, and guardianship of children. Making advance directives needs special skill. Later, the GP, domiciliary teams from genitourinary medicine (GUM) or ID departments, and hospices help with terminal care.

Acute seroconversion As HIV gets more treatable, recognizing this early phase becomes more important.[1] The clinical features are similar to infectious mononucleosis; perform tests if there are unusual signs, eg oral candidiasis, recurrent shingles, leucopenia, or CNS signs (antibody tests may be negative but viral P24 antigen and HIV RNA levels are ↑ in early infection). As ever, the first best 'test' is to take a thorough history. If you *do* identify acute seroconversion illness, get expert help promptly: vigorous anti-HIV combination treatment may be indicated.

1 C Hare 2004 *Curr Infect Dis Rep* **6** 65

Monitoring HIV infection

There is more to monitoring HIV than periodic measurements of the CD4 count. Plasma *HIV RNA levels* strongly predict progression to AIDS and death, whatever the CD4 count. This test typically involves quantitative reverse transcriptase PCR to amplify DNA copies of the target RNA. HIV patients in the lowest quartile of viral load (HIV RNA ≤4530 copies/mL) have an 8% chance of progressing to AIDS in 5yrs compared with 62% in those in the highest quartile (>36,270 copies/mL). Clinical benefit from anti-HIV agents depends not only on improving the *CD4 count* but also from decreasing HIV RNA to undetectable levels. This is now possible with combination therapy.

When to treat HIV infection (UK guidelines)[1]

When to commence anti-HIV treatment is still a controversial issue; no long-term studies (involving clinical endpoints such as death) are available. UK guidelines are that treatment be started in the following circumstances:

- Primary HIV infection.
- Any patient diagnosed with AIDS, or with severe/recurrent HIV-related illness.
- Any patient with CD4 count <200 × 10^6/L.
- Asymptomatic with CD4 count of 200–350 × 10^6/L and a high viral load.
- Asymptomatic with a CD4 count of 200–350 × 10^6/L which is falling rapidly.

CD4 counts and HIV RNA levels should be used to monitor treatment, eg every 3 months. There is an argument for changing treatment if HIV RNA level rebounds (>500 copies/mL on two consecutive tests), if there is a consistent fall in the CD4 count, or if new symptoms occur. The new regimen should include at least two drugs new to the patient. Send resistance tests eg genotyping for HIV reverse transcriptase/protease mutations (if available). **NB:** Multi-drug therapy imposes difficulties both in terms of timing of doses and interactions with other drugs.

1 Recommendations on when to start HIV therapy are constantly evolving. For latest UK guidelines, refer to the British HIV Association (BHIVA) www.bhiva.org.

Antiretroviral agents

This is an expensive luxury for most of the world's HIV patients. In many ways *all* anti-HIV treatment is experimental so perhaps the best question to ask is not *what is the best treatment for HIV* but *which is the most appropriate trial to enter my patient into?* ▶Seek expert help early.

▶HAART (highly active antiretroviral therapy) usually involves combining two nucleoside analogue reverse transcriptase inhibitors (NRTI) with *either* a protease inhibitor (PI) *or* a non-nucleoside reverse transcriptase inhibitor (NNRTI) *or* (in patients with relatively low viral loads) abacavir.[74]

Nucleoside analogue reverse transcriptase inhibitors (NRTI)
- *Zidovudine (Azidothymidine, AZT)* was the first anti-HIV drug. Dose: 250–300mg/12h PO or 1–2mg/kg/4h IV. SE: anaemia, leucopenia, gastrointestinal disturbance, fever, rash, myalgia. Stop treatment if ↑LFT, hepatomegaly, lactic acidosis. CI: anaemia, neutropenia, breast-feeding.
- *Didanosine (DDI; Videx EC®)* Dose: 250mg/24h PO if wt <60kg; 400mg/24h if ≥60kg. SE: pancreatitis, peripheral neuropathy, hyperuricaemia, GI disturbance, retinal and optic nerve changes, liver failure. Stop treatment if significant rise in LFT or amylase. CI: breast-feeding.
- *Lamivudine (3TC)*[75] is probably the best tolerated antiretroviral. Dose: 150mg/12h PO, take without food. SE: see zidovudine, but less common. Stop treatment if ↑LFT, hepatomegaly, lactic acidosis, pancreatitis.
- *Stavudine (D4T)* Dose: 40mg/12h PO if wt ≥60kg; 30mg/12h PO if <60kg. Stop treatment if peripheral neuropathy or ↑LFT.
- *Tenofovir* Dose: 245mg/24h PO. SE: see lamivudine.
- *Abacavir* Dose: 300mg/12h PO. SE: hepatitis, lactic acidosis, hypersensitivity syndrome (3–5%)—rash, fever, vomiting; may be fatal if rechallenged.

Protease inhibitors (PI) slow cell-to-cell spread, and lengthen the time to the first clinical event. PIs are often given with low dose ritonavir (100mg/12hr PO), which appears to enhance drug levels. All PIs are metabolized by the cytochrome P450 enzyme system. They may therefore increase the concentrations of certain drugs by competitive inhibition of their metabolism, if administered concomitantly. PIs appear to be associated with body fat redistribution: increased abdominal fat, breast enlargement, decreased fat under the skin on limbs. Other class specific SE: hyperlipidaemia, hyperglycaemia, insulin resistance, gastrointestinal disturbance.
- *Indinavir* Dose: 800mg/8h PO, 1h before or 2h after a meal. SE: dry mouth, taste disturbance, rash, pruritus, hyperpigmentation, alopecia, nephrolithiasis, anaemia, neutropenia, myalgia, paraesthesiae, ↑LFT.
- *Ritonavir* Dose: 600mg/12h PO. SE: see indinavir.
- *Saquinavir* Dose: 600–1200mg/8h PO. SE: oral ulcers, paraesthesiae, myalgia, headache, dizziness, pruritus, rash, pancreatitis. (Fortovase® is best absorbed form.)
- *Nelfinavir* Dose: 750mg/8h PO. SE: hepatitis, neutropenia, flatulence, ↑CK.
- *Lopinavir/Ritonavir (Kaletra®)* is probably superior to nelfinavir.[77] Dose: 400mg (+100mg ritonavir)/12h PO. SE: see saquinavir.
- *Amprenavir* Dose: 1200mg/12h PO. SE: see saquinavir.

Non-nucleoside reverse transcriptase inhibitors (NNRTI) These may interact with drugs metabolized by the cytochrome P450 enzyme system, which they either induce or inhibit depending on the concomitantly administered drug.[78]
- *Nevirapine* Dose: 200mg/24h for 2wks, then 200mh/12h PO. Resistant mutants emerge readily. SE: Stevens–Johnson syndrome, toxic epidermal necrolysis, hepatitis.
- *Efavirenz* Dose: 600mg/24h PO. SE: rash, sleep disturbance, dizziness. Avoid in pregnancy.

Golden rules in HIV therapy

- Start HAART early, ideally before CD4 count <200 × 10^6/L.
- Explain to patients that regimens are complex and stress the importance of strict adherence. Take time to harmonize pharmacodynamics with the patient's expectations and lifestyle.
- Use three anti-HIV drugs (minimizes replication and cross-resistance).
- Monitor plasma viral load and CD4 count, remembering that what seems like elimination of HIV often turns into reactivation when treatment stops. Aim for undetectable viral loads with 2–4 months of starting HAART. Suspect poor adherence if viral load rebounds.
- If viral load remains high despite good adherence, if there is a consistent fall in CD4 count, or if new symptoms occur, change to a new combination of anti-HIV drugs and send resistance tests eg genotyping for HIV reverse transcriptase/protease mutations (if available).
- Stay informed about new drugs, and new classes of drugs (viral entry inhibitors eg enfuvirtide,[1] integrase inhibitors) that are continuingly emerging.

Making antiretroviral drugs widely available

The WHO-endorsed 'three-by-five' initiative involves training 100,000 workers in using a 'one size fits all' version of antiretroviral therapy. The aim is to provide treatment for an extra three million people by 2005 (WHO 2004).

---

1 Enfuvirtide inhibits viral entry by binding to the HIV-1 envelope glycoprotein gp41. It may be useful in multi-drug resistant HIV. SE: ↑Incidence of bacterial pneumonia, hypersensitivity, injection site reactions. See JP Lalezari 2003 *NEJM* **348** 2175

Sexually transmitted disease (STD)

►Refer early to genitourinary medicine clinic (GUM) for full microbiological investigation and contact tracing and notification. Most clinics see patients immediately during the working day; some offer an on-call service. Avoid giving antibiotics until seen in GUM clinic or at least discussed.

Incidence is rising in England by >10% per year as 'safer sex' practices are being ignored. In 2002, there were >24,000 cases of gonorrhoea, 81,680 cases of genital *Chlamydia*, and 1193 cases of syphilis reported.

Presentation Vaginal or urethral discharge (p588), genital lesions, or HIV (p578). Herpes (p568). Syphilis (p601). *Chlamydia* (*OHCS* p50; often symptomless but may cause infertility or ectopic pregnancy). Genital warts (*OHCS* p592). Salpingitis (*OHCS* p50). Crab lice (*OHCS* p600).

History Ask about timing of last intercourse; contraceptive method; sexual contacts; duration of relationship; sexual practices and orientation; past STDs, menstrual and medical history; antimicrobial therapy.

Examination Detailed examination of genitalia including inguinal nodes and pubic hair. Scrotum, subpreputial space, and male urethra. PR examination and proctoscopy (if indicated); PV and speculum examination.

Tests Refer to GUM clinic. *Urine:* dipstick and MSU for MC+S. *Ulcers:* take swabs for HSV culture (viral transport medium) and dark ground microscopy for syphilis (*T. pallidum*). *Men:* Urethral smear for Gram stain and culture for *N. gonorrhoeae* (send quickly to lab in Stuart's medium); urethral swab for *Chlamydia*. *Women:* High vaginal swab in Stuart's medium for microscopy and culture *Candida, Gardnerella vaginalis*, anaerobes, *Trichomonas vaginalis*); endocervical swab for *Chlamydia trachomatis. Chlamydia* (an obligate intracellular bacteria) is the trickiest STD to diagnose as it is asymptomatic, difficult to culture, and serology may be unhelpful as it cross-reacts with *C. pneumoniae*. Nucleic acid amplification assays (eg urine ligase chain reaction, PCR) are considered good screening tests, with sensitivity >90%. Other tests used include *Chlamydia* antigen and nucleic acid probe assays. *Blood tests:* Syphilis, hepatitis, and HIV serology after full counselling.

Follow-up Arrange to see patients at 1wk and 3 months, with repeat smears, cultures, and syphilis serology.

Scabies (*Sarcoptes scabeii*) Spread is common in families. *Presentation:* Papular rash (on abdomen or medial thigh; itchy at night) + burrows (in digital web spaces and flexor wrist surfaces). *Incubation:* ~6wks (during which time sensitization to the mite's faeces and/or saliva occurs). Penile lesions produce red nodules. *Diagnosis:* Tease a mite out of its burrow with a needle for microscopy. This may fail but if a drop of oil is placed on the lesion, a few scrapes with a scalpel may provide faeces or eggs. *R:* ►Treat all the household. Give written advice (*OHCS* p600). Apply malathion 0.5% liquid (Derbac-M®). Include the head in those <2yrs old, elderly, or immunocompromised. Remember to paint *all* parts, including soles (avoid eyes); wash off after 24h.

Lymphogranuloma *Presentation:* Inguinal lymphadenopathy and ulceration *Causes:* Lymphogranuloma venereum, chancroid (*Haemophilus ducreyi*)[1], or granuloma inguinale (*Calymmatobacterium granulomatis*, ie donovanosis). The latter causes extensive, painless, red genital ulcers and pseudobuboes, ie abscesses near inguinal nodes, with possible elephantiasis ± malignant change. Diagnosis: 'closed safety-pin' inclusion bodies in cytoplasm of histiocytes. Treatment: doxycycline 100mg/12h PO until all lesions epithelialized; alternatives include azithromycin, erythromycin, or tetracycline.

---

1 In the Tropics, chancroid is a common cause of sexually acquired genital ulcers, typically with a granular, yellow base, and ragged edges (± inguinal buboes, which may need draining via a wide-bore needle); the cause is *Haemophilus ducreyi*. WHO recommends erythromycin 500mg/6h PO for 7d, ceftriaxone 250mg IM (1 dose), azithromycin 1g PO (1 dose). Chancroid facilitates spread of HIV.

Chlamydia screening to prevent pelvic inflammatory disease

It has been known for several years that screening for asymptomatic *Chlamydia* infection can decrease the incidence of pelvic inflammatory disease. Large screening programmes are currently in place in countries such as Sweden and the USA. In the UK, the implementation of opportunistic screening of young, sexually active women has been slow due to the logistical difficulties of incorporating such tests into already overburdened GP appointments. One pilot study in the UK showed screening (using the urine ligase chain reaction) to be both feasible and acceptable to patients[1]. Whether national screening will be as straight-forward remains to be seen.

1 M Catchpole 2003 *Sex Transm Infect* **79** 16–27

Vaginal discharge and urethritis

Non-offensive vaginal discharge may be physiological. Most which are smelly or itchy are due to infection. A very foul discharge may be due to a foreign body (eg forgotten tampons, or beads in children).

▶Discharges rarely resemble their classical descriptions.

▶Untreated GU inflammation↑viral shedding of HIV-1 in semen 3-fold.

Thrush *(Candida albicans)* Thrush is the commonest cause of discharge and is classically described as white curds. The vulva and vagina may be red, fissured, and sore. The partner may be asymptomatic. *Risk factors:* Pregnancy, immunodeficiencies, diabetes, the Pill, antibiotics. *Diagnosis:* Microscopy: strings of mycelium or oval spores. Culture on Sabouraud's medium. *Treatment:* A single imidazole pessary, eg clotrimazole 500mg, + cream for the vulva (and partner) is convenient. A single dose of fluconazole 150mg PO is an alternative. Reassure that thrush is not necessarily sexually transmitted. Recurrent thrush: see *OHCS* p48.

Trichomonas vaginalis (TV) Produces vaginitis and a thin, bubbly, fishy smelling discharge. It is sexually transmitted. Exclude gonorrhoea (which may coexist). The motile flagellate may be seen on wet film microscopy, or cultured. *Treatment:* Metronidazole 400mg/12h PO for 5d or 2g PO stat. Treat the partner. If pregnant, use the 5d regimen.

Bacterial vaginosis presents with fishy smelling discharge. The vagina is not inflamed and itch is uncommon. Vaginal pH is >5.5 resulting in alteration of bacterial flora ± overgrowth, eg of *Gardnerella vaginalis*, *Mycoplasma hominis*, peptostreptococci, *Mobiluncus* and anaerobes, eg *Bacteroides* species with too few lactobacillae. There is ↑risk of pre-term labour and amniotic infection if pregnant. *Diagnosis:* Stippled vaginal epithelial 'clue cells' may be seen on wet microscopy. Culture. *Treatment:* *OHCS* p48—eg metronidazole 400mg/12h PO for 5d, or clindamycin cream.

Gonorrhoea *Neisseria gonorrhoea* (gonococcus, GC) can infect any columnar epithelium, eg urethra, cervix, rectum, pharynx, conjunctiva. Incubation: 2–10d. *Symptoms:* ♂: Purulent urethral discharge ± dysuria; or proctitis, tenesmus, ± discharge PR if homosexual. ♀: Usually asymptomatic, but may have vaginal discharge, dysuria, proctitis. Pharyngeal disease is often asymptomatic. *Complications—Local:* Prostatitis, cystitis, epididymitis, salpingitis, Bartholinitis. *Systemic:* Septicaemia, eg with petechiae, hand/foot pustules, arthritis; Reiter's syndrome; endocarditis (rare). *Obstetric:* Ophthalmia neonatorum[ND] (*OHCS* p100). *Long-term:* Urethral stricture, infertility. *Treatment:* One dose of *ciprofloxacin* 500mg PO. Resistance is a problem in ≥10%. Alternatives: *ofloxacin* 400mg PO stat or *cefixime*, eg 400mg PO stat. Treat for chlamydia too (eg doxycycline 100mg/12h PO for 7d, or a single dose of azithromycin 1g PO) as 50% of patients with urethritis or cervicitis will have concomittant *C. trachomatis* infection.[1] Trace contacts. No intercourse or alcohol until cured.

Non-gonococcal urethritis is commoner than GC. Discharge is thinner and signs less acute, but this may not help diagnosis. Women (typically asymptomatic) may have cervicitis, urethritis, or salpingitis (pain, fever, infertility). Rectum and pharynx are not infected. *Organisms:* C. trachomatis (▶special swabs are needed, *OHCS* p50); *Ureaplasma urealyticum*; *Mycoplasma genitalium*; *Trichomonas vaginalis*; *Gardnerella*; Gram –ve and anaerobic bacteria; *Candida*. *Complications:* Similar to local complications of GC. *Chlamydia* may cause Reiter's syndrome and neonatal conjunctivitis. *Treatment:* 1wk of doxycycline 100mg/12h PO. A single dose of azithromycin 1g PO is an alternative where compliance is likely to be problematic. Trace contacts. Avoid intercourse during treatment and alcohol for 4wks.

Non-infective urethritis Traumatic; chemicals; cancer; foreign body.

---

1 Sanford's Guide to Antimicrobial Therapy 2003

When do antibiotic guidelines become outdated?

The emergence of antibiotic resistance amongst pathogens represents one of the main obstacles in the fight against infectious diseases. Antibiotic guidelines, which exist on local, regional, and national levels to ensure optimal therapy, must therefore be continually updated to keep up with evolving pathogen defences. To monitor resistance patterns, sample infective isolates from different UK regions are collected centrally and tested against a variety of antibiotics to determine their sensitivities to the different drugs (as measured by the minimal inhibitory concentration (MIC) of drug required to prevent organism growth in culture). Such results can highlight the need to revise antibiotic guidelines.

589

One example is the emergence of ciprofloxacin resistance amongst *Neisseria gonorrhoeae* isolates in England and Wales. Resistance was found in 9.8% of isolates in 2002, up from 3.1% in 2001 and 2.1% in 2000. National guidelines have aimed for chosen treatments to eliminate gonococcal infection in >95% of patients. Ciprofloxacin, previously the first line drug in the treatment of gonococcal infections, may have to be replaced by cephalosporins in updated antibiotic guidelines for England and Wales.[1]

---

1 KA Fenton 2003 *Lancet* **361** 1867. The BNF recommends cefixine as 1st choice. Pharyngeal infections still require ciprofloxacin or ofloxacin if sensitive.

Miscellaneous Gram positive bacteria

Staphylococci When pathogenic, these are usually *Staph. aureus*. Typically, they cause localized infection of skin, lids, or wounds. Severe infections with *Staph. aureus* include: pneumonia, osteomyelitis, septic arthritis, endocarditis, and septicaemia. Production of β-lactamase which destroys many antibiotics (p542–50) is the main problem. *Staph. aureus* toxins may cause food poisoning (p556) or the toxic shock syndrome toxin (TSST-1): shock, confusion, fever, a rash with desquamation, diarrhoea, myalgia, CPK↑, platelets↓ (associated with the use of hyperabsorbent tampons). *Staph. epidermidis* (*albus*) is increasingly recognized as a pathogen in the immunocompromised, particularly in connection with IV lines or any prosthesis. When isolated from a culture, *Staph. epidermidis* can usually be assumed to be a contaminant. It is often enough to remove the infected line. Deep *Staph.* infections need ≥4wks of flucloxacillin 500mg/6h IV ± removal of foreign bodies, eg prostheses.

Methicillin-resistant Staph. aureus (MRSA) is the big issue in hospital-acquired infection, causing pneumonia, septicaemia, wound infections, and deaths. In the USA, 29% of hospitals have MRSA problems. Carriage rates (eg nasal): 1–10%. Risk factors: HIV, dialysis, being on ITU. MRSA may also be community-acquired. *Management:* Discuss with a microbiologist. Vancomycin or teicoplanin are commonly used, but strains with reduced sensitivity (vancomycin-intermediate *Staph. aureus* (VISA)—↓sensitivity to *both* drugs) have emerged.▣ In such cases, linezolid or quinupristin/dalfopristin (Synercid®) may be effective. Preventive measures:

- Isolate recently admitted patients with suspected MRSA.
- Group all MRSA patients together on 1 ward.
- Wash your hands and your stethoscope!
- Ask about the need for eradication (with *mupirocin*).
- Be meticulous in looking after intravascular catheters when on ITU.
- Surveillance swabs of patients and staff during outbreaks.
- Use gowns/gloves when dealing with infected or colonized patients. Masks may be needed during contact with MRSA pneumonia.

Streptococci Group A streptococci (eg *Strep. pyogenes*) are common pathogens, causing wound and skin infections (eg impetigo, erysipelas, OHCS p590), tonsillitis, scarlet fever[ND], necrotizing fasciitis (p486), toxic shock, or septicaema. Late complications are rheumatic fever and post-streptococcal glomerulonephritis. *Strep. pneumoniae* (pneumococcus, Gram +ve diplococcus) causes pneumonia, otitis media, meningitis, septicaemia, peritonitis (rare). Resistance to penicillin is a problem. *Strep. sanguis*, *Strep. mutans*, and *Strep. mitior* (of the 'viridans' group), *Strep. bovis*, and *Enterococcus faecalis* all cause SBE. *Enterococcus faecalis* also causes UTI, wound infections, and septicaemia. *Strep. mutans* is a very common cause of dental caries. *Strep. milleri* forms abscesses, eg in CNS, lungs, and liver. Most streptococci are sensitive to the penicillins, but *Enterococcus faecalis* and *Enterococcus faecium* may present some difficulties. They usually respond to a combination of ampicillin and an aminoglycoside, eg gentamicin (p547 & p710). Vancomycin-resistant enterococci (VRE) have been reported. Some strains of VRE are sensitive to either teicoplanin or Synercid; all appear to be sensitive to linezolid (p546).[1]

Anthrax[ND] *(Bacillus anthracis)* Occurs in Africa, Asia, China, Eastern Europe, and Haiti. Spread by handling infected carcasses; well-cooked meat poses *no* risk. Terrorists have attempted to use anthrax as a biological weapon.▣ *Presentation:* Common form: local cutaneous 'malignant pustule'. Oedema may be a striking sign ± fever & hepatosplenomegaly. May cause pulmonary or GI anthrax with breathlessness or massive GI haemorrhage (± meningo-encephalitis). *Tests:* CXR may show a widened mediastinum. Gram stain is sometimes diagnostic (Gram +ve rod).

1 There has been a report of a vancomycin-resistant *S. aureus* (VRSA), containing a *vanA* resistance gene identical to that seen in some vancomycin-resistant enterococci. See S Chang 2003 *NEJM* **348** 1342

Treatment: Cutaneous disease: ciprofloxacin 500mg/12h PO for 60d. *Pulmonary or GI anthrax:* Ciprofloxacin 400mg/12h IV with clindamycin 900mg/8h IV + rifampicin 300mg/12h IV. Switch to oral drugs when able; treat for 60d.[1] *Prevention:* Immunization of animals at risk, and enforcement of sound food-handling and carcass-hygiene policies.

Diphtheria[ND] is caused by the toxin of *Corynebacterium diphtheriae*. Presents with tonsillitis ± a pseudomembrane over the fauces and lymphadenopathy ('bull neck'). Further details: see *OHCS* p276. ℞: erythromycin 10–12mg/kg/6h IVI.[2] *Prevention:* 'Adsorbed Diphtheria Vaccine for Adults and Adolescents' 0.5mL × 3 at monthly intervals. Give all close contacts prophylaxis (eg erythromycin 250mg/6h PO for 10d) *before* swab results are known.

Listeriosis is caused by *Listeria monocytogenes*, a Gram +ve bacillus with an unusual ability to multiply at low temperatures. Possible sources of infection include pâtés, raw vegetables, unpasteurized milk, and soft cheeses (brie, camembert, and blue-vein types). It may cause a non-specific 'flu-like illness, pneumonia, meningoencephalitis, ataxia, rash, or PUO, especially in the immuno-compromised, in pregnancy, where it may cause miscarriage or stillbirth, and in neonates. *Diagnosis:* Culture blood, placenta, amniotic fluid, CSF, and any expelled products of conception. ►Take blood cultures in *any pregnant patient with unexplained fever for ≥48h.* Serology, vaginal, and rectal swabs don't help (it may be a commensal here). *Treatment:* Ampicillin IV (erythromycin if allergic) + gentamicin; see p543 & p547 for doses. *Prevention in pregnancy:* • Avoid soft cheeses, pâtés, and under-cooked meat. • Observe 'use by' dates. • Ensure reheated food is piping hot; observe standing times when using microwaves; throw away any left-overs.

Nocardia species cause subcutaneous infection (eg Madura foot) in warm climes. If immunocompromised, it may cause abscesses (lung, liver, cerebral). Microscopy: Branching chains of cocci. *Treatment:* Sulfamethoxazole 3g/12h PO for 6wks; check blood levels if renal failure. Alternative: imipenem.

Clostridia *Cl. perfringens* causes wound infections and gas gangrene ± shock or renal failure after surgery or trauma. *Treatment:* Debridement is essential; benzylpenicillin 1.2–2.4g/6h IV + clindamycin 900mg/8h IV, antitoxin and hyperbaric oxygen may also be used. Amputation may be necessary. *Clostridia* food poisoning (p556). *Cl. difficile:* diarrhoea (the cause of pseudomembranous colitis following antibiotic therapy, p219). *Cl. botulinum:* (Botulism) *Cl. botulinum* toxin blocks release of acetycholine causing descending flaccid paralysis. Botulism is not spread from one person to another. There are 2 adult forms of botulism: food-borne and wound botulism. ►Risk is high in IV drug abusers if heroin is contaminated with *Cl. botulinum.* *Signs:* Afebrile, flaccid paralysis, dysarthria, dysphagia, diplopia, ptosis, weakness, respiratory failure. Autonomic signs: dry mouth, fixed or dilated pupils. *Tests:* Find toxin in blood samples or, in the case of wound botulism, by the identification of *Cl. botulinum* in wound specimens by prompt referral to a reference lab. Samples include: serum, wound pus, swabs in anaerobic transport media (in the UK, phone PHLS, 020 8200 6868.) *Management:* Get help (on ITU). IM botulinum antitoxin works if given early (eg 50,000U of types A and B with 5000U of type E). Also give to those who have ingested toxin but who have not yet developed symptoms. *Cl. botulinum* is sensitive to benzylpenicillin and metronidazole. Out of hours, antitoxin can be got via the CDSC doctor on 020 8200 6868.

Actinomycosis is caused by *Actinomyces israelii*. Usually causes subcutaneous infections, forming chronic sinuses with sulfur granule-containing pus. It commonly affects the area of the jaw (or IUCDs, *OHCS* p62). It may cause abdominal masses (may mimic appendix mass). *Treatment:* Benzylpenicillin (p543) for ≥2wks post-clinical cure. Liaise with surgeons.

---

1 Sanford's Guide to Antimicrobial Therapy 2003 2 Use erythromycin lactobionate form.

Miscellaneous Gram negative bacteria

Enterobacteria Some are normal gut commensals, others environmental organisms. They are the commonest cause of UTI and intra-abdominal sepsis, especially post-operatively and in the acute abdomen. They are also a common cause of septicaemia. Unusually, they may cause pneumonia (especially *Klebsiella*), meningitis, or endocarditis. These organisms are often sensitive to ampicillin and trimethoprim, but in serious infections, use cefuroxime (see also 4th generation cephalosporins, p544) ± an aminoglycoside. *Salmonella* and *Shigella* are discussed on p556 and p596.

Pseudomonas aeruginosa is a serious pathogen, especially in the immuno-compromised and in patients with cystic fibrosis. It causes pneumonia, septicaemia, UTI, wound infection, osteomyelitis, and cutaneous infections. The main problem is its increasing antibiotic resistance. *Treatment:* Piperacillin (p543) or mezlocillin + an aminoglycoside. Ciprofloxacin, ceftazidime, and imipenem (p547) are useful against *Pseudomonas*.

Haemophilus influenzae typically affects unvaccinated children usually <4yrs old. It causes otitis media, acute epiglottitis, pneumonia, meningitis, osteo-myelitis, and septicaemia. In adults it may cause exacerbations of chronic bronchitis. *Treatment:* Unreliably sensitive to ampicillin; cefotaxime is more reliable. Capsulated types tend to be much more pathogenic than non-capsulated types. *Prevention:* Immunization with HiB vaccine (p558) has resulted in a dramatic fall in incidence.

Plague[ND] is caused by *Yersinia pestis*. *Spread:* Fleas of rodents or cats, or droplets from other infected humans. *Incubation:* 1–7d. Bubonic plague presents with lymphadenopathy (buboes). Pneumonic plague may present with lymphadenopathy or a 'flu-like illness leading to dyspnoea, cough, copious, bloody sputum, septicaemia, and a haemorrhagic fatal illness. *Diagnosis:* Phage typing of bacterial culture, or a 4-fold rise in antibodies to F antigen. *Treatment:* Isolate suspects. Streptomycin 15mg/kg/12h IV for 10d. If in 1st trimester of pregnancy, amoxicillin 250–500mg/8h PO; if later in pregnancy, co-trimoxazole 480mg/12h PO; children: co-trimoxazole. Staying at home, quarantine (inspect daily for 1wk), insect sprays to legs and bedding, and avoiding dead animals helps stop spread. *Post-exposure prophylaxis:* doxycycline 100mg/12h PO for 7d. *Prevention:* Vaccines give no *immediate* protection (multiple doses may be needed).

Brucellosis This zoonosis (carried by domestic animals) is common in the Middle East. Typically affects vets or farmers. Cause: *B. melitensis* (the most virulent), *B. abortus*, *B. suis*, or *B. canis*. Symptoms may be indolent and last for years—eg fever (PUO), sweats, malaise, anorexia, vomiting, weight loss, hepato-splenomegaly, constipation, diarrhoea, myalgia, backache, arthritis, sacro-iliitis, rash, bursitis, orchitis, depression. *Complications:* Osteomyelitis, SBE/IE (culture negative), abscesses (liver, spleen, lung), meningoencephalitis. *Diagnosis:* Blood culture (≥6wks but rapid culture systems available, contact lab); serology: if titres equivocal (eg >1 : 40 in non-endemic zones) do ELISA ± immunoradiometric assays; pancytopenia. *Treatment:* Doxycycline 100mg/12h PO for 6 weeks + streptomycin 1g/d IM for 2–3wks (↓relapse rate from 2% to 10% vs >20%). If a child, get expert help.

Whooping cough[ND] is caused by *Bordetella pertussis*. This begins with a prodromal catarrhal phase with fever and cough. After a week or so, the child develops the characteristic paroxysms of coughing and inspiratory whoops. Most children recover without complication, although the illness may last some months. Some, especially the very young, may develop pneumonia (and consequent bronchiectasis) or convulsions and brain damage. *Treatment:* Erythromycin should be given early, if only to limit spread. See *Immunization*, p558.

Pasteurella multocida is acquired via domestic animals, especially cat or dog bites. It can cause cutaneous infections, septicaemia, pneumonia, UTI, or meningitis. *Treatment:* Co-amoxiclav, p543; an IV form is available; the dose, expressed as amoxicillin, is 1g/6–8h IV over 3–4 min.

Yersinia enterocolitica In Scandinavia, this is a common cause of a reactive, asymmetrical polyarthritis of the weight-bearing joints, and, in America, of enteritis. It also causes uveitis, appendicitis, mesenteric lymphadenitis, pyomyositis, glomerulonephritis, thyroiditis, colonic dilatation, terminal ileitis and perforation, and septicaemia. *Diagnosis:* Serology is often more helpful than culture, as there may be quite a time-lag between infection and the clinical manifestations. Agglutination titres >1 : 160 indicate recent infection. *Treatment:* None may be needed or ciprofloxacin 500mg/12h PO for 3–5d.

Moraxella catarrhalis (Gram –ve diplococcus) is an increasingly recognized cause of pneumonia, exacerbations of COPD, otitis media, sinusitis, and septicaemia. *Treatment:* Clarithromycin 500mg/12h PO.

Tularaemia is caused by *Francisella tularensis* (Gram –ve bacillus), which may be acquired by handling infected animal carcasses. It causes rash, fever, malaise, tonsillitis, headache, hepatosplenomegaly, and lymphadenopathy. There may be papules at sites of inoculation (eg fingers).

Complications: Meningitis, osteomyelitis, SBE/IE, pericarditis, septicaemia.

Diagnosis: Contact local microbiologist for advice. Only use laboratories with safety cabinets suitable for dangerous pathogens. Swabs and aspirates must be transported in approved containers. *Treatment:* Gentamicin or streptomycin 7.5–10mg/kg/12h IM for 2wks. Oral tetracycline may be suitable for chemoprophylaxis. *Prevention:* Find the animal vector; reduce human contact with it as far as possible. Vaccination may be possible for high-risk groups.

Cat scratch disease Mostly due to *Bartonella henselae* (a small, curved, pleomorphic, Gram negative rod) or *Afepilis felis*. Think of this when any three of the following coexist: an inoculating cat scratch; regional lymphadenopathy (with –ve lab tests for other causes of lymphadenopathy, p76); positive cat scratch skin test antigen response; or microabscesses in lymph nodes. In HIV-infected patients, the skin lesions may resemble Kaposi's sarcoma. *Treatment:* Usually resolves spontaneously within 1–2 months. One trial found that azithromycin ↑speed of resolution of lymph nodes.⬛ Other drugs that have been used include ciprofloxacin, rifampicin and co-trimoxazole. Usually unresponsive *in vivo* despite susceptibility *in vitro*.

See also **Spirochaetes** p600; **Neisseria.** p368, and **Legionella** p174.

TetanusND

Essence Tetanospasmin, *Clostridium tetani*'s exotoxin, causes muscle spasms and rigidity, cardinal features of tetanus (='to stretch').

Incidence ~50 people/yr in the UK. Mortality: 40% (80% in neonates).

Pathogenesis Spores of *Cl. tetani* live in faeces, soil, dust, and on instruments. A tiny breach in skin or mucosa, eg cuts, burns, ear piercing, banding of piles, may admit the spores. (Diabetics are at especial risk.) Spores may then germinate and make the exotoxin. This then travels up peripheral nerves and interferes with inhibitory synapses.

The Patient *15-25% will have no evidence of recent wounds.* Signs appear from 1d to several months from the (often forgotten) injury. There is a prodrome of fever, malaise, and headache before classical features develop: *trismus* (=lockjaw; Greek trismos = grinding, hence difficulty in opening the mouth); *risus sardonicus* (a grin-like posture of hypertonic facial muscles); *opisthotonus* (arched body with hyperextended neck); *spasms* (which at first may be induced by movement, injections, noise, etc., but later are spontaneous; they may cause dysphagia and respiratory arrest); autonomic dysfunction (arrhythmias and wide fluctuations in BP).

Differential diagnosis is dental abscess, rabies, phenothiazine toxicity, and strychnine poisoning. Phenothiazine toxicity usually only affects facial and tongue muscles; if suspected, give benzatropine 1–2mg IV.

Bad prognostic signs are short incubation, rapid progression from trismus to spasms (<48h), development post-partum or post-infection, and tetanus in neonates and old age.

Treatment Get expert help; use ITU. Monitor ECG + BP. Careful fluid balance.
- Clean/debride wounds, IV penicillin or metronidazole 1g/8h PR for 1wk.
- If tetanus is established, give human tetanus immune globulin (HTIGS) 5000U IV to neutralize free toxin. Local infiltration of 3000U around a suspicious wound is used in some centres. If only horse antitetanus serum (ATS) is available, give a small SC test dose before giving 10,000U IV + 750U per 24h to the cut for 3d. Some advocate intrathecal administration of antitoxin.
- Early ventilation and sedation if symptoms progress.
- Control spasms with diazepam 0.05–0.2mg/kg/h IVI or phenobarbital (=phenobarbitone) 1.0mg/kg/h IM or IV + chlorpromazine 0.5mg/kg/6h IM (IV bolus is dangerous) starting 3h after the phenobarbital. If this fails to control the spasms, paralyse and ventilate (get anaesthetist's help).

Prevention Active immunization with tetanus toxoid is given as part of the 3-stage 'triple' vaccine during the 1st year of life (p558). Boosters are given on starting school and in early adulthood. Once five injections have been given, revaccinate only at the time of significant injury, and consider a final 1-off booster at ~65yrs. *Primary immunization of adults:* 0.5mL tetanus toxoid IM repeated twice at monthly intervals.

Wounds: Any cut merits an extra dose of 0.5mL toxoid IM, unless already fully immune (a full course of toxoid or a booster in last 10yrs). The non-immune will need 2 further injections (0.5mL IM) at monthly intervals. If partially immune (ie has had a toxoid booster or a full course >10yrs previously), a single booster is all the toxoid that is needed.

Human tetanus immunoglobulin: This is required for the partially or non-immune patient (defined above) with dirty, old (>6h), infected, devitalized, or soil-contaminated wounds. Give 250–500 units IM, using a separate syringe and site to the toxoid injection.

▶If immune status is unknown, assume that the patient is nonimmune. Routine infant immunization started in 1961, so many adults are at risk.

▶Hygiene education and wound debridement are of vital importance.

Enteric fever[ND]

Typhoid and paratyphoid are caused by *Salmonella typhi* and *S. paratyphi* (types A, B, and C), respectively. (Other *Salmonella* cause D&V: p556 & p218.) *Incubation:* 3–21d. *Spread:* Faecal–oral. 1% become chronic carriers. *Presentation:* Usually malaise, headache, high fever with relative bradycardia, cough, and constipation (or diarrhoea). CNS signs (coma, delirium, meningism) are serious. Diarrhoea is more common after the 1st week. Rose spots occur on the trunk of 40%, but may be very difficult to see. Epistaxis, bruising, abdominal pain, and splenomegaly may occur. *Tests:* First 10d: blood culture; later: urine/stool cultures. Bone marrow culture has highest yield (infiltration may cause ↓platelets & WCC). LFT↑. Widal test unreliable. DNA probes and PCR tests have been developed, but are not widely available. *Treatment:* Fluid replacement and good nutrition. There is good evidence that fluoroquinolones (eg ciprofloxacin 500mg/12h PO for 6d) are the best antimicrobial treatment for typhoid. Chloramphenicol is still used in many areas: 1g/8h PO until pyrexia diminishes, then 500mg/8h for a week and 250mg/6h to make up 14d (can be shorter). Other alternatives: cefotaxime, azithromycin, or amoxycillin (if fully susceptible). In severe disease, give IV ciprofloxacin or IV cefotaxime for 10–14d. In encephalopathy ± shock, give dexamethasone 3mg/kg IV stat, then 1mg/kg/6h for 48h. Drug resistance is a problem, even with ciprofloxacin, eg due to mutations in the DNA gyrase enzyme of *S. typhi*.[94]
Complications: Osteomyelitis (eg in sickle-cell disease); DVT; GI bleed or perforation; cholecystitis; myocarditis; pyelonephritis; meningitis; abscess. Infection is said to have cleared when 6 consecutive cultures of urine and faeces are –ve. Chronic carriage is a problem; treat if at risk of spreading disease (eg food handlers). Amoxicillin 4–6g/d + probenecid 2g/d for 6wks may work (alternative: ciprofloxacin 500mg/12h PO for 6wks) but cholecystectomy may be needed. *Prognosis:* If untreated, 10% die; if treated, 0.1% die. *Vaccine:* p558.

Bacillary dysentery[ND]

Shigella causes abdominal pain and bloody diarrhoea ± sudden fever, headache, and occasionally neck stiffness. CSF is sterile. UK school epidemics are usually mild (often *S. sonnei*), but imported dysentery may be severe (often *S. flexneri* or *S. dysenteriae*). *Incubation:* 1–7d. *Spread:* Faecal–oral. *Diagnosis:* Stool culture. *Treatment:* Fluids PO. Avoid anti-diarrhoeal drugs. Drugs: ciprofloxacin 500mg/12h PO for 3–5d. Imported shigellosis is often resistant to several antimicrobials: sensitivity testing is important. There may be associated spondyloarthritis (p419).

Cholera[ND]

Caused by *Vibrio cholerae* (Gram negative comma-shaped rod). Pandemics or epidemics may occur, eg 1990s epidemic in S America and Bangladesh (Bengal *Vibrio cholerae* 0139). *Incubation:* From a few hours to 5d. *Spread:* Faecal–oral. *Presentation:* Profuse (eg 1L/h) watery ('rice water') stools, fever, vomiting, and rapid dehydration (the cause of death). *Diagnosis:* Stool microscopy and culture. *Treatment:* Strict barrier nursing. Replace fluid and salt losses meticulously (0.9% saline IVI if shocked), add 20mmol/L K[+] until U&E known (avoid plain Ringer's lactate: it may cause fatal K[+]↓). Oral rehydration with WHO formula (20g glucose/L) is not so effective as cooked rice powder solution (50–80g/L) in reducing stool volume.[95] Its high osmolarity (310mmol/L vs 200mmol/L) is also unfavourable to water absorption. A dose of ciprofloxacin 1g PO may reduce fluid loss.[96] *Prevention:* Only drink boiled or treated water. Cook all food well; eat it hot. Avoid shellfish. Peel all vegetables. Heat-killed vaccine (serovar O1) gives limited protection, and is no longer needed for international travel; newer vaccines are non-standard.[97]

Historical note on the enteric fevers

Typhoid means *like typhus*, τνφοζ (*tuphos* = *smoke*) denoting *stupor, or darkening of the intellect as if wrapped in smoke* (seen in severe typhoid). The provision of clean drinking water and other hygienic measures have lessened the impact of the enteric fevers. But over the centuries, and, even now, in many parts of India and S America, typhoid and typhoid-like illnesses cause significant mortality. Perhaps the most significant such death occurred at noon on 23 April 1851 in Malvern; that of a little-known girl whose death is securely, but circuitously, woven into our consciousness. Her name was Annie Darwin, her father's, Charles. Annie was Charles's favourite fun-loving daughter, and with her lingering enteric death Darwin gave up all belief in a just and moral universe. Thus, unimpeded, his mind was able to frame and compellingly justify the most devastating answer to the oldest question: that we are here by accident, thanks to natural selection, the survival of the fittest, and the 'wasteful, blundering, low & horridly cruel works of nature'.[1]

The next significant death occurred 3 summers later at 40 Broad Street, in the Parish of St James, South London, where a child became ill with diarrhoea at the end of August, 1854—dying on September 2. The mother washed the soiled nappies, disposing of the washings via the house drains. These led to within a few feet of the supply to the Broad Street pump. Both the drain and the pump's well had faulty brickwork allowing the waters to mix. From this confluence sprung the discipline of Public Health, for many of the 500 or so ensuing late summer deaths from cholera clustered around this Broad Street pump, as diagrammed by the local doctor, Dr John Snow. He used his now historic diagrams locating each death to motivate the Board of Guardians of St James's parish during its meeting of Sept 7 '… in consequence of what I said, the handle of the pump was removed the following day'[2]—thereby inaugurating the control of cholera.

These events illustrate two counter-intuitive truths: knowledge of the microscopic cause of a disease is not required for public health measures to be successful (*Vibrio cholerae* was as yet undiscovered)—and, more surprisingly, even the most parochial of Church Councils are capable of prompt and decisive action affecting the lives of millions, when informed by an intelligent doctor in command of his or her facts.

1 A remark of Darwin's in 1856, before starting his *Origin of Species*, and quoted in *Darwin* by Adrian Desmond and James Moore, 1989, Penguin
2 J Snow 1854 *Med Times Gaz* **9** 321, quoted by H Brody 2000 *Lancet* **356** 64

Leprosy[ND]

▶The diagnosis of leprosy (Hansen's disease) must be considered in all who have visited endemic areas who present with painless disorders of skin and nerves. It is not just a tropical disease, and may occur in the USA, eg in Texas, Louisiana, and California, as well as Hawaii and Puerto Rico.

Mycobacterium leprae affects millions of people in the Tropics and subtropics. Since the widespread use of dapsone, and WHO elimination campaigns, prevalence has fallen (from 0.5% to 0.4/10,000 in Uganda; from 11% to 4/10,000 in parts of India). Incidence remains stable, however, at about 800,000 new cases/yr worldwide, many of whom are children.

The Patient The incubation period is months to years, and the subsequent course depends on the patient's immune response. If the immune response is ineffective, '*lepromatous*' or '*multibacillary*' disease develops, dominated by foamy histiocytes full of bacilli, but few lymphocytes. If there is a vigorous immune response, the disease is called '*tuberculoid*' or '*paucibacillary*', with granulomata containing epithelioid cells and lymphocytes, but few or no demonstrable bacilli. Between these poles lie those with 'borderline' disease.

Skin lesions: Hypopigmented anaesthetic macules, papules, or annular lesions (with raised erythematous rims). Erythema nodosum (PLATE 18) occurs in 'lepromatous' disease, especially during the 1st year of treatment.

Nerve lesions: Major peripheral nerves may be involved, leading to much disability. Sometimes a thickened sensory nerve may be felt running into the skin lesion (eg ulnar nerve above the elbow, median nerve at the wrist, or the great auricular nerve running up behind the ear).

Eye lesions: ▶*Refer promptly to an ophthalmologist.* The lower temperature of the anterior chamber favours corneal invasion (so secondary infection and cataract). Inflammatory signs: chronic iritis, scleritis, episcleritis. There may be reduced corneal sensation (V nerve palsy), and reduced blinking (VII nerve palsy) and lagophthalmos (difficulty in closing the eyes; *lagos* is Greek for hare), ± ingrowing eyelashes (trichiasis).

Diagnosis Biopsy a thickened nerve; *in vitro* culture is not possible. As an incidental curio, armadillo (or mouse) foot-pad culture works, but do not taunt your lab by requesting this test! Split skin smears for AFB are +ve in borderline or lepromatous disease. Classification matters as it reflects the biomass of bacilli, influencing treatment: the more organisms, the greater the chance that some will be drug resistant.

Other tests: neutrophilia, ESR↑, IgG↑, false +ve rheumatoid test.

Treatment Ask a local expert about: ● Resistance patterns, eg to dapsone, when ethionamide may (rarely) be needed ● Using prednisolone for severe complications ● Is surgery ± physiotherapy needed as well as drug therapy? In the UK, seek advice from the panel of Leprosy Opinion. In other areas, the administration of some drugs should be supervised (S) whereas others need no supervision (NS). For multibacillary and borderline disease, WHO advises rifampicin 600mg PO monthly (S), dapsone 100mg/24h PO (NS), and clo-fazimine 300mg monthly (S) + 50mg/24h (NS) for 2yrs. In paucibacillary leprosy, rifampicin 600mg monthly (S) and dapsone 100mg/24h (NS) for 6 months. In single skin lesion paucibacillary disease, single-dose therapy (rifampicin 600mg, ofloxacin 400mg, minocycline 100mg, all PO) is advised.

▶Beware sudden permanent *paralysis* from nerve inflammation caused by dying bacilli (± *orchitis*, *prostration*, or *death*); this 'lepra reaction' may be mollified by thalidomide (*NOT* if pregnant). Liaise urgently with a leprologist. Supervised therapy may be problematic as many patients find it hard to attend (nomads, jungle-dwellers). WHO has proposed 'accompanied' multi-drug therapy, where someone close to the patient takes responsibility for ensuring treatment compliance. This strategy is controversial.

Spirochaetes

Lyme disease[101] is a tick-borne infection caused by *Borrelia burgdorferi*. Although originally described in Lyme (Connecticut) it is now widespread, eg New Forest ►Ask: *'Do you remember being bitten by an insect?'* Not all will remember. *Presentation: Erythema chronicum migrans (p428), ± malaise; cognitive impairment; lymphadenopathy; arthralgia (later erosive arthropathy); myocarditis; heart block; meningitis; ataxia; amnesia; cranial nerve palsies; neuropathy; lymphocytic meningoradiculitis (Bannwarth's syndrome). Diagnosis:* Clinical ± serology (if –ve, PCR may help.) *Treatment:* Skin rash: doxycycline 100mg/12h PO (amoxicillin or penicillin V if <8yrs or pregnant) for 14–21d. Later complications: high-dose IV benzylpenicillin, cefotaxime, or ceftriaxone. *Prevention:* Keep limbs covered; use insect repellent; tick collars for pets; check skin often when in risky areas. Vaccination is available eg for those living in high-risk areas. Advice differs on prophylaxis after a tick bites. A single dose of doxycycline 200mg PO given within 72h of a bite is effective prophylaxis; in highly endemic areas, this may be worthwhile (eg if risk is >1%). *Removing ticks:* Suffocate tick with, eg petroleum jelly, then gently remove by grasping close to mouth parts and twisting off; then clean skin.

Endemic treponematoses *Yaws* is caused by *T. pertenue*, which is serologically indistinguishable from *T. pallidum*. It is a chronic granulomatous disease prevalent in children in the rural Tropics. Spread is by direct contact, via skin abrasions, and is promoted by poor hygiene. The primary lesion (an ulcerating papule) appears ~4wks after exposure. Scattered secondary lesions then appear, eg in moist skin, but can be anywhere. These may become exuberant. Tertiary lesions are subcutaneous gummatous ulcerating granulomata, affecting skin and bone. Cardiovascular and CNS complications do not occur. *Pinta* (*T. carateum*) affects only skin; seen in Central and S America. *Endemic non-venereal syphilis (bejel; T. pallidum)* is seen in Third World children, when it resembles yaws. In the developed world, *T. pallidum* causes *syphilis (p601). Diagnosis:* clinical. *Treatment:* procaine penicillin (p543).

Weil's disease[ND] is caused by *Leptospira interrogans* (eg serogroup *L. icterohaemorrhagiae*). Spread is by contact with infected rat urine, eg while swimming. *Presentation:* Fever, jaundice, headache, red conjunctivae, tender legs (myositis), purpura, haemoptysis, haematemesis, or any bleeding. Meningitis, myocarditis, and particularly renal failure may develop. AST rise may be small. *Diagnosis:* Rapid serological assays are replacing the old microscopic agglutination test. Also take blood, urine, and CSF culture (take 4–6wks). *Treat* symptomatically; give doxycycline 100mg/12h PO or, in serious disease, IV benzylpenicillin 600mg/6h for 7d. Prophylaxis (eg doxycycline 200mg/wk PO) may be useful for those at high risk for short periods.

Canicola fever is an aseptic meningitis caused by *Leptospira canicola*.

Relapsing fever[ND] This is caused by *Borrelia recurrentis* (louse-borne) or *B. duttoni* (tick-borne). It typically occurs in pandemics following war or disaster, and may kill millions. *Incubation:* 4–18d. *Presentation:* abrupt onset fever, rigors, and headache. A petechial rash (which may be faint or absent), jaundice, and tender hepatosplenomegaly may develop. Serious complications include myocarditis, hepatic failure, and DIC. Crises of very high fever and tachycardia occur. When the fever abates, hypotension due to vasodilatation may occur and be fatal. Relapses occur, but are milder. *Tests:* Organisms are seen on Leishman-stained thin or thick films. *Treatment:* Tetracycline 500mg PO or 250mg IV as a single dose (but for 10d for *B. duttoni*). Alternative: doxycycline 100mg/12h PO. The Jarisch–Herxheimer reaction (p601) is fatal in 5%: meptazinol 100mg IV slowly is given as prophylaxis with the tetracycline, repeated 30min later (with the chill phase) and during the flush phase (if systolic BP <75mmHg). Delouse the patient and their clothes.[102] Doxycycline (p546) is useful prophylaxis in high-risk groups.

Syphilis—the archetypal spirochaetal (treponemal) disease

▶Any anogenital ulcer is syphilis until proven otherwise. *UK incidence is rising fast, eg >1000 new infections per year.*

Treponema pallidum enters via an abrasion, during sex. All features are due to an endarteritis obliterans. Previously common in merchant seamen and the armed forces, it is now commonest in homosexuals. Incidence has been rising in the UK since the late 1990s, as 'safer-sex' messages are being forgotten or ignored. *Incubation:* 9–90d. Four stages:
- *Primary:* A macule at site of sexual contact becomes a very infectious, painless hard ulcer (*primary chancre*).
- *Secondary:* Occurs 4–8wks after the chancre. Fever, malaise, lymphadenopathy, rash (trunk, face, palms, soles), alopecia, condylomata lata, buccal snail-track ulcers; rarely hepatitis, meningism, nephrosis, uveitis.
- *Tertiary syphilis* follows 2–20yrs latency (when patients are non-infectious): there are *gummas* (granulomas occurring in skin, mucosa, bone, joints, rarely viscera, eg lung, testis).
- *Quaternary syphilis Cardiovascular:* Ascending aortic aneurysm ± aortic regurgitation. *Neurosyphilis: (a) Meningovascular:* Cranial nerve palsies, stroke; *(b) General paresis of insane (GPI):* Dementia, psychoses (fatal untreated; treatment *may* reverse it); *(c) Tabes dorsalis:* Sensory ataxia, numb legs, chest, and bridge of nose, lightning pains ('like a bolt from the blue'), gastric crises, reflex loss, extensor plantars, Charcot's joints (p404). *Argyll Robertson pupil (p82).*

Serology (Two types):
1 *Cardiolipin antibody:* not treponeme-specific. Detectable in primary disease but wanes in late syphilis. Indicates active disease and becomes negative after treatment. *False +ves* (with negative treponemal antibody): pregnancy, immunization, pneumonia, malaria, SLE, TB, leprosy. *Examples:* venereal disease research laboratory (VDRL) slide test, rapid plasma reagin (RPR), Wassermann reaction (WR).
2 *Treponeme-specific antibody:* positive in 1° disease, remains so despite treatment. *Examples:* T. pallidum haemagglutination assay (TPHA), fluorescent treponemal antibody (FTA), T. pallidum immobilization (TPI) test. Non-specific, also +ve in non-venereal yaws, bejel, or pinta.

Other tests In 1° syphilis, treponemes may be seen by *dark ground microscopy* of chancre fluid; serology at this stage is often –ve. In 2° syphilis, treponemes are seen in the lesions and both types of antibody tests are positive. In late syphilis, organisms may no longer be seen, but both types of antibody test usually remain +ve (cardiolipin antibody tests may wane). In neurosyphilis, CSF antibody tests (particularly FTA and TPHA) are +ve. If HIV+ve, serology may be –ve during syphilis reactivation. PCR may help.

Treatment: Procaine penicillin (=procaine benzylpenicillin) 600mg/24h IM for ~28d (14d in early syphilis). Alternative: doxycycline 200mg/12h PO for 28d (100mg/12h PO for 14d in early syphilis). Beware *Jarisch-Herxheimer reaction:* Fever, pulse↑, and vasodilatation hours after the 1st dose of antibiotic. It is thought to be from sudden release of endotoxin. Commonest in 2° disease; most dangerous in 3°. Consider steroids. If HIV+ve, penicillin may not stop neurosyphilis; consult microbiologist. ▶Trace contacts. *Congenital syphilis:* OHCS p98.

PoliomyelitisND

Polio is a highly contagious picornavirus, though only a small proportion of patients develop any illness from the infection. *Spread:* Droplet or faeco–oral.

The Patient: 7 days' incubation, then 2 days' 'flu-like prodrome, leading to a 'pre-paralytic' stage: fever, tachycardia, headache, vomiting, neck stiffness, and unilateral tremor. In <50% of patients this progresses to the paralytic stage: myalgia, lower motor neurone signs, and respiratory failure. *Tests:* CSF: WCC↑, polymorphs then lymphocytes, otherwise normal; paired sera (14 days apart); throat swab & stool culture identify virus. *Natural history:* <10% of those with paralysis die. There may be *delayed progression* of paralysis. *Risk factors for severe paralysis:* Adulthood; pregnancy; post-tonsillectomy; muscle fatigue/trauma during incubation period. *Prophylaxis:* Live vaccine PO (p558). In the tropics, the killed parenteral vaccine may be needed to induce adequate immunity. Adults should be revaccinated when their children are vaccinated.

RabiesND

Rabies is a rhabdovirus spread by bites from any infected mammal, eg bats, dogs, cats, foxes, or raccoons (bites may go unnoticed).

The Patient: Usually 9–90 days' incubation, so give prophylaxis even several months after exposure. Prodromal symptoms include headache, malaise, abnormal behaviour, agitation, fever, and itching at the site of the bite. Progresses to 'furious rabies', eg with water-provoking muscle spasms often accompanied by profound terror (hydrophobia). In 20%, 'dumb rabies' starts with flaccid paralysis in the bitten limb and spreads.

Pre-exposure prophylaxis (eg vets, zoo-keepers, customs officials, bat handlers, travellers): Give human diploid cell strain vaccine (1mL IM, deltoid) on days 0, 7, & 28, and again at 2–3yrs if still at risk.

Treatment if bitten where rabies is endemic (if unvaccinated): ►Seek expert help (UK *virus reference lab,* tel.: 020 8200 4400). Observe the biting animal if possible, to see if it dies (but it is possible that it may not die of rabies before the patient does); asymptomatic carriage occurs but has not (yet) produced rabies in man. Clean the wound. *If previously immunized:* give vaccine (1mL IM) on days 0 and 3. *If previously unimmunized:* give vaccine on days 0, 3, 7, 14, and 28 and human rabies immunoglobulin (20U/kg on day 0; half given IM and half locally infiltrated around wound). Rabies is usually fatal once symptoms begin, but survival has occurred, if there is optimal CNS and cardiorespiratory support. Offer to vaccinate attending staff.

Viral haemorrhagic feversND

Yellow fever: An epidemic arbovirus disease spread by *Aedes* mosquitoes (Brazil, Bolivia, Peru, and Central and West Africa). *Immunization:* p558. *Incubation:* 2–14d. *The Patient:* In mild forms, fever, headache, nausea, albuminuria, myalgia, and relative bradycardia. If severe: 3 days of headache, myalgia, anorexia ± nausea, followed by abrupt fever, a brief remission, then prostration, jaundice (± fatty liver), haematemesis and other bleeding, oliguria. *Mortality:* <10% (day 5–10). *Diagnosis:* ELISA. *Treatment:* Symptomatic.

*Lassa fever*ND, *Ebola virus*ND, *Marburg virus*ND, and *dengue haemorrhagic fever* (DHF) (dengue is the most prevalent arbovirus disease). These diseases may start with sudden-onset headache, pleuritic pain, backache, myalgia, conjunctivitis, prostration, dehydration, facial flushing (dengue), and fever. Bleeding soon supervenes. There may be spontaneous resolution, or renal failure, encephalitis, coma, and death. *Treatment:* Primarily symptomatic; ribavirin is useful in Lassa fever if given early in disease. ►Use special infection control measures (Lassa, Ebola, Marburg); get expert help at once.

Polio: an exercise in prevention

- Pre-1950 distribution was worldwide.
- 12 April 1955: vaccination starts with Salk's inactivated vaccine.
- 1958: Sabin donated his 3 attenuated strains to Chumakov in Moscow, who produced the 3 vaccines, giving them to 15 million people in 1yr.
- 1960s: the 3 vaccines were mixed, to produce a single oral polio vaccine.
- 1988: Estimated 350,000 cases worldwide, occuring in 125 countries. The Global Polio Eradication Initiative, aiming to protect children worldwide through vaccination, is launched. The aim is eradication by year 2000.
- 1991: Transmission interrupted in the Western hemisphere.
- 1993: China starts national immunization days (>80,000,000 children vaccinated in 2 days; in 1994 only 5 cases of virus-confirmed wild polio).
- 1994: WHO declares the Americas polio-free.
- 1997: 1 case of wild polio confirmed in all of the European Region.
- 1999: Only 7090 cases, worldwide.
- 2000: WHO declares the Western Pacific polio-free.
- 2001: Only 483 cases of polio, confined to 10 endemic countries.
- 2002: WHO declares Europe polio-free.
- 2004: Only 6 polio-endemic countries: Afghanistan, India, Niger, Nigeria, and Pakistan.

Any polio seen in the West will now be the very rare kind that may follow vaccination. Half these people will be adult contacts of child vaccinees. In endemic countries, however, the last few cases of polio are proving the most difficult to eradicate. A polio epidemic in India in 2002 led to a rise in new cases to ~1900 worldwide. The original target for the global elimination of polio was ammended to 2005; even this now looks optimistic.

NB: Sabin viruses and their genetic revertants can cause chronic infection in immunodeficient people, who may shed neurovirulent virus in faeces for years. So programmes of oral vaccination should not continue one day longer than necessary to eliminate disease caused by wild virus.

Dengue fever (DF) and dengue haemorrhagic fever (DHF)

There is a global pandemic of this RNA flavivirus, related to poor vector control (*Aedes* mosquitoes), urbanization, and rapid migrations bringing new strains (DEN-2) which become more virulent in those who have had mild dengue. Incidence: $50–100×10^6$/yr; 250,000–500,000/yr get DHF.[1]

Infants typically have a simple febrile illness with a maculopapular rash. Older children/adults have flushing of face, neck, and chest or a centrifugal maculopapular rash from day 3—or a late confluent petechiae with round pale areas of normal skin—also headache, arthralgia, jaundice; hepatosplenomegaly; anuria. *Haemorrhagic signs:* (Unlikely if AST normal). Petechiae, GI, gum or nose bleeds, haematuria; hypermenorrhoea.

Monitor: BP; urine flow; WCC↓; platelets↓; PCV; +ve tourniquet test (>20 petechiae inch^2) + PCV↑ by 20% are telling signs (rapid endothelial plasma leak is the key pathophysiology of DHF). ΔΔ: Chikungunya,[2] measles, leptospirosis, typhoid, malaria. *Exclusion:* If symptoms start >2wks after leaving a dengue-endemic area, or if fever lasts >2wks, dengue can be 'ruled out'. R: Prompt IV resusc., eg Ringer's lactate. ▸▸If shocked (mortality 40%), give a bolus of 15mL/kg; repeat every ½h until BP rises & urine flow >30mL/h.

---

1 M Guzman 2003 *J Clin Virol* 27
2 Haemorrhagic features in Chikungunya virus infections are rare.

Rickettsia and arthropod-borne bacteria

Rickettsia are intracellular bacteria that are carried by host arthropods and invade human mononuclear cells, neutrophils, or blood vessel endothelium (vasculotropic). All the cataclysmic events of the last century (war, revolution, flood, famine, genocide, and overcrowding) have favoured lice infestation. As a result, Rickettsia (in particular typhus) have killed untold millions.

Q fever is caused by *Coxiella burnetii* (100 cases per year in the UK). It is so named because it was first labelled 'query' fever in workers in an Australian abattoir. *Epidemiology:* Occurs worldwide, and is usually rural, with its reservoir in cattle and sheep. The organism is very resistant to drying and is usually inhaled from infected dust. It can be contracted from unpasteurized milk, directly from carcasses in abattoirs, sometimes by droplet spread, and occasionally from tick bites. *Clinical features* Q fever should be suspected in anyone with a PUO or atypical pneumonia. It may present with fever, myalgia, sweats, headache, cough, and hepatitis. If the disease becomes chronic, suspect endocarditis (typically 'culture-negative'). This usually affects the aortic valve, but clinical signs may be absent. It also causes miscarriages and CNS infection. *Investigations:* CXR may show consolidation, eg multilobar or slowly resolving. Liver function tests may be hepatitic and biopsy may show granulomata. Diagnosis is serologically: phase I antigens indicate chronic infection; phase II antigens indicate acute infection. PCR may be used on tissue samples. CSF tests may be needed. *Treatment:* Get expert microbiological help. *Acute:* Tetracycline or doxycycline for 2wks. Minocycline, clarithromycin, ciprofloxacin (in pregnancy) and co-trimoxazole have been used. *Chronic:* Ciprofloxacin + rifampicin for 2yrs ± valve replacement. *Prevention:* Vaccination for those whose occupation places them at high risk.

Bartonellosis is caused by *Bartonella bacilliformis*, a Gram negative, motile, bacillus-like organism which parasitizes RBCs. Spread is by sandflies in the Andes, Peru, Equador, Colombia, Thailand, and Niger. Transient immunosuppression leads to associated infections (eg *Salmonella*). *Incubation:* 10–210 days (average = 60). *Clinical features:* Fever, rashes, lymphadenopathy, hepatosplenomegaly, jaundice, cerebellar syndromes, dermal nodules (verrugas), retinal haemorrhages, myocarditis, pericardial effusion, oedema, and rarely, meningo-encephalomyelitis. *Investigations:* Giemsa-stained blood films. Prolonged incubation of blood cultures. Coomb's negative haemolytic anaemia, and hypochromic, macrocytic red cells with a megaloblastic marrow. CSF pleocytosis. Serological tests exist, but are not widely available. *Treatment:* Responds to penicillin, but chloramphenicol (p596) or ciprofloxacin (500mg/12h PO for 10d) are often used because of its frequent association with salmonelloses. Steroids may be indicated if there is severe fneurological involvement.

Cat scratch disease (p593) is caused by *Bartonella henselae*.

Trench fever is caused by *Bartonella quintana* inoculated from infected louse faeces, not only in soldiers, but also in the homeless, and in alcoholics. *Clinical features:* Fever, headache, myalgia, dizziness, back pain, macular rash, eye pain, leg pain, splenomegaly, and rarely, endocarditis. In HIV-infected patients, the skin lesions may resemble Kaposi's sarcoma. *Investigations:* Blood culture, serology, PCR. *Treatment:* Doxycycline 100mg/12h PO for 15d. *Prognosis:* It is not fatal; it may relapse.

Ehrlichiosis is caused by *Ehrlichia chaffeensis*, an obligate intracytoplasmic Gram –ve organism, related to Rickettsia. It is spread by ticks. *Symptoms:* Fever, headache, anorexia, malaise, abdominal pain, epigastric pain, conjunctivitis, lymphadenopathy, jaundice, rash, confusion, and cervical lymphadenopathy. *Investigations:* Leucopenia, thrombocytopenia, AST↑. Serology and PCR are used for diagnosis. *Treatment:* May respond to doxycycline 100mg/12h PO for 7–14d.

Typhus: the archetypal rickettsial disease

Typhus rickettsia are transmitted between hosts by arthropods. The incubation period is 2–23d.

Pathology Widespread vasculitis and endothelial proliferation may affect any organ and thrombotic occlusion may lead to gangrene.

Clinical features Infection may be mild and asymptomatic or severe and systemic. There may be sudden onset of fever, frontal headache, confusion, and jaundice. With some species, an *eschar* (black scar at the site of the initial inoculation) may be present. A rickettsial rash may be macular, papular, petechial, or haemorrhagic. Investigations may show haemolysis, neutrophilia, thrombocytopenia, clotting abnormalities, hepatitis, renal impairment. Patients die of shock, renal failure, DIC (p650), or stroke.

- *Rocky Mountain spotted fever (R. rickettsii)* is tick-borne and endemic in the Rocky Mountains and the south-eastern states of the USA. The rash begins as macules on the hands and feet and then spreads becoming petechial or haemorrhagic.
- *Tick typhus (R. conorii)* the commonest imported rickettsial disease in the UK (endemic in Africa, the Arabian Gulf, and the Mediterranean). A black eschar may be visible at the site of the infecting bite. The rash starts in the axillae, becoming purpuric as it spreads. *Other features:* conjunctival suffusion; jaundice, deranged clotting, renal impairment.
- *Epidemic typhus (R. prowazeki)* carried by human lice *(Pediculus humanus)* whose faeces are inhaled or pass through skin. It may become latent, and recrudesce later (Brill–Zinsser disease).
- *Murine (endemic) typhus (R. typhi)* is transmitted by fleas from rats to humans. It is more prevalent in warm, coastal ports.
- *Rickettsialpox (R. akari)* Variegate rash: macular, papular, or vesicular.
- *Scrub typhus (Orienta tsutsugamushi)* Most common in SE Asia.

Diagnosis This is difficult as often the picture is non-specific, the organisms are difficult to grow, and the traditional heterophil antibody Weil–Felix test has low sensitivity and specificity. A rise in antibody titre in paired sera is diagnostic. Latex agglutination, indirect immunofluorescence, and ELISAs are available. An accurate, rapid dotblot immunoassay is available for scrub typhus. Skin biopsy may be diagnostic in Rocky Mountain spotted fever.

Treatment Doxycycline 200mg/d PO or tetracycline 500mg/6h PO for 10–14d. Alternative: chloramphenicol 500mg/6h PO or IV for 10–14d. Resistance has been reported in northern Thailand.

Poor prognostic factors Older age, male, Black, G6PD deficiency.

Giardiasis

Giardia lamblia is a flagellate protozoon, which lives in the duodenum and jejunum. It is spread by the faecal–oral route. Risk factors for transmission: travel, immunosuppression, homosexuality, achlorhydria, playgroups, and swimming. Drinking water may become contaminated.

Presentation: Often asymptomatic. Lassitude, bloating, flatulence, abdominal discomfort, loose stools ± explosive diarrhoea are typical. Malabsorption, weight loss, and lactose intolerance may occur.

Diagnosis: Repeated stool microscopy for cysts or trophozoites may be –ve. Duodenal fluid analysis by aspiration or absorption on to a piece of swallowed string (Enterotest®) may be tried. An ELISA test is available. Finally, a trial of therapy may be needed.

Differential diagnosis: Any cause of diarrhoea (p554, p556, p580), tropical sprue (p252), coeliac disease (p252).

Treatment: Scrupulous hygiene. Give metronidazole 500mg/12h PO for ~7d, or 2g/24h for 3d. Alternatives: tinidazole 2g PO once (advise to avoid driving and alcohol) or mepacrine hydrochloride 100mg/8h PO for 5–7d (cheap, but side-effects are common). If treatment fails, check for compliance and consider treating the whole family. If diarrhoea persists, avoid milk as lactose intolerance may persist for 6wks.

Other GI protozoa *Cryptosporidium* (p556), *Microsporidium* and *Isospora* (occur in AIDS, p580), *Balantidium coli*, and *Sarcocystis*.

Amoebiasis

Entamoeba histolytica occurs worldwide. Spread: faecal–oral. Boil water and infected food to destroy cysts. Trophozoites may remain in the bowel or invade extra-intestinal tissues, leaving 'flask-shaped' GI ulcers. Presentation may be asymptomatic, with mild diarrhoea or with severe amoebic dysentery.

Amoebic dysentery[ND] may occur years after the initial infection. Diarrhoea begins slowly, but becomes profuse and bloody. An acute febrile prostrating illness does occur but high fever, colic, and tenesmus are rare. May remit and relapse. *Diagnosis:* stool microscopy shows trophozoites, blood, and pus cells. Faecal antigen detection may also be useful. Serology indicates previous or current infection and may be unhelpful in acute infection. *Differential diagnosis:* Non-pathogenic amoebae (eg *Entamoeba dispar*) are common in the tropics and the cysts are indistinguishable. *Bacillary dysentery* often has a sudden onset and may cause dehydration. Stools are more watery. *Acute ulcerative colitis* has a more gradual onset and the stools are very bloody. Other causes of bloody diarrhoea: p596 & p218.

Amoebic colonic abscess may perforate causing peritonitis.

Amoeboma is an inflammatory mass most often found at the caecum, where it must be distinguished from other RIF masses.

Amoebic liver abscess is usually a single mass in the right lobe, and contains 'anchovy-sauce' pus. There is usually a high swinging fever, sweats, RUQ pain, and tenderness. WCC↑. LFT may be normal or ↑ (cholestatic). 50% have no history of amoebic dysentery. *Diagnosis:* ultrasound/CT ± aspiration; positive serology.

Treatment Metronidazole 800mg/8h PO for 5d for acute amoebic dysentery (active against vegetative amoebae), then diloxanide furoate 500mg/8h PO for 10d to destroy gut cysts (SEs rare). Diloxanide is also best for chronic disease when *Entamoeba* cysts, not vegetative forms, are in stools. Amoebic liver abscess: metronidazole 400mg/8h IV for 10d; repeat at 2wks as needed; aspirate if no improvement within 72h of starting metronidazole; give diloxanide post-metronidazole.

Trypanosomiasis

African trypanosomiasis (sleeping sickness) In West and Central Africa, *Trypanosoma gambiense* causes a slow, wasting illness with a long latent period. In East Africa, *T. rhodesiense* causes a more rapidly progressive illness. Spread by tsetse flies, entering skin following an insect bite. It spreads via the blood to the lymph nodes, spleen, heart, and brain.

Prevalence: ~500,000, nearly all *T. gambiense*. Wars, famine, and other disasters are contributing to an upsurge in African trypanosomiasis. In these destabilized circumstances, population surveillance and control of wild animal populations is being abandoned.

Presentation: A tender, subcutaneous nodule (*T. chancre*) develops at the site of infection. Two stages follow: *Stage I (haemolymphatic):* Non-specific symptoms including fever, rash, rigors, headaches, hepatosplenomegaly, lymphadenopathy, and joint pains. Winterbottom's sign (enlargement of posterior cervical nodes) is a reliable sign, particularly in *T. gambiense* infections. In *T. rhodesiense* infections, this stage may be particularly severe, with potentially fatal myocarditis. *Stage II (meningoencephalitic):* Occurs weeks (in *T. rhodesiense*) or months (in *T. gambiense*) after initial infection. Patients exhibit CNS features, eg convulsions, agitation, and confusion, with later apathy, depression, ataxia, dyskinesias, dementia, hypersomnolence, and coma.

Diagnosis: Microscopy shows trypomastigotes in blood film, lymph node aspirate, or CSF. Serology is only reliable in *T. gambiense* infections.

Treatment: ►Seek expert help.
- Treat anaemia and other infections first.
- Early (pre-CNS) phase: pentamidine isethionate 4mg/kg/d IM for 10d. SE: neutropenia, ↓BP, ↓Ca^{2+}, nephrotoxicity, thrombocytopenia. Alternative: suramin (SE: proteinuria, ↑creatinine).
- CNS disease: melarsoprol, eg '3 by 3' regimen IV: 2–3.6mg/kg/d IV for three doses. Repeat at 7d and once more after 10–21d. SE: pruritus, Jarisch–Herxheimer-like reaction (p600), lethal encephalopathy in up to 10% (abnormal behaviour, fits, coma)—partly preventable with prednisolone (1mg/kg/24h, max 40mg/24h), starting the day before the first injection. Arseno-resistant trypanosomiasis was always fatal until the introduction of difluoromethylornithine (DFMO). Dose example: 100mg/kg/6h IV over 1h for 14d, followed by 75mg/kg/6h for 3–4wks. SE: anaemia, diarrhoea, seizures, leucopenia, hair loss.

American trypanosomiasis (Chagas' disease) is caused by *T. cruzi*. It occurs in Latin America and is spread by triatomine bugs.

The Patient: Acute disease predominantly affects children. An erythematous, indurated nodule (*chagoma*) forms at the site of infection which may then scar. *Signs:* fever, myalgia, rash, lymphadenopathy, hepatosplenomegaly. If the eye is infected, unilateral conjunctivitis and periorbital oedema may occur (*Romaña's sign*). Occasionally death is from myocarditis or meningoencephalitis. In up to 30% of cases, progression to chronic disease occurs after a latency of eg 20yrs. Multiorgan invasion may cause megaoesophagus (dysphagia, aspiration), megacolon (abdominal distension, constipation), or dilated cardiomyopathy (chest pain, heart failure, arrhythmias, syncope, thromboembolism). CNS lesions may occur if HIV +ve.

Diagnosis: Acute disease: trypomastigotes may be seen in or grown from blood, CSF, or lymph node aspirate. Chronic disease: serology (Chagas' IgG ELISA).

Treatment: Unsatisfactory. Nifurtimox 2mg/kg/6h PO after food, or alternatively benznidazole (3.7mg/kg/12h PO for 60d) are used in acute disease (toxic, and only eliminate the parasite in 50%). Chronic disease can only be treated symptomatically. A variety of surgical approaches have been tried.

Trypanosomiasis: the dichotomy between science and health

Typanosomes are of immense research interest. Their defence mechanisms have been studied and their genomes sequenced. It is ironic that the interest in trypanosomes from a basic science perspective is mirrored by the disinterest from a diagnostic and therapeutic perspective. The misfortune of the hundreds of thousands of infected people is only compounded by their fact that they are not commercially viable customers. At the end of the 1990s, no pharmaceutical company would manufacture DFMO for arseno-resistant sleeping sickness in Africa. Agreements signed in 2001 between WHO and two major pharmaceutical companies may serve to rectify this for the next few years, but the lesson that scientific interest does not always benefit the suffering patient must not be ignored.

Leishmaniasis

Leishmania protozoa are intracellular organisms that cause granulomata. They are spread by sandflies and occur in Africa, India, Latin America, the Middle East, and the Mediterranean. Clinical effects reflect: (1) The ability of each species to induce or suppress the immune response, to metastasize, and to invade cartilage, and (2) the speed and efficiency of our own immune response. *L. major*, for example, is the most immunogenic and allergenic of cutaneous Old World *Leishmania*, and causes most necrosis. *L. tropica* is less immunogenic and causes less inflamed, slow-healing sores with relapsing lesions having tuberculoid histology.

Cutaneous leishmaniasis (oriental sore) A major disease affecting >300,000 people mainly in Africa, India, and S America caused by *L. mexicana, L. major*, or *L. tropica*. Lesions develop at the site of the bite, beginning as an itchy papule, from which the crust may fall off to leave an ulcer (*Chiclero's ulcer*). Most heal spontaneously, typically within 3–18 months, with scarring (disfiguring if extensive). *L. mexicana* may cause destruction of the pinna (*Chiclero's ear*).

Diagnosis: Microscopy and culture of aspiration from the edge of the ulcer.

Treatment: Get help. Fluconazole 200mg/d PO for 6wks is effective against *L. major.* Alternatives: miltefosine 2.25mg/kg/d PO for 4wks; sodium stibogluconate (Sb^V, pentavalent antimony) 10mg/kg/12h IV (max 850mg/d) for 28d; paromomycin, eg 14mg/kg/d IM for 60d with 10mg Sb^V/kg/d IM.

Mucocutaneous leishmaniasis is caused by *L. brasiliensis* and occurs in S America. Primary skin lesions may spread to the mucosa of the nose, pharynx, palate, larynx, and upper lip and cause severe scarring. Nasopharyngeal lesions are called *espundia*.

Diagnosis: As the parasites may be scanty, a Leishmanin skin test is often necessary to distinguish the condition from leprosy, TB, syphilis, yaws, and carcinoma. Indirect fluorescent antibody tests and PCR tests are available.

Treatment: Sodium stibogluconate (dose as below). Treatment is unsatisfactory once mucosae are involved, so treat all cutaneous lesions early.

Visceral leishmaniasis (kala-azar) Kala-azar means black sickness and is characterized by dry, warty, hyperpigmented skin lesions. It occurs in Asia, Africa, S America, and the Mediterranean. It is caused by *L. donovani, L. chagasi*, or *L. infantum* (or rarely, 'visceralizing' of *L. tropica*). Incubation: months to years. Protozoa spread via lymphatics from minor skin lesions and multiply in macrophages of the reticuloendothelial system (Leishman–Donovan bodies). There are 30 subclinical cases for every clinical case. ♀ : ♂ ratio > 3 : 1. It is HIV-associated. *Presentation:* see BOX.

Diagnosis: Leishman–Donovan bodies in bone marrow (80%), lymph node or splenic aspirates (95%). Hypersplenism (Hb↓, platelets↓, WCC↓), albumin↓, IgG↑; –ve Leishmanin skin test. Solid-state serology has been developed for field use (K39 antigen). Serology may be –ve if HIV+ve.

Treatment: Seek expert help. WHO regimen: sodium stibogluconate (Sb^V) 20mg/kg/24h IV or IM, up to 850mg/d, for 30d. SE: malaise, cough, substernal pain, prolonged Q–T interval, arrhythmias, anaemia, hepatitis. Regimens are changing as 25% fail to respond or relapse—eg 10mg/kg Sb^V/8h for 10d, without the 850mg limit. Alternative: pentamidine, eg 3–4mg/kg (deep IM) on alternate days, up to 10 doses. SEs may be fatal (BP↓, arrhythmias, glucose↓, diabetes in 4%). Other agents: paromomycin (aminosidine), liposomal amphotericin B (AmBisome®). Miltefosine (50mg/12h PO for 21d) is a promising oral alternative.[1]

Post kala-azar dermal leishmaniasis may occur months or years following successful treatment; lesions resemble leprosy.

1 Further reading: CR Davies 2003 *BMJ* **326** 377–82 and TK Jha 2004 *Clin Infect Dis* **38** 217 [@14469453]

Clinical features of visceral leishmaniasis

Signs & symptoms:
- Fevers 100%
- Sweats 90%
- Rigors 83%
- Burning feet 52%
- Arthralgia 36%

- Splenomegaly 96%
- Fatigue 88%
- Cough 69%
- Insomnia 42%
- Epistaxis 19%

- Weight↓ 95%
- Appetite↓ 87%
- Hepatomegaly 63%
- Abdo pain 42%
- Lymphadenopathy

Complications: Over months to years, emaciation and exhaustion occur, with a protuberant abdomen. Intercurrent infections are common, especially pneumococcal otitis, pneumonia and septicaemia, tuberculosis, measles. Untreated mortality: >80%.

OTM 4e 777

Fungi

Fungi may cause disease by acting as airborne allergens, by producing toxins, or by direct infection. Fungal infection may be superficial or deep, and both are much commoner in the immunocompromised.

Superficial mycoses Dermatophyte infection (*Trichophyton*, *Microsporum*, *Dermatophyton*) causes tinea (ringworm). *Diagnosis:* skin scraping microscopy. *Treatment:* topical clotrimazole 1%. Continue for 14d after healing. If intractable, try itraconazole (100–200mg/24h PO for 7d; SE: D&V; CCF), terbinafine (250mg/24h PO for 4wks) or griseofulvin 0.5–1g/24h (SE: agranulocytosis; SLE).

Candida albicans causes oral (p210) and vaginal (p588) thrush.

Malassezia furfur causes pityriasis versicolor: a macular rash which appears brown on pale skin and pale on tanned skin. *Diagnosis:* microscopy of skin scrapings under Wood's light. *Treatment:* Ketoconazole 200mg/24h PO with food for 7d (also available as a cream); alternatively selenium sulfide lotion.

Some superficial mycoses penetrate the epidermis and cause chronic subcutaneous infections such as Madura foot or sporotrichosis. Treatment is complex and may require amputation of the affected limb.

Systemic mycoses *Aspergillus fumigatus* may precipitate asthma, allergic bronchopulmonary aspergillosis (ABPA), or cause aspergilloma: see p180. Pneumonia and invasive aspergillosis occur in the immunosuppressed. There is some evidence that voriconazole may be superior to amphotericin B in the treatment of invasive aspergillosis.[124]

Systemic *candidiasis* also occurs in the immunocompromised: consider this *whenever* they get a PUO, eg *Candida* UTI in DM or as a rare cause of prosthetic valve endocarditis. Take repeated blood cultures. If the infection does not resolve when the predisposing factor (eg IV line) is removed, the treatment is amphotericin B IV (see p180) or, if not neutropenic, fluconazole 400mg stat then 200mg/d PO. Capsofungin is a newer alternative.[125]

Cryptococcus neoformans causes meningitis or pneumonia. It is commonest in the immunocompromised, eg AIDS, sarcoidosis, Hodgkin's, and those on corticosteroids. The history may be long and there may be features suggesting ICP↑, eg confusion, papilloedema, cranial nerve lesions. *Diagnosis:* Indian Ink CSF staining; blood culture. Cryptococcal antigen is detected in CSF and blood by latex tests. *Treatment:* amphotericin B IV over 4h (Fungizone®) 0.5–0.8mg/kg/d + flucytosine 37.5mg/kg/6h PO until afebrile and culture –ve (eg 6wks; 4 months if meningitis). Adjust flucytosine to give a peak level of 70–80mg/L; trough 30–40mg/L. When culture –ve, start fluconazole 200mg daily PO for 10wks. Response may be monitored clinically and serologically. *If HIV +ve:* See p581 for R̃. It may be necessary to lower CSF pressure by ~50% by removing CSF. Secondary prophylaxis with fluconazole 200mg/d PO is needed until CD4 >150 × 10⁹/L and cryptococcal antigen –ve (p580). GAT[Sanford]2003

Other fungi, mostly from the Americas and Africa, causing deep infection: Histoplasma capsulatum, Coccidioides immitis, Paracoccidioides brasiliensis, and Blastomyces dermatitidis may cause asymptomatic infections, acute or chronic lung disease, or disseminated infection. Acute histoplasma pneumonitis is associated with arthralgia, erythema nodosum (PLATE 18), and erythema multiforme (PLATE 17). Chronic disease, which is commoner with the other 3 fungi, may cause upper-zone fibrosis or radiographic 'coin lesions'. Diagnosis: CXR, serology, culture, and biopsy. These diseases are treated with amphotericin B (above), except *Paracoccidioides* (here use itraconazole 50–100mg/d PO).

Preventing fungal infections This is a goal in the immunocompromised, eg fluconazole 50–400mg/24h after cytotoxics or radiotherapy, preferably started before the onset of neutropenia, and continued for 1wk after WCC returns to normal. Also used as secondary prophylaxis after cryptococcal meningitis in HIV patients.

Candida on ITU: colonization → invasion → dissemination

Not everyone with a positive yeast culture needs treatment: *Candida* is a common commensal (eg on skin, pharynx, or vagina) but if many sites (urine, sputum, or surgical drains) are colonized, risk of invasion rises, particularly when on ITU with known risk factors:[126]

- Prolonged ventilation
- Urinary catheters
- Intravascular lines
- Broad-spectrum antibiotics
- Immunosuppression
- IV nutrition

Invasion implies fungus in normally sterile tissues.

Dissemination involves infection of remote organs via the blood (eg endophthalmitis + fungi in lung or kidney). Consider IV amphotericin (see OPPOSITE) or fluconazole (itraconazole if unresponsive) in these un-equivocal circumstances (especially if your patient is deteriorating):[127]

- A single well-taken +ve blood culture—if risk factors present (above).
- Isolation of *Candida* from any sterile site except urine.
- Yeasts on microscopy on a sterile-site specimen, before culture known.
- Positive histology from normally sterile tissues in those at risk (above).
- Removal/change of IV lines is essential in patients with candidaemia.

▶Consult an ID physician/microbiologist before starting systemic antifungals.

Nematodes (roundworms)

Worldwide, ~1,000,000,000 people are hosts to nematodes (give or take a few hundred million). Many live with us quite peacefully. However, ascariasis can cause GI obstruction, hookworms can stunt growth, necatoriasis can cause debilitating anaemia, and trichuriasis causes dysentery and rectal prolapse. Mass population treatment (eg albendazole 400mg/24h PO for 3d) to school children or immigrants from endemic areas *may* be beneficial.

Necator americanus and *Ankylostoma duodenale (hookworms)* Occur in the Indian subcontinent, SE Asia, Central and N Africa, and parts of Europe. Necator is also found in the Americas and sub-Saharan Africa. Numerous small worms attach to upper GI mucosa, causing bleeding and consequent iron-deficiency anaemia. Eggs are excreted in the faeces and hatch in soil. Larvae penetrate feet, so starting new infections. Oral transmission of *Ankylostoma* may occur. *Diagnosis:* Stool microscopy. *Treatment:* Mebendazole 100mg/12h PO for 3d, and iron.

Strongyloides stercoralis is endemic in the (sub)Tropics. Transmitted percutaneously, it causes rapidly migrating urticaria over thighs and trunk (*cutaneous larva migrans*). Pneumonitis, enteritis, and malabsorption may occur. Chronic signs: diarrhoea, abdominal pain, and urticaria. The worms may take bacteria into the bloodstream, causing Gram negative bacterial septicaemia ± meningitis. *Diagnosis:* Stool microscopy and culture, serology, or duodenal aspiration. *Treatment:* Tiabendazole 25mg/kg/12h (max 1.5g) for 3d—or albendazole 5mg/kg/12h for 3d (recommended doses may not be enough, and 800mg/d PO has been advised for some adults). Ivermectin 0.2mg/kg/24h PO for 72h may be the best for chronic infestations. Hyperinfestation is a problem if immunocompromised (eg on steroids, or, more rarely, in AIDS).

Ascaris lumbricoides occurs worldwide. It looks like (and is named after) the garden worm (*Lumbricus*). An unusual characteristic is that it has 3 finely toothed lips. Transmission is faecal–oral. It migrates through liver and lungs, and settles in the small bowel. It is usually asymptomatic, but death may occur from GI obstruction or perforation. If a worm migrates into the biliary tract, cholangitis or pancreatitis can result. A worm may grow very long (eg 25cm). *Diagnosis:* Stool microscopy shows ova (stained orange by bile); Worms on barium x-rays; eosinophilia (may be absent if immunosuppressed). *Treatment:* Mebendazole 100mg/12h PO for 72h.

Trichinella spiralis occurs worldwide and is transmitted by uncooked pork. It migrates to muscle, causing myalgia, myocarditis, periorbital oedema ± fever. *Treatment:* Albendazole 400mg/12h PO for 8–14d, with concomitant prednisolone 40mg/d PO.

GAT[Sanford] 2003

Trichuris trichiura (whipworm) may cause non-specific abdominal symptoms. *Diagnosis:* Stool microscopy. *Treatment:* Mebendazole.

Enterobius vermicularis (threadworm) is common in temperate climes. It causes anal itch as it leaves the bowel to lay eggs on the perineum. Apply sticky tape to the perineum and identify eggs microscopically. *Treatment:* Mebendazole 100mg PO stat. Repeat at 2wks if ≥2yrs. If aged <2yrs, try piperazine 0.3mL/kg/24h for 7d. Treat the whole family. *Hygiene is more important than drugs* as adult worms die after 6wks. Continued symptoms means *reinfection*.

Toxocara canis Commonest cause of *visceral larva migrans*. Presents with eye granulomas (squint, blindness, pigmentary retinopathy) or visceral involvement (fever, myalgia, hepatomegaly, asthma, cough). *Diagnosis:* Ophthalmoscopy, serology, may require histology. *Treatment:* Tiabendazole or diethylcarbamazine is often unsatisfactory. In ocular disease, visible larvae can sometimes be photocoagulated by laser. *Toxocara* is commonly acquired by ingesting soil contaminated by animal faeces so de-worm pets regularly, and exclude them from play areas.

Filarial infection

This is common—prevalence of lymphatic filariasis: 120 million worldwide.

1 **Onchocerciasis** is caused by *Onchocerca volvulus* and is transmitted by the black fly. It causes river blindness in 72% of some communities in Africa and S America, affecting 17 million worldwide. A nodule forms at the site of the bite, shedding microfilariae to distant skin sites which develop altered pigmentation, lichenification, loss of elasticity, and poor healing. Disease manifestations are mainly due to the localized host response to dead/dying microfilariae. Eye manifestations include keratitis, uveitis, cataract, fixed pupil, fundal degeneration, or optic neuritis/atrophy. Lymphadenopathy and elephantiasis also occur. *Diagnosis:* Visualization of microfilaria in eye or skin snips. Remove a fine shaving of clean, unanaesthetized skin with a scalpel. Put on slide with a drop of 0.9% saline and look for swimming larvae after 30min.

2 **Lymphatic filaria** occur in Asia, Africa, and S America and is transmitted by mosquito vectors. Acute infections cause fever and lymphadenitis. *Wuchereria bancrofti* causes lower limb lymphoedema (elephantiasis) and hydrocoeles. *Brugia malaya* causes elephantiasis below the elbow/knee. *Wuchereria* life cycle: a mosquito bites an infected human → ingested microfilariae develop into larvae → Larvae migrate to mosquito's mouth → Biting of another human → Access to bloodstream → Adult filariae lodge in lymphatic system. *Diagnosis:* Blood film, serology. A rapid immuno-chromatographic fingerprick test has been developed for use in the field. *Complications:* Immune hyperreactivity may cause tropical pulmonary eosinophilia (cough, wheeze, lung fibrosis, high eosinophil counts, IgE↑ and IgG↑). It is a major public health problem and is a WHO target for elimination by the year 2020 (starting with Nigeria, Samoa, and Egypt). The current elimination strategy involves mass treatment with a single yearly dose of 2 drugs for 5yrs: albendazole (400mg) plus *either* ivermectin (200µg/kg) *or* diethylcarbamazine (6mg/kg). An alternative strategy, involving giving diethylcarbamazine-fortified salt to families for 12 months, has also been found to be effective.

3 **Loiasis** is caused by *Loa loa*. It occurs in Africa and is transmitted by the *Chrysops* fly. It causes painful 'Calabar' swellings of the limbs, eosinophilia, and may migrate across the conjunctiva.

Treatment: Seek expert help. Ivermectin is the drug of choice, eg 1 dose of 150µg/kg PO repeated, eg every 6 months for *Onchocerca* (see OHCS p512) or 20µg/kg PO as a single dose for *Wuchereia*. It does not kill adult worms, so repeat treatment may be needed every 6–12 months until adult worms die. Mass treatment campaigns may prevent blindness in some communities, but side-effects may pose problems. Lymphoedema responds to compression garments (hard to use) or benzopyrone (coumarin) 400mg/24h PO.

Wolbachia: a new target for treating filarial infection

Wolbachia are bacterial endosymbionts of the major human filarias. They are essential for the fertility of their nematode hosts and are transmitted transovarially to subsequent generations of worms, in a manner similar to mitochondria. Doxycycline 100mg/day for 6wks has been succesfully used to target these worms in onchocerciasis, interrupting embryogenesis. It may be that *Wolbachia* can be similarly targeted in the treatment of other filarial infections.[1]

1 T Lamb 2004 *J Infect Dis* **189** 120 and A Hoerauf 2003 *BMJ* **326** 207

Cestodes (tapeworms)

Taenia solium (pork tapeworm) infection occurs by eating uncooked pork, or from drinking contaminated water.[1] *T. saginata* is contracted from uncooked beef. Both cause vague abdominal symptoms and malabsorption. Contaminated food and water contain cysticerci which adhere to the gut and develop into adult worms. On swallowing the eggs of *T. solium* they may enter the circulation and disseminate throughout the body, becoming cysticerci within the human host (*cysticercosis*). This tapeworm encysts in muscle, skin, heart, eye, and CNS, causing focal signs. *Subcutaneous cysticercosis* causes palpable subcutaneous nodules in the arms, legs, and chest. *Ocular cysticercosis* causes conjunctivitis, uveitis, retinitis, choroidal atrophy, and blindness.

Neurocysticercosis is the commonest cause of seizures in some places, eg Mexico. Other features: focal CNS signs, eg hemiplegia, odd behavioural, dementia—or no symptoms. Cysticerci may cluster like bunches of grapes ('racemose' form) in the ventricles (causing hydrocephalus) and basal cisterns (causing basal meningitis, cranial nerve lesions, and raised ICP). Spinal cysticerci may cause radicular or compressive symptoms (p350).

Diagnosis: • Stool microscopy and examination of perianal swabs. • Serology: indirect haemagglutination test. • CSF: may show eosinophils in neurocysticercosis, and a CSF antigen test is available. • CT or MRI scan may locate cysts. • SXR and x-rays of soft tissues may show calcified cysts.

Treatment: Seek expert help (*tel:* 0151 708 9393[UK]). Niclosamide 2g PO in 2 doses, separated by 1h. Neurocysticercosis: albendazole 7.5mg/kg/12h PO with food, or praziquantel 17mg/kg/8h PO for 30d. An allergic response to the dying larvae should be covered by dexamethasone 12mg/day PO for 21d. Cimetidine (800mg/d PO) is used to ↑ the concentration of praziquantel. The role of steroids in the routine treatment of neurocysticercosis is controversial. **NB:** If CSF ventricles are involved, you may need to shunt before starting drugs, and drugs may worsen the acute phase of cysticercotic encephalitis. GAT[Sanford]2003 & H Garcia 2004 *NEJM* **350** 249

Diphyllobothrium latum is a fish tapeworm acquired from uncooked fish. It causes similar symptoms to *T. solium*, and is also treated with niclosamide. It is a cause of vitamin B_{12} deficiency.

Hymenolepis nana and *H. diminuta* (dwarf tapeworms) are rarely symptomatic. Treat with niclosamide 2g 1st day, then 1g/24h for 6d. *H. nana* may be treated with a single dose of praziquantel (25mg/kg PO).

Hydatid disease Cystic hydatid disease is a zoonosis caused by ingesting eggs of the dog parasite *Echinococcus granulosus* eg in rural sheep-farming regions. Hydatid is an increasing public health problem in parts of China, Russia, Alaska, Wales, and Japan. *Presentation:* Most cysts are asymptomatic, but liver cysts may present with hepatomegaly, obstructive jaundice, cholangitis, or PUO. Lung cysts may present with dyspnoea, chest pain, haemoptysis, or anaphylaxis. Parasites migrate almost anywhere, eg CNS or it turns up incidentally on CXR. *Diagnosis:* Plain x-ray, ultrasound, and CT of cysts. A reliable serological test has replaced the variably sensitive Casoni intradermal test. *Treatment:* Seek expert help. The drug of choice is albendazole (eg 7.5mg/kg/12h with food; max 800mg/d) for 28d, in 3 cycles. Excise/drain symptomatic cysts. Beware spilling cyst contents (causes anaphylaxis; give praziquantel here). The PAIR approach is commonly used: puncture → aspirate cyst → inject hypertonic saline → reaspirate. Give albendazole pre- and post-drainage to prevent recurrence. (**NB:** Alveolar hydatid is caused by *E. multilocularis*.) GAT[Sanford] 2003

---

1 While eating undercooked pork is the only way to acquire intestinal *T. solium*, any food contaminated by faeces from hosts infected with cysticerci can carry the eggs that may lead to development of cysticercosis. Even vegetarians are therefore at risk. The lack of public awareness of this life cycle poses major obstacles to elimination strategies. See J Sotelo 2003 *BMJ* **326** 511

Diagnosis of cysticercosis

This is by faecal microscopy and examination of perianal swabs.

- Differentiate *T. solium* from *T. saginata* by examining the scolex or a mature proglottid; the eggs are indistinguishable.
- A less technical means of species identification is to ask your patient about *movement* of the worm. If he describes worms vigorously wriggling out of the rectum, they will be *T. saginata*.
- An indirect haemagglutination test is available.
- The CSF may show eosinophils in neurocysticercosis, and a CSF antigen test is available.
- CT or MRI scan may locate cysts. SXR and x-rays of soft tissues of the thigh may show calcified cysts.

Trematodes (flukes)

Schistosomiasis (bilharzia) is the most prevalent disease caused by flukes, affecting 200 million people worldwide. The snail vectors release cercariae which can penetrate the skin, eg during paddling, may cause an itchy papular rash ('swimmer's itch'). The cercariae shed their tails to become schistosomules and migrate via lungs to liver where they grow. ~2wks after initial infestation, there may be fever, urticaria, diarrhoea, cough, wheeze, and hepatosplenomegaly ('Katayama fever'). In ~8wks, mature flukes couple and migrate to resting habitats, ie vesical veins (haematobium) or mesenteric veins (mansoni and japonicum). Eggs released from these sites cause granulomata and scarring. Clinical schistosomiasis is an immunological process on the part of the human host which is known to be due to a type IV hypersensitivity (at least for S. mansoni) to schistosomal eggs.

The Patient is likely to have visited or be from Africa, the Middle East, or Brazil (S. mansoni), and present with abdominal pain and bowel upset, and, later, hepatic fibrosis, granulomatous inflammation, and portal hypertension (transformation into true cirrhosis has not been well-documented). S. japonicum, often the most serious, occurs in SE Asia, tends to affect the bowel and liver, and may migrate to lung and CNS ('travellers' myelitis'). Urinary schistosomiasis (S. haematobium) occurs in Africa, the Middle East, and the Indian Ocean. Signs: frequency, dysuria, haematuria (± haematospermia), incontinence. It may progress to hydronephrosis and renal failure. There is an ↑risk of squamous cell carcinoma of the bladder.

Diagnosis is based on finding eggs in the urine (S. haematobium) or faeces (S. mansoni and S. japonicum) or rectal biopsy (all types). AXR may show bladder calcification in chronic S. haematobium infection. Renal ultrasound identifies renal obstruction, hydronephrosis, thickened bladder wall. Schistosoma ELISA is most sensitive.

Treatment Praziquantel: 40mg/kg PO with food divided into 2 doses separated by 4–6h for S. mansoni & S. haematobium, and 20mg/kg/8h for 1d in S. japonicum. Sudden transitory abdominal pain and bloody diarrhoea may occur shortly after. Oxamniquine is an alternative for S. mansoni infection. Artemether also shows promise, both for prophylaxis in high-risk groups, and as a synergist to praziquantel therapy.[1]

GAT^{sanford} 2003

Fasciola hepatica (liver fluke) is spread by sheep, water, and snails. It causes hepatomegaly, then fibrosis. Presentation: Fever, abdominal pain, diarrhoea, weight↓, jaundice, and eosinophilia. Tests: Stool microscopy, serology. Treatment: Get help. Triclabendazole 10mg/kg PO, 1 dose (may repeat once), or bithionol 30mg/kg/d, max 2g/day IM (15 doses).

Opisthorchis and Clonorchis are liver flukes common in the Far East, where they cause cholangitis, cholecystitis, and cholangiocarcinoma. Tests: Stool microscopy. Treatment: Praziquantel 25mg/kg/8h PO for 1d.

Fasciolopsis buski is a big intestinal fluke ~7cm long causing ulcers or abscesses at the site of attachment. Treatment: as for opisthorchiasis.

Paragonimus westermani (lung fluke) is contracted by eating raw freshwater crabs or crayfish. Parasites migrate through gut and diaphragm to invade the lungs, causing cough, dyspnoea, and haemoptysis. Secondary complications: lung abscess and bronchiectasis. It occurs in the Far East, S America, and the Congo, where it is commonly mistaken for TB (similar clinical and CXR appearances). Tests: Ova in sputum. MRI/CT may disclose CNS/lung lesions. Treatment: Praziquantel (25mg/kg/8h PO for 2d) or bithionol (30–50mg/kg on alternate days PO for 10 days).

---

1 For excellent reviews on schistosomiasis, see AGP Ross 2002 NEJM 346 1212 and D Cioli 2004 Lancet 363 180

Exotic infections

Exotic infections may be *community-acquired* or *nosocomial*, ie acquired in hospital. The increasing prevalence of immunosuppression, both drug induced and innate, and the widespread use of broad-spectrum antibiotics have resulted in an increase in exotic infections. New techniques such as PCR have enabled the identification of more putative infective agents.

History When an infection is suspected (fever, sweats, inflammation, D&V, WCC↑, or *any* unexplained symptom), ask the patient about:
- *Any recent foreign travel?*
- *Previous travel history?*
- *Any foreign bodies, eg hip prosthesis, prosthetic heart valves?*
- *Immunosuppression or risk factors for HIV?*
- *Any necrotic tissues?*
- *Any pets at home?*
- *Any animal or insect bites or scratches?*
- *Any exposure to illness at work?*

Diagnosis Take appropriate cultures (blood, urine, stool, CSF) or swabs as clinically indicated. Liaise early with an infectious diseases physician or microbiologist. Consider CXR, ultrasound, or CT as clinically indicated. If the infection appears to be localized, consider surgical debridement ± drainage. Do not give up if you cannot culture an organism; tests may need to be repeated. Perhaps the organism is 'fastidious' in its nutritional requirement or requires prolonged incubation? Even if culture *is* achieved, it may be that the organism is pathogenic, or it could be a commensal (ie part of the normal flora for that patient). If culture is not possible, look for antibodies or antigen in the serum or other body fluids. It is generally agreed that a 4-fold increase in antibody titres in convalescence (compared with the acute sera) is indicative of recent infection, although not diagnostic. PCR is increasingly being used to make identifications; however, it is far from infallible, and contamination with DNA from the lab or elsewhere is a frequent problem.

Treatment Empirical therapy (p548) may be needed if the patients is ill. *The table opposite is for reference purposes only:* no one can remember *all* the details about even the common infectious diseases, let alone the rare ones. Check with a microbiologist for local patterns of disease and antibiotic sensitivity/resistance. *Antibiotic doses:* Penicillins (p543); cephalosporins (p544); other agents (p546).

Sources J Paul 2003 *OTM* 4e 658; B Currie 2000 *Tr Roy Soc Trop Med Hyg* **94** 301; and S Dorman 2000 *Transfusion* **40** 375

Organism	Site or type of infection	Treatment example
Acanthamoeba	Corneal ulcers	Propamidine + neomycin
Acinetobacter calcoaceticus	UTI; CSF; lung; bone; conjunctiva	Gentamicin
Actinobacillus actinomycetemcomitans	IE; CNS; bone; thyroid; lung Periodontitis; abscesses	Penicillin ± cephalosporin
Actinobacillus lignieresii	CSF; IE; wounds; bone; lymph nodes	Ampicillin ± gentamicin
Actinobacillus ureae	Bronchus; CSF post-trauma; hepatitis	Ampicillin ± gentamicin
Aerococcus viridans	Empyema; UTI; CSF; bone	Penicillin ± gentamicin
Aeromonas hydrophila	IE; CSF; cornea; bone; D&V; liver abscess	Imipenem or ceftriaxone
Afipia broomeae	Marrow; synovium	Co-amoxiclav or cetazidime
Alcaligenes species	Dialysis peritonitis; ear; lung	Penicillin
Arachnia propionica	Actinomycosis; tear ducts; CNS	Penicillin
Arcanobacterium	Throat; cellulitis; leg ulcer	Clindamycin + quinine
Babesia microti (protozoa)	PUO ± haemolysis if old/splenectomized	Gentamicin
Bacillus cereus	Wounds; eye; ear; lung; UTI; IE	Penicillin
Bifidobacterium	Vagina; UTI; IE; peritonitis; lung	Co-trimoxazole?
Bordetella bronchiseptica	URTI; CSF (after animal contact)	Ceftazidime
Burkholderia cepacia, etc (formerly *Pseudomonas*)	Wounds; feet; lungs; IE; CAPD; UTI ecthyma gangrenosa; peritonitis	Clindamycin or gentamicin
Burkholderia pickettii	CSF (formerly a *pseudomonas*)	Cefalosporin
Burkholderia pseudomallei (formerly *Pseudomonas pseudomallei*)	Melioidosis: self-reactivating septic-aemia + multiorgan, protean signs eg in rice-farmers, via water/soil in Pap-ua, Thailand, Vietnam, Torres Straits	Ceftazidime (14d) + Co-trimoxazole or Co-amoxiclav for 3 months
Capnocytophaga ochracea and *C. sputagena*	Oral ulcer; stomatitis; arthritis Blood; cervical abscess	Penicillin or ciprofloxacin
Cardiobacterium hominis	IE (=infective endocarditis)	Penicillin + gentamicin
Chromobacterium violaceum	Nodes; eye; bone; liver; pustules	Erythromycin, chloramphenicol
Citrobacter koseri/diversus	CSF; UTI; blood; cholecystitis	Cefuroxime + gentamicin
Corynebacterium bovis/equi	IE; CSF; otitis; leg ulcer; lung	Erythromycin + rifampicin
Corynebacterium ovis	Joints; liver; muscle; granulomata	Penicillin
Corynebacterium ulcerans	Diphtheria-like ± CNS signs	Penicillin + Diphtheria antitoxin
Cyclospora cayetanensis	Diarrhoea (via raspberries)	Co-trimoxazole
Edwardsiella tarda	Cellulitis; abscesses; BP↓; dysentery via penetrating fish injuries	Cefuroxime + gentamicin
Eikenella corrodens	Sinus; ears; PE post-jugular vein phlebitis (postanginal sepsis) via bites	Penicillin + gentamicin
Erysipelothrix rhusiopathiae	Erysipelas-like (*OHCS* p590); IE	Penicillin
Eubacterium	Wounds; gynaecology sepsis; IE	Penicillin
Flavobacterium meningosepticum	Lungs; epidemic neonatal meningi-tis; post-op bacteraemia	Penicillin
Flavobacterium multivorum	Peritonitis (spontaneous)	Cefuroxime
Gemella haemolysans	IE; meningitis after neurosurgery	Penicillin + gentamicin
Helicobacter cinaedia	Proctitis in homosexual men	Ampicillin or gentamicin
Kingella denitrificans kingae	Throat; larynx; eyelid; joint; skin	Penicillin ± gentamicin
Kurthia bibsonii/sibirica/zopfii	IE (infective endocarditis)	Penicillin
Lactobacillus	Teeth; chorioamnionitis; pyelitis	Cephalosporins, Penicillin
Megasphaera elsdenii	IE (infective endocarditis)	Metronidazole
Mobiluncus curtisii/mulieris	Vagina; uterus; septicaemia in cirrhosis	Cephalosporins or ampicillin
Moraxella osloensis and *M. nonliquefaciens*	Conjunctiva; wound; vagina; UTI; CSF CNS; bone; haemorrhagic stomatitis	Penicillin
Neisseria cani	Wounds from cat bites	Amoxicillin
Neisseria cinerea/mucosa+ *N. subflava*; *N. flavescens*	IE; CNS; bone; post human bites or from peritoneal dialysis	Penicillin, cephalosporin
Pasteurella multocida	Bone; lung; CSF; UTI; pericarditis epiglottitis. Post cat/dog bite	Penicillin
Pasteurella pneumotrophica	Wounds; joints; bone; CSF	Penicillin or ciprofloxacin
Peptostreptococcus magnans	Bone; joint; wound; teeth; face	Penicillin or cephalosporins
Plesiomonas shigelloides	D&V; eye; sepsis post fishbone injury	Ciprofloxacin
Propionibacterium acnes	Face; wounds; CSF shunts; bone; IE liver granuloma (botyromycosis)	Tetracycline or Penicillin
Prototheca wickerhamii/ zopfii = achlorophyllous algae	Subcutaneous granuloma; bursitis Lymphadenitis; nodules; granuloma	Amphotericin or Ketoconazole
Providencia stuartii	UTI; burn or lung infections	Gentamicin
Pseudomonas maltophilia	Wounds; ear; eye; lung; UTI; IE	Co-trimoxazole
Pseudomonas putrefaciens	CSF post CNS surgery/head trauma	Cefotaxime
Rothia dentocariosa	Appendix abscess	Penicillin + gentamicin
Serratia marcescens	Wound; burns; lung; UTI; liver; CSF; bone; IE; red diaper syndrome	Imipenem, ceftazidime, ciprofloxacin
Sphingomonas paucimobilis	Superficial leg ulcer; CSF; UTI	Ceftazidime
Streptococcus bovis	IE if colon cancer; do colonoscopy	Penicillin + gentamicin
Vibrio vulnificus	Wounds; muscle; uterus; fasciitis	Tetracycline, penicillin

621

Haematology[1]

Contents

Relevant pages elsewhere: Transfusion (p464); normal values (p713).

Further reading: D Nathan 1995 *Genes, Blood, and Courage,* Harvard University Press, ISBN 0-674-34473-L. Dayem Saif, introduced when he was a 6-year-old with a stature of a 2-year-old, has an Hb of 1.5g/dL, as low as his chance of survival with thalassaemia. This story about laboratory medicine and its stormy application at the bedside is definitely worth reading when feeling hemmed in by difficult patients, for it demonstrates that there are no difficult patients, only difficult times. The book portrays the vital nature of the doctor–patient relationship, and warns us against labelling people, unless the label is a poem: Dayem is Arabic for *Immortal Sword*.

---

[1] *We thank Dr J Davies who is our Specialist Reader for this chapter.*

On the taking of blood and of holidays

This is not one of those passages about how you should be kind to the patient, explain in full what you are going to do, talk him or her through venepuncture, label the bottles carefully, and make a plan for communicating the results. Be all this virtue as it may, there is something else which needs communicating about the most menial of our tasks: the *act* of taking blood. It is partly to do with the fact that as blood is life, and, because, as Ruskin taught us, 'there is no wealth but life', we are led to the conclusion that what is special about taking blood is that for once *we* are being given something valuable by the patient. What is this wealth? The answer is *time*. For while the blood is flowing into our tube we cannot be disturbed. We are excused from answering our bleeps, and from making polite conversation (a few grunts in reply to patients' enquires about the colour of their blood is quite sufficient)—and we can indulge in that almost unimaginable luxury, at least as far as life on the wards is concerned, of *being alone with our own thoughts*. Thinking of this sacred time as a sort of hypnotic holiday is excellent. For however many nights we have been awoken, and through however many wards we have traipsed to this bedside, this little holiday will be worth an hour's sleep—if our mind is furnished and ready to empty itself of all objectivity. The best sight in haematological practice is, during venepuncture, to watch for those occasions when, owing to some chance characteristic of flow, the jet of blood streaming into our tube breaks up into countless globules, and before coalescing again, these globules jostle together like the overcrowded chain of events which led us to this bedside. During this time, allow your own thoughts to coalesce into a more peaceful order if you can, and let William Blake help you in the task of furnishing your mind to banish objectivity, for he knew some truths about haematology unknown to strictly rational practitioners of this art:

> The Microscope knows not of this nor the Telescope: they alter
> The ratio of the Spectators Organs but leave Objects untouch'd
> For every space larger than a red globule of Mans blood
> Is visionary, and it is created by the Hammer of Los[1]:
> And every space smaller than a Globule of Mans blood opens
> Into eternity of which this vegetable Earth is but a shadow.
> The red Globule is the unwearied Sun by Los created
> To measure Time and Space to mortal Men…

---

1 Los, the *globe of fire*, is a symbol used by Blake to encompass the exultant energy of creation, the poetic imagination, and the burning brightness where all his noble images were pounded out of eternity and compounded into the most compressed verse and art we have (see P Ackroyd 1996 *Blake*, Minerva). These lines are from his poem *Milton*, section 29, lines 17–24, page 516 in OUP's *Blake: Complete Writings*, edited (1925–1969) by Geoffrey Keynes, the surgeon, who, incidentally, led the way to lumpectomy for breast cancer, in preference to the much-hated radical mastectomy.

Anaemia

Anaemia is defined as a low haemoglobin concentration, and may be either due to a low red cell mass, or increased plasma volume (eg in pregnancy). A low Hb (at sea level) is <13.5g/dL for men and <11.5g/dL for women. Anaemia may be due to reduced production or increased loss of RBC and has many causes. These will often be distinguishable by history, examination, and inspection of the blood film.

Symptoms Due to the underlying cause or to the anaemia itself: fatigue, dyspnoea, palpitations, headache, tinnitus, anorexia, dyspepsia, bowel disturbance—and angina if there is pre-existing coronary artery disease.

Signs May be absent even in severe anaemia. Pallor (look at conjunctivae) and retinal haemorrhages. In severe anaemia (Hb <8g/dL), there may be signs of a hyperdynamic circulation, eg tachycardia, murmurs, and cardiac enlargement. Later, heart failure may occur and in this state, rapid blood transfusion may be fatal.

Types of anaemia The first step in diagnosis is to look at the mean cell volume (MCV, *normal MCV is 76-96 femtolitres*, 10^{15} fL = 1L).

Low MCV (microcytic)

- Iron-deficiency anaemia (IDA, most common cause). See p626.
- Thalassaemia (suspect if the MCV is 'too low' for the level of anaemia and the red cell count is raised).
- Congenital sideroblastic anaemia (very rare).

NB: The last 2 are iron-loading conditions and will have serum iron↑; ferritin↑; but a low total iron-binding capacity (TIBC).

Normal MCV (normocytic anaemia)

- Anaemia of chronic disease
- Bone marrow failure
- Renal failure
- Hypothyroidism (or ↑MCV)
- Haemolysis (or ↑MCV)
- Pregnancy

If there is a reduced white cell or platelet count, suspect bone marrow failure and perform a bone marrow biopsy.

High MCV (macrocytic anaemia)

- B_{12} or folate deficiency
- Alcohol
- Liver disease
- Reticulocytosis (eg haemolysis)
- Cytotoxics, eg hydroxyurea (=hydroxycarbamide)
- Myelodysplastic syndromes
- Marrow infiltration
- Hypothyroidism
- Antifolate drugs (eg phenytoin)

Haemolytic anaemias: Do not fall elegantly into the above classification as the anaemia may be normochromic, or, if there are many young (hence larger) RBCs and reticulocytes, macrocytic. Suspect if there is a reticulocytosis (>2% of RBCs; or reticulocyte count >85 × 10^9/L; special stains are needed), mild macrocytosis, haptoglobin↓ (p636), bilirubin↑, and urobilinogen↑. Often mild jaundice (but no bile in the urine).

Blood transfusion Avoid unless Hb dangerously low. The decision will depend on severity and cause. If risk of haemorrhage (eg active peptic ulcer), transfuse up to 8g/dL. In severe anaemia with heart failure, transfusion is vital to restore Hb to safe level, eg 6–8g/dL, but must be done with great care. Give packed cells *slowly* with 10–40mg frusemide (=furosemide) IV/PO with alternate units (dose depends on previous exposure to diuretics; do not mix with blood). Check for rising JVP and basal crepitations. If CCF gets worse, stop and treat. If immediate transfusion is essential, try a 2–3 unit exchange transfusion, removing blood at same rate as it is transfused.

Iron-deficiency anaemia

This is common (seen in up to 14% of menstruating women).

Causes:
- Blood loss, particularly menorrhagia or GI bleeding—from oesophagitis, peptic ulcer, carcinoma, colitis, diverticulitis, or haemorrhoids.
- In the Tropics, hookworm (GI blood loss) is the most common cause.
- Poor diet may cause IDA in babies or children (but rarely in adults), those on special diets, or wherever there is poverty.
- Malabsorption (eg coeliac disease) is a cause of refractory iron-deficiency anaemia.

Signs: Chronic iron-deficiency anaemia: koilonychia (p39), atrophic glossitis, and, rarely, post-cricoid webs (all now rare).

Investigations: Microcytic, hypochromic blood film showing anisocytosis and poikilocytosis (p628). Confirmed by showing serum iron↓ and ferritin↓ (more representative of total body iron) with TIBC↑. If MCV↓, and good history of menorrhagia, oral iron may be started without further tests. Otherwise investigate: faecal occult blood, sigmoidoscopy, barium enema or colonoscopy, gastroscopy, microscope stool for ova. ►*Iron deficiency without an obvious source of bleeding mandates a careful GI workup.*

Treatment: Treat the cause. Oral iron eg ferrous sulfate 200mg/12–8h PO. SE: constipation, black stools. Hb should rise by 1g/dL/week, with a modest reticulocytosis (ie young RBC, p628). Continue until Hb is normal and for at least 3 months, to replenish stores. Parenteral iron is almost never needed. If it is—because oral route is impossible or ineffective, eg patients with functional iron deficiency undergoing haemodialysis and erythropoietin therapy—use intravenous iron and consult the appropriate data sheet.

Refractory anaemia The usual reason that iron-deficiency anaemia fails to respond to iron replacement is that the patient has rejected the pills. Negotiate on concordance issues (p3). Is the reason for the problem GI disturbance (altering the dose of elemental iron may help)? There may be continued blood loss, or malabsorption; or there is misdiagnosis, eg when thalassaemia is to blame.

The anaemia of chronic disease

This is associated with many diseases: eg infection, collagen vascular disease, rheumatoid arthritis, malignancy, renal failure. *Investigations:* Mild normocytic anaemia (eg Hb >8g/dL), TIBC↓ serum iron↓, ferritin normal or↑. *Treatment:* Treat the underlying disease. The anaemia of renal failure is partly due to erythropoietin deficiency and recombinant erythropoietin is effective in raising the haemoglobin level (maintenance dose example: 50–150 units/kg twice weekly—see BNF; SE: 'flu-like symptoms, hypertension, mild rise in the platelet count). It is also effective in raising Hb and improving quality of life in those with malignant disease.[1]

Sideroblastic anaemia

Characterized by dyserythropoiesis and iron loading (bone marrow) and sometimes haemosiderosis (ie endocrine, liver, and cardiac damage). It may be congenital (rare, X-linked) or acquired—usually idiopathic, part of the spectrum of the myelodysplastic disorders, but may follow alcohol or lead excess, myeloproliferative disease, malignancy, malabsorption, or anti-TB drugs. Hypochromic RBCs are seen on the blood film with sideroblasts in the marrow (erythroid precursors with iron deposited in mitochondria in a ring around the nucleus). *Treatment* is supportive; pyridoxine may occasionally be of benefit (eg 10mg/24h PO; higher doses may cause neuropathy); remove the cause if possible. In myelodysplasia erythropoietin, with or without human granulocyte colony stimulating factor (G-CSF) may be effective, although the cost benefit of this approach is controversial.

Interpretation of plasma iron studies

	Iron	TIBC	Ferritin
Iron deficiency	↓	↑	↓
Anaemia of chronic disease	↓	↓	↑
Chronic haemolysis	↑	↓	↑
Haemochromatosis	↑	↓ (or ↔)	↑
Pregnancy	↑	↑	↔
Sideroblastic anaemia	↑	↔	↑

The peripheral blood film

▶Many haematological (and other) diagnoses can be made by careful examination of the peripheral blood film. It is also necessary for interpretation of the FBC indices.

Acanthocytes: RBCs show many spicules (in abetalipoproteinaemia).

Anisocytosis: Variation in size, eg in megaloblastic anaemia, thalassaemia as well as IDA.

Basophilic stippling: of RBCs is seen in lead poisoning, thalassaemia, and other dyserythropoietic anaemias.

Blasts: Nucleated precursor cells (eg in myelofibrosis or leukaemia). They are not normally seen in peripheral blood.

Burr cells: Irregularly shaped cells occurring in uraemia.

Dimorphic picture: A mixture of RBC sizes, eg partially treated iron deficiency, mixed deficiency (Fe with B_{12} or folate deficiency), post-transfusion, sideroblastic anaemia.

Howell-Jolly bodies: Nuclear remnants seen in RBCs post splenectomy; rarely leukaemia, megaloblastic anaemia, iron-deficiency anaemia, hyposplenism (eg coeliac disease, neonates, thalassaemia, SLE, lymphoma, leukaemia, amyloid).

Hypochromia: Less dense staining of RBCs seen in iron-deficiency anaemia, thalassaemia, and sideroblastic anaemia (iron stores unusable).

Left shift: Immature white cells seen in circulating blood in any marrow outpouring, eg infection.

Leucoerythroblastic anaemia: Immature cells (myelocytes and normoblasts) seen in film. Due to marrow infiltration (eg by malignancy), hypoxia, or severe anaemia.

Leukaemoid reaction: A marked reactive leucocytosis. Usually granulocytic, eg in severe infection, burns, acute haemolysis, metastatic cancer.

Myelocytes, promyelocytes, metamyelocytes, normoblasts: Immature cells seen in the blood in leukoerythroblastic anaemia.

Normoblasts: Immature red cells, with a nucleus. Seen in leukoerythroblastic anaemia, marrow infiltration, haemolysis, hypoxia.

Pappenheimer bodies: Granules of siderocytes, eg lead poisoning, carcinomatosis, post splenectomy.

Poikilocytes: Variably shaped cells: seen in iron-deficiency anaemia, myelofibrosis, thalassaemia.

Polychromasia: RBCs of different ages stain unevenly (the young are bluer). This is a response to bleeding, haematinics (eg ferrous sulfate, B_{12}), haemolysis, or dyserythropoiesis.

Reticulocytes: (NR: 0.8–2%; or $<85\times10^9$/L) Young, larger RBCs (contain RNA) signifying active erythropoiesis. Increased in haemolysis, haemorrhage, and if B_{12}, iron or folate is given to marrow that lack these.

Right shift: Hypersegmented polymorphs (>5 lobes to nucleus) seen in megaloblastic anaemia, uraemia, and liver disease.

Rouleaux formation: Red cells stack on each other (the visual 'analogue' of a high ESR—see p670).

Schistocytes: Fragmented RBCs sliced by fibrin bands. Seen in intravascular haemolysis.

Spherocytes: Spherical cells, seen in: haemolysis, hereditary spherocytosis, burns. Look for microangiopathic anaemia, eg DIC (p650), TTP (p282).

Target cells: (also called Mexican hat cells) These are RBCs with central staining, a ring of pallor, and an outer rim of staining seen in liver disease, thalassaemia, or sickle-cell disease—and, in small numbers, in iron-deficiency anaemia.

629

The differential white cell count

Neutrophils $2–7.5 \times 10^9$/L (40–75% of white blood cells: but absolute values are more meaningful than percentages).

Increased in:

- Bacterial infections.
- Trauma; surgery; burns; haemorrhage.
- Inflammation; infarction; polymyalgia; PAN.
- Myeloproliferative disorders. Marked increase in leukaemias.
- Drugs (eg steroids).
- Disseminated malignancy.

Decreased in:

- Viral infections; brucellosis; typhoid; kala-azar; TB.
- Drugs, eg carbimazole; sulfonamides.
- Hypersplenism or neutrophil antibodies (seen in SLE and rheumatoid arthritis)—↑ destruction.
- B_{12} or folate deficiency; in bone marrow failure— ↓ production, p662.

Lymphocytes $1.3–3.5 \times 10^9$/L (20–45%).

Increased in:

- Viral infections, toxoplasmosis; whooping cough; brucellosis
- Chronic lymphatic leukaemia.

Large numbers of abnormal ('atypical') lymphocytes are characteristically seen with EBV infection: these are T-cells reacting against EBV-infected B-cells. They have a large amount of clearish cytoplasm with a blue rim that flows around neighbouring RBCs. Other causes of 'atypical' lymphocytes: see p570.

Decreased in:

- Steroid therapy; SLE; uraemia; legionnaire's disease; HIV infection; marrow infiltration; post chemotherapy or radiotherapy.

T-lymphocyte subset reference values: CD4 count: 537–1571/mm³ (low in HIV infection). CD8 count: 235–753/mm³; CD4/CD8 ratio: 1.2–3.8.

Eosinophils $0.04–0.44 \times 10^9$/L (1–6%). *Increased in:* Asthma/atopy; parasitic infections (especially invasive helminths); PAN; skin disease especially pemphigus; urticaria; malignant disease (including lymphomas and eosinophilic leukaemia); adrenal insufficiency, irradiation; Löffler's syndrome (p728); during the convalescent phase of any infection.

The hypereosinophilic syndrome is seen when there is development of end-organ damage (restrictive cardiomyopathy; neuropathy; hepatosplenomegaly) in association with a raised eosinophil count (>1.5×10^9/L) for more than 6wks.

Monocytes $0.2–0.8 \times 10^9$/L (2–10%).

Increased in: Acute and chronic infections (eg TB; brucellosis; protozoa); malignant disease, including M4 and M5 acute myeloid leukaemia (p654), and Hodgkin's disease; myelodysplasia.

Basophils $0–0.1 \times 10^9$/L (0–1%).

Increased in: Viral infections; urticaria; myxoedema; post splenectomy; CML; UC; malignancy; systemic mastocytosis (urticaria pigmentosa); haemolysis; polycythaemia rubra vera.

Macrocytic anaemia

Macrocytosis (*MCV >96fL*) is a common finding; often due to alcohol (usually without any accompanying anaemia). Although only ~5% are due to B_{12} deficiency, pernicious anaemia is the most common cause of a macrocytic anaemia in Western countries.

Causes of macrocytosis (*MCV >110fL*): Vitamin B_{12} or folate deficiency; drugs, eg hydroxyurea (hydroxycarbamide).

MCV 100-110fL:

- *Drugs: eg alcohol, azathioprine, zidovudine (p584)*
- Marrow infiltration
- Haemolysis
- Liver disease
- Pregnancy
- Hypothyroidism
- Myelodysplasia

Investigations

Blood film: May show hypersegmented polymorphs (B_{12}↓) or target cells (liver disease). *Other tests:* ESR (malignancy), LFT (include γGT), T4, serum B_{12}, and serum folate (or red cell folate). *Bone marrow biopsy* is indicated if the cause is not revealed by the above tests. It is likely to show 1 of these 4 states:

- Megaloblastic—B_{12} or folate deficiency (or cytotoxic drugs). (A megaloblast is a cell in which cytoplasmic and nuclear maturation are out of phase—as nuclear maturation is slow.)
- Normoblastic marrow—liver damage, myxoedema.
- Increased erythropoiesis—eg haemolysis.
- Abnormal erythropoiesis—sideroblastic anaemia, leukaemia, aplasia.

If B_{12} deficiency, consider a *Schilling test* to help to identify the cause. This determines whether a low B_{12} is due to malabsorption (B_{12} is absorbed from the terminal ileum) or to lack of intrinsic factor—by comparing the proportion of an oral dose (1μg) of radioactive B_{12} excreted in urine with and without the concurrent administration of intrinsic factor. (The blood must be saturated by giving an IM dose of 1000μg of B_{12} first.) If intrinsic factor enhances absorption, lack of it (eg pernicious anaemia, p634) is likely to be the cause.

Causes of a low B_{12} Pernicious anaemia (p634); post gastrectomy (no intrinsic factor to ↑absorption from terminal ileum); dietary deficiency (eg vegans); rarely, disease of terminal ileum (where B_{12} is absorbed)—eg Crohn's; resection; blind loops; diverticula; worms (*Dyphyllobothrium*). B_{12} is found in liver and all animal foods. *Body stores:* Sufficient for 3yrs.

Causes of low folate[1]

Poor diet (eg in alcoholics), ↑need (pregnancy, haemolysis, dyserythropoiesis, malignancy, long-term haemodialysis), malabsorption especially coeliac disease, tropical sprue, drugs (phenytoin and trimethoprim). Folate is found in green vegetables, fruit, liver and is synthesized by gut bacteria. *Body stores:* Sufficient for 3 months. Maternal folate deficiency is also linked to neural tube defects in the fetus.

NB: In ill patients with megaloblastic anaemia (eg with CCF), it may be necessary to treat before the results of serum B_{12} and folate are at hand. Use large doses, eg hydroxocobalamin 1mg/24h IM, with folic acid 5mg/24h PO. Blood transfusions are very rarely needed, but see p624.

▶Folate given alone (ie without B_{12}) may precipitate, or worsen, subacute combined degeneration of the spinal cord.

---

1 Homocysteine concentrations in folate-deficient patients can be normalized by folic acid supplementation, which ↑availability of the co-substrate, methyltetrahydrofolate, and drives the pathway for homocysteine remethylation. Other vitamins (B_{12} if B_{12} deficient) may also have a role here. Elderly patients taking vitamin B_6 (at possibly neuropathic doses of 100–200mg/d) showed a 73% ↓ in risk of angina/MI, with an average increase in lifespan of 8 (range 7–17) yrs.   www.txt.co.uk/full.cfm?1011.

Pernicious anaemia

Essence This disease affects all cells of the body and is due to malabsorption of B_{12} resulting from atrophic gastritis and lack of gastric intrinsic factor secretion. In B_{12} deficiency, synthesis of thymidine, and hence DNA, is impaired and consequently red cell production is reduced. In addition, the CNS, peripheral nerves, gut, and tongue may be affected.

Incidence 1 : 1000; ♀ : ♂ = 1.6 : 1, higher incidence if blood group A.

Common features
- Tiredness and weakness (90%)
- Dyspnoea (70%)
- Paraesthesiae (38%)
- Sore red tongue (25%)
- Diarrhoea
- Mild jaundice (lemon tinge to skin)

Other features
- Retinal haemorrhages
- Prematurely grey hair
- Retrobulbar neuritis
- Mild splenomegaly
- Fever
- Neuropsychiatric (dementia)

Subacute combined degeneration of the spinal cord: This may be seen in any cause of a low B_{12}. Posterior and lateral columns are often affected, not always together. Onset is usually insidious with peripheral neuropathy. Joint-position and vibration sense are often affected first (dorsal columns) followed by distal paraesthesiae (neuropathy). If untreated, stiffness and weakness ensue. The classical triad is: • Extensor plantars • Brisk knee jerks • Absent ankle jerks. Less common signs: cognition↓, vision↓, absent knee jerks with brisk ankle jerks and flexor plantars, Lhermitte's sign (p384). Pain and T° sensation may be intact even when joint position sense is severely affected. CNS signs can occur without anaemia.

Associations Thyroid disease (~25%), vitiligo, Addison's disease, carcinoma of stomach (so have a low threshold for endoscopy).

Tests • Hb↓ (3–11g/dL) • MCV >~110fL • Hypersegmented polymorphs • Serum B_{12} is always↓ • WCC & platelets↓ • Megaloblasts in the marrow

Megaloblasts are abnormal red cell precursors in which nuclear maturation is slower than cytoplasmic maturation. Antibodies to parietal cells are found in 90%; there may also be antibodies to intrinsic factor (specific for pernicious anaemia), either at B_{12} binding sites (50%) or at ileal binding sites (35%). A Schilling test (p632) may be appropriate occasionally (expect it to show that <7% of an orally administered dose of labelled B_{12} is excreted—unless concurrent intrinsic factor is given).

Treatment Replenish stores with hydroxocobalamin (B_{12}) 1mg IM alternate days eg for 2wks (or, if CNS signs, until improvement stops). Maintenance: 1mg IM every 2 months for life (child's dose: as for adult). Initial improvement is heralded by a marked reticulocytosis (after 4–5 days, but serum iron falls first). Watch for early hypokalaemia if severely anaemic.

Practical hints Beware of diagnosing pernicious anaemia in those under 40 yrs old: look for GI malabsorption (small bowel biopsy, p252).

1 Watch for hypokalaemia as treatment becomes established.
2 Pernicious anaemia with high output CCF may require exchange transfusion (p624) after blood for FBC, folate, B_{12}, and marrow sampling.
3 As haemopoiesis accelerates on treatment, additional Fe may be needed.
4 WCC and platelet count should normalize in 1wk. Hb rises ~1g/dL per week of treatment.

Prognosis Complete neurological recovery is possible. Most see improvement in the first 3–6 months. Patients do best if treated as soon as possible after the onset of symptoms: don't delay!

An approach to haemolytic anaemia

Haemolysis is the premature breakdown of RBCs. It may occur in the circulation (intravascular) or in the reticuloendothelial system (extravascular). Normal RBCs have a lifespan of ~120d. In sickle-cell anaemia, eg the lifespan may be as short as 5d. If the bone marrow does not compensate sufficiently, a haemolytic anaemia will result.

Causes of haemolysis These are either genetic or acquired.

Genetic:

1 Membrane: hereditary spherocytosis or elliptocytosis.
2 Haemoglobin: sickling disorders (p640), thalassaemia.
3 Enzyme defects: G6PD and pyruvate kinase deficiency.

Acquired:

1 Immune: either isoimmune (haemolytic disease of newborn, blood transfusion reaction), autoimmune (warm or cold antibody mediated), or drug-induced.
2 Non-immune: trauma (cardiac haemolysis, microangiopathic anaemia, p638), infection (malaria, septicaemia), membrane disorders (paroxysmal nocturnal haemoglobinuria, liver disease).

In searching for evidence of significant haemolysis (and, if present, its cause), try to answer these 4 questions:

- *Is there increased red cell breakdown?* Bilirubin↑ (unconjugated), urinary urobilinogen↑, haptoglobin↓ (binds free Hb avidly, and is then removed by the liver, so it is a good marker of haemolysis).
- *Is there increased red cell production?* Eg a reticulocytosis, polychromasia, macrocytosis, marrow hyperplasia.
- *Is the haemolysis mainly extra- or intravascular?* Extravascular haemolysis may lead to splenic hypertrophy. The features of intravascular haemolysis are methaemalbuminaemia, free plasma haemoglobin, haemoglobinuria, low haptoglobin, and haemosiderinuria.
- *Why is there haemolysis?* See below, and p638.

History Ask about family history, race, jaundice, haematuria, drugs, previous anaemia.

Examination Look for jaundice, hepatosplenomegaly, leg ulcers (seen in sickle-cell disease).

Investigation

- FBC, reticulocytes, bilirubin, LDH, haptoglobin, urinary urobilinogen. Films may show polychromasia, macrocytosis, spherocytes, elliptocytes, fragmented cells or sickle cells—and nucleated RBCs if severe.
- Further investigations: *direct Coombs' test* (DCT). This will identify red cells coated with antibody or complement and a positive result usually indicates an immune cause of the haemolysis. The non-immune group are usually identifiable by associated features.
- RBC lifespan may be determined by *chromium labelling* and the major site of RBC breakdown may also be identified. *Urinary haemosiderin* (stains with Prussian Blue) indicates chronic intravascular haemolysis.
- The cause may now be obvious, but further tests may be needed. Membrane abnormalities are identified on the film, and can be confirmed by *osmotic fragility* testing. *Hb electrophoresis* will detect Hb variants. *Enzyme assays* are reserved for situations when other causes have been excluded.

Causes of haemolytic anaemia

Sickle-cell disease See p640.

Hereditary spherocytosis Autosomal dominant RBC membrane defect[?] (RBCs are osmotically fragile). Haemolysis is variable. *Signs:* Splenomegaly ± ↑ risk of gallstones. RBCs show ↑fragility. *Diagnosis:* Hb 8–12g/dL. Osmotic fragility tests. Film: many spherocytes. *Treatment:* Folate replacement; splenectomy if warranted (there are risks with ensuing hyposplenism).

Hereditary elliptocytosis Usually inherited as autosomal dominant. The degree of haemolysis is variable. If needed, splenectomy may help.

Glucose-6-phosphate dehydrogenase deficiency is the commonest RBC enzyme defect. Inheritance is sex-linked with 100 million affected in Africa, the Mediterranean and the Middle/Far East. Neonatal jaundice occurs, but most are symptomless with normal Hb and blood film. They are susceptible to oxidative crises precipitated by drugs (eg primaquine, sulfonamides, ciprofloxacin), exposure to the broad bean *Vicia fava* (favism) or illness. Typically there is rapid anaemia and jaundice with RBC Heinz bodies (denatured Hb stained with methyl violet). *Diagnosis:* enzyme assay. Don't do until some weeks *after* a crisis as young RBCs may have sufficient enzyme to make the results appear normal. *Treatment:* Avoid/remove precipitants; transfusion if severe.

Pyruvate kinase deficiency Usually inherited as autosomal recessive; homozygotes often have neonatal jaundice; later, chronic haemolysis with splenomegaly and jaundice. *Diagnosis:* Enzyme assay. Often well tolerated. There is no specific therapy but splenectomy may help.

Drug-induced immune haemolysis Due to formation of new RBC membrane antigens (eg penicillin in prolonged, high dose), immune complex formation (many drugs, rare), or presence of autoantibodies to the RBC: α-methyldopa, mefenamic acid, L-dopa (rare, Coombs' +ve).

Autoimmune haemolytic anaemia (AHA) *Causes:* warm or cold antibodies. They may be primary (idiopathic) or secondary, usually to lymphoma or generalized autoimmune disease, eg SLE. *Warm AHA:* presents as chronic or acute anaemia. *Treatment:* steroids (± splenectomy). *Cold AHA:* chronic anaemia made worse by cold, often with Raynaud's or acrocyanosis. *Treatment:* keep warm. Blood transfusion is the main therapy, but chlorambucil may help. Mycoplasma and EBV may produce cold agglutinins, but haemolysis is rare.

Paroxysmal cold haemoglobinuria is caused by Donnath–Landsteiner antibody (seen in mumps, measles, chickenpox, syphilis) sticking to RBCs in cold, which causes complement-mediated lysis on rewarming.

Cardiac haemolysis Cell trauma in prosthetic aortic valves. It may indicate valve malfunction.

Microangiopathic haemolytic anaemia (MAHA) Suspect if marked fragmentation ± many microspherocytes on the film. Includes haemolytic-uraemic syndrome, TTP (p282), and pre-eclampsia. Treat underlying disease; blood and fresh frozen plasma (FFP) transfusions, plasma exchange.

Paroxysmal nocturnal haemoglobinuria RBCs are unusually sensitive to complement due to loss of complement-inactivating enzymes on their surface, causing pancytopenia, abdominal pain, or thrombosis (eg Budd–Chiari syndrome, p720) ± haemolysis. *Diagnosis:* Ham's test (*in vitro* acid-induced lysis) or test for GPI[1]-linked antigen loss. *Treatment:* Anticoagulation; blood product replacement; consider stem cell transplant.

Factors exacerbating haemolysis Infection often leads to increased haemolysis. Also parvoviruses (*OHCS* p214) cause cessation of marrow erythropoiesis, ie aplastic anaemia with no reticulocytes (p662).

---

1 GPI = Glucosylphosphatidylinositol.

Sickle-cell anaemia

Sickling disorders are due to the production of abnormal β peptide chains. An amino acid substitution in the gene coding for the β chain (Glu → Val at position 6), results in the production of HbS rather than HbA. Hb A_2 and HbF are still produced. It is common in Black Africans and their worldwide descendants. The homozygote (SS) has sickle-cell *anaemia* (HbSS) and hetero-zygotes (HbAS) have sickle-cell *trait*, which causes no disability (and may protect from *falciparum* malaria) except in hypoxia, eg in unpressurized aircraft or anaesthesia, when veno-occlusive events may occur, so all those of African descent need a sickling test pre-op. Symptomatic sickling occurs in heterozygotes with genes coding other analogous amino acid substitutions (eg HbSC and SD diseases). Homozygotes (CC; DD) have asymptomatic mild anaemia.

Pathogenesis HbS polymerizes when deoxygenated, causing RBCs to sickle. Sickle cells are fragile, and haemolyse; they also block small vessels.

Tests Hb ≈ 6–8g/dL; reticulocytes 10–20%: (haemolysis is variable); ↑Bilirubin. *Electrophoresis:* distinguishes SS, AS states, and other Hb variants. *Film:* all have target cells. Aim for diagnosis *at birth* (cord blood) to aid prompt pneumococcal prophylaxis (vaccine, p172, or penicillin V).

Signs & symptoms *Early:* Anaemia and jaundice, with painful swelling of hands and feet (hand and foot syndrome)—also splenomegaly (rare if >10yrs, as the spleen infarcts). Young sicklers alternate periods of good health with acute crises (below). *Later:* Chronic ill-health (previous crises): ie renal failure; bone necrosis; osteomyelitis; leg ulcers; iron overload from many transfusions. Long-term lung complications—hypoventilation, atelectasis, and lung infiltrates, is partly preventable by incentive spirometry—10 maximal inspirations/2h.

Sickle-cell crises These may be from thrombosis (the aptly named 'painful crises'), haemolysis (rare), marrow aplasia, or sequestration.

Thrombotic crises: Common, often causing severe pain. Precipitated by cold, dehydration, infection, ischaemia, eg muscular exertion. May mimic an acute abdomen or pneumonia. CNS signs: fits, focal signs. Transcranial Doppler can indicate risk of impending stroke (preventable by transfusion). Priapism may occur; if >24h, arrange prompt cavernosus-spongiosum shunting—prevents impotence; priapism also occurs in CML (p656).

Aplastic crises: These are due to parvoviruses, characterized by sudden leth-argy and pallor and few reticulocytes. Urgent transfusion is needed.

Sequestration/hepatic crises: (serious; may need exchange transfusion). Spleen and liver enlarge rapidly from trapped RBCs; signs: RUQ pain, INR/LFT↑, Hb↓↓.

Management of chronic disease

- Consider hydroxyurea (=hydroxycarbamide) if frequent crises.[1]
- Chronic blood transfusion programmes can keep HbS level <30%, but there is a high incidence of development of antibodies to red cell antigens.
- Marrow transplant can be curative, but remains controversial.
- Splenic infarction leads to hyposplenism and appropriate prophylaxis, in terms of antibiotic and immunization should be adopted.
- Febrile children risk septicaemia: repeated admission is avoided by out-patient ceftriaxone (eg 2 doses, 50mg/kg IV on day 0 and 1). Admission may still be needed, eg if Hb <5g/dL; WCC <5 or >30,000 × 10^9/L; severe pain; dehydration; lung infiltration. Seek expert advice.

Prevention Genetic counselling; prenatal tests (*OHCS* p210–12). Parental education can help prevent 90% of deaths from sequestration crises.

---

1 Long-term hydroxyurea causes ↑production of fetal haemoglobin and decreased fibre production via Hb polymerization, with 50% ↓ in both painful crises and episodes of the acute chest syndrome. These effects may result from fewer episodes of bone marrow ischaemia and embolization.

Management of sickle-cell crisis

▶Seek expert help.
- Give *prompt*, generous analgesia, eg with opiates (see p454).
- Crossmatch blood. FBC, reticulocytes, blood cultures, MSU, CXR.
- Rehydrate with IVI and keep warm.
- Give O_2 by mask if P_aO_2 ↓.
- 'Blind' antibiotics (p548) if feverish, after infection screen.
- Measure PCV, reticulocytes, liver, and spleen size twice daily.
- Give blood transfusion if PCV or reticulocytes fall sharply, or if there are CNS or lung complications—when the proportion of sickled cells should be reduced to <30%. This may require urgent exchange transfusion.

The acute chest syndrome entails pulmonary infiltrates involving complete lung segments, causing pain, fever, tachypnoea, wheeze, and cough. It is a serious condition. Incidence: ~0.1 episodes/patient/yr. 13% in the landmark Vichinsky's study needed ventilation, 11% had CNS symptoms, and 9% of those over 20 yrs old died. Prodromal painful crisis occur ~2.5d before any abnormalities on CXR in 50% of patients. The chief causes of the infiltrates are fat embolism from bone marrow, infection with *Chlamydia*, *Mycoplasma*, or virus, and sickled RBCs. *Bronchodilators* (eg salbutamol, p187) have proved to be very effective in 20% having wheezing or obstructive pulmonary function at presentation. *Antibiotics* have an important role. *Take to ITU if* P_aO_2 cannot be kept above 9.2kPa (70mmHg) when breathing air.

Red cell transfusion (C, E, and Kell antigen matched) improves oxygenation, and is as effective as exchange transfusion, which may be best reserved for those who are rapidly deteriorating.   E Vichinsky *NEJM* 2000 **342** 1855

Patient-controlled analgesia (PCA) An example with paediatric doses. First try warmth, hydration, and oral analgesia: ibuprofen 5mg/kg/6h PO (codeine phosphate 1mg/kg/4–8h PO up to 3mg/kg/d may also be tried, but is relatively ineffective). If this fails, see on the ward and offer prompt morphine by IVI—eg 0.1mg/kg. Start PCA with morphine 1mg/kg in 50mL 5% dextrose, and try a rate of 1mL/h, allowing the patient to deliver extra boluses of 1mL when needed. Do respiration and sedation score every ¼h + pulse oximetry if chest/abdominal pain. For further advice, liaise with your local pain clinic service.

Thalassaemia

The thalassaemias are genetic diseases of unbalanced Hb synthesis, as there is underproduction (or no production) of one peptide chain (OPPOSITE). Unmatched globins precipitate, damaging RBC membranes, causing their destruction while still in the marrow. They are common in a band going from the Mediterranean to the Far East.

The β thalassaemias (β^0/β^0, β^+/β^+, or β^+/β^0) are caused by mutations in β-globin genes on chromosome 11, leading to ↓β chain production (β^+) or its absence (β^0). Various combinations of mutations are possible (eg β^0/β^0, β^+/β^+, or β^+/β^0). Severity correlates with genetic deficit. The picture is usually one of severe anaemia presenting in the 1st year, often as failure to thrive. Death may result in 1yr without transfusion. With adequate transfusion, development is reasonably normal but symptoms of iron overload appear after 10yrs as endocrine failure, liver disease, and cardiac toxicity. Death is usually at 20–30yrs due to cardiac siderosis. Long-term infusion of desferrioxamine (=deferoxamine) prevents iron loading. If transfusion is inadequate, there is anaemia with reduced growth and skeletal deformity due to bone marrow hyperplasia, eg bossing of skull. Also splenomegaly, bleeding, and intermittent fever. The film shows very hypochromic, microcytic cells with target cells and nucleated RBCs. HbF ↑↑, HbA_2 variable, HbA absent. Prevalence of carriers: Cypriot 1 : 7; South Italy 1 : 10; Greek 1 : 12; Turkish 1 : 20; English 1 : 100.

β thalassaemia minor (eg β/β^+; heterozygous state): Recognized as MCV <75fL, HbA_2 >3.5% + mild, well-tolerated anaemia (Hb >9g/dL) which may worsen in pregnancy. Elevated HbA_2, slight ↑ HbF. Splenomegaly is rare.

The α thalassaemias The two separate α-globin genes are on chromosome 16. If all 4 α genes are deleted death is *in utero* (Bart's hydrops). If just 1 gene functions, anaemia is mild (+MCV↓). Some patients will have β^+/β^+ thalassaemia too, but less severely, as there are fewer unmatched α chains. α chain deficiency leads to excess β chains and β_4 tetramers (=Hb H; the fetal equivalent) or Hb Barts (physiologically useless γ_4). α^0/α^+ causes haemoglobin H disease with Hb ~8g/dL + hypersplenism. α/α^+ is 'silent'.

Thalassaemia intermedia and Hb variants These cause moderately severe anaemias which are usually transfusion-independent, eg Hb C thalassaemia (1 parent has the Hb C trait, and the other has β^+). Sickle-cell β^0 thalassaemia produces a picture similar to sickle-cell anaemia. HbE trait coupled with β^0 is common in India, and is similar to β^+/β^+ thalassaemia.

Diagnosis FBC, MCV, film, iron, HbA_2, HbF, Hb electrophoresis.

Treatment
- Transfusion to keep Hb >9g/dL.
- Iron-chelators, eg desferrioxamine (compliance may be a problem. Role of oral iron-chelators, eg deferiprone still under study) to protect against cardiac disease & DM, SE: WCC ↓, pruritus, LFTs ↑ scotomata, hearing ↓, risk of Yersinia infection ↑, hypogonadism.
- Large doses of ascorbic acid also increase iron output.
- Splenectomy if hypersplenism exists—give pneumococcal vaccination (p172) ± meningococcal vaccination.
- Folate supplements.
- A histocompatible marrow transplant can offer the chance of a cure.

Prevention Approaches are genetic counselling or antenatal diagnosis using fetal blood or DNA, then 'therapeutic' abortion.

Structure of haemoglobin

Adult haemoglobin (Hb) is a tetramer of 2 α- and 2 β-globin chains each containing a haem group. The three main types of Hb in adult blood are:

Type	Peptide chains	% in adult blood	% in fetal blood
HbA	$\alpha_2\,\beta_2$	97	10–50
HbA$_2$	$\alpha_2\,\delta_2$	2.5	Trace
HbF	$\alpha_2\,\gamma_2$	0.5	50–90

It might be thought that because the molecular details of the thalassaemias are so well worked out they represent a perfect example of the reductionist principle at work: find out *exactly* what is happening *within* molecules, and you will be able to explain all the manifestations of a disease. But this is not so. We have to recognize that two people with the identical mutation at their β loci may have quite different diseases. Co-inheritance of other genes and conditions (eg α thalassaemia) is part of the explanation, as is the efficiency of production of fetal haemoglobin. The reasons lie beyond simple co-segregation of genes promoting the formation of fetal Hb. The rate of proteolysis of excess α-globin chains may also be important—as may mechanisms that have little to do with genetic or molecular events. So the lesson the thalassaemias teach is more subtle than the reductionist one: it is that if you want to understand the *whole* picture, you must look at *every* level: genetic, molecular, physiological, social, and cultural. Each level influences the other, without necessarily determining them.

Further Reading:
See Draw Provan & John G Gribben 1999 *Molecular Haematology*, Blackwell

Bleeding disorders

After injury, 3 processes halt bleeding: vasoconstriction, gap-plugging by platelets, and the coagulation cascade. Disorders of haemostasis fall into these 3 groups. The pattern of bleeding is important—vascular and platelet disorders lead to prolonged bleeding from cuts, and to purpura and bleeding from mucous membranes. Coagulation disorders produce delayed bleeding after injury, into joints, muscle, and the GI and GU tracts.

Vascular defects *Congenital:* Osler–Weber–Rendu syndrome, p732. *Acquired:* senile purpura, angiodysplasia, steroids, trauma/pressure, vasculitis (p424), connective tissue disease, scurvy (perifollicular haemorrhages), and painful bruising syndrome—women who develop tingling under the skin followed by bruising over limbs/trunk, resolving without treatment.

Thrombocytopenia ↓*Production:* marrow failure; megaloblastosis. ↓*Survival:* Immune thrombocytopenic purpura (ITP); viruses; DIC; drugs; SLE; lymphoma; thrombotic thrombocytopenic purpura (TTP, p282); hypersplenism; genetic disease. *Platelet aggregation:* unfractionated heparin in 5% of patients. ITP may be chronic (♀:♂ ≈ 3 : 1) or acute (♀:♂ ≈ 1 : 1, eg in children, OHCS p275, 2wks after infection, with sudden self-limiting purpura). *Cause:* Antiplatelet autoantibodies lead to phagocytic destruction. Chronic ITP runs an indefinite fluctuating course of bleeding, purpura (especially dependent pressure areas), and epistaxis, often in young women. There is no palpable splenomegaly. CNS, conjunctival, and retinal haemorrhage are rare. *Tests:* Antiplatelet IgG autoantibodies +ve and many megakaryocytes in marrow. Also: ANA+ve in 44%; WCC↑ or ↔ ± eosinophilia. If symptomatic or platelets <20 × 10⁹/L, consider prednisolone (start at 1–2mg/kg/d; aim to keep platelets >30 × 10⁹/L—only takes a few days to work) ± splenectomy (cures ≤80%). If fails: immunosuppression, eg azathioprine, ciclosporin, or cyclophosphamide. Platelet transfusions are not used (except during splenectomy or life-threatening haemorrhage). IV immunoglobulin may temporarily raise the platelet count.

Causes of ↓platelet function Marrow diseases/dysplasia, NSAIDs, urea↑.

Coagulation disorders *Congenital:* haemophilia, von Willebrand's p736; *Acquired:* anticoagulants; liver disease; DIC (p650); malabsorption (vit K↓).

- **Haemophilia A** Factor VIII deficiency (inherited as a sex-linked recessive in 1/10,000 ♂ births—often because of a 'flip tip' inversion in the tip of the X chromosome. There is a high rate of new mutations (30% of affected children have no family history). *Presentation* depends on severity and is often early in life or after surgery/trauma—with bleeds into joints and muscle, leading to crippling arthropathy and haematomas with nerve palsies due to pressure. *Diagnose* by ↑KCCT and ↓factor VIII assay. *Management:* Seek expert advice. ***Avoid NSAIDs and IM injections***. Minor bleeding: pressure and elevation of the part. Desmopressin (0.4µg/kg/12–24h IVI in 50mL 0.9% saline over 20min) raises factor VIII levels, and may be helpful.

- **Major bleeds** (eg haemarthrosis) require factor VIII levels to be ↑ to 50% of normal. Life-threatening bleeds (eg obstructing airway) need levels to 100%, eg with virally inactivated lyophilized factor VIII. Genetic counselling: OHCS p212.

- **Haemophilia B (Christmas disease)** Factor IX deficiency (inherited, X-linked recessive); behaves clinically like haemophilia A.

- **Acquired haemophilia** is due to antibodies to factor VIII.

- **Liver disease** produces a complicated bleeding disorder with synthesis of clotting factors↓, absorption of vitamin K↓, and abnormalities of platelet function. *Malabsorption* leads to less uptake of vitamin K (needed for synthesis of factors II, VII, IX, and X). Treatment is parenteral vitamin K (10mg) or FFP for acute haemorrhage.

Anticoagulants See p648. DIC See p650.

The intrinsic and extrinsic pathways of blood coagulation

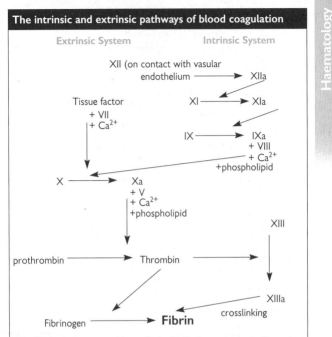

Extrinsic System   Intrinsic System

XII (on contact with vasular endothelium ⟶ XIIa

XI ⟶ XIa

Tissue factor
+ VII
+ Ca²⁺

IX ⟶ IXa
+ VIII
+ Ca²⁺
+phospholipid

X ⟶ Xa
+ V
+ Ca²⁺
+phospholipid

XIII

prothrombin ⟶ Thrombin

XIIIa
crosslinking

Fibrinogen ⟶ **Fibrin**

The fibrinolytic system causes fibrin dissolution and acts via the generation of plasmin. The process starts with the release of tissue plasminogen activator (t-PA) from endothelial cells, a process stimulated by fibrin formation. t-PA converts inactive plasminogen to plasmin which can then cleave fibrin, as well as several other factors. t-PA and plasminogen both bind fibrin thus localizing fibrinolysis to the area of the clot.

Mechanism of fibrinolytic agents

1 *Alteplase* (=rt-PA = Actilyse®; from recombinant DNA) is a fibrinolytic enzyme imitating t-PA, as above. Plasma $t_{1/2} \approx 5$min.

2 *Streptokinase* is a streptococcal exotoxin and forms a complex in plasma with plasminogen to form an activator complex which forms plasmin from unbound plasminogen. Initially there is rapid plasmin formation which can cause uncontrolled fibrinolysis. However, plasminogen is rapidly consumed in the complex and then plasmin is only produced as more plasminogen is synthesized. The activator complex binds to fibrin and so produces some localization of fibrinolysis.

An approach to bleeding

There are 3 sets of questions to be answered:

1 Is there an emergency?—needing resuscitation or immediate referral?
- Is the patient about to exsanguinate (shock, coma, p774-7)?
- Is there hypovolaemia (postural hypotension, oliguria)?
- Is there CNS bleeding (meningism, CNS, and retinal signs)?

2 Why is the patient bleeding? Is bleeding normal, given the circumstances (eg trauma or parturition), or does the patient have a bleeding disorder?
- Is there unexplained bleeding, bruising, or purpura?
- Past or family history of bleeding—trauma, dentistry, surgery? Drugs (warfarin). Alcohol. Liver disease. Recent illness.
- Is the pattern of bleeding indicative of vascular, platelet, or coagulation problems (p644)? Are venepuncture sites bleeding (DIC, p650)? Look for associated conditions (eg with DIC).
- Is a clotting screen abnormal? Check FBC, platelets, INR, KCCT + thrombin time. Consider bleeding time, FDP (below), and factor VIII assay.

3 In the case of a bleeding disorder, what is the mechanism?

Coagulation tests (Sodium citrate tube; false results if under-filled)
- *Prothrombin time (PT):* Thromboplastin is added to test the extrinsic system. PT is expressed as a ratio compared to control [International Normalized Ratio (INR), normal range (NR) = 0.9-1.2]. Prolonged by: coumarins (eg warfarin); vitamin K deficiency; liver disease (as above).
- *Thrombin time:* Thrombin is added to plasma to convert fibrinogen to fibrin. NR: 10-15s, ↑ in heparin treatment, DIC, or afibrinogenaemia.
- *Kaolin cephalin clotting time (KCCT, or APTT, = PTT = partial thromboplastin time):* Kaolin activates the intrinsic system. Normal range 35-45s, prolonged in heparin treatment or haemophilia.

Interpretation

Platelets: If low, do FBC, film, bone marrow biopsy.

INR: If long, look for liver disease or anticoagulant use.

KCCT: If long, consider factor VIII or IX deficiency, or heparin.

Bleeding time: If long, consider von Willebrand's disease (p736), or platelet disorders. Aspirin prolongs the bleeding time.

Disorder[1]	INR	KCCT APTT	Thrombin time	Platelet count	Bleeding time	Notes
Heparin	↑	↑↑	↑↑	↔	↔	
DIC	↑↑	↑↑	↑↑	↓	↑	FDP↑, p650
Liver disease	↑	↑	↔/↑	↔/↓	↔/↑	AST↑
Platelet defect	↔	↔	↔	↔	↑(↑)	
Vit K deficiency	↑↑	↑	↔	↔	↔	
Haemophilia	↔	↑↑	↔	↔	↔	see p644
von Willebrand's	↔	↑↑	↔	↔	↑(↑)	see p736

Special tests may be available (factor assays: ►consult a haematologist).

Management depends on degree of bleeding. If shocked, resuscitate (p778). If bleeding continues, in the presence of a clotting disorder, or a massive transfusion, discuss the need for FFP and platelets with a haematologist. In ITP (p644), steroids ± IV immunoglobulin may be used. Especially in pregnancy (OHCS p142), consult an expert. Is there overdose with anticoagulants (p830)? In haemophiliac bleeds, *consult early* for coagulation factor replacement. *Never give IM injections.*

---

1 After OTS, p215. FDP = fibrin degradation products.

Anticoagulants

The main indications for anticoagulation • DVT; pulmonary emboli.
• Stroke prevention: AF, or prosthetic heart valves. Treat indefinitely.
• Prevention of thromboembolism post-op in high-risk patients (p446).

Anticoagulants *Standard unfractionated (~13,000Da) heparin* (IV or SC). A glycosaminoglycan, which binds antithrombin (an endogenous inhibitor of coagulation), increasing its ability to inhibit thrombin, factor Xa, and IXa. Rapid onset and recovery; used perioperatively and in the treatment of thromboembolic disease (while warfarin is initiated) and unstable angina. Monitor activity using *activated partial thromboplastin time* (APTT).

Low molecular weight (LMW) heparin fragments (5000Da, eg dalteparin, enoxaparin, tinzaparin) Inactivates factor Xa (but not thrombin). T½ is 2–4-fold longer than standard heparin, and response is more predictable, so needs only be given once or twice daily SC, and no monitoring is usually required. Therefore, it can be used in outpatients. *Dose example in prophylaxis:* Dalteparin 2500U SC 2h pre-op +12h post-op, then 5000U daily for 5 days.

SE: Bleeding (at operative site, intracranial, retroperitoneal).

CI: Uncontrolled bleeding/risk of bleeding (eg peptic ulcer); endocarditis.

Warfarin is the most widely used coumarin (use phenindione if warfarin-sensitive). It is used orally once daily as long-term anticoagulation. The therapeutic range is narrow, varying with the condition being treated (see OPPOSITE)—and is measured as a ratio compared with a standard PT (the INR). Warfarin inhibits the reductase enzyme responsible for regenerating the active form of vitamin K, thus producing a state analogous to vit K deficiency *CI:* Peptic ulcer; bleeding disorders; severe hypertension; liver failure; endocarditis; cerebral aneurysms. Use with caution in the elderly and those with past GI bleeds. Use in pregnancy: OHCS p150. In the UK, warfarin tablets are 1mg (brown), 3mg (blue), or 5mg (pink). ▶Interactions: p712.

Others: Ximelagatran, a direct thrombin inhibitor, may provide an alternative to warfarin that does not require monitoring. Fondaparinux is a pentasaccharide Xa inhibitor and may be used in place of LMW heparin .

Beginning anticoagulation • Heparin 5000–10,000iu IV over 5min.
• Then add 25,000iu to 50mL 0.9% saline (=500iu/mL) in a syringe pump.
• Give 1000–2000iu/h IVI (2.8mL/h=1400iu/h). Check APTT at 6h. Institute the 5-d sliding scale below.

Measure APTT every 10h (every 4h if APTT >7, and stop the IVI).

APTT	5–7	4–5	3–4	2½–3	1½–2½	1.2–1.4	<1.2
Change rate (iu/h) by	–500	–300	–100	–50	0	+200	+400

• Alternatively, use low molecular weight heparin. Continue for 6d and until adequately anticoagulated with warfarin.
• Start warfarin 10mg PO at ~18.00 on day 1. Do INR 16h later (let lab know on warfarin). If <1.8 (as is likely) the 2nd dose of warfarin is 10mg at 17.00h (24h after first dose). If >1.8, give warfarin 0.5mg PO at 18.00h.
• Use the sliding scale below to keep INR in the target range. Do INR daily for 5d, then alternate days until stable, then weekly or less often.

INR	<2	2	2.5	2.9	3.3	3.6	4.1
3rd dose	10mg	5mg	4mg	3mg	2mg	0.5mg	0mg
Maintenance	≥6mg	5.5mg	4.5mg	4mg	3.5mg	3mg	*

Miss a dose; give 1-2mg the next day (if INR >4.5, miss 2 doses).
• Stop heparin when INR >2, and tell the lab no longer on heparin.

Antidotes Heparin: consult a haematologist. Stop anticoagulation; if further steps needed, protamine sulfate can counteract heparin: 1mg IVI neutralizes ~90U standard heparin given within 15min. Max dose: 50mg (if exceeded, may itself have anticoagulant effect). Warfarin: see p649.

Warfarin guidelines and target levels for INR

- Prosthetic heart valves. 3–4.9.[22] With higher risk valves (caged ball; tilting disc; mitral and aortic valves), aim perhaps for 4–4.9; with lower risk valves aim for ~3.
- Atrial fibrillation: Aim for 2–3 [23]. Cautious doctors may favour 2.5–3.5 (which offers a margin of error at both ends), particularly if the risk of stroke is low (no diabetes mellitus or past stroke or TIA, no hypertension; aged <65yrs).[24] An alternative (but a slightly less good one) for these low-risk patients is aspirin, particularly if the risk of bleeding is high (serious co-morbidity, or difficulty with monitoring INR).[25]
- Pulmonary embolism and above-knee DVT. Aim for INR of 2–3; 3.5 if recurrent.
- For QALY-based decision analysis on who needs warfarin in AF, see R Thomson 2000 Lancet 355 956

Duration of anticoagulation in DVT/PE (A rough guide)
- 6 weeks if the cause will go away (eg post-op immobility).
- 6 months if no cause found. Recently long-term, low-intensity anti-coagulation with warfarin (INR 1.5–2) has been found to be effective in reducing the risk of recurrence [26]; discuss the benefits/risks with your patients first.
- Indefinitely for identified, enduring causes, eg thrombophilia (p672).

Warfarin overdosage and excessive anticoagulation[27]

INR <6	Reduce warfarin dose or omit.
6–8	Stop warfarin. Restart when INR <5.
>8	If no bleeding: stop warfarin. 0.5–2.5mg vitamin K (oral) if risk factors for bleeding.
Major bleed	Stop warfarin, give prothrombin complex concentrate (≤50units/kg; check with haematologist), or FFP(15mL/kg ≈ 1L for a 70kg man). Give 5mg vit K IV. Get expert help.

Leukaemia and the house officer

Leukaemic patients often fall ill suddenly and deteriorate quickly. Prompt appropriate treatment is essential. Major concerns are infection, bleeding, hyperviscosity (p670). Take non-specific confusion/drowsiness seriously. Do blood cultures. Exclude hypoglycaemia. Measure renal function, LFT, and Ca^{2+}. Check clotting screen. Consider CNS bleeding. CT/MRI of brain if any doubt. Correct any haemostatic defect urgently with platelets/FFP. (See p372 for delirium)

Neutropenic regimen (for patients with a WCC ≤1.0 × 10^9/L)

►Close liaison with a microbiologist and haematologist is essential.

- Full barrier nursing if possible, but simple hand-washing is probably most important. Use a side room.
- Avoid IM injections (danger of an infected haematoma).
- Look for infection (mouth, perineum, axilla, IVI site). Take swabs.
- Check: FBC, platelets, INR, U&E, LFT.
- Take cultures (blood, urine, sputum, Hickman line) and order a CXR.
- Wash perineum after defecation. Swab moist skin with chlorhexidine. Avoid unnecessary rectal examinations. Oral hygiene (eg hydrogen peroxide mouth washes/2h) and Candida prophylaxis are important (p210).
- TPR 4-hrly. High-calorie diet; avoid foods with high risk of microbial contamination. Vases containing cut flowers pose a *Pseudomonas* risk.

Use of antibiotics in neutropenia

- Treat any known infection promptly.
- If T >38.5°C or T >38°C on separate occasions, 1–2h apart, or the patient is toxic, assume septicaemia and start blind broad spectrum antibiotics, eg antipseudomonal penicillin/cephalosporin and aminoglycoside. Vancomycin (p547) may be added if suspected Hickman line sepsis. Check local preferences.
- Continue antibiotics until afebrile for 5d and neutrophils recover (>0.5 × 10^9/L). If fever persists despite antibiotics, consider CMV or fungal infection (eg *Candida* or *Aspergillus*, p612).
- May need to consider treatment for *Pneumocystis* (see p581, eg co-trimoxazole, ie trimethoprim 20mg/kg with sulfamethoxazole 100mg/kg per day PO/IV in 2–4 divided doses). Also remember TB.
- Genetically engineered, recombinant human granulocyte-colony stimulating factor (rhG-CSF, or recombinant human granulocyte macrophage-colony stimulating factor, Gm-CSF) may be used to stimulate neutrophil production. Follow local guidelines, and seek expert advice.

Other dangers *Cell lysis syndrome:* Prevent K^+↑ and urate ↑ after massive destruction of cells, by giving a high fluid intake + allopurinol pre-cytotoxics. For patients at very high risk of cell lysis, eg children with high count ALL, recombinant uricase (rasburicase) may be indicated. Seek local specialist advice. *Hyperviscosity:* If WCC is >100 × 10^9/L WBC thrombi may form in brain, lung, and heart (leucostasis). Avoid transfusing before lowering WCC, eg with hydroxyurea or leukopheresis, as blood viscosity rises (risk of leucostasis ↑). If transfusional vital keep Hb <9g/dL. *Disseminated intravascular coagulation (DIC):* Pathological activation of coagulation mechanisms may occur in malignancy (also infection, trauma, or obstetrics, OHCS p142). Release of procoagulant agents leads to clotting factor and platelet consumption (consumption coagulopathy). Fibrin strands fill small vessels, haemolysing passing RBCs. *Signs:* Extensive bruising, bleeding, eg old venepuncture sites, renal failure, gangrene, bleeding anywhere. *Tests:* Consult lab, as special bottles are used. *Film:* broken RBCs (schistocytes). Platelets↓; PT↑; APTT↑; fibrinogen↓ (correlates best with severity); fibrin degradation products ↑. Blood may not clot in plain bottles. *Treat* the cause where possible; give supportive treatment, eg accurate fluid balance. Give 2 units of FFP IV at once while expert advice is sought. Platelets and blood may be needed. Role of heparin is controversial. The use of all transretinoic acid (ATRA) has significantly reduced the risk of DIC in acute promyelocytic leukaemia (the commonest leukaemia associated with DIC).

Acute lymphoblastic leukaemia (ALL)

Most leukaemias are initiated by specific gene mutations, deletions, or translocation.[1] ALL manifests as neoplastic proliferation of lymphoblasts. The latest WHO organization and classification of tumours divides these disorders into precursor B lymphoblastic leukaemia/lymphoblastic lymphoma and precursor T lymphoblastic leukaemia/lymphoblastic lymphoma. However, the immunological classification used below is still widely applied.

Immunological classification
- *Common (c) ALL:* (~75%) Defined by the presence of CD10. Phenotypically pre-B (ie the cells carry the same surface antigen as the pre-B lymphocyte). Any age may be affected, commonly 2–4-yr-olds. ♂ : ♀ ≈ 1 : 1.
- *T-cell ALL:* Any age but peak in adolescent males, eg presenting with a mediastinal mass and a high WCC.
- *B-cell ALL (Burkitt or Burkitt-like leukaemia):* Rare. Bad prognosis. Immunoglobulins present on blast cells.
- *Null-cell ALL:* Undifferentiated, lacking specific markers above.

Morphological classification The FAB system (French, American, British) divides ALL into 3 types (L1, L2, L3) by microscopic appearance. Although widely used, it provides only limited information compared with other systems.

Signs & symptoms are due to marrow failure: anaemia, infection, and bleeding. Also: bone pain, arthritis, splenomegaly, lymphadenopathy, thymic enlargement, CNS involvement—eg cranial nerve palsies.

Common infections: Zoster, CMV, measles, candidiasis, *Pneumocystis* pneumonia (p580–3), bacterial septicaemia. Consider use of immune serum for patients in contact with measles or zoster when on chemotherapy.

Diagnosis Characteristic cells in blood and bone marrow.

Treatment • *Supportive care:* Blood and platelet transfusions, IV antibiotics (p650) at the first sign of infection.
- *Preventing infections:* The neutropenic regimen (p650); prophylactic antibiotics (eg co-trimoxazole to prevent *Pneumocystis* pneumonia (p580)—but beware: this may worsen neutropenia).
- *Chemotherapy:* As in most leukaemias, patients are entered into national trials. A typical programme is in 4 steps:
  1 *Remission induction:* This may be achieved with vincristine, prenisolone, L-asparaginase, and daunorubicin.
  2 *CNS prophylaxis:* Intrathecal (or high-dose IV) methotrexate; CNS irradiation.
  3 *Consolidation:* High/medium-dose therapy in 'blocks' over several weeks.
  4 *Maintenance:* Prolonged chemotherapy, eg mercaptopurine (daily), methotrexate (weekly), and vincristine + prednisolone (monthly) for 2yrs. Relapse is common in blood, CNS, or testis (so examine these sites at follow-up). Cure rate in children: ~70%. More details: OHCS p190.

Haematological remission means no evidence of leukaemia in the blood, a normal or recovering blood count, and < 5% blasts in a normal regenerating marrow.

Marrow transplant (p654) Consider if poor prognosis. This is the only way to cure those showing t(9;22)—see below.

Quality of life Wigs for alopecia after chemotherapy. Avoid repeated venepuncture by using a Hickman CVP line; a central line with a long, Dacron®-cuffed, subcutaneous portion. **Bad prognosis if:** Adult; male; Philadelphia translocation [t(9;22) (q34:q11)], OHCS p190; presentation with CNS signs or WCC >100 × 10⁹/L; B-cell phenotype. Cure rates for children are 70–90%; for adults only 35% (0–20% if >60yrs old, where there is a 2nd peak in incidence).

The future may lie in tailoring therapy to the exact gene defect. PCR can monitor elimination of affected cells by standard drugs, monoclonal antibodies, gene-targeted retinoids, cytokines, vaccines, or T-cell infusions.

---

1 If this occurs *in utero*, some other promotional postnatal event is required (*Lancet* 1999 **354** 1499)

Acute myeloid leukaemia (AML)

This neoplastic proliferation of blast cells is derived from marrow myeloid elements. It is a very rapidly progressive malignancy (death in ~2 months if untreated; ~20% 3-yr survival after chemotherapy).

Morphological classification now based on WHO histological classification, which is complex and requires specialist interpretation. It recognizes the important prognostic information from cytogenetics and molecular genetics. 5 main types:-

• AML with recurrent genetic abnormalities.
• AML multi-lineage dysplasia.
• AML and myelodysplastic syndromes, therapy related.
• AML not otherwise categorized.
• Acute leukaemias of ambiguous lineage.

Incidence 1 in 10,000/yr. Increases with age. AML is getting more common as a long-term complication of chemotherapy, eg for lymphoma. **Assessment** 3 areas:

Marrow failure	*Leukaemic infiltration*	*Constitutional upset*
Anaemia	Bone pain; tender sternum	Malaise
Infection: often Gram –ve	CNS signs (cord compression, cranial nerve lesions)	Weakness, fever
Bleeding, eg petechiae	Gum, testes, orbit (proptosis)	*Other features:* poly-arthritis; skin/peri-anal
DIC (p650)	Hepatosplenomegaly Lymphadenopathy	involvement

Diagnosis WCC variable. Blast cells may be few in the peripheral blood, so diagnosis depends on bone marrow biopsy. Differentiation from ALL may be by microscopy (the presence of Auer rods), but is usually now based on immunotyping and molecular methods. Cytogenetic analysis (eg type of mutation) may affect treatment recommendations, and helps guide prognosis.

Complications Infection is the major problem, related to both the disease and its treatment. Be alert to septicaemia (p650). Oral infections are common. The place for prophylactic antibiotics is uncertain. Chemotherapy causes ↑plasma urate levels (from tumour lysis)—so give allopurinol with chemotherapy, and keep well hydrated with IV fluids. Big nodes can cause 'mass effects', eg dyspnoea. Leucostasis (p650) may occur if WCC ↑↑: get help.

Treatment *Supportive care:* Blood and platelet transfusions. Side room, IV antibiotics. *Pitfalls in diagnosis of infection:* AML itself causes fever, common organisms present oddly, few antibodies are made, rare organisms—particularly fungi (especially *Candida* or *Aspergillus*).

Chemotherapy is very intensive, resulting in long periods of neutropenia + platelets↓. The main drugs used include daunorubicin, and cytosine arabinoside. Prognosis: overall ~20% long-term survival, but ~40% for younger patients.

654

Bone marrow transplant (BMT) Allogeneic transplants from histocompatible siblings or from unrelated donors (accessed *via* international computer-held databases) or syngeneic transplants from a twin may be indicated in remissions. The idea is to destroy leukaemic cells and the immune system by cyclophosphamide + total body irradiation, and then repopulate the marrow by transplantation from a matched donor infused IVI. BMT allows the most intensive chemotherapy regimens because marrow suppression is not an issue. Cyclosporin (=ciclosporin) ± methotrexate may be used to reduce the effect of the new marrow attacking the patient's body (graft vs host disease). *Complications:* Graft vs host disease (may help explain the curative effect of BMT); infections ; veno-occlusive disease, relapse of leukaemia. *Prognosis:* Allogeneic ~60% long-term survivors. Autologous BMT is intermediate between allogeneic and chemotherapy. The role of reduced intensity conditioned allogeneic transplants is unclear at present. These transplants rely on the immunological effects of allogeneic transplantation (graft vs leukaemia affect) to achieve cure.

Chronic myeloid leukaemia (CML)

CML is characterized by uncontrolled proliferation of myeloid cells. It accounts for 15% of leukaemias. It is a myeloproliferative disorder (p664) having features in common with these diseases: eg splenomegaly (often massive). However, its unique features, see below, mean it is usually considered as a separate entity. It commonly presents with constitutional symptoms. It occurs most often in middle age, with a slight male predominance.

Philadelphia chromosome (Ph¹) A hybrid chromosome comprising translocation between the long arm of chromosome 9 and the long arm of chromosome 22—t(9;22). The Philadelphia chromosome is present in granulocyte, RBC, and platelet precursors in >95% of those with CML. Those without Ph¹ have a worse prognosis. (Some patients have a masked translocation—cytogenetics do not show the Ph¹, but the bcr/abl gene rearrangement is detectable by molecular genetic techniques.)

Symptoms Mostly chronic and insidious, eg weight↓, tiredness, gout, fever, sweats, bleeding, or abdominal pain. 10% are detected by chance.

Signs Splenomegaly, variable hepatomegaly, anaemia, bruising.

Tests WBC ↑↑ (often >100 × 10⁹/L), Hb↓ or normal, platelets variable. Urate and alk phos↑; B₁₂↑. Leucocyte alk phos↓ (on stained film).

Natural history Variable; median survival 3–5yrs; three phases: *chronic*, lasting months or years of few, if any, symptoms → *accelerated phase*, with increasing symptoms, spleen size, and difficulty in controlling counts→*blast transformation*, with features of acute leukaemia ± death.

Treatment See OPPOSITE.

Chronic lymphocytic leukaemia (CLL)

This is a monoclonal proliferation of small lymphocytes—almost always (99%) B-cells. The patient is usually over 40. Men are affected × 2 as often as women. CLL constitutes 25% of all leukaemias.

Staging (*Correlates with survival*)   0 Absolute lymphocytosis >15 × 10⁹/L. I Stage 0 + enlarged lymph nodes. II Stage I + enlarged liver or spleen. III Stage II + anaemia (Hb <11g/dL). IV Stage III + platelets <100 × 10⁹/L.

Symptoms (none in 25%) Bleeding, weight↓, infection, and anorexia.

Signs Enlarged, rubbery, non-tender nodes. Late hepatosplenomegaly.

Film Lymphocytosis may be marked. Often normochromic normocytic anaemia. Autoimmune haemolysis may contribute to this. Thrombocytopenia from marrow infiltration (rarely antiplatelet antibodies).

Complications (1) Autoimmune haemolysis. (2) Infection—bacterial (mostly of respiratory tract, as a result of hypogammaglobulinaemia) or viral (altered cell-mediated immunity). (3) Bone marrow failure.

Natural history Some remain in *status quo* for years, or even regress. Usually nodes slowly enlarge (± lymphatic obstruction). Death is often via infection (pneumococcus, haemophilus, meningococcus, *Candida*, aspergillosis), or transformation to aggressive lymphoma (Richter's syn.).

Treatment *Chemotherapy* is often not needed initially. Chlorambucil is used to ↓lymphocyte count, improve marrow function, and reduce node size. Dose: eg 0.1–0.2mg/kg daily PO. Steroids are used, eg in autoimmune haemolysis.

Radiotherapy: Use for relief of lymphadenopathy or splenomegaly.

Supportive care: Transfusions, prophylactic antibiotics, occasionally IV human immunoglobulin.

Prognosis Often good: depends on stage and molecular/immunological factors (eg ZAP70 or CD38 presence or absence).

Treatment of CML

- Imatinib mesylate (a specific tyrosine kinase inhibitor) has revolutionized the management of CML. It is more effective than the previous gold standard treatment of α-interferon, plus or minus cytarabine in chronic phase patients, in terms of preventing disease progression. It is likely that this will be translated into a survival advantage. The drug is also effective in patients in accelerated phase and blast crises.[1] Imatinib produces high haematological response rates (approximately 80–90%). Cytogenetic remissions are also common, but complete eradication of the Philadelphia clone, as detected by the most sensitive molecular methods is unusual (<5% patients). SE: nausea, vomiting, cramps, oedema, skin rash, cytopenias, abnormal LFT.
- Hydroxyurea (=hydroxycarbamide) may still be used in patients intolerant of Imatinib, or where Imatinib has proved ineffective. Busulfan is very rarely used now.
- Treatment of transformed CML is still problematic. Patients not previously treated with Imatinib may respond temporarily to this agent. Some patients with lymphoblastic transformation may benefit from treatment as for ALL. Treatment of myeloblastic transformation rarely achieves lasting remission and allogeneic transplantation offers the only hope of long-term survival.
- The role of allogeneic transplantation from a HLA matched sibling or unrelated donor is now unclear. Current guidelines suggest that this approach should be used 1st line only for patients in whom transplant related mortality will be very low (<10–15%). Other patients should be offered a trial of imatinib in the first instance.
- The use of α-interferon in CML has declined dramatically with the introduction of imatinib, but α-interferon may still have a role in combination therapy.
- The role of autologous transplantation, if any, in CML, remains to be defined.

1 We recognize that this advice is not congruent with NICE advice issued in 2003—but see L Maness 2004 Curr Hematol Rep 354 [@14695851]

Hodgkin's lymphoma

[Thomas Hodgkin, Guy's,^{UK} 1798–1866]

Lymphomas are malignant proliferations of lymphocytes; histologically divided into Hodgkin's and non-Hodgkin's types. In the former, characteristic cells with mirror-image nuclei occur (Reed–Sternberg cells). ♂:♀ ≈ 2:1; 2 peaks in incidence: young adults and elderly.

Classification (In order of incidence)	Prognosis
Classical Hodgkin's lymphoma	
Nodular sclerosing	Good
Mixed cellularity*	Good
Lymphocyte rich	Good
Lymphocyte-depleted*	Poor

Nodular lymphocyte predominant Hodgkin's lymphoma is now recognized as a separate entity, and behaves as an indolent B-cell lymphoma. *Higher incidence and worse prognosis if HIV +ve.

Symptoms Often presents with enlarged, painless nodes, eg in neck or axillae. 25% have constitutional upset, eg fever, weight loss, night sweats, pruritus, and lethargy. Rarely there may be alcohol-induced pain or features due to mass effects of nodes. The term *Pel-Ebstein fever* implies fever alternating with long periods (15–28 days) of normal or low temperature: it is, at best, rare—and some have called it mythical.[1]

Signs Lymph node enlargement; note position, consistency, mobility, size (in cm), tenderness. Cachexia, anaemia, hepatosplenomegaly.

Tests Lymph node biopsy—diagnosis. FBC, film, ESR, LFTs, LDH, urate, Ca^{2+}, CXR, bone marrow biopsy, CT/MRI thorax, abdo, pelvis. A raised ESR or anaemia indicate a worse prognosis.

Staging (Ann Arbor) Influences treatment and prognosis

I   Confined to single lymph node region.

II   Involvement of two or more regions on the same side of the diaphragm.

III Involvement of nodes on both sides of the diaphragm.

IV Spread beyond the lymph nodes.

Each stage is subdivided into '*A*'—no systemic symptoms other than pruritus; or '*B*'—presence of weight loss >10% in the last 6 months, unexplained fever >38°C, or night sweats. '*B*' indicates more extensive disease. Extranodal disease may be indicated by subscripted '*E*', eg I-A_E.

Treatment Radiotherapy for stages I_A and II_A (eg with ≤3 areas involved). Chemotherapy for II_A with >3 areas involved through to IV_B. Chemotherapy examples: 'ABVD': **A**driamycin, **B**leomycin, **V**inblastine, and **D**acarbazine. More intensive regimens used in poor prognosis or advanced disease. *Peripheral stem-cell transplantation:* Autologous or allogeneic transplantation of blood progenitor cells help restore marrow function after myeloablative therapy—as do agents that stimulate progenitor cells, eg rhG-CSF (Filgrastim® p650).

Complications of treatment: Hypothyroidism; lung fibrosis; other radiation SE (p442). Chemotherapy (p440): nausea, alopecia, infertility in men, infection, and second malignancies, especially AML and non-Hodgkin's lymphoma. Both may produce myelosuppression.

5-year survival Depends on stage and grade: >90% in IA lymphocyte-predominant disease; <40% with IVB lymphocyte-depleted.

Emergency presentations Infection; marrow failure (rare in Hodgkin's); SVC obstruction. This latter presents with: JVP↑, a sensation of fullness in the head, dyspnoea, blackouts, facial oedema. ►An emergency, seek expert help; high-dose corticosteroids (eg dexamethasone 8mg/12h) may also be useful. Is same-day radiotherapy needed? See p436.

1 Pel-Ebstein fever was dismissed by Richard Asher (*Talking Sense*, Pitman), as existing only thanks to its having been exotically named (the 1885 patients of Dr PK Pel had no histology, and fevers in Hodgkin's are *usually* non-specific). Another unfair reason for consigning it to myth is that the paper proving its existence (and its relation to cyclical changes in node size) does not come up in literature searches as Wilhelm *Ebstein* (1836–1912) is spelled *Epstein* throughout (*Cancer* 1975 **36** 2026)

Non-Hodgkin's lymphoma

This includes all lymphomas without Reed–Sternberg cells and is a very diverse group. Most are B-cell proliferations. Not all are centred on lymph nodes (extranodal tissues generating lymphoma include mucosa-associated lymphoid tissue—MALT; gastric MALT is associated with *H. pylori*, and may regress when this is eradicated). The overall incidence of lymphoma has doubled since 1970 (to 1 : 10,000) perhaps from immunosuppression from sunlight exposure, HIV, HTLV-1, EBV, and petrochemicals.

Signs & symptoms • Often symptomless • Lymphadenopathy • Extranodal spread occurs early (30% at presentation), so presentation may be in skin, bone, gut, CNS, or lung • Pancytopenia occurs (marrow dysplasia) • Infection is common • Systemic symptoms as in Hodgkin's lymphoma, p658).
Examine all over. Note nodes (if any is >10cm across, this represents bulk disease and may alter prognosis and management). Do ENT exam if GI lymphoma (GI and ENT lymphoma often co-exist).

Diagnosis & staging As for Hodgkin's (staging less important as 70% have widespread disease at presentation). Do node biopsy & CT/MRI (chest, abdomen, pelvis), FBC, U&E, LFT, LDH. Consider Ba meal/follow through, upper & lower GI endoscopy, cytology of any effusion; CSF cytology if CNS signs.

Histology This is something of a quagmire as classification systems are complex and changing. The current classification is based on the WHO classification of tumours of haemopoietic and lymphoid tissues. Diagnosis and management should be discussed using a multi-disciplinary team, which brings together information available from clinical evaluation, classical histology, immunology, molecular genetics, and imaging.

- Low-grade lymphomas are indolent but incurable. The more aggressive tumours include diffuse large B-cell lymphoma and lymphoblastic lymphomas (analogue of ALL).
- The high-grade types are more aggressive, but long-term cure is achievable. The high grade includes centroblastic, immunoblastic, and lymphoblastic (analogue of ALL).

Survival Worse if the patient is elderly or symptomatic, or there is bulky disease, or anaemia at presentation. Histology is also important. Typical 5-yr survival for treated patients: ~30% for high-grade and >50% for low-grade lymphomas, but the picture is very variable.

Treatment If symptomless and low grade, none may be needed. Chlorambucil or an alternative alkylating agent can control symptoms. Splenectomy may be of benefit in selected sub-groups. Radiotherapy can be used for local bulky disease. Purine analogues (eg fludarabine) are highly effective, either alone or in combination in this group of tumours. Temporary disease control may also be achieved with anti-CD20 monoclonal antibody (Rituximab). For diffuse large B-cell lymphoma, a variant of **CHOP:** **c**yclophosphamide, doxorubicin **h**ydrochloride, vincristine (**O**ncovin®) with **p**rednisolone and infusional anti-CD20 monoclonal antibody (Rituximab) may be used.[1] The addition of rituximab to this regime has produced the first major advance in the treatment of this disorder for 30yrs. **NB:** Only use if full resus facilities are available. Treatment of lymphoblastic lymphoma, Burkitt and Burkitt-like lymphomas, and the rare variants of non-Hodgkin's lymphoma should only be managed in units with particular expertise.

---

1 NICE advice: rituximab is indicated in CD20+ve diffuse large-B-cell lymphoma (DLBCL) at stage II, III, or IV. Do not use if CHOP is contraindicated. DLBCL denotes intermediate- to high-grade lymphomas that are rapidly fatal if untreated but often respond well to intensive chemotherapy. CD20 is a surface marker expressed on most B-cell lymphomas and testing for it is routine. CD20 occurs on normal and malignant B cells, but not on precursor B cells, so obviating long-term B cell depletion. Rituximab kills CD20+ve cells by antibody-directed cytotoxicity ± apoptosis induction. It also sensitizes cells to CHOP.

Pancytopenia, and bone marrow failure

The bone marrow is responsible for haemopoiesis and, in adults, is found in the vertebrae, sternum, ribs, skull, and proximal long bones, although it may expand in some anaemias (eg thalassaemia). All blood cells are thought to arise from an early, pluripotent stem cell, which divides in an asymmetric way to produce a committed progenitor and another stem cell. Committed progenitors then undergo further differentiation before their release as formed elements into the blood.

Bone marrow failure usually produces pancytopenia, often with sparing of lymphocyte count.

Causes of pancytopenia Bone marrow failure, below; hypersplenism; SLE, megaloblastic anaemia, paroxysmal nocturnal haemoglobinuria.

Causes of bone marrow failure

1 Stem cell failure: eg aplastic anaemia (see below).
2 Infiltration: eg malignancy, TB.
3 Fibrosis: eg myelofibrosis.
4 Abnormal differentiation of a genetically damaged clone of cells, eg myelodysplasia, HIV.

Aplastic anaemia

Presentation: Pancytopenia with hypoplastic marrow (ie the marrow stops producing cells). Presents as bleeding, anaemia, or infection.

Causes:
- Cytotoxic drugs/irradiation
- Autoimmune
- Inherited (Fanconi anaemia)
- Drugs (gold)
- Viral (hepatitis)

Incidence: 10–20 per million per year.

Treatment: Support the blood count (see below) while undertaking definitive treatment, which, for the severely affected young patient, is marrow transplantation. Otherwise, cyclosporin (=ciclosporin) and antithymocyte globulin may be effective.

Bone marrow support Red cells survive for ~120d, platelets for an average 8d, and neutrophils for 1–2d so early problems are mainly from neutropenia and thrombocytopenia.

Erythrocytes: A 1-unit transfusion should raise the Hb by ~1–1.5g/dL. See p464. Transfusion may drop the platelet count so it may be necessary to give platelets before and after.

Platelets: Spontaneous bleeding is unlikely if platelets >20 × 10⁹/L, but risk of traumatic bleeds is great if <40 × 10⁹/L. Platelets are stored at 22°C, should not be put in the fridge, and may require irradiation prior to use (eg if marrow transplant, or severely immunosuppressed). Indications for transfusion: counts <10 × 10⁹/L (not in ITP, p644), excessive bleeds, DIC (p650). Cross-matching is not needed but platelets should be ABO compatible (+Rh matched, if of child-bearing age). 4U of fresh platelets should raise the count to >40 × 10⁹/L in an adult. Check the dose required with the lab.

Neutrophils: Use a 'neutropenic regimen' if the count <0.5 × 10⁹/L. See p650. The place of neutrophil transfusions is unclear.

Bone marrow biopsy Ideally an aspirate *and* trephine should be taken, usually from the posterior iliac crest, although aspirates may also be taken from the anterior iliac crest or the sternum. Aspirates should be smeared promptly on to slides (≥8). Thrombocytopenia is rarely a contraindication. Severe coagulation disorders may need to be corrected. Apply pressure afterwards (lie on that side for 1–2h if platelets are low).

The myeloproliferative disorders

These form a group of disorders characterized by proliferation of precursors for myeloid elements—RBCs, WBCs, and platelets. While the cells proliferate, they also retain the ability to differentiate. The 4 disorders share several features, including the fact that all may present with constitutional symptoms such as fever, weight loss, night sweats, itch, and malaise.

Classification is by the cell type which is proliferating[1]:

RBC	→	Polycythaemia rubra vera (PRV).
WBC	→	Chronic myeloid leukaemia (CML, p656).
Platelets	→	Essential thrombocythaemia.
Fibroblasts	→	Primary myelofibrosis (reactive and not part of the malignant clone).

The blood count reflects 2 processes: the *proliferating cell line*—may involve other myeloid elements (eg in PRV, RBC↑; there may also be rises in WBC ± platelets too)—and *marrow fibrosis* which may ↓normal cell numbers.

Polycythaemia may be relative (plasma volume ↓) or absolute (RBC mass↑). *Relative polycythaemia* may be acute and due to dehydration (eg alcohol or diuretics). A more chronic form of relative polycythaemia exists and this is associated with obesity, hypertension, and a high alcohol and tobacco intake. *Absolute polycythaemia* is distinguished by the red cell mass estimation, using radioactive chromium, and may be primary (*polycythaemia rubra vera*) or secondary to hypoxia (eg chronic lung disease or congenital heart disease). Tumours which secrete erythropoietin, particularly renal carcinoma and hepatoma may be associated with polycythaemia.

Polycythaemia rubra vera *Cause:* Neoplasia of a clone from 1 multipotent cell whose erythroid progenitor offspring are unusual in being sensitive, to insulin-like growth factor ± interleukin-3, and in not needing erythropoietin to avoid apoptosis (p395). *Incidence:* 1.5/100,000/yr; peak age: 45–60yrs.

Signs: (determined by hyperviscosity) CNS signs, p670; angina; Raynaud's, p732; itch—typically after a hot bath and ↑RBC turnover (gout). It may also present with bruising, or after a routine FBC. ↑Spleen (in 60%).

Investigations: • ↑PCV • ↑WBC • ↑Platelets or normal • ↓MCV.

Raised red cell mass (>125% of predicted—^{51}Cr studies) and splenomegaly in the presence of normal P_aO_2 provide a diagnosis. Marrow shows erythroid hyperplasia. Leucocyte alk phos (LAP) usually↑ (↓ in CML). B₁₂↑.

Treatment: Refer. Aim to keep PCV <50%, eg by venesection or hydroxyurea (=hydroxycarbamide) if platelet count or WCC is difficult to control. In older patients, consider IV ^{32}P (it is leukaemogenic) or busulfan, ≤4mg/d PO.

Prognosis: Variable; many often remain well for many years but others will die from myelofibrosis, leukaemia, or thrombotic disorders from hyperviscosity and/or malfunctioning platelets. FBC every 3 months (minimum).

Essential thrombocythaemia Platelets ↑↑, eg 500–1000 × 10⁹/L, with abnormal morphology and function, causing bleeding; thrombosis; mononeuritis multiplex, and/or microvascular occlusion. *Treatment:* Hydroxyurea is used to lower platelet count. ^{32}P is used in older patients. Aspirin is useful (esp. if evidence of thrombotic complications). *Other causes of ↑platelet count:* Myeloproliferative or inflammatory disease (eg rheumatoid); bleeding; postsplenectomy. ~50% of those with un-explained ↑platelet count have malignancy.

Myelofibrosis Intense marrow fibrosis with haemopoiesis in the spleen and liver (myeloid metaplasia) causing massive splenomegaly. *Presentation:* Variable: systemic upset, splenomegaly, bone marrow failure. *Film:* Leucoerythroblastic (p628); teardrop RBCs. Hb ↓. Marrow tap: dry. *Treatment:* Supportive (p662): folate. *Other causes of marrow fibrosis:* Any myeloproliferative disorder, lymphoma, secondary carcinoma, TB, leukaemia, irradiation.

---

1 Each may undergo transformation to acute leukaemia.

Myeloma

Myeloma is a neoplastic proliferation of plasma cell with diffuse bone marrow infiltration and focal osteolytic lesions. A monoclonal immunoglobulin band is seen on serum and/or urine electrophoresis.

Incidence 5/100,000. Peak age: 70yrs. Sex ratio equal.

Classification Based on the principal neoplastic cell product:

- IgG   55%
- IgA   25%
- Light chain disease   20%

60% of IgG and IgA myelomas also produce free immunoglobulin (Ig) light chains which are filtered by the kidney and may be detectable as Bence Jones protein (these precipitate on heating and redissolve on boiling). They may cause renal damage and rarely, amyloidosis.

Signs & symptoms • Bone pain/tenderness is common, and often postural, eg back, ribs, long bones, and shoulder—not extremities. (25% have no clinical or x-ray signs of bone disease at presentation.) • Pathological fracture (eg rib) • Lassitude (from anaemia, renal failure, or dehydration via proximal tubule dysfunction, from light chain precipitation) • Pyogenic infection • Amyloidosis • Neuropathy • Signs of hyperviscosity (p670) • Visual acuity↓ ± haemorrhages/exudates on fundoscopy • Bleeding.

Investigations FBC, ESR↑, bone marrow, serum electrophoresis, urine electrophoresis, Ca^{2+}. Alk phos usually normal (unless healing fracture). Non-myeloma immunoglobulins↓; urea, creatinine, urate, and Ca^{2+}↑ in ~40%; β_2-microglobulin (prognostic); bone x-ray: punched-out lesions (pepper-pot skull), osteoporosis. Bone scintigrams may be normal. MRI may be useful particularly in the absence of a spinal disease.

Diagnosis see OPPOSITE.

Treatment *Supportive:* Bone pain, anaemia, and renal failure are the main problems, so give analgesia and transfusion as needed. Advise high fluid intake (important). All patients should receive a bisphosphonate (controls hypercalcaemia, improves bone pain, and reduces osteopenia and risk of fractures). Solitary lesions—radiotherapy produces effective local control of disease and relieves pain.

Chemotherapy: None is curative. 1st line is usually melphalan, either as a 4d course each month, or combined (eg with the ABCM regimen— **A**driamycin, **B**leomycin, **C**yclophosphamide, **M**elphalan). ~60% respond so that the paraprotein level falls before reaching a plateau phase. Treatment is usually stopped at this point, and restarted when the protein level begins to rise (escape phase). High-dose chemotherapy and autologous marrow transplantation improve results. Allogeneic transplantation may be curative in young patients. If hypercalcaemia is a problem, use bisphosphonates (see below and p696). Monitor FBC and paraprotein.

Death is commonly due to infection, renal failure, or haemorrhage.

Survival Worse if urea >10mmol/L or Hb <7.5g/dL. 50% alive at 2yrs.

Problems

1 Ca^{2+}↑↑: p696. Use IV saline 0.9% 4–6L/d with careful fluid balance. Consider steroids, eg hydrocortisone 100mg/8h IV. Intravenous bisphosphonates, eg pamidronate or zolendronate are useful acutely. Maintenance may be either with an IV or oral bisphosphonate.

2 Hyperviscosity (p670), causing cognition ↓, disturbed vision, and bleeding. Plasmapheresis can remove light chains (so helping renal function).

3 Acute renal failure may be precipitated by IVU.

Diagnosing myeloma

Diagnosis requires 1 major and 1 minor criteria to be met, or 3 minor (including the first 2).

Major

- Plasmacytoma on biopsy.
- >30% plasma cells on bone marrow biopsy.
- Monoclonal band on electrophoresis >35g/L for IgG, 20g/L IgA, or >1.0g of light chains excreted in the urine per day.

Minor

- 10–30% plasma cells on bone marrow biopsy.
- Abnormal monoclonal band but levels less than listed above.
- Lytic bone lesions.
- Immunosuppression (other immunoglobulins show reduced levels to <50% normal).

Paraproteinaemia

Paraproteinaemia denotes presence in the circulation of immunoglobulin produced by a single clone of plasma cells or their precursors. The paraprotein is recognized as a sharp M band (M for Monoclonal, not IgM) on serum electrophoresis.[1] There are 6 major categories:

1 *Multiple myeloma:* See p666.
2 *Waldenström's macroglobulinaemia:* This is a lymphoplasmacytoid malignancy producing an IgM paraprotein, lymphadenopathy, and splenomegaly. CNS and ocular symptoms of hyperviscosity may be a presenting feature (p670). Chlorambucil and plasmapheresis[1] (p670) may help.
3 *Primary amyloidosis:* See below.
4 *Monoclonal gammopathy* (benign paraproteinaemia) is common (3% >70yrs) and may be misdiagnosed as myeloma (but paraprotein level is stable and at low levels, marrow plasmacytosis <10%, no lytic bone lesions, and no myeloma-related symptoms).
5 *Paraproteinaemia in lymphoma or leukaemia:* Eg 5% of CLL.
6 *Heavy chain disease:* Production of free heavy chains. α chain disease is the most important, causing malabsorption from infiltration of small bowel wall. It may terminate in lymphoma.

Amyloidosis

This is a disorder characterized by extracellular deposits of an abnormal, degradation-resistant protein called amyloid. Various proteins, under a range of stimuli, may polymerize to form amyloid fibrils, which are detected by +ve staining with Congo Red and by showing apple-green birefringence in polarized light. There are 2 forms: systemic and local.

Systemic:
• Immunocyte dyscrasia (fibrils of immunoglobulin light chain fragments, known as 'AL' amyloid).
• Reactive amyloid ('AA' amyloid—a non-glycosylated protein).
• Hereditary amyloid (eg Type 1 familial amyloid polyneuropathy).

Localized: (rarer) • Bladder • Skin • CNS • Cardiac • Lung • Endocrine.

Types of amyloid *AL amyloid (primary amyloidosis):* ~50% have monoclonal proliferation of plasma cells (eg myeloma); 50% have no coexisting disease. *Symptoms:* Fatigue, weight↓, dyspnoea, faints, paraesthesiae, diarrhoea. *Signs:* Oedema (nephrosis or CCF, a typical cause of death); macroglossia (big tongue); hepatosplenomegaly; carpal tunnel syndrome; purpura around eyes; malabsorption signs (flat villi, p252).

AA amyloid (secondary amyloidosis): This occurs with chronic infections (eg TB, bronchiectasis), inflammation (especially rheumatoid arthritis), and neoplasia. It tends to affect kidneys, liver, and spleen, and commonly presents as proteinuria, nephrosis, and hepatosplenomegaly.

Diagnosis is made after Congo Red staining of affected tissue. The rectum is a favoured site for biopsy (eg +ve in 80%). ~50% have renal impairment at the time of diagnosis. An interesting, but rare, complication of amyloidosis is the intravascular absorption of factor X, causing a long PT and KCCT, and serious coagulopathy.

Treatment is difficult. AA amyloidosis may improve if the primary disease is treated. AL amyloidosis may respond to treatment as for myeloma. Patients with plasma cell myeloma and amyloidosis have a shorter survival than those with myeloma alone.

---

1 Electrophoresis and plasma *pheresis* look as though they should share endings, but they do not: Greek *phoros*=bearing (*esis*=process), but *aphairesis* is Greek for *removal*.

Erythrocyte sedimentation rate (ESR)

The ESR is a non-specific indicator of the presence of disease. It measures the rate of sedimentation of RBCs in anticoagulated blood over 1h. If certain proteins cover red cells, these will stick to each other in columns (the same phenomenon as rouleaux on the blood film, p628)—and so they will fall faster. The ESR rises with age and anaemia. A simple, reliable way to allow for this is to calculate the upper limit of normal, using the Westergren method, to be (for men) age in years ÷ 2. For women, the formula is (years+10) ÷ 2. In those with a slightly abnormal ESR, the best plan is probably to wait a month and repeat the test. The same advice does not hold true for patients with a markedly raised ESR (>100mm/h). In practice, most will have signs pointing to the cause—usually paraproteinaemias, other malignancy (almost always disseminated), connective tissue diseases (eg giant cell arteritis), rheumatoid arthritis, renal disease, sarcoidosis, or infection. There is a group of patients whose vague symptoms would have prompted nothing more than reassurance—were it not for a markedly raised ESR—and in whom there are no pointers to specific disease. The underlying disease (in 1 survey) turned out to include myeloma, giant cell arteritis, abdominal aneurysm, metastatic prostatic carcinoma, leukaemia, and lymphoma. Therefore, it would be wise (after history and examination) to consider these tests: FBC, plasma electrophoresis, U&E and creatinine, PSA, chest and abdominal x-rays, and biopsy of bone marrow or temporal artery.

Some conditions *lower* the ESR, eg polycythaemia, sickle-cell anaemia, and cryoglobulinaemia. Even a slightly raised ESR in these patients should prompt one to ask: *What else is the matter?*

If vacuum ESR tubes (Seditainer) are used, then lower values are recorded compared with the reference method, as follows:

Seditainer:	Reference:	Seditainer:	Reference:	Seditainer:	Reference:
10	11	30	40	50	75
15	18	35	47	55	87
20	25	40	56	60	100
25	32	45	65	65	118

For CRP (an alternative to the ESR), see p702.

Hyperviscosity syndrome

This may occur if the plasma viscosity rises to such a point that the microcirculation is impaired.

Causes: Myeloma (p666), Waldenström's macroglobulinaemia (p668, IgM ↑viscosity more than the same amount of IgG), polycythaemia. High leucocyte counts in leukaemia may also produce the syndrome (leucostasis).

Presentation: Visual disturbance, retinal haemorrhages, headaches, coma, and GU or GI bleeding.

The visual symptoms ('slow-flow retinopathy') may be described as 'looking through a watery car windscreen'. Other causes of slow-flow retinopathy are carotid occlusive disease and Takayasu's disease (p736).

Treatment: Removal of as little as 1L of blood may relieve symptoms. Plasmapheresis may help: in this process, blood is withdrawn and allowed to settle in a container. The supernatant plasma is discarded, and the RBCs returned to the patient after being resuspended in a suitable medium.

The spleen and splenectomy

The spleen was a mysterious organ for many years; we now know that it plays a vital immunological role by acting as a reservoir for lymphocytes, and in dealing with bacteraemias. Splenomegaly is a commonish problem and its causes are divided into *massive* (into the RIF) and *moderate*.

Causes of massive splenomegaly CML, myelofibrosis, malaria (hyper-reactive malarial splenomegaly), leishmaniasis, 'tropical splenomegaly' (idiopathic—Africa, SE Asia), and Gaucher's syndrome.

Moderate splenomegaly: Infection (eg malaria, EBV, endocarditis, TB), portal hypertension, haematological (haemolysis, leukaemia, lymphoma), connective tissue disease (RA, SLE), sarcoidosis, primary antibody deficiency (OHCS p201), CML, idiopathic. *Other causes:* p518.

Splenomegaly can be uncomfortable and may lead to *hypersplenism* (ie pancytopenia as cells become trapped in the spleen's reticuloendothelial system, with symptoms of anaemia, infection, or bleeding). When faced with a mass in the left upper quadrant, it is vital to recognize the spleen: ● It moves with respiration ● It enlarges towards the RIF ● You may feel a notch ● 'You can't get above it' (ie the top margin disappears under the ribs) ● Dull to percussion. Abdominal USS may help. When hunting the cause for enlargement look for lymphadenopathy and liver disease, eg with: FBC, ESR, LFT ± liver, marrow, or lymph node biopsy.

Splenectomy This may be indicated for severe splenic trauma, splenic cysts, splenic (and adjacent organ) tumours, and as part of the treatment of ITP (p644), autoimmune haemolysis, and, occasionally, for the staging of Hodgkin's disease. Postsplenectomy, mobilize early (transient ↑platelets predisposes to thrombi). ►*The main problem post-splenectomy is lifelong increased risk from infection.* Consider those with partial splenectomy also at risk. Reduce this risk by giving:

● Patient-held cards alerting health professionals to the infection risk.
● Pneumococcal vaccine (p172), >2 weeks pre-op to ensure good response. Avoid in pregnancy. Re-immunize every 5–10yrs.
● *Haemophilus influenzae* type b vaccine (p558)±meningococcal vaccine.
● Annual influenza vaccine (p572).
● Prophylactic oral antibiotics (phenoxymethylpenicillin) continuously until aged 16yrs, or for 2yrs postsplenectomy, whichever is longer.
● 'Standby' amoxicillin, to start *at once* if any symptoms of infection present.
● Warnings of risk of severe malaria, and other tropical infections.
● Urgent hospital admission if infection develops despite the above.

Thrombophilia

Thrombophilia (inherited or acquired) is a primary coagulopathy resulting in a propensity to thrombosis. **NB:** thrombocytosis (platelets↑) and polycythaemia also cause thrombosis. It is *not* rare, and it *is* treatable—and needs special precautions in *surgery, pregnancy,* and *enforced inactivity*. Be alert to it in non-haemorrhagic stroke, eg if <60yrs old, thrombosis at <45yrs (or family history). Risk is increased by obesity, immobility, trauma (accidents or surgery), pregnancy, and malignancy.

Inherited[1] *Activated protein C (APC) resistance:* Commonest cause of inherited thrombophilia. Usually associated with a single point mutation in factor V (=FV, ie V Leiden); present in ~5% healthy individuals. Thrombotic risk is increased in preg-nancy and those on oestrogen-containing oral contraceptives (risk ↑ by 30–35-fold in FV:Q heterozygous carriage, and by several 100-fold in homozygous carriage—and screening *might* be appropriate with the newly available modified test for APC resistance). There is ↑ risk of MI. *Prothrombin gene mutation:* High prothrombin levels. ~4% controls and ~20% of patients with venous thrombosis and a positive family history. *Protein C and protein S deficiency:* These vitamin K-dependent factors act together to neutralize factors V and VIII. Heterozygotes deficient for either protein risk thrombosis, and skin necrosis (especially if using oral anticoagulants). Homozygous deficiency for either protein causes neonatal purpura fulminans—fatal, if untreated. *Antithrombin III deficiency:* Less common, affects 1 : 500. Heterozygotes' thrombotic risk is 4-fold greater than protein C or S deficiency. Homo-zygosity is lethal.

Acquired Common causes and unmasking phenomena are new progesterones in the Pill (OHCS p66) and the *antiphospholipid syndrome* when serum antiphospholipid antibodies are found (lupus anticoagulant and/or anticardiolipin antibody)—predisposing to venous and arterial thrombosis, thrombocytopenia, and recurrent fetal loss in pregnant women. Most do not have SLE.

Investigation *Consider special tests if recurrent or unusual thrombosis:*

- Venous thromboembolism <40yrs
- Arterial thrombosis <30yrs
- Skin necrosis (especially if on warfarin)
- Familial thromboembolism
- Recurrent fetal loss
- Neonatal thrombosis

Liaise with a haematologist. Do FBC with platelets; PI; thrombin time; APTT; and fibrinogen concentration. Further tests: APC resistance (ratio), lupus anticoagulant and anticardiolipin antibodies, and looking for antithrombin III and proteins C and S deficiency. Haematologists may recommend looking directly for the V Leiden mutation, and prothrombin gene mutation, eg if already on warfarin, and other results are confusing. Ideally investigate while well, not pregnant, and not anticoagulated.

Treatment Treat acute thromboses with heparin, then warfarin. In antithrombin III deficiency, unusually high doses of heparin may be needed (dose is difficult to determine in those with lupus anticoagulant), so liaise with a haematologist—also in protein C or S deficiency, when skin necrosis may occur. *Prevention:* Counsel as regards the best form of contraception.[2] Advise TED stockings. Risk of recurrent thrombosis following DVT, PE, stroke, or TIA if antiphospholipid antibody +ve is ~30%/yr. Aspirin or warfarin (INR <3) ↓risk to ~20%. If INR >3 on warfarin, excess risk is ~nil. Pregnancy is a problem: warfarin is teratogenic. Get expert help, eg aspirin + heparin (≤10,000U/12h SC for those with ≥2 fetal losses). For those with <2 fetal losses, either giving no treatment or aspirin alone might be appropriate.

Before medium-to-major (especially orthopaedic) surgery, liaise with a haematologist. Antithrombin III/protein C concentrate may be needed, as well as more thorough prophylaxis against post-op thromboses.

---

1 See *Ann Int Med* 2003;**138:**128–34 for a comprehensive review.
2 Note: Screening with blanket exclusion of those with thrombophilia from the Pill is unwise. www.txt.co.uk/full.cfm?1035

Immunosuppressive drugs

As well as being used in leukaemias and cancers, these are used in organ and marrow transplants, rheumatoid arthritis, psoriasis, chronic hepatitis, asthma, giant cell arteritis, polymyalgia, SLE, PAN, and inflammatory bowel and other diseases (so this page could figure in almost any chapter).

Prednisolone Steroids can be life-saving, but a number of points should be taken into consideration before initiating treatment.
- Certain conditions may be made worse by steroids, eg TB, hypertension, osteoporosis, diabetes: here careful monitoring is needed.
- Growth retardation may occur in young patients, and the elderly frequently get more side effects from treatment.
- Interactions: [Prednisolone]↓ by antiepileptics (below) and rifampicin.
- Avoid pregnancy (may cause fetal growth retardation). If breast-feeding and prednisolone >40mg/day, see BNF.

Minimize side effects by using the lowest dose possible for the shortest period of time. Give doses in the morning, and alternate days if possible, to minimize adrenal suppression. Before starting long-term treatment, (>3 weeks, or repeated courses) observe these guidelines:
- Explain about not stopping steroids suddenly. Collapse may result, as endogenous production takes time to restart. ►►See p822.
- Inform about the need to consult a doctor if unwell, and increase the dose of steroid at times of illness/stress (eg flu or pre-op).
- Encourage to carry a steroid card saying dose taken, and the reason.
- You *must* warn patients about the listed side effects if they are receiving long-term treatment (over 6 weeks worth): see BOX.
- Avoid over-the-counter drugs, eg aspirin and ibuprofen (risk of DU etc).
- Prevent osteoporosis if long-term use (p698): exercise, alendronic acid.

Do not stop long-term steroids abruptly as adrenal insufficiency may occur. Once a daily dose of 7.5mg of prednisolone is reached, withdrawal should be gradual. Patients on short-term treatment should be withdrawn gradually if they had repeated courses of steroids, a history of adrenal suppression, greater than 40mg daily, or doses at night.

Azathioprine • SE: peptic ulcer, marrow suppression, WCC↓. Do FBCs.
- *Interactions:* mercaptopurine and azathioprine (which is metabolized to mercaptopurine) are metabolized by xanthine oxidase (XO). So azathioprine toxicity results if XO inhibitors are co-administered (eg allopurinol).

Cyclosporin (=ciclosporin) In transplant patients, 6mg/kg/d may be needed; in rheumatoid arthritis, keep the dose <4mg/kg/d.
- Monitor U&E and creatinine every 2 weeks for the first 3 months, then monthly if dose >2.5mg/kg/d (every 2 months if less than this). ►Reduce the dose if creatinine rises by >30% on 2 measurements *even if the creatinine is still in normal range*. Stop if the abnormality persists.
- Monitor blood levels in transplant patients.
- SE: nephrotoxicity, hepatotoxicity, oedema, gum hyperplasia, tremor, paraesthesiae, BP↑, confusion, seizures, lymphoma, skin cancer.
- Interactions are legion, eg [Ciclosporin]↑ by ketoconazole, diltiazem, verapamil, the Pill, erythromycin. [Ciclosporin]↓ by barbiturates, carbamazepine, phenytoin, rifampicin. Avoid concurrent nephrotoxics: eg gentamicin, concurrent NSAIDs augment hepatotoxicity: monitor LFTs.

Methotrexate An antimetabolite. Inhibits dihydrofolate reductase, which is involved in the synthesis of purines and pyrimidines. • SE: hepatitis, lung fibrosis, CNS signs, teratogenicity • [Methotrexate] ↑ by NSAIDs, aspirin, penicillin, probenecid.

Cyclophosphamide A fungal metabolite. • SE: carcino- and teratogenic, haemorrhagic cystitis.

Side effects of steroid use

System:	Adverse reactions:
Gastrointestinal	Pancreatitis
	Candidiasis
	Oesophageal ulceration
	Peptic ulceration
Musculoskeletal	Myopathy
	Osteoporosis
	Fractures
	Growth suppression
Endocrine	Adrenal suppression
	Cushing's syndrome
CNS	Aggravated epilepsy
	Depression; psychosis
Eye	Cataracts; glaucoma
	Papilloedema
Immune	Increased susceptibility to, and severity of infections, especially chicken pox.

NB: Steroids can also cause fever and leukocytosis; steroids only rarely cause leukopenia.

Explain in terms that patients understand: document this in the notes.

Clinical chemistry[1]

Contents

Relevant pages in other sections: Reference intervals (p710); IV fluids on the surgical wards (p462); acute renal failure (p272, p274).

On being normal in the society of numbers

Laboratory medicine reduces our patients to a few easy-to-handle numbers: this is the discipline's great attraction—and its greatest danger. The normal range (reference interval) is usually that which includes 95% of patients. If variation is randomly distributed, 2.5% of our results will be 'too high', and 2.5% 'too low' on an average day, when dealing with apparently normal people. This statistical definition of normality is the simplest. Other definitions are *normative*—ie stating what an upper or lower limit *should* be. For example, the upper end of the reference interval for plasma cholesterol may be given as 6mmol/L because this is what biochemists state to be the *desired* maximum, while the risk of CHD increases above 5.2mmol/L. 40% of people in some populations will have a plasma cholesterol greater than 6mmol/L and thus may be at increased risk. The WHO definition of anaemia in pregnancy is an Hb of <11g/dL, which makes 20% of mothers anaemic. This 'lax' criterion has the presumed benefit of triggering actions which result in fewer deaths by haemorrhage. So do not just ask 'What is the normal range?'—also enquire about who set the range, for what population, and for what reason.

►Normal values can have hidden historical, social, and political desiderata—just like the normal values novelists ascribe to their characters: '*…Conventions and traditions, I suppose, work blindly but surely for the preservation of the normal type; for the extinction of proud, resolute and unusual individuals… Society must go on, I suppose, and society can only exist if the normal, if the virtuous, and the slightly deceitful flourish, and if the passionate, the headstrong, and the too-truthful are condemned to suicide and to madness. Yes, society must go on; it must breed, like rabbits. That is what we are here for … But, at any rate, there is always Leonora to cheer you up; I don't want to sadden you. Her husband is quite an economical person of so normal a figure that he can get quite a large proportion of his clothes ready-made. That is the great desideratum of life…*' Ford Maddox Ford 1915 *The Good Soldier*, Penguin, p214 & p228

---

[1] We thank Dr R Horvath who is our Specialist Reader for this chapter.

The essence of laboratory medicine

Only do a test if the result will influence management. Make sure you look at the result! Explain to the patient where this test fits in to his or her overall plan of management. ▶Do not interpret laboratory results except in the light of clinical assessment (unless forced to by examiners).

▶If there is disparity: trust clinical judgement and repeat the test.

Reference intervals (normal ranges) are usually defined as the interval, symmetrical about the mean, containing 95% of results on the population studied. The more tests you run, the greater the probability of an 'abnormal' result of no clinical significance: see OPPOSITE.

Artefacts Delayed analysis for plasma potassium (p678).

Anion gap (AG) Reflects unmeasured anions (p682).

Biochemistry results: major disease patterns   (↑ = raised, ↓ = lowered)

Dehydration: Urea↑, albumin↑ (useful to plot change in a patient's condition). Haematocrit (PCV)↑, creatinine↑; also urine volume↓; skin turgor↓.

Renal failure: Creatinine↑, urea↑, AG↑, K^+↑, PO_4^{3-} ↑, HCO_3^- ↓.

Thiazide and loop diuretics: Sodium↓, potassium↓, bicarbonate↑, urea↑.

Bone disease:	Ca^{2+}	PO_4^{3-}	Alk phos
Osteoporosis	Normal	Normal	Normal
Osteomalacia	↓	↓	↑
Paget's	Normal	Normal	↑↑
Myeloma	↑	↑, normal	Normal
Bone metastases	↑	↑, normal	↑
1° Hyperparathyroidism	↑	↓, normal	Normal, ↑
Hypoparathyroidism	↓	↑	Normal
Renal failure (low GFR)	↓	↑	Normal, ↑

Hepatocellular disease: Bilirubin↑, AST↑ (alk phos slightly↑, albumin↓). For details of the differences between AST and ALT, see p255.

Cholestasis: Bilirubin↑, γGT↑↑, alk phos↑↑, AST↑.

Myocardial infarct: AST↑, LDH↑, CK↑, troponin T/I ↑ (p120).

Diabetes mellitus: Glucose↑, (bicarbonate↓ if acidotic).

Addison's disease: Potassium↑, sodium↓.

Cushing's syndrome: May show potassium↓, bicarbonate↑, sodium↑.

Conn's syndrome: May present with potassium↓, bicarbonate↑ (and high blood pressure). Sodium normal or ↑.

Diabetes insipidus: Sodium↑, plasma osmolality↑, urine osmolality ↓ (both hypercalcaemia and hypokalaemia may cause nephrogenic diabetes insipidus).

Inappropriate ADH secretion: Na^+↓ with normal or low urea and creatinine, plasma osmolality ↓. Urine osmolality ↑ (and > than plasma osmolality), urine Na ↑ (>20mmol/L).

Excess alcohol intake: Evidence of hepatocellular disease. Early evidence in γGT ↑, MCV↑, ethanol in blood before lunch.

Some immunodeficiency states: Normal serum albumin but *low* total protein (low as immunoglobulins are missing—also making crossmatching difficult because expected haemagglutinins are absent; OHCS p201).

Life-threatening biochemical derangements See p679.

The laboratory and ward tests

►Laboratory staff like to have contact with you.

A laboratory decalogue

1 Interest someone from the laboratory in your patient's problem.
2 Fill in the request form fully.
3 Give clinical details, not your preferred diagnosis.
4 Ensure that the lab knows who to contact.
5 Label specimens as well as the request form.
6 Follow the hospital labelling routine for crossmatching.
7 Find out when analysers run, especially batched assays.
8 Talk with the lab before requesting an unusual test.
9 Be thoughtful: at 1630h the routine results are being sorted.
10 Plot results graphically: abnormalities show sooner.

Artefacts and pitfalls in laboratory tests

- Do not take blood sample from an arm which has IV fluid running into it.
- Repeat any unexpected result before acting on it.
- For clotting time do not sample from a heparinized IV catheter.
- Serum K^+ is overestimated if sample is old or haemolysed (this occurs if venepuncture is difficult).
- If using Vacutainers, fill *plain* tubes first—otherwise, anticoagulant contamination from previous tubes can cause errors.
- Total calcium results are affected by albumin concentration (p694).
- INR may be overestimated if citrate bottle is underfilled.
- Drugs may cause *analytic* errors (eg prednisolone cross-reacts with cortisol). Be suspicious if results are unexpected.
- Food may affect result, eg bananas raise urinary HIAA (p250).

Using dipsticks Store dipsticks in a closed container in a cool, dry place, not refrigerated. If improperly stored, or past expiry date, do not use. For urine tests, dip the dipstick briefly in urine, run edge of strip along container and hold strip horizontally. Read at the specified time—check instructions for the type of stick. For haematuria, proteinuria, etc., see p258.

Urine specific gravity (SG) can be measured by dipstick. It is not a good measure of osmolality. Causes of low SG (<1.003) are: diabetes insipidus, renal failure. Causes of high SG (>1.025) are: diabetes mellitus, adrenal insufficiency, liver disease, heart failure, acute water loss. Hydrometers underestimate SG by 0.001 per 3°C above 16°C.

Sources of error in interpreting dipstick results

Bilirubin: False +ve: phenothiazines. False –ve: urine not fresh, rifampicin.

Urobilinogen: False –ve: urine not fresh. (Normally present in urine due to metabolism of bilirubin in the gut by bacteria and subsequent absorption.)

Ketones: L-Dopa affects colour (can give false +ve). 3-hydroxybutyrate gives a false –ve.

Blood: False +ve: myoglobin, profuse bacterial growth. False –ve: ascorbic acid.

Urine glucose: Depends on test. Pads with glucose oxidase are not affected by other reducing sugars (unlike Clinitest®) but can give false +ve to peroxide, chlorine; and false –ve with ascorbic acid, salicylate, L-dopa.

Protein: Highly alkaline urine can give false +ve.

Blood glucose: Sticks use enzymatic method and are glucose specific. A major source of error is applying too little blood (a large drop to cover the pad is necessary), and poor timing. Reflectance meters increase precision but introduce new sources of error.

Laboratory results: when to take action NOW

- On receiving a dangerous result, first check the name and date.
- Go to the bedside. If the patient is conscious, turn off any IVI (until fluid is checked: a mistake may have been made) and ask the patient how he or she is. *Any fits, faints, collapses, or unexpected symptoms?*
- Be sceptical of an unexpectedly wildly abnormal result with a well patient. Could the specimens have got muddled up? Is there an artefact? Was the sample taken from the 'drip' arm? (p694). A low calcium, eg may be due to a low albumin (p694). Perhaps the lab is using a new analyser with a faulty wash cycle? ►*When in doubt, repeat the test.*

The values chosen below are somewhat arbitrary and must be taken as a guide only. Many results less extreme than those below will be just as dangerous if the patient is old, immunosuppressed, or has some other pathology such as pneumonia.

Plasma biochemistry (beware electrocardiological ± CNS events, eg fits)

Calcium (corrected for albumin) >3.5mmol/L *If shortening Q–T interval on ECG (p94), then dangerous hypercalcaemia.* See p696.

Calcium (corrected for albumin) <2mmol/L + symptoms such as tetany or long Q–T = *Dangerous hypocalcaemia.* See p694.

Glucose <2mmol/L = *Hypoglycaemia. Glucose 50mL 50% IV if coma.*

Glucose >20mmol/L = *Severe hyperglycaemia. Is parenteral insulin needed?* See p818.

Potassium <2.5mmol/L = *Dangerous hypokalaemia, esp. if on digoxin.*

Potassium >6.5mmol/L = *Dangerous hyperkalaemia.* See p274.

Sodium <120mmol/L = *Dangerous hyponatraemia.* See p690.

Sodium >155mmol/L = *Dangerous hypernatraemia.* See p690.

Blood gases

P_aO_2 <8kPa = *Severe hypoxia. Give O_2.* Go to p192.

pH <7.1 = *Dangerous acidosis. Go to p682 to determine the cause.*

Haematology results

Hb <7g/dL with low mean cell volume (<75fL) or history of bleeding.
   This patient may need urgent transfusion (no spare capacity). See p464.

Platelets <40 × 10^9/L *May need a platelet transfusion; call a haematologist.*

Plasmodium falciparum seen Start antimalarials now. See p562.

ESR >30mm/h + headache *Could there be giant cell arteritis?* See p424.

CSF results

>1 neutrophil/mm^3 *Is there meningitis: usually >1000 neutrophils?* See p368.

Gram stain *Talk to a microbiologist; urgent blind therapy.* See p368.

Conflicting, equivocal, or inexplicable results ►Get prompt help.

Intravenous fluid therapy

(See also p462 & p688.)

If fluids cannot be given orally, they are normally given intravenously. Alternatives are via a central venous line or subcutaneously.

Three principles of fluid therapy

1 Maintain normal daily requirements. About 2500mL fluid containing roughly 100mmol sodium and 70mmol potassium per 24h are required. A good regimen is 2L of 5% dextrose and 1L of 0.9% saline every 30h with 20–30mmol of potassium per litre of fluid. Post-operative patients may need more fluid and more saline depending on operative losses. If the serum sodium is rising, then more dextrose and less saline is required.

2 Replace additional losses. The amount and type of fluid lost is a guide (check fluid charts, drainage bottles, etc.). Remember that febrile patients have increased insensible losses too. In practice, the problem is usually whether to give saline or dextrose. Most body fluids (eg vomit) contain salt, but less than plasma, and thus replacement will require a mixture of saline and dextrose. Shocked patients require resuscitation with saline, or a colloidal plasma expander, eg Dextran® or Haemaccel®, but not dextrose (caution in liver failure, see below). Note that Dextran® interferes with platelet function and may prolong bleeding. Patients with acute blood loss require transfusion with packed cells or whole blood. As a holding measure, colloid or saline may be used while blood is being crossmatched. If more than 1L is required then O-negative or group-specific blood should be used (see p778).

3 Special cases. Patients with *heart failure* are at greater risk of pulmonary oedema if given too much fluid. They also tolerate saline less well since Na^+ retention accompanies heart failure. If IV fluids must be given, use with care. Patients with *liver failure*, despite being oedematous and often hyponatraemic, have increased total body sodium, and saline should not be used in resuscitation; salt-poor albumin solution or blood should be given.

A note on fluids. *0.9% saline ('normal saline')* has about the same sodium content as plasma (150mmol/L) and is isotonic with plasma. *5% dextrose* is isotonic, but only contains 278mmol/L glucose, ie 50g/L (dextrose is glucose), and is a way of giving water, since the liver rapidly metabolizes all the glucose leaving only water. It provides little energy.

More concentrated glucose solutions exist, and may be used in the treatment of hypoglycaemia. They are hypertonic and irritant to veins. Therefore, care in their use is needed, and infusion sites should be inspected regularly, and flushed with saline after use. *Dextrose-saline (one-fifth normal saline)* is also isotonic, containing 30mmol/L of sodium and 4% glucose (222mmol/L). It has roughly the concentration of saline required for normal fluid maintenance, when given 10 hourly. Hypertonic and hypotonic saline solutions are available, but are for specialist use only.

▶Examine patients regularly to assess fluid balance, and look for signs of heart failure (p136), which can result if excess fluid is given. Excessive dextrose infusion may lead to water overload (p690).

▶Daily weighing helps to monitor overall fluid balance, as will fluid balance charts.

Acid–base balance

Arterial blood pH is closely regulated in health to 7.40 ± 0.05 by various mechanisms including bicarbonate, other plasma buffers, and the kidney. Acid–base disorders needlessly confuse many people, but if a few simple rules are applied, then interpretation and diagnosis are easy.

- pH <7.35 is an acidosis; pH >7.45 is an alkalosis.
- CO_2 is an acidic gas (normal concentration 4.7–6.0kPa).
- HCO_3^- is alkaline (normal concentration 22–28mmol/L).
- 1° changes in HCO_3^- are termed *metabolic*, and of CO_2 *respiratory*.

1 Look at the pH: is there an acidosis or alkalosis?
2 Is the CO_2 abnormal? If so, is the change in keeping with the pH (ie if there is an acidosis, is CO_2 raised)? If so it is a *respiratory* problem. If there is no change, or an OPPOSITE one, then the change is compensatory.
3 Is the HCO_3^- abnormal, and if so, is the change in keeping with the pH? If so the problem is a *metabolic* one.

An example
pH 7.05, CO_2 2.0kPa, HCO_3^- 8.0mmol/L.
There is an *acidosis*, and the CO_2 is low, and so is a compensatory change. The HCO_3^- is low, and is thus the cause; ie a *metabolic acidosis*.

Metabolic acidosis *pH↓, HCO_3^- ↓*
To help diagnosis, work out the anion gap (AG)—this estimates unmeasured anions (they are hard to measure directly). It is calculated as the difference between plasma cations (Na^+ and K^+) and anions (Cl^- and HCO_3^-): Normal range: 10–18mmol/L. It is a measure of 'fixed' or organic acids—eg phosphate, ketones, and lactate.

Causes of metabolic acidosis and increased anion gap:
Due to increased production of fixed/organic acids. HCO_3^- falls and unmeasured anions associated with the acids accumulate.
- Lactic acid (shock, infection, hypoxia)
- Urate (renal failure)
- Ketones (diabetes mellitus, alcohol)
- Drugs/toxins (salicylates, biguanides, ethylene glycol, methanol).

Causes of metabolic acidosis and normal anion gap:
Due to loss of bicarbonate or ingestion of H^+ ions (Cl^- is retained).
- Renal tubular acidosis
- Diarrhoea
- Drugs (acetazolamide)
- Addison's disease
- Pancreatic fistulae
- Ammonium chloride ingestion.

Metabolic alkalosis *pH↑, HCO_3^- ↑*
- Vomiting
- K^+ depletion (diuretics)
- Burns
- Ingestion of base.

Respiratory acidosis *pH↓ CO_2↑*
- Any lung, neuromuscular, or physical cause of respiratory failure (p192).

▶Look at the P_aO_2. It will probably be low. Is oxygen therapy required?
▶Use O_2 with care if chronic obstructive pulmonary disease (COPD) is the underlying cause, as too much oxygen may make matters worse (p188).

Respiratory alkalosis *pH↑, CO_2↓*
A result of hyperventilation.
CNS causes: Stroke, subarachnoid haemorrhage, meningitis.
Other causes: Anxiety, altitude, fever, pregnancy, drugs, eg salicylates.
Terminology: To aid understanding, we have used the terms acidosis and alkalosis, where a purist would sometimes have used acid-, alkal-aemia.

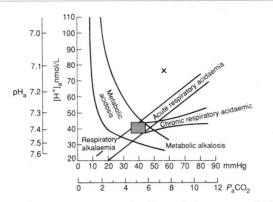

The shaded area represents normality. This method is very powerful. The result represented by point ×, eg indicates that the acidaemia is in part respiratory and in part metabolic. Seek a cause for each.

Kidney function

The kidney controls the elimination of many substances. It also makes erythropoietin, renin, and 1,25-dihydroxycholecalciferol. Filtered sodium is exchanged with potassium and hydrogen ions by exchanges and channels in the distal tubule. Glucose spills over into urine when plasma concentration is above renal threshold for reabsorption (≈10mmol/L, but varies from person to person, and is lower in pregnancy).

Creatinine clearance is a measure of glomerular filtration rate (GFR)—the volume of fluid filtered by glomeruli per minute. About 99% of this fluid is reabsorbed. Creatinine once filtered is only slightly reabsorbed. Thus:

[Creatinine]^{plasma} × creatinine clearance = [creatinine]^{urine} × urine flow rate

To measure creatinine clearance (normal value is ≈125mL/min). Collect urine over 24h. At the start, void and discard urine; from then on, and at end of 24h, void into the bottle. Take sample for plasma creatinine once during 24h. Use formula above. Take care with units. Major sources of error are calculation (eg units) and failure to collect all urine. If urine collection is unreliable, use formula:

$$\text{Creatinine clearance (mL/min)} = \frac{(140 - \text{age in years}) \times (\text{wt in kg})}{72 \times \text{serum creatinine in mg/dL}}$$

For women, multiply above by 0.85. Unreliable if: unstable renal function; very obese; oedematous. For an example adjusting for ideal body weight, see p256. (The protein : creatinine ratio in a spot morning urine is an alternative way to monitor chronic renal decline: see p258.) The conversion factor from μmol/L to mg/dL is 88.4; mg/dL = μmol ÷ 88.4.

Abnormal kidney function

There are three major biochemical pictures.

- **Low GFR** (classic acute renal failure)

  Plasma biochemistry: The following are raised: urea, creatinine, potassium, hydrogen ions, urate, phosphate, anion gap.

  The following are lowered: calcium, bicarbonate.

  Other findings: Oliguria.

  Diagnosis: Low GFR (creatinine clearance).

  Causes: Early acute oliguric renal failure (p272), long-standing chronic renal failure (p276).

- **Tubular dysfunction** (damage to tubules)

  Plasma biochemistry: The following are lowered: potassium, phosphate, urate, bicarbonate. There is acidosis. Urea and creatinine are normal.

  Other findings (highly variable): Polyuria with glucose, amino acids, proteins (lysozyme, β_2-microglobulin), and phosphate in urine.

  Diagnosis: Test renal concentrating ability (p326).

  Cause: Recovery from acute renal failure. Also: hypercalcaemia, hyperuricaemia, myeloma, pyelonephritis, hypokalaemia, Wilson's disease, galactosaemia, heavy metal poisoning.

- **Chronic renal failure:** As GFR reduces, creatinine, urea, phosphate and urate all increase. Bicarbonate (and Hb) decrease(s). Eventually potassium increases and pH decreases. There may also be osteomalacia.

Assessment of renal failure may need to be combined with other investigations to reach diagnosis, eg urine microscopy (p258), radiology (p260), or renal biopsy (in glomerulonephritis), or ultrasound.

Creatinine clearance: a worked example

Suppose:

urine creatinine concentration = u mmol/L;
plasma creatinine concentration = p μmol/L;
24h urine volume = v /mL.

There are 1440min/24h (used below to convert urine flow rate from volume per 24h into volume per minute). $p/1000$ is used to convert micromoles to millimoles.

Creatinine clearance = $u \times v/1440 \div p/1000$ mL/min

$u \times v/p \times 0.7$.

Thus, if: u = 5mmol/L; p = 120μmol/L; v = 2500mL;
creatinine clearance = $5 \times (2500/120) \times 0.7$
= 73mL/min.

Urate and the kidney

Causes of hyperuricaemia High levels of urate in the blood (hyperuricaemia) may result from increased turnover or reduced excretion of urate. Either may be drug-induced.

• *Drugs:* Cytotoxics; thiazides; pyrazinamide.
• *Increased cell turnover:* Lymphoma; leukaemia; psoriasis; haemolysis; muscle death (rhabdomyolysis, p281). *Tumour lysis syndrome:* See p436.
• *Reduced excretion:* Primary gout (p416); chronic renal failure; lead nephropathy; hyperparathyroidism; pre-eclampsia (*OHCS* p96).
• In addition: Hyperuricaemia may be associated with hypertension and hyperlipidaemia. Urate may be raised in disorders of purine synthesis such as the Lesch–Nyhan syndrome (*OHCS* p752).

Hyperuricaemia and renal failure Severe renal failure from any cause may be associated with hyperuricaemia, and very rarely this may give rise to gout. Sometimes the relationship of cause and effect is reversed so that it is the hyperuricaemia that causes the renal failure. This can occur following cytotoxic treatment (*tumour lysis syndrome*), eg in leukaemia; and in muscle necrosis.

How urate causes renal failure In some instances, ureteric obstruction from urate crystals occurs. This responds to retrograde ureteric catheterization and lavage. More commonly, urate precipitates in the renal tubules. This may occur at plasma levels ≥ 1.19 mmol/L.

Prevention of renal failure Before starting chemotherapy, ensure good hydration; consider alkalinization of the urine; and initiate allopurinol (a xanthine oxidase inhibitor), which prevents a sharp rise in urate following chemotherapy. For a specific dosage regimen, see p436. There is a remote risk of inducing xanthine nephropathy.

Treatment of hyperuricaemic acute renal failure Prompt rehydration and alkalinization of the urine after excluding bilateral ureteric obstruction. Once oliguria is established, haemodialysis is required and should be used in preference to peritoneal dialysis.

Gout See p416.

Electrolyte physiology

Most sodium is extracellular and is pumped out of the cell by the sodium pump, in exchange for K^+, which requires energy from ATP.

Osmolarity is the number of osmoles per *litre* of solution.
Osmolality is the number of osmoles per kilogram of solvent (*normal*: 280–300).
A *mole* is the molecular weight expressed in grams.

To estimate plasma osmolality: $2(Na^+ + K^+)$ + Urea + Glucose. If the measured osmolality is greater than this (ie an osmolar gap of >10mmol/L), consider: diabetes mellitus, high blood ethanol, methanol, or ethylene glycol.

Fluid compartments For 70kg man: *total fluid* = 42L (60% body weight). *Intracellular fluid* = 28L (67% body fluid), *extracellular fluid* = 14L (33% body fluid). *Intravascular component* = 5L of blood (3L plasma).

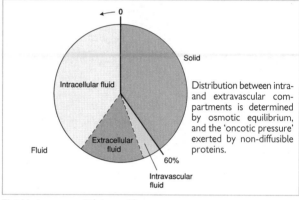

Distribution between intra- and extravascular compartments is determined by osmotic equilibrium, and the 'oncotic pressure' exerted by non-diffusible proteins.

Fluid balance over 24h is roughly:

Input (mL water)	Output (mL water)
Drink: 1500	Urine: 1500
In food: 800	Insensible loss: 800
Metabolism of food: 200	Stool: 200
Total: **2500**	Total: **2500**

Control of sodium *Renin* is produced by the juxtaglomerular apparatus in response to decreased renal blood flow, and catalyses the conversion *angiotensinogen* (a peptide made by the liver) to *angiotensin I*. This is then converted by angiotensin-converting enzyme (ACE, which is located in the lung and blood vessels) to *angiotensin II*. The latter has several important actions including efferent renal arteriolar constriction (so increasing perfusion pressure); peripheral vasoconstriction; and stimulation of the adrenal cortex to produce *aldosterone*, which activates the sodium pump in the distal renal tubule leading to reabsorption of sodium and water from the urine, in exchange for potassium and hydrogen ions.

High GFR (p684) results in high sodium loss.

High renal tubular blood flow and haemodilution decrease sodium reabsorption in the proximal tubule.

Control of water Controlled mainly by sodium concentration. ↑Plasma osmolality causes thirst, and the release of antidiuretic hormone (ADH) from the posterior pituitary which increases the passive water reabsorption from the renal collecting duct, by opening water channels to allow water to flow from the hypotonic luminal fluid into the hypertonic renal interstitium.

Natriuretic peptide

Secretory granules have long been known to exist in the atria, and if homogenized atrial tissue is injected into rats, their urine volume (and Na^+ excretion) rises. This is evidence of endocrine action via the effects of atrial natriuretic peptide (ANP). BNP is a similar hormone originally identified from pig brain (hence the B). Most of the BNP is secreted from ventricular myocardium. Plasma BNP is closely related to left ventricular pressure. In myocardial infarction and left ventricular dysfunction, these hormones can be released in large quantities. Secretion is also increased by tachycardia, glucocorticoids, and thyroid hormones. Vasoactive peptides (endothelin-1, angiotensin II) also influence secretion. ANP and BNP both increase GFR and decrease renal Na^+ resorption; they also decrease preload by relaxing smooth muscle. ANP partly blocks secretion of renin and aldosterone.

BNP as a biomarker of heart failure[1] As plasma BNP reflects myocyte stretch, BNP is used to diagnose heart failure. ↑BNP distinguishes heart failure from other causes of dyspnoea more accurately than left ventricular ejection fraction, ANP, and N-terminal ANP (sensitivity: >90%; specificity: 80–90%). BNP is highest in decompensated heart failure, intermediate in left ventricular dysfunction but no acute heart failure exacerbation, and lowest in those without heart failure or left ventricular dysfunction.

What BNP threshold for diagnosing heart failure? If BNP >100ng/L, this 'diagnoses' heart failure better than other clinical variables or clinical judgement in on-call settings (history, examination, and CXR). BNP can be used to 'rule out' heart failure if <50ng/L (negative predictive value (PV) 96%, ie the chance of BNP being <50ng/L given that heart failure is absent in 96%, see p26). In those with heart failure, BNP is higher in systolic dysfunction than in isolated diastolic dysfunction (eg hypertrophic or dilated cardiomyopathy), and is highest in those with systolic *and* diastolic dysfunction.

Threshold (ng/L)	Sensitivity (%)	Specificity (%)	Positive PV	Negative PV	Accuracy (%)
≥50	97	62	71	96	79
≥80	93	74	77	92	83
≥100	90	76	79	89	83
≥125	87	79	80	87	83
≥150	85	83	83	85	84[2]

BNP increases in proportion to right ventricular dysfunction, eg in primary pulmonary hypertension, cor pulmonale, PE, and congenital heart disease, but rises are less than in left ventricular disorders.

Prognosis in heart failure: The higher the BNP, the higher the cardiovascular and all-cause mortality (independent of age, NYHA class, p137, previous MI and LV ejection fraction). ↑BNP in heart failure is also associated with sudden death. Serial testing may be important: persistently high BNP levels despite vigorous anti-failure treatment predicts adverse outcomes. In one study, those with heart failure randomized to get N-terminal BNP-guided (rather than symptom-guided) therapy had fewer adverse events.

Prognosis in angina and MI: BNP has some prognostic value here (adverse left ventricular remodelling[3]; LV dysfunction; death post-MI).

Prognosis in cor pulmonale/primary pulmonary hypertension: BNP is useful.

Cautions with BNP A BNP >50ng/L does not exclude other coexisting diseases such as pneumonia. Also, assays vary, so liase with your lab.

1 Lemos J 2003 *Lancet* **362** 316 **2** Maisel A N *Engl J Med* 2002 **347** 161
3 Abnormal remodelling (cell slippage producing a more spherical LV + systolic dysfunction) is seen on echo or CT/MRI; it is measured as the *wall motion index* or the *left ventricular end-diastolic volume index* (EDVI, mL/m²). If EDVI ≥5mL/m² ~6 months post-MI (compared with an initial post-MI value), remodelling has occurred. *Sustained* ↑BNP reflects progressive ventricular remodelling long after acute MI. [@9918892] Abnormal remodelling is preventable in CCF by ACE-i and exercise training. [@9918892]

Sodium: hyponatraemia

Signs & symptoms depend on severity and rate of change in serum sodium, and include: confusion, seizures, hypertension, cardiac failure, oedema, anorexia, nausea, muscle weakness.

Diagnosis See tree in diagram OPPOSITE. The key question is: Is the patient dehydrated? History and urine analysis are your guides.

Causes of hyponatraemia (For a full list, see the diagram OPPOSITE.)
- *Diuretics*, especially thiazides.
- *Water excess*, either orally, or as excess 5% dextrose IV.
- *Pseudohyponatraemia*: (1) If serum volume↑ from high lipids or protein, Na^+ falls, but plasma osmolality is ↔. (2) If plasma glucose ≥20mmol/L, make a correction.[1] (3) Na^+ will be ↓ if blood is from an arm with a dextrose IVI.

Management ▶Don't base treatment on plasma Na^+ concentration alone. The presence of symptoms, duration, and state of hydration influence treatment. If possible, correct the underlying cause. If chronic: fluid restriction, or cautious rehydration with saline if dehydrated, is often sufficient if asymptomatic, although demeclocycline may be required. If symptomatic, saline may be given, but do not correct chronic changes rapidly (max 15mmol/d rise in serum sodium). Acute hyponatraemia may be treated with saline infusion and frusemide (=furosemide). *Hypervolaemic hyponatraemia* (cirrhosis, CCF) treat the underlying disorder. *In emergency* (seizures, coma), consider IVI of 0.9% saline or hypertonic saline (eg 1.8% saline) at 70mmol Na^+/h. Aim for a gradual increase in plasma sodium to ≈125mmol/L. Can combine with frusemide (furosemide). Watch for heart failure, and central pontine myelinolysis. ▶Seek expert help.

Syndrome of inappropriate ADH secretion (SIADH) An important, but over-diagnosed, cause of hyponatraemia. The diagnosis requires concentrated urine (sodium >20mmol/L & osmolality >500mosmol/kg) in the presence of hyponatraemia (<125mmol/L) or low plasma osmolality (<260mmol/kg), and the absence of hypovolaemia, oedema, or diuretics.

Causes: Malignancy, eg lung small-cell; pancreas; prostate; lymphoma.
CNS disorders: Meningoencephalitis; abscess; stroke; subarachnoid, subdural haemorrhage; head injury; Guillain–Barré; vasculitis, p424, eg SLE.
Chest disease: TB; pneumonia; abscess; aspergillosis.
Metabolic disease: Porphyria; trauma.
Drugs: Opiates; chlorpropamide; psychotropics; SSRIs; cytotoxics.
Treatment: Treat the cause, fluid restrict, occasionally demeclocycline.

Hypernatraemia

Signs & symptoms Look for thirst, confusion, coma, and fits—with signs of dehydration: dry skin, ↓skin turgor, postural hypotension, and oliguria if water deficient. Laboratory features: ↑PCV, ↑albumin, ↑urea.

Causes Usually due to water loss in excess of sodium loss:
- Fluid loss without water replacement (eg diarrhoea, vomit, burns).
- Incorrect IV fluid replacement (excessive saline).
- Diabetes insipidus (p326). Suspect if large urine volume. This may follow head injury, or CNS surgery, especially pituitary.
- Osmotic diuresis (for diabetic coma, see p818).
- Primary aldosteronism: suspect if BP↑, K^+↓, alkalosis (HCO_3^- ↑).

Management: Give water orally if possible; if not, dextrose 5% IV slowly (~4L/24h) guided by urine output & plasma Na^+. Some authorities recommend 0.9% saline (esp. if hypovolaemic) as this causes less marked fluid shifts and is hypotonic in a hypernatraemic patient. Avoid hypotonic solutions.

---

1 Add ~4.3mmol/L to plasma Na^+ for every 10mmol/L rise in glucose above normal. [@10225241]

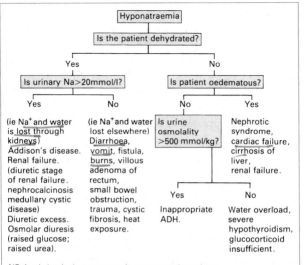

Hyponatraemia

Is the patient dehydrated?

Yes

Is urinary Na>20mmol/l?

Yes

(ie Na⁺ and water is lost through kidneys) Addison's disease. Renal failure. (diuretic stage of renal failure. nephrocalcinosis medullary cystic disease) Diuretic excess. Osmolar diuresis (raised glucose; raised urea).

No

(ie Na⁺ and water lost elsewhere) Diarrhoea, vomit, fistula, burns, villous adenoma of rectum, small bowel obstruction, trauma, cystic fibrosis, heat exposure.

No

Is patient oedematous?

No

Is urine osmolality >500 mmol/kg?

Yes

Inappropriate ADH.

No

Water overload, severe hypothyroidism, glucocorticoid insufficient.

Yes

Nephrotic syndrome, cardiac failure, cirrhosis of liver, renal failure.

NB: in cirrhosis, hyponatraemia may precede oedema.

691

Potassium

General points Most potassium is intracellular, and thus serum potassium levels are a poor reflection of total body potassium. The concentrations of K^+ and H^+ ions in extracellular fluid tend to vary together. This is because these ions compete with each other in the exchange with sodium which occurs across most cell membranes (sodium is pumped out of the cell) and in the distal tubule of the kidney (sodium is reabsorbed from the urine). Thus, if H^+ ion concentration is high, fewer K^+ ions will be excreted into the urine. Similarly K^+ will compete with H^+ for exchange across cell membranes and extracellular K^+ will accumulate. Insulin and catecholamines both stimulate K^+ uptake into cells by stimulating the Na^+/K^+ pump.

Hyperkalaemia

▶A plasma potassium >6.5mmol/L needs urgent treatment (p274) but first ensure that this is not an artefact (eg due to haemolysis inside the bottle).

Signs & symptoms Cardiac arrhythmias. Sudden death. *ECG:* Tall tented T waves; small P wave; wide QRS complex becoming sinusoidal, VF. (see OPPOSITE)

Causes

- Oliguric renal failure
- K^+-sparing diuretics
- Rhabdomyolysis (p281), burns
- Metabolic acidosis (DM)
- Excess K^+ therapy
- Addison's disease (see p312)
- Massive blood transfusion
- Drugs, eg ACE-i, suxamethonium
- Artefact. Haemolysis of sample; delay in analysis—K^+ leaks out of RBCs; thrombocythaemia—platelets leak K^+ as sample clots in tube.

Treatment Treat underlying cause. ▶In emergency, see p824.

Hypokalaemia

If K^+ <2.5mmol/L, urgent treatment is required. Note that hypokalaemia exacerbates digoxin toxicity.

Signs & symptoms Muscle weakness, hypotonia, cardiac arrhythmias, cramps, and tetany. *ECG:* Small or inverted T waves; prominent U wave (after T wave); prolonged P–R interval; depressed ST segment.

Causes

- Diuretics
- Vomiting and diarrhoea
- Pyloric stenosis
- Villous adenoma rectum
- Intestinal fistulae
- Cushing's syndrome/steroids/ACTH
- Conn's syndrome
- Alkalosis
- Purgative and liquorice abuse
- Renal tubular failure (p684)

If on diuretics, then ↑bicarbonate is the best indication that hypokalaemia is likely to have been long-standing. Magnesium may be low, and hypokalaemia is often difficult to correct until magnesium levels are normalized. In hypokalaemic periodic paralysis, intermittent weakness lasting up to 72h appears to be caused by K^+ shifting from extra- to intracellular fluid. See *OHCS* p756. Suspect Conn's syndrome if hypertensive, hypokalaemic alkalosis in someone not taking diuretics (p314).

Treatment *If mild:* (>2.5mmol/L, no symptoms) give oral K^+ supplement (≥80mmol/24h, eg Sando-K® 2 tabs/6–8h). If taking a thiazide diuretic, hypokalaemia >3.0mmol/L rarely needs treating. *If severe:* (<2.5mmol/L, dangerous symptoms) give IV potassium cautiously, not more than 20mmol/h, and not more concentrated than 40mmol/L. Do not give potassium if oliguric.
▶**Never** give potassium as a fast 'stat' bolus dose.

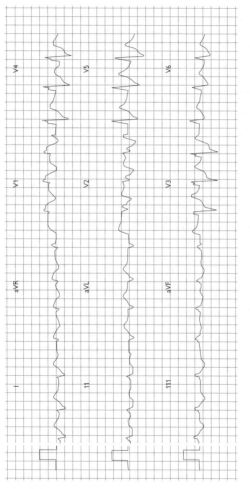

ECG 13—hyperkalaemia—note the flattening of the P-waves, prominent T-waves, and widening of the QRS complex.

Calcium: physiology

General points About 40% of plasma calcium is bound to albumin. Usually it is total plasma calcium which is measured although it is the unbound, ionized portion which is important. Therefore, *adjust total calcium level for albumin as follows:* Add 0.1mmol/L to calcium concentration for every 4g/L that albumin is below 40g/L, and a similar subtraction for raised albumin. However, many factors affect binding (eg other proteins in myeloma, cirrhosis, individual variation) so be cautious in your interpretation. If in doubt over a high calcium, take blood specimens uncuffed (remove tourniquet after needle in vein, but before taking blood sample), and with the patient fasted.

The control of calcium metabolism

- *Parathyroid hormone (PTH):* A rise in PTH causes a rise in plasma Ca^{2+} and a decrease in plasma PO_4^{3-}. This is due to $\uparrow Ca^{2+}$ and $\uparrow PO_4^{3-}$ reabsorption from bone; and $\uparrow Ca^{2+}$ but $\downarrow PO_4^{3-}$ reabsorption from the kidney. PTH secretion enhances active vitamin D formation. PTH secretion is itself controlled by ionized plasma calcium levels.
- *Vitamin D:* Calciferol (Vit D_3), and ergocalciferol (Vit D_2) are biologically identical in their actions. Serum Vit D is converted in the liver to 25-hydroxy Vit D (25(OH) Vit D). In the kidney, a second hydroxyl group is added to form the biologically active 1,25-dihydroxy Vit D (1,25(OH)$_2$ Vit D), also called calcitriol, or the much less active 24,25(OH)$_2$ Vit D. Calcitriol production is stimulated by $\downarrow Ca^{2+}$, $\downarrow PO_4^{3-}$, and PTH. Its actions include $\uparrow Ca^{2+}$ and $\uparrow PO_4$ absorption from the gut; $\uparrow Ca^{2+}$ and $\uparrow PO_4^{3-}$ reabsorption in the kidney; enhanced bone turnover; and inhibition of PTH release. Disordered regulation of 1,25(OH)$_2$ Vit D underlies familial normocalcaemic hypercalciuria which is a major cause of calcium oxalate renal stone formation (p264).
- *Calcitonin:* Made in C-cells of the thyroid, this causes a decrease in plasma calcium and phosphate, but its physiological role is unclear. It is a marker to detect recurrence or metastasis in medullary carcinoma of the thyroid.
- *Thyroxine:* May $\uparrow$plasma calcium although this is rare.
- *Magnesium:* $\downarrow Mg^{2+}$ prevents PTH release, and may cause hypocalcaemia.

Hypocalcaemia

▶Apparent hypocalcaemia may be an artefact of hypoalbuminaemia (above).

Signs & symptoms Tetany, depression, perioral paraesthesiae, carpo-pedal spasm (wrist flexion and fingers drawn together) especially if brachial artery occluded with blood pressure cuff (*Trousseau's sign*), neuromuscular excitability, eg tapping over parotid (facial nerve) causes facial muscles to twitch (*Chvostek's sign*). Cataract if chronic $Ca^{2+}\downarrow$. ECG: Q–T interval$\uparrow$.

Causes It may be a consequence of thyroid or parathyroid surgery. *If phosphate raised,* then either chronic renal failure (p276), hypoparathyroidism, pseudohypoparathyroidism (p308), or acute rhabdomyolysis. If phosphate $\leftrightarrow$ or $\downarrow$ then either osteomalacia (high alkaline phosphatase), over-hydration or pancreatitis. In respiratory alkalosis, the total Ca^{2+} may be normal, but ionized $Ca^{2+}\downarrow$ and the patient may have symptoms because of this.

Treatment If *symptoms are mild,* give calcium 5mmol/6h PO. Do daily plasma calcium levels. ▶For chronic renal failure, see p276. If necessary add alfacalcidol; start at 0.5–1µg/24h PO. If *symptoms are severe,* give 10mL of 10% calcium gluconate (2.25mmol) IVI over 30min (bolus injections are only needed very rarely). Repeat as necessary. If due to respiratory alkalosis, correct the alkalosis.

Hypercalcaemia

Signs & symptoms 'Bones, stones, groans, and psychic moans'. Abdominal pain; vomiting; constipation; polyuria; polydipsia; depression; anorexia; weight loss; tiredness; weakness; BP↑; confusion; pyrexia; renal stones; renal failure; corneal calcification; cardiac arrest. ECG: Q–T interval↓.

Causes & diagnosis Most commonly malignancy (myeloma, bone metastases, PTHrP↑, p308) and 1° hyperparathyroidism. Others include sarcoidosis, vit D intoxication, and familial benign hypocalciuric hypercalcaemia (rare; defect in calcium-sensing receptor). Pointers to malignancy are: ↓albumin, ↓Cl⁻, ↓K⁺, alkalosis, ↓ PO_4^{3-}, ↑alk phos. Other investigations (eg isotope bone scan, CXR, FBC) may also be of diagnostic value.

Treat the underlying cause. If Ca^{2+} >3.5mmol/L, and severe abdominal pain, vomiting, pyrexia, or confusion, aim to reduce calcium as follows:

- Blood tests: Measure U&E, Mg^{2+}, creatinine, Ca^{2+}, PO_4^{3-}, alk phos.
- Fluids: Rehydrate with IVI 0.9% saline, eg 4–6L in 24h as needed. Correct hypokalaemia/hypomagnesaemia (mild metabolic acidosis needs no treatment). This will reduce symptoms, and ↑renal Ca^{2+} loss. Monitor U&E.
- Diuretics: Frusemide (=furosemide) 40mg/12h PO/IV, once rehydrated. Avoid thiazides.
- Bisphosphonates: A single dose of pamidronate (see table, p437) will lower Ca^{2+} over 2–3d. Maximum effect is at 1wk. They inhibit osteoclast activity, and so bone resorption.
- Steroids: Occasionally used, eg prednisolone 40–60mg/d for sarcoidosis.
- Salmon calcitonin: Now rarely used (8U/kg/8h IM). More side effects than bisphosphonates, but quicker onset. Again inhibits osteoclasts.
- Other: Chemotherapy may ↓Ca^{2+} in malignant disease, eg myeloma.

Magnesium

Magnesium is distributed 65% in bone and 35% in cells; plasma concentration tends to follow that of Ca^{2+} and K^+. Magnesium excess is usually caused by renal failure, but rarely requires treatment in its own right.

Magnesium deficiency causes paraesthesiae, fits, tetany, arrhythmias. Digitalis toxicity may be exacerbated. *Causes:* Severe diarrhoea; ketoacidosis; alcohol; total parenteral nutrition (monitor weekly); accompanying hypocalcaemia; accompanying hypokalaemia (especially with diuretics) and hypophosphataemia. *Treatment:* If needed, give magnesium salts, PO or IV (dose example: 8mmol $MgSO_4$ IVI over 3min to 2h, depending on severity; monitor Mg^{2+} often).

Hypermagnesaemia is usually iatrogenic, or excessive antacids. *Features:* Neuromuscular depression, ↓BP, CNS depression, coma.

Zinc

Zinc deficiency This may occur in parenteral nutrition or, rarely, from a poor diet (too few cereals and dairy products; anorexia nervosa; alcoholism). Rarely it is due to a genetic defect. *Signs & symptoms:* Look for red, crusted skin lesions especially around nostrils and corners of mouth. *Diagnosis:* Therapeutic trial of zinc (plasma levels are unreliable as they may be low, eg in infection or trauma, without deficiency).

Selenium

An essential element present in cereals, nuts, and meat. Low soil levels in some parts of Europe and China cause deficiency states. Required for the antioxidant glutathione peroxidase, which ↓harmful free radicals. It is also antithrombogenic, and is required for sperm motility proteins. Deficiency may increase the frequency of neoplasia and atheroma, and may lead to a cardiomyopathy or arthritis. Serum levels are a poor guide. Toxic symptoms may also be found with overenergetic replacement.

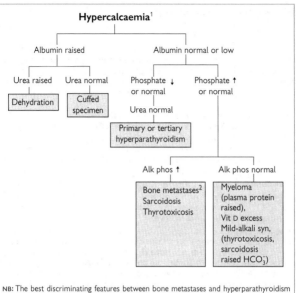

NB: The best discriminating features between bone metastases and hyperparathyroidism (the 2 commonest causes of hypercalcaemia) are low albumin, low chloride, alkalosis (all suggesting metastases). Raised plasma PTH strongly supports hyperparathyroidism.

1 This diagram is only a guide: take in conjunction with the clinical picture.
2 Most common primary: breast, kidney, lung, thyroid, prostate, ovary, colon.

Metabolic bone diseases

1. Osteoporosis

Osteoporosis implies reduced bone density. If trabecular bone is mostly affected, crush fractures of vertebrae are common (accounting for the littleness of little old ladies—and their dowager's hump); if cortical bone is mostly affected, fracture of a long bone is more likely, eg femoral neck: *the* big cause of death and orthopaedic expense, especially in older women. *Prevalence:* 5%. $\female : \male \approx 4 : 1$.

Risk of future osteoporotic fracture is increased if:
- Slender or anorectic
- Smoker or alcoholic
- Prolonged rest; old age
- Hyperparathyroidism
- >5mg/d prednisolone
- Vertebral deformity
- Early menopause
- Cushing's disease
- Malabsorption
- Thyrotoxicosis
- Myeloma
- Amenorrhoea
- Osteoporosis in family
- Primary biliary cirrhosis
- Rheumatoid arthritis
- Hypogonadism
- Past low-trauma fracture
- Mastocytosis (OHCS p602).

Diagnosis: X-ray (easier with hindsight afforded by bone fracture). Serum Ca^{2+}, PO_4^{3-}, and alk phos normal. Bone densitometry (OPPOSITE). Biopsy specimens may be unrepresentative.

Prevention: Exercise: good, Ca^{2+}-rich diet; avoid smoking and excess alcohol. For those at ↑risk, eg on corticosteroids (eg >7.5mg/d of prednisolone), bisphosphonates ↓risk. **NB:** hormone replacement therapy (HRT) can prevent osteoporosis, but the UK Committee on Safety of Medicines (CSM) says that owing to HRT's propensity to cause breast cancer (and other problems) it should no longer be a first-line option for preventing osteoporosis.

Treatment: Ca^{2+}-rich diet.
- *Bisphosphonates* are used for the prevention and treatment of osteoporosis. eg Didronel PMO® (14d of etidronate 400mg/d & 76d of calcium carbonate 1.25g in 90-d cycles), or alendronic acid 10mg/d (SE: abdo pain; nausea; photosensitivity, oesophageal ulcers). ►Explain the need to swallow the pill while remaining upright (for >30min) with plenty of water 20min before breakfast (and any other drugs); stop if dysphagia or pain. A single weekly dose is available (70mg). It is important to maintain a good calcium and vit. D intake, so consider adding a daily supplement.
- *Others:* Vitamin D is effective [?] (watch serum Ca^{2+}). Raloxifene (a selective oestrogen receptor modulator 'SERM') may also ↓ breast cancer risk. Its role is unclear. Calcitonin may be considered; reduces pain post vertebral fracture (now available intra-nasally). Recombinant PTH may soon be available, and seems effective in preventing fractures. [?]

2. Paget's disease of bone

There is increased bone turnover associated with increased numbers of osteoblasts and osteoclasts with resultant remodelling, bone enlargement, deformity, and weakness. Rare in the under-40s. Incidence rises with age (3% over 55yrs old). Commoner in temperate climes, and Anglo-Saxons. It may be asymptomatic or cause pain and enlargement of skull, femur, clavicle—and bowed (*sabre*) tibia—also pathological fractures, nerve deafness (bone overgrowth), and high-output CCF. *X-rays:* Localized enlargement of bone. Patchy cortical thickening with sclerosis, osteolysis, and deformity (*osteoporosis circumscripta* of the skull). Affinity for axial skeleton, long bones, and skull. *Blood biochemistry:* Ca^{2+} and PO_4^{3-} normal; alk phos markedly raised. *Complications:* Bone sarcoma (1% of those affected for >10yrs). Symptoms of nerve compression, eg deafness. *Treatment:* If analgesia fails, alendronic acid (see above) may be tried, to reduce pain and/or deformity. It is more effective than etidronate or calcitonin, and as effective as IV pamidronate. Follow expert advice.

Understanding Dexa bone scan results: WHO osteoporosis criteria

Typical sites examined are the lumbar spine (preferably 3 vertebrae) and hip. Bone mineral density (BMD, in g/cm^2) is compared with that of a young healthy adult. The 'T-score' relates to the number of standard deviations the BMD is from the average. If the T-score is:

>0	BMD is better than the reference.
0 to –1	BMD is in the top 84%: no evidence of osteoporosis.
–1 to –2.5	Osteopaenia, with risk of later osteoporotic complication, so consider preventive measures (see OPPOSITE).
–2.5 or worse	BMD is ≥2.5 standard deviations below the mean value for young adults: osteoporosis is present—severe if there is 1 or more fragility fracture.

An example of a suitable indication for densitometry is before embarking on prednisolone treatment (>6 months, at >7.5mg/d; steroids contribute to osteoporosis by promoting osteoclast bone resorption, and decreasing muscle mass and ↓GI Ca^{2+} absorption).

Benefits of universal screening for osteoporosis are unproven.

Further reading:
See Masud 2000 *BMJ* ii 397 www.bmj.com/cgi/content/full/321/7258/396

3. Osteomalacia

In osteomalacia there is a normal amount of bone but its mineral content is low (there is excess uncalcified osteoid and cartilage). Rickets is the result if this process occurs during the period of bone growth; osteomalacia is the result if it occurs after fusion of the epiphyses.

Forms

Vitamin D deficiency: Due to malabsorption (p252), poor diet, or lack of sunlight.

Renal osteomalacia: Renal failure leads to 1,25-dihydroxycholecalciferol—[1,25(OH)₂vitamin D] deficiency (p694).

Drug-induced: Anticonvulsants may induce liver enzymes, leading to an increased breakdown of 25-hydroxycholecalciferol.

Vitamin D resistance: A number of mainly inherited conditions in which the osteomalacia responds to high doses of vitamin D (see below).

Liver disease: Reduced production of 25-hydroxy vitamin D (25(OH)-vitamin D), and malabsorption of vitamin D, eg cirrhosis (p232).

Tests

Plasma: Mildly $\downarrow$Ca²⁺; $\downarrow$PO₄³⁻; alk phos↑; 25(OH)vitamin D↓, except in resistant cases; in renal failure 1,25(OH)₂vitamin D↓ PTH (p694) high.

Biopsy: Shows incomplete mineralization.

X-ray: Cupped, ragged metaphyseal surfaces (in rickets). In osteomalacia there is a loss of cortical bone; also, apparent partial fractures without displacement may be seen especially on the lateral border of the scapula, inferior femoral neck and medial femoral shaft (Looser's zones).

Signs & symptoms

Rickets: Knock-kneed; bow-legged. Features of hypocalcaemia (p694). Children with rickets are ill.

Osteomalacia: Bone pain; fractures (neck of femur); proximal myopathy (waddling gait), due to $\downarrow$PO₄³⁻ and vitamin D deficiency *per se*.

Treatment Calcium-with-vitamin D (400U) tablets: 1–2 tablets/d.

- If due to malabsorption, give calciferol tablets, up to 1mg (=40,000U) daily or parenteral calciferol, eg 7.5mg monthly.
- If vitamin-D-resistant, give calciferol 10,000 units/24h PO.
- If due to renal disease, give alfacalcidol (1α-hydroxy vitamin D) 1µg/24h PO and adjust dose according to plasma calcium.
- Monitor plasma calcium, initially weekly, and if nausea/vomiting.

▶Vitamin D therapy (esp. alfacalcidol) can cause dangerous hypercalcaemia.

Vitamin D-resistant rickets exists in 2 forms. Type I with low renal 1α-hydroxylase activity, and type II with end organ resistance to 1,25(OH)₂vitamin D, due to a point mutation in the receptor. Both are treated with large doses of 1,25(OH)₂vitamin D (calcitriol).

X-linked hypophosphataemic rickets Dominantly inherited—due to a defect in renal phosphate handling (due to mutations in the PEX or PHEX genes which encode an endopeptidase). Rickets develops in early childhood and is associated with poor growth. Plasma phosphate is low, alkaline phosphatase high, and there is phosphaturia. Treatment is with high doses of oral phosphate, and 1,25(OH)₂vitamin D. Hypophosphataemic osteomalacia may develop in patients consuming phosphate binders, eg aluminium hydroxide, or some rare tumour, and is accompanied by severe muscle weakness.

See also Renal bone disease, p276.

Plasma proteins

Electrophoresis distinguishes a number of bands (see figure OPPOSITE).

Albumin is synthesized in the liver; $t_{\frac{1}{2}} \approx 20d$. It binds *bilirubin*, *free fatty acids*, *calcium*, and some *drugs*. *Low albumin* results in oedema. *Causes:* Liver disease, nephrotic syndrome, burns, protein-losing enteropathy, malabsorption, malnutrition, late pregnancy, artefact (eg from arm with IVI), posture (5g/L higher if upright), genetic variations, malignancy. *High albumin—Causes:* Dehydration; artefact (eg stasis).

α_1 zone: α_1-antitrypsin, thyroxine-binding globulin, and high-density lipoprotein (HDL). α_1-antitrypsin deficiency (autosomal recessive) leads to cirrhosis and emphysema: unopposed phagocyte proteases. Accelerated age-related decline in FEV_1 from a normal of ~35mL/yr to 80mL/yr, exacerbated by smoking. Signs: dyspnoea; weight↓; cor pulmonale; PCV↑; LFT↑ (hepatocytes cannot secrete the protein).

α_2 zone: α_2-macroglobulin, caeruloplasmin, very low density lipoprotein (VLDL, p706), and haptoglobin (p636).

β zone: Transferrin, low-density lipoprotein (LDL), fibrinogen, C3 and C4 complement. Reduced in active nephritis, glomerulonephritis, and SLE.

γ zone: Immunoglobulins, factor VIII, C-reactive protein (CRP), and α-fetoprotein. *Diffusely raised* in: chronic infections, liver cirrhosis, sarcoidosis, SLE, RA, Crohn's disease, TB, bronchiectasis, PBC, hepatitis, and parasitaemia. It is *low* in: nephrotic syndrome, malabsorption, malnutrition, immune deficiency (severe illness, diabetes mellitus, renal failure, malignancy, or congenital).

Paraproteinaemia See p668.

Acute phase response The body responds to a variety of insults with, amongst other things, the synthesis, by the liver, of a number of proteins (normally present in serum in small quantities)—eg α_1-antitrypsin, fibrinogen, complement, haptoglobin, and CRP. An increased density of the α_1- and α_2-fractions, often with a reduced albumin level, is characteristic of conditions such as infection, malignancy (especially α_2-fraction), trauma, surgery, and inflammatory disease.

CRP Levels help monitor inflammation/infection. Normal <8mg/L. Like the ESR, it is raised in many inflammatory conditions, but changes more rapidly; increases in hours and falling within 2–3d of recovery. Therefore, it can be used to follow the response to therapy (eg antibiotics) or disease activity (eg Crohn's disease). CRP values in mild inflammation 10–50mg/L; active bacterial infection 50–200mg/L; severe infection or trauma >200mg/L; see OPPOSITE. CRP levels also predict outcome in patients with cardiovascular disease if measured using a highly sensitive assay. Low risk <1mg/L; moderate risk 1–3; and high risk >3mg/L.

Urinary proteins

If urinary protein loss >0.15g/24h, then pathological. See p258.

Albuminuria Usually caused by renal disease. Microalbuminuria (protein excretion between 3 & 300mg/d may be seen with diabetes or hypertension).

Bence Jones protein consists of light chains excreted in excess by some patients with myeloma (p666). They are not detected by dipsticks and may occur with normal serum electrophoresis.

Haemoglobinuria p638. Myoglobinuria p281. Microalbuminuria (seen in DM; ↑BP; SLE; glomerulonephritis)—see p283 for role in diabetes.

CRP

Marked elevation	Normal-to-slight elevation
Bacterial infection	Viral infection
Abscess	Steroids/oestrogens
Crohn's disease	Ulcerative colitis
Connective tissue diseases (except SLE)	SLE
	Atherosclerosis
Neoplasia	
Trauma	
Necrosis (eg MI)	

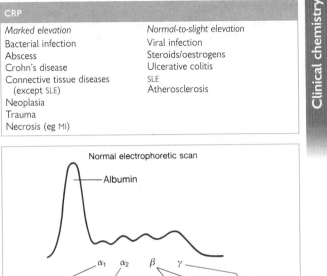

Normal electrophoretic scan

— Albumin

α_1 α_2 β γ

α_1-Antitrypsin α_2 Macroglobulin haptoglobin   Transferrin some LDL β_1 β_2 C_3 Immunoglobulins

Plasma enzymes

▶Reference intervals vary between laboratories.

Raised levels of specific enzymes can be a useful indicator of a disease. However, remember that most can be raised for other reasons too. The major causes of *raised enzymes* are given below. Normal values: see p714.

Alkaline phosphatase

- Liver disease (suggests cholestasis).
- Bone disease (isoenzyme distinguishable, reflects osteoblast activity) especially Paget's, growing children, healing fractures, osteomalacia, metastases, 1° hyperparathyroidism, and renal failure.
- Pregnancy (placenta makes its own isoenzyme).

Alanine-amino transferase (ALT; SGPT)

- Liver disease (suggests hepatocyte damage). Also raised in shock.

α-Amylase

- Acute pancreatitis (Not chronic pancreatitis as little tissue remaining).
- Severe uraemia, diabetic ketoacidosis.

Aspartate-amino transferase (AST; SGOT)

- Liver disease (suggesting hepatocyte damage).
- Myocardial infarction (p120).
- Skeletal muscle damage and haemolysis.

Creatine kinase (CK)

- Myocardial infarction (p120; isoenzyme 'CK-MB'. MI diagnosed if CK-MB>6% total CK, or CK-MB mass >99 percentile of normal).
- Muscle damage (rhabdomyolysis, p281; prolonged running; haematoma; seizures; IM injection; defibrillation; bowel ischaemia; myxoedema; dermatomyositis, p420)—and *drugs* (eg statins—p114 & p706). ▶A raised CK does not necessarily mean an MI.

Gamma-glutamyl transferase (GGT, γGT)

- Liver disease (particularly alcohol-induced damage, cholestasis, drugs).

Lactate dehydrogenase (LDH)

- Myocardial infarction (p120).
- Liver disease (suggests hepatocyte damage).
- Haemolysis, pulmonary embolism, and tumour necrosis.

Tumour markers[7]

Tumour markers are rarely sufficiently specific to be of diagnostic value. Their main value is in monitoring the course of an illness and the effectiveness of treatment. Reference ranges vary between laboratories.

Alpha-fetoprotein ↑In hepatocellular CA (p242), germ cell tumours (not pure seminoma) hepatitis; cirrhosis; pregnancy; open neural tube defects.

CA 125 Raised in carcinoma of the ovary, uterus, breast, and hepatocellular carcinoma. Also raised in pregnancy, cirrhosis, and peritonitis.

CA 15-3 Raised in carcinoma of the breast and benign breast disease.

CA 19-9 Raised in colorectal and pancreatic carcinoma, and cholestasis.

Carcino-embryonic antigen (CEA) ↑In gastrointestinal neoplasms, especially colorectal CA. Also cirrhosis, pancreatitis, and smoking.

Human chorionic gonadotrophin Raised in pregnancy and germ cell tumours. For hydatidiform moles and choriocarcinoma, see *OHCS* p26.

Neurone specific enolase (NSE) Raised in small-cell carcinoma of lung and neuroblastoma.

Placental alkaline phosphatase (PLAP) Raised in pregnancy, carcinoma of ovary, seminoma, and smoking.

Prostate specific antigen (PSA) See BOX.

Prostate specific antigen (PSA)

As well as being a marker of prostate cancer, PSA is (unfortunately) raised in benign prostatic hypertrophy. See prostate cancer (p498) and p499 for advising men who ask for a PSA test. 25% of large benign prostates give PSA up to 10 μg/L; levels may be higher if recent ejaculation; therefore, avoid ejaculation for 24h prior to measurement. Other factors causing raised PSA: recent rectal examination, prostatitis, and UTI (PSA levels may not return to base-line for some months after the latter).[1] Plasma reference interval is age specific, an example of the top end of the reference interval for total PSA is:

Healthy males of age (yrs)	PSA μg/L
40–50	2.5
50–59	3.5
60–69	5.0
70–79	6.5
80–89	7.5

The above is a rough guide only; different labs have different reference ranges, and populations vary. More specific assays, such as free PSA/total PSA index, and PSA density, are also becoming available, which may partly solve these problems. It is shown to illustrate the common problem of interpreting a PSA of ~8—and as a warning against casual requests for PSAs in the (vain) hope of simple answers. The following indicates the proportion of patients with a raised PSA and benign hypertrophy or carcinoma.

	PSA μg/L	
Benign prostatic hypertrophy	<4 in 91%	PSA will be ~50% lower after 6 months on 5α reductase inhibitors (to ↓prostate size, see p496)
	4–10 in 8%	
	>10 in 1%	
Prostate carcinoma	<4 in 15%	
	4–10 in 20%	
	>10 in 65%	

705

1 Up to six months in one study. G Aus 2003 *Urology* **62** 278

Hyperlipidaemia

Cholesterol is a major risk factor for coronary heart disease (CHD). Half the UK population have a serum cholesterol putting them at significant risk of CHD. Do not treat in isolation, assess other risk factors: smoking, BP↑, DM, family history—see *risk equation*, p22. Benefits of treatment must be set against cost, and imposition of diets and tablet-taking (with expensive follow-up plans).

Trial evidence that treating hypercholesterolaemia is worthwhile

- '4S' study.[8] Secondary prevention trial (patients with ischaemic heart disease) using simvastatin ≥20mg/d PO *nocte* in 4444 men aged 35–70 (cholesterol 5.5–8.0mmol/L). Number needed to treat (NNT, p30) to prevent 1 fatal MI was 25 (over 6yrs), and 14 for non-fatal events.
- WOSCOPS.[9] Primary prevention trial in Scotland with over 6500 men (cholesterol >6.5mmol/L), pravastatin 40mg/24h PO *nocte*. NNT to prevent 1 fatal MI was 142 (over 5yrs), and for all cardiac events was 55.
- CARE study.[10] Secondary prevention trial with 40mg of pravastatin/24h PO in >4000 people, post-MI, with 'normal' cholesterol (<6.2mmol/L). NNT for fatalities was 91 (over 5yrs), and for non-fatal MI was 38.
- *HEART PROTECTION STUDY*.[11] Secondary prevention trial with 40mg simvastatin to patients irrespective of cholesterol. NNT for death = 55. No evidence of 'threshold of cholesterol' for benefit.

Who to screen

- CHD or risk↑, eg DM, BP↑.
- Family history of hyperlipidaemia, or CHD before 65yrs old.
- Xanthomata or xanthelasmata.
- Corneal arcus before 50yrs old.

Management[12]

- Exclude familial or 2° hyperlipidaemias. Treat as appropriate.
- Lifestyle advice. Aim for BMI of 20–25. Diet with <10% of calories from saturated fats and plenty of gel-forming fibre (p208). Exercise.
- Treat those with known CHD.
- If *no* CHD, risk tables (p22). ℞ when MI risk is >3%/yr, eg chol >5.5 for 50-yr-old ♂ smoker with DM, LVH & BP↑, but chol >6.9 if no LVH or DM.
- 'Statins' (p114) are first choice; they ↓cholesterol synthesis in the liver (eg *simvastatin* 10–40mg PO at night). CI: porphyria, LFT↑. SE: myositis (stop if CK↑ by ≥10-fold. If any muscle aches, check CK; risk is 1/100,000 treatment yrs[13]); abdominal pain; LFT↑ (stop if AST ≥100U/L).
- 2nd-line therapy: fibrates, eg bezafibrate (useful in familial mixed hyperlipidaemias); cholesterol absorption inhibitors of ezetimibe (useful in combination with a statin to enhance cholesterol reduction); anion exchange resins, eg cholestyramine; & nicotinic acid (HDL↑; LDL↓; SE: severe flushes—aspirin 300mg ½h pre-dose helps this).
- Hypertriglyceridaemia responds best to fibrates, nicotinic acid, or fish oil.

Familial or primary hyperlipidaemias Risk of CHD↑↑ Lipids travel in blood packaged with proteins as lipoproteins. There are four classes: chylomicrons (mainly triglyceride); LDL (mainly cholesterol, the lipid correlating most strongly with CHD); VLDL (mainly triglyceride); HDL (mainly phospholipid, correlating *inversely* with CHD). See table OPPOSITE.

Secondary hyperlipidaemias A result of diabetes mellitus; alcohol abuse; T4↓; renal failure, nephrosis, and cholestasis.

Xanthomata These yellowish lipid deposits may be: eruptive (itchy nodules in crops in hypertriglyceridaemia); tuberous (yellow plaques on elbows and knees); planar—also called palmar (orange-coloured streaks in palmar creases), virtually diagnostic of remnant hyperlipidaemia; or deposits in tendons, eyelids (xanthelasmata), or cornea (arcus).

Primary hyperlipidaemias

Chol = plasma cholesterol mmol/L
Trig = plasma triglyceride (mmol/L); **coloured numerals = WHO** phenotype

Familial hyperchylomicronaemia (lipoprotein lipase deficiency or apoCII deficiency)[I]	Chol <6.5 Trig 10–30 Chylomicrons ↑	Eruptive xanthomata; lipaemia retinalis; hepatosplenomegaly (HSM)
Familial hypercholesterolaemia[II] (LDL receptor defects)	Chol 7.5–16 LDL↑ Trig <2.3	Tendon xanthoma; corneal arcus; xanthelasma
Familial defective apoprotein B-100[IIa]	Chol 7.5–16 LDL↑ Trig <2.3	Tendon xanthoma; arcus; xanthelasma
Polygenic hypercholesterolaemia[IIa]	Chol 6.5–9 LDL↑ Trig <2.3	*The commonest 1° lipidaemia* xanthelasma; corneal arcus
Familial combined hyperlipidaemia[IIb, IV or V]	Chol 6.5–10 LDL↑VLDL↑ Trig 2.3–12 HDL↓	*Next commonest 1° lipidaemia* xanthelasma; arcus
Dysbetalipoproteinaemia (remnant particle disease)[III]	Chol 9–14 IDL↑ Trig 9–14 HDL↓ LDL↓	Palmar striae; tubero-eruptive xanthoma
Familial hypertriglyceridaemia[IV]	Chol 6.5–12 VLDL↑ Trig 3.0–6.0	
Type V hyperlipoproteinaemia	Trig 10–30; chylomicrons	Eruptive xanthoma; lipaemia retinalis; HSM

Primary HDL abnormalities
Hyperalphalipoproteinaemia ↑HDL chol >2
Hypoalphalipoproteinaemia (Tangier disease) ↓HDL chol <0.92

Primary LDL abnormalities
Abetalipoproteinaemia Trig<0.3, Chol<1.3, missing LDL, VLDL and chylomicrons, and fat malabsorption, retinopathy, and acanthocytosis
Hypobetalipoproteinaemia chol<1.5 LDL↓, HDL ↓. Increased longevity

►What are the priorities in treating diet-resistant hyperlipidaemia?

Top priority: *Treat those with known cardiovascular disease.*
2ⁿᵈ priority: *Treat those with DM if risk of CV disease >3% per year.*
3ʳᵈ priority: *Those with a risk of CV disease >3% per year.*

Abbreviations IDL = intermediate-density liproprotein (HDL and LDL denote high and low density, respectively); chol = cholesterol; trig = triglyceride.

The porphyrias

The acute porphyrias are rare genetic diseases caused by errors in the pathway of haem biosynthesis resulting in the toxic accumulation of porphobilinogen and δ-aminolaevulinic acid (porphyrin precursors). Characterized by acute neurovisceral crises, due to the increased production of porphyrin precursors, and their appearance in the urine. Some forms have cutaneous manifestations. Prevalence: 1–2/100,000.

Acute intermittent porphyria A low-penetrant autosomal dominant condition (porphobilinogen deaminase gene); 28% have no family history (*de novo mutations*). ~10% of those with the defective gene have neurovisceral symptoms. Attacks are intermittent, more common in women, and may be precipitated by many drugs (see below). Urine porphobilinogens are raised during attacks and often (50%) between them (the urine may go deep red on standing). Faecal porphyrin levels are normal. There are no skin manifestations.

Variegate porphyria and hereditary coproporphyria Autosomal dominant, characterized by photosensitive blistering skin lesions and/or acute attacks. The former is prevalent in Afrikaners in South Africa. Porphobilinogen is high only in an attack, and other metabolites may be detected in faeces.

Features of an acute attack Colic ± vomiting ± fever ± WCC↑—so mimicking an acute abdomen (anaesthesia can be disastrous here)—also:

- Hypotension
- Hyponatraemia
- Hypokalaemia
- Hypotonia
- Proteinuria
- Psychosis/odd behaviour[1]
- Peripheral neuritis
- Paralysis
- Seizures
- Sensory impairment
- Sight may be affected
- Shock (± collapse).

Drugs to avoid in acute intermittent porphyria are legion (they may precipitate above symptoms ± quadriplegia, see *BNF/OTM*), they include: *alcohol*; *several anaesthetic agents* (barbiturates, halothane); *antibiotics* (chloramphenicol, sulfonamides, tetracyclines); *painkillers* (pentazocine); *oral hypoglycaemics*; *contraceptive pill.*

Treatment of an acute attack
- Remove precipitants, then:
- IV fluids to correct electrolyte imbalance.
- High carbohydrate intake (eg Hycal®) by NG tube if necessary.
- IV haematin is probably the treatment of choice in most centres now.
- Nausea controlled with prochlorperazine 12.5mg IM.
- Sedation if necessary with chlorpromazine 50–100mg PO/IM.
- Pain control with: aspirin, dihydrocodeine, or morphine.
- Seizures can be controlled with diazepam.
- Treat tachycardia and hypertension with propranolol.

Non-acute porphyrias

Porphyria cutanea tarda, *erythropoietic protoporphyria*, and *congenital erythropoietic porphyria* are characterized by cutaneous photosensitivity alone, as there is no overproduction of porphyrin precursors, only porphyrins.

▶Alcohol, lead, & iron deficiency cause abnormal porphyrin metabolism.

▶Offer genetic counselling (*OHCS* p212) to all patients and their families.

---

1 Be sure I looked at her eyes
Happy and proud; at last I knew
Porphyria worshipped me; surprise
Made my heart swell, and still it grew
While I debated what to do.
That moment she was mine, mine, fair,

Perfectly pure and good: I found
A thing to do, and all her hair
In one long yellow string I wound
Three times her little throat around,
And strangled her …
[From *Porphyria's Lover*, Robert Browning]

Reference intervals, etc.

Nomogram for estimating doses of gentamicin

1 Join with a straight line the serum creatinine concentration appropriate to the sex on scale A and the age on scale B. Mark the point at which this line cuts line C.[1]

2 Join with a line the mark on line C and the body weight on line D. Mark the points at which this line cuts lines L and M. These will give the loading and maintenance doses, respectively.

3 Confirm the appropriateness of this regimen at an early stage by measuring serum levels, especially in severe illness and renal impairment.

4 Adjust *dose* if peak concentrations (1h after IM dose; 30min after IV dose) outside the range 5–10mg/L. Trough concentrations (just before dose) above 2mg/L indicate the need for a longer dosage *interval*.

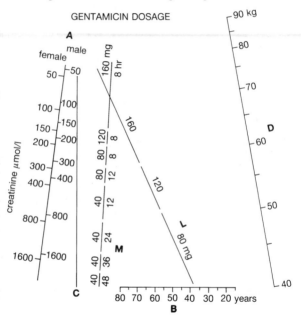

GENTAMICIN DOSAGE

1 Potential for oto- and nephro-toxicity is great if gentamicin is used inappropriately, so use local expert advice/guidelines. The above allows for **thrice daily** doses. Many favour **once daily doses** (eg 5mg/kg/d for a lean person, less if obese)—fewer SEs, ± better bactericidal activity. Meta-analyses back this, provided there is no increase in cardiac output (eg in anaemia; Paget's disease), and the context is not ascites, burns, children, or pregnancy. The big problem is lack of information on calculating and monitoring once-a-day regimens. The *Cooke & Grace* regimen provisionally recommends, for feverish neutropenic adults with serum creatinine <300μmol/L, a starting dose of gentamicin 5mg/kg IVI over 30min. Measure serum trough ~24h later. If OK (<1mg/L), then do twice weekly monitoring. If trough is 1–2mg/L, halve dose, and monitor next trough (ie at 24h). Cooke & Grace stop gentamicin if this level is >2mg/L, eg giving ciprofloxacin instead. Other nomograms exist to optimize dose timing (D Nicolau 1995 *Antimicrob Agents Chemoth* **39** 650); GAT[sanford] recommends a max initial dose of 7mg/kg but this large amount can cause chills and BP↓: http://depts.washington.edu/druginfo/Alerts/dralerts.html. If this is used (get expert help), Parker's *rule of sevens* may help: give 7mg/kg unless obese; check level at 7h; if <7mg/L give gentamicin every 24h. If >7, seek further advice on lengthening the dose interval.

Drug therapeutic ranges in plasma

▶ Ranges should only be used as a guide to treatment.

A drug in an apparently too low concentration may still be clinically useful. Some patients require (and tolerate) levels in the 'toxic' range.

* *Amikacin* peak (1h post IV dose): 20–30mg/L. Trough: <10mg/L.

* *Carbamazepine* Optimal concentration: 20–50μmol/L [4–12mg/L].

* *Clonazepam* trough: 0.08–0.24μmol/L [0.025–0.075mg/L].

* *Digoxin*[1] (6–12h post dose) 1–2.6nmol/L [0.8–2μg/L]. <1.3nmol/L may be toxic if there is hypokalaemia. Signs of CVS toxicity: arrhythmias, heart block. CNS: confusion, insomnia, agitation, seeing too much yellow (xanthopsia), delirium. GI: nausea.

* *Ethosuximide* trough: 300–700μmol/L [40–100mg/L].

* *Gentamicin*[1] Peak—1h post IV dose: 9–18μmol/L [5–10mg/L]. Trough (just before dose): <4.2μmol/L (<2mg/L). Toxic signs: tinnitus, deafness, nystagmus, vertigo, renal failure. See OPPOSITE.

Lithium[1] (12h post dose). Guidelines vary: 0.4–0.8mmol/L is reasonable. *Early* signs of toxicity (Li$^+$ ~1.5mmol/L): tremor, agitation, twitching. *Intermediate:* lethargy. *Late:* (Li$^+$ >2mmol/L) spasms, coma, fits, arrhythmias, renal failure (haemodialysis may be needed). See OHCS p354.

Netilmicin peak—1h post IV dose: 7–12mg/L. Trough <2mg/L.

* *Phenobarbital* Trough: 60–80μmol/L [15–40mg/L].

* *Phenytoin*[1] trough: 40–80μmol/L [10–20mg/L]. Signs of toxicity: ataxia, nystagmus, sedation, dysarthria, diplopia.

Theophylline 10–20mg/mL (55–110μmol/L). (▶ see p795) Take sample 4–6h after starting an infusion (which should be stopped for ~15min just before the specimen is taken). Signs of toxicity: arrhythmias, anxiety, tremor, convulsions.

Tobramycin peak (1h post IV dose): 11–21μmol/L [5–10mg/L]. Trough: ≤4.3μmol/L <2mg/L.

The time since the last dose should be specified on the form.

* Trough levels should be taken just before the next dose.

1 Drugs for which *routine* monitoring is indicated.

Some important drug interactions ▶ see BNF www.bnf.org

Note: '↑' means the effect of the drug in italics is increased (eg through inhibition of metabolism or renal clearance). '↓' means that its effect is decreased (eg through enzyme induction).

Adenosine ↓ by: aminophylline. ↑ by dipyridamole.

Aminoglycosides ↑ by: loop diuretics.

Antidiabetic drugs (any) ↑ by: alcohol, β-blockers, monoamine oxidase inhibitors, bezafibrate. ↓ by: corticosteroids, diazoxide, diuretics, contraceptive steroids, (possibly also lithium).

  Sulfonylureas ↑ by: azapropazone, chloramphenicol, bezafibrate, co-trimoxazole, miconazole, sulfinpyrazone.

  Sulfonylureas ↓ by: rifampicin (nifedipine occasionally).

  Metformin ↑ by: cimetidine. With alcohol: lactic acidosis risk.

Antiretroviral agents (HIV): See p584.

Angiotensin-converting enzyme (ACE) *inhibitors* ↓ effect by: NSAIDs.

Antihistamines (eg terfenadine) Avoid anything which ↑concentrations and risk of arrhythmias, eg erythromycin, other macrolides (eg azithromycin), antifungals, halofantrine, tricyclics, antipsychotics, SSRIs (p334), protease inhibitors (p584), diuretics, β-blockers, antiarrhythmics.

Azathioprine ↑ by: allopurinol.

β-blockers Avoid verapamil; ↓: NSAIDs. Lipophilic β-blockers (eg propranolol) are metabolized by the liver, and concentrations are ↑ by cimetidine. This does not happen with hydrophilic β-blockers (eg atenolol).

Carbamazepine ↑ by: erythromycin, isoniazid, verapamil.

Cimetidine: theophylline↑, warfarin↑, lignocaine (lidocaine)↑, amitriptyline↑, propranolol↑, pethidine↑, phenytoin↑, metronidazole↑, quinine↑.

Contraceptive steroids ↓ by: antibiotics, barbiturates, carbamazepine, phenytoin, rifampicin.

Ciclosporin (=cyclosporin) ↑ by: erythromycin, nifedipine. ↓ by: phenytoin.

Digoxin ↑ by: amiodarone, carbenoxolone and diuretics (as K⁺ levels lowered), quinine, verapamil.

Diuretics ↓ by: NSAIDs—particularly indomethacin (=indometacin).

Ergotamine ↑ by: erythromycin (ergotism may occur).

Fluconazole: Avoid concurrent astemizole or terfenadine.

Lithium ↑ by: thiazide diuretics.

Methotrexate ↑ by: aspirin, NSAIDs.

Phenytoin ↑ by: chloramphenicol, cimetidine, disulfiram, isoniazid, sulfonamides. ↓ by: carbamazepine.

Potassium-sparing diuretics with ACE*-inhibitors:* Hyperkalaemia.

Theophyllines ↑ by: cimetidine, ciprofloxacin, erythromycin, contraceptive steroids, propranolol. ↓ by: barbiturates, carbamazepine, phenytoin, rifampicin. See p795.

Valproate ↓by: carbamazepine, phenobarbital, phenytoin.

Warfarin and *nicoumalone* (=acenocoumarol) ↑ by: alcohol, allopurinol, amiodarone, aspirin, chloramphenicol, cimetidine, ciprofloxacin, co-trimoxazole, danazol, dextropropoxyphene, dipyridamole, disulfiram, erythromycin (and broad-spectrum antibiotics), gemfibrozil, glucagon, ketoconazole, metronidazole, miconazole, nalidixic acid, neomycin, NSAIDs, phenytoin, quinidine, simvastatin (but not pravastatin), sulfinpyrazone, sulfonamides, tetracyclines, thyroxine (=levothyroxine).

Warfarin and *nicoumalone* ↓ by: aminoglutethimide, barbiturates, carbamazepine, contraceptive steroids, dichloralphenazone, griseofulvin, rifampicin, phenytoin, vitamin K.

Zidovudine (AZT) ↑ by: paracetamol (increased marrow toxicity).

IVI solutions to avoid *Dextrose:* Avoid frusemide (=furosemide), ampicillin, hydralazine, insulin, melphalan, quinine.

0.9% saline IVI: Avoid amphotericin, lignocaine, nitroprusside.

Haematology—reference intervals

(For B_{12}, folate, Fe, and TIBC, see p714–17)

Measurement	Reference interval	Your hospital
White cell count (WCC)	4.0–11.0 × 10^9/L	
Red cell count	♂ 4.5–6.5 × 10^{12}/L	
	♀ 3.9–5.6 × 10^{12}/L	
Haemoglobin	♂ 13.5–18.0g/dL	
	♀ 11.5–16.0g/dL	
Packed red cell volume (PCV) or haematocrit	♂ 0.4–0.54L/L	
	♀ 0.37–0.47L/L	
Mean cell volume (MCV)	76–96fL	
Mean cell haemoglobin (MCH)	27–32pg	
Mean cell haemoglobin concentration (MCHC)	30–36g/dL	
Neutrophils	2.0–7.5 × 10^9/L; 40–75% WCC	
Lymphocytes	1.3–3.5 × 10^9/L; 20–45% WCC	
Eosinophils	0.04–0.44 × 10^9/L; 1–6% WCC	
Basophils	0.0–0.10 × 10^9/L; 0–1% WCC	
Monocytes	0.2–0.8 × 10^9/L; 2–10% WCC	
Platelet count	150–400 × 10^9/L	
Reticulocyte count	0.8–2.0%[1] 25–100 × 10^9/L	
Erythrocyte sedimentation rate	Depends on age (p670)	
Prothrombin time (factors I, II, VII, X)	10–14s	
Activated partial thrombo-plastin time (VIII, IX, XI, XII)	35–45s	
D-dimers[2]	<0.5mg/L	

Proposed therapeutic ranges for prothrombin time See p649

713

1 Only use percentages as reference interval if red cell count is normal; otherwise, use the absolute value. Express as a ratio vs control.
2 D-dimer assay may be useful as a screening test for thromboembolic disease see *Lancet* 1999 **353** 190. However, the reference range does depend on the assay—check with your haematology lab.

Reference intervals—*biochemistry*

See p676 for the philosophy of the normal range; see OHCS p292 for children.
Drugs (and other substances) may interfere with any chemical method; as
these effects may be method dependent, it is difficult for the clinician to be
aware of all the possibilities. If in doubt, discuss with the lab.

Substance	Specimen	Reference interval (labs vary, so a guide only)	Your hospital
Adrenocorticotrophic hormone	P	<80ng/L	
Alanine aminotransferase (ALT)	P	5–35iu/L	
Albumin	P[1]	35–50g/L	
Aldosterone	P[2]	100–500pmol/L	
Alkaline phosphatase	P	30–150u/L (adults)	
α-amylase	P	0–180 Somogyi u/dL	
α-fetoprotein	S	<10ku/L	
Angiotensin II	P[2]	5–35pmol/L	
Antidiuretic hormone (ADH)	P	0.9–4.6pmol/L	
Aspartate transaminase	P	5–35iu/L	
Bicarbonate	P[1]	24–30mmol/L	
Bilirubin	P	3–17μmol/L	
BNP (see p689)	P	<50ng/L	
Calcitonin	P	<0.1μg/L	
Calcium (ionized)	P	1.0–1.25mmol/L	
Calcium (total)	P[1]	2.12–2.65mmol/L	
Chloride	P	95–105mmol/L	
[3]Cholesterol (see p676 & p706)	P	3.9–6mmol/L	
VLDL (see p706)	P	0.128–0.645mmol/L	
LDL	P	1.55–4.4mmol/L	
HDL	P	0.9–1.93mmol/L	
Cortisol	P	A.M. 450–700nmol/L midnight 80–280nmol/L	
Creatine kinase (CK)	P	♂ 25–195iu/L ♀ 25–170iu/L	
Creatinine (∝ to lean body mass)	P[1]	70–≤150μmol/L	
Ferritin	P	12–200μg/L	
Folate	S	2.1μg/L	
Follicle-stimulating hormone (FSH)	P/S	2–8u/L in ♀ (luteal); >25u/L in menopause	
Gamma-glutamyl transpeptidase	P	♂ 11–51iu/L ♀ 7–33iu/L	
Glucose (fasting)	P	3.5–5.5mmol/L	
Glycated (glycosylated) Hb	B	2.3–6.5%	
Growth hormone	P	<20mu/L	
HbA₁c (= glycosylated Hb)	B	2.3–6.5%	
Iron	S	♂ 14–31μmol/L ♀ 11–30μmol/L	
Lactate dehydrogenase (LDH)	P	70–250iu/L	
Lead	B	<1.8mmol/L	
Luteinizing hormone (LH) (premenopausal)	P	3–16u/L (luteal)	
Magnesium	P	0.75–1.05mmol/L	

714

1 See *OHCS* p81 for reference intervals in pregnancy.
2 The sample requires special handling: contact the laboratory.
3 Desired upper limit of cholesterol would be ~6mmol/L. In some populations, 7.8mmol/L is the top end of the distribution.

P = plasma (eg heparin bottle); **S** = serum (clotted; no anticoagulant); **B** = whole blood (edetic acid EDTA bottle)

Osmolality	P	278–305mosmol/kg
Parathyroid hormone (PTH)	P	<0.8–8.5pmol/L
Prolactin	P	♂ <450u/L; ♀<600u/L
Prostate specific antigen (PSA)	P	0–4μg/ml, age specific, see p705
Protein (total)	P	60–80g/L
Red cell folate	B	0.36–1.44μmol/L (160–640μg/L)
Renin (erect/recumbent)	P²	2.8–4.5/1.1–2.7pmol/mL/h
Sodium	P¹	135–145mmol/L
Thyroid-binding globulin (TBG)	P	7–17mg/L
Thyroid-stimulating hormone (TSH) NR widens with age, p302	P	0.5–5.7mu/L
Thyroxine (T4)	P	70–140nmol/L
Thyroxine (free)	P	9–22pmol/L
Total iron-binding capacity	S	54–75μmol/L
Triglyceride	P	0.55–1.90mmol/L
Tri-iodothyroinine (T₃)	P	1.2–3.0nmol/L
Troponin T (see p120)	P	<0.1μg/L
Urate	P¹	♂ 210–480μmol/L ♀ 150–390μmol/L
Urea	P¹	2.5–6.7mmol/L
Vitamin B₁₂	S	0.13–0.68nmol/L (>150ng/L)

Arterial blood gases—*reference intervals*

pH: 7.35–7.45 P_aCO_2: 4.7–6.0kPa

P_aO_2: >10.6kPa   Base excess: ±2mmol/L

Note: 7.6mmHg = 1kPa (atmospheric pressure ≈ 100kPa)

Urine reference intervals	*Reference interval*	*Your hospital*
Cortisol (free)	<280nmol/24h	
Hydroxyindole acetic acid	16–73μmol/24h	
Hydroxymethylmandelic acid (HMMA, VMA)	16–48μmol/24h	
Metanephrines	0.03–0.69μmol/mmol creatinine (or <5.5μmol/day)	
Osmolality	350–1000mosmol/kg	
17-oxogenic steroids	♂ 28–30μmol/24h ♀ 21–66μmol/24h	
17-oxosteroids (neutral)	♂ 17–76μmol/24h ♀ 14–59μmol/24h	
Phosphate (inorganic)	15–50mmol/24h	
Potassium	14–120mmol/24h	
Protein	<150mg/24h	
Sodium	100–250mmol/24h	

Useful addresses (for those in the UK)

For *addresses of disease-specific organizations*, see the Health Information Line (below, or www.patient.org.uk/); for *poisons information services* see p826

British Diabetic Association/Diabetes (UK) 10 Queen Ann St, London W1M 0BD (020 7323 1531)

British Medical Association (BMA) BMA House, Tavistock Square, London WC1H 9JP (020 7387 4499)

Bureau of Hygiene and Tropical Medicine Keppel St, London WC1E 7HT (020 7636 8636)

Central Public Health Lab 61 Colindale Av, London NW9 5HT (020 8200 4400)

Committee on Safety of Medicines Freepost, London SW8 5BR

Communicable Disease Surveillance Centre (for up-to-date advice on travel health needs) 61 Colindale Avenue, London NW9 5HT (020 8200 6868)

Disabled Living Foundation (Advice on aids and equipment to help the disabled) 380–384 Harrow Rd, London W9 2HU (020 7289 6111)

Evidence-based medicine Cochrane Centre (01865 516300)

NHS Centre for Reviews and Dissemination (01904 433707)

Central Health Outcomes Unit DoH (020 7972 2000)

Centre for Health Economics (01904 433645)

Centre for Evidence-based Medicine (01865 221321)

Bandolier (01865 226863); INTERNET: www.jr2.ox.ac.uk/Bandolier

UK clearing house—Health Outcomes (0113 233 3940)

General Medical Council 178 Great Portland St, London W1W 5JE (020 7580 7642)

Health Information Line (for a wide range of information for doctors and patients, and addresses of disease-specific organizations) 0800 665544

Liverpool School of Tropical Medicine Pembroke Place, Liverpool L3 5QA (0151 708 9393)

Malaria Reference Laboratory (for advice on malaria prophylaxis) 020 7636 8636 (for advice on treatment ring 020 7387 4411)

Medic-Alert Foundation 12 Bridge Wharf, 156 Caledonian Rd, London N1 9UD (020 7833 3034)

Medical Defence Union (UK) 3 Devonshire Place, London W1N 2EA (020 7486 6181 and 0800 716376, fax 0161 491 1420)

Medical and Dental Defence Union 144 West George St, Glasgow (0141 332 6646)

Medical Foundation for the Care of Victims of Torture 96–98 Grafton Rd, Kentish Town, London NW5 3EJ (020 7813 7777) www.torturecare.org.uk

Medical Protection Society 50 Hallam St, London W1N 6DE (020 7637 0541)

Multiple Sclerosis Society 25 Effie Road, London SW6 1EE (020 7736 6267)

National Counselling Service for Sick Doctors (0870 241 0535)

The Patients' Association (an advice service for patients) PO Box 935, Harrow (0845 608 4455)

Transplant service (UK) (Can these organs be used?) 0117 9507 777

The internet is older than most doctors, being of the same vintage as, say, penicillin—is used more often than penicillin, and is having just as profound effects on medicine. During the time it takes you to read this page, your better-connected patients may have checked out your latest prescription and be wondering why it does not tally with the recommendations of Guatamalan Guidelines on Gynaecomastia, or the National Institute for Clinical Excellence's Treatise on Toxoplasmosis. Our patients have time and motivation, whereas we have little time and our motivation may be flickering. This can seem threatening to the doctor who sees himself/herself as a dispenser of wisdom and precious remedies. It is less threatening if we consider ourselves to be in partnership with our patients. The evidence is that those who use the internet to question their therapy receive a better service.

If all this makes you depressed don't give up: you don't have to get connected immediately. The chances are that someone in your team is more familiar with the technology than you. Ask her if she will be your Knowledge Information Officer for a while. The answer will probably be 'Yes'. If everyone says 'No', then you are probably ahead of your team. So go to your local librarian, and ask his advice, get some training, and then offer yourself as your team's Knowledge Information Officer . If no one asks you any questions, your team is either sleeping or dead (all organisms and organizations have information needs)—or you are not available at the right time (get yourself an e-mail address and teach the team how to send you messages).

How to use a Knowledge Information Officer Their role is to answer your clinical questions. Can tetanus toxoid cause purpura? Is there a connection between knee pain and constipation? Frame your questions as simply as possible. You are not asking him whether it is likely that this patient's purpura is due to last week's tetanus vaccine, just if it is a reported happening. You maintain clinical responsibility and use the knowledge you are given to frame appropriate management.

Useful sources for Knowledge Information Officers *A basic starter kit:*

• *Drugs:* eMIMS (more up to date than *eBNF*, but see the *What's new* section at www.bnf.org); *eMIMS* contains many Data Sheets and additional information; free and updated monthly (needs *Windows* 95 or *NT* or higher).

• *Differential diagnoses* (eg what causes chest pain, knee pain, and urea↑?) and *rare diseases*—try Oxford Clinical Mentor (www.emispdp.com) contains this book, *OHCS*, and the Oxford Handbook of Clinical Rarities—so we must declare an interest here.)

• *Abstracts of research:* Medline free, www.ncbi.nlm.nih.gov/entrez/query.fcgi?db = PubMed. Searches can be limited: eg angina [therapy] AND jones [author] AND (1999 [date published] OR 2000 [date published]). Note use of upper case AND/OR. For advanced advice on using Medline, see *OHCS* p447.

• *Full-text online peer-reviewed material:* www.bmj.com (free).

• *Meta-analyses:* www.update-software.com/Scripts/ssserver.exe (Cochrane library).

If you *are* your team's Knowledge Information Officer, decide how to categorize, store, and retrieve the knowledge you import and export. Time-management consultants tell us that the main time-waster is, for most organizations, chasing items you know are there but seem lost. Manual systems and bursting filing cabinets are not the answer: linked hard disks and searchable databases probably are.

Eponymous syndromes

See also *OHCS* p742–58

Alice in Wonderland syndrome (Todd's syndrome) Disturbance of one's view of oneself ± fast-forwarding of intrapsychic time. Can occur in epilepsy, migraine, or infectious mononucleosis.

Arnold–Chiari malformation The cerebellar tonsils and medulla are malformed and herniate through the foramen magnum. This may cause progressive hydrocephalus with mental retardation, optic atrophy and ocular palsies, and spastic paresis of the limbs. It may also cause syringomyelia (p404) or focal cerebellar and brainstem signs such as ataxia, dysphagia, oscillopsia, and nystagmus. There may be an association with bony abnormalities of the base of the skull (basilar impression). MRI is better than CT in aiding diagnosis.

Baker's cyst Posterior herniation of capsule of the knee joint leads to escape of synovial fluid into one of the posterior bursae, stiffness and knee swelling (transilluminable popliteal space). *Tests:* Ultrasound. *Differential:* DVT (may coexist). *Treatment:* Aspiration is possible, but recurrence is common.

Barrett's oesophagus[1] In chronic reflux oesophagitis (p216), squamous mucosa shows metaplastic change and the squamocolumnar junction (*ora serrata*) migrates upwards. The length affected may be a few cm only or all the oesophagus. It carries a 40-fold ↑risk of adenocarcinoma.
Symptoms: • Retrosternal pain, radiating to neck, worsened by hot or cold foods • Dysphagia • Vomiting • Haematemesis • Melaena.
Once diagnosed, endoscopic surveillance programmes vary depending on age and general health; there is little evidence that they have ↓deaths from oesophageal cancer. *Management* depends on what histology is found on biopsy. *If pre-malignant changes are found*, some advocate oesophageal resection especially in younger, fit patients; others favour frequent endoscopic ultrasound monitoring ± epithelial laser/photodynamic ablation. Photodynamic therapy (PDT) involves light-induced activation of an orally administered photosensitizer such as 5-aminolaevulinic acid which causes the accumulation of protoporphyrin IX in GI mucosal cells. Local laser light then causes necrosis, which is confirmed by finding squamous re-epithelialization. PDT remains experimental. *If no pre-malignant changes are found*, regular endoscopy + biopsy, and intensive antireflux measures including long-term proton pump inhibitors are used, but exactly who to screen and when is not clear.

Bazin's disease Localized areas of fat necrosis with ulceration and an indurated rash, characteristically on adolescent girls' legs. Originally thought to be a form of skin TB, but cases unrelated to tuberculosis have been seen.

Behçet's disease A multiorgan inflammatory disease associated with HLA-B51 and thromboses. ♂:♀ ≈ 2:1. *Joints:* Arthritis. *Eyes:* Pain, vision↓, floaters, iritis, hypopyon, retinal vein occlusion. *Mouth, scrotum, labia:* Painful ulcers (heal by scarring). *Gut:* Colitis. *Skin signs:* PLATE 22. *CNS:* Meningoencephalitis, ICP↑, brainstem signs, dementia, myelopathy, encephalopathy, cerebral vein thrombosis. *Treatment:* Colchicine, steroids (topical ± oral), ciclosporin, chlorambucil, and interferon-α have all been used.

Berger's disease (IgA nephropathy) The commonest glomerulonephritis (p268) in the West—causing episodic haematuria that may coincide with viral infections. IgA is deposited in glomeruli; microscopy shows mesangial proliferation. Heavy proteinuria & hypertension indicate a poor prognosis. ~17% go on to end-stage renal failure. Secondary IgA nephropathy may be associated with ankylosing spondylitis, coeliac disease, and HIV. *Treatment:* Steroids, ACE inhibitors, dietary fish oil, tonsillectomy, and renal transplantation all have a role.

Bickerstaff's brainstem encephalitis Progressive cranial nerve dysfunction, ataxia, coma, and apnoea may lead to a (reversible) brain death picture (but no *macrostructural* damage). Plasmapheresis may help.

---

[1] For a review of Barrett's oesophagus, see SJ Spechler 2002 *NEJM* **346** 836

Eponyms are so-called because they take their names from their chief protagonists (either doctors or patients). They are the sole route to medical fame: 'if one was a drunkard and one's name was Johnny Walker one could form a society called *Alcoholics Eponymous*'. Alan Bennett

Consult the index for eponymous covered in other chapters.
For biographical details, see www.whonamedit.com

ECG of Brugada syndrome

Note the unusual morphology of the raised ST segments in V1–3. This inherited condition predisposes to fatal arrhythmias, eg ventricular fibrillation, typically in young males, and is preventable by using an implantable defibrillator. ►*Consider primary electrical cardiac disease in all those with unexplained syncope.* Relatives of those with sudden unexplained death may undergo unmasking of arrhythmias by IV ajmaline tests—but some results are false +ve. Use judgment in subjecting those with ST abnormalities but no symptoms to electrophysiological studies, right ventricular myocardial biopsy, and MRI. Sequencing of the SCN5A locus may identify the R367H missense mutation in affected families.[1]

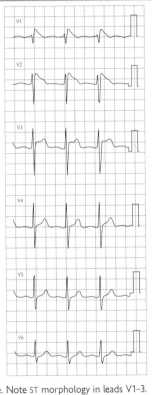

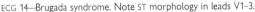

ECG 14—Brugada syndrome. Note ST morphology in leads V1–3.

719

1 J Ahn 2004 *Circulation* **109** 1463; ECG by kind permission of Dr Shayashi

Bornholm disease (Devil's grip) Coxsackie B virus causes chest and abdominal pain, typically with rhinitis. ΔΔ: MI, acute abdomen. *Treatment:* Analgesics. *Prognosis:* Recovery in 2wks.   [Bornholm Island, Denmark]

Brown-Séquard syndrome A lesion in one (lateral) half of the cord (eg hemisection) causes ipsilateral spastic paralysis and joint position sense loss below the lesion. There is ipsilateral analgesia and thermoanaesthesia at the level of the lesion, but there is contralateral loss of these modalities a few segments below the lesion (because of the pattern of decussation in the cord). Also: brisk reflexes, ↑tone ipsilaterally, sphincter disturbance. *Causes:* trauma, neoplasia, MS, degenerative disease, HTLV-1, *Gnathostoma spinigerum* (nematode).   [Charles Brown-Séquard, 1817-94]

Budd–Chiari syndrome Hepatic vein obstruction (eg thrombosis, tumour) presents with acute epigastric pain and shock, or insidious portal hypertension, ascites, jaundice, and cirrhosis. The Pill, pregnancy-related disease, malignancy, and nocturnal haemoglobinuria (p730) are typical causes. Also PRV, thrombophilia, platelets↑, IVC membranes. Ultrasound + hepatic vein Dopplers may be diagnostic. Surgery ± balloon dilatation may be indicated. Anticoagulate (lifelong) unless there are varices. In IVC blockage, a meso-atrial shunt may be used. Consider liver transplant if necrosis/fibrosis on biopsy.

Buerger's disease (Thromboangiitis obliterans) This is inflammation of arteries, veins, and nerves with thrombosis in the middle sized arteries eg in ♂ cigarette smokers. It may lead to gangrene. The underlying cause is unknown, but may involve hyperhomocysteinaemia.

Caplan's syndrome This is rheumatoid arthritis with necrotic lung granulomata in coal miners. These cause cough, dyspnoea, and haemoptysis. CXR: bilateral nodules (0.5–5cm). *Treatment:* Steroids (after excluding TB).

Charcot–Marie–Tooth syndrome (Peroneal muscular atrophy) This starts at puberty with foot drop and weak legs. The peroneal muscles are the first to atrophy, then hands, and then the arms. Sensation is usually diminished, as are reflexes. The most common form, CMT1A (caused by mutations in the PMP22 myelin gene on chromosome 17), is inherited in an autosomal dominant manner; other forms may be autosomal recessive or sex-linked. It is seldom *totally* incapacitating. Hand pain/paraesthesiae may respond to nerve release.

Creutzfeldt–Jakob disease (CJD; scrapie-like spongiform encephalopathy) The cause is a prion, ie a protein (PrPSc), which is an altered form of a normal protein (PrPc) that can cause the normal protein to transform into the abnormal prion protein (hence its infectivity). ↑PrPSc leads to CNS and tiny cavities. In *genetically determined forms* (Gerstmann–Sträussler syndrome), it is thought that the 'normal' protein is abnormally unstable and readily transforms to PrPSc. *Infection* with prions may occur via meat products, causing 'variant' type disease (vCJD). The route of infection appears to have started when the prion that causes scrapie in sheep crossed to cows, causing bovine spongiform encephalopathy (BSE). Mechanically recovered meat became contaminated with CNS tissue from BSE cows, thus entering the human food chain leading to vCJD. Other possible routes of infection include: surgical instruments (?dental instruments in touch with nerve roots), corneal transplants, and hormones made from human pituitaries. Normal sterilizing does not completely inactivate it. *Signs:* (after a long incubation), dementia, focal CNS signs, myoclonus, vision↓. *Tests:* tonsil/olfactory biopsy; CSF gel electrophoresis. *Treatment:* none proven to be effective. *Prevention:* International regulations aimed at limiting the spread of BSE, the transmission of BSE prions to humans, and human-to-human prion transmission, will hopefully halt the spread of this disease.

Crigler–Najjar syndrome An inherited cause of unconjugated hyperbilirubinaemia that presents in the first days of life with jaundice ± CNS signs. The cause is a genetic mutation leading to abolition of bilirubin UDP-glucuronosyltransferase (UGT) activity. *Treatment:* Liver transplant before irreversible kernicterus develops. Phototherapy can keep bilirubin levels down while awaiting transplant.

The fine line between fame and infamy

After his neurological experiments. Brown-Séquard proclaimed that he had discovered the secret of perpetual youth after injecting himself with a concoction of testicular blood, seminal fluid, and testicular extracts from dogs and guinea pigs. In the 1880s over 12,000 doctors were queuing up for his special extracts, which they used on their patients in various ways. He gave the extracts away free, provided that results of their use were reported back to him. 314 out of 405 cases of tabes were improved, and his own urinary flow rate improved by 25%. Endocrinologists never forgave him for bringing their science into disrepute—but, to this day, no one really knows whether he discovered anything of any practical use. ⏻₉

Signs which may distinguish 'variant' CJD from 'old' CJD:

- An early age at presentation (median 29 years; range 16–48 years).
- Prolonged duration of illness (median 14 months; range 11–21 months).
- Emotional features are an early sign (anxiety, withdrawal, apathy, agitation, a permanent look of fear in the eyes, depression, personality change, lack of awareness of surroundings, insomnia).
- Hallucinations and delusions may occur—before akinetic mutism.
- Sensory disturbance (cold legs, foot pain hyperaesthesia, dysaesthesia).
- Paresis of upwards gaze ± cortical blindness.
- Dysphagia and incontinence may occur.
- Involuntary movements (myoclonus, chorea) ± dysarthria may occur early in the disease.
- Normal EEG (standard CJD has a characteristic spike and wave pattern).
- MRI *may* show a characteristic signal in the posterior thalamic area. CT is normal in both forms of the illness, and CSF tests detecting 14-3-3 protein cannot be relied on (and are +ve in new and standard variant).
- Homozygosity for methionine at codon 129 of the PRP gene has been found in every case of vCJD so far.

Curtis–Fitz-Hugh syndrome Chlamydial perihepatitis, usually in sexually active women. It may simulate biliary pain and cause peritonitis with ascites.

Devic's syndrome (Neuromyelitis optica) This may be a variant of multiple sclerosis (but there are different imaging features on MRI). There is demyelination of the optic nerves, chiasm, and the cord. *Treatment:* Azathioprine is often used to suppress attacks, as opposed to treatments such as β-interferon in MS. *Prognosis* is variable, and complete remission may occur.

Dressler's syndrome This develops 2–10wks after an MI or heart surgery. It is thought that myocardial necrosis stimulates the formation of autoantibodies against heart muscle. *The Patient:* He or she may suffer recurrent fever and chest pain, ± pleural and pericardial rub (from serositis). Cardiac tamponade may occur, so avoid anticoagulants. *Treatment:* Steroids and anti-inflammatory agents are used.

Dubin–Johnson syndrome A familial trait which leads to failure of excretion of conjugated bilirubin. It is caused by a point mutation in a gene coding for a canalicular transport protein. There is intermittent jaundice with pain in the right hypochondrium. It does not cause hepatomegaly. *Tests:* Alk phos ↔; bile in the urine. Liver biopsy shows diagnostic pigment granules.[10]

Dupuytren's contracture Palmar fascia contracts so that the fingers (eg right 5th finger) cannot extend. There is nodular thickening of the connective tissue over the 4th & 5th fingers. See PLATE 23. *Prevalence:* ~10% of ♂ >65yrs (> if +ve family history). *Associations:* Smoking, alcohol use, heavy manual labour, trauma, DM, phenytoin, Peyronie's, AIDS. It may be a marker of disturbed metabolism of free radicals derived from O_2: ischaemia (the primary event) → increased xanthine oxidase activity → reduced oxygen → superoxide free radicals → fibroblast proliferation → Type III collagen → palmar fibrosis. Allopurinol (binds xanthine oxidase) has been observed to reduce symptoms—but surgery is often needed.

Ekbom's syndrome (Restless legs) There is an irresistible desire to move the legs when in bed, ± unpleasant leg sensations. *Pathogenesis:* ?basal ganglia malfunction. *Treatment:* Dopamine agonists are commonly used; benzodiazepines eg clonazepam (1–4mg PO nocte) may also help. Ekbom also described 'delusional parasitosis': eg 'I am invaded by parasites.'[11]

Fabry's disease An X-linked disorder (single base substitutions or big rearrangements) of glycolipid metabolism due to ↓levels of lysosomal α-galactosidase A. Globotriaosylceramide is deposited in the skin (angiokeratoma corporis diffusum), kidneys, and vasculature. Most die in the 5th decade. *Cardiac signs:* infarction, angina, ↓P–R, arrhythmias, LVH, CCF, mitral valve lesions, congestive or obstruction cardiomyopathies. *Treatment:* Biweekly infusions of recombinant human α-galactosidase A are safe and effective.[12]

Fanconi anaemia (autosomal recessive) Aplastic anaemia with an increased susceptibility to acute myeloid leukaemia. Most patients also have neurological (eg congenital deafness, IQ↓), skeletal (eg absent radii, short stature, microcephaly, syndactyly), or other somatic abnormalities (eg cryptorchidism, skin pigmentation). Several genes have been implicated.[13]

Felty's syndrome This is rheumatoid arthritis (long-standing) + splenomegaly + WCC↓; also recurrent infections; hypersplenism (causing anaemia ± platelets↓); lymphadenopathy; pigmentation; skin ulcers. Rh factor: ↑↑. Splenectomy may improve neutropenia. [Augustus Felty, 1934]

Foster Kennedy syndrome Optic atrophy of 1 eye with papilloedema of the other, from a mass (meningioma, hydatid, plasmacytoma) on a frontal lobe's underside, on the side of the optic atrophy. [F Kennedy, 1884-1952]

Friedreich's ataxia (eg autosomal recessive) Cause: expansions of the trinucleotide repeat GAA in the X25 (frataxin) gene. Spinocerebellar tracts degenerate causing cerebellar ataxia, dysarthria, nystagmus, and dysdiadochokinesis. Loss of corticospinal tracts occurs (∴weakness and plantars ↑↑)

Features distinguishing Devic's disease from multiple sclerosis[1]

	Devic's disease	Multiple sclerosis
Course	May be monophasic or relapsing	Relapsing usually; see p384
Attack severity	Usually severe	Often mild
Respiratory failure	~30% of cases due to cervical myelitis	Rare
MRI head	Usually normal	Many periventricular white-matter lesions
MRI cord	Multiple, small, peripheral lesions	Extensive central lesions
CSF oligoclonal bands	Absent	Present
Permanent disability	Usually attack-related	Usually in late progressive disease
Coexistent autoimmune disease	Present in up to 50%	Uncommon

1 BG Weinshenker 2003 *Lancet* **361** 889

and nerve damage, so the tendon reflexes are paradoxically depressed (differential diagnosis p351). There is dorsal column degeneration, hence loss of postural sense. Pes cavus and scoliosis occurs. Cardiomyopathy may cause CCF. Typical age at death: ~50yrs. *Treatment:* There is no cure; surgery may provide symptomatic relief for musculoskeletal problems. Treat any CCF.

Froin's syndrome CSF protein↑ and xanthochromia with normal cell count, seen in CSF below a block in cord compression. *[Georges Froin, 1874]*

Gardner's syndrome (Autosomal dominant) Variant of familial adenomatous polyposis, caused by mutations in the APC gene. Features include multiple premalignant colon polyps, benign bone exostoses, epidermal cysts, dermoid tumours, fibromas, and neurofibromas. *Fundoscopy:* Black spots (congenital hypertrophy of retinal pigment epithelium) and helps detect carriers of the gene before symptoms develop. *Onset:* ~20yrs, eg with mass effect (eg obstructed ureters) or bloody diarrhoea. Careful follow-up is needed. Subtotal colectomy + fulguration of polyps may prevent malignancy. Endoscopic polypectomy with long-term sulindac therapy has been tried to postpone prophylactic colectomy. [■]

Gélineau's syndrome (Narcolepsy) The patient, usually a young man, succumbs to irresistible attacks of inappropriate sleep ± vivid hallucinations, cataplexy (sudden hypotonia), and sleep paralysis (paralysis of speech + willed movement on waking, while fully alert, *OHCS* p390). *Putative mechanism:* Genetic mutations lead to loss of hypothalamic hypocretin-containing neurones, possibly via autoimmune destruction. [■] *Associations:* encephalitis; head injury; MS; HLA DR2. *Treatment:* Methylphenidate (*OHCS* p207) 10mg PO after breakfast and lunch. This amphetamine may cause dependence ± psychosis. Modafinil (~200mg PO as a single daily dose before noon) may be better. SE: anxiety, aggression, dry mouth, euphoria, insomnia, BP↑, dyskinesia, alk phos↑.

Gerstmann's syndrome Finger agnosia, left/right disorientation, dysgraphia, and acalculia. Although these do not occur together more often than predicted by chance, when they do, they suggest a dominant parietal lesion.

Gilbert's syndrome This inherited metabolic disorder is quite a common cause of *unconjugated* hyperbilirubinaemia, due to decreased bilirubin UDP-glucuronosyltransferase enzyme activity. Prevalence is estimated at 1–2%. The onset is shortly after birth, but it may be unnoticed for many years. Liver biopsy is normal, but should rarely be required clinically. Jaundice occurs during intercurrent illness. A rise in bilirubin on fasting or after IV nicotinic acid can confirm the diagnosis. Prognosis is excellent. *[Nicolas Gilbert, 1901]*

Gilles de la Tourette syndrome *Presentation:* (♂:♀ ≈ 4:1) Waxing and waning motor and phonic tics (p352; mean age of onset: 6.4yrs), blinking, nodding, stuttering ± irrepressible, explosive, occasionally obscene verbal ejaculations/gestures ± anger control problems and attention-deficit disorder. There may be a witty, innovatory, phantasmagoric picture, 'with mimicry, antics, playfulness, extravagance, impudence, audacity, dramatizations, surreal associations, uninhibited affect, speed, 'go', vivid imagery and memory, and hunger for stimuli'; also grunting, sniffing, throat-clearing, twirling, nipping people, obscene gestures (copropraxia), repeating self and others (palilalia, echolalia), repeating others' movements (echopraxia). *Pathogenesis:* Probably an inherited developmental disorder causing basal ganglia disinhibition. Group A β-haemolytic streptococcal infection *may* have a role in triggering symptoms, in a manner similar to Sydenham's chorea (p144). *Associations:* Obsessive–compulsive disorder, attention-deficit hyperactivity disorder. *Treatment:* Neuroleptics eg haloperidol (eg 1.5mg/8h PO), pimozide, or respiridone—if the patient wants help. [■] *[Georges Gilles de la Tourette]*

Goodpasture's syndrome Proliferative glomerulonephritis with lung symptoms (haemoptysis) caused by antibasement membrane antibodies (binding kidney's basement membrane and the alveolar membrane). *Tests:* CXR: infiltrates, often in the lower zones. Kidney biopsy: crescentic nephritis. Many

die in the first 6 months. *Treatment:* Vigorous immunosuppressive treatment and plasmapheresis (p670) may help. [Ernest Goodpasture, 1919]

Guillain–Barré polyneuritis *Incidence:* 1–2/100,000/yr. *Signs:* A few weeks after surgery, 'flu vaccine,☛ or infection (URTI, mycoplasma, zoster, HIV, CMV, EBV, *Campylobacter jejuni*) an ascending neuropathy occurs (?from cell-mediated hypersensitivity to myelin ± antibody-mediated demyelination). In 40%, no cause is found. It may advance fast, affecting all limbs at once. Unlike other neuropathies, *proximal* muscles are more affected, and trunk, respiratory, and cranial nerves (esp. VII) may be affected. Sensory symptoms are common (eg backache) but signs are usually hard to detect. It is the progressive respiratory involvement that is the chief danger. Chronic inflammatory demyelinating polyradiculopathy (CIDP) is a variant of Guillain–Barré, characterized by a slower onset and recovery. *Tests:* Nerve conduction studies and electromyography; vital capacity 4 hourly. CSF: protein↑ (eg by 10g/L) ± lymphocyte count↑ *Treatment:* Respiratory involvement requires transfer to ITU. ►*Ventilate sooner rather than later*, eg if FVC <1.5L; P_aO_2 <10kPa; P_aCO_2 >6kPa. Immunoglobulin 0.4g/kg/24h IV for 5d is often preferred to the option of plasma exchange. *Prognosis:* Good; ~85% make a complete or nearly complete recovery. 10% are unable to walk alone at 1yr. *Complete paralysis is compatible with complete recovery. Mortality:* 10%. *Lancet 2004 181*

Henoch–Schönlein purpura (HSP) This presents with purpura (ie purple spots/nodules which do not disappear on pressure—signifying intradermal bleeding) often over buttocks and extensor surfaces. There may be associated urticaria and duodenojejunitis. The typical patient is a boy. There may be a nephritis (+ crescents, in one-third of patients—an IgA nephropathy—we could think of HSP as being a systemic version of Berger's p718), joint involvement, abdominal pain (±intussusception), which may mimic an 'acute abdomen'. The fault lies in the vasculature; the platelets are normal. It often follows respiratory infection. *Treatment:* Nephritis may respond to the same treatments as Berger's disease (p718). *Prognosis:* good. *Complications* (worse if adult): GI bleeds, ileus, haemoptysis ± renal failure (both rare).

Horner's syndrome Pupil constriction (miosis), sunken eye (enophthalmos), ptosis and ipsilateral loss of sweating (anhydrosis) due to interruption of the face's sympathetic supply, eg at the brainstem (*demyelination; vascular disease*), cord (*syringomyelia*), thoracic outlet (*Pancoast's tumour*, p732), or on the sympathetic nerves' trip on the internal carotid artery into the skull (*carotid aneurysm*), and thence to the orbit. [Johann Horner, 1869]

Huntington's chorea is an autosomal dominant condition (gene on chromosome 4) with full penetrance, due to expansions of a CAG trinucleotide repeat. Onset is usually in middle age, so the child of an affected parent lives under a Damocles' sword, having a 50% chance of becoming affected. Genetic tests are available. Signs are insidious, then progressive, eg chorea → irritability → dementia ± seizures → death. *Pathology:* Too few corpus striatum GABA-nergic & cholinergic neurones. *Treatment:* (p66) None prevents progression. Offer counselling to patient and family.[17] [George Huntington, 1872]

Jervell–Lange-Nielsen syndrome (autosomal recessive) An inherited disorder of ventricular repolarization, which causes prolonged QT^c interval, bilateral deafness, and a predisposition to syncope, seizures, and sudden death. Mutations in a K^+ channel regulatory subunit may be responsible.[18]

Kaposi's sarcoma (KS) This indolent sarcoma is either derived from capillary endothelial cells or from fibrous tissue associated with a serologically identifiable human γ-herpes virus (KSHV = HHV-8). It presents as purple papules or plaques on skin and mucosa (any organ). It metastasizes to lymph nodes. 4 types: (1) Classic, affecting elderly Eastern European and Mediterranean men, possibly with associated lymphoedema. Good prognosis. (2) Endemic (Central Africa), featuring peripheral, slow-growing lesions with rare visceral involvement. (3) KS in patients undergoing immunosuppression eg organ transplant

Diagnostic criteria in typical Guillain–Barré polyneuritis[1]

Features required for the diagnosis:
Progressive weakness of all 4 limbs
Areflexia

Features excluding the diagnosis:
Purely sensory symptoms
Diagnosis of: – myasthenia
– botulism
– poliomyelitis
– diphtheria
– porphyria
– toxic neuropathy

Features strongly supporting diagnosis:
Progression over up to 4wks
Near symmetry of symptoms
Sensory symptoms/signs only mild
Bilateral facial weakness
Recovery starts ~2wks after
the period of progression has
finished
Autonomic dysfunction
Absence of fever at onset
CSF protein ↑ with
CSF WCC <10 × 10⁶/L
Typical electrophysiological tests

Rarer features: Papilloedema (? from ↓CSF resorption), dysautonomia (p390), Miller Fisher syndrome (ataxia, ophthalmoplegia, areflexia). The purpose of this table is to give a checklist to use when considering diagnosing Guillain–Barré syndrome.

1 See M Bersudsky 2000 *Neuromuscul Disord* **10** 182 & A Hahn 1998 *Lancet* **352** 635

recipients. This tends to be aggressive, with visceral involvement. (4) KS in HIV +ve patients (particularly in homosexual men), where it is diagnostic of AIDS (p578), and carries a very poor prognosis. Pulmonary KS may present as breathlessness. Lymphatic obstruction predisposes to cellulitis. *Diagnosis* is by biopsy. *Treatment* (extensive or unsightly disease): local radiotherapy, IFN-α, and chemotherapy with doxorubicin, bleomycin, vinblastine, paclitaxel, and dacarbazine have been tried. In single lesion classic KS, surgical excision may be curative.[19]   [Moricz Kaposi, 1887]

Klippel–Trenaunay syndrome A triad of port-wine stain, varicose veins, and limb hypertrophy. Usually sporadic, though a few families exhibiting autosomal dominant inheritance have been reported.[20]

Korsakoff's syndrome ↓Ability to acquire new memories, eg after Wernicke's encephalopathy, due to thiamine deficiency (eg in alcoholics). The patient may have to relive his grief each time he hears of the death of a friend. He will confabulate to fill in the gaps in his memory. *Treatment:* See Wernicke's, p738.   [Sergei Korsakoff (more accurately transliterated Korsakov), 1887]

Langerhans'-cell histiocytosis (Histiocytosis X) Monoclonal proliferation, and single- or multi-organ infiltration, by Langerhans' cells. Organs affected can include lung, bone, skin, pituitary, liver, spleen, lymph nodes, and thyroid. A lethal leukaemia-like picture may be seen in infants. *Diagnosis:* Biopsy shows lytic aggregates of eosinophils, plasma cells, and histiocytes. ^{99m}Tc radionucleotide imaging may highlight lesions. *Treatment:* bone surgery, steroids, cytotoxics, and radiotherapy have all been used. See OHCS p748.[21]

Leriche's syndrome Absent femoral pulses, intermittent claudication of buttock muscles, pale cold legs, and impotence. It is due to aortic occlusive disease (eg a saddle embolism at its bifurcation).   [René Leriche, 1940]

Löffler's eosinophilic carditis Restrictive cardiomyopathy + eosinophilia (eg 120×10^9/L). These infiltrate many organs. It may be an early stage of tropical endomyocardial fibrosis and overlaps with idiopathic hypereosinophilic syndrome (HES), but is distinct from eosinophilic leukaemia. *Signs:* increasing heart failure (75%) ± mitral regurgitation (49%) ± heart block. *Treatment:* Digoxin + diuretics often only help if the eosinophilia is suppressed, eg by prednisolone or hydroxyurea (=hydroxycarbamide).[22]

Löffler's syndrome (Pulmonary eosinophilia) Allergic eosinophil infiltration of the lungs. Allergens include: *Ascaris lumbricoides, Trichinella spiralis, Fasciola hepatica, Strongyloides, Ankylostoma, Toxocara canis,* sulfonamides, hydralazine, and nitrofurantoin. Often symptomless, and the diagnosis is suggested by an incidental CXR (diffuse fan-shaped shadows)—or there may be cough, fever, and an eosinophilia (eg 20%). *Treatment:* Eradicate allergens. If idiopathic, steroids are tried.   [Wilhelm Löffler, born 1887]

Lown–Ganong–Levine syndrome A preexcitation syndrome, similar to Wolf–Parkinson–White (WPW: p128), characterized by a short P–R interval (<0.12 sec), occurence of supraventricular tachycardia (but not AF/flutter), and a *normal* QRS complex (as opposed to the δ-waves of WPW). The cause is not completely understood, but may be due to paranodal fibres that bypass all or part of the atrioventricular node.[23]

728 **McArdle's glycogen storage disease** (Type V) Caused by myophosphorylase deficiency (do muscle biopsy). Inheritance: autosomal recessive. Stiffness follows exercise. Venous blood from exercised muscle shows low levels of lactate and pyruvate. There may be myoglobinuria. *Treatment:* Aerobic exercise is beneficial, but avoid extreme exertion. A high-protein diet may help.[24]

Mallory–Weiss tear Vomiting *causes* haematemesis via an oesophageal tear.

Marchiafava–Bignami syndrome Alcoholism induces corpus callosum degeneration ± unilateral dysgraphia, apraxia, alexia, dementia, mutism, dysarthria, ↑tone, fits, ataxia, tremor, apathy. *Diagnosis:* MRI.[25]

Marchiafava–Micheli syndrome (Paroxysmal nocturnal haemoglobinuria) This haemopoietic stem cell disease with intravascular haemolysis, haemoglobinuria, cytopenia, and thrombi is due to a mutation in an X-linked gene (PIG-A). Marrow transplantation is a curative option.

Marfan's syndrome Autosomal dominant connective tissue disease, caused by mutations of the fibrillin-1 (FBN1) gene (15q21.1) causing abnormal synthesis, secretion, or matrix incorporation of fibrillin (a glycoprotein in elastic fibres). *Major criteria* (diagnostic eg if >2 with +ve family history): lens dislocation (the unsupported iris shimmers); aortic dissection/dilatation (β-blockers appear to slow this); dural ectasia (below); and skeletal features, eg arachnodactyly (long spidery fingers), armspan > height. During pregnancy, risk of aortic incompetence/dissection rises. Echo screening may be helpful. Homocystinuria may give a similar picture. Many people have *minor signs* (eg high-arched palate, scoliosis, joint hypermobility, pectus deformity), so genetic tests are often tried, but are problematic (intragenic heterogeneity). More helpful may be MRI looking for dural ectasia (enlargement of the neural canal, anywhere along its length, eg with widening of neural foramina, ± anterior meningocele).

| *Marfan's*^{autosomal dominant} | vs | *Homocystinuria* cystathione β-synthetase deficiency; a rare autorecessive causing early vasculopathy |

Marfan's (autosomal dominant) vs *Homocystinuria* (cystathione β-synthetase deficiency; a rare autorecessive causing early vasculopathy)

Marfan's	*Homocystinuria*
• Upwards lens dislocation	• Downwards dislocation
• Aortic incompetence	• Heart rarely affected
• Normal mentality	• Mental retardation
• Scoliosis, flat feet, herniae	• Recurrent thromboses; osteoporosis
• Life expectancy is ~halved from cardiovascular risks	• +ve urine cyanide-nitroprusside test
	• Response to pyridoxine

Meckel's diverticulum *Prevalence:* ≤2%. ≤2 inches long, and >2 feet from the ileocaecal valve, it contains gastric and pancreatic tissue, and can cause occult GI pain and bleeding. *Diagnosis:* radionucleotide scan; laparotomy.

Meigs' syndrome The association of a pleural effusion (transudate) with a benign ovarian fibroma or thecoma ± ascites.   [Joseph Meigs, 1937]

Ménétrier's disease Hyposecretion of gastric acid, gross mucosal hypertrophy with folds ≤4cm high, epigastric pain, GI bleeding, protein loss from the stomach, ↓gastric motility, oedema, weight↓, D&V, due to trophic effects of a hormone, or to regurgitation of small bowel contents through an incompetent pylorus. Gastric cancer may follow. *Treatment:* May respond to *H. pylori* eradication therapy.   [Pierre Ménétrier 1859-1935]

Meyer–Betz syndrome (Paroxysmal myoglobinuria) Muscle necrosis causes muscle tenderness, (±weakness, swelling, bruising), chills, pallor, fever, WCC↑, LFT↑, DIC, P_aO_2↓, and BP↓. Urine changes: pink→brown (as more myoglobin is excreted)→anuria. *Diagnosis:* Muscle biopsy, CPK↑, serum myoglobin↑.

Mikulicz's syndrome A variant of Sjögren's syndrome with dry mouth, epithelial salivary gland hyperplasia, blocking of ducts, and symmetrical enlargement. Lacrimal glands also enlarge.   [Johann von Mikulicz-Radecki, 1892]

Milroy's syndrome (Lymphoedema praecox) An inherited malfunction of the lymphatics causing asymmetric swelling of young girls' legs. *Management:* • Reassure (it is benign; ≤10% progress to the other leg). • Treat any infection actively. • Good foot hygiene. • If support stockings do not help, try a Lymphapress® device for active compression at night. Surgery with skin grafts is very rarely needed for 'elephantiasis leg'.

Münchausen's syndrome The patient gains hospital admissions via deception, feigning illness, hoping for a laparotomy (*laparotimophilia migrans*), or by bleeding (*haemorrhagica histrionica*) or with curious fits (*neurologica diabolica*) or false heart attacks (*cardiopathia fantastica*). Munchausen-by-proxy entails injury to a dependent person by his or her carer (eg mother) to gain medical attention. Covert video surveillance is an ethically problematic tool which may be necessary for diagnosis.

Nelson's syndrome If bilateral adrenalectomy is performed, feedback inhibition of ACTH is removed. Browning of the skin due to this excess ACTH production is known as Nelson's syndrome.

Ogilvie's syndrome Acute functional ('pseudo') colonic obstruction caused by: malignant retroperitoneal infiltration; spine fracture; U&E↑. A contrast enema or colonoscopy allows decompression, and excludes mechanical causes. Correct U&E. Neostigmine is also effective, suggesting parasympathetic suppression is to blame.[27] Caecal exteriorization is rarely needed.

Ortner's cardiovocal syndrome Recurrent laryngeal nerve palsy from a large left atrium (eg via mitral stenosis) or aortic dissection.

Osler–Weber–Rendu syndrome (Hereditary haemorrhagic telangiectasia) Punctiform lesions on mucous membranes cause epistaxis or GI bleeds. Big AV malformations cause high-output heart failure. Hepatic telangiectasia can cause cirrhosis. Inheritance: autosomal dominant.[28]

Paget's disease of breast is intra-epidermal spread of an intraductal cancer. Any red, scaly lesion around the nipple should suggest Paget's disease: do a biopsy. ►Never diagnose eczema of the nipple without a biopsy. *Treatment:* Mastectomy (or possibly radiotherapy).[29]   [Sir James Paget, 1874]

Pancoast's syndrome Apical lung cancer + ipsilateral Horner's (p726), from invasion of the cervical sympathetic plexus. Also shoulder/arm pain (brachial plexus invasion C8–T2) ± hoarse voice/bovine cough (unilateral recurrent laryngeal nerve palsy and vocal cord paralysis).   [Henry Pancoast, 1932]

Parinaud's syndrome (Dorsal midbrain syndrome) Upward gaze palsy with pseudo-Argyll Robertson pupils (p82). Causes include hydrocephalus and pineal tumours.

Peutz–Jeghers' syndrome Germline mutations of gene LKB1 cause mucocutaneous dark freckles on lips, oral mucosa, lips, face, palm, & soles ± GI obstruction, bleeds, or polyps. *Malignant change:* in ≤3%, typically with duodenal polyps. *Treatment:* Usually conservative or local excision. **NB:** hamartomas are an excessive focal overgrowth of normal, mature cells in an organ composed of identical cellular elements.

Peyronie's disease Penile fibrosis leads to angulation, making coitus most inconvenient. *Associations:* Dupuytren's (p722); atheroma. *Treatment:* Surgery and prostheses aid penetration. Shock wave therapy and iontophoresis may also help.[30] Oral therapies eg tamoxifen, vitamin E, colchicine, or acetyl-L-carnitine, are useful in early disease.[31]   [François de la Peyronie, 1743]

Pott's syndrome This is spinal TB. Rare in the West, this tends to affect young adults, causing pain, and stiffness of *all* back movements. ESR↑. Abscess formation and cord compression may occur, leading to paraplegia, and bowel and bladder dysfunction. Disc spaces may be affected in isolation or with vertebral involvement either side (usually anterior margins early). *X-rays:* narrow disc spaces and vertebral osteoporosis early, with bone destruction leading to wedging of vertebrae later. Whereas in the thoracic spine paraspinal abscesses are seen on x-ray and kyphosis on examination, with lower thoracic or lumbar involvement, abscess formation may be by psoas muscle in the flank, or in the iliac fossa. T10–L1 are most commonly affected. *R:* Anti-TB drugs (p566).   [Sir Percival Pott, 1779]

Prinzmetal (variant) angina Angina occurring at rest, due to coronary artery spasm, causes ECG shows ST elevation. *Treatment:* As for ordinary angina (p118); nifedipine is said to be particularly useful. *Association:* Circle of Willis occlusion from intimal thickening (*moyamoya disease*).

Raynaud's syndrome This is episodic digital ischaemia, precipitated by cold or emotion. Fingers ache and change colour: pale → blue → red. It may be idiopathic (Raynaud's *disease*—prevalence: 3–20%; ♀:♂ >1:1, or have an underlying cause (Raynaud's *phenomenon*). *Tests:* Exclude an underlying cause (see BOX). *Treatment:* Keep warm (eg electrically heated mittens) ; stop smoking. Nifedipine 5–20mg/8h PO helps some as may losartan, prazosin, or fluoxetine. Sympathectomy may help in those with severe

Conditions in which Raynaud's phenomenon may be exhibited[1]		
Scleroderma; SLE	Rheumatoid arthritis	Thoracic outlet obstruction
Trauma	Arteriosclerosis	Use of vibrating tools
Leukaemia	Thrombocytosis	Mixed cryoglobulinaemia
Cold agglutinins	Drugs; PRV (p664)	Monoclonal gammopathies

1 Patient information on Raynaud's is available from 112 Crewe Road, Alsalgar, Cheshire, ST7 2JA.
For a review of Raynaud's phenomenon, see FM Wigley 2002 *NEJM* **347** 100

disease. Iloprost, eg starting at 0.5ng/kg/min IVI (available via Schering for named patients) may salvage digits with ulcers ± near-gangrene; effects last ≤16wks. Relapse is common.

Refsum's syndrome (autosomal recessive) Polyneuritis, nerve deafness, night blindness (pigment retinopathy), cerebellar ataxia, ichthyosis, cardiomyopathy, anosmia + ↑CSF protein. Phytanic acid ↑in fat, liver, kidneys, and nerves. The cause is usually a mutation of the gene coding for the peroxisomal enzyme phytanoyl-CoA hydroxylase. *Tests:* Plasmalogens (a kind of phospholipid)↓, plasma phytanic acid & pipecolic acid↑. *Treatment:* Restrict foods containing phytanic acid; plasmapheresis.

Romano–Ward syndrome (autosomal dominant) A mutation in a K^+ channel subunit causes a predisposition towards ventricular tachyarrythmias, syncope, and sudden death.

Rotor syndrome Defective excretion of conjugated bilirubin, producing cholestatic jaundice. Inheritance is probably autosomal recessive.

Sister Mary Joseph nodule An umbilical metastatic deposit from an intra-abdominal malignancy.

Sjögren's syndrome This is the association of a connective tissue disease (rheumatoid arthritis in 50%) with keratoconjunctivitis sicca (↓lacrimation causing dry eyes) or xerostomia (↓salivation causing dry mouth). Lymphocytes and plasma cells infiltrate secretory glands (also lungs and liver) causing fibrosis. The connective tissue disease is often severe (rheumatoid factor is always +ve). Anti-Ro (SSA) and anti-La (SSB) antibodies are variably present. Gland biopsy shows sialadenitis. Involvement of other glands is common causing dyspareunia, dry skin, dysphagia, otitis media, and pneumonia. *Other features:* neuropathy, renal involvement, hepatosplenomegaly, + an association with other connective tissue disorders, renal tubular acidosis, drug reactions, lymphoma, and ↓well-being (headaches, GI symptoms, concentration↓). *Tests:* Conjunctival dryness may be quantified by putting a strip of filter paper under the lower lid and measuring the distance along the paper that tears are absorbed (Schirmer's test); <10mm in 5min is +ve. *Treatment:* Hypromellose (artificial tears) ± occlusion of the punctum which drains tears. Xerostomia may respond to frequent cool drinks, or artificial saliva spray. Novel therapies include topical ciclosporin A for ocular complications, topical human interferon for oral complications, and tumour necrosis factor (TNF) inhibitors for systemic disease.[32]   [Henrik Sjögren, 1933]

Stevens–Johnson syndrome Drugs (sulfonamides, penicillin, sedatives), viruses or other infection (eg orf, *herpes simplex*), neoplasia or other systemic disease induce a systemic illness with fever, arthralgia, myalgia ± pneumonitis and conjunctivitis. Vesicles develop in mucosa of mouth, GU tract, ± conjunctivae. The skin develops typical target lesions of erythema multiforme, often on the palms. They may blister in the centre. The signs may also include polyarthritis and diarrhoea. *Treatment:* The disease is usually self-limiting, so supportive care (eg calamine lotion for the skin) will usually suffice. Steroids (systemic & eye-drops) were once used, but results from trials have been variable, so ask a dermatologist and ophthalmologist. Ciclosporin has also been used with some success, but IV immunoglobulin is not helpful.[33] *Prognosis:* Mortality ~5%. The illness may be severe for the 1st 10d before resolving over 30d. Damage to the eyes may persist and at worst, blindness may result.[34]

Sturge–Weber syndrome (Encephalotrigeminal angiomatosis) The association of a trigeminal port wine stain on the face (haemangioma) with contralateral focal fits. There may also be glaucoma, exophthalmos (p305), strabismus, optic atrophy, and spasticity with a ↓IQ. Fits are caused by a corresponding capillary haemangioma in the brain. *Tests:* Skull x-ray shows cortical calcification, but angiography is usually normal. MRI with gadolinium

contrast may show pial angiomata. *Treatment:* Laser therapy can remove facial port wine stains. Anticonvulsants are indicated for seizures; hemispherectomy may be required if seizures are refractory to therapy.

Takayasu's arteritis (Aortic arch syndrome) Idiopathic arteritis causes narrowing of the 1st few cm of the innominate, carotid, and subclavian arteries with the adjacent aorta, as well as renal arteries. *The Patient* is typically a woman 20–40yrs old. Eyes—vision↓, cataracts, atrophy of the iris, optic nerve, and retina. CNS—hemiplegia, headache, vertigo, syncope, convulsions. CVS—pulselessness; systolic murmurs above and below the clavicle; aortic regurgitation; aortic aneurysm. Renal—BP↑. *Diagnosis:* ESR >40mm/h (if disease is active); aortography (invasive or via CT/MRI). *R:* Prednisolone (starting example: 40mg/24h PO); angioplasty ± stenting, or reconstructive surgery/endarterectomy may be tried. *10yr survival:* ~90%. [Mikito Takayasu, 1908]

Tietze's syndrome (Idiopathic costochondritis) Localized pain/tenderness in costal cartilage enhanced by motion, coughing, or sneezing. The 2nd rib is most often affected. The diagnostic key is *localized* tenderness which is marked (flinches on prodding). *Treatment:* Simple analgesia, eg aspirin. Its importance is that it is a benign cause of what at first seems to be alarming, eg cardiac, pain. In lengthy illness, local steroid injections may be used.

Todd's palsy Focal CNS signs (eg hemiplegia) following a seizure. The patient seems to have had a stroke, but recovers in <24h. [Robert Todd, 1856]

Vincent's angina Mouth infection with ulcerative gingivitis from *Borrelia vincentii* (a spirochaete) + fusiform bacilli (Gram –ve, nonsporing variously called *Bacteroides* or *Fusobacteria*). Try penicillin V 250mg/6h & metronidazole 400mg/8h PO. ΔΔ: oral lymphoma.

Von Hippel–Lindau syndrome This predisposition to renal cysts ± carcinomas, phaeochromocytoma, and haemangioblastoma (in lateral lobes of the cerebellum) ± aneurysms and tortuosities of retinal vessels, leading to subretinal haemorrhages presents in young adults with headache, dizziness, unilateral ataxia, or blindness. The culprit gene acts by binding elongin A.

Von Willebrand's disease (vWD) Von Willebrand's factor (vWF) has 3 roles in clotting: to bring platelets into contact with exposed subendothelium; to make platelets bind to each other, and to bind to factor VIII (protecting it from destruction in the liver after release from hepatocytes). There are >22 types of vWD, some of which are:
Type I: (Commonest) Autosomal dominant deficiency (↓levels) of vWF.
Type II: Abnormal vWF with lack of high molecular weight multimers.
Type III: Undetectable vWF levels (autosomal recessive with gene deletions).
Type Normandy: Impaired vWF-VIII binding (mutations in VIII-binding domains of vWF cause an autosomal recessive mimic of haemophilia A).
Signs: Bruising; mucocutaneous bleeding; menorrhagia; ↑bleeding post tooth extraction. Asymptomatic in one-third of Type I. *Tests:* Liaise with a haematologist. APTT↑ VIIIC↓; INR & platelets ↔. *Treatment:* (p644) Get expert help. Factor VIII cryoprecipitate; vasopressin. Avoid NSAIDs. The Pill increases vWF.

Wallenberg's lateral medullary syndrome This relatively common syndrome comprises lesions to multiple CNS nuclei, caused by posterior inferior

cerebellar artery occlusion. Features include dysphagia and dysarthria (IX and X nuclei), vomiting (nucleus ambiguus), vertigo (vestibular nucleus) with ipsilateral cerebellar ataxia (inferior cerebellar peduncle), ipsilateral Horner's syndrome (descending autonomic fibres), loss of pain, and temperature sensation on the ipsilateral face (V nucleus) and contralateral limbs (lateral lemniscus). There is no limb weakness as the pyramidal tracts are unaffected.

In the rare *medial medullary syndrome*, vertebral or anterior spinal artery occlusion causes contralateral weakness (pyramidal tract) and loss of position sense (medial lemniscus), with ipsilateral tongue paralysis (XII nucleus).

Waterhouse–Friederichsen's syndrome and meningococcaemia (Haemorrhage into the adrenal cortex with a fulminant necrotizing meningo-coccaemia, causing purpura, rash, fever, meningitis, coma, and DIC). There is shock as normal vascular tone requires cortisol to set activity of alpha and beta adrenergic receptors—and aldosterone is needed to maintain extracellular fluid volume. Sepsis is only one cause of adrenal haemorrhage; others are coagulopathy states, pregnancy diseases, shock, and other stresses. It is best to think of meningococcal endotoxin as a potent initiator of inflammatory and coagulatory cascades. *Treatment:* ▶▶Antibiotics eg ceftriaxone 2g/12h IV, hydrocortisone 200mg/4h IV, and get expert help for renal failure and DIC—difficult and controversial; antithrombin III (AT-III) may help; heparin is ineffective if AT-III levels are low. See BOX for novel therapies.

Weber's syndrome Ipsilateral 3rd-nerve palsy with contralateral hemiplegia, due to midbrain infarction after occlusion of the paramedian branches of the basilar artery (which supplies the cerebral peduncles).

Wegener's granulomatosis A potentially fatal granulomatous vasculitis. *Diagnostic criteria:*
• Necrotizing granulomas in respiratory tract
• Generalized necrotizing arteritis
• Glomerulonephritis.
Any organ *may* be involved, eg nasal ulcers, epistaxis, rhinitis, sinus involvement, otitis media (± sensorineural deafness/vertigo), multiple cranial nerve lesions, oral ulcers, gum hypertrophy ± bleeding and microabscesses, lung symptoms and variable shadows on CXR (eg multiple nodules), hypertension and glomerulitis. The patient is also systemically ill. A 'saddle-nose' deformity is a feature sometimes seen in Wegener's.[1] *Eye signs* (seen in 50%): proptosis ± ptosis (orbital granuloma), conjunctivitis, corneal ulcers, episcleritis, scleritis, uveitis, retinitis. *Tests:* cANCA (p421) helps diagnostically and in disease monitoring. Cytology from sputum/BAL may show atypical cells that can be confused with bronchial carcinoma. *Treatment:* High-dose steroids, backed up by cyclophosphamide, has revolutionized prognosis. Continuous oral cyclophosphamide is more effective than pulsed IV regimens at inducing sustained remission, but also causes more side effects. *Pulsed dose example:* 3 pulses of 500mg cyclophosphamide IV separated by 7d with mesna to ↓cyclo-phosphamide-induced chemical cystitis. Severe renal disease may benefit from plasma exchange. Localized lung disease has been treated with just steroids ± co-trimoxazole.

Wernicke's encephalopathy Thiamine (vitamin B_1) deficiency, often occurring in alcoholics, with a classical triad of ophthalmoplegia (external recti commonly), ataxia, and confusion. Other eye signs such as nystagmus, ptosis, abnormal pupillary reactions, and altered consciousness may occur. Consider this diagnosis in all those with any of the above signs: it may present with headache, anorexia, vomiting, and confusion. *Causes:* Alcoholism, eating disorders, malnutrition, and prolonged vomiting associated with chemotherapy can all cause ↓thiamine. Wernicke's can be precipitated by glucose administration to a thiamine-deficient patient. *Tests:* Red cell transketolase↓; plasma pyruvate↑. *Treatment:* Urgent thiamine to prevent irreversible Korsakoff's syndrome (p728). Dose examples: thiamine 200–300mg/24h PO; maintainance: 25mg/24h PO. This regimen is generally safe, but risks undertreatment, so if the oral route is impossible or there is danger of rapid progression to irreversible Korsakoff's syndrome (often the case), give Pabrinex® 2–3 pairs of high-potency ampules/8h IV over 10min for ≤2d, then daily for 5–7d. An IM (gluteal) preparation is available (dose example: 1 pair/12h IM for up to 7d). Have resuscitation facilities to hand as anaphylaxis can occur. [Karl Wernicke, 1875]

---

1 Common causes of a 'saddle-nose' deformity are trauma, and iatrogenic (eg post-rhinoplasty). The rarer causes, which are popular with some finals examiners, include Wegener's, syphilis, and leprosy.

New approaches to meningococcaemia[1]

(Offered here more as possibilities than as recommended treatments; they may provide an extra option in serious cases):

Extracorporeal membrane oxygenation May help cardiorespiratory failure.

Terminal fragment of human bactericidal/permeability-increasing protein ($rBPI_{21}$): This endotoxin-binding part of neutrophil azure granules can ↓cytokines. 1 trial found $rBPI_{21}$ conferred no significant reduction in mortality, but mortality *was* lower in those who received the entire infusion course.[37]

Heparin with protein C concentrate Protein C is a naturally occurring anti coagulant, and deficiency (which occurs in meningococcaemia) leads to intravascular thrombosis. It can reverse coagulopathy and appears to decrease mortality in severe sepsis.[38]

Plasmapheresis (± fresh frozen plasma/cryoprecipitate) *may* remove cytokines and *may* help by correcting acidosis, though the only randomized trial found no mortality benefit.[39]

Thrombolysis may help limb reperfusion.

Other targets for novel therapies include interleukin 6, which is a pleiotropic cytokine produced during meningococcal infection, and is thought to be the mediator of myocardial depression.[2]

739

1 For a review of severe meningococcal sepsis in children, covering most of these novel interventions, see PB Baines 2003 *Br J Anaesthesia* **90** 72–83
2 N Pathan 2004 *Lancet* **363** 203

Whipple's disease[1] A cause of GI malabsorption (p252) which usually occurs in men >50yrs old—caused by *Tropheryma whippelii* (a Gram +ve rod).

General/GI features: Weight↓; diarrhoea; abdominal pain; arthralgia (chronic, migratory, seronegative arthropathy affecting mainly peripheral joints); fever; skin hyperpigmentation; lymphadenopathy; clubbing; pleurisy; oedema; anaemia; hepato/splenomegaly.

Eye signs: Uveitis, scotomata, papilloedema.

Cardiac signs: BP↓; ascites; pericarditis; SBE/IE (typically culture –ve); heart block; coronary arteritis.

CNS signs (in 10%): Dementia, ophthalmoplegia, and facial myoclonus are typical (if all together, they are highly suggestive). Also scotomata, meningitis, and seizures ± hypothalamic syndrome (insomnia, hyperphagia, polydipsia).

Tests: Jejunal biopsy shows intact villi, but the cells of the lamina propria are replaced by macrophages which contain PAS +ve glycoprotein granules. Similar cells are found in nodes, spleen, and liver. Immunohistochemistry can aid diagnosis, as can PCR. MRI is useful in identifying CNS involvement. *R:* One option is initial parenteral penicillin and streptomycin for 2wks then oral co-trimoxazole for 1yr. Shorter courses risk relapse with CNS features. Ceftriaxone is an alternative for the initial IV therapy.   *[George Whipple, 1907]*

Zellweger syndrome (autosomal recessive) A rare leukodystrophy characterized by decreased/absent peroxisomes. It is a severe form of infantile Refsum's syndrome, and exhibits similar biochemical abnormalities (p734). Clinical features include developmental delay; craniofacial abnormalities; glaucoma; cataract; hepatomegaly; renal cysts; hypotonia. A number of causative genes (eg *PEX1*) have been identified.

Zollinger–Ellison syndrome This is the association of peptic ulcer with a gastrin-secreting pancreatic adenoma (or simple islet cell hyperplasia). Gastrin excites excessive acid production which can produce many ulcers in the duodenum and stomach. Rarely, adenomas are located in the stomach or duodenum. 50–60% are malignant, 10% are multiple and 30% of cases are associated with multiple endocrine adenomatosis (MEN type I, p309). One-third of those with sporadic gastrinomas have a mutation in the MEN1 gene.[40]

Incidence: 0.1% of patients with duodenal ulcer disease. Suspect in those with multiple peptic ulcers resistant to drugs, particularly if there is associated diarrhoea and steatorrhoea or a family history of peptic ulcers (or of islet cell, pituitary, or parathyroid adenomas).

Tests: Raised fasting serum gastrin level (>1000pg/mL) *when not on acid-reduction therapy*; there may also be a raised basal gastric acid output of >15mmol/h (the latter test is of less importance). The secretin stimulation test is useful in suspected cases with only mild hypergastrinaemia.

Treatment: Proton pump inhibitors (PPIs) such as lanzoprazole and omeprazole (p214) are more effective than H_2-blockers. These PPIs bind irreversibly with parietal cell potassium hydrogen ATP-ase. SE: headaches, rash, diarrhoea. Dose of omeprazole: 20mg/24h–60mg/12h PO (start with 60mg/d and adjust according to response). Measuring intragastric pH helps determine the best dose (aim to keep pH at 2–7; a daily dose of 60mg typically achieves this). The hazards of long-term use are unknown. Ask an expert about the possibility of excising the tumour after location by ultrasound, CT scans, or angiography, provided there is not already disseminated malignancy (usually in the liver). Some say that surgery should be reserved for when medical treatment fails. Others suggest that all those with sporadic (ie not MEN1-associated) gastrinomas, but no hepatic metastases, should be offered surgery.[41] *Prognosis:* 5-year survival with metastases: ~20%.

1 For a review of Whipple's disease, see T Marth 2003 *Lancet* **361** 239

Practical procedures[1]

Contents

There is no substitute for learning by experience. Often it is wiser to wait for someone to come and carry out an urgent procedure than to try for the first time by oneself—but some procedures must occasionally be performed at once.

[1] We thank Dr F Poyner who is our Specialist Reader for this chapter.

Nasogastric (Ryle's) tubes

These tubes are passed into the stomach *via* either the nose or the mouth, and drain externally. Sizes: 16 = large, 12 = medium, 10 = small.

Uses:

- To empty the stomach (pre-op, or in acute pancreatitis, or paralytic ileus).
- For irreversible dysphagia (eg motor neurone disease).
- For feeding ill patients (use a special fine-bore tube).

Passing the tube Nurses are experts and will ask you (who may never have passed one) to do so only when they fail—so the first question to ask is: 'Have you asked the charge-nurse from the ward next door?'

- Wear non-sterile gloves and a nurse's apron to protect from those 'rich encrustations' so often found on our clothes after a few days on the wards.
- Explain the procedure. Take a new, cool (hence less flexible) tube.
- Use the tube, by holding it against the patient's head, to estimate the length required to get from the nostril to the back of the throat.
- Place lubricated tube in nostril with its natural curve promoting passage down, rather than up. Right nostril is often easier than the left. Advance towards occiput (not upwards).
- When the tip is estimated to be entering the throat, rotate the tube by ~180° to discourage passage into the mouth.
- Advance the tube into the oesophagus during a swallow—and thence into the stomach. *If this fails:* Try the other nostril, then oral insertion.
- Secure with tape to the nose. Use litmus paper (are the contents gastric, ie acid?)
- Either spigot the tube, or allow to drain into a dependent catheter bag secured to the patient's clothing (zinc oxide tape around tube to form a flap, safety pin through flap). ▶Do not agree to plans to pass the tube under anaesthesia: the great danger is fatal inhalation of vomit on induction.

Complications

- Pain, or, rarely:
- Loss of electrolytes
- Oesophagitis
- Tracheal or duodenal intubation
- Necrosis: retro- or nasopharyngeal
- Perforation of the stomach

Placing IV cannulae ('drips')

► Try to avoid IVIs, as infections at the IVI site can cause real problems.

1 Set up a tray Swab to clean skin. Find: 3 cannulae; syringe + 1mL 1% lidocaine; 3 fine needles (orange); cotton-wool to stop bleeding from unsuccessful attempts; tape to fix cannula; elastoplast; flush.

2 Set up a 'drip'-stand with first bag of fluid (carefully checked with a nurse); 'run through' a giving-set (a nurse will show you how).

3 Ask a nurse to help until you are experienced. Nurses prefer helping rather than changing the bed clothes because of spilt blood.

4 Explain procedure to patient. Place the tourniquet around the arm.

5 Search hard for the best vein (palpable, not merely visible). Don't be too hasty. Rest the arm below the level of the heart to aid filling. Ask them to clench and unclench their fist.

6 Sit comfortably—with the patient lying (prevents most faints).

7 Tap the vein to make it prominent. Avoid sites spanning joints.

8 Place a paper towel under arm to soak up any blood.

9 Clean the skin Use local anaesthetic (or Emla® cream): it is kinder, and studies show that it *does* work. Use a fine needle to raise a bleb of lidocaine, like a nettle sting, just to the vein's side. Wait 15s. Insertion skill is best shown at the bedside by an expert.

After it is in: (1) Connect fluid tube; check flow. (2) Fix cannula firmly with tape. (3) Bandage a loop of the tube to the arm. If the 'drip' is across a joint, use a splint. (4) Check the flow speed. Write a fluid chart (p462). Does the nurse understand it? (5) Explain that no needle is left in the arm, but that care needs to be taken. (6) Adding heparin to the IVI makes drips last longer (>30h in 1 study): give 500U/500mL; it is incompatible with phenytoin, aminoglycosides, & amiodarone; SE: platelets↓. (7) When the 'drip' comes down, remove the cannula. (A patient once asked at follow-up if he still needed 'this green plastic thing on my hand'.)

If you fail after three attempts ►Shocked patients need fluid quickly: if you are having trouble putting in a 'drip', call your senior. The advice below assumes that the 'drip' is not immediately life-saving.

Experienced doctors can forget they had to learn. Ask to be taught and for help when you need it. Is this the right needle for the right job? What is the 'drip' for? If the patient may need blood quickly, use a large size (eg brown; green is suitable for slow IVIs—or even pink if the veins are fragile). *If the IVI really is needed*, proceed as follows:
- Explain to the patient that veins are difficult.
- Fetch a bowl of warm water. This gives you time to calm down.
- Immerse the patient's arm in the warm water for 2min.
- Use a blood pressure cuff at 80mmHg as a tourniquet—and try again.
- Alternatively, a small amount of GTN paste over the vein may enlarge it.

If you still cannot get the 'drip' in You are now downcast, so call your senior—it may hurt your pride but there is nothing that makes your registrar happier than to succeed with a 'drip' where you have failed. Calling him could make both you and your patient happy. Not many things do that! If you are too frightened of your senior, ask another house officer—they are much more likely to succeed than you at this juncture. If you cannot find anyone to help, have a coffee and return an hour later. Veins are capricious: they come and go.

'The drip has tissued' Ask yourself:
- Is there fluid in bag and giving-set?
- Inspect the cannula: take bandage off.
- Is the 'drip' still needed?
- Are the control taps open?
- Are there kinks in the tube?

Inflamed drip sites need prompt re-siting of the drip. If site is healthy, gently infuse a 2mL syringe of 0.9% saline through the cannula. If resistance prevents this, the 'drip' needs resiting. (Needle-stick injury: see p582.)

Catheterizing bladders

Catheters *Size* (in French gauge): 12 = small; 16 = large. Usually a 12 or 14 is right. Use the smallest you can. Latex is soft; *simplastic* firmer. A *silastic* (silicone) catheter may be used long term, but costs more. *Shape: Foley* is typical; *coudé (elbow) catheters* have an angled tip to ease around prostates but are more risky. *Teeman* catheters have tapered ends for a similar reason. *Condom catheters*♂ (Paul's tubing) have no in-dwelling parts, and are preferred by nurses and patients (less pain, less restriction of movement), even though they may leak and fall off.[2]

Catheter problems: • Infection (don't use antibiotics unless systemically unwell). Consider bladder irrigation, eg 0.9% saline or chlorhexidine 0.02% (may irritate). • *Bladder spasm* may be painful. Try reducing the water in the balloon or using anticholinergic drugs, eg propantheline 15mg/8h PO.

Methods of catheterizing bladders

1 *Per urethram* This route is used to relieve urinary retention, to monitor urine output in critically ill patients, or to collect urine for diagnosis uncontaminated by urethral flora. It is *contraindicated* in urethral injury (eg pelvic fracture) and acute prostatitis. Catheterization introduces bacteria into the bladder, so aseptic technique is essential. Women are often catheterized by nurses but you should be able to catheterize patients of either sex.

- Lie the patient supine in a well-lit area: women with knees flexed and hips abducted with heels together. Use a gloved hand to prep urethral meatus in a pubis-to-anus direction, holding the labia apart with the other hand. With un-circumcised men, retract the foreskin to 'prep' the glans; use a gloved hand to hold the penis still and off the scrotum. The hand used to hold the penis or labia should not touch the catheter (use forceps if needed).
- Put sterile lidocaine 2% gel on the catheter tip and ≤10mL into the urethra (≤5mL if ♀). In men, stretch the penis perpendicular to the body to eliminate any urethral folds that may lead to false passage.
- Use steady *gentle* pressure to advance the catheter. Significant obstructions encountered should prompt withdrawal and reinsertion. With prostatic hypertrophy, a *coudé* tip catheter may get past the prostate.
- Insert to the hilt; wait until urine emerges before inflating the balloon. Remember to check the balloon's capacity before inflation. Pull the catheter back so that the balloon comes to rest at the bladder neck.
- Remember to reposition the foreskin in un-circumcised men to prevent massive oedema of the glans after the catheter is inserted.

Self-catheterization This is a good, safe way of managing chronic retention from a neuropathic bladder (eg in multiple sclerosis, diabetic neuropathy, spinal tumour). Never consider a patient in difficulties from a big residual volume to be too old, young, or disabled to learn. 5-yr-old children can learn the technique, and can have their lives transformed—so motivation may be excellent. There may be *fewer* UTIs as there is no residual urine—and less reflux obstructive uropathy. Assessing suitability entails testing sacral dermatomes: a 'numb bum' implies ↓ sensation of a full bladder; higher sensory loss may mean catheterization will be painless. Get help from your continence adviser who will be in a position to teach the patient or carer that

catheterizations must be gentle, particularly if sensation is lacking, and must number >4/d ('always keep your catheter with you; don't wait for an urge before catheterizing').

2 Suprapubic catheterization is sometimes necessary and may be preferred. Ensure the bladder is distended; then clean the skin. Infiltrate with local anaesthetic down to the bladder, nick the skin, and then insert the catheter down vertically above the symphysis pubis. When urine is draining, advance the catheter over the trocar and tape it down securely.

Ascitic tap

Ascites may be sampled to provide a cytological or bacterial diagnosis, eg to exclude spontaneous bacterial peritonitis. Before starting ensure that you know the patient's prothrombin time or INR. If it is abnormal, seek help before proceeding.

- Place the patient flat and tap out the ascites, marking a point where fluid has been identified, avoiding scars or vessels.
- Clean the skin. May need some local anaesthetic.
- Insert a 21G needle on a 20mL syringe into the skin and advance while aspirating until fluid is withdrawn.
- Remove the needle and apply a sterile dressing.
- Send fluid for microscopy, culture, chemistry (protein), and cytology.

Diagnostic aspiration of a pleural effusion

- Percuss the upper border of the pleural effusion and choose a site 1 or 2 intercostal spaces below it (usually posteriorly or laterally).
- Mark the spot and then clean the area with an antiseptic solution.
- Infiltrate down to the pleura with 5–10mL of 1% lidocaine.
- Attach a 21G needle to a syringe and insert it just above the upper border of the rib below the mark (avoids neurovascular bundle). Aspirate whilst advancing the needle.
- Draw off 10–30mL of pleural fluid.

Send fluid to the lab for *chemistry* (protein, glucose, pH, LDH, amylase); *bacteriology* (microscopy and culture, auramine stain, TB culture); *cytology* and, if indicated, *immunology* (rheumatoid factor, ANA, complement).

Pleural biopsy

This is usually performed in patients with a pleural effusion when analysis of pleural fluid has not provided an underlying diagnosis. It should not be performed on the ward in patients without an effusion as this requires a different approach. This procedure requires some practice, so if you are inexperienced, ask a senior doctor to assist you.

- Place the patient in an upright position on the edge of the bed, arms resting on a pillow on a bed-table to provide support.
- Identify the upper border of the pleural effusion posteriorly or laterally and mark an intercostal space 1–2 ribs below this.
- Clean the skin with an antiseptic solution and apply sterile drapes.
- Infiltrate down to the pleura with 5–10mL of 1% lidocaine.
- Check that you are in the correct space by aspirating pleural fluid.
- Make a deep skin incision 0.5cm wide immediately above the upper border of the rib below the chosen intercostal space (avoids neurovascular bundle).
- Carefully advance the Abrams' needle through the incision until a 'give' is felt as you enter the pleural space.
- Open the needle by twisting the trocar. Check that fluid can be aspirated.
- Manoeuvre the open needle so that the cutting notch is caught on the pleura—pull the needle back slightly at an angle to the chest wall—then close the needle and withdraw. A slight tug may be required at this stage.
- Withdraw the needle in expiration and repeat.
- Place the tissue samples in the appropriate media for histological and microbiological examination. Send to the lab for microscopy, culture, and histology.
- Withdraw the needle, and apply a sterile dressing, occasionally a single suture may be required.
- Perform a post-procedure CXR.

Inserting a chest drain[3]

See also p196 and p798.

- Sterile procedure.
- Have the x-rays or CT-scans available to confirm location for chest drain insertion.
- Preparation: trolley with dressing pack, iodine, needles, 10mL syringe, 20mL 1% lignocaine (=lidocaine), scalpel (N°15), suture, chest drain (eg 10–14F, if trauma or haemothorax larger gauge eg 28–30F) drainage bottle, connection tubes, sterile H$_2$O, tape. Incontinence pad under patient. Swab extensively.
- Choose insertion site:[4] 4th–6th intercostal space, anterior to mid-axillary line—the 'safe triangle' (see OPPOSITE). A more posterior approach eg the 7th space posteriorly may be required to drain a loculated effusion, and occasionally the 2nd intercostal space in the mid-clavicular line may be used for apical pneumothoraces—however, both approaches tend to be less comfortable.
- Infiltrate down to pleura with 10–20mL of 1% lidocaine. Check that either air or fluid can be aspirated from the proposed insertion site—if not **do not** proceed. Wait 3min.
- Make 2cm incision above 6th rib, to avoid neurovascular bundle under 5th rib. Bluntly dissect with forceps down to pleura. Puncture pleura with scissors/forceps. If large bore tube (>24F), then sweep a finger inside chest to clear adherent lung and exclude (eg in blunt abdominal trauma) stomach in the chest!
- Before inserting the drain, remove the metal trochar completely; introduce the drain *atraumatically* using forceps to advance it.
- Advance the tip upwards to the apex (or base if draining an effusion). Stop when you meet resistance. Then attach the drain via the tubing to the underwater seal. Ensure that the longer tube within the bottle is underwater and bubbling with respiration. If patient is to be moved to another hospital, substitute Heimlich flutter valve or drainage bag with flap valve for underwater drain. You should never clamp chest drains inserted for pneumothoraces. Clamping is occasionally used when pleural effusions are being drained to control the rate of drainage and prevent expansion pulmonary oedema.[5]
- With large/medium bore tubes, the incision should be closed with a mattress suture or suture across the incision. Purse string sutures are no-longer recommended as they may lead to scarring and increased wound pain.
- Fix the drain with a second suture tied around the tube like a 'Roman gaiter'. Secure the drain with tape (eg 'Sleek®') to prevent it from slipping.
- Request CXR to check the position of the drain. Give analgesia (PO/IM).

▸▸ Relieving a tension pneumothorax

- Aim: to release air from the pleural space. In a tension pneumothorax air is drawn into the intra-pleural space, with each breath, but cannot escape due to a valve-like effect of the tiny flap in the parietal pleura. The increasing pressure progressively embarrasses the heart and the other lung.
- 100% oxygen.

- Insert a large bore IV cannula (eg Venflon®) through an intercostal space anywhere on the affected side. Usually 2nd intercostal space in the mid-clavicular line. Remove the stylet, which will allow the trapped air to escape, usually with an audible hiss.
- Tape securely.
- Proceed to formal chest drainage immediately.

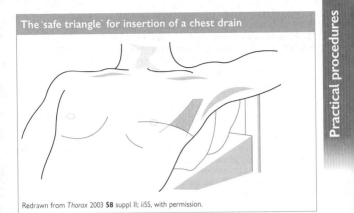

The 'safe triangle' for insertion of a chest drain

Redrawn from *Thorax* 2003 **58** suppl II; ii55, with permission.

Lumbar puncture (LP)

Contraindications • Bleeding diathesis • Cardiorespiratory compromise • Infection at site of needle insertion, and most importantly: • ↑Intracranial pressure (suspect if very severe headache, ↓level of consciousness with falling pulse, rising BP, vomiting, focal signs, or papilloedema), give urgent treatment as needed; discuss urgently with relevant clinician with a view to CT scan. CT is not infallible, so be sure your indication for LP is strong.

Method Explain to the patient *what* sampling CSF entails, *why* it is needed, that *co-operation* is vital, and that they can *communicate with you* at all stages.

• Place the patient on his or her left side, with the back on edge of bed, fully flexed (knees to chin). Avoid allowing the patient to slump.
• Landmarks: plane of iliac crests through L4. In adults, the spinal cord ends at the L1, 2 disc. Mark L4, 5 or L3, 4 intervertebral space, eg by a *gentle* indentation of a thumb-nail on the overlying skin (better than a ballpoint pen mark, which might be erased by the sterilizing fluid).
• Wash hands. Don a mask and sterile gloves.
• Sterilize the back with tincture of iodine unless allergic.
• Open the spinal pack. Check manometer fittings. Have 3 plain sterile tubes and 1 fluoride (for glucose) tube ready.
• Inject 0.25–0.5mL 1% lidocaine under skin at marked site.
• Wait 1min, then insert spinal needle (22G, stilette in place) through the mark aiming towards umbilicus. Feel resistance of spinal ligaments, and then the dura, then a 'give' as the needle enters the subarachnoid space. **NB:** Keep the needle's bevel facing *up*, parallel with dural fibres.
• Withdraw stilette. Wait for CSF.
• Measure CSF pressure with manometer.
• Catch fluid in three sequentially numbered bottles (<5–10mL total). Consider taking and privately reserving a labelled sample in case of accident!
• Remove needle and apply dressing. Send CSF promptly for microscopy, culture, protein, and glucose (do plasma glucose too). If applicable, also send for: cytology, fungal studies, TB culture, virology (including Herpes PCR), syphilis serology, oligoclonal bands (with serum sample for comparison) if multiple sclerosis suspected. Is there xanthochromia (p362)?
• Lying flat for >1h is traditionally advised (probably unnecessary), checking CNS observations and BP regularly. Post-LP headache is partly preventable by reducing CSF leakage by using finer needles shaped to part the dura rather than cut it: see OPPOSITE.

CSF composition *Normal values:* Lymphocytes <5/mm³; polymorphs 0; protein <0.4g/L; glucose >2.2mmol/L (or ≥50% plasma level); pressure <200mmCSF. *In meningitis:* See p368–9. *In multiple sclerosis:* See p384.

Bloody tap: This is an artefact due to piercing a blood vessel, which is indicated (unreliably) by fewer red cells in successive bottles, and no yellowing of CSF (xanthochromia). To estimate how many white cells (*W*) were in the CSF before the blood was added, use the following:

$$W = \text{CSF WCC} - [\text{blood WCC} \times \text{CSF RBC} \div \text{blood RBC}]$$

If the patient's blood count is normal, the rule of thumb is to subtract from the total CSF WCC (per µL) one white cell for every 1000 RBCs. To estimate the true protein level, subtract 10mg/L for every 1000 RBCs/mm³ (be sure to do the count and protein estimation on the same bottle). Note: High protein levels in CSF make it appear yellow.

Subarachnoid haemorrhage: Xanthochromia (yellow supernatant on spun CSF). Red cells in equal numbers in all bottles (unreliably). RBCs will excite an inflammatory response (eg CSF WCC raised), most marked after 48h.

Raised protein: Meningitis; MS; Guillain–Barré syndrome. *Very raised CSF protein:* Spinal block; TB; or severe bacterial meningitis.

Post-LP headache

Risk: ~30%, typically occurring within 24h of LP, with resolution over hours to 2wks (mean: 3–4d). Patients describe a constant, dull, ache bilaterally which is more frontal than occipital. The most characteristic symptom is of *positional exacerbation*—worse when upright and usually pain-free when recumbent. There may be mild meningism or nausea. The pathology is thought to be continued leakage of CSF from the puncture site and intracranial *hypo*tension.

Prevention: Use the smallest spinal needle that is practical (22G) and keep the bevel aligned as described OPPOSITE. *Blunt* needles (more expensive!) can reduce risk, perhaps from 30% to 5%—and are recommended[8] (ask an anaesthetist about supply). Collection of CSF takes too long (>6min) if needles smaller then 22G are used.[7]

Treatment: Despite years of anecdotal advice to the contrary, *none* of the following have ever been shown to be a risk factor: position during or after the procedure; hydration status before, during, or after; amount of CSF removed; immediate activity or rest post-LP. *Time* is a consistent healer. For severe or prolonged headaches, ask an anaesthetist to do a *blood patch*. This is a careful injection of 20mL of autologous venous blood into the epidural space previously punctured (said to 'clog-up the hole'). Immediate relief occurs in 95%.

NB: Post-LP brain MRI scans often show diffuse meningeal enhancement with gadolinium. This is thought to be a reflection of increased blood flow secondary to intracranial hypotension. Interpret these scans with caution and in the context of the patient's clinical situation.

Method of defining the interspace between the 3rd and 4th lumbar vertebrae

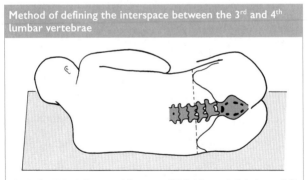

After Vakil and Udwadia *Diagnosis and Management of Medical Emergencies* 2nd edn, OUP, Delhi.

Cardioversion/defibrillation

- Indications: ventricular fibrillation/tachycardia, fast AF (p130), supraventricular tachycardias if other treatments (p130–32) have failed or there is haemodynamic compromise.
- Aim: to completely depolarize the heart using a direct current.
- Unless critically unwell, conscious patients require a general anaesthetic.
- Procedure (*for monophasic defibrillators*): do not wait for a crisis before familiarizing yourself with the defibrillator.
  - Set the energy level (eg 200J for ventricular fibrillation or ventricular tachycardia; 100J for atrial fibrillation; 50J for atrial flutter).
  - Place conduction pads (eg Littmann™ Defib Pads) on chest, 1 over apex (p64) and 1 below right clavicle (less chance of skin arc than jelly).
  - **Make sure no one else is touching the patient or the bed**.
  - Press the button(s) on the electrode(s) to give the shock.
  - Watch ECG. Repeat the shock at a higher energy if necessary.
- **NB:** For AF and SVT, it is necessary to synchronize the shock on the R-wave of the ECG (by pressing the 'SYNC' button on the machine). This ensures that the shock does not initiate a ventricular arrhythmia. *If the SYNC mode is engaged in VF, the defibrillator will not discharge!*
- It is only necessary to anaesthetize the patient if conscious.
- After giving the shock, monitor ECG rhythm. Consider anticoagulation, as the risk of emboli is increased. Get an up-to-date 12-lead ECG.

▶In children, use 2J/kg, then 4J/kg in VF/VT; if >10kg, use *adult* paddles; OHCS p311.

Cricothyroidotomy

Essence An emergency procedure to overcome upper airway obstruction above the level of the larynx.

Indications Upper airway obstruction when endotracheal intubation not possible, eg irretrievable foreign body; facial oedema (burns, angio-oedema); maxillofacial trauma; infection (epiglottitis).

Procedure Lie the patient supine with neck extended (eg pillow under shoulders). Run your index finger down the neck anteriorly in the midline to find the notch in the upper border of the thyroid cartilage: just below this, between the thyroid and cricoid cartilages, is a depression—the cricothyroid membrane.

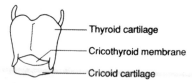

— Thyroid cartilage

— Cricothyroid membrane

— Cricoid cartilage

a. *Needle cricothyroidotomy:* Pierce the membrane with large-bore cannula (14G) attached to syringe: withdrawal of air confirms position lidocaine may or may not be required). Slide cannula over needle at 45° to skin in sagittal plane. Use a Y-connector or improvise connection to O_2 supply and give 15L/min: use thumb on Y-connector to allow O_2 in over 1s and CO_2 out over 4s ('transtracheal jet insufflation'). Preferred method in children <12yrs. Will only sustain life for 30–45min before CO_2 builds up.

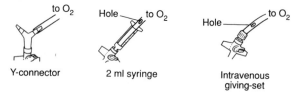

to O_2 Hole ⎯ to O_2 Hole ⎯   to O_2

Y-connector   2 ml syringe   Intravenous
giving-set

b. *Mini-Trach II®:* This contains a guarded blade, introducer, 4mm uncuffed tube (slide over introducer) with ISO connection and binding tape. Patient can breathe spontaneously or be ventilated via bag (high resistance). Will sustain for 30–45min.

c. *Surgical cricothyrotomy:* Smallest tube for prolonged ventilation is 6mm. Introduce high-volume low-pressure cuff tracheostomy tube through horizontal incision in membrane.

Complications Local haemorrhage; posterior perforation of trachea ± oesophagus; laryngeal stenosis if membrane over-incised in childhood; tube blockage; subcutaneous tunnelling.

▶**NB:** Needle and Mini-Trach® are temporary measures pending formal tracheostomy.

Emergency[1] needle pericardiocentesis

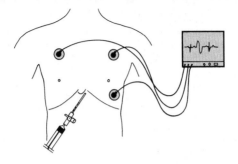

- Get your senior's help (for whom this may serve as an *aide-mémoire*).
- Equipment: 20mL syringe, long 18G cannula, 3-way tap, ECG monitor, skin cleanser.
- If time allows, use aseptic technique, and, if conscious, local anaesthesia and sedation, eg with midazolam: titrate up to 0.07mg/kg IV—start with 2mg over 1min, 1mg in elderly—antidote: flumazenil 0.2mg IV over 15s, then 0.1mg every 60s, up to 1mg in total.
- Ensure you have IV access and full resuscitation equipment to hand.
- Introduce needle at 45° to skin just below and to left of xiphisternum, aiming for tip of left scapula. Aspirate continuously and watch ECG. Frequent ventricular ectopics or an injury pattern (ST segment↓) on ECG imply myocardium breached—withdraw slightly.
- Evacuate pericardial contents through the syringe and 3-way tap. Removal of only a small amount of fluid (eg 20mL) can produce marked clinical improvement. If you are not sure whether the fluid you are aspirating is pure blood (eg on entering a ventricle), see if it clots (heavily bloodstained pericardial fluid does not clot), or measure its PCV.
- You can leave the cannula *in situ* temporarily, for repeated aspiration. If there is reaccumulation, pericardiectomy may be needed.
- Send fluid for microscopy and culture, as needed, including tests for TB.

Complications: laceration of ventricle or coronary artery (± subsequent haemopericardium); aspiration of ventricular blood; arrhythmias (ventricular fibrillation); pneumothorax; puncture of aorta, oesophagus (± mediastinitis), or peritoneum (± peritonitis).

---

1 Procedures used by cardiologists for elective pericardiocentesis may differ, involving the use of guide-wires, screening, and catheters.

Aspiration of a pneumothorax

- Identify the 2nd intercostal space in the midclavicular line (or 4–6th intercostal space in the midaxillary line) and infiltrate with 1% lidocaine down to the pleura overlying the pneumothorax.
- Insert a 16G cannula into the pleural space. Remove the needle and connect the cannula to a 3-way tap and a 50mL syringe. Aspirate up to 2.5L of air (50mL × 50). Stop if resistance is felt, or if the patient coughs excessively.
- Request a CXR to confirm resolution of the pneumothorax. If successful, consider discharging the patient and repeating the CXR after 24h to exclude recurrence, and again after 7–10d. Advise to avoid air travel for 6 weeks after a normal CXR. Diving should be permanently avoided.
- If aspiration is unsuccessful (significant, symptomatic pneumothorax), insert an intercostal drain (see p750). Other indications for intercostal drain insertion: recurrent pneumothorax <24h after aspiration; haemopneumothorax; mechanically ventilated patients; traumatic pneumothorax; patients that need to be transferred by air.

Subclavian venous cannulation

Subclavian venous cannulae may be inserted to provide a measurement of the central venous pressure, to administer certain drugs (eg amiodarone), or for intravenous access. They are not without hazards—infection, pneumothorax, haemothorax, so decide whether the patient requires one first, and then ask for help if you are inexperienced.

• Position the patient flat, with 1 pillow. Head-down tilt may help if volume depleted.
• Wash hands, don a gown and sterile gloves. This is an aseptic procedure.
• Clean the area with chlorhexidine or iodine solution (unless allergic to these), and apply sterile drapes.
• Assemble the catheter, and flush all the lumina with saline.
• Identify the insertion point: 1cm below the junction of the medial third and lateral ⅔ of the clavicle. Nick the skin with a scalpel.
• Using a green needle inject 5–10mL of 1–2% lidocaine under the skin and into the subcutaneous tissues, down to the clavicle.
• Using the introducer needle, and an appropriate syringe, partly filled with saline, puncture the skin and advance the needle to the clavicle. Once you hit the clavicle, move the needle under the clavicle and aim for the opposite sternoclavicular joint. This methods reduces the risk of puncturing the pleura. Aspirate as you advance the needle and you should be able to cannulate the subclavian vein. When in the vein you should be able to easily aspirate blood.
• Remove the syringe, keeping the needle still and insert the guide-wire. Remove the needle over the wire but **never** let go of the wire or it may all enter the vein, making removal very difficult. The wire should advance with ease, if it does not, remove the wire, check that you can still aspirate blood and alter the angle of the needle or position of the bevel.
• Next, feed the dilator over the wire. Often twisting it slightly will facilitate its insertion. **NB:** Always have 1 hand on the wire.
• Remove the dilator and feed the catheter over the wire, remembering to have the end of the wire in your hand before the tip of the catheter enters the skin.
• Feed the catheter into the vein, remove the wire, and check that blood can be aspirated through each lumen.
• Flush each lumen, and then stitch the catheter in place.
• Order a CXR to check the position of the catheter and exclude a pneumothorax.
• If a cannula is found to be located in the internal jugular vein, it must be withdrawn and another re-inserted.

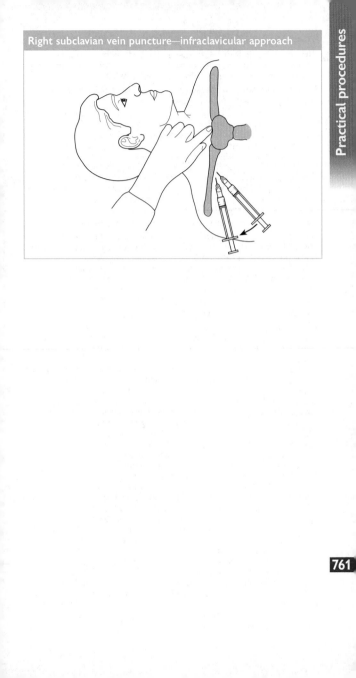

Right subclavian vein puncture—infraclavicular approach

Inserting a temporary cardiac pacemaker

Often it is wiser to liaise with a specialist pacing centre to arrange prompt, definitive pacing than to try temporary pacing, which often has complications (eg infection; air embolism), which may delay a definitive procedure.[?]

Possible indications in the acute phase of myocardial infarction

- Complete AV block: –with inferior MI (right coronary artery occlusion) pacing may only be needed if symptomatic; *spontaneous recovery may occur.*
  – with anterior MI (representing massive septal infarction).
- Second degree block: – Wenckebach (p127) implies decremental AV node conduction; may respond to atropine in inferior MI; pace if anterior MI.
  – Type 2 block is usually associated with distal fascicular disease and carries high risk of complete heart block, so pace in both types of MI.
- First degree block: observe carefully: 40% develop higher degrees of block.
- Bundle branch block: pace prophylactically if evidence of trifascicular disease (p98) or non-adjacent bifascicular disease.
- Sino-atrial disease + serious symptoms: pace unless responds to atropine.

Other indications where temporary pacing may be needed

- Pre-op: if surgery is required in patients in any of the categories above (whether or not MI has occurred), do 24h ECG; liaise with the anaesthetist.
- Drug poisoning, eg with β-blockers, digoxin, or verapamil.
- Symptomatic bradycardia, uncontrolled by atropine or isoprenaline.
- Suppression of drug-resistant VT and SVT (overdrive pacing; do on ITU).
- Asystolic cardiac arrest with P-wave activity (ventricular standstill).
- During or after cardiac surgery—eg around the AV node or bundle of His.

Method and technique for temporary pacing Learn from an expert.

- Preparation: monitor ECG; have a defibrillator to hand; check that a radiographer with screening equipment is present. Create a sterile field and ensure that the pacing wire fits down the cannula easily. Insert a peripheral cannula.
- Insertion: place the cannula into the subclavian or internal jugular vein (p760). If this is difficult, access to the right atrium can be achieved *via* the femoral vein. Pass the pacing wire through the cannula into the right atrium. It will either pass easily through the tricuspid valve or loop within the atrium. If the latter occurs, it is usually possible to flip the wire across the valve with a combined twisting and withdrawing movement. Advance the wire slightly. At this stage the wire may try to exit the ventricle through the pulmonary outflow tract. A further withdrawing and rotation of the wire will aim the tip at the apex of the right ventricle. Advance slightly again to place the wire in contact with the endocardium. Remove any slack to ↓risk of subsequent displacement.
- Checking the threshold: connect the wire to the pacing box and set the 'demand' rate slightly higher than the patient's own heart rate and the output to 3V. A paced rhythm should be seen. Find the pacing threshold by slowly reducing the voltage until the pacemaker fails to stimulate the tissue (pacing spikes are no longer followed by paced beats). The threshold should be less than 1V, but a slightly higher value may be acceptable if it is stable—eg after a large infarction.

- Setting the pacemaker: set the output to 3V or over 3 times the threshold value (whichever is higher) in 'demand' mode. Set the rate as required. Suture the wire to the skin, and fix with a sterile dressing.
- Check the position of the wire (and exclude pneumothorax) with a CXR.
- Recurrent checks of the pacing threshold are required over the next few days. The formation of endocardial oedema can be expected to raise the threshold by a factor of 2–3.

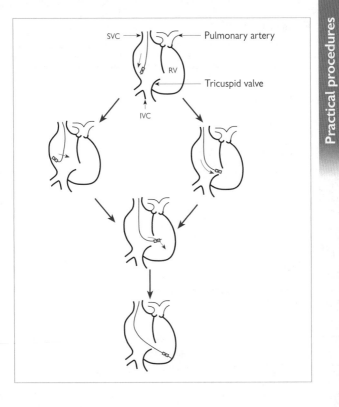

SVC
Pulmonary artery
RV
Tricuspid valve
IVC

Emergencies[1]

Don't go so fast: we're in a hurry! Talleyrand to his coachman

Many diseases may present as emergencies, but if you know about the following, you will be very unlucky to lose a patient from a disease not listed here, on a general medical take, provided you remember to ask for help.

Emergencies covered in other chapters See front end-papers.

In OHCS—Paediatrics: Life support and cardiac arrest (OHCS p310–11); is he seriously ill? (OHCS p175); epiglottitis (OHCS p276). *Adults:* The major disaster (OHCS p796) Trauma (OHCS p678–p740); drowning (OHCS p682); ectopic pregnancy (OHCS p24); eclampsia (OHCS p96); amniotic fluid embolus (OHCS p143); obstetric shock (OHCS p106); glaucoma (OHCS p494); pre-hospital care/first aid (OHCS p780–p802).

Sources include: BMJ; NEJM; Oxford Handbook of Acute Medicine, OUP.

---

1 *We thank Dr F Poyner (Specialist Reader) & Specialist Readers from other chapters.*

Introduction to emergencies

There is nothing more intoxicating than spending a day saving lives, but as night creeps on, and you start losing more patients than you should, despair can hit with the force of ice. It is no comfort to know that you are now wiser and older (by 100yrs). So when you find yourself washing your hands between one death and the next, for one second be honest with yourself, and write of your errors and sorrows on the surface of the water—a few temporary ambiguous squiggles framing your thoughts and the life that is lost. This is not about audit and accountability (this comes later: now you need to fortify yourself to survive this onslaught)—so, in case a manager is looking over your shoulder, pull the plug, and as the water flows away, know that it mingles with the rising tide of our own failings at the bedside, through which we have surfaced—no doubt a little faster than we should. At your next bedside you may do better if you can buy time: time to take a history, time to think, and time to ask. To buy this precious time, support vital functions, as follows.

Preliminary assessment (primary survey)

Airway   Protect cervical spine, if injury possible.

Assessment: any signs of obstruction? Ascertain patency

Management: establish a patent airway.

Breathing   Assessment: determine respiratory rate, check bilateral chest movement, percuss and auscultate.

Management: if no respiratory effort, treat as arrest (p766), intubate and ventilate. If breathing compromised, give high concentration O_2, manage according to findings, eg relieve tension pneumothorax.

Circulation   Assessment: check pulse and BP; is he peripherally shutdown?; check capillary refill; look for evidence of haemorrhage.

Management:
– if no cardiac output, treat as arrest (p766)
– if shocked, treat as on p778.

Disability   Assess 'level of consciousness' with AVPU score (alert? responds to voice? to pain? unresponsive?); check pupils: size, equality, reactions. *Glasgow Coma scale*, if time allows.

Exposure   Undress patient, but cover to avoid hypothermia.

Quick history from relatives may assist with diagnosis: *Events* surrounding onset of illness, evidence of overdose/suicide attempt, any suggestion of trauma? *Past medical history:* Especially diabetes, asthma, COPD, alcohol, opiate or street drug abuse, epilepsy or recent head injury; recent travel. *Medication:* Current drugs. *Allergies.*

Once ventilation and circulation are adequate, you may have bought enough time to carry out history, examination, investigations, and appropriate management in the usual way.

▶▶Cardiorespiratory arrest

Ensure safety of patient and yourself. Confirm diagnosis (unconscious, apnoeic, absent carotid pulse).

Causes MI; PE; trauma; tension pneumothorax, electrocution; shock; hypoxia; hypercapnia; hypothermia; U&E imbalance; drugs, eg digoxin.

Basic life support Shout for help. Ask someone to call the arrest team and bring the defibrillator. Note the time. Precordial thump (in witnessed arrests; recheck carotid pulse). Begin CPR as follows (ABC):

Airway: Head tilt (if no spine injury) + chin lift/jaw thrust. Clear the mouth.

Breathing: Give 2 breaths, each inflation ~2s long. Use specialized bag and mask system (eg Ambu® system) if available and 2 resuscitators present. Otherwise, mouth-to-mouth breathing.

Chest compressions: Give 15 compressions to 2 breaths (15 : 2). CPR should not be interrupted except to give shocks or to intubate. Use the heel of hand with straight elbows. Centre over the lower third of the sternum. Aim for 5cm compression at 100/min.

Advanced life support For algorithm & details, see OPPOSITE. Notes:
- Place defibrillator paddles on chest as soon as possible and set monitor to read through the paddles if delay in attaching leads. Assess rhythm: is this VF/pulseless VT? The following assumes monophasic defibrillator.
- In VF/VT, defibrillation must occur without delay: 200;200;360J.
- Asystole and electromechanical dissociation (synonymous with pulseless electrical activity) are rhythms with a poorer prognosis than VF/VT, but potentially remediable (see box OPPOSITE). Treatment may be life-saving.
- Obtain IV access and intubation if possible.
- Look for reversible causes of cardiac arrest, and treat accordingly.
- Check for pulse if ECG rhythm compatible with a cardiac output.
- Reassess ECG rhythm. Repeat defibrillation if still VF/VT. All shocks 360J.
- Send someone to find the patient's notes and the patient's usual doctor. These may give clues as to the cause of the arrest.
- If IV access fails, adrenaline, atropine, and lidocaine may be given down the tracheal tube but absorption is unpredictable. Give 2–3 times the IV dose diluted in ≥10mL 0.9% saline followed by 5 ventilations to assist absorption. Intracardiac injection is not recommended.

When to stop resuscitation: No general rule, as survival is influenced by the rhythm and the cause of the arrest. In patients without myocardial disease, do not stop until core temperature is >33°C and pH and potassium are normal. Consider stopping resuscitation after 20min if there is refractory asystole or electromechanical dissociation.

After successful resuscitation:
- 12-lead ECG; CXR, U&Es, glucose, blood gases, FBC, CK/troponin.
- Transfer to coronary care unit/ITU.
- Monitor vital signs.
- Whatever the outcome, explain to relatives what has happened.

When 'do not resuscitate' may be a valid decision (UK DoH guidelines)
- If a patient's condition is such that resuscitation is unlikely to succeed.
- If a mentally competent patient has consistently stated or recorded the fact that he or she does not want to be resuscitated.
- If the patient has signed an advanced directive forbidding resuscitation.
- If resuscitation is not in a patient's interest as it would lead to a poor quality of life (often a great imponderable!). ▶*Ideally, involve patients & relatives in the decision **before** the emergency.* When in doubt, resuscitate.

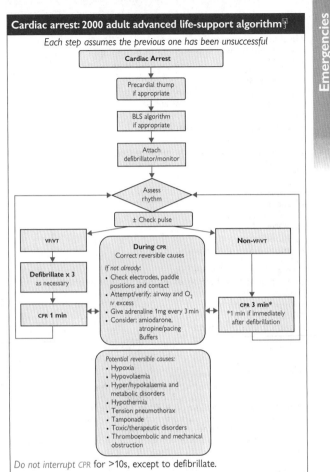

Cardiac arrest: 2000 adult advanced life-support algorithm

Each step assumes the previous one has been unsuccessful

Cardiac Arrest

Precardial thump if appropriate

BLS algorithm if appropriate

Attach defibrillator/monitor

Assess rhythm

± Check pulse

VF/VT

Defibrillate x 3 as necessary

CPR 1 min

During CPR
Correct reversible causes

If not already:
- Check electrodes, paddle positions and contact
- Attempt/verify: airway and O_2 IV excess
- Give adrenaline 1mg every 3 min
- Consider: amiodarone, atropine/pacing Buffers

Non-VF/VT

CPR 3 min*
*1 min if immediately after defibrillation

Potential reversible causes:
- Hypoxia
- Hypovolaemia
- Hyper/hypokalaemia and metabolic disorders
- Hypothermia
- Tension pneumothorax
- Tamponade
- Toxic/therapeutic disorders
- Thromboembolic and mechanical obstruction

Do not interrupt CPR for >10s, except to defibrillate.

Resistant VF/VT consider:

- Amiodarone 300mg IV (peripherally if no central access). A further 150mg may be given, followed by an infusion of 1mg/min for 6h, then 0.5mg/min for 6h.
- Alteratives to amiodarone are:
  - Lidocaine 100mg IV; can repeat once; then give 2–4mg/min IVI.
  - Procainamide 30mg/min IV to a total dose of 17mg/kg.
- Seek expert advice from a cardiologist.

Asystole with P waves: Start external pacing (percutaneous transthoracic pacing through special paddles). Use endocardial pacing if experienced pacer is available. If unavailable, use atropine 0.6mg/5min IV while awaiting further help.

Treat acidosis with good ventilation. Sodium bicarbonate may worsen intra-cellular acidosis and precipitate arrhythmias, so use only in severe acidosis after prolonged resuscitation (eg 50mL of 8.4% solution by IVI).

Headache: differential diagnosis

No signs on examination
- Tension headache
- Migraine
- Cluster headache
- Post-traumatic
- Drugs (nitrates, calcium channel antagonists)
- Carbon monoxide poisoning or anoxia

Signs of meningism?
- Meningitis (may not have fever or rash)
- Subarachnoid haemorrhage

Decreased conscious level or localizing signs?
- Encephalitis/meningitis
- Stroke
- Cerebral abscess
- Subarachnoid haemorrhage
- Tumour
- Subdural haematoma
- TB meningitis

Papilloedema?
- Tumour
- Malignant hypertension
- Benign intracranial hypertension
- Any CNS infection, if prolonged (eg >2wks)—eg TB meningitis

Others
- Temporal arteritis (ESR↑)
- Glaucoma
- Paget's disease (Alk Phosp ↑↑↑)
- Sinusitis
- Altitude sickness
- Cervical spondylosis

Worrying features or 'red flags'[1]
- First and worst headache—*subarachnoid haemorrhage*
- Thunderclap headache—*subarachnoid haemorrhage;* (p364 for other causes).
- Unilateral headache and eye pain—*cluster headache, acute glaucoma*
- Unilateral headache and ipsilateral symptoms—*migraine, tumour, vascular*
- Cough-initiated headache—*raised ICP/venous thrombosis*
- Persisting headache ± scalp tenderness in over 50s—*temporal arteritis*
- Headache with fever or neck stiffness—*meningitis*
- Change in the pattern of 'usual headaches'
- Decreased level of consciousness

Two other vital questions:
- Where have you been? (malaria)
- Might you be pregnant? (eclampsia; especially if proteinuria and BP↑)

1 Adapted from C Hawkes 2002 Hosp Med **63** 732–42

Breathlessness: emergency presentations

Wheezing?
- Asthma
- COPD
- Heart failure
- Anaphylaxis

Stridor? (Upper airway obstruction)
- Foreign body or tumour
- Acute epiglottitis
- Anaphylaxis
- Trauma, eg laryngeal fracture

Crepitations?
- Heart failure
- Pneumonia
- Bronchiectasis
- Fibrosis

Chest clear?
- Pulmonary embolism
- Hyperventilation
- Metabolic acidosis, eg diabetic ketoacidosis (DKA)
- Anaemia
- Drugs, eg salicylates
- Shock (may cause air hunger, p778)
- Central causes

Others
- Pneumothorax—pain, increased resonance
- Pleural effusion—'stony dullness'

Chest pain: differential diagnosis

First exclude any potentially life-threatening causes, by virtue of history, brief examination, and limited investigations. Then consider other potential causes. For the full assessment of cardiac pain, see p92 & p120.

Life-threatening
- Acute myocardial infarction
- Angina/acute coronary syndrome
- Aortic dissection
- Tension pneumothorax
- Pulmonary embolism
- Oesophageal rupture

Others
- Pneumonia
- Empyema
- Chest wall pain
  - Muscular
  - Rib fractures
  - Bony metastases
  - Costochondritis
- Pleurisy
- Gastro-oesophageal reflux
- Pericarditis
- Oesophageal spasm
- Herpes zoster
- Cervical spondylosis
- Intra-abdominal
  - Cholecystitis
  - Peptic ulceration
  - Pancreatitis
- Sickle-cell crisis

Before discharging patients with undiagnosed chest pain, be sure in your own mind that the pain is not cardiac (this pain is usually dull, may radiate to jaw, arm, or epigastrium, and is usually associated with exertion). Do CXR, ECG, FBC, U&E, and 'cardiac' enzymes, including troponin T (p93 & p120). Discuss options with a colleague, and the patient. Don't simply turn people out on to the street.

▶Just because the patient's chest wall is tender to palpation, doesn't mean the cause to the chest pain is musculoskeletal. Make sure you have excluded all potential life-threatening causes.

Coma

Definition *Unrousable unresponsiveness.*

Causes of coma

Metabolic: Drugs, poisoning, eg carbon monoxide, alcohol, tricyclics

Hypoglycaemia, hyperglycaemia (ketoacidotic, or HONK, p820)

Hypoxia, CO_2 narcosis (COPD)

Septicaemia

Hypothermia

Myxoedema, Addisonian crisis

Hepatic/uraemic encephalopathy

Neurological: Trauma

Infection meningitis (p368); encephalitis, eg Herpes simplex give IV aciclovir if the slightest suspicion (p568), *tropical:* malaria (▸▸p810; do thick films), typhoid, rabies, trypanosomiasis

Tumour: cerebral/meningeal tumour

Vascular, subdural/subarachnoid haemorrhage, stroke, hypertensive encephalopathy

Epilepsy: non-convulsive status (p373) or post-ictal state

Immediate management see OPPOSITE (and coma CNS exam, p776)

- Assess airway, breathing, and circulation. Consider intubation if GCS <8. Support the circulation if required (ie IV fluids). Give O_2 and treat any seizures. Protect the cervical spine.
- Check blood glucose in all patients. Give 50mL 50% dextrose IV immediately if presumed hypoglycaemia.
- IV thiamine if any suggestion of Wernicke's encephalopathy.
- IV naloxone for opiate intoxication (may also be given IM or via ET tube); IV flumazenil for benzodiazepine intoxication *if* airway compromised.

Examination

- Vital signs are vital—obtain full set, including temperature.
- Signs of trauma—haematoma, laceration, bruising, CSF/blood in nose or ears, fracture 'step' deformity of skull, subcutaneous emphysema, 'panda eyes'.
- Stigmata of other illnesses: liver disease, alcoholism, diabetes, myxoedema.
- Skin for needle marks, cyanosis, pallor, rashes, poor turgor.
- Smell the breath (alcohol, hepatic fetor, ketosis, uraemia).
- Meningism (p368) ▸but do *not* move neck unless cervical spine is cleared.
- Heart/lung exam for murmurs, rubs, wheeze, consolidation, collapse.
- Abdomen/rectal for organomegaly, ascites, bruising, peritonism, melaena.
- Are there any foci of infection (abscesses, bites, middle ear infection?)
- Any features of meningitis: neck stiffness, rash, focal neurology?
- Note the *absence* of signs, eg no pin-point pupils in a known heroin addict, or a diabetic patient whose breath does *not* smell of acetone.

Quick history from family, ambulance staff, bystanders: Abrupt or gradual onset? How found—suicide note, seizure? If injured, suspect cervical spinal injury and do not move spine (*OHCS* p726). Recent complaints—headache, fever, vertigo, depression? Recent medical history—sinusitis, otitis, neurosurgery, ENT procedure? Past medical history—diabetes, asthma, ↑BP, cancer, epilepsy, psychiatric illness? Drug or toxin exposure (especially alcohol or other recreational drugs)? Any travel?

Taking stock The diagnosis may be clear, eg hyperglycaemia, alcohol excess, drug poisoning, uraemia, pneumonia, hypertensive, or hepatic encephalopathy (p230). If there are localizing CNS signs and no history of trauma, and there is no fever, the diagnosis is only *probably* stroke. In all undiagnosed coma patients or in those with focal neurological signs, a CT scan is very helpful. A lumbar puncture may be needed for meningitis (p368) or subarachnoid haemorrhage (p362).

Management of coma[1]

ABC of life support

↓

O_2, IV access

↓

Stabilize cervical spine

↓

Blood glucose (eg BM stix)

↓

Control seizures

↓

Consider IV glucose, thiamine, naloxone, or flumazenil

↓

Brief examination, obtain history

↓

Investigations

ABG, FBC, U&E, LFT, ESR, CRP

Ethanol, toxic screen, drug levels

Blood cultures, urine culture, consider malaria

CXR

↓

Reassess the situation and plan further investigations

1 *Check pupils every few minutes during the early stages,* particularly if trauma is the likely cause. Doing so is the quickest way to find a localizing sign (so helpful in diagnosis, but remember that false localizing signs *do* occur)—and observing *changes* in pupil behaviour (eg becoming fixed and dilated) is the quickest way of finding out just how bad things are.

The Glasgow coma scale (GCS)[4]

This gives a reliable, objective way of recording the conscious state of a person. It can be used by medical and nursing staff for initial and continuing assessment. It has value in predicting ultimate outcome. 3 types of response are assessed:

Best motor response This has 6 grades:

6 Carrying out request ('obeying command'): The patient does simple things you ask (beware of accepting a grasp reflex in this category).

5 Localizing response to pain: Put pressure on the patient's fingernail bed with a pencil then try supraorbital and sternal pressure: purposeful movements towards changing painful stimuli is a 'localizing' response.

4 Withdraws to pain: Pulls limb away from painful stimulus.

3 Flexor response to pain: Pressure on the nail bed causes abnormal flexion of limbs—decorticate posture.

2 Extensor posturing to pain: The stimulus causes limb extension (adduction, internal rotation of shoulder, pronation of forearm)—decerebrate posture.

1 No response to pain.

Note that it is the best response of any limb which should be recorded.

Best verbal response This has 5 grades:

5 Oriented: The patient knows who he is, where he is and why, the year, season, and month.

4 Confused conversation: The patient responds to questions in a conversational manner but there is some disorientation and confusion.

3 Inappropriate speech: Random or exclamatory articulated speech, but no conversational exchange.

2 Incomprehensible speech: Moaning but no words.

1 None.

Record level of best speech.

Eye opening This has 4 grades:

4 Spontaneous eye opening.

3 Eye opening in response to speech: Any speech, or shout, not necessarily request to open eyes.

2 Eye opening in response to pain: Pain to limbs as above.

1 No eye opening.

An overall score is made by summing the score in the 3 areas assessed. Eg: no response to pain + no verbalization + no eye opening = 3. Severe injury, GCS ≤8; moderate injury, GCS 9–12; minor injury, GCS 13–15.

NB: An abbreviated coma scale, AVPU, is sometimes used in the initial assessment ('primary survey') of the critically ill:

• A = alert
• V = responds to vocal stimuli
• P = responds to pain
• U = unresponsive

Some centres score GCS out of 14, not 15, omitting 'withdrawal to pain'.
NB: The GCS scoring is different in young children.

The neurological examination in coma

This is aimed at locating the pathology in 1 of 2 places. Altered level of consciousness implies either (1) a diffuse, bilateral, cortical dysfunction (usually producing loss of awareness with normal arousal) or (2) damage to the ascending reticular activating system (ARAS) located throughout the brainstem from the medulla to the thalami (usually producing loss of arousal with unassessable awareness). The brainstem can be affected directly (eg pontine haemorrhage) or indirectly (eg compression from trans-tentorial or cerebellar herniation secondary to a mass or oedema).

- Level of consciousness; describe using *objective* words.
- Respiratory pattern—Cheyne–Stokes (p66), hyperventilation (acidosis, hypoxia, or rarely, neurogenic), ataxic or apneustic (breath-holding) breathing (brainstem damage with grave prognosis).
- Eyes—almost all patients with ARAS pathology will have eye findings.

Visual fields—in light coma, test fields with visual threat. No blink in 1 field suggests hemianopsia and contralateral hemisphere lesion.

Pupils *Normal direct & consensual* = intact midbrain. *Midposition (3-5mm) non-reactive ± irregular* = midbrain lesion. *Unilateral dilated & unreactive ('fixed')* = 3rd nerve compression. *Small, reactive* = pontine lesion ('pinpoint pontine pupils') or drugs. *Horner's syndrome* (p726) = ipsilateral lateral medulla or hypothalamus lesion, may precede uncal herniation. Beware patients with false eyes or who use eye drops for glaucoma.

Extraocular movements (EOMs)—observe resting position and spontaneous movement; then test the vestibulo-ocular reflex (VOR) with either the *Doll's-head manoeuvre* (normal if the eyes keep looking at the same point in space when the head is quickly moved laterally or vertically) or *ice water calorics* (normal if eyes deviate towards the cold ear with nystagmus to the other side). If present, the VOR exonerates *most* of the brainstem from the VII nerve nucleus (medulla) to the III (midbrain). *Don't move the head unless the cervical spine is cleared.*

Fundi—papilloedema, subhyaloid haemorrhage, hypertensive retinopathy, signs of other disease (eg diabetic retinopathy).

- Examine for CNS asymmetry (tone, spontaneous movements, reflexes).

▸▸Shock

Essence Circulatory failure resulting in inadequate organ perfusion. *Generally* systolic BP is <90mmHg. Signs: pallor, pulse↑, capillary return↓ (press a nailbed), air hunger, oliguria. Causes are either *pump failure* or *peripheral circulation failure*.

Pump failure

- **Cardiogenic shock**
- **Secondary:** *pulmonary embolism, tension pneumothorax, cardiac tamponade.*

Peripheral circulation failure

- **Hypovolaemia:**
  Bleeding: trauma, ruptured aortic aneurysm, ruptured ectopic pregnancy. *Fluid loss:* Vomiting (eg GI obstruction), diarrhoea (eg cholera), burns, pools of sequestered (unavailable) fluids ('third spacing', eg in pancreatitis). *Heat exhaustion* may cause hypovolaemic shock (also hyperpyrexia, oliguria, rhabdomyolysis, consciousness↓, hyperventilation, hallucination, incontinence, collapse, coma, pin-point pupils, LFTs↑, and DIC, p650).
- **Anaphylaxis**
- **Sepsis:** Gram –ve (or +ve) septicaemic shock from endotoxin-induced vasodilatation may be sudden and severe, with shock and coma but no signs of infection (fever, WCC↑).
- **Neurogenic:** eg post-spinal surgery.
- **Endocrine failure:** Addison's disease or hypothyroidism; see p822.
- **Iatrogenic:** Drugs, eg anaesthetics, antihypertensives.

Assessment ▸ABC.

- *ECG:* rate, rhythm, ischaemia?
- *General:* cold and clammy—cardiogenic shock or fluid loss. Look for signs of anaemia or dehydration—skin turgor, postural hypotension? Warm and well perfused, with bounding pulse—septic shock. Any features suggestive of anaphylaxis—history, urticaria, angio-oedema, wheeze?
- *CVS:* usually tachycardic (unless on β-blocker, or in spinal shock—*OHCS* p728) and hypotension. But in the young and fit or pregnant women, the systolic BP may remain normal, although the *pulse pressure* will narrow, with up to 30% blood volume depletion. Difference between arms—aortic dissection?
- *JVP or central venous pressure:* If raised, cardiogenic shock likely.
- *Check abdomen:* any signs of trauma, or aneurysm? Any evidence of GI bleed?—check for melaena.

Management ▸If BP unrecordable, call the cardiac arrest team.

See opposite for general management. Specific measures:

- **Anaphylaxis:** p780.
- **Cardiogenic shock:** p788.
- **Septic shock:** (if no clue to source, p548): IV cefuroxime 1.5g/8h (after blood culture) or gentamicin (p710; do levels; reduce in renal failure) + antipseudomonal penicillin, eg ticarcillin (as Timentin® p543, max dose 3.2g/4h IVI). Give colloid, or crystalloid, by IVI. Refer to ITU if possible for monitoring ± inotropes (eg dopamine in 'renal' dose of 2–5μg/kg/min IVI).
- **Hypovolaemic shock:** Fluid replacement: saline or colloid initially; if bleeding use blood; risks and benefits: see p464. Titrate against BP, CVP, urine output. Treat the underlying cause. If severe haemorrhage, exsanguinating, or more than 1L of fluid required to maintain BP, consider using group-specific blood, or O Rh–ve blood (p464). Correct electrolyte abnormalities. Acidosis often responds to fluid replacement.
- **Heat exposure (heat exhaustion):** tepid sponging + fanning; avoid ice and immersion. Resuscitate with high-sodium IVI, such as 0.9% saline ± hydrocortisone 100mg IV. Dantrolene seems ineffective. Chlorpromazine 25mg IM may be used to stop shivering. Stop cooling when core temperature <39°C.

Management of shock

If BP unrecordable, call the cardiac arrest team
↓
ABC (including high-flow O$_2$)
↓
Raise foot of the bed
↓
IV access × 2 (wide bore; get help if this takes >2min)
↓
Identify and treat underlying cause
↓
Infuse crystalloid *fast* to raise BP
(unless cardiogenic shock)
↓
Seek expert help early
↓
Investigations
FBC, U&E, ABG, glucose, CRP
Cross-match and check clotting
Blood cultures, urine culture, ECG, CXR
Others: lactate, echo, abdominal CT, USS
↓
Consider arterial line, central venous line, and
bladder catheter (aim for a urine flow >30mL/h)
↓
Further management
Treat underlying cause if possible
Fluid replacement as dictated by BP, CVP, urine output
Don't overload with fluids if cardiogenic shock
If persistently hypotensive, consider inotropes

NB: *Remember that higher flow rates can be achieved through peripheral lines than through 'standard' gauge central lines.*

If cause unclear: ℞ *as hypovolaemia—most common cause, and reversible.*

Ruptured abdominal aortic aneurysm: aim for a systolic BP of ~90mmHg.

SIRS, sepsis, and related syndromes

The pathogenesis of sepsis and septic shock is becoming increasingly understood. The 'systemic inflammatory response syndrome' (SIRS) is thought to be a central component, involving cytokine cascades, free radical production, and the release of vasoactive mediators. SIRS is defined as the presence of 2 or more of the following features:[5]
• Temperature >38°C or <36°C   • Tachycardia >90 bpm
• Respiratory rate >20 breaths/min or P_aCO_2 <4.3 kPa
• WBC >12 × 10^9/L or <4 × 10^9/L, or >10% immature (band) forms

Related syndromes include:

Sepsis: SIRS occurring in the presence of infection.

Severe sepsis: Sepsis with evidence of organ hypoperfusion eg hypoxaemia, oliguria, lactic acidosis, or altered cerebral function.

Septic shock: Severe sepsis with hypotension (systolic BP <90mmHg) despite adequate fluid resuscitation, or the requirement for vasopressors/inotropes to maintain blood pressure.

Septicaemia was used to denote the presence of multiplying bacteria in the circulation, but has been replaced with the definitions above.[6]

779

▸▸Anaphylactic shock

Type I IgE-mediated hypersensitivity reaction. Release of histamine and other agents causes: capillary leak; wheeze; cyanosis; oedema (larynx, lids, tongue, lips); urticaria. More common in atopic individuals. An *anaphylactoid reaction* results from direct release of mediators from inflammatory cells, without involving antibodies, usually in response to a drug, eg N-acetylcysteine.

Common precipitants
- Drugs, eg penicillin, and contrast media in radiology
- Latex
- Stings, eggs, fish, peanuts, strawberries, semen

Signs and symptoms
- Itching, erythema, urticaria, oedema
- Wheeze, laryngeal obstruction, cyanosis
- Tachycardia, hypotension

Management of anaphylaxis[7]

Secure the airway—give 100% O_2
Intubate if respiratory obstruction imminent
↓
Remove the cause; raising the feet may help restore the circulation
↓
Give adrenaline IM
0.5mg (ie 0.5mL of 1 : 1000)
Repeat every 5min, if needed as guided by BP, pulse, and respiratory function, until better
↓
Secure IV access
↓
Chlorpheniramine[1] 10mg IV and hydrocortisone 200mg IV
↓
IVI (0.9% saline, eg 500mL over ¼h; up to 2L may be needed)
Titrate against blood pressure
↓
If wheeze, treat for asthma (p794)
May require ventilatory support
↓
If still hypotensive, admission to ITU and an IVI of adrenaline may be needed ± aminophylline (795) and nebulized salbutamol (795): get expert help.

Further management
- Admit to ward. Monitor ECG.
- Continue chlorpheniramine[1] 4mg/6h PO if itching.
- Suggest a 'Medic-alert' bracelet naming the culprit allergen (p716).
- Teach about self-injected adrenaline (eg 0.3mg, Epipen®) to prevent a fatal attack.
- Skin-prick tests showing specific IgE help identify which allergens to avoid.[8]

Note
▸▸Adrenaline (=epinephrine) is given IM and NOT IV unless the patient is severely ill, or has no pulse. The IV dose is **different:** 100μg per min—titrating with the response. This is 1mL of **1 : 10,000 solution** per minute. Stop as soon as a response has been obtained.

If on a β-blocker, consider salbutamol IV in place of adrenaline.

---

1 New name: chlorphenamine.

Acute myocardial infarction

A common medical emergency, and prompt appropriate treatment saves lives and myocardium. If in doubt, seek immediate help. Diagnosis: p120.

Pre-hospital management

Arrange an emergency ambulance. Aspirin 300mg PO (unless clear contraindication). Analgesia, eg morphine 5–10mg IV + metoclopramide 10mg IV (avoid IM injections, as risk of bleeding with thrombolysis). Sublingual GTN unless hypotensive.

Management See OPPOSITE for acute measures.

Thrombolysis effective in reducing mortality if given early. Greatest benefit is seen if given <12h of the onset of chest pain, but some benefit up to 24h. The British Heart Foundation advises that the time from onset of pain to thrombolysis should be <90min (<60min if possible).

Indications for thrombolysis: Presentation within *12h* of chest pain with:
• ST elevation >2mm in 2 or more chest leads or
• ST elevation >1mm in 2 or more limb leads or
• Posterior infarction (dominant R waves and ST depression in V_1–V_3)
• New onset left bundle branch block.

Presentation within *12–24h* if continuing chest pain and/or ST elevation.

Thrombolysis contraindications: (consider urgent angioplasty instead)
• Internal bleeding
• Prolonged or traumatic CPR
• Heavy vaginal bleeding
• Acute pancreatitis
• Active lung disease with cavitation
• Recent trauma or surgery (<2wks)
• Cerebral neoplasm
• Severe hypertension (>200/120mmHg)
• Suspected aortic dissection
• Previous allergic reaction
• Pregnancy or <18wks postnatal
• Severe liver disease
• Oesophageal varices
• Recent head trauma
• Recent haemorrhagic stroke

Relative CI: History of severe hypertension; peptic ulcer; history of CVA; bleeding diathesis; anticoagulants.

Streptokinase (SK) is the usual thrombolytic agent. Dose: 1.5 million units in 100mL 0.9% saline IVI over 1h. SE: nausea; vomiting; haemorrhage; stroke (1%); dysrhythmias. Any hypotension usually responds to slowing down or stopping the infusion. Also watch for allergic reactions and anaphylaxis (rare). Do not repeat unless it is within 4d of the first administration.

Alteplase (rt-PA) may be indicated if the patient has previously received SK (>4d) or reacted to SK. Accelerated rt-PA has benefit if given within 6h, especially in younger patients with anterior MI. Standard rt-PA is given to patients presenting at 6–12h. *Tenecteplase* is given by bolus injection (over 10sec), which in some cases may be an advantage. Dose 500–600µg/kg.

Complications
• Recurrent ischaemia or failure to reperfuse (usually detected as persisting pain and ST-segment elevation in the immediate aftermath of thrombolysis): additional analgesia, GTN, β-blocker, consider re-thrombolysis or do angioplasty if increased or new ST segment elevation.
• Stroke.
• Pericarditis: analgesics, try to avoid NSAIDs.
• Cardiogenic shock: see p788 and heart failure: see p786.

Right ventricular infarction
• Confirm by demonstrating ST elevation in RV3/4, and/or echo. **NB:** RV4 means that V_4 is placed in the right 5th intercostal space in the midclavicular line.
• Treat hypotension and oliguria with fluids.
• Avoid nitrates and diuretics.
• Intensive monitoring and inotropes may be useful in some patients.

Management of an acute MI

Attach ECG monitor and record a 12-lead ECG

↓

High-flow O_2 by face mask (caution, if COPD)

↓

IV access

Bloods for FBC, U&Es, glucose, lipids, cardiac enzymes (p121)

↓

Brief assessment

History of cardiovascular disease; risk factors for IHD

Contraindications to thrombolysis?

Examination: pulse, BP, JVP, cardiac murmurs, signs of heart failure, peripheral pulses, scars from previous cardiac surgery

↓

Aspirin 300mg chewed (unless already given by GP/paramedics)

↓

Morphine 5–10mg IV + antiemetic, eg metoclopramide 10mg IV

↓

GTN sublingually 2 puffs or 1 tablet as required

↓

β-blocker, eg atenolol 5mg IV (unless asthma or left ventricular failure)

↓

Thrombolysis see OPPOSITE

↓

CXR

Do not delay thrombolysis while waiting unless aneurysm suspected

↓

Consider glucose, insulin, and potassium infusion for patients with diabetes mellitus (DIGAMI regimen[1])

↓

Consider DVT prophylaxis

↓

Continue medication except calcium channel antagonists (unless specific indication)

↓

For further management: see p124

▶If pain is uncontrolled, especially if continuing ST elevation, consider re-thrombolysis with rt-PA (no bolus), tenecteplase, or rescue angioplasty.

---

1 *Note on the role of glucose, potassium, and insulin infusion (GKI) in acute MI.* Use of GKI in acute MI has gone in and out of vogue. Evidence for insulin infusion in whatever form in diabetic patients is more clear, and this should probably be part of our 'best care' management. More recently, interest has focused on the role of such infusions in non-diabetic patients, and meta-analyses do suggest benefit. A recent well-conducted trial (below) examined the use of GKI in patients with a suspected acute MI (patients also received thrombolysis). This showed clear benefit, with a large reduction in total mortality. Side-effects are minimal and costs low. But before this is introduced into practice, it needs to be confirmed, and various regimens compared. The mechanism of benefit is unclear, but protection from the harmful effects of toxic free fatty acids may be important. R Diaz 1998 *Circulation* **98** 2227 [@9867443]

Acute coronary syndrome (ACS) (without ST-elevation)

ACS includes unstable angina, evolving myocardial infarction (MI), and non-Q wave or subendocardial MI. Although the underlying pathology is similar, management differs and, therefore, ACS is usually divided into 2 classes:

• *ACS with ST segment elevation* or new LBBB (acute MI see p782).
• *ACS without ST segment elevation* (unstable angina or non-Q wave MI).

ACS is associated with a greatly increased risk of MI (up to 30% in the 1st month). Patients should be managed medically until symptoms settle. They are then investigated by angiography with a view to possible angioplasty or surgery (CABG).

Assessment

Brief history: previous angina, relief with rest/nitrates, history of cardiovascular disease, risk factors for IHD.

Examination: pulse, BP, JVP, cardiac murmurs, signs of heart failure, peripheral pulses, scars from previous cardiac surgery.

Investigations ECG: ST depression; flat or inverted T waves; or normal. FBC, U&E, glucose, lipids, cardiac enzymes. CXR.

Measurement of cardiac troponins helps predict which patients are at risk of a cardiac event, and who can be safely discharged early. Note that 2 different forms of troponin are measured: troponin T and troponin I: they have different reference intervals (consult your lab).

Management

▶See OPPOSITE for acute management
▶For management of ACS with ST-elevation, see p782.

The aim of drug therapy is twofold:

1 Anti-ischaemic, eg β-blocker, nitrate, calcium channel antagonist.
2 Antithrombotic, eg aspirin, low molecular weight heparin, abciximab, which interfere with platelet activation, and so reduce thrombus formation.

Further measures:
• Wean off *glyceryl trinitrate* (GTN) infusion when stabilized on oral drugs.
• Stop heparin when pain-free for 24h, but give at least 3–5d therapy.
• Check serial ECGs and cardiac enzymes for 2–3d.
• Address modifiable risk factors: smoking, hypertension, hyperlipidaemia, diabetes.
• Gentle mobilization.

▶*If symptoms recur, refer to a cardiologist for urgent angiography and angioplasty or CABG.*

Prognosis Overall risk of death ~1–2%, but ~15% for refractory angina despite medical therapy. Risk stratification can help predict those most at risk and allow intervention to be targeted at those individuals. The following are associated with an increased risk:
• Haemodynamic instability: hypotension, pulmonary oedema
• T-wave inversion or ST segment depression on resting ECG
• Previous MI
• Prolonged rest pain
• Older age
• Diabetes mellitus.

Indications for consideration of invasive intervention:
• Poor prognosis, eg pulmonary oedema
• Refractory symptoms
• Positive exercise tolerance tests (ETT) at low workload
• Non-Q wave MI.

Acute management of ACS without ST-segment elevation

Admit to CCU and monitor closely
↓
High-flow O_2 by face mask
↓
Analgesia:
eg morphine 5–10mg IV + metoclopramide 10mg IV
↓
Nitrates: GTN spray or sublingual tablets as required
↓
Aspirin: 300mg PO (unless contraindicated)
reduces risk of MI and death
↓
β-blocker: eg metoprolol 50–100mg/8h or atenolol 50–100mg/24h
If β-blocker contraindicated (asthma, COPD, LVF, bradycardia, coronary artery spasm), give rate-limiting calcium antagonist (eg verapamil [1] 80–120mg/8h PO, or diltiazem 60–120mg/8h PO)
↓
Low molecular weight heparin
(eg enoxaparin 1mg/kg/12h or dalteparin 120u/kg/12h SC)
Alternatively: unfractionated heparin 5000U IV bolus then IVI
Check APTT 6-hourly. Alter IVI rate to maintain APTT at 1.5–2.5 times control
↓
IV nitrate if pain continues
(eg GTN 50mg in 50mL 0.9% saline at 2–10mL/h)
titrate to pain, and maintain systolic BP >100mmHg
↓
Record ECG while in pain
↓

High-risk patients

(persistent or recurrent ischaemia, ST-depression, diabetes, ↑troponin)
Infusion of a GPIIb/IIIa antagonist (eg tirofiban) and, ideally, urgent angiography. Addition of clopidogrel may also be useful
↓
Optimize drugs: β-blocker; Ca^{2+} channel antagonist; ACE-i nitrate. Intensive statin regimens, *starting at top dosages*, may decrease long- and short-term mortality/adverse events, eg by stabilizing plaques.[2,3]
↓
▶*If symptoms fail to improve, refer to a cardiologist for urgent angiography ± angioplasty or CABG*

Low-risk patients

*(no further pain, flat or inverted T-waves, or normal ECG, **and** negative troponin)*
May be discharged if a repeat troponin is negative.
Treat medically and arrange further investigation eg stress test, angiogram.

1 Do not use verapamil and a β-blocker together (can cause asystole).
2 Comparing intensive & moderate lipid lowering with statins after ACS. N=4162. Cannon C NEJM 2004
3 Intensive statin therapy—a sea change in cardiovascular prevention. Topol E NEJM 2004 [@15007110]

▸▸Severe pulmonary oedema (X-RAY PLATE 2)

Causes
- Cardiovascular—usually left ventricular failure—post-MI, or ischaemic heart disease. Also mitral stenosis, arrhythmias, and malignant hypertension.
- ARDS (p190, any cause, eg trauma, malaria, drugs), look for predisposing factors, eg trauma, post-op, sepsis. *Is aspirin overdose or glue-sniffing/drug abuse likely?* Ask friends/relatives.
- Fluid overload.
- Neurogenic, eg head injury.

Differential diagnosis Asthma/COPD, pneumonia, and pulmonary oedema are often hard to distinguish, especially in the elderly, where that may co-exist. Do not hesitate to treat all 3 simultaneously (eg with salbutamol nebulizer, frusemide (=furosemide) IV, diamorphine, amoxicillin—p542).

Symptoms Dyspnoea, orthopnoea (eg paroxysmal), pink frothy sputum. NB: drugs; other illnesses (recent MI/COPD or pneumonia).

Signs Distressed, pale, sweaty, pulse↑, tachypnoea, pink frothy sputum, pulsus alternans, JVP↑, fine lung crackles, triple/gallop rhythm (p44), wheeze (cardiac asthma). Usually sitting up and leaning forward. Quickly examine for possible causes.

Investigations
- CXR (X-RAY PLATE 2)—cardiomegaly, signs of pulmonary oedema: look for shadowing (usually bilateral), small effusions at costophrenic angles, fluid in the lung fissures, and Kerley B lines (linear opacities).
- ECG—signs of MI.
- U&E; 'cardiac' enzymes, ABG.
- Consider echo.

Management

Begin treatment before investigations. See OPPOSITE.

Monitoring progress: BP; heart rate; cyanosis; respiratory rate; JVP; urine output, ABG.

Once stable and improving:
- Daily weights; BP and pulse/6h. Repeat CXR.
- Change to oral frusemide or bumetanide.
- If on large doses of loop diuretic, consider the addition of a thiazide (eg bendrofluazide (=bendroflumethiazide) or metolazone 2.5–5mg daily PO).
- ACE-i if left ventricular failure—also consider echo. If ACE-i contraindicated, consider hydralazine and nitrate.
- Also consider β-blocker and spironolactone.
- Is the patient suitable for cardiac transplantation?
- Consider digoxin ± warfarin, especially if AF.

Management of heart failure

Sit the patient upright

↓

Oxygen
100% if no pre-existing lung disease

↓

IV access and monitor ECG
Treat any arrhythmias, eg AF (p126-32)

↓

Investigations while continuing treatment
see OPPOSITE

↓

Diamorphine 2.5–5mg IV slowly
Caution in liver failure and COPD

↓

Frusemide[1] 40–80mg IV slowly
Larger doses required in renal failure

↓

GTN spray 2 puffs SL or 2 × 0.3mg tablets SL
Don't give if systolic BP <90mmHg

↓

Necessary investigations, examination, and history

↓

If systolic BP ≥100mmHg, start a nitrate infusion
eg isosorbide dinitrate 2-10mg/h IVI; keep systolic BP ≥90mmHg

↓

If the patient is worsening: further dose of frusemide 40–80mg
Consider ventilation (invasive or non-invasive eg CPAP; get help)
or increasing nitrate infusion
Alternatively venesect 500mL blood (rarely done)

↓

If systolic BP <100mmHg, treat as cardiogenic shock (p788),
ie consider a Swan-Ganz catheter and inotropic support

↓

If systolic BP is >180mmHg, consider treating for hypertensive LVF
(p142)

1 = furosemide.

▸▸Cardiogenic shock

This has a high mortality. ▸ Ask a senior physician's help both in formulating an *exact* diagnosis and in guiding treatment.

Cardiogenic shock is shock caused primarily by the failure of the heart to maintain the circulation. It may occur suddenly, or after progressively worsening heart failure.

Causes

- Arrhythmias
- Cardiac tamponade
- Tension pneumothorax
- Myocardial infarction
- Myocarditis; myocardial depression (drugs, hypoxia, acidosis, sepsis)
- Valve destruction (endocarditis)
- Pulmonary embolus
- Aortic dissection

Management

If the cause is myocardial infarction prompt revascularization (thrombolysis or acute angioplasty) is vital; ▸▸ see p782[1] for indications and contraindications.

- Manage in Coronary Care Unit, if possible.
- Investigation and treatment may need to be done concurrently.
- See OPPOSITE for details of management.
- *Investigations* ECG, U&E, CK, ABG, CXR, echo. If indicated, CT thorax (aortic dissection) and V̇/Q̇ scan or pulmonary angiogram for PE.
- *Monitor* CVP, BP, ABG, ECG; urine output. Do a 12-lead ECG every hour until the diagnosis is made. Consider a Swan–Ganz catheter to assess pulmonary wedge pressure and cardiac output, and an arterial line to monitor pressure. Catheterize for accurate urine output.

Cardiac tamponade

Essence: Pericardial fluid collects → intrapericardial pressure rises → heart cannot fill → pumping stops.

Causes: Trauma, lung/breast cancer, pericarditis, myocardial infarct, bacteria, eg TB. *Rarely:* Urea↑, radiation, myxoedema, dissecting aorta, SLE.

Signs: Falling BP, a rising JVP, and muffled heart sounds = Beck's triad; JVP↑ on inspiration (Kussmaul's sign); pulsus paradoxus (pulse fades on inspiration). Echocardiography may be diagnostic. CXR: globular heart; left heart border convex or straight; right cardiophrenic angle <90°. ECG: electrical alternans (p158).

Management: This can be very difficult. Everything is against you: time, physiology, and your own confidence, as the patient may be too ill to give a history, and signs may be equivocal—but bitter experience has taught us not to equivocate for long.

▸▸ Request the presence of your senior at the bedside (do not make do with telephone advice). With luck, prompt pericardiocentesis (p757) brings swift relief. While awaiting this, give O₂, monitor ECG, and set up IVI. Take blood for group and save.

1 SHOCK trial 2003 V Menon *Congest Heart Fail* **9** 35. NNT for acute angioplasty = 5.

Management of cardiogenic shock

Oxygen
Titrate to maintain adequate arterial saturations
↓
Diamorphine 2.5–5mg IV for pain and anxiety
↓
Investigations and *close monitoring*
(see OPPOSITE)
↓
Correct arrhythmias (p126–p130), U&E abnormality
or acid–base imbalance
↓
Optimize filling pressure
if available measure pulmonary capillary wedge pressure (PCWP)

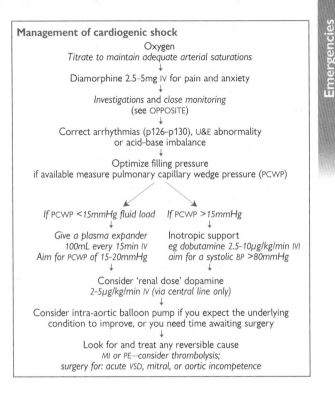

If PCWP *<15mmHg fluid load*   *If* PCWP *>15mmHg*
↓   ↓
Give a plasma expander   *Inotropic support*
100mL every 15min IV   *eg dobutamine 2.5–10µg/kg/min IVI*
Aim for PCWP of 15–20mmHg   *aim for a systolic BP >80mmHg*
↓
Consider 'renal dose' dopamine
2–5µg/kg/min IV (via central line only)
↓
Consider intra-aortic balloon pump if you expect the underlying
condition to improve, or you need time awaiting surgery
↓
Look for and treat any reversible cause
MI or PE—consider thrombolysis;
surgery for: acute VSD, mitral, or aortic incompetence

▸▸Broad complex tachycardia

ECG shows rate of >100bpm and QRS complexes >120ms (>3 small squares on ECGs done at the standard UK rate of 25mm/s).

Principles of management

If in doubt, treat as ventricular tachycardia (the commonest cause).

Identify the underlying rhythm and treat accordingly.

Differential

- Ventricular tachycardia (VT) including torsade de pointes
- SVT with aberrant conduction, eg AF, atrial flutter
- Pre-excited tachycardias, eg AF, atrial flutter, or AV re-entry tachycardia with underlying WPW (p128).

(NB: Ventricular ectopics should not cause confusion when occurring singly; but if >3 together at a rate of >120, this constitutes VT.)

Identification of the underlying rhythm may be difficult, seek expert help. Diagnosis is based on the history: if IHD/MI the likelihood of a ventricular arrhythmia is >95%, a 12-lead ECG, and the lack of response to IV adenosine (p128).

ECG findings in favour of VT:
- Fusion beats or capture beats (ECG p133)
- Positive QRS concordance in chest leads
- Marked left axis deviation or rightwards axis
- AV dissociation (occurs in 25%) or 2:1 or 3:1 AV block
- QRS complex >160ms
- Any atypical bundle-branch-block pattern.

Management Give high-flow O_2 by mask and monitor O_2 saturations.
- Connect patient to a cardiac monitor and have a defibrillator to hand
- Assess CVS: consciousness↓, BP <90, oliguria, angina, pulmonary oedema.
- Obtain 12-lead ECG (request CXR) and obtain IV access.

If haemodynamically unstable
- Synchronized DC shock (see European Resuscitation Guidelines p767)
- Correct any hypokalaemia and hypomagnesaemia: 60mmol KCl at 30mmol/h, and 5mL 50% magnesium sulphate over 30min)
- Follow with amiodarone 150mg IV over 10min
- For refractory cases procainamide or sotalol may be considered.

If haemodynamically stable
- Correct hypokalaemia and hypomagnesaemia: as above
- Amiodarone 150mg IV over 10 min. Alternatively lidocaine 50mg (2.5mL of 2% solution) IV over 2min, repeated every 5min upto 200mg.
- If this fails, use synchronized DC shock.

After correction of VT
- Establish the cause (via the history and tests above)
- Maintenance anti-arrhythmic therapy may be required. If VT occurs after MI, give IV amiodarone or lidocaine infusion for 12–24h; if 24h after MI, also start oral anti-arrhythmic: sotalol (if good LV function) or amiodarone (if poor LV function)
- Prevention of recurrent VT: surgical isolation of the arrhythmogenic area or implantation of tiny automatic defibrillators may help.

Ventricular fibrillation (ECG p135.) Use non-synchronized DC shock (there is no R wave to trigger defibrillation, p754): see European Resuscitation Guidelines (p767).

Ventricular extrasystoles (ectopics) are the commonest post-MI arrhythmia but they are also seen in healthy people (often >10/h). Patients with frequent ectopics post-MI have a worse prognosis, but there is no evidence that anti-dysrhythmic drugs improve outcome, indeed they may increase mortality.

Torsade de pointes: A form of VT, with a constantly varying axis, often in the setting of long-QT syndromes (ECG p133). This can be congenital or acquired, eg from drugs (eg some anti-dysrhythmics, tricyclics, antimalarials, newer antipsychotics and terfenadine). Torsade in the setting of congenital long-QT syndromes can be treated with high doses of β-blockers.

In acquired long-QT syndromes, stop all predisposing drugs, correct hypokalaemia, and give $MgSO_4^{2+}$ (1–4g IV). Alternatives include: overdrive pacing or isoprenaline IVI to increase heart rate.

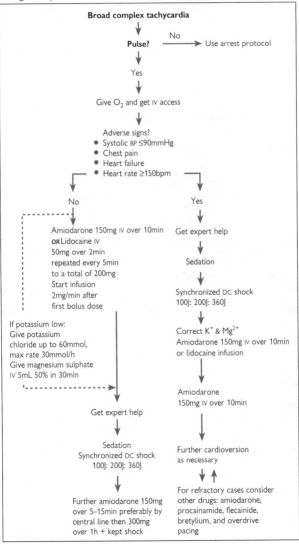

Broad complex tachycardia

↓

Pulse? — No → Use arrest protocol

↓

Yes

↓

Give O_2 and get IV access

↓

Adverse signs?
- Systolic BP ≤90mmHg
- Chest pain
- Heart failure
- Heart rate ≥150bpm

No / Yes

No:
Amiodarone 150mg IV over 10min
OR Lidocaine IV
50mg over 2min
repeated every 5min
to a total of 200mg
Start infusion
2mg/min after
first bolus dose

If potassium low:
Give potassium
chloride up to 60mmol,
max rate 30mmol/h
Give magnesium sulphate
IV 5mL 50% in 30min

Get expert help

↓

Sedation
Synchronized DC shock
100J: 200J: 360J

↓

Further amiodarone 150mg
over 5–15min preferably by
central line then 300mg
over 1h + kept shock

Yes:
Get expert help

↓

Sedation

↓

Synchronized DC shock
100J: 200J: 360J

↓

Correct K^+ & Mg^{2+}
Amiodarone 150mg IV over 10min
or lidocaine infusion

↓

Amiodarone
150mg IV over 10min

↓

Further cardioversion
as necessary

↓↑

For refractory cases consider
other drugs: amiodarone,
procainamide, flecainide,
bretylium, and overdrive
pacing

791

▸▸Narrow complex tachycardia

ECG shows rate of >100bpm and QRS complex duration of <120ms (<3 small squares on ECGs done at the standard UK rate of 25mm/s).

Differential diagnosis

- Sinus tachycardia: normal P-wave followed by normal QRS.
- *Atrial tachyarrhythmias:* Rhythm arises in atria, AV node is a bystander.
  Atrial fibrillation (AF): absent P-wave, irregular QRS complexes.
  Atrial flutter: atrial rate ~260–340bpm. Saw-tooth baseline, due to continuous atrial electrical activity. Ventricular rate often 150bpm (2 : 1 block).
  Atrial tachycardia: abnormally shaped P-waves, may outnumber QRS.
  Multifocal atrial tachycardia: 3 or more P-wave morphologies, irregular QRS complexes.
- *Junctional tachycardia:* AV-node is part of the pathway. P-wave either buried in QRS complex or occurring after QRS complex.
  AV nodal re-entry tachycardia.
  AV re-entry tachycardia, includes an accessory pathway, eg WPW (p128).

Principles of management See algorithm OPPOSITE.

- If the patient is compromised, use DC cardioversion.
- Otherwise, identify the underlying rhythm and treat accordingly.
- Vagal manoeuvres (carotid sinus massage, Valsalva manoeuvre) transiently increase AV block, and may unmask an underlying atrial rhythm.
- If unsuccessful use adenosine which causes transient AV block. It has a short half-life (10–15s) and works in 2 ways:
  - by transiently slowing ventricles to show the underlying atrial rhythm,
  - by cardioverting a junctional tachycardia to sinus rhythm.

Give 6mg IV bolus into a large vein, followed by saline flush, while recording a rhythm strip. If unsuccessful, give 12mg, 12mg then 12mg at 2min intervals. Warn about SE: transient chest tightness, dyspnoea, headache, flushing. CI: asthma, $2^{nd}/3^{rd}$-degree AV block or sinoatrial disease (unless pacemaker). *Interactions:* potentiated by dipyridamole, antagonized by theophylline.

Specifics *Sinus tachycardia:* Identify and treat underlying cause.

Supraventricular tachycardia: If adenosine fails, use verapamil 5–10mg IV over 2–3min. **NB:** NOT if on a β-blocker. If no response, a further 5mg IV over 3min (if age <60yrs). Alternatives: atenolol 5mg IV or sotalol 20–120mg IV (over 10min); or amiodarone. If unsuccessful, use DC cardioversion.

Atrial fibrillation/flutter: Manage along standard lines (p130).

Atrial tachycardia: Rare; may be due to digoxin toxicity: withdraw digoxin, consider digoxin-specific antibody fragments. Maintain K^+ at 4–5mmol/L.

Multifocal atrial tachycardia: Most commonly occurs in COPD. Correct hypoxia and hypercapnia. Consider verapamil if rate remains >110bpm.

Junctional tachycardia: Where anterograde conduction through the AV node occurs, vagal manoeuvres are worth trying. Adenosine will usually cardiovert a junctional rhythm to sinus rhythm. If it fails or recurs, β-blockers (or vera-pamil—**not** with β-blockers, digoxin, or class I agents such as quinidine). If this does not control symptoms, consider radiofrequency ablation.

Wolff–Parkinson–White (WPW) syndrome (ECG p131.) Caused by con-genital accessory conduction pathway between atria and ventricles. Resting ECG shows short P–R interval and widened QRS complex due to slurred up-stroke or 'delta wave'. 2 types: WPW type A (+ve δ wave in V_1), WPW type B (–ve δ wave in V_1). Patients present with SVT which may be due to an AVRT, (p128) pre-excited AF, or pre-excited atrial flutter. Risk of degeneration to VF and sudden death. Ɍ flecainide, propafenone, sotalol, or amiodarone. Refer to cardiologist for electrophysiology and ablation of the accessory pathway.

Narrow complex tachycardia
(Supraventricular tachycardia)

↓

Give O₂ and get IV access

↓

Vagal manoeuvres
(caution, if possible digoxin toxicity,
acute ischaemia, or carotid bruit)

↓

Adenosine 6mg bolus injection[1]
Repeat if necessary every 1–2min
using 12mg, then 12mg, then 12mg
(ATP is an alternative)

↓

Atrial
fibrillation
(>130bpm)

Seek expert help ←

↓

Adverse signs?
Hypotension: BP ≤90mmHg
Chest pain
Heart failure
Impaired consciousness
Heart rate ≥200bpm

No ↓   Yes ↓

No:

Choose from:
- Esmolol: 40mg IV over 1min
  + infusion 4mg/min
  (IV injection can be repeated
  with increments of infusion
  to 12mg/min)
- Digoxin: max IV dose 500µg
  over 30min ×2
- Verapamil: 5–10mg IV over 2min
- Amiodarone: 300mg over IV
  1h; may be repeated once
  if necessary via a central
  line if possible
- Overdrive pacing—not AF

Yes:

Sedation

↓

Synchronized
cardioversion
100J: 200J: 360J

↓

Amiodarone 150mg IV
over 10min
then 300mg
over 1h if necessary
preferably by central
line, and repeat
cardioversion

1 Consult *BNF* if on dipyridamole or has had a heart transplant.

▶▶Acute severe asthma[11]

▶The severity of an attack is easily underestimated.

▶An atmosphere of calm helps.

Presentation Acute breathlessness and wheeze.

History Ask about usual and recent treatment; previous acute episodes and their severity and best peak expiratory flow rate (PEFR). Have they been admitted to ITU?

Differential diagnosis Acute infective exacerbation of COPD, pulmonary oedema, upper respiratory tract obstruction, pulmonary embolus, anaphylaxis.

Investigations PEF—but may be too ill; arterial blood gases; CXR (to exclude pneumothorax, infection); FBC; U&E.

Assessing the severity of an acute asthmatic attack

Severe attack:
- Unable to complete sentences
- Respiratory rate >25/min
- Pulse rate >110 beats/min
- Peak expiratory flow <50% of predicted or best

Life-threatening attack:
- Peak expiratory flow <33% of predicted or best
- Silent chest, cyanosis, feeble respiratory effort
- Bradycardia or hypotension
- Exhaustion, confusion, or coma
- Arterial blood gases: normal/high P_aCO_2 >5kPa (36mmHg)
  P_aO_2 <8kPa (60mmHg)
  low pH, eg <7.35

Treatment ▶Life-threatening or severe asthma, see OPPOSITE.
- Salbutamol 5mg nebulized with oxygen.
- If PEF remains <75%, repeat salbutamol and give prednisolone 30mg PO.
- Monitor oxygen saturation, heart rate, and respiratory rate.

Discharge

Patients, before discharge, must have:
- Been on discharge medication for 24h.
- Had inhaler technique checked.
- Peak flow rate >75% predicted or best with diurnal variability <25%.
- Steroid and bronchodilator therapy.
- Own a PEF meter and have management plan.
- GP appointment within 1wk.
- Respiratory clinic appointment within 4wks.

Drugs used in acute asthma

Salbutamol (β_2-agonist) *SE:* Tachycardia, arrhythmias, tremor, K$^+$↓.

Aminophylline (Inhibits phosphodiesterase; ↑[cAMP]). *SE:* pulse↑; arrhythmias, nausea, seizures. The amount of IVI aminophylline may need altering according to the individual patient: always check the BNF. Monitor ECG.
- *Factors which may necessitate reduction of dose:* Cardiac or liver failure, drugs which increase the half-life of aminophylline, eg cimetidine, ciprofloxacin, erythromycin, contraceptive steroids.
- *Factors which may require ↑dose:* Smoking, drugs which shorten the half-life, eg phenytoin, carbamazepine, barbiturates, rifampicin.
- ▶Aim for plasma concentration of 10–20µg/mL (55–110µmol/L). Serious toxicity (BP↓, arrhythmias, cardiac arrest) can occur at concentrations ≥25µg/mL. Measure plasma K$^+$: theophyllines may cause K$^+$↓. Don't load patients already on oral preparations.

Immediate management of acute severe asthma[12]

Assess severity of attack (see above). Warn ITU if attack severe.

Start treatment immediately (prior to investigations).
- Sit patient up and give high-dose O_2 in: 100% via non-rebreathing bag.
- Salbutamol 5mg (or terbutaline 10mg) plus ipratropium bromide 0.5mg nebulized with O_2.
- Hydrocortisone 100mg IV or prednisolone 30mg PO or both if very ill.
- CXR to exclude pneumothorax.

If life-threatening features (above) present:
- Inform ITU, and seniors.
- Add magnesium sulphate ($MgSO_4$) 1.2–2g IV over 20min.
- Give salbutamol nebulizers every 15min, or 10mg continuously per hour.

Further management

If improving
- 40–60% O_2.
- Prednisolone 30–60mg/24h PO.
- Nebulized salbutamol every 4h.
- Monitor peak flow and oxygen saturations.

▶▶If patient not improving after 15–30min
- Continue 100% O_2 and steroids.
- Hydrocortisone 100mg IV or prednisolone 30mg PO if not already given.
- Give salbutamol nebulizers every 15min, or 10mg continuously per hour.
- Continue ipratropium 0.5mg every 4–6h.

▶▶If patient still not improving
- Discuss with seniors and ITU.
- Repeat salbutamol nebulizer every 15min.
- $MgSO_4$ 1.2–2g IV over 20min, unless already given.
- Consider aminophylline; if not already on a theophylline, load with eg 5mg/kg IVI over 20min,[1] then 500µg/kg/h, eg in a small adult: 750mg/24h; large adult 1200mg/24h. Adjust dose according to plasma theophylline, if available. Do levels if infusion lasts >24h. Alternatively, give salbutamol IVI, eg 3–20µg/min. IPPV may be required.
- If no improvement, or life-threatening features are present, consider transfer to ITU, accompanied by a doctor prepared to intubate.

Monitoring the effects of treatment
- Repeat PEF 15–30min after initiating treatment.
- Pulse oximeter monitoring: maintain S_aO_2 >92%.
- Check blood gases within 2h if: initial P_aCO_2 was normal/raised or initial P_aO_2 <8kPa (60mmHg) or patient deteriorating.
- Record PEF pre- and post-β-agonist in hospital at least 4 times.

Once patient is improving
- Wean down and stop aminophylline over 12–24h.
- Reduce nebulized salbutamol and switch to inhaled β-agonist.
- Initiate inhaled steroids and stop oral steroids if possible.
- Continue to monitor PEF. Look for deterioration on reduced treatment and beware early morning dips in PEF.
- Look for the cause of the acute exacerbation and admission.

795

---

1 British Thoracic Society advice 2003 *Thorax* **58** sup 1 page 1.

Acute exacerbations of COPD

Common medical emergency especially in winter. May be triggered by viral or bacterial infections.

Presentation Increasing cough, breathlessness, or wheeze. Decreased exercise capacity.

History Ask about usual/recent treatments (especially home oxygen), smoking status, and exercise capacity (may influence a decision to ventilate the patient).

Differential diagnosis Asthma, pulmonary oedema, upper respiratory tract obstruction, pulmonary embolus, anaphylaxis.

Investigations
- Peak expiratory flow (PEF)—but may be too ill.
- Arterial blood gases.
- CXR to exclude pneumothorax and infection.
- FBC; U&E; CRP.
- ECG.
- Blood cultures (if pyrexial).
- Send sputum for culture.

Management
- Look for a cause, eg infection, pneumothorax.
- See OPPOSITE for acute management.
- Prior to discharge, liaise with GP regarding steroid reduction, domiciliary oxygen (p188), smoking, pneumococcal & 'flu vaccinations (p172).

Treatment of stable COPD: See p188 for further information.

Non-pharmacological:	Stop smoking, encourage exercise, treat poor nutrition or obesity, influenza, vaccination.
Pharmacological:	
• Mild	Short-acting β_2-agonist or ipratropium PRN.
• Moderate	Regular short-acting β_2-agonist and/or ipratropium. Consider corticosteroid trial.
• Severe	Combination therapy with regular short-acting β_2-agonist and ipratropium. Consider corticosteroid trial (p189). Assess for home nebulizers.

More advanced disease:
- Consider pulmonary rehabilitation in moderate/severe disease.
- Consider long-term oxygen therapy if P_aO_2 <7.3kPa (p188).
- Indications for surgery: recurrent pneumothoraces; isolated bullous disease; lung volume reduction surgery (selected patients).
- Assess social circumstances and support required. Identify and treat depression.
- Air travel may be hazardous if P_aO_2 <6.7kPa; check availability of O_2.

Management of acute COPD

Controlled oxygen therapy
Start at 24–28%; vary according to ABG.
Aim for a P_aO_2 >8.0kPa with a rise in P_aCO_2 <1.5kPa

↓

Nebulized bronchodilators:
Salbutamol 5mg/4h and ipratropium 500μg/6h

↓

Steroids
IV hydrocortisone 200mg and oral prednisolone 30–40mg

↓

Antibiotics:
Use if evidence of infection, eg amoxicillin 500mg/8h PO, p172

↓

Physiotherapy to aid sputum expectoration

↓

If no response:
Repeat nebulizers and consider IV aminophylline[1]

↓

If no response:

1. Consider nasal intermittent positive pressure ventilation
(NIPPV) if respiratory rate >30 or pH <7.35.
It is delivered by nasal mask and a flow generator

↓

2. Consider intubation[2] & ventilation if pH <7.26 and P_aCO_2 is rising

↓

3. Consider a respiratory stimulant drug, eg doxapram
1.5–4mg/min IV SE: agitation, confusion, tachycardia, nausea
Only for patients who are not suitable for mechanical ventilation
A short-term measure only

Oxygen therapy

- The greatest danger is hypoxia, which probably accounts for more deaths than hypercapnia. *Don't leave patients severely hypoxic.*
- However, in some patients, who rely on their hypoxic drive to breathe, too much oxygen may lead to a reduced respiratory rate, and hypercapnia, with a consequent fall in conscious level.
- Therefore, care is required with O_2, especially if there is evidence of CO_2 retention. Start with 24–28% O_2 in such patients. Reassess after 30min.
- Monitor the patient carefully. Aim to raise the P_aO_2 above 8.0kPa with a rise in P_aCO_2 <1.5kPa.
- In patients without evidence of retention at baseline use 28–40% O_2, but still monitor and repeat ABG.

797

1 Aminophylline: Do not give a loading dose to patients on maintenance methylxanthines (theophyllines/aminophylline). Load with 250mg over 20min, then infuse at a rate of ~500μg/kg/h. Check plasma levels if given for >24h. ECG monitoring is required.
2 A decision to ventilate will depend on the patient's premorbid state—exercise capacity, home oxygen, and comorbidity. Ask about this information before you need to make this decision.

►►Pneumothorax (X-RAY PLATE 6)

►►Tension pneumothorax requires immediate relief (see below). Do not delay management by obtaining a CXR.

Causes Often spontaneous (especially in young thin men) due to rupture of a subpleural bulla. Other causes: asthma; COPD; TB; pneumonia; lung abscess; carcinoma; cystic fibrosis; lung fibrosis; sarcoidosis; connective tissue disorders (Marfan's syndrome, Ehlers–Danlos syndrome); trauma; iatrogenic (subclavian CVP line insertion, pleural aspiration or biopsy, percutaneous liver biopsy, positive pressure ventilation).

Clinical features *Symptoms:* There may be no symptoms (especially in fit young people with small pneumothoraces) or there may be sudden onset of dyspnoea and/or pleuritic chest pain. Patients with asthma or COPD may present with a sudden deterioration. Mechanically ventilated patients may present with hypoxia or an increase in ventilation pressures. *Signs:* reduced expansion, hyper-resonance to percussion and diminished breath sounds on the affected side. *With a tension pneumothorax, the trachea will be deviated away from the affected side and the patient will be very unwell.*

Investigations ►A CXR *should not be performed if a tension pneumothorax is suspected, as it will delay immediate necessary treatment.* Otherwise, request an expiratory film, and look for an area devoid of lung markings, peripheral to the edge of the collapsed lung (X-RAY PLATE 6). Ensure the suspected pneumothorax is not a large emphysematous bulla. Check ABG in dyspnoeic patients and those with chronic lung disease.

Management Depends on whether it is a primary or secondary (underlying lung disease) pneumothorax, size and symptoms—see OPPOSITE.
• Pneumothorax due to trauma or mechanical ventilation requires a chest drain.
• Aspiration of a pneumothorax, see p758.
• Insertion and management of a chest drain, see p750.

Surgical advice: Arrange if: bilateral pneumothoraces; lung fails to expand after intercostal drain insertion; 2 or more previous pneumothoraces on the same side; or history of pneumothorax on the opposite side.

►►Tension pneumothorax (X-RAY PLATE 6)

This is a medical emergency.

Essence: Air drawn into the pleural space with each inspiration has no route of escape during expiration. The mediastinum is pushed over into the contralateral hemithorax, kinking and compressing the great veins. Unless the air is rapidly removed, cardiorespiratory arrest will occur.

Signs: Respiratory distress, tachycardia, hypotension, distended neck veins, trachea deviated away from side of pneumothorax. Increased percussion note, reduced air entry/breath sounds on the affected side.

Treatment:

►►To remove the air, insert a large-bore (14–16G) needle with a syringe, partially filled with 0.9% saline, into the 2nd intercostal interspace in the midclavicular line on the side of the suspected pneumothorax. Remove plunger to allow the trapped air to bubble through the syringe (with saline as a water seal) until a chest tube can be placed. Alternatively, insert a large-bore venflon in the same location.

►►Do this *before* requesting a CXR.

Then insert a chest drain. See p750.

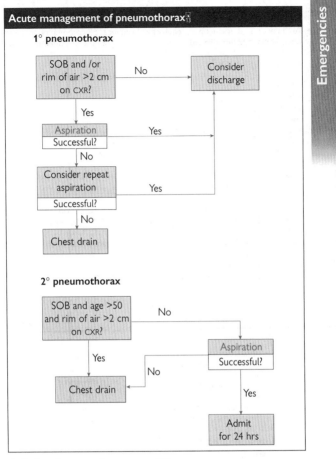

Acute management of pneumothorax[13]

1° pneumothorax

SOB and /or rim of air >2 cm on CXR? — No → Consider discharge

Yes ↓

Aspiration / Successful? — Yes →

No ↓

Consider repeat aspiration / Successful? — Yes →

No ↓

Chest drain

2° pneumothorax

SOB and age >50 and rim of air >2 cm on CXR? — No →

Yes ↓

Aspiration / Successful?

No ← → Chest drain

Yes ↓

Admit for 24 hrs

Aspiration of a pneumothorax: ►►see p758.

Intercostal tube drainage: For insertion, see p750.
- Use a small tube (10–14F) unless blood/pus is also present.
- Never clamp a bubbling tube.
- Tubes may be removed 24h after the lung has re-expanded and air leak has stopped (ie the tube stops bubbling). This is done during expiration or a valsalva manoeuvre.
- If the lung fails to re-expand within 48h, or if there is a persistent air leak, specialist advice should be obtained, as suction or surgical intervention may be required.
- If suction is required, high volume, low pressure (–10 to –20cm H_2O) systems are required.

Pneumonia (X-RAY PLATE 5 & 8)

An infection of the lung parenchyma. Incidence of community-acquired pneumonia is 12 per 1000 adults. Of these, 1 will require hospitalization, and mortality in these patients is still 10%.

Common organisms
- *Streptococcus pneumoniae* is the commonest cause (60–75%).
- *Mycoplasma pneumoniae* (5–18%).
- *Staphylococcus aureus.*
- *Haemophilus influenzae.*
- *Legionella* species and *Chlamydia psittaci.*
- Gram-negative bacilli, often hospital-acquired or immunocompromised, eg *Pseudomonas* especially in those with COPD.
- Viruses including influenza account for up to 15%.

Symptoms
- Fever, rigors, malaise, anorexia, dyspnoea, cough, purulent sputum (classically 'rusty' with pneumococcus), haemoptysis, and pleuritic chest pain.

Signs
- Fever, cyanosis, herpes labialis (pneumococcus), confusion, tachypnoea, tachycardia, hypotension, signs of consolidation (diminished expansion, dull percussion note, increased tactile vocal fremitus/vocal resonance, bronchial breathing), and a pleural rub.

Investigations
- CXR (X-RAY PLATE 5 & 8).
- Oxygen saturation arterial blood gases if S_aO_2 <92% or severe pneumonia.
- FBC, U&E, LFT, CRP, atypical serology.
- Blood and sputum cultures.
- Pleural fluid may be aspirated for culture.
- Bronchoscopy and bronchoalveolar lavage if the patient is immunocompromised or on ITU.

Severity
Core adverse features 'CURB' score[14]:
- Confusion (abbreviated mental test ≤8);
- Urea >7mmol/L;
- Respiratory rate ≥30/min;
- BP <90/60mmHg).

A score >2 indicates severe pneumonia. Other features increasing the risk of death are: age ≥50yrs; co-existing disease; bilateral/multilobar involvement; P_aO_2 <8kPa or S_aO_2 <92%.

Management See OPPOSITE.

Complications

Pleural effusion, empyema, lung abscess, respiratory failure, septicaemia, pericarditis, myocarditis, cholestatic jaundice, renal failure.

Management of pneumonia

Oxygen to maintain P_aO_2 >8kPa
caution if history of COPD

↓

Treat hypotension and shock: see p778

↓

Investigations
see OPPOSITE

↓

Antibiotics
see BELOW

↓

Intravenous fluids may be required
(anorexia, dehydration, shock)

↓

Analgesia for pleuritic chest pain, eg paracetamol 1g/6h or NSAID

↓

Some patients may need intubation and a period of ventilatory support

Antibiotics See p173 for recommendation regarding specific organisms.

Community-acquired

Mild	*Streptococcus pneumoniae* *Haemophilus influenzae* *Mycoplasma pneumoniae*	Amoxicillin 500mg–1.0g/8h PO + erythromycin[1] 500mg/6h PO or fluoroquinolone if IV required: ampicillin 500mg/6h + erythromycin[1] 12.5mg/kg/6h IVI
Severe	As above	Co-amoxiclav IV or cephalosporin IV (eg Cefuroxime 1.5g/8h IV) AND erythromycin[1] as above
Atypical	*Legionella pneumophilia*	Clarithromycin 500mg/12h PO/IVI ± rifampicin
	Chlamydia species	Tetracycline
	Pneumocystis carinii	High-dose co-trimoxazole

Hospital acquired

	Gram −ve bacilli Pseudomonas Anaerobes	Aminoglycoside (p710) IV + antipseudomonal penicillin IV or 3rd gen cephalosporin IV

Aspiration

	Strep. pneumoniae Anaerobes	Cefuroxime 1.5g/8h IV + metronidazole 500mg/8h IVI

Neutropenic patients

	Gram +ve cocci Gram −ve bacilli	Aminoglycoside IV + antipseudomonal penicillin IV or 3rd gen cephalosporin IV
	Fungi (p180)	Consider antifungals after 48h

3rd gen = 3rd generation, eg cefotaxime, p710

801

1 Clarithromycin 500mg PO/IVI is an alternative.

▸▸Massive pulmonary embolism (PE)

▸Always suspect pulmonary embolism (PE) in sudden collapse 1–2wks after surgery. Death rate in England and Wales: 30,000–40,000/yr.

Mechanism Venous thrombi, usually from DVT, pass into the pulmonary circulation and block blood flow to lungs. The source is often occult.

Risk factors
- Malignancy
- Surgery—especially pelvic
- Immobility
- The Pill (there is also a slight risk attached to HRT)
- Previous thromboembolism and inherited thrombophilia, see p672

Prevention Early post-op mobilization is the simplest method; consider:
- Antithromboembolic stockings.
- Low molecular weight heparin prophylaxis SC.
- Avoid contraceptive pill if at risk, eg major or orthopaedic surgery.
- Recurrent PEs may be prevented by anticoagulation, vena caval filters are of limited use, and should be combined with anticoagulation.

Signs and symptoms
- Acute dyspnoea, pleuritic chest pain, haemoptysis, and syncope.
- Hypotension, tachycardia, gallop rhythm, JVP↑, loud P_2, right ventricular heave, pleural rub, tachypnoea, and cyanosis, AF.

Classically, PE presents 10d post-op, with collapse and sudden breathlessness while straining at stool—but PE may occur after any period of immobility, or with no predisposing factors. Breathlessness may be the only sign. Multiple small emboli may present less dramatically with pleuritic pain, haemoptysis, and gradually increasing breathlessness.

▸Look for a source of emboli—especially DVT (is a leg swollen?).

Investigations
- *U&E, FBC,* baseline clotting.
- *ECG* (commonly normal or sinus tachycardia); right ventricular strain pattern V1–3 (p98), right axis deviation, RBBB, AF, may be deep S-waves in I, Q-waves in III, inverted T-waves in III ('S_I Q_{III} T_{III}').
- *CXR*—often normal; decreased vascular markings, small pleural effusion. Wedge-shaped area of infarction.
- *ABG:* hyperventilation + gas exchange↓: P_aO_2↓, P_aCO_2↓, pH often↑, p168.
- *CT* pulmonary angiography is sensitive and specific in determining if emboli are in pulmonary arteries. If helical CT is unavailable, a *ventilation-perfusion ($\dot{V}/\dot{Q}$) scan* can aid diagnosis. If $\dot{V}/\dot{Q}$ scan is equivocal, pulmonary angiography or bilateral venograms may help.
- *D-dimer* blood test, ↑ if thrombosis present. May help in excluding a PE.

Management See OPPOSITE for immediate management.
- Try to prevent further thrombosis with compression stockings.
- Heparin should be given for ≥5d, and until INR >2. Then stop.
- If obvious remedial cause, 6wks' treatment with warfarin may be sufficient. Otherwise, continue for at least 3–6 months (long-term if recurrent emboli, or underlying malignancy).
- Is there an underlying cause, eg thrombophilic tendency (p672), malignancy (especially prostate, breast, or pelvic cancer), SLE, or polycythaemia?

▸If good story and signs, make the diagnosis. Start treatment (OPPOSITE) before definitive investigations: most PE deaths occur within 1h.

Management of massive pulmonary embolism

Oxygen, 100%

↓

Morphine 10mg IV with antiemetic
if the patient is in pain or very distressed

↓

►If critically ill, consider immediate surgery

↓

IV access and start heparin
either unfractionated heparin 10,000U IV bolus,
then 15–25U/kg/h IVI as guided by APTT (p648)
or low molecular weight heparin, eg tinzaparin 175U/kg/24h SC

↓

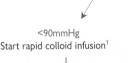
What is the systolic BP?

<90mmHg
Start rapid colloid infusion[1]

↓

If BP still↓ after 500mL colloid,
dobutamine 2.5–10µg/kg/min IV;
aim for systolic BP >90mmHg

↓

If BP still↓, consider noradrenaline

↓

If the systolic BP <90mmHg after
30–60min of standard treatment,
clinically definite PE and no CI
(p782), consider thrombolysis.[2]

>90mmHg
Start warfarin
10mg/24h PO (p648)

↓

Confirm diagnosis

1 Controversial, but some authorities say it is best to infuse plasma-expanding fluids even if CVP↑, to maintain BP & organ perfusion, see *Concise OTM* (OUP, 2000) page 151—but see Task Force on PE, European Society Cardiology *Eur Heart J* 2000 **21** 1301
2 A standard regimen is: **Loading dose:** streptokinase 250,000U IVI over 30min.
Maintenance dose: streptokinase 100,000U/h IVI for 12–72h, according to response. **Or** rt-PA (alteplase) 10mg IV over 1–2min followed by 90mg IV over 2h; max 1.5mg/kg if patient <65kg.

▸▸Acute upper gastrointestinal bleeding

Causes

Common: • Gastric/duodenal ulcer • Gastritis • Mallory–Weiss tear (oesophageal tear due to vomiting) • Oesophageal varices • Portal hypertensive gastropathy • Drugs: NSAIDs, aspirin, thrombolytics, anticoagulants.

Rarer: • Haemobilia • Nose bleeds (swallowed blood) • oesophageal/gastric malignancy • Oesophagitis • Angiodysplasia • Haemangiomas • Ehlers–Danlos or Peutz–Jeghers' syndrome (p732) • Bleeding disorders • Aorto-enteric fistula (in those with an aortic graft).

Signs & symptoms Haematemesis, or melaena, dizziness (especially postural), fainting, abdominal pain, dysphagia? Postural hypotension, hypotension, tachycardia (not if on β-blocker), ↓JVP, ↓urine output, cool and clammy, signs of chronic liver disease (p232); telangiectasia or purpura; jaundice (biliary colic + jaundice + melaena suggests haemobilia). **NB:** Ask about previous GI problems, drug use, and alcohol intake.

Management *Assess whether patient is in shock:*
• Cool & clammy to touch (especially nose, toes, fingers) ↓capillary refill.
• Pulse >100bpm
• JVP <1cm H_2O
• Systolic BP <100mmHg
• Postural drop
• Urine output <30mL/h.

If not shocked: Insert 2 big cannulae; start slow saline IVI to keep lines patent; check bloods and monitor vital signs + urine output. Aim to keep Hb >8g/dL. **NB:** Hb may not fall until circulating volume is restored.

If shocked: See OPPOSITE for management

Variceal bleeding: Resuscitate then proceed to urgent endoscopy for banding or sclerotherapy. Give octreotide 50µg/h IVI for 2–5d. Terlipressin may also be used. If massive bleed or bleeding continues, pass a Sengstaken–Blakemore tube p231. A bleed is the equivalent of a large protein meal so start treatment to avoid hepatic encephalopathy (p227). Esomeprazole 40mg PO may also be helpful in preventing stress ulceration.

Endoscopy Within 4h if you suspect variceal bleeding; within 12–24h if shocked on admission or significant comorbidity. Endoscopy can identify the site of bleeding, estimate the risk of rebleeding (rebleeding doubles mortality) and can be used to administer treatment. *Risk of rebleeding:* Active arterial bleeding seen (90% risk); visible vessel (70% risk); adherent clot/black dots (30% risk). *No site of bleeding identified:* Bleeding site missed on endoscopy; bleeding site has healed (Mallory–Weiss tear or Dieulafoy's lesion); nose bleed (swallowed blood); site distal to 3rd part of the duodenum (Meckel's diverticulum, colonic site).

Rebleeds Serious event: 40% of patients who rebleed will die. If 'at risk' maintain a high index of suspicion. If a rebleed occurs, check vital signs every 15min and call senior cover. To prevent rebleeding in endoscopically-proven high risk cases, IVI omeprazole has been tried, eg 80mg followed by an infusion of 8mg/h for 72h, then 20mg/24h PO for 8wks.[16]

Signs of a rebleed:
• Rising pulse rate.
• Falling JVP ± decreasing hourly urine output.
• Haematemesis or melaena.
• Fall in BP (a late and sinister finding) and decreased conscious level.

Acute drug therapy Following successful endoscopic therapy in patients with **major** ulcer bleeding, IV omeprazole (80mg stat followed by 8mg/h for 72h) is recommended. There is no firm evidence to support the use of somatostatin or antifibrinolytic therapy in the majority of patients.

Immediate management if shocked

Protect airway and keep NBM
↓
Insert two large-bore cannulae *14-16G*
↓
Draw bloods
FBC, U&E, LFT, glucose, clotting screen
Cross-match 6 units
↓
Give high-flow O_2
↓
Rapid IV colloid infusion
Up to 1L
↓
If remains shocked, give blood
Group specific or O Rh-ve until cross-match done
↓
Otherwise slow saline infusion[1]
To keep lines open
↓
Transfuse as dictated by haemodynamics
↓
Correct clotting abnormalities
Vitamin K, FFP, platelet concentrate
↓
Set up CVP line to guide fluid replacement
Aim for >5cm H_2O CVP may mislead if there is ascites or CCF
A Swan-Ganz catheter may help
↓
Catheterize and monitor urine output
Aim for >30mL/h
↓
Monitor vital signs every 15min until stable, then hourly
↓
Notify surgeons of all severe bleeds
↓
Urgent endoscopy for diagnosis ± control of bleeding

Poor prognostic signs:

- Age >60
- Bradycardia or rate >100bpm
- Chronic liver disease
- Significant co-morbidity

- Systolic BP <100mmHg
- Bleeding diathesis
- Consciousness level↓

1 Avoid saline in patients with decompensated liver disease (ascites, peripheral oedema) as it worsens ascites, and despite a low serum sodium, patients have a high body sodium. Use whole blood, or salt-poor albumin for resuscitation, and 5% dextrose for maintenance.

Acute liver failure

Fulminant liver failure is assumed to be potentially reversible. Therefore, treatment is supportive and designed to buy time for the patient's liver to regenerate.

Management
- Seek expert help. Is transfer to a liver unit appropriate? see p231.
- Nurse with a 20° head-up tilt in ITU.
- Treat the cause if known (eg paracetamol overdose, p832).
- Caution with secretions and blood if hepatitis suspected.
- Check blood glucose 1–4 hourly and give 50mL 50% dextrose IV if <3.5mmol/L. Give 10% dextrose IV, 1L/12h to avoid hypoglycaemia.
- NGT to avoid aspiration and remove any blood (bleeding varices) from stomach. Protect the airway with an endotracheal tube.
- Monitor temperature; pulse; RR; BP; pupils; urine output.
- Daily lab blood glucose; INR; U&E; LFT; blood cultures, and EEG. The INR (or PT) is the best measure of liver synthetic function.
- Avoid FFP unless bleeding or undergoing a surgical procedure. Some centres give vitamin K daily. Platelet transfusions may be required if thrombocytopaenic and bleeding.
- Daily weights (ascites).
- Minimize absorption of nitrogenous substances and worsening of coma by restricting protein and emptying the bowel with lactulose and magnesium sulfate enemas. Aim for 2 soft stools/day.
- Consider neomycin 1g/6h PO to reduce numbers of bowel organisms.
- Consider N-acetylcysteine. Even in non-paracetamol liver failure, this can improve oxygenation and clotting profiles.
- Watch renal function carefully. Terlipressin may help if deterioration is due to hepatorenal syndrome. Consider haemodialysis if water overload or acute renal failure develops.
- Reduce acid secretion and risk of gastric stress ulcers, eg with cimetidine IV or a proton pump inhibitor (p214). Cimetidine dose by slow IV injection: 200mg over >5min; may be repeated every 8h (or use IVI in 0.9% saline).
- Avoid sedatives (but diazepam is used for seizures), or other drugs with hepatic metabolism (see BNF).
- Treat sepsis aggressively, and don't forget the risk of spontaneous bacterial peritonitis.

NB: Attempts to correct acid–base balance are often harmful.

▸▸MeningitisND

▶**Do not** delay treatment, it may save a life.

▶Make sure the referring GP gives a dose of antibiotic (parenteral benzylpenicillin, eg 1.2g IM/IV before sending the patient to you if possible.

Presentation
- Headache
- Meningism: neck stiffness, photophobia, Kernig's sign, headache
- Conscious level ↓, coma
- Petechial (non-blanching) rash—may only be 1 or 2 spots
- Seizures (~20%)
- Focal neurological signs (~20%)

Common organisms
- Meningococcus
- Pneumococcus
- *Haemophilus influenzae* (especially children)
- *Listeria monocytogenes*

Management
- Careful examination: pay attention to neurology; look for rashes; assess GCS.
- If shocked, resuscitate with fluids and oxygen.
- If ICP raised, summon help immediately and inform neurosurgeons.
- Start antibiotics (below) immediately.

Investigations
- U&E, FBC, LFT, glucose, coagulation screen.
- Blood culture, throat swabs (one for bacteria, one for virology), stool culture for viruses.
- Lumbar puncture (p752) if safe. Don't forget to measure the opening pressure! **Contraindications** are: suspected intracranial mass lesion, focal signs, papilloedema, trauma, or middle ear pathology. Major coagulopathy. Send samples for MC&S, gram stain, protein estimation, glucose, and to virology.
- CT head before LP if mass lesion or raised ICP suspected.
- CXR.

Antibiotics
Local policies vary. If in doubt ask. The following are suggestions only, where the organism is unknown:
- <50yrs: ceftriaxone 2g IV over >2mins as 1 daily dose.
- >50yrs: ceftriaxone 2g IV over >2mins daily + ampicillin 2g IV/4h (for *Listeria*).
- Aciclovir if encephalitis suspected.
- Once organism isolated, seek urgent microbiological advice.

Further measures
- There is some evidence that high dose steroids may reduce neurological complications. Therefore, some centres recommend the administration of dexamethasone 10mg IV before or with the 1st dose of antibiotics (but do not delay giving antibiotics), then every 6h for 4d. Avoid in patients with shock.
- General supportive measures.
- Remember meningitis is a notifiable disease.
- Inform local public health officer for contact tracing.
- Antibiotic prophylaxis for family and close contacts (depends on the organism—ask a microbiologist). See p370.

Typical CSF in meningitis

	Pyogenic	Tuberculous	Viral ('aseptic')
Appearance	Often turbid	Often fibrin web	Usually clear
Predominant cell[1]	Polymorphs	Mononuclear	Mononuclear
Cell count/mm^3	eg 90–1000+	10–1000/mm^3	50–1000/mm^3
Glucose	<½ plasma	<½ plasma	>½ plasma
Protein (g/L)	>1.5	1–5	<1
Organisms	In smear and culture	Often absent in smear	Not in smear or culture

(There are no hard-and-fast rules)

1 ≤5 lymphocytes/mm^3 may be normal, as long as there are no neutrophils. If bloody tap, red cell count may be less in each successive bottle and the CSF WCC will be high. The true CSF white count can be estimated by subtracting 1 white cell for every 1000 RBC. Normal protein: 0.15–0.45g/L. Normal CSF glucose: 2.8–4.2mmol/L (↓by: bacterial, fungal, mumps or carcinomatous meningitis, herpes encephalitis, hypoglycaemia, sarcoid, CNS vasculitides—OTM 4e, 955).
The predominant cell type may be lymphocytes in TB, listerial, and cryptococcal meningitis. Normal opening pressure: 7–18cmCSF; in meningitis, it may be >40 (typically 14–30cmCSF).

Cerebral abscess

Suspect this in any patient with ICP↑, especially if there is fever or ↑WCC. It may follow ear, sinus, dental, or periodontal infection; skull fracture; congenital heart disease; endocarditis; bronchiectasis.

Signs: Seizures, fever, localizing signs, or signs of ↑ICP. Coma. Signs of sepsis elsewhere (eg teeth, ears, lungs, endocarditis).

Investigations: CT/MRI (eg 'ring-enhancing' lesion); ↑WBC, ↑ESR; biopsy.

Treatment: Urgent neurosurgical referral; treat ↑ICP (p816). If frontal sinuses or teeth are the source, the likely organism will be *Strep. milleri* (microaerophilic), or oropharyngeal anaerobes. In ear abscesses, *B. fragilis* or other anaerobes are most common. Bacterial abscesses are often peripheral; toxoplasma lesions (p580) are deeper (eg basal ganglia). Remember the possibility of underlying immunosuppression.

Cerebral malaria

Falciparum malaria is one of the great killers—principally because it is swift and difficult to treat: so get expert help in anyone who could have travelled abroad particularly in the last few months, who is feverish with clouding of consciousness. But remember: fever is not a constant feature of malaria, and signs may be unusual if prophylaxis has been given, and is partly effective. The central event in severe *Falciparum* malaria is sequestration of parasitized erythrocytes in the microvasculature of vital organs. Death rate: ~1 million deaths per year, worldwide.[18]

Diagnosis See p560. What is the parasite count? Key prognostic factors: plasma bicarbonate, creatinine. Shock (algid malaria), metabolic acidosis, hypoglycaemia, renal failure, and acute respiratory distress syndrome (ARDS, p190) may also be presentations.

Treatment Take advice. Transfer to ITU, give quinine (dihydrochloride) 20mg salt /kg IV over 4h, then after 8h give 10mg/kg (max 700mg) over 4h every 8h (or give by constant IVI of 30mg/kg/d after loading dose[1]). Give IV until the patient can swallow; complete the course orally. Monitor for hypoglycaemia. In some countries, artesunate (2.4mg/kg IM or IV stat followed by 1.2mg/kg at 12h then daily) or artemether (3.2mg/kg followed by 1.6mg/kg daily) is available. These are as effective as quinine. In the UK, eg artemether is only available on a named patient basis: get local advice, but do not wait for an ideal drug to arrive when there is a reasonable alternative to hand: delay may result in death.[19]

If swallowing OK & no complications (shock; ARDS, renal failure) give either:

a) Artemether-lumefantrine (80/480mg twice daily for 3d with food).

b) Malarone® (atovaquone + proguanil; 4 tabs once daily for 3d with food).

c) Quinine (600mg salt/8h PO for 7d), with either doxycyline 200mg daily or clindamycin 600mg/12h for 7d PO.

1 Do not give loading doses if the patient has already definitely had quinine, quinidine or mefloquine in last 24h. Warn about tinnitus. In some countries, IV quinine is not available; quinidine gluconate is an alternative, eg a loading dose of 10mg/kg over 1–4h then 0.02mg/kg/min IVI by pump for 72h or until the patient can swallow. ECG monitoring is essential when quinidine is given (not needed for quinine). Stop or ↓infusion if BP↓ or QTc prolonged by >25% (p84). For further details, see A Omari 2004 *BMJ* **328** 154

ITU monitoring in cerebral malaria

- Fluid requirements vary widely; careful fluid management is critical. Haemofilter early if renal failure. Ventilate early if pulmonary oedema.
- Consider exchange transfusion in very seriously ill patients if feasible.
- Monitor blood lactate (or bicarbonate) and glucose: quinine may cause hypoglycaemia. Also do LFTs and clotting studies and cross-match blood if haematocrit <20%.
- Repeated U&E (and arterial blood gases if ARDS).
- Arrange repeated skilled microscopy to monitor the parasite counts.[20]

Expect a >75% decrease in the parasite count by 48h of treatment.

▸▸Status epilepticus

This means seizures lasting for >30min, or repeated seizures without intervening consciousness. Mortality and the risk of permanent brain damage increase with the length of attack. Aim to terminate seizures lasting more than a few minutes as soon as possible (<20min).

Status usually occurs in known epileptics. If it is the 1st presentation of epilepsy, the chance of a structural brain lesion is high (>50%). Diagnosis of tonic–clonic status is usually clear. Non-convulsive status (eg absence status or continuous partial seizures with preservation of consciousness) may be more difficult: look for subtle eye or lid movement. For other signs, see p373. An EEG can be very helpful. ▸Could the patient be pregnant (any pelvic mass)? If so, eclampsia (OHCS p96) is the likely diagnosis, check the urine and BP: call a senior obstetrician—immediate delivery may be needed.

Investigations

- Bedside glucose, the following tests can be done once R has started.
- Glucose, blood gases, U&E, Ca^{2+}, FBC, ECG.
- Consider anticonvulsant levels, toxicology screen, LP, culture blood and urine, EEG, CT, carbon monoxide level.
- Pulse oximetry, cardiac monitor

Treatment See OPPOSITE. Basic life support—and these agents:

1 Lorazepam ~4mg as a slow bolus (≤2min) into a large vein. Beware respiratory arrest during the last part of the injection. Have full resuscitation facilities to hand for all IV benzodiazepine use. (Alternative: diazepam as Diazemuls® but it is less long-lasting—give 10mg IV over 2min; if needed, repeat at 5mg/min, until seizures stop or 20mg given—or significant respiratory depression occurs). The rectal route is an alternative for diazepam if IV access is difficult.[1]

While waiting for this to work, prepare other drugs. If fits continue …

2 Phenytoin infusion: 15mg/kg IVI, at a rate of ≤50mg/min. (Don't put diazepam in same line: they don't mix.) Beware BP↓ and do not use if bradycardic or heart block. Requires BP and ECG monitoring. 100mg/6–8h is a maintenance dose (check levels). If fits continue …

3 Diazepam infusion: 100mg in 500mL of 5% dextrose; infuse at about 40mL/h (3mg/kg/24h). Close monitoring, especially respiratory function, is vital. It is most unusual for seizures to remain unresponsive following this. If they do, allow the idea to pass through your mind that they could be pseudoseizures (p730), particularly if there are odd features (pelvic thrusts; resisting attempts to open lids and your attempts to do passive movements; arms and legs flailing around).

4 Dexamethasone 10mg IV if vasculitis/cerebral oedema (tumour) possible.

5 General anaesthesia expert guidance on ITU.

As soon as seizures are controlled, start oral drugs (p380). Ask what the cause was, eg hypoglycaemia, pregnancy, alcohol, drugs, CNS lesion or infection, hypertensive encephalopathy, inadequate anticonvulsant dose (p378).

---

1 Diazepam Rectubes®: give 0.5mg/kg stat dose—eg ~3 10mg tubes PR (respiratory problems at this dose are *very* rare: all survived). If your back is still against the wall with no response after 10min, try 1 last 10mg tube. Halve dose if elderly. *For children's Stesolid® regimen* (it is different), see *OHCS* p266.

Management of status epilepticus

Open and maintain the airway, lay in recovery position
Remove false teeth if poorly fitting, insert oral/nasal airway, intubate if necessary

↓

Oxygen, 100% + suction (as required)

↓

IV access and take blood
*U&E, LFT, FBC, glucose (eg BM test®), calcium,
Toxicology screen if indicated, anticonvulsant levels*

↓

Thiamine 250mg IV over 10min if alcoholism or malnourishment suspected. Unless glucose known to be normal IV glucose 50mL 50%

↓

Correct hypotension with fluids

↓

Slow IV bolus phase—to stop seizures: eg lorazepam 4mg

↓

IV infusion phase: If seizures continue, start phenytoin, 15mg/kg IVI, at a rate of ≤50mg/min. Monitor ECG and BP. 100mg/6–8h is a maintenance dose (check levels). Alternative: diazepam infusion: 100mg in 500mL of 5% dextrose; infuse at ~40mL/h as opposite

↓

General anaesthesia phase: Continuing seizures require expert help with paralysis and ventilation with continuous EEG monitoring in ITU

▶*Never spend longer than 20min on someone with status epilepticus without having help at the bedside from an anaesthetist.*

▸▸Head injury

▸If the pupils are unequal, diagnose rising intracranial pressure (ICP), eg from extradural haemorrhage, and summon urgent neurosurgical help (p366). Retinal vein pulsation at fundoscopy helps exclude ICP↑.

Initial management (See OPPOSITE.) Write full notes. Record times.
- Involve neurosurgeons at an early stage, especially with comatosed patients, or if raised ICP suspected.
- Examine the CNS. Chart pulse, BP, T°, respirations + pupils every 15min.
- Assess anterograde amnesia (loss from the time of injury, ie post-traumatic) and retrograde amnesia—its extent correlates with the severity of the injury, and it never occurs without anterograde amnesia.
- Nurse semi-prone if no spinal injury; meticulous care to bladder & airway.

Who needs a CT head?
If any of the following are present, a CT is required immediately:
- GCS<13 at any time, or GCS 13 or 14 at 2h following injury
- Focal neurological deficit
- Suspected open or depressed skull fracture, or signs of basal skull fracture
- Post-traumatic seizure
- Vomiting >once
- Loss of consciousness AND any of the following
  - Age ≥65
  - Coagulopathy
  - 'Dangerous mechanism of injury' eg RTA, fall from great height
  - Antegrade amnesia of >30min.

When to ventilate immediately:
- Coma ≤8 on Glasgow coma scale (GCS; p776)
- P_aO_2 <9kPa in air (<13kPa in O_2) or P_aCO_2 >6kPa
- Spontaneous hyperventilation (P_aCO_2 <3.5)
- Respiratory irregularity.

Ventilate before neurosurgical transfer if:
- Deteriorating level of consciousness
- Bilateral fractured mandible
- Bleeding into mouth, eg skull base fracture
- Seizures.

Risk of intracranial haematoma in adults
Fully conscious, no skull fracture = <1 : 1000
Confused, no skull fracture = 1 : 100
Fully conscious, skull fracture = 1 : 30
Confused, skull fracture = 1 : 4

Criteria for admission
- Difficult to assess (child; post-ictal; alcohol intoxication).
- CNS signs; severe headache or vomiting; fracture.
- Loss of consciousness does **not** require admission if well, and a responsible adult is in attendance.

Drowsy trauma patients (GCS <15 to >8) smelling of alcohol: Alcohol is an unlikely cause of coma if plasma alcohol <44mmol/L. If unavailable, estimate blood alcohol level from the osmolar gap, p688. If blood alcohol ≈ 40mmol/L, osmolar gap ≈ 40mmol/L. Never assume signs are just alcohol.

Complications *Early:* extradural/subdural haemorrhage, seizures.
Late: subdural, p366; seizures; diabetes insipidus; parkinsonism; dementia.

Indicators of a bad prognosis Increasing age, decerebrate rigidity, extensor spasms, prolonged coma, hypertension, P_aO_2↓ (on blood gases), T° >39°C. 60% of those with loss of consciousness of >1 month will survive 3–25yrs, but may need daily nursing care.

For *Spinal cord injury & Persistent vegetative states*, see OHCS (p726–32 & p733).

Immediate management plan

ABC

↓

Oxygen, 100%
Intubate and hyperventilate if necessary
NB: *beware of a cervical spine injury*

↓

Stop blood loss and support circulation
Treat for shock if required (p778)

↓

Treat seizures with diazepam

↓

Assess level of consciousness (GCS)
Antegrade and retrograde amnesia

↓

Rapid examination survey

↓

Investigations
U&Es, glucose, FBC, blood alcohol, toxicology screen, ABG & clotting

↓

Neurological examination

↓

Brief history
When? Where? How? Had a fit? Lucid interval? Alcohol?

↓

Evaluate lacerations of face or scalp
*Palpate deep wounds with sterile glove to check for
step deformity. Note obvious skull/facial fractures[1]*

↓

Check for CSF leak, from nose (rhinorrhoea) or ear
Any blood behind the ear drum?
*If either is present, suspect basilar skull fracture: do CT
Give tetanus toxoid, and refer at once to neurosurgeons*

↓

Palpate the neck posteriorly for tenderness and deformity
*If detected, or if the patient has obvious head injury,
or injury above the clavicle with loss of consciousness,
immobilize the neck and get cervical spine radiographs*

↓

Radiology
As indicated: cervical spine, chest x-rays; CT of head

815

---

1 Periorbital (raccoon sign), or postauricular (Battle sign) ecchymoses.

▶▶Raised intracranial pressure (ICP↑)

There are 3 types of cerebral oedema:
- Vasogenic: ↑ capillary permeability—tumour, trauma, ischaemia, infection.
- Cytotoxic—cell death, from hypoxia.
- Interstitial (eg obstructive hydrocephalus).

Because the cranium defines a fixed volume, brain swelling quickly results in ↑ICP which may produce a sudden clinical deterioration. Normal ICP is 0–10mmHg. The oedema from severe brain injury is probably both cytotoxic and vasogenic.

Causes
- Primary or metastatic tumours.
- Head injury.
- Haemorrhage (subdural, extradural, subarachnoid; intracerebral, intraventricular).
- Meningoencephalitis; brain abscess.
- Hydrocephalus; cerebral oedema; status epilepticus.

Signs & symptoms
- Headache; drowsiness; vomiting; seizures. History of trauma.
- Listlessness; irritability; drowsiness; falling pulse and rising BP (Cushing's response); coma; Cheyne–Stokes respiration; pupil changes (constriction at first, later dilatation—do not mask these signs by using agents, such as tropicamide, to dilate the pupil to aid fundoscopy).
- Papilloedema is an unreliable sign, but venous pulsation at the disc may be absent (absent in ~50% of normal people, but *loss* of it is a useful sign).

Investigations
- U&E, FBC, LFT, glucose, serum osmolality, clotting, blood culture, CXR
- CT head
- Then consider lumbar puncture if safe. Measure the opening pressure!

Treatment
The goal is to ↓ICP and avert secondary injury. Urgent neurosurgery is required for the definitive treatment of ↑ICP from focal causes (eg haematomas). This is achieved via a craniotomy or burr hole. Also, an ICP monitor (or bolt) may be placed to monitor pressure. Surgery is generally *not* helpful following ischaemic or anoxic injury.

Holding measures are listed OPPOSITE.

Herniation syndromes *Uncal herniation* is caused by a lateral supratentorial mass which pushes the ipsilateral inferomedial temporal lobe (uncus) through the temporal incisura and against the midbrain. The 3rd nerve, travelling in this space, gets compressed causing a dilated ipsilateral pupil, then ophthalmoplegia (a fixed pupil localizes a lesion poorly but is 'ipsilateralizing'). This may be followed (quickly) by contralateral hemiparesis (pressure on the cerebral peduncle) and coma from pressure on the ascending reticular activating system (ARAS) in the midbrain.

Cerebellar tonsil herniation is caused by ↑pressure in the posterior fossa forcing the cerebellar tonsils through the foramen magnum. Ataxia, VI nerve palsies, and +ve Babinskis (upgoing plantars) occur first, then loss of consciousness, irregular breathing, and apnoea. This syndrome may proceed very rapidly given the small size of, and poor compliance in, the posterior fossa.

Subfalcian (cingulate) herniation is caused by a frontal mass. The cingulate gyrus (medial frontal lobe) is forced under the rigid falx cerebri. It may be silent unless the anterior cerebral artery is compressed and causes a stroke— eg contralateral leg weakness ± abulia (lack of decision-making).

Immediate management plan

ABC
↓

Correct hypotension and treat seizures
↓

Brief examination, history if available
Any clues, eg meningococcal rash, previous carcinoma
↓

Elevate the head of the bed to 30°–40°
↓

If intubated, hyperventilate to ↓P_aCO_2 (eg to 3.5kPa)
This causes cerebral vasoconstriction and reduces ICP almost immediately
↓

Osmotic agents (eg mannitol) can be useful *pro tem* but
may lead to rebound ↑ICP after prolonged use (~12–24h)
*Give 20% solution 1-2g/kg IV over 10-20min (eg 5mL/kg). Clinical effect is
seen after ~20min and lasts for 2-6h. Follow serum osmolality—aim for
about 300mosmol/kg but don't exceed 310*
↓

Corticosteroids are *not* effective in reducing ICP
except for oedema surrounding tumours
eg dexamethasone 10mg IV and follow with 4mg/6h IV/PO
↓

Fluid restrict to <1.5L/d
↓

Monitor the patient closely, consider monitoring ICP
↓

Aim to make a diagnosis
↓

Treat cause or exacerbating factors
eg hyperglycaemia, hyponatraemia
↓

Definitive treatment if possible

▸▸Diabetic ketoacidosis (DKA)

Hyperglycaemic ketoacidotic coma only occurs in type I diabetes: it may be the mode of presentation, eg a 1–3-day history of gradual decline into dehydration, acidosis, and coma. Precipitants include: infection, surgery, MI, non-compliance, or wrong insulin dose. The diagnosis requires ketosis and acidosis (pH <7.3).

Signs & symptoms
- Polyuria, polydipsia, lethargy, anorexia, hyperventilation, ketotic breath, dehydration, vomiting, abdominal pain, coma.

Investigations
- Lab glucose, U&E, HCO_3^-, amylase, osmolality, ABG, FBC, blood cultures.
- Urine tests: ketones, MSU; CXR.
- To estimate plasma osmolarity: 2[Na$^+$] + [urea] + [glucose] mmol/L.

Pitfalls in diabetic ketoacidosis
- *Plasma glucose* is usually high, but not always, especially if insulin continued.
- *High WCC* may be seen in the absence of infection.
- *Infection:* often there is no fever. Do MSU, blood cultures, and CXR. Start broad-spectrum antibiotics early if infection is suspected.
- *Creatinine:* some assays for creatinine cross-react with ketone bodies, so plasma creatinine may not reflect true renal function.
- *Hyponatraemia* is common, due to osmolar compensation for the hyperglycaemia. ↑ or ↔ [Na$^+$] indicates severe water loss. As treatment commences Na$^+$ rises as water enters cells. Na$^+$ is also low due to an artefact; corrected plasma [Na$^+$] = Na$^+$ + 2.4[(glucose −5.5)/5.5].
- *Ketonuria* does not equate with ketoacidosis. Normal individuals may have up to ++ketonuria after an overnight fast. Not all ketones are due to diabetes—consider alcohol if glucose normal. Test plasma with Ketostix® or Acetest® to demonstrate ketonaemia.
- *Recurrent ketoacidosis:* blood glucose may return to normal long before ketones are removed from the blood, and a rapid reduction in the amount of insulin administered may lead to lack of clearance and return to DKA. This may be avoided by maintaining a constant rate of insulin, eg 4–5U/h IVI, and co-infusing dextrose 10–20% to keep plasma glucose at 6–10mmol/L—the extended insulin regimen.
- *Acidosis* but without gross elevation of glucose may occur, but consider overdose (eg aspirin) and lactic acidosis (in elderly diabetics).
- *Serum amylase* is often raised (up to ×10) and non-specific abdominal pain is common, even in the absence of pancreatitis.

Management See OPPOSITE. Dehydration is more life-threatening than hyperglycaemia—so its correction takes precedence.
- Monitor potassium, glucose, creatinine, HCO_3^-, hourly initially. Aim for a fall in glucose of 5mmol/h, and correction of the acidosis. The use of venous HCO_3^-, as a guide to progress, may prevent the need for repeated arterial blood gas sampling. K$^+$ disturbance may cause dysrhythmias.
- Flow chart of vital signs, conscious level, urine output, and ketones; insert catheter if no urine passed for >4h. Monitoring CVP may sometimes be helpful in guiding fluid replacement.
- Find and treat infection (lung, skin, perineum, urine after cultures).
- Give heparin 5000U/8h (or low molecular weight version) SC until mobile.
- Change to SC insulin when ketones are ≤1+ and eating (p293).

NB: If acidosis is severe (pH <7), some give IV bicarbonate (eg 1mL/kg of 8.4% over 1h, and recheck arterial pH); others never give it because of effects on the Hb-dissociation curve and cerebral circulation—discuss with senior.

Complications Cerebral oedema, aspiration pneumonia, hypokalaemia, hypomagnesaemia, hypophosphataemia, thromboembolism.

▸Talk with the patient: ensure there are no further preventable episodes.
Other emergencies: Hyperosmolar non-ketotic coma & hypoglycaemia: p820.

Management plan

IV access and start fluid (0.9% saline IVI) replacement immediately

↓

Check plasma glucose: usually >20mmol/L
if so give 4–8U soluble insulin IV

↓

Investigations
Lab glucose, U&E, HCO$_3^-$, osmolality, blood gases, FBC, blood culture
Urine tests: ketones, MSU; CXR

↓

NG tube only if nauseated/vomiting/unconscious

↓

Insulin sliding scale (below)

↓

Continue fluid replacement, K$^+$ replacement

↓

Check glucose and U&E, HCO$_3^-$ regularly (hourly initially)

↓

What precipitated the coma?

Fluid replacement

- Give 1 litre (L) of 0.9% saline stat. Then, typically, 1L over the next hour, 1L over 2h, 1L over 4h, then 1L over 6h
- Use dextrose saline or 5% dextrose when blood glucose is <15mmol/L
- Those >65yrs or with CCF need less saline more cautiously

Potassium replacement

- Total body potassium is invariably low, and plasma K$^+$ falls as K$^+$ enters cells with treatment
- Don't add K$^+$ to the first bag, less will be required in renal failure or oliguria. Check U&Es hourly initially, and replace as required:

Serum K$^+$ (mmol/L)	Amount of KCl to add per litre of IV fluid:
<3.0	40mmol
3–4	30mmol
4–5	20mmol

Sliding scale of insulin via IVI pump in diabetic ketoacidosis

Add 50U soluble insulin (Actrapid/Humulin-S) to 50mL saline in a syringe (1U/mL)		
Hourly glucose result	*Soluble insulin*	*If infection or insulin resistance (p295)*
0–3.9	0.5U/h	1U/h
4–7.9	1	2
8–11.9	2	4
12–16.0	3	6
>16mmol/L	4	8

If no pump, load with 10U IM, then give 4–6U/h IM while glucose is >14mmol/L

▸▸ Other diabetic emergencies

Hypoglycaemic coma Usually *rapid* onset; may be preceded by odd behaviour (eg aggression), sweating, pulse↑, seizures.

Management: Give 20–30g dextrose IV eg 200–300ml of 10% dextrose. This is preferable to 50–100mL 50% dextrose which harms veins. Expect prompt recovery. Glucagon 1mg IV/IM is nearly as rapid as dextrose but will not work in drunk patients. Dextrose IVI may be needed for severe prolonged hypoglycaemia. Once conscious, give sugary drinks and a meal.

Hyperglycaemic hyperosmolar non-ketotic (HONK) coma Only those with type-2 diabetes are at risk of this. The history is longer (eg 1wk), with marked dehydration and glucose >35mmol/L. Acidosis is absent as there has been no switch to ketone metabolism—the patient is often old, and presenting for the first time. The osmolality is >340mosmol/kg. Focal CNS signs may occur. The risk of DVT is high, so give *full* heparin anticoagulation (p648).

Rehydrate over 48h with 0.9% saline IVI, eg at ½ the rate used in ketoacidosis. Wait an hour before giving any insulin (it may not be needed, and you want to avoid rapid changes). If it is needed, 1U/h might be a typical initial dose. Look for the cause, eg MI, or bowel infarct.

Hyperlactataemia is a rare but serious complication of DM (eg after septicaemia or biguanide use). Blood lactate: >5mmol/L. Seek expert help. Give O_2. Treat any sepsis vigorously.

▸▸ Thyroid emergencies

Myxoedema coma *Signs & symptoms:* Looks hypothyroid (p306); >65yrs; hypothermia; hyporeflexia; glucose↓; bradycardia; coma; seizures.

History: Prior surgery or radioiodine for hyperthyroidism.

Precipitants: Infection; myocardial infarction; stroke; trauma.

Examination: Goitre; cyanosis; heart failure; precipitants.

Treatment: Preferably in intensive care.
- Take venous blood for: T3, T4, TSH, FBC, U&E, cultures, cortisol.
- Take arterial blood for P_aO_2.
- Give high-flow O_2 if cyanosed. Correct any hypoglycaemia.
- Give T3 (triiodothyronine) 5–20µg a IV slowly. Be cautious: this may precipitate manifestations of undiagnosed ischaemic heart disease.
- Give hydrocortisone 100mg/8h IV—vital if pituitary hypothyroidism is suspected (ie no goitre, no previous radioiodine, no thyroid surgery).
- IVI 0.9% saline. Be sure to avoid precipitating LVF.
- If infection suspected, give antibiotic, eg cefuroxime 1.5g/8h IVI.
- Treat *heart failure* as appropriate (p138).
- Treat *hypothermia* with warm blankets in warm room. Beware complications (hypoglycaemia, pancreatitis, arrhythmias). See p836.

Further therapy: T3 5–20µg/4–12h IV until sustained improvement (eg ~2–3d) then thyroxine (T4=levothyroxine) 50µg/24h PO. Continue hydrocortisone. Give IV fluids as appropriate (hyponatraemia is dilutional).

Hyperthyroid crisis (thyrotoxic storm) *Sign & symptoms:* Severe hyperthyroidism: fever, agitation, confusion, coma, tachycardia, AF, D&V, goitre, thyroid bruit, 'acute abdomen' picture.

Precipitants: Recent thyroid surgery or radioiodine; infection; MI; trauma.

Diagnosis: Confirm with technetium uptake if possible, but do not wait for this if urgent treatment is needed.

Treatment: Enlist expert help from an endocrinologist. See OPPOSITE.

Management plan for thyrotoxic storm

IVI 0.9% saline, 500mL/4h. NG tube if vomiting.

↓

Take blood for: T3, T4, cultures (if infection suspected).

↓

Sedate if necessary (eg chlorpromazine 50mg PO/IM).

↓

If no contraindication, give propranolol 40mg/8h PO (maximum IV dose: 1mg over 1min, repeated up to 9 times at ≥2min intervals).

↓

High-dose digoxin may be needed to slow the heart, eg 1mg over 2h IVI.

↓

Antithyroid drugs: carbimazole 15–25mg/6h PO (or via NGT, if needed). After 4h give Lugol's solution 0.3mL/8h PO for 1wk to block thyroid.

↓

Hydrocortisone 100mg/6h IV or dexamethasone 4mg/6h PO.

↓

Treat suspected infection with eg cefuroxime 1.5g/8h IVI.

↓

Adjust IV fluids as necessary; cool with tepid sponging ± paracetamol.

↓

Continuing treatment: After 5d reduce carbimazole to 15mg/8h PO. After 10d stop propranolol and iodine. Adjust carbimazole (p304).

▸▸Addisonian crisis

Signs & symptoms may present in shock (tachycardia; peripheral vasoconstriction; postural hypotension; oliguria; weak; confused; comatose)—typically (but not always!) in a patient with known Addison's disease, or someone on long-term steroids who has forgotten to take tablets. An alternative presentation is with hypoglycaemia.

Precipitating factors: Infection, trauma, surgery.

Management: If suspected, treat before biochemical results.
- Take blood for cortisol (10mL heparin or clotted) and ACTH if possible (10mL heparin, to go straight to laboratory).
- Hydrocortisone sodium succinate 100mg IV stat.
- IVI: use a plasma expander first, for resuscitation, then 0.9% saline.
- Monitor blood glucose: the danger is hypoglycaemia.
- Blood, urine, sputum for culture.
- Give antibiotics (eg cefuroxime 1.5g/8h IVI).

Continuing treatment
- Glucose IV may be needed if hypoglycaemic.
- Continue IV fluids, more slowly. Be guided by clinical state.
- Continue hydrocortisone sodium succinate 100mg IV/IM every 6h.
- Change to oral steroids after 72h if patient's condition good. The tetracosactrin (=tetracosactide) test is impossible while on hydrocortisone.
- Fludrocortisone is needed only if hydrocortisone dose <50mg/d and the condition is due to adrenal disease.
- Search for the cause, once the crisis is over.

▸▸Hypopituitary coma

Usually develops gradually in a person with known hypopituitarism. Rarely, the onset is rapid due to infarction of a pituitary tumour (pituitary apoplexy)—as symptoms include headache and meningism, subarachnoid haemorrhage is often misdiagnosed.

Presentation: Headache; ophthalmoplegia; consciousness↓; hypotension; hypothermia; hypoglycaemia; signs of hypopituitarism (p318).

Tests: T4; cortisol; TSH; ACTH; glucose. Pituitary fossa CT/MRI.

Treatment:
- Hydrocortisone sodium succinate 100mg IV/6h.
- Only after hydrocortisone begun: T3 10µg/12h PO.
- Prompt surgery is needed if the cause is pituitary apoplexy.

▸▸Phaeochromocytoma emergencies

Stress, abdominal palpation, parturition, general anaesthetic, or contrast media used in radiography may produce dangerous *hypertensive crises* (pallor, pulsating headache, hypertension, feels 'about to die').

Treatment ▸Get help.
- Phentolamine 2–5mg IV. Repeat to maintain safe BP.
- Labetalol is an alternative agent (p142).
- When BP controlled, give phenoxybenzamine 10mg/24h PO (increase by 10mg/d as needed, up to 0.5–1mg/kg/day PO); SE: postural hypotension; dizziness; tachycardia; nasal congestion; miosis; idiosyncratic marked BP drop soon after exposure. The idea is to increase the dose until the blood pressure is controlled and there is no significant postural hypotension. A β₁-blocker may also be given at this stage.
- Surgery is usually done electively after a period of 4–6wks to allow full alpha blockade and volume expansion. When admitted for surgery the phenoxybenzamine dose is increased until significant postural hypotension.

Acute renal failure (ARF)—management

▶Seek expert help promptly: BP, urinary sediment, serum K^+, creatinine, and ultrasound **must** be rapidly known. Have them to hand. See p272.

Definition Acute (over hours or days) deterioration in renal function, characterized by a rise in serum creatinine and urea, often with oliguric or anuria.

Causes⬚
- Hypovolaemia
- Low cardiac output
- Sepsis
- Drugs
- Obstruction (p266)
- Other eg hepatorenal syndrome (p231), vasculitis (p424).

Investigations
- U&E, Ca^{2+}, PO_4^{3-}, FBC, ESR, CRP, INR, LFT, CK, LDH, protein electrophoresis, hepati-tis serology, autoantibodies (p421), blood cultures.
- Urgent urine microscopy and cultures. White cell casts suggest infection, but are seen in interstitial nephritis, and red cell casts an inflammatory glomerular condition (p268).
- USS of the renal tract.
- ECG, CXR.

Management See OPPOSITE for acute measures. Underlying principles are:
1 **Treat precipitating cause** Treat acute blood loss with blood transfusion, and sepsis with antibiotics (p548). ARF is often associated with other diseases that need more urgent treatment. For example, someone in respiratory failure *and* renal failure may need to be managed on ITU, not a renal unit, to ensure optimal management of the respiratory failure.
2 **Treat life-threatening hyperkalaemia** See OPPOSITE.
3 **Treat pulmonary oedema, pericarditis, and tamponade** (p788) Urgent dialysis may be needed. If in pulmonary oedema, and no diuresis, consider removing a unit of blood, before dialysis commences.
4 **Treat volume depletion** if necessary. Resuscitate quickly; then match input to output. Use a large-bore line in a large vein (central vein access can be risky in obvious volume depletion).
5 **Treat sepsis**
6 **Further care**
- Has obstruction been excluded? ▶Examine for masses PR and *per vaginam*; arrange urgent ultrasound; is the bladder palpable? Bilateral nephrostomies relieve obstruction, provide urine for culture, and allow anterograde pyelography to determine the site of obstruction.
- If worsening renal function but dialysis independent, consider renal biopsy.
- Diet: high in calories (2000–4000kcal/d) with adequate high-quality protein. Consider nasogastric feeding or parenteral route if too ill.

Prognosis Depends on cause (ATN mortality: surgery or trauma—60%, medical illness—30%, pregnancy—10%). Oliguric ARF is worse than non-oliguric—more GI bleeds, sepsis, acidosis, and higher mortality.

Urgent dialysis if :
- K^+ persistently high (>6.0mmol/L).
- Acidosis (pH <7.2).
- Pulmonary oedema and no substantial diuresis.
- Pericarditis. (In tamponade (p788), only dialyse *after* pressure on the heart is relieved.)
- High catabolic state with rapidly progressive renal failure.

Management

Catheterize to assess hourly urine output, and establish fluid charts
↓

Assess intravascular volume BP, JVP, skin turgor, fluid
balance sheet, weight, CVP, attach to cardiac monitor
consider inserting a central venous cannula
↓

Investigations *(see OPPOSITE)*
↓

Identify and treat hyperkalaemia—see below
Use a cardiac monitor
↓

If dehydrated
Fluid challenge: 250–500mL of colloid or saline over 30min
↓

Reassess
Repeat if still fluid depleted. Aim for a CVP of 5–10cm H_2O
↓

Once fluid replete, continue fluids at 20mL + previous hour's
urine output per hour
↓

If volume overloaded. Consider urgent dialysis
A nitrate infusion, frusemide[1] or 'renal dose' dopamine may help in the
short term, especially to make space for blood transfusion etc.
but does not alter outcome
↓

Correct acidosis with sodium bicarbonate, eg 50mL of 8.4% IV
↓

If clinical suspicion of sepsis, take cultures, then treat vigorously
Do not leave possible sources of sepsis (eg IV lines) in situ if not needed
↓

Avoid nephrotoxic drugs, eg NSAIDs, ACE-inhibitors, care
with gentamicin. Check Data Sheet for all drugs given.

Hyperkalaemia

The danger is ventricular fibrillation. A K^+ >6.5mmol/L will usually require urgent treatment, as will those with ECG changes:
• Tall 'tented' T-waves ± flat P-waves ± increased P-R interval (see p693).
• Widening of the QRS complex—leading eventually, and dangerously, to a sinusoidal pattern and VF/VT.

Treatment:
• 10mL calcium gluconate (10%) IV over 2min, repeated as necessary if severe ECG changes. This provides cardio-protection. It does not change serum potassium levels.
• Insulin + glucose, eg: 20U soluble insulin + 50mL of glucose 50% IV. Insulin moves K^+ into cells.
• Nebulized salbutamol (2.5mg) also makes K^+ enter cells.
• Polystyrene sulfonate resin (eg Calcium Resonium®, 15g/8h in water) orally or, if vomiting makes the PO route problematic, as a 30g enema (followed by colonic irrigation, after 9h, to remove K^+ from the colon).
• Dialysis.

1 Frusemide = furosemide.

Acute poisoning—general measures

Diagnosis mainly from history. The patient may not tell the truth about what has been taken. Use *MIMS Colour Index*, *eMIMS* images, BNF descriptions, or the computerized system 'TICTAC' (ask pharmacy) to identify tablets and plan specific treatment. Clues may become apparent:

• *Fast or irregular pulse:* Salbutamol, antimuscarinics, tricyclics, quinine, or phenothiazine poisoning.
• *Respiratory depression:* Opiate or benzodiazepine toxicity.
• *Hypothermia:* Phenothiazines, barbiturates.
• *Hyperthermia:* Amphetamines, MAOIs, cocaine, or ecstasy (p831).
• *Coma:* Benzodiazepines, alcohol, opiates, tricyclics, or barbiturates.
• *Seizures:* Recreational drugs, hypoglycaemic agents, tricyclics, phenothiazines, or theophyllines.
• *Constricted pupils:* Opiates or insecticides (organophosphates, p831).
• *Dilated pupils:* Amphetamines, cocaine, quinine, or tricyclics.
• *Hyperglycaemia:* Organophosphates, theophyllines, or MAOIs.
• *Hypoglycaemia:* Insulin, oral hypoglycaemics, alcohol, or salicylates.
• *Renal failure:* Salicylate, paracetamol, or ethylene glycol.
• *Metabolic acidosis:* Alcohol, ethylene glycol, methanol, paracetamol, or carbon monoxide poisoning—p830.
• ↑*Osmolality:* Alcohols (ethyl and methyl); ethylene glycol. See p682.

Management See OPPOSITE for a general guide to management
• *Take blood* as appropriate (p828). Always check paracetamol and salicylate levels.
• *Empty stomach* if appropriate (p828).
• *Consider specific antidote* (p830) or oral activated charcoal (p828).
• *If you are not familiar with the poison* get more information. The *Data Sheet Compendium* SPC is useful. If in doubt how to act, phone the Poisons Information Service: in the UK phone 0870 600 6266.

Continuing care Measure temperature, pulse, BP, and blood glucose regularly. Use a continuous ECG monitor. If unconscious, nurse semi-prone, turn regularly, keep eyelids closed. A urinary catheter will be needed if the bladder is distended, or renal failure is suspected, or forced diuresis undertaken. Take to ITU, eg if respiration↓.

Psychiatric assessment Be sympathetic despite the hour! Interview relatives and friends if possible. Aim to establish:
• *Intentions at time:* Was the act planned? What precautions against being found? Did the patient seek help afterwards? Does the patient think the method was dangerous? Was there a final act (eg suicide note)?
• *Present intentions.*
• *What problems* led to the act: do they still exist?
• *Was the act* aimed at someone?
• Is there a *psychiatric disorder* (depression, alcoholism, personality disorder, schizophrenia, dementia)?
• What are his *resources* (friends, family, work, personality)?

The assessment of suicide risk: The following increase the chance of future suicide: original intention was to die; present intention is to die; presence of psychiatric disorder; poor resources; previous suicide attempts; socially isolated; unemployed; male; >50yrs old. See OHCS p338.

Referral to psychiatrist: This depends partly on local resources. Ask advice if presence of psychiatric disorder or high suicide risk.

Common law or the Mental Health Act: (in England and Wales) may provide for the detention of the patient against his or her will: see OHCS p398.

Emergency care

ABC, clear airway
↓
Consider ventilation (if the respiratory rate is <8/min, or P_aO_2
<8kPa, when breathing 60% O_2, or the airway is at risk, eg GCS < 8)
↓
Treat shock (p778)
↓
If unconscious, nurse semi-prone

Further management
↓
Assess the patient
↓
History from patient, friends, or family is vital
↓
Features from the examination may help (see OPPOSITE)
↓
Investigations
Glucose, U&E, FBC, LFT, INR, ABG, ECG, paracetamol, and salicylate levels
Urine/serum toxicology, specific assays as appropriate
↓
Monitor
$T°$, pulse & respiratory rate, BP, O_2 saturations, urine output ± ECG
↓
Treatment
Supportive measures: may need catheterization
↓Absorption: consider gastric lavage ± activated charcoal, see p828
Specific measures, see p828; for antidotes, see p830
Consider naloxone if ↓conscious level and pin-point pupils

Acute poisoning—specific points

Plasma toxicology For all unconscious patients, paracetamol and aspirin levels and blood glucose are required. The necessity of other assays depends on the drug taken and the index of suspicion. Be guided by the poisons information service. More common assays include: digoxin; methanol; lithium; iron; theophylline. Toxicological screening of urine, especially for recreational drugs, may be of use in some cases.

Gastric lavage In general only of use if presentation within 1h of poisoning, and if a potentially toxic dose of a drug has been taken. Lavage beyond this time frame may make matters worse. ►*Do not empty stomach* if petroleum products or corrosives such as acids, alkalis, bleach, descalers have been ingested (*exception:* paraquat), or if the patient is unconscious or unable to protect their airway (unless intubated). ►Never induce vomiting.

Gastric emptying and lavage If comatosed, or no gag reflex, ask for an anaesthetist to protect airway with cuffed endotracheal tube. If conscious, get verbal consent.

- Monitor O_2 by pulse oximetry. See p168.
- Have suction apparatus to hand and working.
- Position the patient in left lateral position.
- Raise the foot of the bed by 20cm.
- Pass a lubricated tube (14mm external diameter) via the mouth, asking the patient to swallow.
- Confirm position in stomach—blow air down, and auscultate over the stomach.
- Siphon the gastric contents. Check pH with litmus paper.
- Perform gastric lavage using 300–600mL tepid water at a time. Massage the left hypochondrium.
- Repeat until no tablets in siphoned fluid.
- Leave activated charcoal (50g in 200mL water) in the stomach unless alcohol, iron, Li^+, or ethylene glycol ingested.
- When pulling out tube, occlude its end (prevents aspiration of fluid remaining in the tube).

Activated charcoal reduces the absorption of many drugs from the gut when given as a single dose of 50g with water, eg salicylates, paracetamol. It is given in repeated doses (50g 4hourly) to increase elimination of some drugs from the blood, eg carbamazepine, dapsone, theophyllines, quinine, digoxin, phenytoin, phenobarbitone (phenobarbital), & paraquat. Lower doses are used in children.

Help on the web UK GPs and other NHS workers and departments may register with **toxbase** at www.spib.axl.co.uk for free up-to-date toxicological advice.

Some specific poisons and their antidotes

Benzodiazepines Flumazenil (for respiratory arrest) 200µg over 15s; then 100µg at 60s intervals if needed. Usual dose range: 300–600µg IV over 3–6min (up to 1mg; 2mg if on ITU). May provoke fits.

β-blockers Severe bradycardia or hypotension. Try atropine up to 3mg IV. Give glucagon 2–10mg IV bolus + 5% dextrose if atropine fails (± an atropine infusion of 50µg/kg/h). If unresponsive, consider pacing or an aortic balloon pump.

Co-proxamol Dextropropoxyphene (long-acting opiate + paracetamol, p832). Respiratory depression (use naloxone) & dysrhythmias may occur.

Cyanide This fast-killing poison has affinity for Fe^{3+}, and inhibits the cytochrome system, ↓aerobic respiration. *3 phases:* • Anxiety ± confusion • Pulse↑ or ↓ • Fits ± shock ± coma. *Treatment:* ▶▶100% O_2, GI decontamination; if consciousness↓ give dicobalt edetate 300mg IV over 1–5min, then 50mL 50% dextrose IV. Repeat up to twice. *Get expert help.* See p835.

Carbon monoxide Despite hypoxaemia skin is pink (or pale), not blue as carboxyhaemoglobin (COHb) displaces O_2 from Hb binding sites. *Symptoms:* Headache, vomiting, pulse↑, tachypnoea, and, if COHb >50%, fits, coma, & cardiac arrest. ▶▶Remove the source. Give 100% O_2. Metabolic acidosis usually responds to correction of hypoxia. If severe, anticipate cerebral oedema. Give mannitol IVI (p817). Confirm diagnosis with a heparinized blood sample (COHb >10%) quickly as levels may soon return to normal. Monitor ECG. *Hyperbaric O_2 may help: discuss with the poisons service if is or has been unconscious, pregnant, COHb >20%, or failing to respond.*

Digoxin *Symptoms:* Cognition↓, yellow-green visual halos, arrhythmias, nausea, & anorexia. If serious arrhythmias are present, correct hypokalaemia, and inactivate with digoxin-specific antibody fragments (Digibind®). If load or level is unknown, give 20 vials (800mg)—adult or child >20kg. Consult Data Sheet/SPC. Dilute in water for injections (4mL/38mg vial) and 0.9% saline (to make a convenient volume); give IVI over ½h, via a 0.22µm-pore filter. If the amount of digoxin ingested is known, the data-sheet/SPC will tell you how many vials of Digibind® to give, eg if 25 tabs of 0.25mg ingested, give 10 vials; if 50 tabs, give 20 vials; if 100 tabs, give 40 vials.

Heavy metals Enlist expert help.

Iron Desferrioxamine (=deferoxamine) 15mg/kg/h IVI; max 80mg/kg/d. **NB:** gastric lavage if iron ingestion in last hour; consider whole bowel irrigation.

Oral anticoagulants If major bleed, treat with vitamin K, 5mg slow IV; give prothrombin complex concentrate 50U/kg IV (or if unavailable, fresh frozen plasma 15mL/kg IVI). For abnormal INR with no (or minimal) bleeding, see BNF. If it is vital that anticoagulation continues, enlist expert help. Warfarin can normally be restarted within 2–3d.

NB: Coagulation defects may be delayed for 2–3d following ingestion.

Opiates (Many analgesics contain opiates.) Give naloxone eg 0.8–2mg IV; repeat every 2min until breathing adequate (it has a short $t_{\frac{1}{2}}$, so it may need to be given often or IM; max 10mg). Naloxone may precipitate features of opiate withdrawal—diarrhoea and cramps which will normally respond to diphenoxylate and atropine (Lomotil®—eg 2 tablets/6h PO). Sedate as needed (see p15). High-dose opiate misusers may need methadone (eg 10–30mg/12h PO) to combat withdrawal. Register opiate addiction (*OHCS* p362), and refer for help.

Phenothiazine poisoning (eg chlorpromazine) No specific antidote. *Dystonia (torticollis, retrocollis, glossopharyngeal dystonia, opisthotonus)*: try benzatropine 1–2mg IV/IM. Treat *shock* by raising the legs (± plasma expander IVI, or dopamine IVI if desperate). Restore body temperature. *Monitor ECG*. Avoid lignocaine (=lidocaine) in dysrhythmias. Use diazepam IV for prolonged fits in the usual way (p812). *Neuroleptic malignant syndrome* consists of: hyperthermia, rigidity, extrapyramidal signs, autonomic dysfunction (labile BP, pulse↑, sweating, urinary incontinence), mutism, confusion, coma, WCC↑, CPK↑; it may be treated with cooling. Dantrolene has been tried (p450).

Carbon tetrachloride poisoning this solvent, used in many industrial processes, causes vomiting, abdominal pain, diarrhoea, seizures, coma, renal failure, and tender hepatomegaly with jaundice and liver failure. IV acetylcysteine may improve prognosis. Seek expert help.

Organophosphate insecticides inactivate cholinesterase—the resulting increase in acetylcholine causes the SLUD response: salivation, lacrimation, urination, and diarrhoea. Also look for sweating, small pupils, muscle fasciculation, coma, respiratory distress, and bradycardia. *Treatment*: Wear gloves; remove soiled clothes. Wash skin. Take blood (FBC & serum cholinesterase activity). Give atropine IV 2mg every 10min till full atropinization (skin dry, pulse >70, pupils dilated). Up to 3 days' treatment may be needed. Also give pralidoxime 30mg/kg slowly IV (in the UK, the poisons information service will tell you how to get it; it is diluted with ≥10mL water for Injections). Repeat as needed every 30min; max 12g in 24h. Even if fits are not occurring, diazepam 5–10mg IV seems to help.

Paraquat poisoning (Found in weed-killers.) This causes D&V, painful oral ulcers, alveolitis, and renal failure. Diagnose by urine test. Give activated charcoal *at once* (100g followed by a laxative, then 50g/3–4h, ± antiemetic). ▶Get expert help. Avoid O₂ early on (promotes lung damage).

Ecstasy poisoning Ecstasy is a semi-synthetic, hallucinogenic substance (MDMA, 3,4-methylenedioxymethamphetamine). Its effects range from nausea, muscle pain, blurred vision, amnesia, fever, confusion, and ataxia to tachyarrhythmias, hyperthermia, hyper/hypotension, water intoxication, DIC, K⁺↑, acute renal failure, hepatocellular and muscle necrosis, cardiovascular collapse, and ARDS. There is no antidote and treatment is supportive. Management depends on clinical and lab findings, but may include:

- Administration of activated charcoal and monitoring of BP, ECG, and temperature for at least 12h (rapid cooling may be needed).
- Monitor urine output and U&E (renal failure p274), LFT, creatinine kinase, platelets, and coagulation (DIC p650). Metabolic acidosis may benefit from treatment with sodium bicarbonate.
- Anxiety: diazepam 0.1–0.3mg/kg PO. Max IV does over 2min.
- Narrow complex tachycardias in adults: consider metoprolol 5–10mg IV.
- Hypertension can be treated with nifedipine 5–10mg PO or phentolamine 2–5mg IV. Treat hypotension conventionally (p778).
- Hyperthermia: attempt to cool, if rectal T° > 39°C. Consider dantrolene 1mg/kg IV (may need repeating: discuss with your senior and a poisons unit, p826). Hyperthermia with ecstasy is akin to serotonin syndrome, and propranolol, muscle relaxation and ventilation may be needed.[23]

Snakes (adders) *Anaphylaxis p780. Signs of envenoming*: BP↓ (vasodilatation, viper cardiotoxicity) D&V; swelling spreading proximally within 4h of bite; bleeding gums or venepuncture sites; anaphylaxis; ptosis; trismus; rhabdomyolysis; pulmonary oedema. *Tests*: WCC↑; clotting↓; platelets↓; U&E; urine RBC↑; CK↑; P_aO_2↓, ECG. *Management*: Avoid active movement of affected limb (so use splints/slings). Avoid incisions and tourniquets. ▶Get help.[24] Is antivenom indicated (IgG from venom-immunized sheep)?—eg 10mL IV over 15min (adults **and** children) of *European Viper Antiserum* (from Farillon) for adder bites; have adrenaline (=epinephrine) to hand—p780. Monitor ECG. For foreign snakes, see BNF.

Salicylate poisoning

Children: *OHCS* p254

Aspirin is a weak acid with poor water solubility. It is present in many over-the-counter preparations. Anaerobic metabolism and the production of lactate and heat are stimulated by the uncoupling of oxidative phosphorylation. Effects are dose-related, and potentially fatal:

• 150mg/kg: mild toxicity • 250mg/kg: moderate • >500mg/kg: severe toxicity.

Signs & symptoms Unlike paracetamol, many early features. Vomiting, dehydration, hyperventilation, tinnitus, vertigo, sweating. Rarely; lethargy or coma, seizures, vomiting, ↓BP and heart block, pulmonary oedema, hyperthermia. Patients present initially with respiratory alkalosis due to a direct stimulation of the central respiratory centres and then develop a metabolic acidosis. Hyper- or hypoglycaemia may occur.

Management *General:* p826. Correct dehydration. Gastric lavage if within 1h, activated charcoal (may be repeated, but is of unproven value).

• Paracetamol and salicylate level, glucose, U&E, LFT, INR, ABG, HCO_3^-, FBC. Salicylate level may need to be repeated after 2h, due to continuing absorption if a potentially toxic dose has been taken.

• Levels over 700mg/L are potentially fatal.

• Monitor urine output, and blood glucose. If severe poisoning: salicylate levels, blood pH, and U&E. Consider urinary catheter and monitoring urine pH. Beware hypoglycaemia.

• Correct any metabolic acidosis with 1.26% HCO_3^- (sodium bicarbonate).

• If plasma level >500mg/L (3.6mmol/L), consider alkalinization of the urine , eg 1.5L 1.26% HCO_3^- with 40mmol KCl IV over 3h. Aim to make the **urine** pH 7.5–8.5. **NB:** monitor serum K^+ as hypokalaemia may occur.

• Consider dialysis if plasma level >700mg/L, and if renal or heart failure, seizures, severe acidosis, or persistently ↑plasma salicylate. ECG monitor.

• Discuss any serious cases with the local toxicological service or national poisons information service.

Paracetamol poisoning

150mg/kg, or 12g in adults may be fatal. However, prompt treatment can prevent liver failure and death. ►1 tablet of paracetamol = 500mg.

Signs & symptoms None initially, or vomiting ± RUQ pain. Later: jaundice and encephalopathy from liver damage (the main danger) ± renal failure.

Management *General measures* p826, lavage if >12g (or >150mg/kg) taken within 1h. Give activated charcoal if <8h since ingestion. Specific measures:

• Glucose, U&E, LFT, INR, ABG, HCO_3^- , FBC. Blood level at 4h post-ingestion.

• If <8h since overdose and plasma paracetamol is above the line on the graph OPPOSITE, start N-acetylcysteine.

• If >8h and suspicion of large overdose (>7.5g) err on the side of caution and start acetylcysteine, stopping it if paracetamol level below the treatment line and INR and ALT are normal.

• Acetylcysteine is given by IVI: 150mg/kg in 200mL of 5% dextrose over 15min. Then 50mg/kg in 500mL of 5% dextrose over 4h. Then 100mg per kg/16h in 1L of 5% dextrose. Rash is a common SE: treat with chlorpheniramine (=chlorphenamine), and observe; do not stop unless anaphylaxis, ie shock, vomiting, wheeze occurs (≤10%). An alternative is methionine 2.5g/4h PO for 16h (total: 10g), but absorption is unreliable if there is vomiting. Benefit is lessened by concurrent charcoal.

• If ingestion time is unknown, or it is staggered, or presentation is >15h from ingestion, treatment *may* help. ►Get advice.

• The graph may mislead if HIV+ve (hepatic glutathione↓), or if long-acting paracetamol has been taken, or if pre-existing liver disease or induction of liver enzymes has occurred. ►Beware glucose↓; ward-test hourly; INR/12h.

• Next day do INR, U&E, LFT. If INR rising, continue acetylcysteine until <1.4.

• If continued deterioration, discuss with the liver team.

Do not hesitate to get expert advice. *Criteria for transfer to a specialist unit:*
- *Encephalopathy* or *ICP↑*. Signs of CNS oedema: BP >160/90 (sustained) or brief rises (systolic >200mmHg), bradycardia, decerebrate posture, extensor spasms, poor pupil responses. ICP monitoring can help, p816.
- *INR* >2.0 at <48h—or >3.5 at <72h (so measure INR every 12h). Peak elevation: 72–96h. LFTs are *not* good markers of hepatocyte death. If INR is *normal* at 48h, the patient may go home.
- *Renal impairment* (creatinine >200µmol/L). Monitor urine flow. Daily U&E and serum creatinine (use haemodialysis if >400µmol/L).
- *Blood pH* <7.3 (lactic acidosis → tissue hypoxia). • *Systolic BP* <80mmHg.

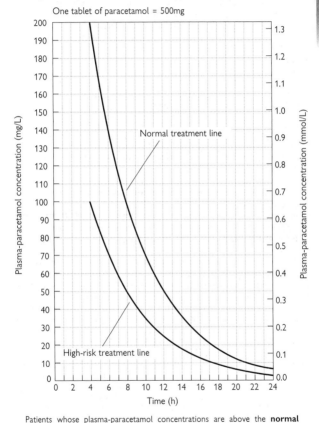

One tablet of paracetamol = 500mg

Patients whose plasma-paracetamol concentrations are above the **normal treatment line** should be treated with acetylcysteine by intravenous infusion (or, provided the overdose has been taken **within 10–12h**, with methionine by mouth). Patients on enzyme-including drugs (eg carbamazepine, phenobarbital, phenytoin, rifampicin, and alcohol) or who are malnourished (eg in anorexia, in alcoholism, or those who are HIV-positive) should be treated if their plasma-paracetamol concentrations are above the **high-risk treatment line**. (We thank Dr Alun Hutchings for permission to reproduce this graph.)

▸▸Burns

Resuscitate and arrange transfer for all major burns. (>25% partial thickness in adult and >20% in children). Assess site, size, and depth of the burn. Referral is still warranted in cases of full thickness burns >5%, partial thickness burns >10% in adults or >5% in children or the elderly, burns of special sites, chemical and electrical burns and burns with inhalational injury.

Assessment *Burn size* is important to assess (see table) as it influences the magnitude of the inflammatory response (vasodilatation, increased vascular permeability) and thus the fluid shift from the intravascular volume. The fluid must be estimated to calculate fluid requirements. Ignore erythema.

Burn depth determines healing time/scarring; assessing this may be hard, even when experienced. The big distinction is whether the burn is partial thickness (painful, red, and blistered) or full thickness (insensate/painless and white/grey). **NB:** burns can evolve, particularly over the 1st 48h.

Resuscitation *Airway:* Beware of upper airway obstruction developing if hot gases inhaled. Suspect if history of fire in enclosed space, soot in oral/nasal cavity, singed nasal hairs of hoarse voice. A flexible laryngo/bronchoscopy is useful. Involve anaesthetists early and consider early intubation.

Breathing: Exclude life-threatening chest injuries (eg tension pneumothorax) and constricting burns. Give 100% O_2 if carbon monoxide poisoning is suspected (mostly from history, may have cherry-red skin, measure carboxy-haemoglobin (COHb) and compare to nomograms). With 100% O_2 $t_{1/2}$ of COHb falls from 250min to 40min (consider hyperbaric oxygen if pregnant; CNS signs; >20% COHb). SpO_2 measured by pulse oximeter is unreliable. Do escharotomy if thoracic burns impair chest excursion (*OHCS* p689).

Circulation: Partial thickness burns >10% burns in a child and >15% in adults require IV fluid resuscitation. Put up 2 large-bore (14G or 16G) IV lines. Do not worry if you have to put these through burned skin, intraosseous access is valuable in infants (see *OHCS*). Secure them well: they are literally lifelines.

Use a *burns calculator*[25] flow chart or a formula, eg: *Parkland formula* (popular): 4 × weight (kg) × % burn=mL Hartmann's solution in 24h, half given in 1st 8h.

Muir and Barclay formula: [weight (kg) × %burn]/2 =mL colloid (eg Haemaccel®) per unit time. Time periods are 4h, 4h, 4h, 6h, 6h, and 12h.

Either formula is acceptable but must use appropriate fluid ie crystalloid for Parkland not colloid. **NB:** a meta-analysis (somewhat flawed[26]) suggests the use of colloid (albumin) can cause ↑ mortality (slightly); it is also expensive. Replace fluid from the time of burn, not from the time first seen in hospital.

Formulae are only guides: adjust IVI according to clinical response and urine output; aim for >0.5mL/kg/h (>1mL/kg/h in children), ~50% more in electrical burns & inhalation injury. Monitor T° (core & surface); catheterize the bladder.

Treatment Do *not* apply cold water to extensive burns: this may intensify shock. If transferring to a burns unit, do not burst blisters or apply any special creams as this can hinder assessment. Simple saline gauze or Vaseline® gauze is suitable; cling film is useful as a temporary measure and relieves pain. Use morphine in IV aliquots and titrate for good analgesia. Ensure tetanus immunity. Antibiotic prophylaxis is not routine.

Definitive dressings There are many dressings for partial thickness burns, including biological (pigskin, cadaveric skin), synthetic (Mepitel®, Duoderm®) and silver sufadiazine cream (Flamazine®). Major full thickness burns benefit from early tangential excision and split-skin grafting as the burns wound is a major source of inflammatory cytokines causing SIRS (systemic inflammatory response syndrome)[27] and from an ideal medium for bacterial growth.

Smoke inhalation

Initially there is laryngospasm that leads to hypoxia and straining (leading to petechiae), then hypoxic cord relaxation leads to true inhalation injury. Free radicals, cyanide compounds, and carbon monoxide accompany thermal injury. Cyanide compounds (generated from burning plastic in particular) bind reversibly with ferric ions in enzymes, so stopping oxidative phosphorylation, causing dizziness, headaches, and seizures. Tachycardia and dyspnoea soon give way to bradycardia and apnoea. Carbon monoxide is generated later in the fire as oxygen is depleted; the COHb level does not correlate well with the severity of poisoning.

▶▶ 100% O_2 is given to elute both cyanide and CO.

▶▶ Involve ICU/anaesthetists early: early ventilation may be useful, consider repeated bronchoscopic lavage.

▶▶ Enrole expert help in cyanide poisoning, there is no single regimen suitable for all situations. Clinically mild poisoning may be treated by rest, O_2, and amyl nitrite 0.2–0.4mL via an Ambu® bag. IV antidotes may be used for moderate poisoning: sodium thiosulphate is a common first choice. More severe poisoning may require eg hydroxocobalamin, sodium nitrite, and dimethylaminophenol.

Lund & Browder charts[1]

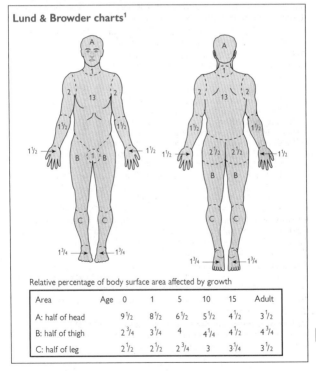

Relative percentage of body surface area affected by growth

Area	Age	0	1	5	10	15	Adult
A: half of head		$9^1/2$	$8^1/2$	$6^1/2$	$5^1/2$	$4^1/2$	$3^1/2$
B: half of thigh		$2^3/4$	$3^1/4$	4	$4^1/4$	$4^1/2$	$4^3/4$
C: half of leg		$2^1/2$	$2^1/2$	$2^3/4$	3	$3^1/4$	$3^1/2$

1 Accurate but time-consuming compared with the 'Rule of nines': arm: 9%; front of trunk 18%; head & neck 9%; leg 18%; back of trunk 18%; perineum 1%. This generally overestimates burn area (better than underestimating). It is even accurate for those <10 years old.

Hypothermia

▶*Have a high index of suspicion and a low-reading thermometer.* Most patients are elderly and do not complain, or feel, cold—so they have not tried to warm themselves up. In the young, hypothermia is usually either from cold exposure (eg near-drowning), or it is secondary to impaired level of consciousness (eg following excess alcohol or drug overdose).

Definition Hypothermia implies a core (rectal) temperature <35°C.

Causes In the elderly hypothermia is often caused by a combination of:
• Impaired homeostatic mechanisms: usually age-related.
• Low room temperature: poverty, poor housing.
• Disease: Impaired thermoregulation (pneumonia, MI, heart failure).
• Reduced metabolism (immobility, hypothyroidism, diabetes mellitus).
• Autonomic neuropathy (p390, eg diabetes mellitus, Parkinson's).
• Excess heat loss (psoriasis). Cold awareness ↓ (dementia, confusion).
• Increased exposure to cold (falls, especially at night when cold).
• Drugs (major tranquillizers, antidepressants, diuretics). Alcohol.

The patient *How frozen I then became: I did not die, yet nothing of life remained.*[1] So don't assume that if vital signs seem to be absent, the patient must be dead: rewarm (see below) and re-examine. If T° <32°C, this sequence may occur: ↓BP → coma → bradycardia → AF → VT → VF. The abdomen can feel 'colder than clay'. If >32°C, there may simply be pallor ± apathy.

Diagnosis Check oral or axillary T°. If ordinary thermometer shows <36.5°C, use a low-reading one PR. Is the rectal temperature <35°C?

Tests Urgent U&E, plasma glucose, and amylase. Thyroid function tests; FBC; blood cultures. Consider blood gases. The ECG may show J-waves.

Treatment
• Ventilate if comatose or respiratory insufficiency.
• Warm IVI (for access or to correct electrolyte disturbance).
• Cardiac monitor (both VF and AF can occur during warming).
• Consider antibiotics for the prevention of pneumonia (p174). Give these routinely in patients over 65yrs with a temperature <32°C.
• Consider urinary catheter (to assess renal function).
• *Slowly rewarm.* Do not reheat too quickly, causing peripheral vasodilatation, shock, and death. Aim for a rise of ½°C/h. Old, conscious patients should sit in a warm room taking hot drinks. Thermal blankets may cause too rapid warming in old patients. The first sign of too rapid warming is falling BP. Treat by allowing patient to cool down slightly.
• Rectal temperature, BP, pulse, and respiratory rate every ½ hour.

NB: Advice is different for victims of sudden hypothermia from immersion. Here, eg if there has been a cardiac arrest, and T° <30°C, mediastinal warm lavage, peritoneal or haemodialysis, and cardiopulmonary bypass (no heparin if trauma) may be needed (*OHCS* p682).

Complications Arrhythmias (if there is a cardiac arrest continue resuscitating until T° >33°C, as cold brains are less damaged by hypoxia); pneumonia; pancreatitis; acute renal failure; intravascular coagulation.

Prognosis Depends on age and degree of hypothermia. If age >70yrs and T° <32°C then mortality >50%.

Before hospital discharge Anticipate problems. *Will it happen again? What is her network of support?* Review medication (*could you stop tranquillizers?*). *How is progress to be monitored?* Liaise with GP/social worker.

---

1 In the last round of the 9th circle of *Hell*, Dante tells how those betraying their benefactors are encased in ice (*canto XXXIV*) 'Com'io divenni allor gelato e fioco...Io non mori e non rimasi vivo.'

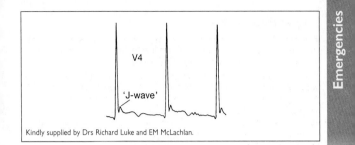

Kindly supplied by Drs Richard Luke and EM McLachlan.

Major disasters

Planning All hospitals have a detailed *Major Accident Plan*, but additionally the tasks of key personnel can be distributed on individual *Action Cards*.

At the scene Call the police; tell them to take command.

Safety: Is paramount—your own and others. Be visible (luminous monogrammed jacket) and wear protective clothing where appropriate (safety helmet; waterproofs; boots; respirator in chemical environment).

Triage: See OHCS p787. Label RED if will die in a few mins if no treatment. YELLOW = will die in ~2h if no treatment; GREEN = can wait. (BLUE = dead).

Communications: Are essential. Each emergency service will dispatch a control vehicle and will have a designated incident officer for liaison. Support medical staff from hospital report to the medical incident officer—he is usually the first doctor on the scene: his job is to assess then communicate to the receiving hospital the number and severity of casualties, to organize resupply of equipment and to replace fatigued staff. He must resist temptation to treat casualties as this compromises his role.

Equipment: Must be portable and include: intubation and cricothyrotomy set; intravenous fluids (colloid); bandages and dressings; chest drain (+flutter valve); amputation kit (when used, ideally 2 doctors should concur); drugs— *analgesic:* morphine; *anaesthetic:* ketamine 2mg/kg IV over >60s (0.5mg/kg is a powerful analgesic without respiratory depression); limb splints (may be inflatable); defibrillator/monitor; ± pulse oximeter.

Evacuation: Remember: with immediate treatment on scene, the priority for evacuation may be reduced (eg a tension pneumothorax— RED—relieved can wait for evacuation—becomes YELLOW), but those who may suffer by delay at the scene must go first. Send any severed limbs to the same hospital as the patient, ideally chilled—but not frozen.

At the hospital a 'major incident' is declared. The *first receiving* hospital will take most of the casualties; the *support* hospital(s) will cope with overflow and may provide mobile teams so that staff are not depleted from the first hospital. A control room is established and the medical coordinator ensures staff have been summoned, nominates a triage officer, and supervises the best use of inpatient beds and ITU/theatre resources.

Blast injury may be caused by domestic (eg gas explosion) or industrial (eg mining) accidents or by terrorist bombs. Death may occur without any obvious external injury (air emboli). Injury occurs in 6 ways:

1 **Blast wave** A transient (milliseconds) wave of overpressure expands rapidly producing cellular disruption, shearing forces along tissue planes (submucosal/subserosal haemorrhage) and re-expansion of compressed trapped gas—bowel perforation, fatal air embolism.

2 **Blast wind** This can totally disrupt a body or cause avulsive amputations. Bodies can be thrown and sustain injuries on landing.

3 **Missiles** Penetration or laceration from missiles are by far the commonest injuries. Missiles arise from the bomb or are secondary, eg glass.

4 **Flash burns** These are usually superficial and occur on exposed skin.

5 **Crush** Injuries: beware sudden death or renal failure after release.

6 **Psychological injury** Eg post-traumatic stress disorder (OHCS p347).

Treatment Approach the same as any major trauma OHCS p684. Rest and observe any suspected of exposure to significant blast but without other injury. Gun-shot injury: see OHCS p679.

838

Source: I Greaves 1999 *Pre-hospital Medicine*, Arnold; S Mellor *Recent Advances is Surgery* 14, Churchill Livingstone, London 1991 53–68

Index

Manual indexes have limitations: use our *intelligent electronic index* in our electronic product (Mentor www.emispdp.com) for exploring and explaining *combinations* of signs, symptoms, and test results.

(►For drugs, consult the disease you want to treat rather than the drug name.)

841

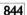

863

864

866

Useful doses for the new house officer

▶These pages outline typical adult doses, and the commoner side-effects, of medications that a new house officer will be called upon to prescribe. If in any doubt, consult an appropriate drug formulary (eg British National Fomulary, BNF, http://www.bnf.org).

Drug	Dose and frequency	Notes
Analgesics	(see p454 for more details on analgesia)	
Aspirin	300–900mg/4–6h PO, max. 4g/24h	SE of NSAIDs: gastritis; bronchospasm; hypersensitivity. CI: GI ulcer/bleeding; NSAID-induced asthma; coagulopathy. Avoid aspirin in children (risk of Reye's syndrome).
Diclofenac	50mg/8h PO/PR	
Ibuprofen	400mg/6h PO, max. 2.4g/24h	
Paracetamol	0.5–1g/4–6h PO, max 4g/24h	Avoid if hepatic impairement.
Codeine phosphate	30–60mg/4h PO/IM max. 240mg/24h	Patients with chronic pain (eg malignancy) may require higher doses. SE of opioids: nausea and vomiting; constipation; drowsiness; hypotension; respiratory depression, dependence. CI: Acute respiratory depression, acute alcoholism. Use carefully in head injury, as may hinder neurological assessment.
Dihydrocodeine tartrate	30mg/4–6h PO, OR 50mg/4–6h IM/SC	
Meptazinol	200mg/3–6h PO, OR 50–100mg/2–4h IM/IV	
Oxycodone	5mg/6h PO	
Pethidine	50–100mg/4h PO/IM/SC	
Tramadol	50–100mg/4h PO/IM/IV	
Morphine	5–10mg/4h PO/IM/SC	
Antibiotics	(see p542–548)	
Antiemetics		
Cyclizine	50mg/8h PO/IM/IV	
Metaclopramide	10mg/8h PO/IM/IV	May cause extrapyramidal SE, especially in young adults.
Ondansetron	8mg/8h PO, or 4mg IM/IV	
Antihistamines		
Chlorpheniramine	10–20mg IM/IV, maximum 40mg/24h OR 4mg/6h PO	SE of antihistamines: Drowsiness; urinary retention; dry mouth; blurred vision; GI disturbance; arrhythmias. Drowsiness is less commoner with newer drugs eg cetirizine, fexofenadine.
Cetirizine	5–10mg/24h PO	
Levocetirizine	5mg/24h PO	
Fexofenadine	120–180mg/24h PO	
Loratadine	10mg/24h PO	
Desloratadine	5mg/24h PO	
Gastric acid reducing drugs		
Cimetidine	400mg/6–12h PO	SE of H$_2$-blockers: GI disturbance; ↑LFTs.
Ranitidine	150mg/12h PO	
Omeprazole	20–40mg/24h PO	SE of PPIs: GI disturbance; hypersensitivity. ▶Acid-reducing drugs may mask symptoms of gastric cancer; use with care in middle-aged patients.
Esomeprazole	20–40mg/24h PO	
Lansoprazole	15–30mg/24h PO	
Pantoprazole	20–40mg/24h PO	

Drug	Dose and frequency	Notes
Heparins	(see p648 for more details on anticoagulation)	
Unfraction-ated heparin	*DVT prophylaxis:* 5000U/12h SC	SE of heparins: bleeding; thrombocytopenia; hypersen-sitivity; hyperkalaemia; osteo-porosis after prolonged use. CI: coagulopathy; peptic ulcer; recent cerebral bleed; recent trauma or surgery; active bleeding.
Enoxaparin	*DVT prophylaxis:* 20–40mg/24h SC. *DVT/PE treatment:* 1.5mg/kg/24h SC until warfarinized. *Unstable angina:* 1mg/kg/12h SC for 2–8d	
Tinzaparin	*DVT prophylaxis:* 3500–4500U/24h SC. *DVT/PE treatment:* 175U/kg/24h SC until warfarinized.	
Dalteparin	*DVT prophylaxis:* 2500–5000U/24h SC. *DVT/PE treatment:* 200U/kg/d SC (18,000U/24h maximum). *Unstable angina:* 120U/kg/12h SC (up to 10,000U/12h maximum) for 5–8d.	
Hypnotics		
Temazepam	10–20mg PO at night	SE: Drowsiness; dependence. Zopicolone also causes bitter taste and GI disturbances. CI: Respiratory depression; myasthenia.
Zopiclone	3.75–7.5mg PO at night	
Tranquilizers		
Haloperidol	2–5mg IM/IV initially, then every 4–8h till response, maximum 18mg in total.	SE: Extrapyramidal effects, sedation, hypotension, anti-muscarinic effects, neurolep-tic malignant syndrome.
Others		
Digoxin	(see p100)	
Naloxone	*In opiate overdose:* 0.8–2mg IV repeated every 2–3min to a maximum of 10mg if respiratory function does not improve. *To reverse opiate-induced respiratory depression:* 100–200µg IV every 2min.	SE: tachycardia; fibrillation. Can precipitate opiate with-drawl.
Flumazenil	*To reverse benzo-diazepines:* 200µg IV over 15s, then 100µg every 60s if required, up to 1mg maximum.	SE: convulsions (esp. in epi-leptics); nausea and vomiting; flushing. Avoid if patient has a life-threatening illness con-trolled by benzodiazepines (eg status epilepticus).

UK adult basic life-support algorithm[1]

The algorithm assumes that only one rescuer is present, with no equipment. (If a defibrillator is to hand, get a rhythm readout, and defibrillate, as opposite, as soon as possible.)

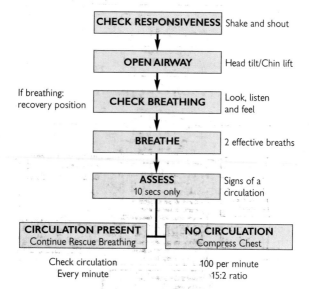

CHECK RESPONSIVENESS Shake and shout

↓

OPEN AIRWAY Head tilt/Chin lift

↓

If breathing: recovery position

CHECK BREATHING Look, listen and feel

↓

BREATHE 2 effective breaths

↓

ASSESS 10 secs only Signs of a circulation

↓

CIRCULATION PRESENT Continue Rescue Breathing

Check circulation Every minute

NO CIRCULATION Compress Chest

100 per minute 15:2 ratio

Send or go for help as soon as possible according to guidelines

Managing the airway
- You open the airway by tilting the head and lifting the chin—but only do this if there is no question of spinal trauma.
- Use a close-fitting mask if available, held in place by thumbs pressing downwards either side of the mouthpiece; palms against cheeks.

Chest compressions
- Cardiopulmonary resuscitation (CPR) involves compressive force over the lower sternum with the heal of the hands placed one on top of the other, directing the weight of your body through your vertical, straight, arms.
- Depth of compression: ~4cm.
- Rate of compressions: 100/min.

Remember that these are guidelines only, and that the exact circumstances of the cardiorespiratory arrest will partly determine best practice. The guidelines are also more consensus-based than evidence based (p24), and are likely to be adapted from time to time, for example, as consensus develops about the best recovery position—eg semi-lateral position, with under-most arm either straight at the side, in dorsal position, or in the ventral position cradling the head with the upper-most arm crossing it (more stable, but possible risk to arm blood flow).[2]

1 www.resus.org.uk/pages.blsalgo.pdf **79** 151 2 A Handley 1993 *Resuscitation* **26** 93-95

Postscript

This book contains quotations, some of them slightly adapted, from works by: René Belletto, Hans Bellmer, Jorge Luis Borgès, Michel Butor, Italo Calvino, Agatha Christie, Gustave Flaubert, Sigmund Freud, Alfred Jarry, James Joyce, Franz Kafka, Michel Leiris, Malcolm Lowry, Thomas Mann, Gabriel García Marquez, Harry Mathews, Herman Melville, Vladimir Nabokov, Georges Perec, Roger Price, Marcel Proust, Raymond Queneau, François Rabelais, Jacques Roubaud, Raymond Roussel, Stendhal, Lawrence Sterne, Theodore Sturgeon, Jules Verne, Unica Zürn.

Translator's Note

This translation contains quotations, occasionally somewhat modified, from published translations done by Robert Baldick, Anthony Bonner, Max Brod, J. M. Cohen, Ernest Jones, Anthony Kerrigan, Terence Kilmartin, Alban Krailsheimer, H. T. Lowe-Porter, Dmitri Nabokov, Vladimir Nabokov, Sir Malcolm Pasley, Alastair Reid, Francis Steegmuller, Helen Temple, Norman Thomas di Giovanni, Ruthven Todd, J. A. Underwood, Sir Thomas Urquhart, William Weaver, Barbara Wright.

Chapters 27 and 74 of *Life A User's Manual* have appeared previously, in *Grand Street* (New York), Autumn 1983, and in *Fiction International* (San Diego), 1985, in translations by Harry Mathews, which are reused here, with minor modifications, with the kind permission of the translator.

This translation is gready indebted to Ela Bienenfeld, Eugen Helmle, Bianca Lamblin, and Harry Mathews: without their help and encouragement I would have made many more errors than I have done.

My thanks go also to all those who have answered queries, solved puzzles, and helped with the material production of this translation: Jacques Beaumatin, Alexander Bellos, Philip Bennett, Vera Brice, Graham Chesters, Julian Kinderlerer, Una Kelly, Andy Leak, Susan Lendrum, Terry Lewis, Sylvia Richardson and especially Sarah Asquith, Ruth Sharman, Dorothy Straight, and Willy Wauquaire.

DB
Sheffield-Manchester-
Princeton, 1986-2007

THE HISTORY OF VINTAGE

The famous American publisher Alfred A. Knopf (1892–1984) founded Vintage Books in the United States in 1954 as a paperback home for the authors published by his company. Vintage was launched in the United Kingdom in 1990 and works independently from the American imprint although both are part of the international publishing group, Random House.

Vintage in the United Kingdom was initially created to publish paperback editions of books acquired by the prestigious hardback imprints in the Random House Group such as Jonathan Cape, Chatto & Windus, Hutchinson and later William Heinemann, Secker & Warburg and The Harvill Press. There are many Booker and Nobel Prize-winning authors on the Vintage list and the imprint publishes a huge variety of fiction and non-fiction. Over the years Vintage has expanded and the list now includes both great authors of the past – who are published under the Vintage Classics imprint – as well as many of the most influential authors of the present.

For a full list of the books Vintage publishes, please visit our website
www.vintage-books.co.uk

For book details and other information about the classic authors we publish, please visit the Vintage Classics website
www.vintage-classics.info

www.vintage-classics.info